Encyclopedia of Otolaryngology, Head and Neck Surgery

Stilianos E. Kountakis

Editor

Encyclopedia of Otolaryngology, Head and Neck Surgery

Volume 2

D–H

With 1451 Figures and 341 Tables

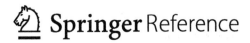

Editor
Stilianos E. Kountakis
Department of Otolaryngology-Head and Neck Surgery
Medical College of Georgia
Augusta, GA, USA

ISBN 978-3-642-23498-9   ISBN 978-3-642-23499-6 (eBook)
ISBN 978-3-642-23500-9 (print and electronic bundle)
DOI 10.1007/978-3-642-23499-6
Springer Heidelberg New York Dordrecht London

Library of Congress Control Number: 2012954535

Printed on acid-free paper

Springer is part of Springer Science+Business Media (www.springer.com)

To all my fellows, residents and students for they give meaning to my academic career.
To my wonderful wife Eleni and children Eftihia, Emmanuel, Nikoleta and Alexandra for their continued support.

Stilianos E. Kountakis, MD, PhD
Professor

Foreword

"The Encyclopedia of Otolaryngology-Head and Neck Surgery is a brilliant concept brought to fruition by Stilianos Kountakis and his colleagues. The contributors and their offerings are current and extremely well planned. In reviewing the format of this reference source, it is amazing how easy it is to navigate and find exactly the information you seek. There is no doubt in my mind that physicians at all levels- from medical students to senior surgeons- will use this resource to obtain critical information quickly. I will recommend it as a reference to all in my department. I congratulate Professor Kountakis on this outstanding offering!!"

January 2013

Harold C. Pillsbury, MD
Chapel Hill, NC, USA

Preface

Otolaryngology-Head and Neck Surgery is the medical and surgical specialty addressing disorders of the head and neck in both adult and pediatric populations. The anatomy and physiologic functions of this region are diverse and require knowledge of all aspects of medicine. They also require understanding of surgical techniques that include microscopic-minimally invasive procedures, in addition to the performance of large resections, while predicting the aftermath required for reconstruction. The goal of the encyclopedia is to serve as a single and comprehensive source of all the information that is requisite to all health care practitioners and students of the specialty.

The vast amount of information included in the encyclopedia is divided into 5 volumes across otorhinolaryngology-head and neck surgery, in line with the subspecialties of general otolaryngology, head and neck surgery, pediatric otolaryngology, otology-neurotology and facial plastics and reconstructive surgery. All section editors are internationally recognized otolaryngologists with experience in publishing. They are experts and leaders in their respective fields, with advanced knowledge of all scientific and clinical issues currently discussed in the literature. Each section editor in turn recruited experienced authors from all over the world who contributed to structured topics and all entries are supported by published references. Thus, all information included in the encyclopedia is from credible sources and was carefully screened for accuracy.

The strength of the encyclopedia is its online availability and quick search features for definitions and more in-depth information. Key words are hyperlinked to provide a getaway to numerous referenced manuscripts, journals and books until all information on the queried subject is exhausted.

February 2013

Stilianos E. Kountakis, MD
Editor-in-Chief

Acknowledgments

I wholeheartedly thank all section editors for their leadership and hard work toward the completion of the encyclopedia of Otolaryngology, Head and Neck Surgery. Without their commitment and dedication this project would not be possible.

Stilianos E. Kountakis, MD, PhD
Editor-in-Chief

I wish to extend a deep debt of gratitude to my long time friend, Stil Kountakis, the Editor-in-Chief of the Encyclopedia. Stil and I have been co-Rhinologists on the Board of the American Rhinologic Society and I have a great deal of respect for him. Stil chose me to develop the General/Rhinologic Section of the Encyclopedia and I hope that the section provides up to date, detailed information to all Otolaryngologists and Rhinologists.

I also want to extend my sincere appreciation to my co-editors, Drs. Rich Lebowitz, Calvin Wei and Seth Lieberman. Dr Lebowitz is the Academic Vice Chair of Otolaryngology at New York University Medical Center and a Rhinologist. Dr Wei has just completed a 2 year fellowship with Drs Kennedy and Palmer and Dr. Lieberman is presently a fellow with Dr. Roy Casiano. My gratitude is also extended to all authors for their contributions. They have, across the board, provided the Encyclopedia with specialized information in their respective field of interest. The Encyclopedia is unmatched in the depth and breath of subject material and is truly unique.

Lastly, I would like to thank all of the editorial and administrative staff at Springer for their hard work and dedication to the project.

Joseph B. Jacobs
General Otolaryngology

As Section Editor, I would like to acknowledge the assistance of Dr. Ravi Samy for his efforts, who greatly facilitated the identification of essay authors, and for whose help I am personally very grateful for.

Brian J. McKinnon
Otology-Neurotology

I would like to thank my co-editor, Dr. Kristen Otto, for her leadership on this project and her dedication to its completion. She completed the overwhelming majority of the work while balancing a busy academic head and neck-microvasular practice and her duties as a spouse and a mother of three young children. The joy in my career stems from watching such outstanding young faculty members blossom in their academic careers. I would like to thank all of the essay authors who so willing and graciously shared their precious time and knowledge to help educate current and future providers with the ultimate goal of improvement in the quantity and quality of life for our patients. I would particularly like to thank the many faculty members and residents in the Department of Otolaryngology and Communicative Sciences at the University of Mississippi Medical Center who went above and beyond to pitch in to make the project a success.

Scott P. Stringer
Head and Neck Surgery

The 'Pediatric Otolaryngology' section in Encyclopedia of Otolaryngology, Head and Neck Surgery is a user-friendly text directed at clinicians treating children with ear, nose and throat disorders. It provides an overview of the main aspects of pediatric otolaryngology and highlights the many areas that have seen significant progress. It is both comprehensive but easy to read and reference. In addition, the many pictures and videos will aid the reader in understanding some of the more complex facets of care in the pediatric head and neck.

The care of children with ear, nose and throat problems has become more complex over the last 20 years. With this, pediatric otolaryngology has emerged as a recognized subspecialty within otolaryngology-head and neck surgery. This section reflects these changes and covers the breath of the subspecialty including management of ear infections, sleep disorders, cochlear implantation, airway management and many more topics. It is designed to be both a source of succinct information but also a reference text for use by busy clinicians.

We would like to extend our thanks to the many authors who have devoted an extensive amount of time and energy to the development of this book. We would also like to thank Springer and the editorial team for their commitment to publishing this book. This book would have remained an unfulfilled dream if not for the support of our spouses Iona Pereira and Lauren Mitchell and our children Karen, Nicola, Rachel, Dalia, Ariella, Gabi and Liam who allowed us the many nights and weekends spent writing and editing this section.

Kevin D. Pereira and Ron B. Mitchell
Pediatric Otolaryngology

A general acknowledgement to all who contributed to the facial plastic section.

Ira D. Papel and Kofi Derek O. Boahene
Facial Plastic and Reconstructive Surgery

I would like to thank my friends and colleagues, in particular the faculty and residents in the Department of Otolaryngology at New York University School of Medicine, who contributed their time, effort and expertise to this project. Special thanks are in order to Dr. Seth Lieberman and Dr. Calvin Wei; without their work the completion of this venture would not have been possible. I would also like to thank Dr. Stil Kountakis for his stewardship throughout the process, and Dr. Joseph Jacobs for inviting me to participate. Finally, as always, thank you to my wife, Lisa.

Richard A. Lebowitz
General Otolaryngology

About the Editor

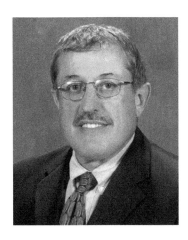

Dr. Stilianos E. Kountakis received his undergraduate degree in Chemical Engineering from the University of Houston and his medical degree from the University of Texas-Houston. He completed his training in Otolaryngology-Head and Neck Surgery at the University of Texas-Houston affiliated hospitals in 1993. After his training Dr. Kountakis stayed on as a faculty at the University of Texas-Houston Medical School until 1999, when he was appointed the Director of Rhinology-Sinus Surgery at the University of Virginia in Charlottesville, Virginia. Dr. Kountakis joined the faculty at Georgia Health Sciences University (Medical College of Georgia), effective July 1, 2003 as Professor of the Department of Otolaryngology and as the Chief of the Division of Rhinology - Sinus Surgery. He is also the Director of the Otolaryngology Residency Program and the Director of the Rhinology Fellowship at the institution.

Dr. Kountakis' research interests include clinical, physiological, genetic and immune-basic science parameters of chronic sinusitis and medical-surgical outcomes. His research interests also include development of a staging and classification system of chronic sinusitis. He has received multiple honors and awards including the Certificate of Honor by the American Academy of Otolaryngology-Head & Neck Surgery and the Golden Mirror Teaching Award by the American Rhinologic Society. He has served as an oral examiner of the American Board of Otolaryngology and has been recognized by the Best Doctors in America for several years. Dr. Kountakis is also recognized in the Top Doctors category of the US News and World Report.

Dr. Kountakis has published extensively, has edited multiple books, is on the editorial and review boards of multiple journals and serves as an associate editor of the International Forum of Allergy & Rhinology. Among his many other professional activities, Dr. Kountakis is a Fellow of the American Academy of Otolaryngology - Head and Neck Surgery, the American College of Surgeons, and the American Rhinologic Society. Dr. Kountakis has served as President of the American Rhinologic Society and the Georgia Society of Otolaryngology-Head and Neck Surgery and has held senior leadership positions within the Georgia Health Sciences University, the Physicians Practice Group (Chair of the Foundation) and the Medical Center.

Section Editors

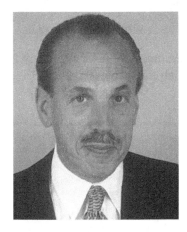

Joseph B. Jacobs Department of Otolaryngology, NYU Langone Medical Center, New York, NY, USA

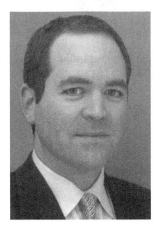

Richard A. Lebowitz Department of Otolaryngology-Head and Neck Surgery, New York University School of Medicine, NYU Langone Medical Center, New York, NY, USA

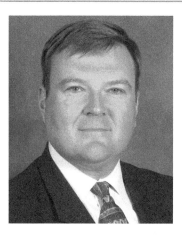

Brian J. McKinnon Department of Otolaryngology-Head and Neck Surgery, Georgia Health Sciences University, Augusta, GA, USA

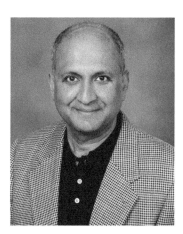

Kevin D. Pereira Department of Otorhinolaryngology-HNS, University of Maryland School of Medicine, Baltimore, MD, USA

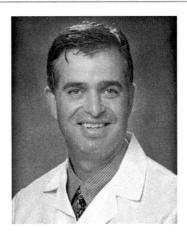

Ron B. Mitchell Otolaryngology and Pediatrics, University of Texas Southwestern Medical Center, Children's Medical Center Dallas, Dallas, TX, USA

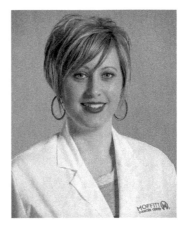

Kristen J. Otto Head and Neck, Moffitt Cancer Center, Tampa, Florida, USA

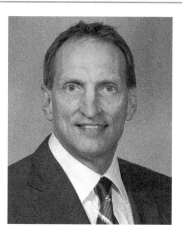

Scott P. Stringer Department of Otolaryngology and Communicative Sciences, University of Mississippi Medical Center, Jackson, MS, USA

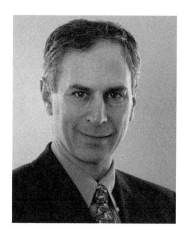

Ira D. Papel The Johns Hopkins Medical Institutions, Division of Facial Plastic Surgery, Department of Otolaryngology-Head and Neck Surgery, Baltimore, Maryland, USA

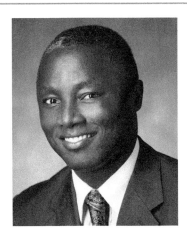

Kofi Derek O. Boahene Department of Otolaryngology-Head and Neck Surgery, Johns Hopkins University School of Medicine, Baltimore, MD, USA

Contributors

Walid Mohamed Abdellatif Cairo University Hospitals, Cairo, Egypt

Jihad Achkar Division of Laryngology, Department of Otology and Laryngology, Mass Eye and Ear Infirmary/Harvard Medical School, Boston, MA, USA

Oliver F. Adunka Division of Otology/Neurotology/Skull Base Surgery, Department of Otolaryngology-Head and Neck Surgery, University of North Carolina at Chapel Hill, Chapel Hill, NC, USA

Garima Agarwal Department of Otorhinolaryngology-Head and Neck Surgery, University of Texas Medical School at Houston, Houston, TX, USA

Sumit K. Agrawal London Health Sciences Centre - University Campus, London, ON, Canada

Shema Ahmad Department of Medicine/Endocrinology, Division of Endocrinology, University of Mississippi Medical Center, Jackson, MS, USA

Amir Ahmadian Department of Neurosurgery, University of South Florida, Tampa, FL, USA

Daniel S. Alam Department of Facial Plastic and Reconstructive Surgery, Head and Neck Institute, Cleveland Clinic Foundation, Cleveland, OH, USA

Aurash S. Alemi Department of Head and Neck Surgery, University of California, San Fransisco, CA, USA

Ashlin Alexander Department of Otolaryngology, NYU Medical Center, New York, NY, USA

Scott T. Allen Uniformed Services, University of Health Sciences School of Medicine, Bethesda, MD, USA

Cargill H. Alleyne Jr. Department of Neurosurgery, Medical College of Georgia at Georgia Health Sciences University, Augusta, GA, USA

Yaser Alrajhi Walter Mackenzie Center, University of Alberta Hospital, Edmonton, AB, Canada

Jeremiah A. Alt Oregan Health Science Universtiy, Portland, OR, USA

Kenneth W. Altman Department of Otolaryngology, The Mount Sinai School of Medicine, New York, NY, USA

Bryan T. Ambro Otolaryngology-Head and Neck Surgery, University of Maryland Medical Center, Baltimore, Baltimore, MD, USA

Milan R. Amin Department of Otolaryngology-Head and Neck Surgery, New York University Langone Medical Center, New York, NY, USA

Kal Ansari Walter Mackenzie Center, University of Alberta Hospital, Edmonton, AB, Canada

Department of Otrolaryngology, University of Alberta, Edmonton, AB, Canada

Patrick J. Antonelli Department of Otolaryngology-Head and Neck Surgery, University of Florida, Gainesville, FL, USA

Stephanie Moody Antonio Eastern Virginia Medical School, Department of Otolaryngology, Sentara Norfolk General Hospital, Norfolk, VA, USA

Rachel Appelblatt Department of Oral and Maxillofacial Surgery, New York University College of Dentistry, New York, NY, USA

Ellis M. Arjmand Department of Otolaryngology, University of Cincinnati, Cincinnati Children's Hospital Medical Center, Ear and Hearing Center Cincinnati, Cincinnati, OH, USA

Demetri Arnaoutakis Otolaryngology-Head and Neck Surgery, University of Florida, College of Medicine, Gainesville, FL, USA

Bruce Ashford Department of Head & Neck Surgery, Liverpool Hospital, Liverpool, Sydney, NSW, Australia

Jean Ashland Department of Speech, Language & Swallowing Disorders and Reading Disabilities, Massachusetts General Hospital, Boston, MA, USA

Mary G. Ashmead Department of Otolaryngology and Communicative Sciences, University of Mississippi Medical Center, Jackson, MS, USA

Ihab Atallah Department of Otolaryngology-Head and Neck Surgery, University Hospital of Grenoble, Grenoble, France

Arnaud Attye Department of Otolaryngology-Head and Neck Surgery, Otology/Neurotology Unit, University Hospital of Grenoble, Grenoble, France

Service ORL. Hôpital A. Michallon, Grenoble, France

Department of Neuroradiology, University Hospital of Grenoble, Grenoble, France

Verica Avramovic Institute of Histology, University of Nis, Nis, Serbia

Alba Miranda Azola Department of Otolaryngology-Head and Neck Surgery Resident, University of Maryland Medical Center, Baltimore, MA, USA

Karam Badran Department of Otolaryngology-Head and Neck Surgery, University of California, Irvine Medical Center, Orange, CA, USA

Kenneth Bagwell Albert Einstein College of Medicine, Bronx, NY, USA

Cristina M. Baldassari Department of Otolaryngology, Eastern Virginia Medical School, Norfolk, VA, USA

Thomas J. Balkany Department of Otolaryngology-Head and Neck Surgery, University of Miami Miller School of Medicine, University of Miami Ear Institute, Miami, FL, USA

Pete S. Batra Department of Otolaryngology-Head and Neck Surgery, University of Texas Southwestern Medical Center, Dallas, TX, USA

Saba Battelino Department of Otorhinolaryngology and Cervicofacial Surgery, University Medical Centre, Ljubljana, Slovenia

Rodrigo Bayon Department of Otolaryngology-Head and Neck Surgery, University of Iowa Hospitals & Clinics, Iowa City, IA, USA

Timothy J. Beacham Department of Anesthesiology, University of Mississippi, Jackson, MS, USA

Adam M. Becker Division of Otolaryngology-Head and Neck Surgery, Department of Surgery, Duke University School of Medicine, Durham, NC, USA

Diana Bell Department of Pathology, University of Texas MD Anderson Cancer Center, Houston, TX, USA

Eric E. Berg University of Texas – Southwestern School of Medicine, Dallas, Texas, Georgia

Daniel M. Beswick University of Pittsburgh, Pittsburgh, PA, USA

Scott E. Bevans Department of Otolaryngology, Madigan Healthcare System, Tacoma, WA, USA

Feriyl Bhaijee Department of Pathology, University of Mississippi Medical Center, Jackson, MS, USA

Rita G. Bhatia Miller School of Medicine, University of Miami, Miami, FL, USA

Nishant Bhatt Department of Otolaryngology-Head and Neck Surgery, Georgia Health Sciences University, Augusta, GA, USA

Anil Bhavsar Department of Radiology & Otolaryngology, University of Cincinnati, Cincinnati, OH, USA

Sanjiv Kumar Bhimrao Division of Otolaryngology-Head and Neck Surgery, University of British Columbia, Vancouver, BC, Canada

Amit D. Bhrany Department of Otolaryngology-Head and Neck Surgery, Facial Plastic and Reconstructive Surgery, University of Washington, Seattle, WA, USA

Lana Kovač Bilić Department for ENT and Head and Neck Surgery, University Hospital Center Zagreb, Zagreb, Croatia

Eric Bissada Department of Otolaryngology-Head and Neck Surgery, University of Toronto, Toronto, ON, Canada

Samra S. Blanchard Division of Pediatric Gastroenterology, University of Maryland, School of Medicine, Baltimore, MD, USA

Nikolas H. Blevins Department of Otolaryngology-Head and Neck Surgery, Stanford University, Stanford, CA, USA

Jason D. Bloom Division of Facial Plastic and Reconstructive Surgery, Department of Otolaryngology, New York University School of Medicine, New York, NY, USA

Kofi Derek O. Boahene Department of Otolaryngology-Head and Neck Surgery, Johns Hopkins University School of Medicine, Baltimore, MD, USA

Roman Bošnjak Department of Neurosurgery, University Medical Centre, Ljubljana, Slovenia

Emily F. Boss Division of Pediatric Otolaryngology, Department of Otolaryngology-Head and Neck Surgery, The Johns Hopkins University School of Medicine, Baltimore, MD, USA

Sean Boutros Houston Plastic and Craniofacial Surgery, Houston, TX, USA

Jennings R. Boyette Department of Otolaryngology-Head and Neck Surgery, University of Arkansas for Medical Sciences, Little Rock, AR, USA

Srećko Branica Department for ENT and Head and Neck Surgery, University Hospital Center Zagreb, Zagreb, Croatia

Amy Brenski Otolaryngology, Head and Neck Surgery, Division of Pediatric Otolaryngology, Children's Medical Center Dallas, University of Texas Southwestern, Dallas, TX, USA

Todd M. Brickman Department of Otolaryngology-Head and Neck Surgery, Louisiana State University School of Medicine-Health Science Center, New Orleans, LA, USA

Edward G. Brooks Departments of Pediatrics and Internal Medicine, University of Texas, Health Science Center at San Antonio, San Antonio, TX, USA

David K. Brown Communication Sciences Research Center, Cincinnati Children's Hospital Medical Center, Cincinnati, OH, USA

Departments of Otolaryngology and Communication Sciences and Disorders, University of Cincinnati, Cincinnati, OH, USA

Jimmy James Brown Department of Otolaryngology-Head and Neck Surgery, Georgia Health Sciences University, Augusta, GA, USA

Seth M. Brown Department of Surgery, Division of Otolaryngology, The Connecticut Sinus Institute, University of Connecticut, Farmington, CT, USA

Justin M. Broyles Department of Plastic and Reconstructive Surgery, The Johns Hopkins Hospital, Baltimore, MD, USA

Carrie M. Bush Department of Otolaryngology, Medical College of Georgia, Augusta, GA, USA

John F. Caccamese Jr. Department of Oral-Maxillofacial Surgery, R. Adams Cowley Shock Trauma Center, University of Maryland Children's Hospital, University of Maryland Medical Center, Baltimore, MD, USA

Ron Caloss Oral and Maxillofacial Surgery & Pathology, School of Dentistry, University of Mississippi Medical Center, Jackson, MS, USA

Steven B. Cannady Department of Otolaryngology, SUNY Downstate Medical Center, Brooklyn, NY, USA

Robert M. Cannon University of Mississippi School of Medicine, Jackson, MS, USA

John P. Carey Department of Otolaryngology-Head and Neck Surgery, Johns Hopkins University School of Medicine, Baltimore, MD, USA

Simon Carr Department of Otorhinolaryngology, Bradford Royal Infirmary, Bradford, UK

Ryan C. Case Department of Otolaryngology-Head and Neck Surgery, University of Mississippi School of Medicine, University of Mississippi Medical Center, Jackson, MS, USA

Roy R. Casiano Department of Otolaryngology, Miller School of Medicine, University of Miami, Miami, FL, USA

Margaretha L. Casselbrant Division of Pediatric Otolaryngology, Children's Hospital of Pittsburgh, University of Pittsburgh, Pittsburgh, PA, USA

Johnathan E. Castaño Department of Otolaryngology-Head and Neck Surgery, West Virginia University School of Medicine, Robert C. Byrd Health Sciences Center South, Morgantown, WV, USA

Jimmy Caudell Moffitt Cancer Center, Tampa, FL, USA

J. Brett Chafin Division of Pediatric Otolaryngology-HNS, Nemours Children's Clinic, Jacksonville, FL, USA

Michael J. Chandler NYU Langone School of Medicine, New York, NY, USA

Rakesh Chandra Department of Otolaryngology-Head and Neck Surgery, Northwestern University – Feinberg School of Medicine, Chicago, IL, USA

Ravi Chandran Oral and Maxillofacial Surgery & Pathology, School of Dentistry, University of Mississippi Medical Center, Jackson, MS, USA

C. Y. Joseph Chang Texas Ear Center and Department of Otorhinolaryngology, University of Texas – Houston Medical School, Houston, TX, USA

Mitchell H. Charap New York University School of Medicine, New York, NY, USA

Katrina Chaung Northwestern Sinus & Allergy Center, Feinberg School of Medicine, Department of Otolaryngology-Head and Neck Surgery, Northwestern University, Chicago, IL, USA

Brian S. Chen Department of Otolaryngology, Madigan Healthcare System, Tacoma, WA, USA

Herbert Chen Section of Endocrine Surgery, Department of Surgery, School of Medicine, University of Wisconsin, Madison, WI, USA

Si Chen New York University School of Medicine, New York, NY, USA

Neil N. Chheda Department of Otolaryngology, University of Florida, Gainesville, FL, USA

Wade W. Chien Department of Otolaryngology-Head and Neck Surgery, Johns Hopkins University School of Medicine, Baltimore, MD, USA

Lynn L. Chiu-Collins Facial Plastic Surgery, San Francisco Plastic Surgery & Laser Center, San Francisco, CA, USA

Sydney Ch'ng Sydney Head & Neck Cancer Institute, Royal Prince Alfred Hospital, Camperdown, Sydney, NSW, Australia

Eugene A. Chu Facial Plastic and Reconstructive Surgery, Rhinology, Skull Base Surgery, Kaiser Permanente, Department of Otolaryngology-Head and Neck Surgery, Downey, CA, USA

Benjamin West Cilento Texas Facial Plastic Surgery & Rhinology, The Woodlands, TX, USA

Martin J. Citardi Department of Otorhinolaryngology-Head and Neck Surgery, University of Texas Medical School at Houston, Houston, TX, USA

Texas Skull Base Physicians and Texas Sinus Institute, Houston, TX, USA

Francisco J. Civantos University of Miami Miller, School of Medicine, Miami, FL, USA

Cheryl Clark Department of Otolaryngology and Feist-Weiller Cancer Center, Louisiana State University Health Sciences Center - Shreveport, Shreveport, LA, USA

Jonathan R. Clark Sydney Head and Neck Cancer Institute, Royal Prince Alfred Hospital, Camperdown, Sydney, NSW, Australia

Marc A. Cohen Department of Otolaryngology-Head and Neck Surgery, University of Toronto, University Health Network/Toronto General Hospital, Toronto, ON, Canada

Candice C. Colby Emory University School of Medicine, Atlanta, GA, USA

Ryan Collar Department of Otolaryngology-Head and Neck Surgery, Johns Hopkins University School of Medicine, Baltimore, MD, USA

Brett T. Comer Department of Otolaryngology-Head and Neck Surgery, Community Howard Regional Health, Kokomo, IN, USA

George S. Conley Department of Otolaryngology-Head and Neck Surgery, University of Pittsburgh, Pittsburgh, PA, USA

Minas Constantinides Division of Facial Plastic and Reconstructive Surgery, Department of Otolaryngology, School of Medicine, NYU Langone Medical Center, New York University, New York, NY, USA

Christina Cooper Neuro Rehab & Balance Centre, Kettering Health Network, Centerville, OH, USA

Rebecca Cornelius Department of Radiology & Otolaryngology, University of Cincinnati, Cincinnati, OH, USA

Maura K. Cosetti Department of Otolaryngology, New York University School of Medicine, New York, NY, USA

James V. Crawford Department of Otolaryngology, Madigan Healthcare System, Tacoma, WA, USA

Karen M. Crews University of Mississippi Medical Center, Jackson, MS, USA

Robin E. Criter Special Education & Communication Disorders, University of Nebraska-Lincoln, Lincoln, NE, USA

Calhoun D. Cunningham III Carolina Ear & Hearing Clinic, P.C., Raleigh, NC, USA

David Darrow Eastern Virginia Medical School, Norfolk, VA, USA

Terence M. Davidson Division of Otolaryngology-Head and Neck Surgery, University of California, San Diego, San Diego, CA, USA

Krsto Dawidowsky Department for ENT and Head and Neck Surgery, University Hospital Center Zagreb, Zagreb, Croatia

John M. DelGaudio Department of Otolaryngology-Head and Neck Surgery, Emory University School of Medicine, Atlanta, GA, USA

Michael DeMarcantonio Eastern Virginia Medical School, Norfolk, VA, USA

Todd Demmy Department of Thoracic Surgery, Roswell Park Cancer Institute, Buffalo, NY, USA

Craig Derkay Department of Otolaryngology-Head and Neck Surgery, Children's Hospital of the King's Daughters, Eastern Virginia Medical School, Norfolk, VA, USA

Ari DeRowe Pediatric Otolaryngology Unit, Dana-Dewek Children's Hospital, Tel Aviv Sourasky Medical Center, Tel Aviv University, Sackler School of Medicine, Tel-Aviv, Israel

Shruti N. Deshpande Department of Communication Sciences and Disorders, University of Cincinnati- College of Allied Health Sciences, Cincinnati, OH, USA

G. Paul Digoy Department of Otorhinolaryngology, University of Oklahoma, Oklahoma City, OK, USA

Christine T. Dinh Department of Otolaryngology-Head and Neck Surgery, Leonard M. Miller School of Medicine Jackson Memorial Hospital, University of Miami, Miami, FL, USA

Carol Dinnes Massachusetts General Hospital, Revere and Chelsea Healthcare Centers, Department of Speech-Language, Swallowing Disorders and Reading Disabilities, Revere/Chelsea, MA, USA

Benjamin J. Dixon Department of Otolaryngology, Head and Neck Surgery, University of Toronto, Toronto, ON, Canada

Hamid Djalilian Department of Otolaryngology-Head and Neck Surgery, University of California, Irvine Medical Center, Orange, CA, USA

Eric J. Dobratz Department of Otolaryngology, Eastern Virginia Medical School, Norfolk, VA, USA

Kelley Dodson Department of Otolaryngology-Head and Neck Surgery, Virginia Commonwealth University, Richmond, VA, USA

Joni K. Doherty Center for Neural Tumor Research, House Research Institute, Los Angeles, CA, USA

Kimberly A. Donnellan Department of Facial Plastic and Reconstructive Surgery, IMC Otolaryngology Facial Plastic and Reconstructive Surgery, Mobile, AL, USA

John L. Dornhoffer Department of Otolaryngology-Head and Neck Surgery, University of Arkansas for Medical Sciences, Little Rock, AR, USA

Richard L. Doty Department of Otorhinolaryngology-Head and Neck Surgery, Smell and Taste Center, University of Pennsylvania School of Medicine, University of Pennsylvania Medical Center, Philadelphia, PA, USA

Angela E. Downes Department of Neurosurgery, University of South Florida, Tampa, FL, USA

Leonid Drozhinin Department of Radiology, New York University School of Medicine, New York, NY, USA

Georges Dumas Department of Otolaryngology-Head and Neck Surgery, Otology/Neurotology Unit, University Hospital of Grenoble, Grenoble, France

Service ORL. Hôpital A. Michallon, Grenoble, France

Honey E. East Department of Medicine/Endocrinology, Division of Endocrinology, University of Mississippi Medical Center, Jackson, MS, USA

Ardalan Ebrahimi Sydney Head and Neck Cancer Institute, Camperdown, NSW, Australia

David J. Eisenman Department of Otorhinolaryngology-Head and Neck Surgery, University of Maryland School of Medicine, Baltimore, MD, USA

Oleksandr Ekshyyan Department of Otolaryngology and Feist-Weiller Cancer Center, Louisiana State University Health Sciences Center - Shreveport, Shreveport, LA, USA

Ravindhra G. Elluru Department of Otolaryngology, Cincinnati Children's Hospital and University of Cincinnati College of Medicine, Cincinnati, OH, USA

Jeffrey S. Epstein Foundation for Hair Restoration, University of Miami, Miami, FL, USA

Boban M. Erovic Department of Otolaryngology-Head and Neck Surgery, Wharton Head and Neck Program, University Health Network, Princess Margaret Hospital, Toronto, ON, Canada

Francesco T. Mangano D. O. F.A.C.O.S. Division of Pediatric Neurosurgery, Cincinnati Children's Hospital Medical Center, Cincinnati, OH, USA

Samer Fakhri Department of Otorhinolaryngology-Head and Neck Surgery, University of Texas Medical School at Houston, Houston, TX, USA

Texas Skull Base Physicians and Texas Sinus Institute, Houston, TX, USA

Carole Fakhry Department of Otolaryngology-Head and Neck Surgery, Johns Hopkins School of Medicine, Baltimore, MD, USA

Marcela Fandiño Departments of Otolaryngology-Head and Neck Surgery and Diagnostic Imaging, University of Toronto, Toronto, ON, Canada

Te-Yung Fang Cathay General Hospital, Taipei, Taiwan

Rola Farah Department of Communication Sciences and Disorders, College of Allied Health Sciences, University of Cincinnati, Cincinnati, OH, USA

Callum Faris Department of Otolaryngology, Southampton University Hospitals, Southampton, Hampshire, UK

Roger W. Farmer Miller School of Medicine, University of Miami, Miami, FL, USA

Tarik Farrag Department of Otolaryngology, Medical College of Georgia, Augusta, GA, USA

Girish Fatterpekar Department of Radiology, New York University School of Medicine, New York, NY, USA

Jose N. Fayad House Clinic, Los Angeles, CA, USA

House Clinic and Department of Histopathology, University of Southern California, House Ear Institute, Los Angeles, CA, USA

Leah M. Feazel Division of Infectious Diseases, School of Medicine, University of Colorado, Aurora, CO, USA

Berrylin J. Ferguson Department of Otolaryngology, University of Pittsburgh, Pittsburgh, PA, USA

Rui P. Fernandes Division of Oral and Maxillofacial Surgery, College of Medicine, University of Florida, Jacksonville, FL, USA

Robert L. Ferris Department of Otolaryngology Head Neck Surgery, University of Pittsburgh, Pittsburgh, PA, USA

Ramón E. Figueroa Department of Radiology, Georgia Health Sciences University, Augusta, GA, USA

Jonathan D. Finder School of Medicine, University of Pittsburgh, Pittsburgh, PA, USA

Nathaniel von Fischer Department of Radiology, University of Cincinnati, Cincinnati, OH, USA

David Fisher Auckland City Hospital, Auckland, New Zealand

Andrew J. Fishman Departments of Otolaryngology & Neurosurgery, Northwestern University Feinberg School of Medicine, Chicago, IL, USA

Gadi Fishman Pediatric Otolaryngology, Dana Children's Hospital, Department of Otolaryngology-Head and Neck Surgery and Maxillofacial Surgery, Sourasky Tel-Aviv Medical Center, Affiliated to the Tel-Aviv University, Tel-Aviv, Israel

Kenneth E. Fleisher Department of Oral and Maxillofacial Surgery, New York University College of Dentistry, New York, NY, USA

Department of Surgery, NYU Langone Medical Center, New York, NY, USA

M. Taylor Fordham Otolaryngology-Head and Neck Surgery, College of Medicine, Medical University of South Carolina, Charleston, SC, USA

Steven J. Frampton Poole Hospital NHS Foundation Trust, Poole, Dorset, UK

Cancer Sciences Division, University of Southampton, Southampton, Hampshire, UK

Christine B. Franzese Department of Otolaryngology and Communicative Sciences, University of Mississippi Medical Center, Jackson, MS, USA

Jeremy L. Freeman Mount Sinai Hospital, Toronto, ON, Canada

Marvin P. Fried Department of Otorhinolaryngology-Head and Neck Surgery, Montefiore Medical Center, Albert Einstein College of Medicine, Bronx, NY, USA

David R. Friedland Department of Otolaryngology and Communication Sciences, Division of Otology and Neuro-otologic Skull Base Surgery, Medical College of Wisconsin, Milwaukee, WI, USA

Adva B. Friedman Department of Otolaryngology-Head and Neck Surgery, University of Arkansas for Medical Sciences, Arkansas Children's Hospital, Little Rock, AR, USA

Michael Friedman Advocate Illinois Masonic Medical Center, Chicago ENT an Advanced Center for Specialty Care, Chicago, IL, USA

Department of Otolaryngology and Bronchoesophagology, Rush University Medical Center, Chicago, IL, USA

Denby K. Fukuda Otology/Neurotology Otolaryngology Division, Tripler Army Medical Center, Honolulu, HI, USA

Christopher E. Fundakowski Department of Otolaryngology-Head and Neck Surgery, University of Miami, Leonard M. Miller School of Medicine, Miami, FL, USA

David Furgiuele Department of Anesthesiology, NYU Langone Medical Center, New York University, New York, NY, USA

Mark J. Furin The Vancouver Clinic, Vancouver, WA, Canada

Alexis D. Furze Private Practice Facial Plastic and Reconstructive Surgery, Newport Beach, CA, USA

Arun K. Gadre University Surgical Associates, Louisville, KY, USA

Thomas J. Gal Department of Otolaryngology-Head and Neck Surgery, University of Kentucky, Chandler Medical Center, Lexington, KY, USA

Diogo Galheigo New York University School of Medicine, New York, NY, USA

Anthony W. Gannon Division of Endocrinology, Metabolism and Diabetes, Department of Internal Medicine, University of Mississippi Medical Center, Jackson, MS, USA

Eric A. Gantwerker Department of Otolaryngology-Head and Neck Surgery, University of Cincinnati, Cincinnati, OH, USA

Brian C. Gartrell Department of Surgery, Division of Otolaryngology, University of Wisconsin Hospital and Clinics, Madison, WI, USA

Jaime Gateno Department of Oral and Maxillofacial Surgery, The Methodist Hospital, Houston, TX, USA

Department of Surgery, Weill Medical College of Cornell University, New York, NY, USA

Cindy Gauger Division of Pediatric Hematology-Oncology, Nemours Children's Clinic, Jacksonville, FL, USA

Rachel A. Georgopoulos School of Medicine, Stony Brook University, East Setauket, NY, USA

Melissa Ghiringhelli Massachusetts General Hospital, Revere and Chelsea Healthcare Centers, Department of Speech-Language, Swallowing Disorders and Reading Disabilities, Revere/Chelsea, MA, USA

Paul Gidley Department of Head and Neck Surgery, University of Texas M. D. Anderson Cancer Center, Houston, TX, USA

Douglas A. Girod Department of Otolaryngology-Head and Neck Surgery, University of Kansas School of Medicine, Kansas City, KS, USA

Jack Gladstein Department of Pediatrics and Neurology, University of Maryland School of Medical, Baltimore, MD, USA

Robert S. Glickman Department of Oral and Maxillofacial Surgery, New York University Medical Center/Bellevue Hospital Center, New York, NY, USA

Department of Surgery, NYU Langone Medical Center, New York, NY, USA

Michael B. Gluth Department of Otolaryngology-Head and Neck Surgery, University of Arkansas for Medical Sciences, Little Rock, AR, USA

John C. Goddard House Clinic, Los Angeles, CA, USA

Andrew N. Goldberg Department of Otolaryngology-Head and Neck Surgery, University of California, San Francisco, CA, USA

David P. Goldstein Department of Otolaryngology-Head and Neck Surgery, Wharton Head and Neck Program, University Health Network, Princess Margaret Hospital, Toronto, ON, Canada

Nathan Gonik Department of Otorhinolaryngology-Head and Neck Surgery, Albert Einstein College of Medicine, Bronx, NY, USA

Jorge E. González Bloomsburg University of Pennsylvania, Bloomsburg, PA, USA

Mitchell Gore Department of Otolaryngology-Head and Neck Surgery, University of North Carolina at Chapel Hill, Chapel Hill, NC, USA

Katherine Green School of Medicine, Department of Otolaryngology, University of Colorado, Children's Hospital Colorado, Aurora, CO, USA

Alan R. Grimm Department of Otolaryngology and Communicative Sciences, University of Mississippi Medical Center, Jackson, MS, USA

Jonathan M. Grischkan Department of Otolaryngology, Nationwide Children's Hospital, The Ohio State University, Columbus, OH, USA

William Grist Department of Otolaryngology, Emory University School of Medicine, Atlanta, GA, USA

Samuel P. Gubbels Department of Surgery, Division of Otolaryngology, University of Wisconsin Hospital and Clinics, Madison, WI, USA

Patrick J. Gullane Department of Otolaryngology, University of Toronto, Toronto, ON, Canada

Reena Gupta Voice and Swallowing Center, Osborne Head and Neck Institute, Los Angeles, CA, USA

Sachin Gupta Division of Facial Plastic & Reconstructive Surgery, Department of Otolaryngology, New York University School of Medicine, New York, NY, USA

Vishal Gupta Head and Neck – Plastic Reconstructive Surgery, Roswell Park Cancer Institute, Buffalo, NY, USA

Richard K. Gurgel Department of Otolaryngology-Head and Neck Surgery, Stanford University, Stanford, CA, USA

Rudolf Hagen Department of Otorhinolaryngology, Plastic, Aesthetic and Reconstructive Head and Neck Surgery, University of Wuerzburg, Wuerzburg, Germany

Mari Hagiwara Department of Radiology, New York University School of Medicine, New York, NY, USA

Craig Hamilton Advocate Illinois Masonic Medical Center, Chicago ENT an Advanced Center for Specialty Care, Chicago, IL, USA

Joseph K. Han Department of Otolaryngology-Head and Neck Surgery, Division of Rhinology and Endoscopic Sinus & Skull Base Surgery, Eastern Virginia Medical School, Norfolk, VA, USA

J. Edward Hartmann Georgia Health Sciences, University/Medical College of Georgia, Augusta, GA, USA

George T. Hashisaki Department of Otolaryngology-Head and Neck Surgery, University of Virginia Health System, Charlottesville, VA, USA

David S. Haynes The Otology Group of Vanderbilt, Vanderbilt University Medical Center, Nashville, TN, USA

Sabrina M. Heman-Ackah School of Medicine, University of North Carolina, Chapel Hill, NC, USA

Selena E. Heman-Ackah Department of Otolaryngology-Head and Neck Surgery, New York University, New York, NY, USA

Maggie Hendrickson Dizziness and Balance Disorder Lab, University of Nebraska-Lincoln, Lincoln, NE, USA

Oswaldo A. Henriquez Department of Otolaryngology-Head and Neck Surgery, School of Medicine, Emory University, Atlanta, GA, USA

Bjorn Herman Department of Otolaryngology Head and Neck Surgery, University of Miami Miller School of Medicine, Miami, FL, USA

Ronna Hertzano Department of Otorhinolaryngology-Head and Neck Surgery, University of Maryland School of Medicine, Baltimore, MD, USA

Amy C. Hessel Department of Head and Neck Surgery, M. D. Anderson Cancer Center, The University of Texas, Houston, TX, USA

Barry E. Hirsch Department of Otolaryngology, Eye & Ear Institute, UPMC, Pittsburgh, PA, USA

Stephen Q. Hoang Department of Anesthesiology and Pain Management, UT Southwestern Medical Center Dallas, Children's Medical Center Dallas, Dallas, TX, USA

Brian Ho Department of Otolaryngology, Georgia Health Sciences University, Augusta, GA, USA

Tang Ho Department of Otorhinolaryngology-Head and Neck Surgery, University of Texas Health Science Center at Houston, Houston, TX, USA

Michael E. Hoffer Department of Otolaryngology, Spatial Orientation center, Naval Medical Center, San Diego, CA, USA

Julie A. Honaker Department of Special Education and Communication Disorders, University of Nebraska-Lincoln, Lincoln, NE, USA

Gia E. Hoosien Department of Otolaryngology-Head and Neck Surgery, University of Miami, Leonard M. Miller School of Medicine, Miami, FL, USA

Drew M. Horlbeck Department of Surgery, Division of Pediatric Otolaryngology, Nemours Children's Clinic, Jacksonville, FL, USA

Lisa Houston Department of Audiology, UC Physicians ENT, Cincinnati, OH, USA

Sun Hsieh Medical College of Georgia, Georgia Health Sciences University, Augusta, GA, USA

Matthew A. Hubbard Department of Otolaryngology-Head and Neck Surgery, University of Virginia Health System, Charlottesville, VA, USA

Anthony Hughes Department of Otolaryngology, Medical College of Georgia, Georgia Health Sciences University, Augusta, GA, USA

Jacob Hunter Department of Otorhinolaryngology-Head and Neck Surgery, Albert Einstein College of Medicine, New York, USA

Inna Husain Department of Otolaryngology-Head and Neck Surgery, Feinberg School of Medicine, Northwestern University, Chicago, IL, USA

Sara Immerman Department of Otolaryngology, NYU Medical Center, New York, NY, USA

Jonathan C. Irish Department of Otolaryngology, Head and Neck Surgery, University of Toronto, Toronto, ON, Canada

Princess Margaret Hospital, Toronto, ON, Canada

Seth Isaacs Cincinnati Sinus Institute, Group Health Associates, Cincinnati, OH, USA

Brandon Isaacson Otolaryngology-Head and Neck Surgery, University of Texas Southwestern Medical Center, Dallas, TX, USA

Amal Isaiah Department of Otorhinolaryngology-HNS, University of Maryland School of Medicine, Baltimore, MD, USA

Mark Izzard Auckland City Hospital, Auckland, New Zealand

Alexis Jackman Hope Department of Otorhinolaryngology, Albert Einstein College of Medicine/Montefiore Medical Center, Bronx, NY, USA

Lance E. Jackson Ear Institute of Texas, San Antonio, TX, USA

Howard S. Jacobs Department of Pediatrics, University of Maryland School of Medical, Baltimore, MD, USA

Hachem Jammal Department of Surgery, Tawam Hospital, Al Ain, UAE

Tanima Jana Department of Otolaryngology, University of Mississippi Medical Center, Jackson, MS, USA

Michael P. Janjigian New York University School of Medicine, New York, NY, USA

Eric M. Jaryszak Children's Ear, Nose, and Throat Associates, Orlando, FL, USA

Gina D. Jefferson Department of Otolaryngology and Communicative Sciences, University of Mississippi Medical Center, Jackson, MS, USA

Anita Jeyakumar Department of Otolaryngology-Head and Neck Surgery, Louisiana State University School of Medicine-Health Science Center, New Orleans, LA, USA

Christopher M. Johnson Department of Otolaryngology, Spatial Orientation center, Naval Medical Center, San Diego, CA, USA

Romaine F. Johnson Department of Otolaryngology-Head and Neck Surgery, UT Southwestern Medical Center at Dallas, Dallas, TX, USA

Daekeun Joo Department of Surgery, Division of Otolaryngology-Head and Neck Surgery, Loma Linda University Medical Center, Loma Linda, CA, USA

Randy Jordan Department of Otolaryngology and Communicative Sciences, University of Mississippi Medical Center, Jackson, MS, USA

Gary D. Josephson Division of Pediatric Otolaryngology-HNS, Nemours Children's Clinic, Jacksonville, FL, USA

Jeb M. Justice Division of Otolaryngology-Head and Neck Surgery, University of Utah, Salt Lake City, UT, USA

Abdul Aleem Kadar Otolaryngology-Head and Neck Surgery, Jinnah Postgraduate Medical Centre, Karachi, Sindh, Pakistan

Mohan Kameswaran Department of Implant Otology, Madras ENT Research Foundation (P) Ltd, Chennai, Tamil Nadu, India

Alex Kane Department of Plastic Surgery, University of Texas Southwestern Medical Center, Dallas, TX, USA

Gerald T. Kangelaris Department of Otolaryngology-Head and Neck Surgery, University of California, San Francisco, San Francisco, CA, USA

Seth J. Kanowitz Department of Otolaryngology, Morristown Medical Center, Morristown, NJ, USA

Elina Kari House Ear Clinic, Los Angeles, CA, USA

Alexandre Karkas Clinique Universitaire Oto–Rhino–Laryngologie, Centre Hospitalier Universitaire A. Michallon, Grenoble, France

Department of Otolaryngology-Head and Neck Surgery, Otology/Neurotology Unit, University Hospital of Grenoble, Grenoble, France

Service ORL. Hôpital A. Michallon, Grenoble, France

Tom T. Karnezis Division of Otolaryngology-Head and Neck Surgery, University of California, San Diego, San Diego, CA, USA

Jack M. Kartush Michigan Ear Institute, Farmington Hills, MI, USA

David M. Kaylie Department of Otolaryngology, Duke University Medical Center, Durham, NC, USA

Robert W. Keith Department of Communication Sciences and Disorders, College of Allied Health Sciences, University of Cincinnati, Cincinnati, OH, USA

Robert Kern Northwestern Sinus & Allergy Center, Feinberg School of Medicine, Department of Otolaryngology-Head and Neck Surgery, Northwestern University, Chicago, IL, USA

Bradley W. Kesser Department of Otolaryngology-Head and Neck Surgery, University of Virginia Health System, Charlottesville, VA, USA

Majid A. Khan Division of NeuroRadiology, University of MS Medical Center, Jackson, MS, USA

Mumtaz J. Khan Head & Neck Institute, Cleveland Clinic Foundation, Cleveland, OH, USA

Alexander Kiderman Neuro-Kinetics, Inc., Pittsburgh, PA, USA

Michael M. Kim Division of Facial Plastic & Reconstructive Surgery, Department of Otolaryngology-Head and Neck Surgery, Oregon Health & Science University, Portland, OR, USA

Paul D. Kim Department of Surgery, Division of Otolaryngology-Head and Neck Surgery, Loma Linda University Medical Center, Loma Linda, CA, USA

Department of Otolaryngology, Loma Linda School of Medicine, Loma Linda, CA, USA

Charles P. Kimmelman Otolaryngology Head and Neck Surgery, Weill Cornell Medical Center, New York, NY, USA

Emma V. King Poole Hospital NHS Foundation Trust, Poole, Dorset, UK

Cancer Sciences Division, University of Southampton, Southampton, Hampshire, UK

Todd T. Kingdom Department of Otolaryngology-Head and Neck Surgery, School of Medicine, University of Colorado, Aurora, CO, USA

Usha Kini Department of Pathology, St John's Medical College, Bangalore, Karnataka, India

Liat Kishon-Rabin Communication Disorders Department, Sackler Faculty of Medicine, Tel-Aviv University, Tel Aviv, Israel

Adam M. Klein Department of Otolaryngology-Head and Neck Surgery, Emory University School of Medicine, Atlanta, GA, USA

Micah L. Klumpp Department of Otolaryngology, LSU Health Sciences Center, Our Lady of the Lake Hearing and Balance Center, Baton Rouge, LA, USA

Christian A. Koch Department of Medicine/Endocrinology, Division of Endocrinology, University of Mississippi Medical Center, Jackson, MS, USA

Harold Kolodney Jr. Department of Otolaryngology and Communicative Sciences, The University of Mississippi Medical Center, Jackson, MS, USA

Russell W. H. Kridel Department of Otolaryngology-Head and Neck Surgery, Division of Facial Plastic Surgery, University of Texas Health Sciences Center, Houston, Texas, USA

Kumaresh Krishnamoorthy ENT and Head & Neck Surgery & Neurotology, Dr Kumaresh ENT Care, Bangalore, India

Jeffrey B. Krutoy Department of Oral and Maxillofacial Surgery, New York University Medical Center/Bellevue Hospital Center, New York, NY, USA

Jeffery J. Kuhn Otology/Neurotology, Department of Otolaryngology-Head and Neck Surgery, Naval Medical Center Portsmouth, Portsmouth, VA, USA

Maggie A. Kuhn Department of Otolaryngology-Head and Neck Surgery, New York University Langone Medical Center, New York, NY, USA

Ronald B. Kuppersmith The Texas Institute for Thyroid and Parathyroid Surgery, Texas ENT and Allergy, College Station, TX, USA

Joe Walter Kutz Jr. Otolaryngology-Head and Neck Surgery, University of Texas Southwestern Medical Center, Dallas, TX, USA

Anil K. Lalwani Department of Otolaryngology-Head and Neck Surgery, New York University, New York, NY, USA

John T. Lam Department of Pathology, University of Mississippi Medical Center, Jackson, MS, USA

Paul R. Lambert Department of Otolaryngology-Head and Neck Surgery, College of Medicine, Medical University of South Carolina, Charleston, SC, USA

Deidre R. Larrier Texas Children's Hospital, Houston, TX, USA

L. Frederick Lassen Department of Otolaryngology, Lakeview Medical Center, Suffolk, VA, USA

Adrienne M. Laury Department of Otolaryngology-Head and Neck Surgery, Emory University School of Medicine, Atlanta, GA, USA

Amy Lawrason Division of Otolaryngology, Department of Head and Neck Surgery, University of Connecticut Health Center, Farmington, CT, USA

Cathy L. Lazarus Thyroid Head and Neck Cancer Research Center, Thyroid Head and Neck Cancer Foundation, Department of Otolaryngology, Beth Israel Medical Center, New York, NY, USA

Richard A. Lebowitz Department of Otolaryngology-Head and Neck Surgery, New York University School of Medicine, NYU Langone Medical Center, New York, NY, USA

Judy Washington Lee Division of Facial Plastic and Reconstructive Surgery, Department of Otolaryngology, School of Medicine, NYU Langone Medical Center, New York University, New York, NY, USA

Kenneth Lee Diagnostic Pathology Unit, Concord Repatriation General Hospital, Concord, Sydney, NSW, Australia

Nancy Lee Department of Radiation Oncology, Memorial Sloan-Kettering Cancer Center, New York, NY, USA

Shanjean Lee Duke University Medical Center, Durham, NC, USA

Christopher E. Lee Department of Otolaryngology and Communicative Sciences, University of Mississippi School of Medicine, Jackson, MS, USA

Edward R. Lee Medical College of Wisconsin, Milwaukee, WI, USA

Kenneth H. Lee Department of Otolaryngology-Head and Neck Surgery, University of Texas Southwestern Medical Center at Dallas, Dallas, TX, USA

Steve C. Lee Department of Otolaryngology-Head Neck Surgery, Loma Linda University School of Medicine, Loma Linda, CA, USA

Jason M. Leibowitz Department of Otolaryngology Head and Neck Surgery, University of Miami Miller School of Medicine, Miami, FL, USA

Lori A. Lemonnier Department of Otolaryngology, Temple University, Philadelphia, PA, USA

Randy Leung Department of Otolaryngology-Head and Neck Surgery, Northwestern University, Feinberg School of Medicine, Barrie, ON, Canada

Randal Leung The Royal Victorian Eye and Ear Hospital, The University of Melbourne, Melbourne, VIC, Australia

Marci H. Levine Department of Oral and Maxillofacial Surgery, New York University College of Dentistry, New York, NY, USA

Timothy S. Lian Department of Otolaryngology-Head and Neck Surgery, Louisiana State University Health Sciences Center-Shreveport, Shreveport, LA, USA

Seth Lieberman School of Medicine, Department of Otolaryngology, New York University Langone Medical Center, New York, NY, USA

Rui Jun Lin Division of Otolaryngology-Head and Neck Surgery, University of British Columbia, Vancouver, BC, Canada

James Lin Department of Otolaryngology, Kansas University Medical Center, Kansas City, KS, USA

LindauRobert H. III Univeristy of Nebraska Medical Center, Omaha, NE, USA

Nebreska Methodist Estabrook Cancer Center, Omaha, NE, USA

Philip Littlefield Division of Otology/Neurotology, Walter Reed Military Medical Center Bethesda, Bethesda, MD, USA

Stephanie Lockhart UC Health, Otolaryngology-Head and Neck Surgery, Cincinnati, OH, USA

John P. Loh Department of Radiology, NYU School of Medicine, New York, NY, USA

Irene Low Department of Anatomical Pathology, PathWest, Sir Charles Gairdner Hospital, Nedland, Perth, WA, Australia

Amber Luong Department of Otorhinolaryngology-Head and Neck Surgery, University of Texas Medical School at Houston, Houston, TX, USA

Texas Skull Base Physicians and Texas Sinus Institute, Houston, TX, USA

Michael D. Lupa Department of Otolaryngology, Emory University, Atlanta, GA, USA

Lawrence R. Lustig Department of Otolaryngology-Head and Neck Surgery, University of California, San Francisco, San Francisco, CA, USA

Sofia Lyford-Pike Department of Otolaryngology, Johns Hopkins University School of Medicine, Baltimore, MD, USA

Hossein Mahboubi Department of Otolaryngology-Head and Neck Surgery, University of California, Irvine Medical Center, Orange, CA, USA

Anjali Malkani Department of Pediatric Gastroenterology and Nutrition, University of Maryland, School of Medicine, Baltimore, MD, USA

Pavan S. Mallur Department of Otology and Laryngology, Harvard Medical School, Boston, MA, USA

Beth Israel Deaconess Medical Center, Boston, MA, USA

Alex Mammen Medical College of Georgia, Department of Ophthalmology, Georgia Health Sciences University, Augusta, GA, USA

Li-Xing Man Department of Otolaryngology-Head and Neck Surgery, University of Rochester School of Medicine and Dentistry, University of Rochester Medical Center, Rochester, NY, USA

Ellen M. Mandel Division of Pediatric Otolaryngology, Children's Hospital of Pittsburgh, University of Pittsburgh, Pittsburgh, PA, USA

Jeffrey Marino Division of Otolaryngology, Department of Head and Neck Surgery, University of Connecticut Health Center, Farmington, CT, USA

Jonathan Mark Department of Otolaryngology, Eastern Virginia Medical School, Norfolk, VA, USA

John C. Mason Department of Otolaryngology, University of Virginia, Charlottesville, VA, USA

Douglas E. Mattox Department of Otolaryngology-Head and Neck Surgery, School of Medicine, Emory University, Atlanta, GA, USA

Haggi Mazeh Section of Endocrine Surgery, Department of Surgery, School of Medicine, University of Wisconsin, Madison, WI, USA

J. Seth McAfee Department of Otolaryngology-Head and Neck Surgery, Division of Rhinology and Endoscopic Sinus & Skull Base Surgery, Eastern Virginia Medical School, Norfolk, VA, USA

John E. McClay University of Texas at Southwestern Medical School, Dallas, TX, USA

Scott McClintick Department of Otolaryngology-Head and Neck Surgery, University of Iowa Hospitals & Clinics, Iowa City, IA, USA

John T. McElveen Jr. Carolina Ear & Hearing Clinic, P.C., Raleigh, NC, USA

Brian J. McKinnon Department of Otolaryngology-Head and Neck Surgery, Georgia Health Sciences University, Augusta, GA, USA

Caitlin P. McMullen Department of Otorhinolaryngology, Albert Einstein College of Medicine/Montefiore Medical Center, Bronx, NY, USA

Beth McNulty Department of Surgery, Otolaryngology-Head and Neck Surgery, University of Louisville, Louisville, KY, USA

Theodore R. McRackan Vanderbilt University Medical Center, Nashville, TN, USA

Mahesh Mehta University of Mississippi Medical Center, Jackson, MS, USA

Jeremy D. Meier Department of Otolaryngology-Head and Neck Surgery, Medical University of South Carolina, Charleston, SC, USA

Maria Cecilia Melendres Department of Pediatrics, Johns Hopkins University, Baltimore, MD, USA

Thuy-Anh Melvin Department of Otolaryngology-Head and Neck Surgery, Johns Hopkins School of Medicine, Baltimore, MD, USA

Yusuf Menda Departments of Radiology, University of Iowa Hospitals and Clinics, Iowa City, IA, USA

Cédric Mendoza Department of Otolaryngology-Head and Neck Surgery, Otology/Neurotology Unit, University Hospital of Grenoble, Grenoble, France

Service ORL. Hôpital A. Michallon, Grenoble, France

Department of Neuroradiology, University Hospital of Grenoble, Grenoble, France

Caroline Mesmer Department of Otolaryngology, Naval Medical Center, San Diego, CA, USA

Aaron M. Metrailer Department of Otolaryngology-Head and Neck Surgery, University of Arkansas for Medical Sciences, Little Rock, AR, USA

Ted A. Meyer Department of Otolaryngology-Head and Neck Surgery, Medical University of South Carolina, Charleston, SC, USA

Jozef Mierzwinski Department of Otolaryngology, Children's Hospital of Bydgoszcz, Bydgoszcz, Poland

Dragan Mihailovic Institute of Pathology, University of Nis, Nis, Serbia

Anthony A. Mikulec Department of Otolaryngology, Saint Louis University School of Medicine, St. Louis, MO, USA

Dusan Milisavljevic University ORL Clinic, Nis, Serbia

Sean M. Miller Department of Otolaryngology, Saint Louis University School of Medicine, St. Louis, MO, USA

Lloyd B. Minor Department of Otolaryngology-Head and Neck Surgery, Johns Hopkins University School of Medicine, Baltimore, MD, USA

D. Mistry ENT Department, Bradford Royal Infirmary, Bradford, West Yorkshire, UK

Ron B. Mitchell Otolaryngology and Pediatrics, University of Texas Southwestern Medical Center, Children's Medical Center Dallas, Dallas, TX, USA

Robert Mlynski Department of Otorhinolaryngology, Plastic, Aesthetic and Reconstructive Head and Neck Surgery, University of Wuerzburg, Wuerzburg, Germany

Anne M. Mooney NYU Sleep Disorders Center, New York, NY, USA

NYU Langone Medical Center and NYU School of Medicine, New York, NY, USA

Charles E. Moore Department of Otolaryngology-Head and Neck Surgery, Emory University School of Medicine, Atlanta, GA, USA

Howard S. Moskowitz Department of Otolaryngology-Head and Neck Surgery, Johns Hopkins, Baltimore, MD, USA

Badr Eldin Mostafa Department of Otorhinolaryngology-Head and Neck Surgery, Faculty of Medicine, Ain-Shams University, Nasr City, Cairo, Egypt

Patrick D. Munson Department of Surgery, Division of Otolaryngology, University of South Dakota School of Medicine, Sanford Children's Hospital, Sioux Falls, SD, USA

Craig S. Murakami Department of Otolaryngology-Head and Neck Surgery, Virginia Mason Medical Center, University of Washington, Seattle, WA, USA

Andrew H. Murr Department of Otolaryngology-Head and Neck Surgery, University of California, San Francisco School of Medicine, San Francisco, CA, USA

Ryan Murray Division of Otolaryngology, Department of Surgery, Nemours/Alfred I. duPont Hospital for Children, Wilmington, DE, USA

Department of Otolaryngology-Head and Neck Surgery, Jefferson Medical College, Thomas Jefferson University, Philadelphia, PA, USA

Wojciech K. Mydlarz Department of Otolaryngology-Head and Neck Surgery, Johns Hopkins University School of Medicine, Baltimore, MD, USA

Natalya Nagornaya Miller School of Medicine, University of Miami, Miami, FL, USA

Maja Nahtigal Department of ORL and MFS, University Clinical Center Maribor, Maribor, Slovenia

J. Rie Nakayama Tripler Army Medical Center, Honolulu, HI, USA

Iman Naseri Division of Otolaryngology, College of Medicine, University of Florida, Jacksonville, FL, USA

Cherie-Ann O. Nathan Department of Otolaryngology and Feist-Weiller Cancer Center, Louisiana State University Health Sciences Center - Shreveport, Shreveport, LA, USA

Ilka C. Naumann Michigan Ear Institute, Farmington Hills, MI, USA

Chetan S. Nayak Department of Otolaryngology-Head and Neck Surgery, University of Miami Leonard M. Miller School of Medicine, Miami, FL, USA

Ravi C. Nayar Department of Otolaryngology and Head and Neck Surgery, St John's Medical College Hospital, Bangalore, Karnataka, India

Matthew Ng Department of Surgery, Division of Otolaryngology, University of Nevada School of Medicine, Las Vegas, NV, USA

Tam Nguyen Department of Otolaryngology-Head and Neck Surgery, University of Virginia Health System, Charlottesville, VA, USA

Todd A. Nichols Division of NeuroRadiology, University of MS Medical Center, Jackson, MS, USA

Grace L. Nimmons Departments of Otolaryngology-Head and Neck Surgery, University of Iowa Hospitals and Clinics, Iowa City, IA, USA

Jennifer Nolan Walter Reed National Military Medical Center, Bethesda, MD, USA

Daniel Novakovic Sydney Voice and Swallowing, St Leonards, Sydney, NSW, Australia

Ajani G. Nugent Department of Otolaryngology-Head and Neck Surgery, Emory University, Atlanta, GA, USA

M. Elizabeth Oates Department of Radiology, University of Kentucky, College of Medicine, Lexington, KY, USA

Brendan P. O'Connell Department of Otolaryngology-Head and Neck Surgery, College of Medicine, Medical University of South Carolina, Charleston, SC, USA

Miriam O'Leary Department of Otolaryngology, Tufts Medical Center, Boston, MA, USA

Eric R. Oliver Department of Otolaryngology-Head and Neck Surgery, Wake Forest University School of Medicine, Winston-Salem, NC, USA

Sepehr Oliaei Department of Otolaryngology-Head and Neck Surgery, University of California Irvine, Orange, CA, USA

Robert A. Ord Department of Oral-Maxillofacial Surgery, R. Adams Cowley Shock Trauma Center, Greenebaum Cancer Center, University of Maryland Medical Center, Baltimore, MD, USA

Richard R. Orlandi Division of Otolaryngology-Head and Neck Surgery, University of Utah, Salt Lake City, UT, USA

James A. Owusu Department of Otolaryngology-Head and Neck Surgery, University of Minnesota, Minneapolis, MN, USA

Pia Pace-Asciak Gordon and Leslie Diamond Health Care Centre, Department of Otolaryngology, UBC, Vancouver, BC, Canada

Nitin A. Pagedar Departments of Otolaryngology-Head and Neck Surgery, University of Iowa Hospitals and Clinics, Iowa City, IA, USA

Michael N. Pakdaman Department of Otolaryngology-Head and Neck Surgery, University of Texas Health Science Center at Houston, Houston, TX, USA

Richard N. Palu Section of Ophthalmic Plastic and Reconstructive Surgery, New York University Medical Center, New York, NY, USA

Kourosh Parham Division of Otolaryngology, Department of Head and Neck Surgery, University of Connecticut Health Center, Farmington, CT, USA

Sanjay R. Parikh Division of Pediatric Otolaryngology, Department of Otolaryngology-Head and Neck Surgery, Seattle Children's Hospital, University of Washington School of Medicine, Seattle, WA, USA

Albert H. Park Division of Otolaryngology-ENT Head and Neck Surgery, Department of Surgery, University of Utah, Salt Lake City, UT, USA

Steven Y. Park Department of Otorhinolaryngology, Montefiore Medical Center, Bronx, NY, USA

William J. Parkes Division of Otolaryngology, Department of Surgery, Nemours/Alfred I. duPont Hospital for Children, Wilmington, DE, USA

Department of Otolaryngology-Head and Neck Surgery, Jefferson Medical College, Thomas Jefferson University, Philadelphia, PA, USA

Lorne S. Parnes London Health Sciences Centre – University Campus, London, ON, Canada

Department of Otolaryngology, University of Western Ontario, London, ON, Canada

Rajan Patel Department of Otolaryngology, Auckland City Hospital, University of Auckland, Auckland, New Zealand

Sohil H. Patel Department of Radiology, New York University School of Medicine, New York, NY, USA

Kavita Malhotra Pattani Otolaryngology, Head and Neck Surgical Oncology, MD Anderson Cancer Center Orlando, Orlando, FL, USA

Benjamin C. Paul Division of Facial Plastic and Reconstructive Surgery, Department of Otolaryngology, New York University, School of Medicine, New York, NY, USA

Gidley Paul Department of Head and Neck Surgery, University of Texas M. D. Anderson Cancer Center, Houston, TX, USA

Christine Pearson Midwestern University Medical School, Downers Grove, IL, USA

Angela Peng Department of Otolaryngology-Head and Neck Surgery, Virginia Commonwealth University, Richmond, VA, USA

Kevin D. Pereira Department of Otorhinolaryngology-HNS, University of Maryland School of Medicine, Baltimore, MD, USA

Sunita Pereira Division of Newborn Medicine, Department of Pediatrics, Tufts Medical Center, Boston, MA, USA

Ronen Perez Department of Otolaryngology-Head and Neck Surgery, Shaare Zedek Medical Center affiliated with the Hebrew University School of Medicine, Jerusalem, Israel

Katherine Perry Otolaryngology-Head and Neck Surgery, University of Maryland Medical Center, Baltimore, Baltimore, MD, USA

Daniel Petrisor Division of Oral and Maxillofacial Surgery, College of Medicine, University of Florida, Jacksonville, FL, USA

Karen T. Pitman Department of Otolaryngology, University of Mississippi Medical Center, Jackson, MS, USA

Steven D. Pletcher Department of Otolaryngology-Head and Neck Surgery, University of California, San Francisco, CA, USA

Bidyut Pramanik Department of Radiology, NYU Langone Medical Center, New York, NY, USA

John Drew Prosser Department of Otolaryngology, Georgia Health Sciences University, Augusta, GA, USA

Neil Prufer Department of Otolaryngology, The Mount Sinai School of Medicine, New York, NY, USA

John Puetz Department of Pediatrics, Division of Pediatric Hematology and Oncology, Cardinal Glennon Children's Medical Center, Saint Louis University, St. Louis, MO, USA

Patricia Purcell Department of Otolaryngology-Head and Neck Surgery, University of Washington, Seattle, WA, USA

Max Pusz Department of Otolaryngology-Head and Neck Surgery, Walter Reed National Military Medical Center, Bethesda, Bethesda, MD, USA

S. Raghunandhan Department of Implant Otology, Madras ENT Research Foundation (P) Ltd, Chennai, Tamil Nadu, India

Chris Raine ENT Department, Bradford Royal Infirmary, Bradford, West Yorkshire, UK

Ryan Raju Department of Otorhinolaryngology, University of Oklahoma, Oklahoma City, OK, USA

Vijay R. Ramakrishnan Department of Otolaryngology-Head and Neck Surgery, School of Medicine, University of Colorado, Aurora, CO, USA

P. L. Ramchandani Department of Oral and Maxillofacial Surgery, Poole Hospital NHS Foundation Trust, Poole, Dorset, UK

Mitchell J. Ramsey Otology/Neurotology Otolaryngology Division, Tripler Army Medical Center, Honolulu, HI, USA

Darron M. Ransbarger Department of Otolaryngology-Head and Neck Surgery, Loma Linda University Medical Center, Loma Linda, CA, USA

Nidhi Rawal Department of Pediatric Gastroenterology and Nutrition, University of Maryland, Baltimore, MD, USA

Janez Rebol Department of Otorhinolaryngology, University Clinical Center Maribor, University Maribor, Maribor, Slovenia

Bhavya Rehani Department of Radiology, University of Cincinnati, Cincinnati, OH, USA

Susie Rhee Department of Surgery, Medical College of Georgia, Georgia Health Sciences University, Augusta, GA, USA

Matthew Richardson Department of Otolaryngology-Head and Neck Surgery, University of Mississippi Medical Center, Jackson, MS, USA

Jeremy N. Rich Department of Otolaryngology-Head and Neck Surgery, Walter Reed National Military Medical Center, Bethesda, MD, USA

Gresham T. Richter Department of Otolaryngology-Head and Neck Surgery, University of Arkansas for Medical Sciences, Arkansas Children's Hospital, Little Rock, AR, USA

Alejandro Rivas Vanderbilt University Medical Center, Nashville, TN, USA

Arnaldo L. Rivera Department of Otolaryngology-Head and Neck Surgery, Walter Reed National Military Medical Center, Bethesda, MD, USA

Carlos M. Rivera-Serrano Department of Otolaryngology, Facial Nerve Center, School of Medicine, University of Pittsburgh Medical Center, Pittsburgh, PA, USA

Department of Surgery, Division of Plastic Surgery, University of Florida College of Medicine, Gainesville, FL, USA

Michael H. Rivner Department of Neurology, Georgia Health Sciences University, Augusta, GA, USA

Derek Robinson Department of Otolaryngology-Head and Neck Surgery, University of Virginia Health System, Charlottesville, VA, USA

Corrie E. Roehm Division of Otolaryngology, Department of Head and Neck Surgery, University of Connecticut Health Center, Farmington, CT, USA

Pamela C. Roehm Department of Otolaryngology-Head and Neck Surgery, New York University, New York, NY, USA

Department of Otolaryngology, New York University School of Medicine, New York, NY, USA

J. Thomas Roland Jr. Department of Otolaryngology, New York University School of Medicine, New York, NY, USA

Peter Sargent Roland Department of Otolaryngology-Head and Neck Surgery, UT - Southwestern Medical Center, University of Texas Southwestern, Dallas, TX, USA

Tara L. Rosenberg Department of Otolaryngology and Communicative Sciences, University of Mississippi Medical Center, Jackson, MS, USA

Stephen Rothstein Department of Otolaryngology, New York University Langone Medical Center, New York, NY, USA

Lorne Rotstein Division of General Surgery, Department of Surgery, University Health Network, Princess Margaret Hospital, Toronto, ON, Canada

Patricia A. Rush Hearing and Speech Services, Flowood, MS, USA

Matthew W. Ryan Department of Otolaryngology, University of Texas, Southwestern Medical Center at Dallas, Dallas, TX, USA

Babak Sadoughi Laryngology/Neurolaryngology, New York Center for Voice and Swallowing Disorders, Head & Neck Surgical Group, St. Luke's-Roosevelt Hospital Center, Bronx, NY, USA

Christian Samuelson Advocate Illinois Masonic Medical Center, Chicago ENT an Advanced Center for Specialty Care, Chicago, IL, USA

Zoukaa B. Sargi Department of Otolaryngology-Head and Neck Surgery, University of Miami Miller School of Medicine, Miami, FL, USA

Johnathan Sataloff Department of Otolaryngology-Head and Neck Surgery, Drexel University College of Medicine, Philadelphia, PA, USA

Robert T. Sataloff Department of Otolaryngology-Head and Neck Surgery, Drexel University College of Medicine, Philadelphia, PA, USA

Natasha Savage Department of Pathology and Anatomical Sciences, Georgia Health Sciences University, Augusta, GA, USA

Anna M. Sawka Division of Endocrinology, Department of Medicine, University Health Network, Princess Margaret Hospital, Toronto, ON, Canada

Barry M. Schaitkin Department of Otolaryngology, Facial Nerve Center, School of Medicine, University of Pittsburgh Medical Center, Pittsburgh, PA, USA

Joseph Scharpf Cleveland Clinic Foundation, Cleveland, OH, USA

David A. Schessel Neurotology Section, Division of Otolaryngology Head and Neck Surgery, Stony Brook University, East Setauket, NY, USA

Sébastien Schmerber Department of Otolaryngology-Head and Neck Surgery, Otology/Neurotology Unit, University Hospital of Grenoble, Grenoble, France

Service ORL. Hôpital A. Michallon, Grenoble, France

Otology, Neurotology and Auditory Implants Department, University Hospital of Grenoble CHU A. Michallon, Grenoble, France

Daniel S. Schneider Microvascular/Facial Plastic Surgery, Oregon Health & Science University, Portland, USA

James Seaward Department of Plastic Surgery, University of Texas Southwestern Medical Center, Dallas, TX, USA

Brent A. Senior Department of Otolaryngology-Head and Neck Surgery, University of North Carolina at Chapel Hill, Chapel Hill, NC, USA

Gonca Sennaroglu Audiology Section, Department of Otolaryngology, Hacettepe University Medical Faculty, Ankara, Turkey

Levent Sennaroglu Department of Otolaryngology, Hacettepe University Medical Faculty, Ankara, Turkey

Jeremy Setton Department of Radiation Oncology, Memorial Sloan-Kettering Cancer Center, New York, NY, USA

Melanie W. Seybt Department of Otolaryngology, Medical College of Georgia, Georgia Health Sciences University, Augusta, GA, USA

Manish D. Shah Department of Otolaryngology-Head and Neck Surgery, University of Toronto, Toronto, ON, Canada

Ojas A. Shah Department of Otolaryngology, Cincinnati Children's Hospital and University of Cincinnati College of Medicine, Cincinnati, OH, USA

Udayan K. Shah Division of Otolaryngology, Department of Surgery, Nemours/Alfred I. duPont Hospital for Children, Wilmington, DE, USA

Department of Otolaryngology-Head and Neck Surgery, Department of Pediatrics, Jefferson Medical College, Thomas Jefferson University, Philadelphia, PA, USA

Kerwin F. Shannon Sydney Head & Neck Cancer Institute, Royal Prince Alfred Hospital, Camperdown, Sydney, NSW, Australia

Douglas Shaw Sydney Head and Neck Cancer Institute, Camperdown, NSW, Australia

LaGuinn Sherlock Department of Otolaryngology-Head and Neck Surgery, University of Maryland, School of Medicine, Baltimore, MD, USA

Sirikishan Shetty Department of Ophthalmology, Medical College of Georgia School of Medicine, Georgia Health Sciences University, Augusta, GA, USA

Mike C. Sheu Division of Facial Plastic and Reconstructive Surgery, Department of Otolaryngology, New York University School of Medicine, New York, NY, USA

Edward Shin The New York Eye and Ear Infirmary, New York, NY, USA

Shelly I. Shiran Department of Radiology, Tel Aviv Sourasky Medical Center, Affiliated with Tel Aviv University Sackler School of Medicine, Tel Aviv, Israel

Jack A. Shohet Shohet Ear Associates Medical Group, Inc., Newport Beach, CA, USA

Nael Shoman Division of Otolaryngology, University of Saskatchewan Saskatoon, Saskatchewan, Canada

Anwer Siddiqi Department of Pathology, University of Mississippi Medical Center, Jackson, MS, USA

James D. Sidman Children's Hospitals and Clinics of Minnesota, University of Minnesota, Minneapolis, MN, USA

Kathleen C. Y. Sie Department of Otolaryngology-Head and Neck Surgery, University of Washington, Seattle, WA, USA

Childhood Communication Center, Seattle Children's Hospital, Seattle, WA, USA

Bianca Siegel Department of Otorhinolaryngology-Head and Neck Surgery, Albert Einstein College of Medicine, Bronx, NY, USA

Rodrigo C. Silva Department of Otolaryngology-Head and Neck Surgery, University of Florida, Gainesville, FL, USA

Natalie Silver University of Kentucky, Lexington, KY, USA

Joshua B. Silverman Department of Otolaryngology, SUNY Downstate Medical Center, Brooklyn, NY, USA

Alfred Simental Department of Otolaryngology-Head Neck Surgery, Loma Linda University School of Medicine, Loma Linda, CA, USA

Michael C. Singer Department of Otolaryngology, Medical College of Georgia, Georgia Health Sciences University, Augusta, GA, USA

Praby Singh Division of Otolaryngology-Head and Neck Surgery, Walter Mackenzie Center, University of Alberta Hospital, Edmonton, AB, Canada

Matthew Sitton Department of Otolaryngology and Communication Sciences, Division of Otology and Neuro-otologic Skull Base Surgery, Medical College of Wisconsin, Milwaukee, WI, USA

David F. Smith Division of Pediatric Otolaryngology, Department of Otolaryngology-Head and Neck Surgery, The Johns Hopkins University School of Medicine, Baltimore, MD, USA

Timothy L. Smith Oregon Sinus Center, Department of Otolaryngology-Head and Neck Surgery, Oregon Health and Science University, Portland, OR, USA

Steven E. Sobol Division of Otolaryngology, The Children's Hospital of Philadelphia, Philadelphia, Pennsylvania

Arturo Solares Department of Otolaryngology, Medical College of Georgia, Augusta, GA, USA

Zachary M. Soler Department of Otolaryngology-Head and Neck Surgery, Medical University of South Carolina, Charleston, SC, USA

Alla Solyar Coastal Ear, Nose and Throat, Neptune, NJ, USA

Hwa J. Son Department of Otolaryngology-Head and Neck Surgery, Division of Neurotology, University of Cincinnati, Cincinnati, OH, USA

Philip Song Division of Laryngology, Department of Otology and Laryngology, Mass Eye and Ear Infirmary/Harvard Medical School, Boston, MA, USA

Hinrich Staecker Department of Otolaryngology-Head and Neck Surgery, University of Kansas Medical Center, Kansas City, KS, USA

James A. Stankiewicz Department of Otolaryngology-Head and Neck Surgery, Loyola University School of Medicine, Maywood, IL, USA

Ivona Stankovic University of Nis, Nis, Serbia

Milan Stankovic EAONO, University ORL Clinic Nis, Nis, Serbia

Chelsea Steele University of Mississippi Medical Center, Jackson, MS, USA

Jeffrey Steiner Department of Anesthesiology and Pain Management, UT Southwestern Medical Center Dallas, Children's Medical Center Dallas, Dallas, TX, USA

Margie N. Sutton Ear Institute of Texas, San Antonio, TX, USA

Monica J. Sutton University of Mississippi Medical Center, Jackson, MS, USA

Peter Szmuk Department of Anesthesiology and Pain Management, UT Southwestern Medical Center Dallas, Children's Medical Center Dallas, Dallas, TX, USA

Salvatore Taliercio Eastern Virginia Medical School, Department of Otolaryngology, Sentara Norfolk General Hospital, Norfolk, VA, USA

Bruce K. Tan Department of Otolaryngology-Head and Neck Surgery, Northwestern University – Feinberg School of Medicine, Chicago, IL, USA

Zachary H. Taxin NYU Sleep Disorders Center, New York, NY, USA

George M. Taybos Department of Otolaryngology and Communicative Sciences, University of Mississippi Medical Center, Cancer Institute, Jackson, MS, USA

Chris Sanders Taylor Department of Neurological Surgery, University of Cincinnati, Cincinnati, OH, USA

David Taylor Midwestern University Medical School, Downers Grove, IL, USA

Shelley Segrest Taylor Department of Otolaryngology and Communicative Sciences, The University of Mississippi Medical Center, Jackson, MS, USA

John F. Teichgraeber Department of Pediatric Surgery, The University of Texas Health Science Center at Houston, Houston, TX, USA

David J. Terris Department of Otolaryngology, Medical College of Georgia, Georgia Health Sciences University, Augusta, GA, USA

Belachew Tessema Department of Surgery, Division of Otolaryngology, The Connecticut Sinus Institute, University of Connecticut, Farmington, CT, USA

Thunchai Thanasumpun Department of Otolaryngology-Head and Neck Surgery, University of Texas Southwestern Medical Center, Dallas, TX, USA

Jenna Theriault London Health Sciences Centre - University Campus, London, ON, Canada

Dilip A. Thomas Department of Ophthalmology, Medical College of Georgia School of Medicine, Georgia Health Sciences University, Augusta, GA, USA

Sarah Elizabeth Bailey Department of Otolaryngology andCommunicative Sciences, University of Mississippi Medical Center, Jackson, MS, USA

Dilip A. Thomas Medical College of Georgia, Department of Ophthalmology, Georgia Health Sciences University, Augusta, GA, USA

Jennifer Thompson University of Kansas Medical Center, Kansas City, KS, USA

Robert J. Tibesar Pediatric Otolaryngology-Facial Plastic Surgery, Pediatric ENT Associates, Children's Hospitals and Clinics of Minnesota and University of Minnesota, South Minneapolis, MN, USA

Shelby Topp Department of Otolaryngology, Naval Medical Center San Diego, San Diego, CA, USA

Betty S. Tsai Vanderbilt University Medical Center, Nashville, TN, USA

Ralph Tufano Department of Otolaryngology-Head and Neck Surgery, Johns Hopkins School of Medicine, Baltimore, MD, USA

Samir S. Undavia Department of Otolaryngology-Head and Neck Surgery, Division of Facial Plastic Surgery, University of Texas Health Sciences Center, Houston, Texas, USA

Tulio A. Valdez Connecticut Children's Medical Center – Otolaryngology-Head and Neck Surgery, University of Connecticut, Hartford, CT, USA

Jessica Van Beek-King Department of Otolaryngology, Georgia Health Sciences University, Augusta, GA, USA

John R. Vender Department of Neurosurgery, Medical College of Georgia, Georgia Health Sciences University, Augusta, GA, USA

Vickie Verea Department of Anesthesiology, NYU Langone Medical Center, New York University, New York, NY, USA

Allan D. Vescan Department of Otolaryngology-Head and Neck Surgery, University of Toronto, Toronto, ON, Canada

Vani Vijayakumar Department of Radiology, University of Mississippi Medical Center, Jackson, MS, USA

Craig R. Villari Department of Otolaryngology-Head and Neck Surgery, Emory University School of Medicine, Atlanta, GA, USA

Hade D. Vuyk Department of Otolaryngology & Facial Plastic Reconstructive Surgery, Tergooi Hospitals, Blaricum, Netherlands

Michael Wajda Department of Anesthesiology, NYU Langone Medical Center, New York University, New York, NY, USA

Thomas J. Walker Department of Otolaryngology-Head and Neck Surgery, Miller School of Medicine, University of Miami, Miami, FL, USA

Susan B. Waltzman New York University Cochlear Implant Center, New York University School of Medicine, New York, NY, USA

Rohan R. Walvekar Louisiana State University Health Sciences Center, New Orleans, LA, USA

Matthew J. Ward Cancer Sciences Division, University of Southampton, Southampton, Hampshire, UK

Oshri Wasserzug Department of Otolaryngology-Head and Neck Surgery and Maxillofacial Surgery, Tel-Aviv Medical Center, Affiliated to the Tel-Aviv University, Tel-Aviv, Israel

Mark K. Wax Department of Otolaryngology-Head and Neck Surgery, Oregon Health and Science University, Portland, OR, USA

Thomas J. Way University of Kentucky, Lexington, KY, USA

Calvin Wei Department of Otorhinolaryngology-Head and Neck Surgery, University of Pennsylvania School of Medicine, Philadelphia, PA, USA

Jessica Weiss Division of Otolaryngology, Department of Head and Neck Surgery, University of Connecticut Health Center, Farmington, CT, USA

Kevin C. Welch Department of Otolaryngology-Head and Neck Surgery, Loyola University School of Medicine, Maywood, IL, USA

Brian D. Westerberg Division of Otolaryngology-Head and Neck Surgery, University of British Columbia, Vancouver, BC, Canada

Otology & Neurotology, St. Paul's Rotary Hearing Clinic, Vancouver, BC, Canada

David R. White Department of Otolaryngology-Head and Neck Surgery, Medical University of South Carolina, Charleston, SC, USA

Lauren C. White Department of Otolaryngology-Head and Neck Surgery, Georgia Health Sciences University, Augusta, GA, USA

W. Matthew White Department of Otolaryngology, NYU Medical Center, New York, NY, USA

Eric P. Wilkens Department of Anesthesiology, Albert Einstein Medical College, New York, NY, USA

Eric P. Wilkinson House Ear Clinic, Los Angeles, CA, USA

WilliesKanye Section of Plastic Surgery, Department of Surgery, Medical College of Georgia, Georgia Health Sciences University, Augusta, GA, USA

Sarah K. Wise Department of Otolaryngology-Head and Neck Surgery, Emory University School of Medicine, Atlanta, GA, USA

Department of Otolaryngology, Emory University, Atlanta, GA, USA

Ian J. Witterick Departments of Otolaryngology-Head and Neck Surgery and Diagnostic Imaging, University of Toronto, Toronto, ON, Canada

Amanda K. Wolfe Department of Special Education and Communication Disorders, University of Nebraska-Lincoln, Lincoln, NE, USA

Sarin Wongprasartsuk Division of Otolaryngology-Head and Neck Surgery, University of British Columbia, Vancouver, BC, Canada

Peak Woo Department of Otolaryngology, The Mount Sinai School of Medicine, New York, NY, USA

Aaron Wood Department of Otorhinolaryngology-Head and Neck Surgery, University of Maryland School of Medicine, Baltimore, MD, USA

Erika Woodson Head and Neck Institute, Cleveland Clinic Foundation, Cleveland, OH, USA

James J. Xia Department of Pediatric Surgery, The University of Texas Health Science Center at Houston, Houston, TX, USA

Department of Oral and Maxillofacial Surgery, The Methodist Hospital, Houston, TX, USA

Department of Surgery, Weill Medical College of Cornell University, New York, NY, USA

Robin Yang Department of Oral-Maxillofacial Surgery, University of Maryland Medical Center, Baltimore, MD, USA

Patricia J. Yoon School of Medicine, Department of Otolaryngology, University of Colorado, Children's Hospital Colorado, Aurora, CO, USA

Christopher York University of Texas, Southwestern Medical Center, Dallas, TX, USA

Ramzi Younis Department of Otolaryngology-Head and Neck Surgery, Leonard M. Miller School of Medicine Jackson Memorial Hospital, University of Miami, Miami, FL, USA

A. Samy Youssef Department of Neurosurgery, University of South Florida, Tampa, FL, USA

Patrick P. Youssef Department of Neurosurgery, Medical College of Georgia, Georgia Health Sciences University, Augusta, GA, USA

Eugene Yu Department of Otolaryngology-Head and Neck Surgery, Mount Sinai Hospital, Toronto, ON, Canada

Princess Margaret Hospital University Health Network, Toronto, ON, Canada

Jack C. Yu Section of Plastic Surgery, Department of Surgery, Medical College of Georgia, Georgia Health Sciences University, Augusta, GA, USA

Sancak Yuksel Department of Otorhinolaryngology-Head and Neck Surgery, University of Texas Medical School at Houston, Houston, TX, USA

Issa Jason Zeidan Department of Otolaryngology, Medical College of Georgia, Augusta, GA, USA

Melbourne, FL, USA

Daniel M. Zeitler Department of Otolaryngology-Head and Neck Surgery, University of Miami Miller School of Medicine, University of Miami Ear Institute, Miami, FL, USA

Denver Ear Associates, Denver, CO, USA

Karen B. Zur Department of Otorhinolaryngology-Head and Neck Surgery, The Children's Hospital of Philadelphia, Perelman School of Medicine, The University of Pennsylvania, Philadelphia, PA, USA

D

Decompression Illness

▶ Barotrauma and Decompression Sickness

Decompression Sickness

▶ Barotrauma and Decompression Sickness

Deep Neck Infection

▶ Imaging for Parapharyngeal Space Masses: Parapharyngeal Space Infection

Deep Neck Infections

Reena Gupta
Voice and Swallowing Center, Osborne Head and Neck Institute, Los Angeles, CA, USA

Definitions

Fascia: a sheet of fibrous tissue that lies deep to the skin or invests muscles and various body organs.

Ludwig's angina: cellulitis of the floor of the mouth, usually due to dental infection. Most often, the affected teeth are third molars, and the organism is streptococcal bacteria. Airway compromise occurs due to posterior and superior displacement of the tongue from the expanding floor of mouth.

Necrotizing fasciitis: a severe deep neck infection that occurs in the elderly or immunocompromised patient. The infection causes liquefaction necrosis and defies fascial barriers, causing rapid tissue death and neurovascular compromise.

Introduction

Deep neck infections are infections or abscesses that occur in the deep fascial layers and spaces of the neck. While the incidence of deep neck infections has decreased with the advent of antibiotics, they still represent a significant clinical problem. Perhaps in part because of the decline in frequency, deep neck infections are difficult to recognize, and diagnosis is often delayed until further in the course of the disease.

The term "deep neck" refers to a collection of fascia-enclosed spaces in the neck. These fascial layers include the superficial, middle, and deep layers of the deep cervical fascia (also called the investing layer of the deep cervical fascia). It excludes the superficial cervical fascia, a layer that encloses the muscles of the scalp and face as well as the platysma (Bailey 2006).

The connections between the deep fascial layers and other anatomic structures result in the formation of several deep neck spaces, specifically the parapharyngeal, submandibular, sublingual, retropharyngeal, danger, prevertebral, masticator, peritonsillar, parotid, carotid, and anterior visceral spaces (Cummings 2010). An infection begins within

S.E. Kountakis (ed.), *Encyclopedia of Otolaryngology, Head and Neck Surgery*, DOI 10.1007/978-3-642-23499-6,
© Springer-Verlag Berlin Heidelberg 2013

a single space, but can spread into other spaces via lymphatics, blood vessels, and along fascial planes. Some spaces are not fully isolated from others, and thus, infection may spread directly between these regions. Appropriate treatment of a deep neck infection therefore requires a thorough understanding of these fascial planes and fascial connections.

Dental infections are the most common precursors of deep neck infections, followed by oropharyngeal infections, although predominance of pathology may vary according to geography and socioeconomic factors (Larawin et al. 2006).

Deep neck infections often present subtly, and effective treatment is further compromised by the potential occurrence of serious complications. Airway compromise, mediastinal involvement, erosion into major vessels, and intracranial extension have been known to occur as complications of deep neck infections (Larawin et al. 2006). Treatment is further complicated by the density of important neurovascular structures in the head and neck and may involve sacrifice of any number of these structures. Treatment and outcome are dictated by the originating source, type of organism, and presence of complications.

Anatomy

The superficial layer of deep cervical fascia circumscribes the neck. Its attachments include the superior nuchal ligament, the ligamentum nuchae of the cervical vertebrae, the mastoid process, the zygomatic arch, the hyoid, the clavicle, the acromion, and the spine of the scapula. It encloses the sternocleidomastoid and trapezius muscles as well as the muscles of mastication. The superficial layer of the deep cervical fascia also encloses parotid and submandibular glands. It forms the stylomandibular ligament and contributes to the lateral aspect of the carotid sheath.

The middle layer of deep cervical fascia is divided into visceral and muscular divisions. The muscular division surrounds the strap muscles, including the sternohyoid, sternothyroid, thyrohyoid, and omohyoid. The visceral division envelops the buccinator, and pharyngeal constrictors muscles. It also surrounds the larynx, trachea, esophagus, thyroid, and parathyroid and forms the pretracheal fascia. Finally, the middle layer contributes to the buccopharyngeal fascia and the medial aspect of the carotid sheath.

The deep layer of the deep cervical fascia is divided into the alar and prevertebral fascia. The prevertebral layer encloses the paraspinal and scalene muscles. It also encompasses the cervical vertebrae and contributes to the posterior carotid sheath. The alar layer covers the sympathetic trunk and separates the retropharyngeal and danger spaces. When the orientation of the layers of the cervical fascia are understood, it is easier to appreciate how they relate to form the deep spaces of the neck.

The parapharyngeal space is also referred to as the lateral pharyngeal space, the pterygomaxillary space, and the pharyngomaxillary space. It is shaped like an inverted pyramid with its base at the skull base. It ends inferiorly with its apex at the lesser cornu of the hyoid bone. Medially, it is bounded by the pharyngeal constrictors and laterally by the fascia overlying the mandible, medial pterygoids, and parotid gland. The prevertebral division of the deep layer of the deep cervical fascia forms the posterior border. The parapharyngeal space is conceptually divided into two spaces by a line between the medial pterygoid plate and the styloid process. The anterior compartment is referred to as the prestyloid compartment and contains the internal maxillary artery, inferior alveolar nerve, lingual nerve, and the auriculotemporal nerve. The posterior compartment is called the poststyloid compartment and contains the carotid sheath and the glossopharyngeal, accessory, and hypoglossal nerves as well as the sympathetic chain. The parapharyngeal space is continuous with the retropharyngeal space, the submandibular space, and the masticator space. This space is involved with infections of the tonsils, pharynx, dentition, salivary glands, or mastoid abscesses. These infections may cause trismus, drooling, dysphagia, and odynophagia.

The submandibular and sublingual spaces function as a single space. Superiorly, the floor of mouth limits these spaces, and inferiorly, the digastric muscle and hyoid bone form the lower boundary. The mandible limits the space laterally. The sublingual and submaxillary spaces are the two subdivisions of this space. The mylohyoid muscle divides the two, although the division is somewhat arbitrary as infectious processes easily track behind the posterior border of the mylohyoid to involve both subdivisions. Infections in this space tend to originate in the dentition or from the submandibular gland. Ludwig's angina refers to cellulitis of this space causing elevation of the floor of mouth. This pushes the tongue superiorly and posteriorly, compromising the airway.

The retropharyngeal space extends from the skull base to the mediastinum at the tracheal bifurcation and is really a potential space between the middle and deep layers of the deep cervical fascia. This space is typically involved when the parapharyngeal space is involved due to a lateral connection between the two. In children, a persistent lymph node in this space is often involved due to upper respiratory infections. In adults, infections are usually due to trauma or foreign bodies. Infections in the nose, adenoids, nasopharynx, or sinuses may also track into this space.

The danger space is so called because the loose areolar tissue in this space is little barrier to the spread of infection into the posterior mediastinum and to the diaphragm. This space lies between the retropharyngeal space and the prevertebral space, and therefore, infections in either of these spaces may spread into the danger space. The superior limit of this space is the skull base.

The prevertebral space extends from the clivus to the coccyx. It contains dense areolar tissue as well as paraspinous, prevertebral, and scalene muscles, the brachial plexus, and the phrenic nerve. Vertebral body infections and penetrating injuries are the primary means of involvement of this space.

The masticator space contains the mandible and the muscles of mastication as well as the third portion of the trigeminal nerve, the ramus and body of the mandible, and the inferior alveolar vessel and nerve. It is located anterolateral to the parapharyngeal space and medial to the masseter.

The peritonsillar space is located between the palatine tonsil and the superior constrictor muscle, the anterior and posterior tonsillar pillars, and the posterior tongue. Involvement of this space from a tonsillar process often results in trismus, pain, odynophagia, and palatal asymmetry.

The parotid space is formed by the superficial layer of the deep cervical fascia, which splits to surround the parotid gland. The superior aspect is open and communicates with the prestyloid compartment of the parapharyngeal space. It contains the parotid gland, the external carotid artery, the posterior facial vein, and the facial nerve. Parotitis due to dehydration or poor oral hygiene may precipitate an infection of this space.

The carotid space is a potential space within the carotid sheath that contains the carotid artery, internal jugular vein, vagus nerve, and sympathetic postganglionic fibers. Parapharyngeal space infections may spread into the carotid space or the space may be directly involved from trauma such as intravenous drug use.

The anterior visceral space is also called the pretracheal space and extends from the thyroid cartilage to the superior mediastinum. It contains the pharynx, esophagus, larynx, trachea, and thyroid gland and is formed by the visceral division of the middle layer of the deep cervical fascia. Trauma, endoscopic instrumentation, or foreign bodies may result in infections of this space, causing odynophagia, fever, and possible airway obstruction.

Etiology

Odontogenic infections are the most common precipitating source of deep neck infections and are the source in over 40% of cases (Parhiscar et al. 2001). Other sources include sialadenitis, upper respiratory infections, trauma (including intravenous drug use or instrumentation during oral surgical procedures), superinfected congenital lesions (such as branchial cleft cysts or thyroglossal duct cysts), acute mastoiditis, foreign body, and necrotic malignant lymphadenopathy, among others (Bailey 2006). In as many as 20% of cases of deep neck infections, no source is found. In children, tonsillitis and pharyngitis are the leading causes of cervical lymphadenitis, while acute rhinosinusitis can lead to retropharyngeal lymphadenitis.

Once infection is initiated, it may spread through lymphatics, blood vessels, or along fascial planes throughout the neck spaces. Regional lymphadenopathy may also suppurate, resulting in a deep neck infection. Without antibiotic intervention, a phlegmon forms which eventually organizes into an abscess.

These infections are polymicrobial in 90% of cases, with aerobic and anaerobic organisms that represent oropharyngeal flora (Ungkanont et al. 1995). Streptococci species, predominantly alpha hemolytic, are the most common organisms found in cultures of deep neck abscesses. However, anaerobic bacteria are very common and are likely underestimated in frequency due to difficulty in culturing them. In cases where the host is immunocompromised, such as HIV-positive patients or patients with diabetes, relatively benign organisms can cause the severe deep neck infection, necrotizing fasciitis. Here, bacteria travel aggressively through fascial planes, usually far beyond the original insult and what is apparent on physical exam.

Atypical organisms, such as *Actinomyces* and *Mycobacterium tuberculosis*, may also cause these infections. Increasingly, methicillin-resistant *Staphylococcus aureus* (MRSA) is seen in community-acquired infections (Thomason et al. 2007).

Clinical Presentation

The diagnosis of a deep neck infection is made difficult by a subtle presentation. Often, the primary disease process (i.e., tooth abscess) is considered responsible for all presenting signs because the symptoms of the primary infection and a deep neck infection overlap (i.e., odynophagia, fever, etc.). Further, due to the deep location of the infection, surface findings may be absent. It is only with progression of disease that signs become apparent enough that diagnosis is obvious.

Fever, pain, and swelling are the most common symptoms. Other symptoms are related to the space that is involved. These may include neck pain, trismus, shortness of breath, hoarseness, ear pain, and dysphagia (Bottin et al. 2003). Slight torticollis might be present due to paraspinal muscle inflammation. As complications develop, symptoms referable to these complications manifest (i.e., spiking fevers in a patient with internal jugular vein thrombophlebitis with septic embolization).

A well-taken history can clarify the clinical presentation if it elicits recent pharyngitis, trauma, intravenous drug use, dental work, sinusitis, or otitis. Often, a preceding history of treatment with antibiotics, steroids, or nonsteroidal anti-inflammatories (NSAIDs) is present. A high index of suspicion should be maintained in patients such as these, particularly if they are immunosuppressed (i.e., HIV/AIDS, tuberculosis, diabetes, hepatitis). This latter group is at a much greater risk for infection with atypical organisms and rapidly progressive disease (Bottin et al. 2003).

Diagnosis

A complete examination of the head and neck is critical to determine if a deep neck infection exists and to find the offending primary source. Even subtle areas of fluctuance, crepitance, or tenderness in the neck suggest an underlying deep neck infection. Erythema or warmth of the skin, without a skin lesion or process to explain cellulitis, is also a sign of a deep neck infection. During a thorough head and neck exam, attention to detail is critical. Oropharyngeal evaluation should be accompanied by an assessment for trismus. Dental examination must not be overlooked, as this is the most common source of deep neck infections. This includes visual inspection and palpation of the alveola and floor of mouth.

A complete cranial nerve examination may reveal findings that suggest progression of infection. Additionally, the presence of Horner's syndrome (ptosis, miosis, facial anhidrosis) indicates sympathetic involvement. Flexible fiber-optic laryngoscopy is a critical part of the exam, both to assess for a primary source and to verify airway patency. This is particularly important if clinical suspicion justifies radiographic evaluation, prior to transport for imaging which requires supine positioning. Airway compromise may be seen in infections of the peritonsillar, retropharyngeal, parapharyngeal, submandibular, and pretracheal spaces.

Laboratory tests often demonstrate an elevated white blood cell count, although in cases of immunosuppression, this marker is significantly less useful. Blood chemistry should be performed to assess serum glucose, particularly in diabetics.

When clinical suspicion exists, plain radiography should not be overlooked as a first step. A Panorex may be obtained to evaluate dentition, particularly in patients with poor dental hygiene or those with a recent history of oral surgical intervention. Lateral neck radiographs may also demonstrate foreign bodies, subcutaneous air, and vertebral body erosion. Chest radiography may detect pneumomediastinum. In children, lateral plan films may demonstrate thickening of the prevertebral tissue, suggesting retropharyngeal infection or thickening of the epiglottis and arytenoids, indicating epiglottitis (Cummings 2010).

This may be followed by computed tomography (CT) with intravenous contrast, which allows differentiation of cellulitis from abscess and can aid in determining the extent of disease. Physical exam alone results in incorrect identification of the space involved in 70% of cases making CT scanning critical

(Crespo et al. 2004). If an abscess is identified, the CT scan also enables surgical planning by demonstrating the location of the collection as well as its proximity to neurovascular structures.

Care must be taken to ensure imaging extends to the mediastinum. The danger space, immediately posterior to the retropharyngeal space extends from the skull base to the diaphragm. This space is filled with loose areolar tissue, which provides no resistance to the spread of infection. Retropharyngeal, parapharyngeal, or prevertebral space infections may easily spread to the danger space. Complete imaging to the level of the diaphragm is required in these cases to fully delineate the extent of disease.

It is important to note that in cases of necrotizing fasciitis, CT scan often does not predict the true extent of disease. CT findings of fascial plane dissection or areas of fluid collection that defy fascial compartments may be seen. Subcutaneous emphysema is seen in approximately half of these cases. These signs may not be present, however, and an alternative means of diagnosis must be employed when clinical suspicion is high. These may include surgical exploration or local cut-down procedure (Lee et al. 2010).

Certain anatomic areas are better evaluated using magnetic resonance imaging (MRI), including the intracranial cavity, parotid, and prevertebral space. Due to the duration of the exam and the potential discomfort of a patient with dyspnea or dysphagia, this exam should be used judiciously.

Ultrasound may also be utilized, particularly for pediatric patients given the concern of radiation exposure. This modality also offers the ability to obtain sample material to guide antibiotic treatment and may also prove therapeutic (Duque et al. 2007).

Differential Diagnosis

The most important element in diagnosis of deep neck infection is determining the extent of disease. Often, symptoms are vague and can be attributed to a detectable primary infection, such as tonsillitis causing severe odynophagia, fevers, and leukocytosis. Symptoms disproportionate to the clinical exam, findings in an immunocompromised patient, or a clinical exam consistent with cellulitis warrant consideration of a deep neck infection. The pain of tumor metastasis may mimic a deep neck infection. However, few other clinical entities are easily mistaken with deep neck infections.

Treatment

As with any inflammatory process involving the head and neck, securing the airway is of primary importance. Flexible laryngoscopy aids in airway assessment and allows the caregiver to determine the likelihood of successful intubation. Intubation is not restricted to orotracheal intubation; nasotracheal intubation is a viable and often preferable option. Extreme caution should be exercised during intubation attempts. A stable airway, when instrumented, can rapidly become edematous, precipitating airway crisis. Also, an abscess in the upper airway can be ruptured during intubation attempts, causing aspiration of abscess contents, resulting in airway obstruction or death.

Tracheostomy wisely minimizes the potential for airway compromise in cases of deep neck infection where flexible laryngoscopy demonstrates impingement of the airway. If the airway examination confirms a 50% or greater luminal patency at the glottic or supraglottic level and airway symptoms are mild, medical therapy alone may be sufficient while under monitored care (Cummings 2010). However, if surgical intervention is expected to result in prolonged airway edema and intubation, elective tracheotomy should be considered. Tracheostomy should also be performed if the airway is restricted more than 50%. In these cases, tracheostomy under local anesthesia is advisable.

These patients require fluid resuscitation as well as management of concurrent medical conditions, such as diabetes. Antibiotics must be instituted immediately and should be broad spectrum initially; modification may occur after culture and sensitivity results are obtained. Antibiotic choice may need to include coverage for *Pseudomonas* in cases of otologic infection, sinus etiology, or nosocomial infections, as this organism is more common in these cases. Anaerobic coverage should be widened in cases of severe odontogenic infections (Cummings 2010).

Surgical drainage is the mainstay of management of deep neck infections. However, in patients with small retropharyngeal or parapharyngeal fluid collections and without respiratory compromise, nonsurgical management can be attempted for 48 h. Failure to improve after 48 h mandates surgical intervention (Plaza Mayor et al. 2001). Also, pediatric patients with retropharyngeal abscesses should be observed for improvement while receiving IV antibiotics prior to incision and drainage. Patients not fitting into these categories, particularly if there are impending complications, and patients who have failed a trial of IV antibiotics should undergo surgical incision and drainage.

Needle aspiration may be utilized for small abscesses within lymph nodes or when an infection is suspected to be caused by a congenital cyst. In these cases, a 16- or 18-gauge intravenous catheter may be advanced under negative pressure until the abscess cavity is reached. The needle may then be removed, leaving the catheter in for saline flush. Image guidance may be utilized when this is unsuccessful.

Retropharyngeal abscesses and peritonsillar abscesses may be approached transorally, with caution to protect the airway from accidental spillage of pus into the airway after incision of the abscess wall.

Both needle drainage of a suspected congenital cyst and transoral drainage of a peritonsillar abscess may be followed by definitive removal of the cyst or tonsil when the acute infection has resolved.

All other circumstances require traditional surgical incision and drainage. The typical surgical approach involves a transcervical incision for wide exposure. This enables protection of intact neurovascular structures as well as thorough visualization of abscess limits. Once exposed, the abscess contents must be cultured and the cavity copiously irrigated. The area must be examined thoroughly to ensure all reaches of the infectious process have been identified and cleared. After debridement of infected material, the wound may be left open with a drain or packing material.

IV antibiotics should be continued until the patient is improving and afebrile for 48 h. After this time, the regimen may be changed to oral antibiotics.

Complications

Because of the high density of critical neurovascular structures in the head and neck and the large distance the deep neck spaces traverse, complications can be devastating.

The most severe and immediately concerning is airway compromise. Tracheal compression occurs rapidly in the presence of an expanding collection and surrounding inflammation. Aspiration may also cause airway compromise and may occur when a retropharyngeal abscess perforates or during intubation attempts.

Vascular complications include thrombosis or rupture of the great vessels. Lemierre's syndrome is internal jugular vein thrombophlebitis and is most often caused by *Fusobacterium necrophorum*, a Gram-negative bacillus. It most commonly follows pharyngitis and is marked by fever, lethargy, neck tenderness, and septic emboli (Golpe et al. 1999). Cavernous sinus thrombosis may also occur from retrograde spread of infection from the paranasal sinuses or upper dentition. Fever, orbital pain, proptosis, dilated pupil with a sluggish papillary light reflex, and restricted extraocular mobility are seen (Cummings 2010).

Mediastinitis is a direct consequence of spread along the retropharyngeal and prevertebral planes of the neck. Pleuritic pain, hypoxia, tachycardia, and dyspnea result and imaging may reveal a pleural effusion or mediastinal widening. Thoracotomy is often needed due to the involvement of multiple compartments. When the mediastinum is involved, surgical exploration and drainage significantly reduces mortality over cervical drainage alone (Corsten et al. 1997).

Necrotizing fasciitis has been discussed and is a severe deep neck infection often seen in elderly or immunocompromised patients. As with most deep neck infections, odontogenic sources are most common. Mixed flora, including aerobic and anaerobic flora, are seen. Patients typically have a rapidly progressive cellulitis with neck edema and may have subcutaneous crepitus. CT scan will demonstrate widespread hypodensities without peripheral enhancement, which represents liquefaction necrosis. Treatment involves operative debridement, critical care support, broad-spectrum antibiotics, and management of immunocompromising conditions. Postoperatively, wounds should be left open for wet-to-dry dressing changes and to continue to monitor the margins of disease.

References

Bottin R, Marioni G, Rinaldi R et al (2003) Deep neck infection: a present-day complication. A retrospective review of 83 cases (1998–2001). Eur Arch Otorhinolaryngol 260:576–579

Corsten MJ, Shamji FM, Odell PF et al (1997) Optimal treatment of descending necrotizing mediastinitis. Thorax 52:702–708

Crespo AN, Chone CT, Fonseca AS et al (2004) Clinical versus computed tomography evaluation in the diagnosis and management of deep neck infection. Sao Paulo Med J 122:259–263

Duque CS, Guerra L, Roy S (2007) Use of intraoperative ultrasound for localizing difficult parapharyngeal space abscesses in children. Int J Pediatr Otorhinolaryngol 71:375–378

Gadre A, Gadre K (2006) Infections of the deep spaces of the neck. In: Bailey B, Johnson JT (eds) Head & neck surgery – otolaryngology, 4th edn. Lippincott Williams & Wilkins, Philadelphia, pp 665–682

Golpe R, Marin B, Alonso M (1999) Lemierre's syndrome (necrobacillosis). Postgrad Med J 75:141–144

Larawin V, Naipao J, Dubey SP (2006) Head and neck space infections. Otolaryngol Head Neck Surg 135:889–893

Lee JW, Immerman SB, Morris LG (2010) Techniques for early diagnosis and management of cervicofacial necrotizing fasciitis. J Laryngol Otol 124:759–764

Oliver ER, Gillespie MB (2010) Deep neck space infections. In: Flint P, Haughey BH, Lund VJ, Niparko JK, Richardson MA, Robbins KT, Thomas JR (eds) Cummings otolaryngology: head & neck surgery, 5th edn. Mosby Elsevier, Philadelphia, pp 201–208

Parhiscar A, Har-El G (2001) Deep neck abscess: a retrospective review of 210 cases. Ann Otol Rhinol Laryngol 110: 1051–1054

Plaza Mayor G, Martínez-San Millán J, Martínez-Vidal A (2001) Is conservative treatment of deep neck space infections appropriate? Head Neck 23(2):126–133

Thomason TS, Brenski A, McClay J et al (2007) The rising incidence of methicillin-resistant *Staphylococcus aureus* in pediatric neck abscesses. Otolaryngol Head Neck Surg 137:459–464

Ungkanont K, Yellon RF, Weissman JL et al (1995) Head and neck space infections in infants and children. Otolaryngol Head Neck Surg 112:375

Deep Neck Space Infections

Craig R. Villari and Charles E. Moore
Department of Otolaryngology-Head and Neck Surgery, Emory University School of Medicine, Atlanta, GA, USA

Synonyms

Parapharyngeal abscess; Peritonsillar abscess; Retropharyngeal abscess

Definition

Deep neck space infection: an infection, usually bacterial, within the neck, deep to the superficial layer of the cervical fascia.

Etiology

In the pediatric setting, tonsillitis and resultant spread remains the most common source of deep neck infections (Vasan 2008). In adults, most infections are odontogenic in nature or are the result of intravenous drug abuse (Weed et al. 2005). Other etiologies include infection of congenital structures (thyroglossal duct cysts, branchial cleft cysts, or laryngoceles), trauma, infected necrotic lymph nodes or tumor beds, trauma, and spread from contiguous sources of infection (Vasan 2008; Weed et al. 2005).

Key to identification of a deep neck space infection is understanding the roles of the cervical fascia and the lymphatic drainage. The head and neck have a rich lymphatic drainage system that terminates in the deep cervical chains. These lymphatic channels allow for local spread of infection.

Knowledge of these anatomic planes aids in understanding the patient's presentation and can help guide treatment. The cervical fascia can be divided into the superficial and deep cervical layers. The superficial cervical fascia envelops the muscles of facial expression and the platysma. The deep cervical fascia envelopes deeper structures (Vasan 2008).

The deep cervical fascial layer can be further divided into the superficial deep, middle deep, and the deep deep fascial layers. The superficial deep layer envelops the parotids and submandibular glands as well as the trapezius and sternocleidomastoid muscles. The middle deep layer primarily invests the strap muscles, thyroid, pharynx, larynx, trachea, and esophagus. The deep deep layer encompasses the deep prevertebral musculature, vascular and neural components (Vasan 2008).

There are two planes of deep deep cervical fascia posterior to the esophagus. This bilayered setup forms a potential space between these two planes that continues from skull base to mediastinum. This region known as the "danger space" allows deep cervical infection to spread down into the mediastinum (Vasan 2008).

In immunocompetent patients, pathologic isolates from deep neck space infections tend to be laden with staphylococcal and streptococcal species. Immunosuppressed patients can be susceptible to a myriad of microbiologic agents ranging from mycobacterial and enterobacter species to *Toxoplasma gondii*, *Pneumocystis carinii*, or *Bartonella henslae* (Lin et al. 2008).

Clinical Presentation

Patient presentation varies on many factors but depends most heavily on the affected fascial contents. Infections involving only the superficial cervical fascia may cause local inflammation but rarely elicit a systemic response. More rostral infections within the superficial and middle layers of the deep cervical fascia can result in systemic sepsis such as Ludwig's angina, and peritonsillar, submandibular, or sublingual abscesses (Weed et al. 2005).

Peritonsillar abscesses are characterized by tonsillar fullness with caudal deviation of the tonsil, contralateral uvular deviation, halitosis, trismus, inability to handle secretions, dysphagia, and a muffled hot potato voice (Vasan 2008). Submandibular and sublingual space infections can present in a similar fashion to peritonsillar abscesses but tend not to have trismus (the muscles of mastication are rarely involved) and will obviously not deviate the position of the tonsil. Consequently, these particular infections can present as local inflammation and/or a mass palpable either intraorally or through the use of bimanual examination. It is important to differentiate these submandibular and sublingual space infections from infections of the glands themselves which are covered elsewhere in this text. Ludwig's angina is a diffuse, tense swelling of the sublingual and submandibular spaces (Vasan 2008). Usually odontogenic in nature, symptoms can quickly progress from localized swelling of the floor of the mouth to diffuse swelling to complete obstruction of the airway by an edematous, inflamed base of the tongue. Airway patency and control must always be of paramount importance when evaluating a patient with concern for Ludwig's angina (Vasan 2008; Weed et al. 2005).

Infection of the more caudal middle deep and deep deep cervical plains can result in parapharyngeal and retropharyngeal pathology. Parapharyngeal space infections are classified by further anatomic compartmentalization. The prestyloid or muscular compartment of the parapharyngeal space lies anteriorly; infections here can lead to significant trismus as the medial and lateral pterygoids will be affected (Johnson 2008). The posterior compartment is the post-styloid or neurovascular compartment; infections of this space can lead to thrombosis of the internal jugular vein and resulting septic embolisms (Johnson 2008). Infection of

the parapharyngeal space can generally be manifested by dysphagia, trismus, a medial bulge along the lateral pharyngeal wall, and cranial nerve involvement which can, in turn, lead to tongue paralysis, hoarseness, and Horner's syndrome.

Retropharyngeal space infections lie between the middle deep and deep deep cervical fascial layers. This space contains lymph nodes and lymphatic channels that tend to be infected by nasopharyngeal pathogens (Vasan 2008). Infections of this space can elicit symptoms similar to infections of the peritonsillar space, but there may also be cervical rigidity. Great concern must be paid to infections of the retropharyngeal space given the proximity of this space to the "danger zone." Infections in this potential space can easily track to the mediastinum (Vasan 2008). Signs or symptoms of retropharyngeal space infection in conjunction with any hemodynamic instability, chest pain, or shortness of breath should warrant appropriate escalation of the patient workup and treatment.

All three layers of the deep cervical fascia coalesce to help create the carotid sheath. This sheath also creates a potential avenue of spread from the skull base to thorax. Infections of this space can lead to neurologic changes secondary to inflammation of the vagus nerve leading to hoarseness. Additionally, torticolis may result secondary to inflammation of the overlying sternocleidomastoid muscle (Vasan 2008).

Diagnostics

Although a thorough history and physical examination are the obligate first diagnostic studies that should be obtained, evaluation of the respiratory status for airway compromise must be assessed and ruled out before any further investigation is started. Important aspects of the patient history taking should address recent history of head and neck or odontogenic infections or procedures, recent trauma, history of IV drug abuse, and history of immunosuppression. The physical examination should begin with an assessment of airway status. A complete head and neck examination should be completed. Fiber-optic flexible laryngoscopy may be warranted to assess for potential airway compromise and to plan for intubation if necessary.

Once the history and physical reinforce the diagnosis of a deep neck space infection, further workup can commence. Basic laboratory work can help assess for leukocytosis. Three radiologic modalities may be useful in diagnosis. Ultrasound examination is a relatively safe and fast means of assessing cystic masses. Lateral neck films can demonstrate widening of the prevertebral tissues and have been found to be 83% sensitive in diagnosing pediatric deep neck space infections. Key references are normal thickness of 7 mm at C2 and 14 mm (pediatric) or 22 mm at C6 (Weed et al. 2005). Plain film chest x-rays are useful if there is concern for mediastinal spread of infection though concern of this sequelae would likely push the physician to order a computed tomography (CT) scan.

Computed tomography can be extremely beneficial but may not be indicated in some deep neck space infections. Diagnosis of a peritonsillar abscess, for instance, is a clinical diagnosis. If there is suspicion of a deeper abscess or continuity into the thorax, CT is indicated and can be utilized for surgical planning. Magnetic resonance imaging (MRI) can provide incredible imaging of neck soft tissues and vasculature, but it is much more expensive and time intensive than CT examination.

Differential Diagnosis

Deep neck space infections are usually bacterial in nature but other infectious etiologies are possible. With an immunocompromised patient, pathogens like *Toxoplasma gondii*, and *Pneumocystis carinii* should be considered. For patients with long-standing lymphadenitis that has not responded to appropriate antibiotic treatment, atypical mycobacterium including tubercular disease should be considered. Other granulomatous diseases like *Bartonella henselae* (cat-scratch fever) may also present as long-standing cervical lymphadenopathy in both the immunocompetent and immunocompromised population (Weed et al. 2005; Lin et al. 2008).

Prophylaxis

Prophylaxis against these infections is difficult given the prevalence of the likely pathogens in normal nasopharyngeal and oropharyngeal flora. For appropriate patients with Human Immunodeficiency Virus (HIV), antiretroviral medication should be utilized to minimize susceptibility to opportunistic infections.

Therapy

Airway management supersedes all other concerns. If needed, intubation or tracheotomy must be completed before further treatment can progress. Once a safe airway is established, conservative therapy should be utilized whenever possible. Initial treatment with antibiotics is appropriate for a vast majority of cases.

Intravenous (IV) antibiotics and hydration can be started as soon as a diagnosis is made. Antibiosis should target streptococcal and staphylococcal pathogens; clindamycin or ampicillin-sulbactam can be started and easily converted to equivalent oral medications when appropriate. If methicillin-resistant *Staphylococcus aureus* is suspected, vancomycin may be added. For immunocompromised patients, ticarcillin-clavulanate or clindamycin with ceftzidime should be utilized as a first-line regimen (Weed et al. 2005).

Surgical management should be entertained when there is airway compromise, when conservative measures fail (lack of response to IV antibiotics for 48 h), with deep abscesses, or with signs of systemic sepsis. Physical examination and available imaging help guide the surgical approach (Weed et al. 2005). Both extraoral and intraoral approaches can be used but one should remember that normal anatomy will likely be distorted secondary to inflammation and edema. Surgical planning should minimize risk to vascular and nervous structures and informed consent should highlight structures and functions being placed at risk by the given approach. Once the abscess is surgically encountered, the contents should be sampled and sent for microbiologic review. At a minimum, specimen(s) should be sent for gram stain, cultures (aerobic, anaerobic, and acid-fast bacilli), and susceptibilities. Additional pathologic review can be utilized when indicated. All loculations within the abscess should be obliterated with blunt dissection and the wound should be thoroughly irrigated. A drain can be placed to allow percutaneous drainage of the wound for postoperative monitoring.

The patient can be transitioned to sensitivity-guided IV and then oral antibiotics once clinically stable and afebrile for at least 48 h (Weed et al. 2005). Management is expectant thereafter unless a complication has occurred.

Prognosis

Complications do arise from deep neck infections. Jugular thrombosis, carotid rupture, mediastinitis, and necrotizing fasciitis are all poor outcomes associated with deep neck space infections. Jugular thrombosis can result in showering of septic emboli and can lead to cerebrovascular accidents in patients with a patent foramen ovale. Rupture of the carotid is lethal in over 30% of cases (Weed et al. 2005). Mediastinitis is possible when infection passes caudally through various potential spaces in the neck; extension into the thorax may necessitate thoracic surgery and debridement. Cervical necrotizing fasciitis is identified by erythema without clearly demarcated edges, subcutaneous emphysema, and pale anesthetic skin that can progress to severe diffuse blistering. Immediate surgical intervention and continued debridement is necessary but patients still carry a significant mortality rate (Weed et al. 2005). When caught early and treated appropriately, prognosis is excellent for deep neck space infections with full recovery expected in almost all patients.

References

Johnson JT (2008) Deep neck abscesses. In: Myers EN (ed) Operative otolaryngology: head and neck surgery, 2nd edn. Saunders Elsevier, Philadelphia
Lin DT, Deschler DG (2008) Neck Masses. In: Lalwani AK (ed) Current diagnosis & treatment: otolaryngology head and neck surgery, 2nd edn. McGraw Hill Medical, New York
Vasan NR (2008) Neck spaces and fascial planes. In: Lee KJ (ed) Essential otolaryngology: head and neck surgery, 9th edn. McGraw Hill Medical, New York
Weed HG, Forrest LA (2005) Deep neck infection. In: Cumming CW et al (eds) Cummings otolaryngology: head and neck surgery, 4th edn. Elsevier Mosby, Philadelphia

Deep Neck Trauma

▶ Penetrating Neck Trauma

Deep Plane Face-lift

Benjamin West Cilento
Texas Facial Plastic Surgery & Rhinology,
The Woodlands, TX, USA

Synonyms

Composite face-lift/rhytidectomy; Deep plane rhytidectomy; Sub-SMAS face-lift/rhytidectomy

Definition

A rhytidectomy which is performed in the plane deep to the superficial musculoaponeurotic system (▶ Superficial Musculoaponeurotic System (SMAS)) and superficial to the parotidomasseteric fascia. It is designed to reposition the ptotic tissues of the neck, jawline, and midface with equal effect and have a longer duration than standard face-lifts. In contradistinction to less invasive SMAS tightening procedures, the deep plane face-lift more effectively treats the midface and nasolabial fold region as well as the neck and jowls and is generally thought to have more natural, longer-lasting results.

Purpose

In order to understand the deep plane face-lift as an advanced technique of surgical rejuvenation, it is important to begin with a brief description of the evolution of the ▶ rhytidectomy from its inception. In the first 50 years of the twentieth century, it became clear that undermining and redraping the skin of the face and neck could drastically diminish the effects of age-related changes in the lower face. Although skin tightening improved the neckline, the results were short lived and did nothing for the nasolabial fold region, creating disparity between the neck, lower face, and midface. Despite these short-lived, modest results, the "skin only" procedure remained the procedure of choice until platysmal redraping was described by Tord Skoog in 1968. This "new" procedure was based on subplatysmal dissection and redraping of the platysma/skin unit to improve the jawline and lower face. Although it constituted a major improvement in these areas over the skin-only lift, it created a disparity between midface/neck and jawline/lower face.

This was followed shortly thereafter by Mitz and Peyronies's description of the SMAS in 1976. Once surgeons realized that it was possible to reposition the inelastic tissues deep to the skin, SMAS lifting techniques quickly became the new standard face-lifting paradigm. SMAS techniques (plication, imbrication, or excision) offered better, longer-lasting results than the skin-only techniques but still had the problem of disparity between jawline and midface. In the 1980s, Sam Hamra, MD, began exploring different planes of dissection in the neck and midface regions. His triplane rhytidectomy published in 1984 described a preplatysmal neck dissection, advancing the cervical platysma anteriorly and the skin posteriorly in a sliding fashion better defining both the neck and jawline. This led him to apply the same principles to the midface by separating the muscles of facial movement from the tissues being repositioned. This "deep plane" face-lift helped diminish the disparity between the nasolabial fold, jawline, and neck and was rapidly adopted and refined by many surgeons around the world. Calvin M Johnson, Jr., MD, was an early advocate of the procedure and helped to refine and popularize the technique. The author trained with Dr. Johnson and it is his techniques, with some personal modifications, that are presented here in text and video.

Principle

Relevant Anatomy: The key to understanding the deep plane face-lift is an intimate knowledge of the anatomy of the midface and malar region. Any surgeon attempting to incorporate the deep plane face-lift into his repertoire should undertake a detailed study of the relevant anatomical reports published recently. While a complete discussion of the anatomic relationships is beyond the scope of this text, certain key features bear mentioning.

The SMAS warrants specific mention since it is the structure upon which all modern face-lifts are based. Understanding the anatomical relationships of the SMAS is vital both to safely dissect in the deep plane and to understand the benefits and limitations of proper repositioning. Since the first description of the SMAS

by Mitz and Peyronie, techniques involving SMAS manipulation have become the standard for face-lift surgery. It is defined as the superficial fibromuscular layer of the face and neck investing the mimetic musculature, including the platysma, orbicularis oculi, occipitofrontalis, zygomatici, and levator labii superioris. It is thicker laterally over the parotid where a distinct tissue plane is sometimes difficult to discern but it tapers medially as the deep plane dissection is carried anterior to the parotid. It is here that the branches of the facial nerve can be seen exiting the substance of the parotid and spreading over the surface of the masseter muscle. This sometimes causes fear in surgeons as they begin their exploration of the deep plane. However, the parotido-masseteric fascia remains superficial to the nerves and serves as a protective layer during the remainder of the dissection. As long as this investing fascia remains intact there is little fear of damage to the nerves below it. The SMAS is considered to have an extensive domain, just how extensive varies somewhat depending on the source. It is generally agreed upon that the SMAS is in continuity with the muscular layer of the lower cheek and neck known as the platysma. It is this continuity which allows a sling-like redraping of the sagging structures of the neck, jawline, and cheek as one relatively uninterrupted complex during the conduct of any SMAS-based face-lift. Most authors also agree that the galea aponeurotica is the suprazygomatic extension of the SMAS.

There are several notable points when considering the facial nerve during any face-lift and the deep plane is no exception. An intimate understanding of the course of the facial nerve is important when performing a deep plane face-lift. As the main trunk of the nerve divides into its five main branches it is protected by the body of the parotid gland. It is after they exit the gland at its anterior border that these branches become vulnerable as they become more superficial (Fig. 1). The most vulnerable nerves are not the buccal branches that are exposed during dissection of the deep plane but rather the frontal and marginal branches due to their lack of anastomotic connections. The frontal branch of the facial nerve is most susceptible to injury as it courses over the zygomatic arch. Here, it is generally considered to reside in a zone of probability bounded by imaginary lines 2.0 cm posterior to the bony orbital rim and 1.8 cm anterior to the superior auricular attachment. In this

Deep Plane Face-lift,
Fig. 1 Relevant facial nerve
anatomy in the deep plane
(From Azzizzadeh et al.
(2007), Fig. 8.2, p. 126); The
video with modifications and
figures were published in
Master Techniques in Facial
Rejuvenation, Azzizadeh,
Murphy and Johnson, Jr,
Chapter 2, Pages 28-29,
Copyright Elsevier 2007

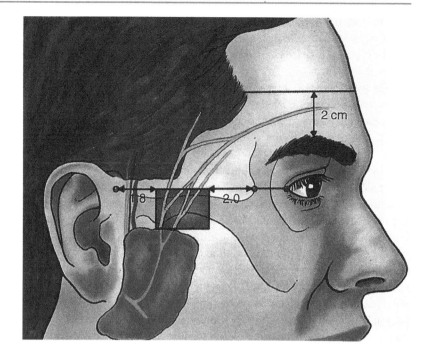

zone, the nerve lies just superficial to the subcutaneous fat and theoretically is vulnerable to injury when entering the deep plane (Fig. 2).

The rami mandibularis or marginal mandibular branches of the facial nerve are also vulnerable to injury during deep plane dissection. The nerve courses deep to the platysma approximately 2–4 cm below the mandible until a point approximately 2.0 cm lateral to the corner of the mouth at which point it becomes more superficial (Fig. 3). The deep plane dissection is carried out deep to the platysma and therefore has the greatest theoretical potential to cause injury to the marginal branch due to its occupation of this plane. For this reason, dissection in the deep plane is generally carried out to the inferior border of the mandible and to the posterior edge of the platysma but no further.

The Great Auricular Nerve is a sensory nerve composed of branches of spinal nerves C2 and C3 and originating from the cervical plexus. It provides sensory innervation for the skin of the external ear, lower cheek, and upper neck variably. The main trunk wraps around the posterior edge of the sternocleidomastoid (SCM) muscle and extends superoanteriorly across its surface superficial to the platysma until it reaches the posterior edge of the parotid gland where it divides into posterior and anterior branches. It is during its traverse

of the upper part of the SCM that it is most vulnerable to injury during a face-lift since the skin and platysma can be adherent to the SCM in this area. Making sure that dissection is carried out in the appropriate plane ensures that the nerve is protected during elevation of the skin flap posterior to the ear and inferiorly into the neck.

Being in the appropriate plane is key in all phases of the deep plane face-lift. Once the surgeon is comfortable with the anatomy of key structures, safety can be ensured by paying attention to dissection planes and boundaries. For example, in the lower face, sub-SMAS dissection can safely proceed medially up to the facial artery and vein. Anterior to these structures there is increased risk to the now superficial branches of the facial nerve. Likewise, identification of the zygomaticus major muscle and, to a lesser degree, the orbicularis oris muscle is an important part of the operation. The zygomaticus major muscle can reliably be found at its insertion into the anterior face of the body of the zygoma, approximately 1 cm anterior and superior to the zygomatic notch. Because the mimetic muscles are innervated on their deep surface, dissection into the midface is carried out superficial to the zygomaticus major and orbicularis oris muscles to the level of the melolabial fold.

Deep Plane Face-lift,
Fig. 2 Location of the frontal
branch of the facial nerve.
Printed with permission:
Larrabbee and Makielski,
Surgical Approaches to the
Face, Lippincott Williams and
Wilkins (2004)

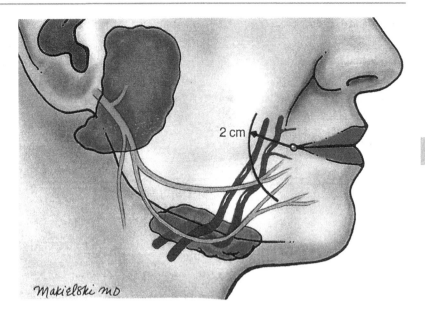

D

The retaining ligaments of the face are also structures that bear mention in a discussion of the deep
plane face-lift. It is the release of these ligaments that
allows repositioning of the skin muscle flaps. Although
many of the fat compartments of the midface and
cheek have condensations that are named as cutaneous
ligaments, our dissection is concerned primarily with
the zygomatic, mandibular, and masseteric ligaments.
The zygomatico-cutaneous ligaments, first described
by McGregor, insert on the inferior edge of the zygomatic arch and anterior aspect of the body of the
zygoma, extend through the malar fat pad, suspending
it over the malar eminence, and attach to the skin. An
artery and sensory nerve accompany the ligamentous
strands of these ligaments and will need to be cauterized and cut during the release of this structure sometimes called McGregor's Patch. It is this ligamentous
complex that becomes lax with age causing midface
ptosis and accentuation of the melolabial/nasolabial
fold and it must be released in order to allow redraping
of the skin. Care should be taken in its release however
as a zygomatic branch of the facial nerve lies immediately deep to the ligament and is vulnerable to injury if
planes are not respected.

In the lower face, there are two main retaining
ligaments, one osseocutaneous (anterior) and one
fasciocutaneous (posterior). The mandibulo-cutaneous
ligament is an osseocutaneous ligament inserting on
the parasymphyseal mandible and attaching the

overlying skin inferior to the depressor anguli oris
and interdigitating with the platysma. It is generally
thought that this ligament should be left intact as an
anchor point against which the platysma/skin complex
is pulled to counteract jowling. The masseteric ligament is a fasciocutaneous ligament that arises from the
anterior border of the masseter muscle and radiates
attachments to the overlying skin. It is these fibers
that weaken with age and rotate inferomedially to
accentuate the labiomandibular crease.

No discussion of pertinent anatomy would be complete without a brief discussion of facial vasculature
relevant to the deep plane dissection. There are three
concentric vascular arcades that supply the layers of
the face involved in the deep plane dissection, the
lateral, middle, and medial arcades. This is a very
important concept when raising a skin flap in a skin-
only or SMAS face-lift since the skin flap is a random
flap whose blood supply becomes more tenuous the
more medial it is raised. Raising the flap in the deep
plane avoids this tenuous blood supply.

Procedure: The details of this procedure are very
similar to those of Dr. Calvin Johnson, MD, as
published in "Master Techniques in Facial Rejuvenation," Saunders 2007, with some exceptions. First, the
patient is positioned on the operative table in a supine
position. The head of the bed is rotated 90°–180° in
order to allow access to the vertex of the head. In
general, I perform all face-lifts under general

Deep Plane Face-lift,
Fig. 3 Location of the
Marginal Branch of the facial
nerve with respect to
surrounding anatomy and
landmarks. Printed with
permission: Larrabbee and
Makielski, Surgical
Approaches to the Face,
Lippincott Williams and
Wilkins (2004)

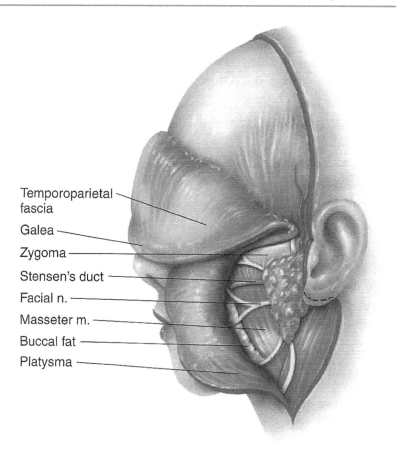

Temporoparietal fascia

Galea

Zygoma

Stensen's duct

Facial n.

Masseter m.

Buccal fat

Platysma

anesthesia for comfort and safety but many physicians use local with sedation and this is certainly acceptable.

After the patient is properly sedated and intubated, the hair is prepared for surgery. A disposable clipper is used to shave a small amount of hair in the temporal tuft and in the postauricular hairline. Regular tan colored masking tape is then used to tape the hair back applied as a single encircling band about 1 cm back from the hairline. I avoid wrapping the tape too tight and putting tension on the scalp and distorting the incision line. The proposed incision lines are marked out at this point with a violet surgical marker as shown in (Figs. 4 and 5). Two areas of discussion are the temporal tuft and postauricular hairline. In general, I use the "hair-sparing" incision as shown in Fig. 5. A gently curved incision extending through the sideburn hair beveled with the hair roots provides excellent camouflage and appropriate vectors for vertical and posterior lifting. As the incision approaches the superior attachment of the auricle it forms a "bird's beak"

for approximately 1 cm over the ears attachment before descending in the native preauricular crease. As the incision descends, it can either continue in a pretragal or post-tragal position depending on the relative prominence of the tragus and depth of the preauricular crease. The more prominent the tragus, the less I like to use a post-tragal incision because it tends to accentuate this prominence. In most cases, the crease is adequate to hide the incision. As the incision descends it curves around the lobule and is brought slightly onto the conchal bowl as it approaches its superior aspect and then extends posteriorly toward the hairline. The posterior extension of this incision is drawn out in a line bisecting the angle between the lower hairline and a line extending posteriorly from the superior aspect of the conchal bowl.

Once the incisions are marked, the subdermal plane is injected with an appropriate amount of lidocaine (0.5%) and epinephrine (1:200,000). The entire face, neck, perioral, and postauricular region are then

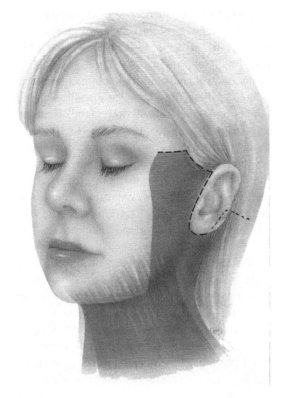

Deep Plane Face-lift, Fig. 4 Location of the incisions involved in the deep plane face-lift. (Azzizzadeh et al. (2007), Fig. 8.11, p. 130); The video with modifications and figures were published in Master Techniques in Facial Rejuvenation, Azzizadeh, Murphy and Johnson, Jr, Chapter 2, Pages 28-29, Copyright Elsevier 2007

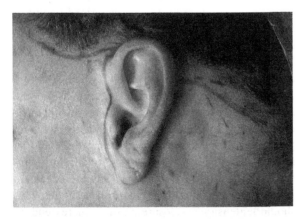

Deep Plane Face-lift, Fig. 5 Pre auricular incisions sparing the temporal tuft of hair (Azzizzadeh et al. (2007), Fig. 8.4, p. 128); The video with modifications and figures were published in Master Techniques in Facial Rejuvenation, Azzizadeh, Murphy and Johnson, Jr, Chapter 2, Pages 28-29, Copyright Elsevier 2007

prepped in standard surgical fashion leaving the endotracheal tube external to the drapes and covered with a sterile sheath. This allows for easy access to the submental region and free movement of the tube for flexibility during dissection. During the procedure, the endotracheal tube may be anchored to the inside of the cheek, or the teeth of the mandible, or remain without anchor if appropriate care is taken to ensure proper placement is maintained. Like Dr. Johnson, I use a No. 10 blade for all incisions because the larger blade length makes true incisions easier. Once the incisions are made, skin flaps are raised in the subdermal plane using a transillumination technique in order to ensure the proper depth of dissection is maintained. Although the surgeon can start at any point along the incision, I usually start at the bird's beak portion of the preauricular incision. As the flap is raised the surgical field is kept relatively dark while the flap is illuminated with the overhead surgical lights. This transillumination creates a distinct color at the correct depth of dissection which can be used to maintain the correct flap thickness throughout the procedure. Retraction is just as important as lighting when dissecting superficially and in the deep plane. This is why it is so important to have an excellent assistant to apply countertension while raising flaps. It should be noted that once a few centimeters of skin have been undermined with the fine scissors, I switch to bear claw retractors and blunted face-lift scissors to continue in the same plane. This dissection is carried out to 5 or 6 cm from the incision line as seen in the video. Anteriorly, this translates to the malar eminence and inferiorly the flap is elevated to the angle of mandible. Once progress reaches the angle of mandible, the dissection deepens to incorporate the subdermal fat of the neck. At this point, transillumination is abandoned in favor of a lighted retractor to allow for extended retraction in combination with illumination. By sharp and blunt dissection just lateral to the angle of the mandible, the fibers of the platysma are uncovered and a supraplatysmal plane is developed and carried anteriorly to the midline. This dissection usually requires extra long scissors to reliably reach the midline and spreading is done perpendicular to the surface of the platysma. Dissection in the neck is carried superiorly to the lower border of the mandible and inferiorly to a variable extent depending on the degree of neck rhytids and redundant skin. After the preplatysmal plane is fully developed, fat can be directly excised from the flap to help contour the neckline as necessary.

Once the subdermal and preplatysmal flaps are elevated, attention is turned to the deep plane. I prefer to enter the deep plane along a line starting 1 cm superior and 2 cm anterior to the angle of mandible and extending superiorly to the body of the zygoma just anterior to notch. After incising along this line with a number 10 blade, the deep plane is entered over the parotid gland for ease and safety. The lighted retractor is again used in combination with retraction from the assistant to help with separation and dissection of the deep plane. As appropriate tension/counter-tension is applied to the SMAS in this area, the parotidomasseteric fascia falls away easily exposing the deep plane. Quite often, branches of the facial nerve can be seen radiating out from the anterior edge of the parotid gland and running along the floor of the dissection while strands of the platysma run across the roof, denoting the deep side of the SMAS. Although dissection in the deep plane can be accomplished with a blunt scissor with perpendicular spreads, the preferred method is to use a number 10 blade in a pushing fashion to peel the fascial attachments from the undersurface of the SMAS. This inferior aspect of the deep plane dissection extends anteriorly to within a couple of centimeters of the oral commissure and inferiorly to the inferior border of the mandible to protect the marginal branch. It is important throughout the dissection of the deep plane to remain at the appropriate depth; the tendency is to become too superficial which will compromise the structural integrity of the SMAS.

After the inferior dissection has progressed to the appropriate degree, attention is turned to the superior aspect of the deep plane dissection. The superior end of the incision extends slightly anterior to the notch of the zygoma. It is at this point that the edge of the incision is grasped between the teeth of the lighted retractor and the surgeons finger and placed under tension. The deep plane is entered and immediately the dissection is advanced over the body of the zygoma. The zygomaticus major muscle is identified at its insertion on the face of the zygoma approximately 1 cm anterior and superior to the notch. Once identified, the zygomaticus major provides a safe plane of dissection extending to the nasolabial fold since

facial nerve branches are deep to this structure. Sometimes the lateral edge of the orbicularis muscle comes into the plane of dissection superiorly and can be confused with the zygomaticus major. Any confusion between the two can be alleviated by noting the relative depth of dissection. The orbicularis is superficial and the zygomaticus is found deep in the dissection at its zygomatic attachment. Using the No 10 blade in a pushing fashion, dissection is continued superficial to the zygomaticus major muscle to within a centimeter of the nasolabial fold. At this point, the deep plane dissection consists of two well-developed tunnels with an intervening bridge of slightly more dense tissue. Using these two well-developed planes as a guide, and under appropriate tension and counter-tension, the tunnels are connected by confidently dissecting through the bridge of tissue using the number 10 blade as before. Once the dissection extends to within a centimeter of the nasolabial fold, the buccal fat pad can be addressed. I do not usually disturb buccal fat since it is sometimes difficult to gauge the effect it will have on contour and symmetry. Also, to access the buccal fat requires deepening the plane of dissection and putting the facial nerve branches at risk. However, now that the deep plane dissection is complete on one side, the process is duplicated on the other side before any suspension sutures are placed. After both sides have been dissected, attention is then turned to the submental region.

Not every patient needs dissection in the submental plane, however most patients undergoing a deep plane lift have significant relaxation and anterior drooping of the platysma requiring platysmaplasty and varying degrees of direct excision or liposuction of fat deposits. When necessary, the submental dissection is performed after the deep planes have been fully elevated and before the suspension has been performed. A 1 cm incision in the submental crease is made and a preplatysmal plane is elevated and immediately joined with the bilateral preplatysmal dissections already created. When the medial edges of the platysma are identified, any redundancies are resected as necessary and the edges are sutured together using buried 4-0 prolene sutures. This should be a tensionless closure and should not extend too inferiorly as it interferes with laryngeal structures. After the platysma is trimmed and sutured, the fat in the submental region can be addressed but with caution. Fat removal in this area should be carried out conservatively since the defects from excessive removal are exceedingly hard to fix. At this point, the bilateral deep plane flaps are lifted superiorly and slightly posterior and sutured with buried 3-0 prolene sutures under minimal tension. There are many variations in trimming and securing the deep plane but in all cases care should be taken not to excessively thin or perforate the flap and to avoid asymmetric tension while suturing the two halves.

Once the deep plane flaps are secured, number 8 round drains are placed under the skin flap through postauricular incisions and the skin is then trimmed and sutured in place as well. The direction of pull for the skin is the same as for the deep plane flap, superoposterior. The tailoring is started at the temporal tuft with a tacking suture placed at the superior aspect of the auricle. A second key suspension suture is placed at the posterosuperior edge of the auricle, lifting the skin flap to its final position. With the skin tacked in place, the skin along the preauricular crease is trimmed. It is important to be very conservative with skin removal in the region of the ear lobe as excessive tension in this region gives rise to pixie deformity. The skin is then trimmed in the posterior hairline and the wound is stapled closed. Finally, excess skin is tailored posteriorly. Staples are used in the posterior hairline, and the temporal tuft, while 5-0 ethilon is used to close the preauricular skin and absorbable sutures behind the ear. After closure is complete, all wounds are covered with bactroban ointment and telfa pads and a bulky cotton bandage completely surrounds the face. A layer of coban or some other snug fitting material is then wrapped around the outside of the bulky cotton to complete the pressure dressing.

Indication

The goal of any rhytidectomy is to counteract the effects of aging by resuspending ptotic tissues in a more youthful position. Aging is a process of cellular senescence that causes loss of volume as much as a reduction of structural support. The combination of these two factors acting in concert, leads to the telltale signs of aging in various regions of the face. The malar fat pad atrophies and descends over time leading to deepening of the nasolabial fold and a hollowing of the lid-cheek margin or a tear trough deformity. Loss of volume of the buccal fat pad, descent and weakening of the platysma, and bony resorption lead to jowling and submental banding. A good preoperative assessment will highlight these changes in any given patient. With that said, the ideal candidate for a deep plane face-lift is a middle-aged female/male with medium to thin skin, strong jawline and prominent zygomatic complex, low facial adipose content, and midface ptosis and jowling as the predominant features of their aging pattern.

Contraindication

In general, patients in poor health should refrain from cosmetic surgery. Absolute contraindications include patients graded as class IV and V by the American Society of Anesthesiologists (ASA). This classification system delineates patients with severe comorbidities and helps the surgeon weigh out the risks of undergoing surgery on any given patient. No cosmetic procedure is worth risking the life of a patient.

Smoking is considered a relative contraindication despite the adverse affect it has on skin flap survival and increased hematoma formation. It is a relative contraindication because cessation a month before and after surgery significantly reduces these risks. Diseases and conditions that impair wound healing are also considered relative contraindications since they can compromise the outcome. Long-term steroid use, diabetes mellitus, connective tissue disorders such as Ehler Danlos, and genetic conditions such as Dyskeratosis Congenita are a few examples of strong relative contraindications.

Advanced age in general should not be an absolute contraindication to performing a face-lift. The healthy but elderly population deserve the same opportunities as everyone else.

Complications

Hematoma- Hematomas generally occur in the first 12 h postoperatively. Because of this, it is advisable to have the patient remain in a facility overnight or be close by so that they can be checked on the morning after surgery. The generally quoted rate of hematoma formation in face-lifts in general is 0.3–15% and is increased with preoperative hypertension. The rate reported for deep plane face-lifts is 2.2% but none of these occurred in the deep plane itself.

Skin Loss – Occurs very rarely but the incidence is higher in patients who smoke or have compromised blood supply for other reasons.

Hypertrophic scarring – Usually occurs in the postauricular region and is treated with judicious use of Kenalog 40 injections with a 30 gauge needle and lessens drastically with time.

Nerve Injury – It is tempting to think of the deep plane face-lift as somehow more dangerous to the facial nerve branches than other types of face-lifts. However, in the author's experience there is no greater risk to the facial nerve than any other type of face-lift. Kamer has reported no cases of facial nerve injury in 2,600 cases and Dr. Johnson has also no documented cases of nerve injury since starting the deep plane as his main form of face-lift (unpublished data). Reports in the literature vary according to surgeon and technique from 0.4% to 2.6%. The most commonly injured nerve is the Great Auricular Nerve and the motor nerve most vulnerable to injury is the frontal and marginal branches of the facial nerve.

Cross-References

▶ Retaining Ligaments of Face
▶ Superficial Musculoaponeurotic System (SMAS)

References

Azzizzadeh B, Murphy MR, Johnson CM (2007) Master techniques in facial rejuvenation. Saunders, Philadelphia
Hamra ST (1990) The deep plane rhytidectomy. Plast Reconstr Surg 86:53–61
Hamra ST (1993) Composite rhytidectomy. Quality Medical, St. Louis
Larrabbee WF, Makielski KH (2004) Surgical anatomy of the face, 2nd edn. Lippincott W and W, Philadelphia
Papel ID et al (2009) Facial plastic and reconstructive surgery, 3rd edn. Thieme, New York
Trueswell WH (2009) Surgical facial rejuvenation. Thieme, New York

Deep Plane Rhytidectomy

▶ Deep Plane Face-lift

Deep Space Neck Infection

▶ Pediatric Neck Infections

Delay of Flap

Lynn L. Chiu-Collins[1], Jeffrey S. Epstein[2] and Eugene A. Chu[3]
[1]Facial Plastic Surgery, San Francisco Plastic Surgery & Laser Center, San Francisco, CA, USA
[2]Foundation for Hair Restoration, University of Miami, Miami, FL, USA
[3]Facial Plastic and Reconstructive Surgery, Rhinology, Skull Base Surgery, Kaiser Permanente, Department of Otolaryngology-Head and Neck Surgery, Downey, CA, USA

Synonyms

Delay phenomenon; Flap delay; Surgical delay; Vascular delay

Definitions

Surgical interruption of a portion of the blood supply in a preliminary stage prior to tissue transfer.

Principle

Surgical delay is a perfusion preconditioning technique in reconstructive soft tissue flap surgery. In this technique, the flap's vascular supply is partially disrupted in a separate procedure prior to a subsequent transfer procedure.

Purpose

The purpose of the technique is to allow for enhanced flap length and viability in reconstruction. Flap delay has been used for nearly 500 years in reconstructive surgery for reliably transferring a greater amount of harvested tissue than one would be able to otherwise

(Myers and Cherry 1967). The method of delaying the flap involves incising the borders of the flap with or without partial subcutaneous elevation and leaving it in situ for a duration of time, usually 10–14 days (Milton 1969), at which time delay is thought to have its maximum effect. After the period of delay, the flap is fully elevated and transposed. Delayed flaps have been shown to have better survival than similar flaps that are raised and transposed primarily.

Mechanism

The mechanism for flap delay, though studied in depth, remains unclear. Studies suggest that the ischemia acts as a stimulus for increased tissue perfusion via vascular changes ranging from the effects of denervation, to the dilation of vessels, to changes in metabolism and new blood vessel formation.

Changes in Sympathetic Tone
In the 1970s, experimental animal data demonstrated increased flap survival with either denervation alone (leaving the vascular supply intact) or devascularization alone (leaving the innervation intact). In the latter theory, sympathetic nerves are divided, allowing the release of norepinephrine and subsequent vasoconstriction and relative ischemic effects. This stage lasts for up to 30 h. Upon delayed flap elevation, the hyperadrenergic state abates when the nerve endings are depleted of norepinephrine, and vasodilation ensues, thus increasing the blood supply and tissue viability (Finseth and Cutting 1978; Cutting et al. 1981; Pearl 1981; Banbury et al. 1999). Finseth and Cutting assessed flap delay in a rat neurovascular island flap, by dividing the artery, vein, and nerve. Division of all three resulted in the greatest flap survival, and division of the vein alone had the least benefit. Numerous authors have reported similar findings in various models consistent with these findings of vasodilation in the first 2–3 days after flap elevation (Sasaki and Pang 1984; Pang et al. 1986; Jonsson et al. 1988).

Dilation and Reorientation of Vessels
Choke vessels are the small anastomotic vessels between adjacent angiosomes. They are not associated with a main source artery. Dilation of choke vessels has been demonstrated in flap delay and are independent of the increased blood flow due to sympathectomy alone (Callegari et al. 1992; Taylor et al. 1992; Morris and Taylor 1995). Reorientation of vessels has also been observed (Barker et al. 1999).

Changes in Metabolism
Ischemic preconditioning has also been studied as a mechanism of flap delay. Preconditioned tissues demonstrate decreased energy requirements, altered energy metabolism, improved electrolyte homeostasis, less-reactive oxygen species, reduced release of activated neutrophils, reduced apoptosis, and better perfusion, resulting in an increase of the ischemic tolerance of tissues (Ghali et al. 2007).

Neovascularization
Ghali et al. thoroughly reviewed the role of angiogenesis and adult vasculogenesis in flap delay (Ghali et al. 2007). His group studied vasculogenesis in a flap delay model and demonstrated bone marrow–derived endothelial progenitor cell recruitment to ischemic tissue within 72 h (Tepper et al. 2005). Recruitment was directly proportional to the level of tissue ischemia. Growth factors, like VEGF, were released during ischemia, with subsequent mobilization of endothelial progenitor cells from the bone marrow. By day 14 after flap elevation, these endothelial progenitor cell clusters coalesced into vascular cords, becoming vessels by day 21. The suggestion is that hypoxia alters the vascular endothelium in ischemic tissue to isolate endothelial progenitor cells in regions where neovascularization is needed (Lineaweaver et al. 2004).

Proximal Versus Distal Flap Delay
Tissue flap survival in proximal flap delay versus distal flap delay has also been studied. Since flap necrosis most often occurs at the distal end of a flap, it is often assumed that the delay of the distal flap alone contributes to flap survival. Cutting demonstrated in a porcine tissue model that when the proximal portion of a flap is delayed, flap survival is significantly improved. Distal delay alone showed the poorest survival, and delay of the entire flap, both proximal and distal portions, showed the best survival (Cutting et al. 1980).

Nonsurgical Flap Delay
Flap delay is generally surgical in nature, and hence necessitates an operation. Nonsurgical alternatives to delaying a flap have also been studied.

Studies on delay of flaps using laser have been promising in human subjects. Using flashlamp-pumped pulsed-dye laser at a wavelength of 585 nm, it was demonstrated that laser delay is as effective as surgical delay and that laser delay by lasering lateral borders leads to dilation and longitudinal rearrangement of the existing vessels rather than angiogenesis, whereas laser delay by lasering the entire surface results in delay effect by inducing angiogenesis due to activation and degranulation of the mast cells (Ercocen et al. 2003). Another group found that CO_2 and Erbium: YAG lasers are as effective as surgery for delay of skin flaps in the rat model (Reichner et al. 2003).

Chemical delay has also been studied as an alternative to surgical delay. In a rat skin flap model, although not as effective as the surgical delay procedure, the topical combination of nicoboxil and nonivamide proved to be of significant value in order to ameliorate ischemic necrosis in experimental skin flaps. Due to its ease and safety in application, this ointment may prove clinically useful in selected situations, especially when combined with an additional postoperative treatment (Huemer et al. 2009). Another group studied the use of an epinephrine-loaded microsphere delivery system in a rat model. Statistically similar results in comparison to surgical delay were obtained by chemical delay initiated by epinephrine-loaded microspheres. Chemical delay is less invasive, less time-consuming, and far more cost-effective compared with its surgical alternative. This chemical delay model lends further support to the role of relative hypoxia as the primary promoter of the delay phenomenon (Karacaoglu et al. 2002).

Indications

Flap delay improves flap survival, increases the length-to-width ratio in random pattern flaps, and allows for the reliable transfer of greater volumes of tissue in axial pattern flaps. Thus, in cutaneous local flaps, delay can be accomplished by incisions around the planned flap territory or by partial undermining of the flap before it is returned to its native bed. In myocutaneous or other composite flaps with multiple named source vessels, flap delay can be achieved by division of some of these named vessels, leaving the flap territory supplied principally by the vessel on which the flap is to be based.

Although the increasing use of microvascular free flaps has obviated the need to use flaps relying on the delay phenomenon, the delay technique still has a role in frequently used flaps, including forehead, scalp, groin, and local flaps.

Within the field of head and neck surgery, multiple reconstructive flaps can benefit from delay, such as the pectoralis myocutaneous flap (Attinger et al. 1996), the paramedian forehead flap, and the temporoparietal-occipital flap. The paramedian forehead flap as a delayed flap will be discussed here. Although less frequently used today, the temporoparietal-occipital (TPO) pedicle flap is also a particularly illustrative example used in treatment for male pattern baldness (Epstein and Kabaker 1997).

Paramedian Forehead Flap

The forehead flap is a useful application of the delay concept. The paramedian forehead flap has become our workhorse flap for large nasal reconstruction. The axial design, based on a single supratrochlear artery, is a reliable option for large, subtotal, and total nasal reconstruction. Some have also suggested that the paramedian forehead flap has a robust random blood supply and could survive even when the supratrochlear artery is not present (McCarthy et al. 1985). Modifications of the paramedian forehead flap, like a narrower pedicle and more inferior cut near the eyebrow have provided greater effective length, especially in comparison to the older median forehead flap. Although the paramedian forehead flap is an effective option for nasal reconstruction, some cases like in heavy smokers require greater length and more flap viability even still.

Delay of the paramedian forehead flap has been suggested in the past for gaining flap length or viability in the case of inner lining reconstruction, a relatively distant recipient site, or complicated revision (Schreiber and Mobley 2011; Menick 2012). A recent case report on a 71-year-old male 4-pack-per-day smoker demonstrated excellent flap survival and nasal reconstruction using a vascular delayed paramedian forehead flap (Kent and Defazio 2011). The patient was not able to reduce his smoking habits prior to surgery. In the case report, after confirming the location of the supratrochlear artery, the horizontal dimension of the flap was increased by 4 mm to allow freshening of the edges after the delay. In typical fashion, the vertical limbs of the flap were incised down through the frontalis muscle, and the flap was elevated off the loose areolar tissue.

After hemostasis was reached, the flap was sutured back into its donor site using 4-0 nylon running suture. On day 14, the patient returned for execution of the usual Stage 1 of the forehead flap. After 4 weeks, the flap was divided and inset uneventfully, and later follow-up showed a healthy flap.

Temporoparietal-Occipital Flap

The TPO flap is one example of a scalp-rotation flap procedure for treatment of fronto-temporal male-pattern baldness. Despite technological advances in hair grafting, the TPO flap still remains an option for patients who want pronounced results in a short period of time and are able to tolerate multiple stage, more invasive surgery. Compared to grafting techniques, scalp flaps offer unsurpassed hair density (Epstein and Kabaker 1997). The TPO flap is not ideal for patients with significant vertex balding since the TPO does not address that area and may actually make the contrasting baldness more apparent. Various iterations of scalp rotation flaps have been discussed in the literature; however, the technique that yields the most reliable and favorable result is the twice-delayed TPO flap. When compared to the singly-delayed temporoparietal flap, the twice-delayed TPO flap yields twice the length and breadth of flap (Williams and Lam 2003). It is a massive flap with a length-to-width ratio of 7:1 (Ende and Kabaker 2010). Originally described by Juri (1975) and popularized by Kabaker (1978, 1979; Kabaker et al. 1986), the twice-delayed TPO flap or "Juri flap" can offer dense hair-bearing tissue coverage of up to 4 cm in width, spanning the entire frontal hairline. The natural progression of the patient's fronto-temporal hair recession usually is not an issue. However, if hair behind the TPO flap inset becomes too sparse, a second, contralateral TPO flap can be planned for after 6–12 months from the final inset of the first flap. Alternatively, grafting techniques may also be used to help fill in the naked scalp.

The TPO flap is an axial pattern flap in the proximal aspect and a random flap in the distal aspect. The proximal two-thirds are based on the posterior branch of the superficial temporal artery (STA), and the distal one third is based randomly on the postauricular and occipital arteries. After the surgeon and patient establish the desired hairline, the flap is carefully planned.

The TPO flap is usually 3–4 cm wide and 23–25 cm long (Epstein and Kabaker 1997). It should be noted that in its final inset position, the distal two thirds of the flap will make up the new hairline and the proximal one third will sit behind the hairline. Thus, the peak of the flap should be fashioned at the junction of the middle and distal two thirds (Kabaker 1979).

The first delay procedure is essentially the creation of a bipedicle flap with random pattern posterior circulation that is provided by the perforating vessels of the occipital artery (Ende and Kabaker 2010). At the start of the first stage of the operation, the proximal flap is mapped out using intraoperative Doppler study of the posterior branch of the STA. An unraveled 4×4 gauze is used to measure the distance of the proposed, new hairline and the flap length designed accordingly. Two superoposteriorly aimed parallel incisions will be made in the temporal area to establish the pedicle base. The posterior incision is positioned starting 4 cm above the anterior aspect of the auricular helix. The anterior incision is positioned starting at a point 30°–45° above the horizontal plane, and 4 cm away from the first incision, thus establishing the width of the pedicle. Both incisions are carried posteriorly along the axis of the posterior branch of the STA toward the occiput. The distal portion of the flap typically does not pass the midline of the occiput (Fig. 1). After flap length and design have been confirmed, the proximal two thirds of the flap are raised from its bed in the subgaleal plane and immediately returned to its native position and secured back in position.

After 1 week, the second stage is undertaken. Here, the distal one third is now elevated and returned to its native position. Care should be taken not to disturb the proximal two thirds of the flap.

After 1 more week, the whole flap is lifted and transposed into its new position. Integrity of the flap should be inspected here. Venous congestion or poor arterial flow can warrant further delay by another week if needed (Williams and Lam 2003). Doppler analysis may be helpful here as well. The proposed hairline is incised in an irregular fashion and with a 45° bevel and the recipient site bed prepared for the transposition. The intervening bridge of scalp tissue is excised to accommodate the flap inset. The flap is secured into its new position and the donor site closed. Extensive undermining of the scalp and neck is required to minimize wound tension. A dog-ear typically forms at the pedicle base and is addressed several weeks later.

Delay of Flap, Fig. 1 Design of the temporoparietal occipital flap. The flap is fashioned around the posterior branch of the superficial temporal artery. The posterior incision starts 4 cm above the anterior aspect of the auricular helix. The anterior incision starts at a point 30°–45° above the horizontal plane, and 4 cm away from the first incision. In the first delay, the proximal two thirds of the flap are raised from its bed and immediately returned to its native position. In the second delay, the distal one third is elevated and returned. In the final stage, the whole flap is lifted and transposed into its new position

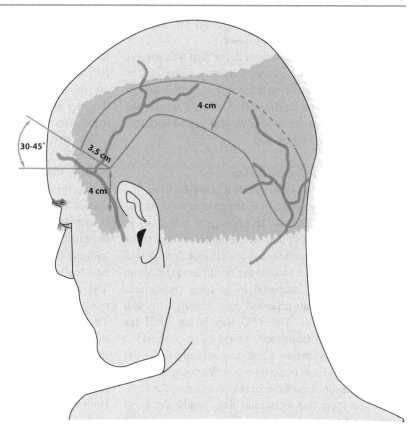

Favorable long-term results have been studied in the literature (Epstein and Kabaker 1996). Frank flap necrosis fortunately is extremely rare. Also rare, are a few cases of minimal distal flap loss. Fortunately, this can heal completely by secondary intention. Future excision or grafting can help improve the appearance of the wound (Williams and Lam 2003). Unnatural density of the hairline may occur since the TPO hair quality is so robust. Micrografts and minigrafts can help irregularize and soften the transition zone.

Contraindications

Patients who are unable to tolerate multiple stages or are unlikely to follow up.

Advantages/Disadvantages

Delay may be performed in pedicled flaps as well as in random areas of free flaps.

The main disadvantage of delaying the flap is the requirement of multiple procedures.

Acknowledgments The authors would like to thank Eden Palmer for her illustration in this work.

Cross-References

▶ Free Flaps
▶ Local Flaps
▶ Regional Flaps
▶ Rotational Flaps
▶ Transposition Flap

References

Attinger CE, Picken CA et al (1996) Minimizing pectoralis myocutaneous flap loss with the delay principle. Otolaryngol Head Neck Surg 114(1):148–157. Official Journal of American Academy of Otolaryngology-Head and Neck Surgery

Banbury J, Siemionow M et al (1999) Muscle flaps' triphasic microcirculatory response to sympathectomy and denervation. Plast Reconstr Surg 104(3):730–737

Barker JH, Frank J et al (1999) An animal model to study microcirculatory changes associated with vascular delay. Br J Plast Surg 52(2):133–142

Callegari PR, Taylor GI et al (1992) An anatomic review of the delay phenomenon: I. Experimental studies. Plast Reconstr Surg 89(3):397–407; discussion 417-398

Cutting C, Bardach J et al (1980) Skin flap delay procedures: proximal delay versus distal delay. Ann Plast Surg 4(4):293–296

Cutting CB, Bardach J et al (1981) Haemodynamics of the delayed skin flap: a total blood-flow study. Br J Plast Surg 34(2):133–135

Ende KH, Kabaker SS (2010) Hair restoration: medical and surgical techniques, Elsevier. Cummings Otolaryngology Head and Neck Surgery, Chapter 26, 2008

Epstein JS, Kabaker SS (1996) Scalp flaps in the treatment of baldness: long term results. Dermatol Surg 22:45–50

Epstein JS, Kabaker SS (1997) Has technology killed the flap? Am J Cosmet Surg 14(2):133–136

Ercocen AR, Kono T et al (2003) Efficacy of the flashlamp-pumped pulsed-dye laser in nonsurgical delay of skin flaps. Dermatol Surg 29(7):692–699; discussion 699. Official Publication for American Society for Dermatologic Surgery [et al.]

Finseth F, Cutting C (1978) An experimental neurovascular island skin flap for the study of the delay phenomenon. Plast Reconstr Surg 61(3):412–420

Ghali S, Butler PE et al (2007) Vascular delay revisited. Plast Reconstr Surg 119(6):1735–1744

Huemer GM, Froschauer SM et al (2009) A comparison of pretreatment with a topical combination of nonivamide and nicoboxil and surgical delay in a random pattern skin flap model. J Plast Reconstr Aesthetic Surg 62(7):914–919

Jonsson K, Hunt TK et al (1988) Tissue oxygen measurements in delayed skin flaps: a reconsideration of the mechanisms of the delay phenomenon. Plast Reconstr Surg 82(2):328–336

Juri J (1975) Use of parieto-occipital flaps in the surgical treatment of baldness. Plast Reconstr Surg 55(4):456–460

Kabaker S (1978) Experiences with parieto-occipital flaps in hair transplantation. Laryngoscope 88(1 Pt 1):73–84

Kabaker SS (1979) Juri flap procedure for the treatment of baldness. 2 year experience. Arch Otolaryngol 105(9):509–514

Kabaker SS, Kridel RW et al (1986) Tissue expansion in the treatment of alopecia. Arch Otolaryngol Head Neck Surg 112(7):720–725

Karacaoglu E, Yuksel F et al (2002) Chemical delay: an alternative to surgical delay experimental study. Ann Plast Surg 49(1):73–80; discussion 82–71

Kent DE, Defazio JM (2011) Improving survival of the paramedian forehead flap in patients with excessive tobacco use: the vascular delay. Dermatol Surg 37:1362–1364

Lineaweaver WC, Lei MP et al (2004) Vascular endothelium growth factor, surgical delay, and skin flap survival. Ann Surg 239(6):866–873; discussion 873-865

McCarthy JG, Lorenc ZP et al (1985) The median forehead flap revisited: the blood supply. Plast Reconstr Surg 76(6):866–869

Menick FJ (2012) An approach to the late revision of a failed nasal reconstruction. Plast Reconstr Surg 129(1):92e–103e

Milton SH (1969) The effects of "delay" on the survival of experimental pedicled skin flaps. Br J Plast Surg 22(3):244–252

Morris SF, Taylor GI (1995) The time sequence of the delay phenomenon: when is a surgical delay effective? an experimental study. Plast Reconstr Surg 95(3):526–533

Myers MB, Cherry G (1967) Augmentation of tissue survival by delay: an experimental study in rabbits. Plast Reconstr Surg 39(4):397–401

Pang CY, Forrest CR et al (1986) Augmentation of blood flow in delayed random skin flaps in the pig: effect of length of delay period and angiogenesis. Plast Reconstr Surg 78(1):68–74

Pearl RM (1981) A unifying theory of the delay phenomenon–recovery from the hyperadrenergic state. Ann Plast Surg 7(2):102–112

Reichner DR, Scholz T et al (2003) Laser flap delay: comparison of erbium: YAG and CO_2 lasers. Am Surg 69(1):69–72

Sasaki GH, Pang CY (1984) Pathophysiology of skin flaps raised on expanded pig skin. Plast Reconstr Surg 74(1):59–67

Schreiber NT, Mobley SR (2011) Elegant solutions for complex paramedian forehead flap reconstruction. Facial Plast Surg Clin North Am 19(3):465–479

Taylor GI, Corlett RJ et al (1992) An anatomic review of the delay phenomenon: II. Clinical applications. Plast Reconstr Surg 89(3):408–416; discussion 417-408

Tepper OM, Capla JM et al (2005) Adult vasculogenesis occurs through in situ recruitment, proliferation, and tubulization of circulating bone marrow-derived cells. Blood 105(3):1068–1077

Williams EF, Lam SM (2003) Comprehensive facial rejuvenation: a practical and systematic guide to surgical management of the aging face. Lippincott Williams & Wilkins, Philadelphia

Delay Phenomenon

▶ Delay of Flap

Dental Caries (Radiation Caries)

Shelley Segrest Taylor
Department of Otolaryngology and Communicative Sciences, The University of Mississippi Medical Center, Jackson, MS, USA

Definition

Decalcification and dental decay that result from a radiation-induced decrease in quantity and quality of saliva.

Cross-References

▶ Dental Evaluation in Head and Neck Cancer Patient

Dental Evaluation in Head and Neck Cancer Patient

Shelley Segrest Taylor
Department of Otolaryngology and Communicative Sciences, The University of Mississippi Medical Center, Jackson, MS, USA

Introduction

Head and neck cancer treatment requires a multidisciplinary team approach. Members of the treatment team are composed of an otolaryngologist, a head and neck surgeon, a medical oncologist, a radiation oncologist, a radiologist, a pathologist, a speech pathologist, and a oral/dental oncologist. The intraoral side effects of resection surgery and the cancericidal dosages of radiation and/or chemotherapy are critical patient management considerations for physicians and dentists in the treatment of the head and neck cancer patient. Once the treatment modality has been determined, an early referral from the radiation oncologist to an oral oncologist or an adequately trained dentist for evaluation and proper timing of treatment is necessary. The integration of dental care prior to the initiation of radiation and/or chemotherapy will reduce management complications, dramatically improve the quality of life, and best serve the health and well-being of the patients that are involved. Treatment of the head and neck cancer patient will likely involve a combination of therapies; therefore, it is imperative to reach optimal oral health. The goal of dental treatment is to obtain a disease-free oral cavity prior to beginning chemotherapy and/or radiation therapy and maintain oral health during and after completion of treatment. The incorporation of an adequately trained dentist into the overall cancer treatment plan will improve the dental health of the patient and help to decrease the incidence of any unwanted oral side effects, therefore promoting a lifetime of oral health (Carl 1993).

Dental Management before Radiation Treatment

A comprehensive oral and dental assessment should be performed and dental treatment then incorporated into the overall cancer treatment plan to prevent and aid in the management of any adverse effects of radiation therapy. The effects of radiation therapy in the head and neck cancer patient can range from acute to long-term or chronic complications. The acute effects include bacterial and fungal infection, oral mucositis, altered salivary gland function, and taste alteration. Patients often also experience long-term side effects ranging from radiation caries, xerostomia, dysgeusia/ageusia, and muscular/cutaneous fibrosis to alterations in vascularity in soft tissue and bone, the latter of these leading to soft tissue necrosis and osteoradionecrosis (Peterson 2000).

Once a dental referral has been made, the treating dentist should consult with the appropriate physicians for proper timing and coordination of dental care with the patient's cancer treatment plan. When chemotherapy and/or radiotherapy is to be employed, it is generally in the patient's best interest to complete any dental treatment, especially oral surgery, prior to the initiation of cancer therapy. A minimum of 2 weeks (14 days), 21 days is ideal, is needed for adequate healing of the oral tissues between oral surgery and the initiation of radiation therapy (Marx and Johnson 1987). The dentist must have knowledge of the regions of the jaws that will be receiving radiation and the doses that are to be delivered, therefore aiding in the prediction of the areas that are more at risk of soft tissue and bone necrosis. Knowing this information, a timely dental treatment plan is fabricated, reducing the likelihood of the development of osteoradionecrosis as well as other unwanted side effects of cancer therapy.

Before a patient begins chemotherapy and/or radiotherapy for head and neck cancer, a comprehensive oral and dental evaluation including any pertinent radiographs is performed by an oral oncologist or an adequately trained dentist. A thorough hard and soft tissue examination, complete periodontal charting, and a panoramic radiograph are essential in determining the presence of pathology that should be addressed prior to undergoing radiation therapy. Dental pathology can be of pulpal or periapical origin or can affect the supporting structures of the tooth, which is known as periodontal disease. The dental practitioner must also evaluate the presence of plaque, calculus, and past dental hygiene practices of the patient, thus predicting motivation and future compliance with impeccable dental hygiene to prevent future caries. If patient motivation with oral hygiene is low, then full mouth dental extractions is the optimal treatment.

After performing a detailed oral and dental evaluation as well as interpreting the panoramic radiograph, it is necessary that any teeth that are nonrestorable be extracted at least a minimum of 2 weeks (14 days), 21 days is ideal, prior to radiation therapy. Teeth that are identified as having moderate to advanced periodontal disease are to be extracted. Extractions are also indicated for third molars that are partially erupted and exposed to the oral environment. Third molars presenting in this fashion are at risk of developing pericoronitis, which is characterized as soft tissue inflammation surrounding a partially erupted third molar that often leads to infection. Other forms of oral surgery such as alveoloplasty for corrections of edentulous prominences and excision of dentoalveolar pathosis should be performed at the earliest time possible prior to initiating cancer therapy. It is also important to remove any source of irritation such as calculus, sharp teeth, and current prostheses that are being worn. Head and neck radiation or chemotherapy agents can cause severe and painful side effects to the oral mucosa. Patients should be advised not to wear any dental prostheses when undergoing therapy. When evaluating teeth which will be maintained, all carious lesions are to be excavated and amalgam or composite restorative material is placed to assist in caries control.

In some patient cases, radiation therapy must be initiated as soon as possible due to the size and growth rate of the tumor. In these circumstances, dental surgery should not be done during radiation treatment, but delayed until after treatment has ended and the patient has somewhat recovered. Dental extractions or any oral surgery should be delayed at least 3 weeks after radiotherapy has been completed. Changes within the bone may worsen over time, so treatment should not be delayed an excess amount of time.

Other scenarios exist that should be considered when planning for radiation therapy. Preradiotherapy extractions are also to be considered for maxillary or mandibular teeth with no opposing teeth to prevent supraeruption. Teeth with periapical radiolucent lesions or active periapical disease that are within the field of planned radiation should be extracted

(Hancock et al. 2003). Teeth outside the field of radiation that have necrotic pulpal tissue may have root canal treatment, but all treatment must be completed at least a minimum of 2 weeks (14 days), 21 days is ideal, prior to the initiation of radiation therapy. Orthodontic bands or appliances should be removed before treatment, eliminating all sources of trauma.

Radiotherapy results in a decrease in the quantity and quality of saliva, consequently promoting decalcification of remaining teeth and dental decay. Patients with salvageable teeth are to be placed into an intensive oral hygiene program which includes: dental prophylaxis and oral hygiene instructions every 3–6 months, proper tooth brushing two times daily with a fluoride toothpaste, proper use of dental floss daily, and the fabrication of fluoride trays. Alginate impressions are taken on maxillary and mandibular arches which have remaining teeth that are not indicated for extractions. Fluoride trays are then fabricated for the daily application of fluoride gel to aid in the prevention of dental caries. Fluoride gel in the form of 0.4% stannous fluoride or 1.1% sodium fluoride is applied in the gel carrier in a ribbon form. The fluoride trays are to be worn daily for 5 min. Stringently applied oral hygiene regimens will assist in minimizing the effects from therapy, therefore reducing the probability that there will be a disruption in radiotherapy and the survival rate is thereby enlarged (Barasch and Safford 1993).

As a result of dental management, partial or complete edentulism is inevitable. Many patients inquire about time frames for fabrication of dental prostheses. If prostheses are to be fabricated at the end of radiation treatment, all preprosthetic surgery must be completed at least 2 weeks (14 days), 21 days is ideal, prior to initiation of radiation treatment. This will aid in preventing bone and soft tissue necrosis. Dental prostheses fabrication should not be initiated until 4–6 months after radiation has been completed.

Dental Management with Chemotherapy Agents

Patients being treated for head and neck cancer with high dose chemotherapy agents are at risk for many oral complications. Xerostomia, mucositis, and a decrease in saliva quantity are common occurrences in these patients, but pain, bleeding, infection, and diminish in taste acuity can occur as well (Raber-Durlacher et al. 2004). (Please refer to the section on Complications of Cancer Treatment Therapy. Most of these complications occur in both radiation and chemotherapy treatments and are managed similarly.) Comprehensive oral and dental evaluations with the appropriate dental radiographs are imperative to diagnose dental problems before the start of chemotherapy treatment. The same guidelines should be followed as the patient who is undergoing radiation therapy. Chemotherapy can be the primary treatment for some cancers or used as an adjunct. Head and neck cancer patients are often treated with a concomitant treatment; thus, with any treatment regimen, it is appropriate to achieve optimal oral health prior to the initiation of cancer therapy.

Preceding the initiation of chemotherapy, it is best to eliminate all sources of trauma and infection. Teeth which have been categorized as nonrestorable and symptomatic teeth with periapical radiolucencies are to be extracted. If the patient reports that no symptoms are present, then extractions can wait until after chemotherapy. Partially erupted third molars are to be extracted if there is a likelihood that pericoronitis will develop. Pericoronitis is characterized as soft tissue inflammation surrounding a partially erupted third molar that often leads to infection.

Proper oral hygiene should be demonstrated to the patient and enforced. A dental prophylaxis is to be performed every 3–6 months with proper oral hygiene instructions. If mild periodontal disease is present, then scaling and root planings are preferred as these teeth do not have to be extracted prior to chemotherapy. Patients who currently wear dental prostheses should be instructed not to wear them during treatment, which eliminates all sources of trauma.

Chemotherapy agents can cause myelosuppression and immunosuppression, which places the patient at risk for infection. The source of infection often results from the presence of poor dentition present in the oral cavity. Thrombocytopenia also occurs in patients receiving chemotherapy agents; consequently, platelet counts must be evaluated to minimize the risk of excessive postoperative bleeding. It must be realized that chemotherapy treatment may be initiated prior to achieving proper oral health due to cancer staging and advancement. Dialogue between the medical oncologist and the oral oncologist (dentist) or dental practitioner must be communicated to achieve a proper time frame between chemotherapy and dental extractions.

Complications of Cancer Treatment Therapy

Mucositis

Mucositis is an undesirable complication of head and neck radiation, myelosuppressive chemotherapy, and stem cell transplantation. It is characterized as the damage that occurs to the mucosal lining of the gastrointestinal tract with the oral and oropharyngeal mucosa being particularly affected. It is the most common cause of pain during cancer treatment with troublesome sequelae such as severe pain, risk of local and systemic infection, risk of compromised oral and pharyngeal function, and oral bleeding, therefore leading to further hospital care and increases in healthcare costs (Greenberg et al. 2008).

Affecting nearly all head and neck radiation and chemotherapy patients, oral mucositis is a frequent and debilitating side effect that can become a dose-limiting toxicity resulting in the slowing or the discontinuity of cancer therapies among some patients. Mucositis is multifactorial and a biologically complex event beginning with an inflammatory/vascular event and epithelial phase, then followed by ulceration and bacterial colonization, and finally ending with healing (Sonis et al. 2004). The first clinical signs usually begin in the second week after the initiation of radiation therapy and usually diminish weeks after therapy has ended. The mucosa will have a red appearance due to the hyperemia/epithelial thinning or assume a white presence as a result of epithelial hyperplasia/hypertrophy and intraepithelial edema. Ulceration of the oral tissues with pseudomembrane formation compromises oral hygiene practices, which further complicates oral mucositis (Greenberg et al. 2008).

Management of Oral Mucositis

When caring for patients that have radiation- or chemotherapy-induced oral mucositis, basic oral care, oral care protocols/patient education, and palliative care should be communicated. Oral hygiene regimens reduce the amount of oral microbial flora, which minimizes soft tissue infection and reduces symptoms of pain that are cancer induced. Patient education is of the utmost importance. Knowledge about oral complications that occur as a result of cancer therapy should be communicated to patients including what to expect and how to cope. Palliative care includes the use of systemic analgesics, mouthwashes containing mixtures of different agents, coating agents, and topical anesthetics/analgesics (Rubenstein et al. 2004).

An emphasis on proper oral hygiene is a necessity to patients receiving chemotherapy and radiation treatment. The severity of mucositis can be reduced with good oral hygiene (McGuire et al. 2006). Brushing twice a day and flossing daily is recommended. Chlorhexidine has shown no positive influence on the effects of oral mucositis (Barasch et al. 2006). Bland oral rinses, topical anesthetics, and coating agents can aid in the palliation of mild to moderate mucositis. Saline, sodium bicarbonate, and water rinses aid in mucosal moisturizing and lubrication. Topical anesthetics such as lidocaine, benzocaine, "magic mouth rinses" (compounded rinses which include lidocaine, diphenhydramine, Amphojel, and nystatin), and Benzydamine (not approved by the FDA) are recommended for the progression of mucositis. Mucosal surface protectants are available, but limited in clinical research effectiveness. If patients need more than bland rinses for mild to moderate pain control, then nonsteroidal anti-inflammatory drugs are recommended. The advantages of NSAIDS include analgesic properties, low cost, and over-the counter availability. To aid in the prevention of dry lips, lip lubricants are very beneficial. For more severe cases of mucositis, opioids are recommended, but providers must be aware that tolerance to these drugs can be developed (Sonis 2008).

Xerostomia

Xerostomia is a debilitating side effect of head and neck radiation and many chemotherapy regimens. Patients presenting with a decrease in salivary flow are more at risk for rampant dental caries, periodontal disease, and common oral infections. It is imperative for the dental practitioner to educate patients on the side effects of xerostomia and perform thorough examinations before the start of treatment. Past oral hygiene practices of the patient must be considered, therefore indicating proper maintenance of the remaining dentition during and after cancer therapy. It is in the best interest of the patient to extract all remaining teeth whether in the field of radiation or not if oral hygiene compliance is a potential problem. Patients undergoing radiation treatment for head and neck cancer usually report signs of xerostomia a couple of weeks following start of therapy, although signs can be continual and infinite for some patients (Torres et al. 2002). Radiation damage to the acinar cells in the salivary glands and diminish in quantity of saliva results in a thick, ropey, and tacky consistency that is aggravating and troublesome to patients (Makkonen et al. 1986). Patients often report that food particles are more inclined to stick to the remaining teeth or edentulous tissues and are not easily washed away during meals.

Management of Xerostomia

Management of patients reporting xerostomia includes fabrication of fluoride gel carriers to prevent future dental decay, dispensing of antibacterial solutions, use of oral moisturizers, saliva substitutes, and prescription sialagogues (Epstein et al. 2001).

Constant moistening of the tissues can simply be achieved by sipping and swishing with water periodically throughout the day. A regimen such as this is mandatory for patients suffering from hyposalivation. The use of sugarless gum can also help stimulate some salivary function. Pilocarpine is a sialagogue that shows benefit for stimulating salivary function. Other sialagogues that have been studied are bethanechol and cevimeline, which aid in hyposalivation. Oral moisturizers and saliva substitutes are other options that are available (Greenspan 1990).

Osteoradionecrosis

Osteoradionecrosis is a debilitating complication that is associated with head and neck radiation therapy. Patients must be educated before starting their cancer therapy of the devastating side effects that can result, accordingly preparing patients should a complication occur. Head and neck radiation therapy induces vascular and cellular changes as well as a decrease in the amount of oxygen that is available in the tissues, resulting in bone and soft tissue that is incapable of healing when a stimulus is presented. Catalysts include dental extractions, trauma, and periodontal disease, wearing of denture prostheses, or impromptu lesions that develop with no apparent source. Patients who develop osteoradionecrosis have complaints of pain and often a production of a pathologic jaw fracture, subsequently a jaw resection may be inevitable. Soft tissue necrosis can also evolve on any site of the oral tissue. These should be monitored periodically to eliminate a possible cancer recurrence due to the ulcerative presentation.

Several factors must be evaluated when assessing the risk of radiation-induced osteonecrosis. Radiation doses, the field of radiation, the number of fractions, the length of posttreatment time, and edentulism versus dentulism must considered. There is no transparent answer as to who will develop this debilitating side affect, but patients are more at risk with higher doses and higher number of fractions of radiation. Occurrence of osteoradionecrosis is more likely in the mandible than the maxilla and patients who are dentulous have a higher risk of developing osteoradionecrosis than patients who are edentulous prior to beginning radiation therapy (Silverman 2003). The risk of development of radiation-induced osteonecrosis is an endless battle for both the patient and the practitioner. Responses to radiotherapy vary from patient to patient, patients and practitioners should realize that a significant number of patients will develop this complication as a result of the inability of the irradiated tissues to replenish normal cellular turnover.

Management of Osteoradionecrosis

Head and neck cancer patients should have all nonrestorable teeth extracted at least 14 days, although 21 days is optimal, prior to the start of radiation therapy, subsequently reducing the risk of osteoradionecrosis (Marx and Johnson 1987). Once radiation therapy has ceased, patients should periodically be monitored and followed by a dentist. Oral hygiene always is emphasized with the utmost importance. Clinical examinations and radiographs are a necessity in diagnosing adverse events that can occur. For patients who present with a bony sequestrum, analgesics can be used for pain control and antibiotic therapy is recommended if swelling is present. If oral surgery is inevitable for treatment, then it is best for the patient to undergo 20–30 sessions of hyperbaric oxygen before the surgical procedure is performed. A negative aspect of hyperbaric oxygen often presents the problem of cost and time, therefore dental extractions sometimes must be performed without hyperbaric oxygen therapy. In this case, patients should prophylactically be covered with antibiotics prior to the extractions and post extractions. Prilocaine is recommended as the local anesthetic of choice and an atraumatic surgical technique with periodic follow-up visits is required (Maxymiw et al. 1991).

Radiation Caries

Demineralization and the promotion of dental decay is a complication that is associated with head and neck radiation therapy. Proper oral hygiene should be emphasized to patients and the use of fluoride gel carriers demonstrated. This is a lifelong commitment that is addressed before the start of cancer therapy. Dental caries are the result of the decrease in saliva and the change that occurs within the composition of the teeth. Moistening of the tissues with water and the use of saliva substitutes can help to decrease the incidence of dental disease.

Hypogeusia/Ageusia/Dysgeusia

Partial (hypogeusia) or complete (ageusia) loss of taste acuity is a complication that can result from chemotherapy and radiotherapy to the head and neck region. Alterations in taste (dysgeusia) awareness can also occur. These complications in taste awareness are the result of radiation damage to the taste buds or the decrease in salivation, but often only lasting for a short time with recovery in a couple of months. Permanent alterations can occur in some cases (Silverman 2003).

As a result, patients often experience a loss of appetite, consequently leading to a decrease in weight. Vitamins that include elemental zinc can be beneficial in amplifying taste acuity. Recommendations are 50–100 mg of elemental zinc taken daily (Silverman et al. 1983).

Trismus

Trismus is a complication that can result from radiation therapy to the head and neck. The development of limited opening occurs due to contraction of the masticatory muscles and the temporomandibular joint. Trismus can occur secondarily to fibrosis. Radiation doses and fields that include the pterygoids are the more likely cause. (Dijkstra et al. 2006). Patients who develop limited opening can perform daily mandibular exercises to stretch the masticatory muscles and decrease muscular fibrosis. Tongue blades are often prescribed to increase opening, but if a patient develops severe fibrosis, there may be no benefit.

Candidiasis

Candida albicans is a fungal infection that affects most patients who have undergone head and neck radiation therapy. The quantity changes in saliva are associated with the presence of this infection (Rossie et al. 1987).

Patients often report pain being associated. Treatment includes use of systemic or topical antifungal agents. Systemic agents such as Ketoconazole or fluconazole can be prescribed and appear to be more effective. Topical agents such as nystatin or clotrimazole can be used if patients have difficulty in swallowing as a result of mucositis.

Surgical Considerations

When indicated for the treatment of head and neck cancer, the surgical approach is intended to eliminate malignant and adjacent tissue, therefore removing all cancerous cells. Dental rehabilitation is planned with the head and neck surgeon at the time of initial diagnosis; therefore the surgeon, the dental practitioner, and the patient have a thorough understanding of the potential outcomes (See ▶ Maxillofacial Prosthetics for Head and Neck Defects).

References

Barasch A, Safford MM (1993) Management of oral pain in patients with malignant diseases. Compendium 14(11): 1376, 1378–1382, 1384

Barasch A, Elad S, Altman A et al (2006) Antimicrobials, mucosal coating agents, anesthetics, analgesics and nutritional supplements for alimentary tract mucositis. Support Care Cancer 14:528–532

Carl W (1993) Local radiation and systemic chemotherapy: preventing and managing the oral complications. J Am Dent Assoc 124(3):119–123

Dijkstra PU, Huisman PM, Roodenburg JLN (2006) Criteria for trismus in head and neck oncology. Int J Oral Maxillofac Surg 35:337–342

Epstein JB, Robertson M, Emerton S et al (2001) Quality of life and oral function in patients treated with radiation therapy for head and neck cancer. Head Neck 23:389–398

Greenberg MS, Glick M, Ship JA (2008) Burkett's oral medicine, 11th edn. BC Decker, Hamilton, pp 177–187

Greenspan D (1990) Management of salivary gland dysfunction. Natl Cancer Inst Monogr 9:159–161

Hancock PJ, Epstein JB, Sadler GR (2003) Oral and dental management related to radiation therapy for head and neck cancer. J Can Dent Assoc 69(9):585–590

Makkonen TA, Tenovuo J, Vilja P et al (1986) Changes in the protein composition of whole saliva during radiotherapy on patients with oral oropharyngeal cancer. Oral Surg Oral Med Oral Pathol 62:270–275

Marx RE, Johnson RP (1987) Studies in the radiobiology of osteoradionecrosis and their clinical significance. Oral Surg Oral Med Oral Pathol 64:379–390

Maxymiw W, Wood RE et al (1991) Postradiation dental extractions without hyperbaric oxygen. Oral Surg Oral Med Oral Pathol 72:270–274

McGuire DB, Correa MEP, Johnson J, Wienandts P (2006) The role of basic oral care and good clinical practice principles in the management of oral mucositis. Support Care Cancer 14:541–547

Peterson DE (2000) Oral problems in supportive care: no longer an orphan topic? Support Care Cancer 8:347–348

Raber-Durlacher JE, Barasch A, Peterson DE et al (2004) Oral complications and management considerations in patients treated with high-dose chemotherapy. Support Cancer Ther 1(4):219–229

Rossie KM, Taylor J, Beck FM et al (1987) Influence of radiation therapy on oral Candida albicans colonization: a quantitative assessment. Oral Surg Oral Med Oral Pathol 64:698–701

Rubenstein EB, Peterson DE, Schubert M (2004) Clinical practice guidelines for the prevention and treatment of cancer therapy-induced oral and gastrointestinal mucositis. Cancer 100(9 Suppl):2026–2046

Silverman S Jr (2003) American cancer society atlas of clinical oncology oral cancer, 5th edn. BC Decker, Hamilton, pp 120–127

Silverman JE, Weber CW, Silverman S Jr et al (1983) Zinc supplementation and taste in head and neck cancer patients undergoing radiation therapy. J Oral Med 38:14–16

Sonis S (2008) Management of oral mucositis pain. In: Oral health in cancer therapy. A guide for health care professionals, 3rd edn. Dental Education Oncology Program, San Antonio, Monograph

Sonis ST, Elting LS, Keefe D et al (2004) Perspectives on cancer therapy-induced mucosal injury. Cancer 100(9 Suppl):1995–2025

Torres SR, Peixoto CB, Caldas DM (2002) Relationship between salivary flow rates and Candida counts in subjects with xerostomia. Oral Surg Oral Med Oral Pathol Oral Radiol Endod 93:149–154

Dermatochalasis

Michael M. Kim
Division of Facial Plastic & Reconstructive Surgery, Department of Otolaryngology-Head and Neck Surgery, Oregon Health & Science University, Portland, OR, USA

Definition

Dermatochalasis is an excess of skin of the upper or lower eyelid. Dermatochalasis of the upper eyelids can cause visual field obstruction and/or age-related changes that may be treated by various blepharoplasty techniques. Visual field obstruction can be measured by visual field testing and may be a prerequisite for the procedure to be deemed functional versus aesthetic.

Dermoids

▶ Heterotopias, Teratoma, and Choristoma

Developmental Anatomy

▶ Embryology of Ear (General)

Developmental Central Auditory Processing Disorders

Rola Farah[1], David K. Brown[2,3] and Robert W. Keith[1]
[1]Department of Communication Sciences and Disorders, College of Allied Health Sciences, University of Cincinnati, Cincinnati, OH, USA
[2]Communication Sciences Research Center, Cincinnati Children's Hospital Medical Center, Cincinnati, OH, USA
[3]Departments of Otolaryngology and Communication Sciences and Disorders, University of Cincinnati, Cincinnati, OH, USA

Synonyms

Auditory processing disorder (APD); Central auditory processing disorder – [(C)APD]

Definition

Introduction
The definition of (Central) Auditory Processing Disorder (C)APD has been controversial through the years since the term auditory processing was introduced in 1954. Consequently, the nature of the disorder and the best diagnostic and treatment procedures were debatable. Four position statements by professional bodies in the field of audiology provided definitions and are outlined here.

1. Consensus Report by the American Speech-Language Hearing Association (ASHA 1996)
   "Central auditory processing disorder (CAPD) is an observed deficiency in one or more of the following behaviors: sound localization and lateralization, auditory discrimination, auditory pattern recognition, temporal aspects of audition; including temporal resolution, temporal masking, temporal integration, and temporal ordering, auditory performance decrements with competing acoustic signals and auditory performance decrements with degraded acoustic signals. The auditory system mechanisms and processes responsible for the above listed behaviors are presumed to apply to nonverbal as well as verbal signals and have neurophysiological as well as behavioral correlates.

   For some persons, CAPD is presumed to result from the dysfunction of processes and mechanisms dedicated to audition; for others, CAPD may stem from some more general dysfunction, such as an attention deficit or neural timing deficit that affects performance across modalities. It is also possible for CAPD to reflect coexisting dysfunctions of both sorts."

2. Report of the Consensus Conference on APD in Children (Jerger and Musiek 2000)
   "An auditory processing disorder (APD) can be broadly defined as a deficit in the processing of information that is specific to the auditory modality. The problem may be exacerbated in unfavorable acoustic environments. It may be associated with difficulties in listening, speech understanding, language development and learning."

3. Technical Report by the American Speech-Language Hearing Association (ASHA 2005)
   "(Central) Auditory Processing [(C)AP] refers to the efficiency and effectiveness by which the central nervous system (CNS) utilizes auditory information. Narrowly defined, (C)AP refers to the perceptual processing of auditory information in the CNS and the neurobiologic activity that underlies that processing and gives rise to electrophysiologic auditory potentials." "(C)APD is best viewed as a deficit in the neural processing of auditory

stimuli that may coexist with, but *is not the result of*, dysfunction in other modalities."

4. Practice Guidelines for (C)APD by the American Academy of Audiology (AAA 2010)

   The definition of (C)APD by the American Academy of Audiology (2010) builds on ASHA's 2005 definition and states that "(C)APD refers to difficulties in the perceptual processing of auditory information in the central nervous system and the neurobiologic activity that underlies that processing and gives rise to the electrophysiologic auditory potentials."

   The guidelines also refer to the accumulating evidence supporting the presence of (C)APD as a "true" clinical disorder and provide evidence connecting known pathologies of the Central Auditory Nervous System (CANS) with abnormalities in behavioral and electrophysiological measures.

Clinical Features

Children with (C)APD demonstrate a pattern of difficulties with poor performance in one or more of the following skills: sound localization and lateralization, auditory discrimination, auditory pattern recognition, temporal aspects of audition; including temporal resolution, temporal masking, temporal integration, and temporal ordering, auditory performance decrements with competing acoustic signals and auditory performance decrements with degraded acoustic signals (ASHA 2005).

Behaviors associated with the above-mentioned skills include: difficulty understanding in the presence of background noise or in reverberant acoustic environments, inconsistent or inappropriate responses to requests for information, difficulty following rapid speech, frequent requests for repetition and/or rephrasing of information, difficulties following directions, difficulty maintaining auditory attention, a tendency to be easily distracted, and academic difficulties, including reading, spelling, and/or learning problems (Keith 2009; AAA 2010).

Other common reported and/or observed symptoms include: poor listening skills, difficulty learning through the auditory modality, weak auditory memory span for commands and sequences, difficulty understanding muffled or distorted speech, deficits with auditory integration, reduced tolerance to loud noise,

hypersensitivity to sounds, and poor speech recognition in noise (Keith 2009).

It is rare to observe all clinical symptoms in all children with (C)APD due to the complex, intrinsic nature of the CANS and the extensive interaction between its structures. Furthermore, there is a substantial overlap of these behaviors with those usually seen in other cognitive and linguistic disorders like learning disabilities, ADHD, and developmental language delay. The presence of one or more of these behaviors should be considered carefully since they are not exclusive to (C)APD and should put the child in the category of "at-risk of APD."

Prevalence

The prevalence of (C)APD in school-age children has been estimated as 2–5%. The dearth of more accurate prevalence numbers is due to the lack of a "gold standard," controversies in defining and diagnosing (C)APD, and the different criteria used to include children. Furthermore, the variance in prevalence estimates might be due to the heterogeneity of this population and the mild cases of (C)APD which go undetected in children who learn to compensate in different ways.

Etiology

In some cases, the etiology underlying (C)APD may be identified in the presence of neurological conditions, delayed maturation of the central nervous system (CSN), or peripheral hearing loss such as early ► chronic otitis media. There is some speculation that (C)APD has a genetic link similar to dyslexia, but that fact is yet to be proven. Children with exceptionally low birth weight (e.g., below 1,000 g) who have language and learning problems are likely to be at risk for (C)APD. Auditory deprivation due to history of ► acute and chronic otitis media with effusion in children has been linked to higher incidence of difficulties on central auditory processing tasks. Many cases of (C)APD show atypical hemispheric asymmetry in auditory signal neural representation, ineffective interhemispheric transmission of auditory information, and inexact neural synchrony (Bellis 2007). However, in most cases, the etiology for (C)APD remains undetermined.

In adults, several factors are known to involve the central auditory nervous system (CANS) and cause an auditory processing disorder such as tumors of the CANS affecting auditory areas. Brain tumors interfering with the central auditory pathway can lead to ear deficits and dysfunction in auditory processing. Other impairments associated with APD include: alcoholism, multiple sclerosis (MS), Alzheimer's disease, and psychiatric disorders. Of recent interest is the growing awareness of auditory processing disorders in persons who experience traumatic brain injury from blunt or penetrating head injury from sports, automobile, or war injuries.

Comorbidity of (C)APD and ADHD, Learning Disabilities and Language Impairment

The relationship between (C)APD and attention deficit hyperactivity disorder (ADHD), Learning Disabilities and Language Impairment has been extensively investigated. Frequently, subjects diagnosed with (C)APD demonstrate difficulties in language, learning, and other higher-order functions. Similarly, (C)APD is seen in subjects diagnosed with ADHD, language impairment, and learning disabilities.

The overlap of symptoms and clinical manifestation challenges professionals to attain clinical diagnosis. For example, the main symptoms observed in children with (C)APD include difficulty listening in background noise, difficulty following oral instructions, poor listening skills, deficits in auditory divided/selective and sustained attention, difficulties in academics, poor auditory association skills, inattention, and distractibility. The major signs observed in children with ADHD include inattention, distractibility, hyperactivity, academic difficulties, poor listening skills, restlessness, impulsiveness, interruptions, and difficulty hearing in background noise (Chermak 2007). Therefore, while distractibility is a dominant feature of ADHD and difficulty listening in noise is a dominant feature of (C)APD, there is substantial overlap of behaviors in the two groups. Nevertheless, it is important to differentiate between the two when possible, since (C)APD is not treated with stimulant medication while ADHD may be.

The complex organization of the brain plays a major role in the comorbidity of (C)APD and Language, Learning, ADHD, and other higher-order disorders.

The brain is non-modular in nature, therefore a dysfunction in shared or contiguous neuroanatomical loci can affect several different functions. There are auditory-specific areas in the brain but the neurons contained in such areas respond primarily, but not exclusively to auditory signals. There are additional areas in the brain, not auditory-specific, which are connected to the auditory neurons along the central auditory pathways. Many of these brain areas support higher-order functions and are associated with attention and motor control while involved in the underlying patho physiology of ADHD (Chermak 2007). The shared physiologic and neurologic loci results in similar clinical manifestations which deem the differential diagnosis complex and challenging.

The CANS integrity is critical to auditory functions including spoken language processing and the processing of many other complex signals (ASHA 1996) but the integrity of other systems is mandatory in order to execute auditory as well as motivation, attention, and learning tasks. Thus, one can imagine that a dysfunction in the auditory system might affect attention (bottom-up), since attention is driven by accurate processing and integration of incoming sensory stimulation. On the other hand, impaired attention to auditory signals might cause an auditory processing dysfunction (top-down).

Similarly, (C)APD is frequently associated with language impairment and learning disabilities. Language acquisition requires an intact processing of acoustic information among other factors. Once the acoustic signal reaches the auditory cortex, other processes come into play to attach meaning and comprehend the incoming acoustic signal by means of the linguistic system. Any dysfunction through this hierarchy can lead to different symptoms associated with both auditory processing disorders and/or language impairment/learning disability. In spite of this, not every child diagnosed with (C)APD has language and/or learning difficulties and auditory processing might be intact in children diagnosed with language and/or learning difficulties. The effect of certain auditory deficits may be diverse for different populations and different auditory deficits might cause different functional profiles (ASHA 2005). In other words, even though some children with language impairment or learning disability may exhibit auditory processing deficiencies in processing the spoken language, it cannot be assumed that (C)APD is causing their difficulties unless it is proven through auditory diagnostic measures. The heterogeneity in the effects of (C)APD and language impairment/learning disability, along with overlapping symptoms in all groups, causes the clinicians to face a tremendous challenge while conducting assessments. This fact delineates the need for multidisciplinary team approach that scrutinizes the nature and basis of the difficulties observed in each child suspected of having (C)APD.

Screening for (C)APD

A full assessment for (C)APD is a lengthy procedure that requires multiple sessions by a multidisciplinary team. To avoid unnecessary referrals and effective identification of (C)APD, screening methods are indispensable. Screening procedures obtain initial information that could lead to the identification of children who are "at-risk" for (C)APD and reduce the number of inappropriate referrals for diagnostic assessment (Bellis 2003). The screening process involves efficient and methodical examination of auditory behaviors and listening skills as well as communication and different levels of function in the CANS (Bellis 2003). (C)APD screening can be carried out by audiologists, speech-language pathologists, psychologists, and other health professionals using measures sensitive to identifying auditory function deficiencies (ASHA 2005).

The main characteristics needed for a good screening measure are high sensitivity (the ability to detect (C)APD when it is present) and good specificity (the ability to rule out (C)APD when it does not exist). While there is no universally accepted screening test for (C)APD, a number of approaches are in general use. One such approach is the "HQT," which includes an adequate history, a valid questionnaire, and a screening test. If the screening tool identifies an individual at risk for (C)APD, they should be referred for a comprehensive diagnostic evaluation.

Case History: A comprehensive case history can provide crucial information about the possible etiology, site of dysfunction within the CANS and the test battery needed to uncover the dysfunction. Furthermore, the case history can reveal other sensory deficiencies, which might confound the results if not addressed and can guide the diagnosis and intervention needed (AAA 2010). The American Academy of Audiology (AAA 2010) recommends that the case history

should probe the areas of auditory and/or communication difficulties experienced by the individual, any family history of hearing loss and/or central auditory processing deficits, and the individual's medical history. The medical history should inquire about their birth, otologic, neurologic, and general health history, medications, speech and language development, behavioral, educational and/or work history, the existence of any known comorbid conditions, including cognitive, intellectual, and/or medical disorders, social development, and linguistic and cultural background.

Questionnaire: Screening tools include questionnaires and checklists designed to identify individuals at risk for (C)APD who should be referred to a comprehensive diagnostic evaluation. Typically, caregivers or teachers are asked to fallout a questionnaire or a checklist aiming to get relevant information from people who know the child.

Screening Tests: One of the screening tools available is the Children's Auditory Performance Scale (CHAPS), a 25-item scale that utilizes a scaling continuum related to the child's auditory behaviors. Another is The Children's Home Inventory for Listening Difficulties (CHILD), which includes the assessment of listening skills at home. This survey is completed by a parent and can be used with children from age 3 through 12. Other available surveys are The Listening Inventory (TLI), the Listening Questionnaire; however, these tools have not been validated and usually have poor specificity (AAA 2010). In the past, the SCAN-C and SCAN-A tests of auditory processing disorders have been widely used but more recently the SCAN-3 Tests of Auditory Processing Disorders for Children, Adolescents, and Adults (Keith 2009) is among the most widely used tools for screening and diagnosing (C)APD.

Assessment and Diagnosis of (C)APD

Assessment refers to the process of gathering information and data about the child in diverse domains in order to determine functional abilities. It is usually carried out by a multidisciplinary team including audiologist, speech-language pathologist, psychologist, educators, physicians, and parents. This multidisciplinary approach is critical to define the functional deficits of the child. Diagnosis, on the other hand, refers to the identification and classification of the specific dysfunction by using specific diagnostic measures. Since (C)APD is an auditory disorder, the diagnostic process falls under the responsibility of the audiologist (ASHA 2005).

Once the child has been identified by the screening process as being at risk for(C)APD, further testing needs to be done to determine the presence and type of the disorder. This is achieved by using diagnostic tests to delineate the specific dysfunctions in the central auditory nervous system.

Due to the complexity, redundancy, and unique organization of the brain and CANS, heterogeneity is seen in the effect of (C)APD on different individuals. Consequently, consideration should be given when choosing the test battery appropriate for the individual. A test battery approach, which is geared toward the specific complaints of the individual and the information obtained through the case history, is essential. When choosing among the different tests available, it is crucial to tailor the battery to meet the child's chronological and developmental age; language, mental, and cognitive ability; attention; fatigue; memory; and motivation. All of these factors can influence the test outcomes and render the interpretation of its results questionable, if not taken into consideration.

Tests for (C)APD

Diagnosis of (C)APD relies on administration and interpretation of a sensitive and specific behavioral and electrophysiological test battery as well as integrating the results with a comprehensive case history and assessment outcomes. The audiologist should choose the test battery which shows both sensitivity and specificity to lesions and dysfunction of the CANS as well as validity to test the different levels (brainstem, cortical, or interhemispheric) or interactions in the CANS as well as different auditory processes. The test battery should include tests which are proven to be sensitive to CANS lesions while assessing the different auditory processes and the different levels of the CANS. Further considerations include the subject's age; some behavioral and electrophysiological tests for (C)APD require a minimal age for testing children (AAA 2010) due to the normal maturation course of the CANS. The minimal age for testing is typically 7 years or a cognitive ability consistent with this age.

Several tests are available for the diagnosis of (C)APD. Due to the complexity of the CANS, no single test is sufficient to assess the individual's auditory processing ability. Different tests are utilized to assess the various complex auditory processes and it is the audiologist's responsibility to construct the best possible test battery. However, consensus is missing as to which tests should be included in the test battery. There are two broad categories of tests including "behavioral" (where the subject actively responds to the signal by repeating it) and "electrophysiological" (where the subject listens either actively or passively and evoked potentials are recorded from the auditory pathways of the brainstem and cortex).

Behavioral Tests
These tests are categorized by different classification approaches. One of the most popular approaches suggests categorization according to the auditory processes that underlie the normal functioning of the CANS (Bellis 2003; ASHA 2005; AAA 2010). Accordingly, tests are categorized as follows:

Dichotic Listening Tests
The dichotic listening test (DLT) is a behavioral, noninvasive test which has been used widely to examine language dominance, maturation of the central auditory nervous system, and interruption in cortical auditory functions in diverse population groups (Table 1). Various dichotic tests have been developed over the years using different auditory stimuli with varying difficulty and linguistic load (e.g., digits, nonsense syllables, words, spondees, and sentences). In the DLT, different verbal stimuli are presented to the two ears simultaneously and the subject is requested to repeat what was heard. Instructions to the subject or administration modes (Keith and Anderson 2007) vary based on the specific test used and can fall into seven distinct modes. The most popular administration modes included frequently in the behavioral test battery to diagnose (C)APD are divided attention or *free recall*, where the subject reports everything heard in both ears in any order. Divided attention mode is utilized in the dichotic digits test testing for binaural integration. Divided attention with pre-cued direction is where the subject reports everything heard starting with the right ear and then reporting both stimuli starting with the left ear. This administration mode is usually used with the

Developmental Central Auditory Processing Disorders, Table 1 Tests used to assess the different categories of auditory processing and what auditory processing function each test assesses

Test category	Selected tests	Auditory processes
Dichotic listening tests	Dichotic digits	Binaural integration and binaural separation. Hemispheric dominance and maturation of the neural pathways of the auditory nervous system pathways
	Dichotic consonant vowels	
	Competing words	
	Staggered spondaic words	
	Competing sentences	
	Synthetic sentence identification-contralateral competing message	
Monaural low-redundancy tests	Low-pass filtered speech tests: e.g., filtered words (FW) subtest	Auditory closure
	Speech-in-noise tests, e.g., auditory figure ground (AFG) subtest, SSI – ICM subtest	Auditory figure/ground
		Auditory closure
	Time-compressed speech tests, e.g., words, sentences	Auditory closure
Temporal patterning/ ordering and temporal processing	Random gap detection test (RGDT)	Temporal resolution
	Duration pattern test (DPT)	Duration discrimination, temporal ordering
	Frequency pattern test (FPT)	Frequency discrimination, temporal ordering
Binaural interaction	Masking level difference (MLD)	Binaural interaction

competing words subtest of the SCAN test battery (Keith 2009). Finally, in the directed attention mode the subject is instructed to repeat what was heard in one ear and disregard what was heard in the other ear. An example is the competing sentences subtest of the SCAN test battery.

A significant body of research has shown that in the majority of right-handed subjects, more correct responses are reported from the right ear. This finding is termed the right ear advantage (REA) and it is assumed to derive from two well-established aspects of human brain organization: (1) left hemisphere dominance for language in the vast majority of right-handed individuals, and (2) greater robustness of contralateral (right to left or left to right) as opposed to ipsilateral (right to right or left to left) pathways of information transmission (Fig. 1). When the DLT yields more correct responses from the left ear (left ear advantage – LEA) possible explanations include right hemisphere dominance for language and mixed dominance or inefficient transmission between the two hemispheres.

The interpretation of dichotic tests results can be generalized as follows:
For typical normal young subjects, a right ear advantage is present, and is greater as linguistic content

increases from digits to sentences. It is also present for both divided attention (free recall) and directed attention administration modes. After age 13 years, the right ear advantage for all dichotic listening tests is minimal or no ear advantage is present for any of the dichotic measures, regardless of test instruction (divided attention or directed attention) or linguistic content.

Patients with auditory processing disorders show poor overall performance with enhanced right ear advantage on directed ear listening with right ear first and enhanced left ear advantage on directed ear listening with left ear first. Abnormal findings could manifest as a Left ear advantage under all listening conditions or errors in the ear opposite a hemispheric lesion.

Abnormal dichotic test results confirm the presence and extent of injury to the auditory pathways and the diminished auditory processing abilities of the affected person. Similar to the functional tests of auditory processing, abnormal dichotic performance indicates the need to identify and institute appropriate remediation programs.

Among the most common dichotic listening tests in the test battery for (C)APD are the dichotic digits test (DDT), the competing words subtest of SCAN

Developmental Central Auditory Processing Disorders, Fig. 1 The Dichotic Listening model (From "Dichotic Listening Tests" by R. W. Keith and J. Anderson in Handbook of (Central) Auditory Processing Disorders: Auditory Neuroscience and Diagnosis, Volume 1 (p. 209) by F. E. Musiek and G. D. Chermak (Eds.). Copyright © 2007 Plural Publishing, Inc. All rights reserved. Used with permission)

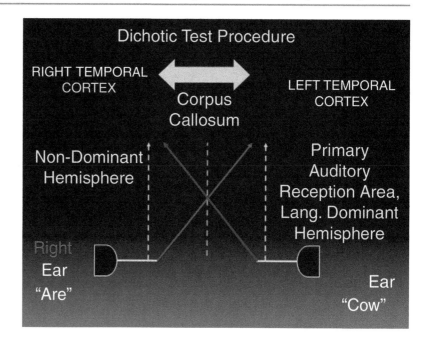

(Keith 2009), the staggered spondee word test (SSW), and the competing sentences of the SCAN and Willeford batteries. Central auditory lesions have a prominent effect on dichotic tests performance. It has been shown that the DLTs are sensitive to cortical and corpus callosal dysfunction and to a lesser extent, the brainstem. Reduced performance scores in the ear contralateral to the lesioned hemisphere have been reported and reduced performance scores in the ipsilateral ear have been attributed to compromised callosal function. Atypical performance in both ears have been reported as reflecting either dysfunction in both hemispheres or dysfunction of one hemisphere and the collosal relay (Bellis 2003; Keith and Anderson 2007). Auditory processes assessed by the DLT are binaural integration (i.e., integrating different signals from both ears) and binaural separation (i.e., separating the incoming signals while paying attention only to one ear).

Monaural Low-Redundancy Speech Tests
Monaural low-redundancy tests are used to assess auditory closure and auditory figure/ground skills (Table 1). Their basis relies on the interaction between extrinsic and intrinsic redundancy. Extrinsic redundancy of the speech signal occurs due to overlapping acoustic and linguistic cues. Acoustic cues like frequency, intensity, and timing interact with linguistic cues like semantic, syntactic, phonemic, and

morphological cues to build up the extrinsic redundancy of the speech signal. Intrinsic redundancy, on the other hand, refers to the complex structural and functional organization of the CANS whereby serial and parallel processing of information takes place. Normal listeners can compensate on the reduced extrinsic redundancy (degraded/distorted speech signal) when the intrinsic redundancy (normal functioning CANS) is intact.

In monaural low-redundancy speech tests, electroacoustical modifications are made to the speech signal by means of temporal (time), intensity, or frequency modifications that reduce the extrinsic redundancy of the signal. If intrinsic redundancy is reduced due to CANS dysfunction, then auditory closure will be hard to achieve. Altering the speech signal will be challenging to individuals with (C)APD while their performance might be normal with appropriate and ideal listening environments.

Commercially available monaural low-redundancy speech tests can be categorized into four categories:

Low-Pass Filtered Speech Tests The *low-pass filtered speech tests* utilize monosyllabic low-pass filtered words. The Willeford battery for diagnosing (C) APD in children aged 5–10 years old, includes lists of consonant-nucleus-consonant (CNC) words filtered with a 500 Hz cutoff frequency at a rate of 18 dB per octave. The SCAN-3 test battery (Keith 2009), which is widely used clinically, includes the filtered words (FW) subtest intended for children between 5 and 12 years. It consists of 20 monosyllabic words presented to each ear that are low-pass filtered at 750 Hz at a roll-off of 32 dB per octave. The raw scores are then converted into standard scores. The low-pass filtered speech tests are known to be moderately sensitive to temporal lobe lesions and even less to brainstem and interhemispheric dysfunction (Bellis 2003).

Speech-in-Noise Tests Speech-in-noise tests consist of speech signals embedded in background noise with varying signal-to-noise ratios (SNR). Standardized speech-in-noise tests include the auditory figure ground (AFG) subtest of the SCAN-3 test battery, which assesses the child's ability to understand words presented with speech babble from different speakers. The SNR included in the SCAN-3 test battery are 0 dB, +8 dB, and +12 dB indicating that the words are presented at an equal intensity, or either 8 and 12 dB higher than the speech babble (noise). Another test is the synthetic sentence identification with ipsilateral competing message (SSI-ICM), which contains synthetic sentences presented at a fixed intensity in competition with connected discourse (story telling) with varying SNR. The sentences are meaningless, but the subject has to read them and report the number of the sentence heard, thus limiting its application to children who can read. The third test of speech-in-noise tests is the Pediatric Speech Intelligibility (PSI), which is an adaptation of the (SSI-ICM) test for the pediatric population between ages 3–6 years. It includes simple words and sentences with competition and the child is asked to point to the picture corresponding to the word/sentence heard from a closed set. The sensitivity of speech-in-noise tests is considered to be marginal-moderate to various CANS disorders.

Time-Compressed Speech Tests In this category of test, the temporal characteristics of the signal are altered while leaving the spectral features unchanged. The subject is asked to achieve auditory closure with an altered and rapidly changing speech signal. In general, as the signal's compression ratio increases (from 45% to 65%), the performance will decrease even with normal hearing subjects. Reverberation, defined as sound persistence in an enclosed space, could be added to reduce the extrinsic redundancy even more

and challenge the task of achieving auditory closure. Time-compressed speech signal is highly sensitive to diffuse pathology of the primary auditory cortex and the temporal lobe. Pediatric norms were reported for monosyllabic words (Bellis 2003) with 45% time compression and for sentences (Keith 2002) with (0%, 40%, and 60%) time compression.

Temporal Patterning/Ordering and Temporal Processing Tests

Temporal patterning/ordering tests involve the ability to discriminate frequency or duration and to recognize patterns of auditory stimuli (Table 1). Among the most popular tests in this category is the *duration pattern test (DPT)*. In this test, a 1,000 Hz auditory signal with two different durations (short – 250 ms and long – 500 ms) is presented to the subject in different combinations (i.e., short-long-short, long-long-short), and the subject is instructed to report the pattern heard, both verbally and by humming. Another test in this category is the *frequency pattern test (FPT)*. The FPT has a similar procedure to the DPT except that the auditory stimuli differ in frequency not duration. Two auditory stimuli with low (880 Hz) and high (1,122 Hz) frequencies are presented in different combination (i.e., high-low-low, high-high-low) and the subject is instructed to report the pattern verbally and by humming.

In both tests, if the subject is unable to respond verbally, the test is considered to indicate a possible lesion of the corpus callosum that enables intrahemispheric transfer of information, or to a lesion in the left hemisphere. If the subject is unable to hum the pattern, the test is considered to indicate a possible lesion in the right hemisphere; which is responsible for processing nonverbal stimuli.

Temporal processing ability is crucial to almost all tasks requiring auditory processing. It requires the ability to analyze acoustic signals over time; thus it is critical to the perception of speech and music. To evaluate specific temporal processes, several paradigms are used including:

Gap detection: the subject's ability to detect a short silent interval embedded in the acoustic signal

Auditory fusion: the subject's ability to perceive two signals as one based on the silent gap duration between them

Two-tone ordering: the subject's ability to verify the order of two tones based on the silent gap duration needed

Forward and backward masking: the effect of noise proceeding (forward) or following (backward) on the threshold needed to detect the signal

Commercially available tests of auditory temporal processing include the random gap detection test (RGDT). This test measures the ability to detect whether there was one stimulus or two based on different silent gap interval durations between the two stimuli (from 0 to 40 ms). The gap detection threshold is the smallest gap that can be detected between the two stimuli. RGDT is sensitive to cortical lesions, particularly temporal lobe dysfunction.

Binaural Interaction Tests

Tests of binaural interaction assess the ability of the CANS to integrate acoustic information efficiently from both ears, when the information presented is disparate in terms of intensity, timing, or frequency (Table 1). The listener needs to integrate the information in order to receive the whole message. Tests of binaural fusion are considered to evaluate function of the auditory pathways of the brainstem.

The most clinically used test to assess binaural interaction is the *masking level difference (MLD)* test. In this test, tonal or speech stimuli are presented to both ears along with broadband masking noise under two conditions: homophasic condition, where both the signal and the noise are presented in phase or antiphasic, where the signal and the noise are presented out of phase. The difference score between the two conditions is referred to as the masking level difference. This test is known to be sensitive to brainstem lesions.

Electroacoustic Procedures Electroacoustic procedures are used to rule out pathologies or dysfunction of the middle ear and cochlea. Acoustic signals are recorded from within the ear canal as a response to acoustic stimuli, and include:

▶ Otoacoustic emissions(OAEs): evoked OAEs use a stimuli in the ear canal to generate a low level sound in the cochlea which is recorded with a microphone placed in the external ear canal. OAEs are thought to be the response of the outer hair cells in the cochlea.

Acoustic immittance measures like tympanography, acoustic reflex and acoustic reflex decay. The acoustic reflex threshold (ART) refers to the minimal sound intensity needed to cause minimal mobility change of the middle ear in relation to the eardrum. Clinically, it is utilized to detect lower brainstem lesions. Acoustic reflex decay refers to the reduction of the stapedial muscle reflex movement in response to a signal presented 10 dB above the ART threshold for 10 s.

Electrophysiologic   Procedures Electrophysiological measures assess the neural functioning of the CANS in a noninvasive and objective way. These measures are beneficial when testing young children or other hard-to-test patients as the response does not rely on the subject's cooperation nor does not require a behavioral response from the patient. Moreover, electrophysiological measures complement the behavioral assessment of (C)APD especially when confounding factors like motivation, cognitive ability, distractibility, and intelligence exist. These measures include:

The ▶ *auditory brainstem response (ABR)* is an early latency response that occurs in the first 10 ms after the onset of the stimulus and assesses the integrity of the brainstem auditory pathway. Using tonal or speech stimuli ABR is sensitive to space-occupying lesions of the VIIIth nerve and to auditory neuropathy. The ABR is not typically sensitive to lesions involving higher order auditory deficits, however, one out of ten children diagnosed with (C)APD by behavioral methods demonstrate abnormal click-evoked ABR. Higher sensitivity has been reported for speech-evoked ABR in the diagnosis of (C)APD and in assessing intervention outcomes.

The *middle latency response (MLR)* occurs from 10 to 50 ms following stimulus onset. Its neural generators include the thalamocortical pathways including the primary auditory cortex. The MLR reaches adult values by 10 years of age. The response can be elicited by tones and speech signals and can be affected by sleep states. The implication for (C)APD is assumed either by presence or absence of the response or by comparing the response recorded from the patient's right versus left side(intrasubject comparisons). The sensitivity of MLR in (C)APD diagnosis is still under investigation due to the variability of response in the normal hearing population (AAA 2010).

Cortical evoked potentials occur beyond 50 ms poststimulus onset as a response to both speech and nonspeech signals. These include, but are not limited to, the *late latency response (LLR), P300 and mismatch negativity (MMN)* (ASHA 2005).

The generators of the different cortical evoked potentials are not definite but they involve the auditory cortex, thalamus, and higher order structures associated with attention and integrative functions of the brain. LLRs are distinguished by a negative peak (N1) occurring around 90 ms poststimulus followed by a positive peak (P1) at about 180 ms poststimulus onset. Complete maturation of the LLR does not occur until adolescence. P300 is the large positive wave arising at approximately 300 ms poststimulus on set. The P300 requires attentional and discrimination resources from the patient while attending to an oddball paradigm of frequent and deviant stimuli embedded within. Adult-like values of P300 appear during the mid-teenage years. MMN waveform is an event-related potential elicited with an oddball paradigm and is the difference wave resulting from the subtraction of the deviant wave from the standard wave. It is a negative wave occurring at approximately 200 ms and unlike P300; is a passive response that does not need the patient's attentional resources. MMN is present and robust in school-aged children.

Applying cortical evoked potentials clinically must be considered with caution. Research is lacking on the sensitivity and specificity of these evoked potentials for (C)APD diagnosis, normative data is needed and accepted protocols must be developed. Moreover, integrating cortical evoked potential in the diagnostic process for (C)APD requires special equipment not readily available in most clinics. However, the power of electrophysiological tests is accentuated when testing children for whom the behavioral test battery cannot be administered due to age limitations, or if the behavioral test battery provides inconclusive information or when behavioral measures are not available in the patient's native language.

Interpretation of Central Auditory Processing Test Results

Central Auditory Processing test results should provide information about the presence or absence of the disorder, hence providing the diagnosis of (C)APD. If the diagnosis is established, the question remains as to what underlying processes are affected. Furthermore, test results should help to delineate site-of-lesion dysfunction when possible. Finally, differential diagnosis should be addressed to differentiate (C)APD from other look-alike disorders, which share overlapping symptoms.

Several approaches are used to diagnose (C)APD, some clinics utilize absolute or norm-based interpretation (ASHA 2005; AAA 2010). This approach compares the child's performance on tests relative to normative data and cutoff scores. The criterion used for the diagnosis of (C)APD is a score of two standard deviations or more below the mean for at least one ear on at least two different behavioral tests (ASHA 2005; AAA 2010). This approach should be implemented with care as not all behavioral tests are standardized on large groups of normal peers. There are also inconsistencies and other confounding factors, like motivation, distractibility, or higher order disorders, which might contaminate the test results. A child is considered to have (C)APD if they perform poorly (>two standard deviations from the mean) on one test but shows inconsistency in the response patterns (i.e., right ear advantage in one test and left ear advantage on other test), or if they perform poorly on one test only (scores fall below three standard deviations from the mean) and have additional functional difficulty in everyday activities evident.

Other approaches suggest the use of inter-test and intra-test analysis. In inter-test analysis, comparison of patterns observed between tests in the test battery provides direction toward the diagnosis while in intra-test analysis, comparison of patterns within a test, like ear difference in the presence of symmetrical hearing sensitivity, provides the evidence for the diagnosis. After the diagnosis is established, it is important to scrutinize the nature of the auditory deficits in order to design an appropriate intervention strategy tailored to the specific deficits observed. Table 2 illustrates the auditory processes, their definition, importance, and the (C)APD tests affected by a deficit in that process.

Site-of-Lesion Patterns Analysis

Pattern analysis helps to guide the interpretation of tests results. When a clear pattern is revealed, it helps to rule out other higher-order factors (e.g., attention, cognition, memory, motivation). These factors might affect performance but are known to have a more global effect on test results without clear patterns. When a child demonstrates difficulties in all tests of (C)APD, it should argue for other causes and not for dysfunction in all brain areas responsible for auditory processing (Bellis 2003).

The CANS is a highly complex and redundant system. Along with the non-modular nature of the brain

Developmental Central Auditory Processing Disorders, Table 2 Auditory processes, definition, their role in auditory processing and the (C)APD tests affected

Process assessed	Definition	Importance	Deficit performance
Binaural separation	Attending to one ear while ignoring competing signals in the other ear	Hearing and processing speech in noise	Dichotic tests requiring report from one ear, e.g., dichotic sentences
Binaural integration	Attending to auditory signals presented to both ears at the same time	Hearing and processing speech in noise	Dichotic tests requiring report from both ears, e.g., dichotic words, dichotic digits
Monaural separation/auditory closure	Filling in missing pieces of the signal when the input is degraded, distorted, or embedded in noise	Speech understanding in background noise or in unclear communication situations	Low-pass filtered speech
			Time-compressed speech
			Speech in noise tests
Temporal patterning/ordering	Discrimination of auditory signals	Speech understanding	Frequency pattern test
	Sequencing signals over time	Language comprehension	Duration pattern test
		Recognizing prosody, rhythm, and stress	
Temporal processing	Resolving acoustic signals occurring rapidly	Perception of speech and music	Gap detection
Auditory discrimination	Discrimination among the spectrotemporal features of the acoustic signal	Discriminating similar sounding phonemes/words	Affects many tests
		Distinguishing prosodic elements of the signal	
Binaural interaction	Integrating disparate information from both ears		Masking level difference (MLD)
			Localization tasks

organization, it is difficult to determine with certainty the precise site of dysfunction. However, patterns in the behavioral test battery characterizing deficits in different CANS levels should be considered.

Brainstem dysfunction is characterized by poor performance on the Masking Level Difference (MLD) test, the Synthetic Sentence Identification with Ipsilateral Competing message (SSI-ICM), and the staggered spondaic words (SSW) test. Lateralization and localization may be poor and deficits on most tests ipsilaterally are possible. Auditory Brainstem Response (ABR) and Acoustic Reflex (AR) are sensitive to brainstem dysfunction and might be abnormal.

Left hemisphere dysfunction (the primary auditory cortex) is indicated by poor performance on dichotic speech tests and tests of monaural separation/auditory closure, bilaterally or contralateral to the language dominant hemisphere. Tests include low-pass filtered speech test, time-compressed speech test, and speech in noise tests. Tests of temporal patterning might show poor performance bilaterally but only when linguistic labeling of the pattern is required (e.g., low-high-low on test of frequency patterns).

Right hemisphere dysfunction is typical and left (contralateral) ear deficits are expected on dichotic speech tests, deficits on temporal patterning tests (both linguistic labeling and humming) and poor nonspeech discrimination is expected. On the other hand, normal performance is expected on tests of temporal processing and monaural low-redundancy speech tests.

Interhemispheric dysfunction is usually revealed by a poor performance in the left ear on dichotic speech tests along with deficit performance on temporal patterning (frequency/duration patterns) tests in the linguistic labeling condition only. Typically, the humming condition is preserved and normal performance on monaural low-redundancy speech tests and binaural interaction tests is expected.

Intervention and Management of (C)APD

Intervention for (C)APD should be initiated immediately following the diagnosis and should be complemented by the assessment findings from a multidisciplinary team. In order to exploit the neuroplasticity feature of the brain, which is dependent on stimulation, a comprehensive, multidisciplinary, individualized plan for management should be executed (ASHA 2005).

Three basic components must be incorporated in any comprehensive management plan for (C)APD. These include *environmental modifications*, *direct remediation techniques* based on the specific deficits apparent in the diagnostic test battery, and providing *compensatory strategies* premeditated to capitalize on the use of auditory information by improving listening skills.

Environmental modifications can be implemented through a combination of different approaches to facilitate access to auditory information. By enhancing the incoming signal and improving the listening environment, children with auditory processing difficulties may gain better access to auditory information. These approaches include assessing the classroom/home acoustics and reducing noise and reverberation when possible through covering reflective surfaces like walls, floor, and ceilings, using absorption materials and improving the signal-to-noise ratio (SNR). Additionally, noise sources must be reduced or eliminated when possible. Preferential seating is recommended while taking into consideration the importance of seating in a way where the teacher's face is visible to the child and noise sources are as far as possible. Finally, some children with (C)APD might benefit from assistive listening devices (FM or infrared systems). Children who perform poorly on monaural low-redundancy tests and on dichotic listening tests might benefit the most from the use of this technology, since these tests resemble the effect of noise, and degraded speech on the child's performance. Caution must be taken when recommending the use of assistive listening devices since not all children with (C)APD benefit from this additional help and since the use of these devices might increase reliance on improved SNR, thus causing some kind of sensory deprivation when the child does not interact with the outside world. It is also crucial to monitor the child's performance and the benefit they receive from the assistive listening device.

Direct remediation techniques target the deficient auditory processes and mechanisms and employ auditory training programs specific to the child's

difficulties. It relies on neuroplasticity theories which suggest that stimulating the brain can result in functional improvements. Auditory training can be applied to improve auditory discrimination skills, temporal processing, temporal patterning, binaural interaction, and dichotic listening and auditory closure. For instance, if the behavioral test battery reveals deficits in temporal processing, then auditory training of temporal processing is used with the child. Examples of auditory training tasks targeting auditory closure include missing word/syllable exercises and examples of auditory training tasks targeting binaural separation/integration include dichotic listening training and localization training.

Computerized therapy using specific software is also available. It provides the advantage of an engaging format with the use of multisensory stimulation and generous feedback and reinforcement. However, most importantly, computerized therapy gives the child an opportunity for intensive, adaptive, and efficient training (AAA 2010). It is important to note that not all children diagnosed with (C)APD will benefit from these computer-assistive programs and the application of this kind of training as well as any kind of auditory training should be individualized.

Compensatory Strategies for children with(C)APD include learning active listening skills; using whole body listening techniques (Bellis 2003), which involve physically preparing the body to be alert and ready to listen, directing attention to the speaker's face and avoiding excessive movement that might distract the child's attention away from the speaker. Metacognitive strategies involve the active thinking of the child of how to improve listening, communication, and learning through incorporating self-instruction, self-regulation, and problem solving and use drawing to illustrate the concept behind the message. Metalinguistic strategies on the other hand include language rules training; learning to understand discourse cohesion devices like adversative terms (e.g., but, moreover, however), additives (e.g., and), and referents (e.g., pronouns).Other strategies include formal schema induction and content schemata. Instructional compensations like scheduling breaks through the day/class and while doing homework after class, reducing assignment time, extending test time and using tests with multiple choice can help the child overcome the auditory processing load. All compensatory strategies need to be applied and practiced in different situations so the child will be capable of using them when needed.

In summary, all three components are needed to build a comprehensive intervention plan for children with (C)APD: *environmental modifications, direct remediation techniques*, and *compensatory strategies*. All three will help alleviate the effect of auditory processing deficits and provide better chances for children with (C)APD to succeed.

Cross-References

▶ Auditory Brainstem Response (ABR)
▶ OAEs
▶ Otitis Media with Effusion

References

American Academy of Audiology (2010) Diagnosis, treatment and management of children and adults with central auditory processing disorder. http://www.audiology.org/resources/documentlibrary/Documents/CAPD%20Guidelines%208-2010.pdf. Accessed 3 May 2011
American Speech-Language-Hearing Association (2005) (Central) auditory processing disorders [Technical report]. http://www.asha.org/docs/html/TR2005-00043.html. Accessed 3 May 2011
American Speech-Language-Hearing Association (1996) Central auditory processing: current status of research and implications for clinical practice. Am J Audiol 5:41–54
Bellis TJ (2003) Assessment and management of central auditory processing disorders in the educational setting: from science to practice, 2nd edn. Thomson Learning, Clifton Park
Bellis TJ (2007) Differential diagnosis of (central) auditory processing disorder in older listeners. In: Musiek FE, Chermak GD (eds) Handbook of (central) auditory processing disorder: auditory neuroscience and diagnosis, vol 1. Plural Publishing, San Diego, pp 319–346
Chermak GD (2007) Differential diagnosis of (central) auditory processing disorder and attention deficit hyperactivity disorder. In: Musiek FE, Chermak GD (eds) Handbook of (central) auditory processing disorder: auditory neuroscience and diagnosis, vol 1. Plural Publishing, San Diego, pp 365–394
Jerger J, Musiek F (2000) Report of the consensus conference on the diagnosis of auditory processing disorders in school-aged children. J Am Acad Audiol 11(9):467–474
Keith RW (2002) Standardization of the time compressed sentence test. J Educ Audiol 10:15–20
Keith R (2009) SCAN-3 for children: tests for auditory processing disorders. Pearson Education, SanAntonio
Keith R, Anderson J (2007) Dichotic listening tests. In: Musiek FE, Chermak GD (eds) Handbook of (central) auditory processing disorder: auditory neuroscience and diagnosis, vol 1. Plural Publishing, San Diego, pp 207–230

Deviated Nasal Septum

Seth J. Kanowitz
Department of Otolaryngology, Morristown Medical Center, Morristown, NJ, USA

Definition

Nasal septum: A midline nasal structure containing cartilage and bone lined by nasal mucosa that supports the external nose and divides the left and right nasal cavities.

Deviated nasal septum: Septum that impinges upon the nasal airway and causes nasal airflow obstruction.

Concha bullosa: A pneumatized middle turbinate that may impinge upon the middle meatus or nasal airway and contribute to nasal airflow obstruction.

Basic Characteristics

Anatomy

The nasal septum is a central structure composed of multiple layers designed to support the external nose, aid in nasal airflow resistance, and contribute to sense of smell. While it is considered to be a singular structure, it is composed of multiple layers in multiple planes. The outer soft tissue, or lining, of the nasal septum consists of respiratory mucosa. Underlying the mucosa is either perichondrium anteriorly or periosteum posteriorly, which also provides the rich vascular supply to the mucosa. Anteriorly, the cartilaginous nasal septum is formed by the quadrangular cartilage, which derives its name from its shape in the sagittal plane. The most anterior portion of the quadrangular cartilage is supported by the medial crus of the lower lateral cartilages, which help form the shape of the nostrils. Just posterior to this, the membranous septum which is an area that is actually devoid of any cartilaginous support structures and forms a bridge of soft tissue between the most anterior (caudal) portion of the septum and the paired medial crus. Inferiorly, the quadrangular cartilage sits in a bony groove called the nasal crest, which is formed by the maxilla anteriorly and palatine bone posteriorly. The bony posterior portion of the nasal septum is formed by the perpendicular plate of the ethmoid bone superiorly and the vomer inferiorly. The perpendicular plate of the ethmoid bone articulates with the sphenoid rostrum posteriorly, the quadrangular cartilage anteriorly, and the roof the ethmoid superiorly. The vomer articulates with the sphenoid rostrum posteriorly, the quadrangular cartilage anteriorly, the nasal crest inferiorly, and the perpendicular plate of the ethmoid superiorly. All together, these structures form a partition that divides the nasal cavity into left and right sides. The bony and cartilaginous portions of the septum articulate with each other at a juncture that has connective tissue, thus forming a joint.

The nasal septum has a rich blood supply due to the confluence of vasculature from the external (EC) and internal carotid (IC) artery systems. Anteriorly, the nasal septum is supplied by the EC from septal branches of the sphenopalatine artery (SPA), greater palatine artery, descending palatine artery, and superior labial artery. Posteriorly, the nasal septum is supplied by the EC from the posterior septal nasal artery branch of the SPA. The IC contributes to septal blood supply from terminal branches of the anterior and posterior ethmoid arteries. Kisselbach's plexus, located within Little's area, refers to the confluence of vasculature within the most anterior portion of the nasal septum.

The nasal septum receives its nervous supply from the branches of the trigeminal nerve (CN V) and the olfactory nerve (CN I). Superiorly, the septal mucosa has fibers from the olfactory nerve that traverse the cribriform plate through multiple foramina. The posterior inferior half of the septal mucosa receives fibers from maxillary division of the trigeminal nerve (CN V2) via the nasopalatine nerve. The anterior inferior half of the septal mucosa receives its innervation from the ophthalmic division of the trigeminal nerve (CN V1) via the anterior ethmoid nerve branches of the nasociliary nerve (Fettman et al. 2009).

Symptoms of Septal Deviation

Deviation of the nasal septum commonly causes nasal obstruction. Airflow through the nose is directed above the head of the inferior turbinate and then through the middle meatus before passing posteriorly and inferiorly through the choanae into the nasopharynx. Nasal airflow is a combination of both laminar and turbulent flow, with the ratio of turbulent to laminar airflow contributing to the sensation of nasal obstruction (Watkins and Chandra 2009). Deviations of the nasal

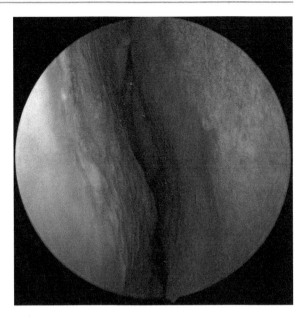

Deviated Nasal Septum, Fig. 1 Septal deviation impinging upon the internal nasal valve with limited visualization of the vertical strut of the middle turbinate

septum contribute to increased turbulent airflow through the nasal cavity, leading to increased airway resistance and the perception of nasal obstruction. The obstruction may occur on the same side as the deviation due to overall narrowing of cross-sectional area of the nasal airway, impingement upon the internal nasal valve, or narrowing of the nasal vestibule due to deviation of the medial crus of the lower lateral cartilages (Fig. 1). However, nasal obstruction can also occur on the contralateral, or concave, side of the deviation as well due to compensatory hypertrophy of the inferior turbinate mucosa or the presence of an aerated middle turbinate (concha bullosa) blocking the nasal airway (Fig. 2). As a result, patient with a deviated septum may complain of bilateral nasal obstruction. The deviation may also cause epistaxis due to turbulent nasal airflow, causing a drying effect of the attenuated septal mucosa, rhinosinusitis due to impingement upon the middle turbinate and/or lateral nasal wall with subsequent narrowing of the middle meatus, and less often a sense of unilateral pain and pressure when other sources of headache have been ruled out. Sometimes, a deviated nasal septum is found as an incidental finding on routine physical exam or imaging studies in an asymptomatic patient and thus does not warrant treatment.

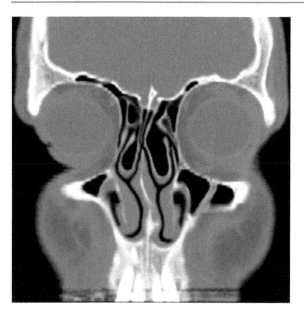

Deviated Nasal Septum, Fig. 2 Bilateral concha bullosa impinging upon the middle meatus and nasal airway with deviation of the nasal septum to the *right*

Etiology of Septal Deviation

Deviation of the nasal septum is either congenital or acquired. Common theories for congenital deviated septum include birth canal trauma as well as development of the septum at varying rates subsequently causing compressive forces within the fixed bony framework of the maxillofacial skeleton. Given the pliable nature of the nasal septum, these forces cause the septum to deviate. While forceps delivery may cause incidental compression of the nasal bones and septum, deviated nasal septum has also been described in caesarean section. Positioning head and facial skeleton in utero may also eventually cause deviation of the nasal septum.

Most, if not all, forms of acquired septal deviations are the result of traumatic injury. Blunt force injury to the nose can cause the septum to shift, bend, or fracture dependent upon the nature of the injury. The presence of connective tissue within the bony-cartilaginous junction as well as the membranous septum allows the septum to bend without actually fracturing or completely dislocating. In other rare instances, the septum may be deviated due to unilateral nasal pathology (i.e., sinonasal tumors) that pushes the nasal septum to the opposite side. Finally, a deviated nasal

septum may result from surgical procedures where the nasal septum is inadvertently shifted to create access to the skull base (i.e., transsphenoidal pituitary surgery).

Evaluation and Management of Septal Deviation

Patients who present with symptoms of nasal obstruction should be evaluated for the presence of a deviated nasal septum. Evaluation of the nasal septum begins with observation of the external nose including size, shape, and symmetry for the purposes of documentation and potential contributing factors. For instance, a patient may in fact have a deviated septum; however, if they also have a depressed nasal bone or upper lateral cartilage due to a traumatic event, then correction of the septal deformity alone may lead to less than optimal long-term results. The next portion of the exam involves anterior rhinoscopy with a nasal speculum and headlight to visualize the caudal septum, inferior nasal turbinates, and internal nasal valve. The internal nasal valve forms the narrowest portion of the nasal airway and is bordered by the caudal septum, anterior tip of the inferior turbinate, and the ipsilateral upper lateral cartilage in the coronal plane. It is also important to observe the patient during respiration to rule out the presence of dynamic obstructions that occur as a result of weak lower lateral cartilages and supporting connective tissue within the soft tissue envelope of the nose. Although addressed elsewhere in this book, the inferior turbinates should be examined as a source of nasal obstruction, as turbinate surgery is often performed in conjunction with septoplasty. Nasal endoscopy is paramount to completely evaluate the patient with nasal obstruction and a suspected deviated nasal septum, as anterior rhinoscopy only allows visualization of the most caudal portion of the nasal septum (Goyal and Hwang 2007). Mid- to posterior septal deviations or spurs may not be apparent on anterior rhinoscopy, especially when patient has concomitant inferior turbinate hypertrophy obscuring adequate illumination (Fig. 3). Visualization of the middle turbinate to evaluate for the possibility of a concha bullosa is also important as this may require surgical intervention as well. Finally, endoscopic visualization of the entire septum, middle meatus, and nasopharynx is necessary to rule out other causes of nasal obstruction such as septal perforation, rhinosinusitis, sinonasal polyps, sinonasal neoplasms, adenoid hypertrophy, choanal atresia, and nasopharynx neoplasms.

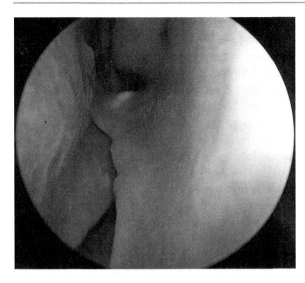

Deviated Nasal Septum, Fig. 3 Right-sided septal spur impinging upon the decongested right inferior turbinate and lateral nasal wall with attenuated mucosa overlying the apex of the spur

In many patients with a deviated septum, a trial of topical nasal steroid or antihistamine sprays is usually warranted in conjunction with nasal saline irrigation. This is performed in an effort to reduce mucosal edema throughout the nasal cavity. However, this is not mandatory in all cases as some patients may have a significant septal deviation that nearly occludes the nasal airway without any other signs or symptoms of mucosal inflammation. In these patients, nasal sprays are unlikely to deposit within the obstructed nostril and may even lead to mucosal dryness, crusting, and bleeding. Management of allergies and rhinosinusitis in those patients suspected of concurrently suffering from these disease entities is also important prior to surgical intervention on the nasal septum.

Computed tomography (CT) of the sinuses may sometimes be helpful in patients with a deviated nasal septum. When significant narrowing of the middle meatus or lateralization of the middle turbinate exists as a result of a septal deviation, or when a concha bullosa is suspected, preoperative radiographic visualization of the nasal airway and paranasal sinuses may assist in surgical planning and management. Additionally, when the posterior nasal cavity cannot be visualized with an endoscope due to a significant septal deviation, it is important to evaluate for the presence of other sinonasal pathology more posterior to the deviation. However, preoperative CT

scanning is *not* mandatory to make the diagnosis of a deviated nasal septum causing nasal airway obstruction, and its use is determined on a case-by-case basis.

Surgical Technique

After induction of general anesthesia and topical decongestion of the nasal mucosa, the nasal septum is injected in the subperichondrial and subperiosteal plane with an anesthetic and hemostatic agent such as 1% lidocaine with 1:100,000 epinephrine. Not only does this assist with immediate postoperative pain control and intraoperative hemostasis, but also the injection of fluid into the proper space allows for hydrodissection of the mucoperichondrial and mucoperiosteal septal flap (Ketcham and Han 2010). An incision is then made along the caudal margin of the quadrangular cartilage through the membranous septum (hemitransfixion incision) or approximately 1–2 cm posterior to the columella along the quadrangular cartilage (Killian incision) based upon the area of deviation (anterior cartilaginous vs. posterior bony) and surgeon preference. The side of the incision (left vs. right) is also surgeon dependent. A mucoperichondrial flap is then elevated using a combination of a Cottle and/or Freer elevator. Identification of the proper subperichondrial plane will lead to an avascular dissection and easier visualization of the nasal septum in a nearly bloodless surgical field. Elevation of the flap may be assisted with the use of a rigid endoscope (Sautter and Smith 2009; Chung et al. 2007). Performing broad elevation while using the endoscope is paramount to prevent a narrow field of vision within the flap (Fig. 4). The transition zone at the bony-cartilaginous junction is somewhat tethered and thus care must be taken not to perforate the flap in this region. Additionally, the flap is often tethered inferiorly at the transition between the quadrangular cartilage and bony maxillary crest by decussating fibers that divide the perichondrium of the cartilage from the periosteum of the bone. Sharp dissection of these fibers with sharp tip scissors often facilitates a smooth transition of the flap at this point. Once a unilateral flap has been elevated, it is protected with a nasal speculum. When encountering a septal spur, it may be necessary to tunnel under the spur with a Cottle elevator and eventually join the flap at the apex of the spur. The mucosa at the apex of the spur is often extremely attenuated and thus perforating the flap at this point is not uncommon. A vertical crossover

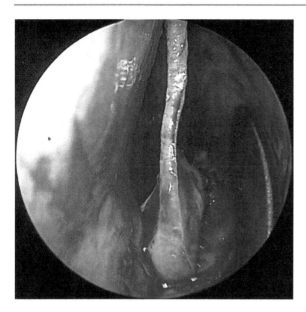

Deviated Nasal Septum, Fig. 4 Endoscopic view of the cartilaginous nasal septum with the elevated septal flaps displaced laterally by freer elevator

incision is then made in the quadrangular cartilage with a septal button or ophthalmic crescent knife in order to access the contralateral side. It is important to leave a cartilaginous caudal and dorsal "L-strut" of at least 1 cm to prevent disruption of nasal tip support and collapse of the nasal dorsum. A similar mucoperichondrial and mucoperiosteal flap is then elevated on the contralateral side, and the flaps are protected with an appropriately sized nasal speculum.

With proper flap elevation, hemostatic injections, and controlled hypotension, bleeding should be minimal. Resection of the deviated portions of cartilage begins using Ballenger swivel knife to remove a strip of quadrangular cartilage. This cartilage can be saved for replacement at the end of the case or for reconstructive purposes. Additional portions of cartilage and/or bone can then be removed with a combination of the open Jansen-Middleton forceps or Takahashi forceps. Sometimes, simply disarticulating the cartilaginous septum from the bony-cartilaginous junction or the maxillary crest may correct the deformity by releasing the deforming forces. The cartilage may also be scored with a knife on its concave side to release the forces causing the convex deformity on the opposite side. When resecting more posterior bony deviations, it is important to first disconnect them from the perpendicular plate of the ethmoid bone using sharp

dissection with open Jansen-Middleton forceps or endoscopic scissors, as rocking or removing posterior deviations without first performing this maneuver can lead to CSF leak. The bony septum does not provide nasal support and thus conservative resection is not necessary. Endoscopic visualization within the flaps can also be performed, and resection can be performed with a variety of endoscopic instruments such as thru-cutting forceps or endoscopic scissors. When deviations involve the bony maxillary crest, sharp dissection with a 3- or 4-mm osteotome assists with resection.

Once the resection has been completed, the flaps are replaced in the midline, and reinspection of the nasal cavity is performed with a headlight or rigid nasal endoscope to verify adequate resection and nasal airway patency. The incision (hemitransfixion or Killian) is then closed with 4-0 chromic gut suture, and the flaps are coapted in a quilting manner with 4-0 plain gut suture on a straight Keith needle. A septal stapler may also be employed to coapt the flaps. A variety of nasal-septal splints may be employed (open lumen Doyle nasal splint) to help stabilize the septum in the midline, coapt the flaps, and limit synechiae formation when turbinate surgery is performed in conjunction with septoplasty. The use of a nasal splint is strictly surgeon preference. The quilting suture and/or nasal-septal splints help reduce fluid and blood collection between the flaps and allow the patient to recover without the discomfort of nasal packing.

Postoperative Care

Septoplasty is almost always performed on an outpatient basis. Patients are usually instructed to begin saline irrigations the day after surgery to help remove crusts, coagulum, and mucous from the nasal cavity. Routine use of postoperative nasal packing has not been shown to reduce complications or improve long-term outcomes and is associated with increased patient discomfort (Dubin and Pletcher 2009). If stents are employed to help limit synechiae formation, especially when concurrent turbinate surgery is performed, the surgeon removes them within 3–7 days after surgery on a case-by-case basis. An antistaphylococcal antibiotic may also be employed to help limit bacterial contamination of the stents and subsequent crusting. Pain should be managed accordingly. Patients are instructed to avoid any nose blowing, strenuous activity, or anticoagulants for at least 1 week after surgery. Any topical nasal sprays used for management of allergic rhinitis are also withheld during the first post-operative week as they may cause discomfort and drying of the nasal cavity mucosa. During the first postoperative visit, nasal crusts and coagulum are removed from the nasal cavity with a variety of suctions or nasal instruments to help improve nasal airflow. Nasal endoscopy may also be performed to help assess healing and nasal patency. Cleaning of the nasal cavity is especially important when turbinate surgery is performed in conjunction with septoplasty and helps limit long-term synechiae formation. Commercially available nasal moisturizing products may also be employed in the perioperative period to assist with nasal hygiene and mucosal hydration.

Outcomes

The long-term benefit of septal surgery for nasal obstruction has been validated by several studies. Stewart et al. evaluated 59 patients undergoing septal surgery for symptoms of nasal obstruction for at least 3 months after failing a trial of medical therapy for 4 weeks (Stewart et al. 2004). Patients underwent septoplasty with or without concomitant turbinate surgery as determined by the treating surgeon. The Nasal Obstruction Septoplasty Effectiveness (NOSE) scale was employed to assess disease specific quality of life (QOL). There was a significant improvement in NOSE scores for all patients at 3 months, with these results remaining stable at 6 months. In addition, the authors demonstrated high patient satisfaction rates and a statistically significant decrease in use of oral decongestants and nasal steroids 3 months after surgery. Siegel et al. evaluated 161 patients undergoing septal surgery with or without concomitant turbinate surgery and/or external nasal surgery with validated measures of general health (Short Form-12) and nasal-specific health (Nasal Health Survey) (Siegel et al. 2000). Assessments were made preoperatively and again at 6 and 12 months postoperatively. At a mean of 9 months follow-up, both symptoms and medication subscores of the Nasal Health Survey demonstrated significant improvement.

Cross-References

▶ Aesthetic Subunits of Nose
▶ Alar Retraction
▶ Allergic Rhinitis
▶ Nasal and Sinus Trauma

▶ Nasal Valve
▶ Radiologic Evaluation/Diagnostic Imaging of Paranasal Sinuses and Chronic Rhinosinusitis

References

Chung BJ, Batra PS, Citardi MJ, Lanza DC (2007) Endoscopic septoplasty: revisitation of the technique, indication, and outcomes. Am J Rhinol 21(3):307–311

Dubin M, Pletcher SD (2009) Postoperative packing after septoplasty: it is necessary? Otolaryngol Clin North Am 42:279–285

Fettman N, Sanford T, Sindwani R (2009) Surgical management of the deviated septum: techniques in septoplasty. Otolaryngol Clin North Am 42:241–252

Goyal P, Hwang PH (2007) Septal and turbinate surgery. In: Rhinologic and sleep apnea techniques, vol 5. Springer, Berlin/Heidelberg, pp 49–60

Ketcham AS, Han JK (2010) Complications and management of septoplasty. Otolaryngol Clin North Am 43:897–904

Sautter NB, Smith TL (2009) Endoscopic septoplasty. Otolaryngol Clin North Am 42:253–260

Siegel NS, Gliklich RE, Taghizadeh F, Chang Y (2000) Outcomes of septoplasty. Otolaryngol Head Neck Surg 122:228–232

Stewart MG, Smith TL, Weaver EM et al (2004) Outcomes after nasal septoplasty: results from the nasal obstruction septoplasty effectiveness (NOSE) study. Otolaryngol Head Neck Surg 130:283–290

Tami TA, Kuppersmith RB, Atkins JA (2010) A clinical evaluation of bioresorbable staples for mucoperichondrial flap coaptation in septoplasty. Am J Rhinol Allergy 24:137–139

Watkins JP, Chandra RK (2009) The stuffy nose. In: Rhinology and facial plastic surgery, vol 14. Springer, Berlin/Heidelberg, pp 165–179

Device Failure

▶ Cochlear Implantation, Revision – Adult
▶ Surgical Devices (Cochlear Implantation, Revision – Pediatric)

Diagnostic Aspiration

▶ Fine Needle Aspiration for Head and Neck Tumors

Diagnostic Hearing Evaluation

▶ Audiometry

Differential Diagnosis of Adult Neck Masses

Tara L. Rosenberg
Department of Otolaryngology and Communicative
Sciences, University of Mississippi Medical Center,
Jackson, MS, USA

Introduction

Otolaryngologists and primary care providers frequently encounter adult patients with neck masses. The differential diagnosis is quite extensive, but the best way to help refine this list is by initially performing a thorough history and physical examination. Further evaluation of the mass by biopsy or imaging is also warranted in many situations. For example, an adult patient over 40 years of age with a persistent neck mass should raise concerns for malignancy, and appropriate evaluation for such should ensue.

One common pneumonic used to help formulate a differential diagnosis is "KITTENS," which is described in Pasha's book, Otolaryngology: Head and Neck Surgery Clinical Reference Guide. This pneumonic stands for K – congenital, I – infectious/inflammatory/ iatrogenic, T – trauma, T – toxic, E – endocrine, N – neoplasms, S – systemic diseases. The following discussion is not intended to be a complete list of differential diagnoses, but this is intended to help one formulate a differential diagnosis through a methodical approach for each adult patient who presents with a neck mass. Each of these diagnoses is discussed in much greater detail in other entries in this encyclopedia.

Congenital

Congenital or developmental anomalies can present as neck masses in adults. The most common congenital neck anomaly is a thyroglossal duct cyst. It is usually identified as a midline cystic mass inferior to the hyoid bone that elevates with swallowing or tongue protrusion. Most of them are diagnosed before 20 years of age. However, approximately 7% of adults still have this anomaly. In adults, this cystic mass may, though rarely, contain the patient's only functional thyroid tissue. Therefore, computed tomography (CT) scan or ultrasound of the neck should be obtained to confirm the presence of a thyroid gland. Also, about 1% of adults with thyroglossal duct cysts have foci of carcinoma within the cyst. Treatment for a thyroglossal duct cyst is surgical excision.

Branchial cleft cysts are usually found in late childhood or early adulthood. They may not become apparent until they become inflamed during an upper respiratory infection. They are usually lateral neck masses, but the level depends on what type of branchial cleft cyst is present. Treatment includes surgical excision of the cyst and tract, if one exists.

Ranulas are mucous retention cysts of the floor of the mouth. They usually arise from the sublingual gland and are called plunging ranulas if they extend through the mylohyoid muscle and into the neck. Plunging ranulas may present as a neck mass that fluctuates in size and is soft and compressible on physical examination. Treatment is excision.

Lymphangiomas rarely present in adulthood. Most are diagnosed before 3 years of age. They usually present as a painless, compressible, soft neck mass, most commonly in the posterior triangle of the neck. CT of the neck with contrast or magnetic resonance imaging (MRI) of the neck is useful to evaluate the mass. Treatment varies but may include resection, though this is very difficult and involves a high rate of recurrence.

Infectious/Inflammatory

Cervical lymphadenopathy can be caused by many viral infections including human immunodeficiency virus (HIV), Epstein-Barr virus (EBV), cytomegalovirus (CMV), and toxoplasmosis. Size and extent of lymphadenopathy should be documented at each clinic visit. If the lymphadenopathy does not resolve with treatment of the underlying cause, fine-needle aspiration (FNA) can be performed to further evaluate the mass.

Bacterial infections can also lead to cervical lymphadenitis, which may turn into a neck abscess. Neck abscesses can occur from salivary or dental infections, spread of more superficial infections, penetrating trauma, or other causes such as infected thyroglossal duct cyst or branchial cleft cyst. Historical information suggestive of infection is usually described by the patient, and examination often reveals a tender, fluctuant mass with overlying erythema, edema, induration, and warmth to touch. CT scan of the neck with contrast can be helpful in localizing the infection and determining its extent if clinically necessary. Treatment involves antibiotic therapy and surgical drainage, depending on the size and location of the abscess and its response to antibiotic therapy. In adults, an inflamed necrotic lymph node may present as a neck abscess, so history, physical examination, and imaging are critical if malignancy is suspected.

Acute and chronic sialadenitis can lead to a neck mass in the area of the involved salivary gland. In the acute sialadenitis setting, the affected gland is swollen and painful, and there may be systemic symptoms of infection. Some risk factors include known sialolithiasis, dehydration, recent surgery or dental procedure, and elderly age. Physical examination reveals an enlarged salivary gland with tenderness to palpation, and possible local erythema, induration, edema, warmth, and fluctuance if an abscess has formed. Intraoral examination reveals purulent or inspissated secretions expressed from the involved gland's duct. Also, if sialolithiasis or another mass causing obstruction of the involved salivary duct is present, there may be a palpable mass in the duct on bimanual exam. Treatment of acute sialadenitis includes antibiotic therapy, hydration, warm compresses, sialogogues, massaging the involved gland in the direction of the duct, draining the abscess if present, and relieving the obstruction of the gland by the indicated method.

Chronic sialadenitis is usually caused by chronic salivary duct stenosis or obstruction from sialolithiasis or another mass. This leads to salivary gland enlargement and fibrosis from chronic inflammation. There may also be chronic pain of the involved gland with repeated episodes of local pain and swelling. Physical examination is similar to that described for acute sialadenitis, but there are usually no signs of abscess or acute infection, rather, an enlarged, tender salivary gland with possible palpable mass near the duct. The important part of chronic sialadenitis is identifying the cause of the chronic obstruction (most commonly sialolithiasis). CT scan of the neck with contrast is usually indicated to help identify the cause, although ultrasound is another useful option for imaging. Treatment to relieve the obstruction is indicated. In the setting of sialolithiasis, there are several options for treatment depending on the size and location of the obstruction.

Cat scratch disease, tuberculous lymphadenitis, and atypical/nontuberculous mycobacterial infection can cause a neck mass or cervical lymphadenopathy. After diagnosis, cat scratch disease and tuberculous lymphadenitis are usually able to be treated with the appropriate antibiotic/antitubercular therapy. However, atypical or nontubercular mycobacterial infections are primarily treated with excision of the involved lymph node due to resistance to antitubercular drug therapy.

Epidermal cysts on the neck are soft, compressible masses that may have puncta in the center. If they are inflamed, they may be erythematous and tender. Management includes treatment of the infection followed by complete surgical excision.

Trauma

Some neck masses secondary to trauma include a hematoma, pseudoaneurysm or arteriovenous fistula, and laryngocele. History and physical exam are again key in their diagnosis. A recent hematoma may have overlying ecchymosis and be soft or tense on palpation. Older, well-organized hematomas may be firm from fibrosis. Small hematomas will resolve spontaneously over time. However, if the neck hematoma is expanding or causing airway compression, it requires emergent surgical exploration and drainage.

Shearing or penetrating trauma to the neck may result in formation of a pseudoaneurysm or arteriovenous fistula, though the presentation is usually delayed. On exam, one can often appreciate a thrill and audible bruit. Treatment is usually surgical ligation.

Laryngoceles can result from repeated use of musical instruments such as a trumpet or may result from repeated glassblowing. They may lead to hoarseness, dysphagia, or globus sensation. The mass on exam can be soft and compressible and is filled with fluid and air. Flexible laryngoscopy may be beneficial in diagnosis. Definitive treatment is surgical excision.

Toxic

Graves disease, toxic nodular goiters, and toxic thyroid adenomas can lead to thyrotoxicosis, which is caused by high concentrations of thyroid hormones. This is more likely to happen in females, and Graves disease is the most common disease responsible for this condition.

Endocrine

Thyroid and parathyroid pathology can present as neck masses in adults. This can include multiple types of thyroid cancer, benign thyroid nodules, multinodular goiters, cysts, parathyroid adenomas, parathyroid hyperplasia, or, rarely, parathyroid carcinoma.

Neoplasms

Several neoplasms of the head and neck can present in adulthood as a neck mass. These may be benign or malignant, but any adult patient over 40 years of age who presents with a neck mass should raise concerns for malignancy.

Malignant neoplasms of the head and neck may present as a neck mass due to cervical lymph node metastasis. Squamous cell carcinoma is the most common malignancy of the upper aerodigestive tract, and it may present in this way. However, there are many other malignancies of the head and neck (such as skin malignancies) that may present in a similar fashion. As always, thorough history and physical examination are important. Flexible laryngoscopy is also important in localizing the primary site of the malignancy if in the upper aerodigestive tract, and it helps identify second primaries if present.

Other neoplasms of the head and neck may present as a neck mass due to the site of the primary tumor. Examples include salivary gland neoplasms, thyroid neoplasms, lymphoma, neurogenic/vascular tumors, and even lipomas.

Systemic Diseases

Several granulomatous diseases may present as a neck mass in an adult. An example is sarcoidosis, which is most common in African-American females. This may present with cervical lymphadenopathy in 25–50%. However, most are asymptomatic and present as hilar lymphadenopathy incidentally found on chest x-ray. Histopathology classically shows non-caseating granulomas, among other findings.

Fine-Needle Aspiration

FNA is the standard of care in the diagnostic workup of most adult patients with a neck mass. This biopsy is especially helpful since it is highly sensitive and specific for neoplasia. It can also be used to obtain cultures, Gram stain, and smears for masses suspicious for infectious etiology. FNA should not be attempted on pulsatile or suspected vascular lesions.

Imaging

In most situations, the best initial imaging study to obtain in an adult patient with a neck mass is a CT scan of the neck with contrast. MRI can occasionally add more anatomical information for soft tissue masses, but this is not usually required to make the correct diagnosis. It can be helpful in some situations, such as evaluating patients with a thyroid mass that extends into the mediastinum. This is because iodine in CT contrast is metabolized in the thyroid gland and can interfere with the timing of radioactive iodine ablation. However, ultrasound of the thyroid is the imaging modality of choice in most patients with a thyroid mass.

Conclusions

The differential diagnosis for an adult with a neck mass is very extensive. The approach to each patient should be methodical with attention paid to the importance of a thorough history and physical examination. Forming a differential diagnosis is critical in each situation. The description from Pasha's book, Otolaryngology: Head and Neck Surgery Clinical Reference Guide, which is reviewed above using the "KITTENS" method, can be helpful in this process.

Cross-References

▶ Benign Salivary Gland Neoplasms
▶ Congenital Cysts, Sinuses, and Fistulae
▶ Fine Needle Aspiration for Head and Neck Tumors
▶ Follicular Thyroid Cancer
▶ Granulomatous Disorders
▶ Head and Neck Manifestations of AIDS
▶ Imaging Cystic Head and Neck Masses
▶ Parapharyngeal Space Tumors
▶ Parathyroid Imaging
▶ Primary Neck Neoplasms
▶ Salivary Gland Malignancies
▶ Thyroiditis
▶ Unknown Primary Squamous Cell Carcinoma of Neck
▶ Well-Differentiated Thyroid Cancer

References

Cummings CW, Flint PW, Harker LA et al (2005a) Differential diagnosis of neck masses. In: Otolaryngology – head and neck surgery, 4th edn. Elsevier Mosby, Philadelphia, PA, pp 2540–2553

Cummings CW, Flint PW, Harker LA et al (2005b) Overview of diagnostic imaging of the head and neck. In: Otolaryngology – head and neck surgery, 4th edn. Elsevier Mosby, Philadelphia, PA, pp 25–92

McGuirt WF (1999) The neck mass. In: Kaye KS and Kaye D (eds) Medical clinics of North America: Otolaryngology for the Internist 83:1, pp 220–234

Pasha R (2006) Otolaryngology – head and neck surgery clinical reference guide, 2nd edn. Plural Publishing, San Diego, CA, pp 206–213, 248–249, 288–289

Rosenberg TL, Brown JJ, Jefferson GD (2010) Evaluating the adult patient with a neck mass. In: Ryan MW (ed) Medical clinics of North America: Otolaryngology for the Internist 94:5, pp 1017–1029

Shahan FF, Johnson KJ, Zitelli JA et al (2006) Management of benign facial lesions. In: Bailey BJ, Johnson JT (eds) Otolaryngology – head and neck surgery, 4th edn. Lippincott Williams and Wilkins, Philadelphia, PA, p 2732

Difficult Airway

▶ Emergency Airways
▶ Emergent Airway

Difficult Intubation

▶ Emergent Airway

Difficult Ventilation

▶ Emergent Airway

Diotic Summation

Abdul Aleem Kadar
Otolaryngology - Head & Neck Surgery, Jinnah Postgraduate Medical Centre, Karachi, Sindh, Pakistan

Definition

Doubling of perceptual loudness accompanied by increased sensitivity to differences in intensity and frequency leading to improvement in speech intelligibility under both quiet conditions and in noise.

Cross-References

▶ Bone-Anchored Hearing Aids (BAHAs)

Diplopia

▶ Sinus Surgery, Complications

Direct Acoustical Cochlear Stimulator (DACS)

▶ Implantable Hearing Devices

Direct Bone Stimulator

▶ Bone-Anchored Hearing Aid in Single-Sided Deafness
▶ Bone-Anchored Hearing Aids in Conductive and Mixed Hearing Loss

Direct Cochlear Nerve Action Potential (CNAP)

Amir Ahmadian, Angela E. Downes and A. Samy Youssef
Department of Neurosurgery, University of South Florida, Tampa, FL, USA

Definition

Direct measurement CN VIII action potential is a near-field technique that is recorded after electrodes are placed directly on the nerve. This produces high amplitude signals, therefore requiring minimal signal averaging which equates to nearly real-time recording. The response latency is affected (increased) with nerve stretching.

Cross-References

▶ Cranial Nerve Monitoring – *VIII, IX, X, XI*

Directed Parathyroidectomy

▶ Minimally Invasive Parathyroid Surgery

Disorders of Pinna, Relapsing Polychondritis

D. Mistry and Chris Raine
ENT Department, Bradford Royal Infirmary,
Bradford, West Yorkshire, UK

Definition

Relapsing polychondritis (RPC) is a rare disease associated with inflammation in cartilaginous tissue (especially hyaline cartilage) throughout the body. The pinna is most commonly affected. Histological examination of affected structures reveals chondritis with a mixed inflammatory cell infiltrate (O'Connor Reina et al. 1999). Later, there is cartilage destruction with fibrous tissue replacement (Clark et al. 1992).

Clinical Aspects

The incidence of RPC is estimated to be 3.5 cases per million. The female to male ratio is roughly equal and mean age at diagnosis is 40–60 years (Kent et al. 2004). Pediatric cases have been described (Belot et al. 2010). Most cases of RPC occur in whites (Kent et al. 2004).

The clinical course of RPC may be indolent over many years or short and aggressive (Clark et al. 1992).

The pathogenesis of RPC remains unknown, although the observed immune abnormalities have led to RPC being classified as an autoimmune disease (Kent et al. 2004). Many patients have antibodies to type 2 collagen (O'Connor Reina et al. 1999; Clark et al. 1992) as well as collagens IX and XI (O'Connor Reina et al. 1999).

It has been postulated that the pathogenesis of RPC begins with an insult that induces the exposure of connective tissue or cell membrane epitopes, which can lead to an immune response. This insult may be due to nutrient vasculature damage, trauma, toxic, chemical or infectious agents, and also antigenic mimicry between an infectious agent and a connective tissue antigen. Ongoing inflammation would perpetuate enzymatic and oxygen metabolite–mediated connective tissue degradation (Lahmer et al. 2010).

Clinical Presentation

The commonest presenting sign is auricular chondritis (43%) (Clark et al. 1992). It is bilateral in 95% of cases and over the lifetime of the disease, occurs in 88% of cases (McAdam et al. 1976). The onset may be acute or subacute, and the affected auricles appears swollen and diffusely erythematous with sparing of the non-cartilaginous earlobes (Kent et al. 2004). The inflammation may last for days or weeks. If the inflammation affects the EAM, hearing may be compromised. A relapsing and remitting course can eventually lead to a floppy ear or cauliflower deformity (Kent et al. 2004).

The next most common presenting symptoms and signs are arthritis (32%), laryngotracheal symptoms (23%), nasal chondritis (21%), and ocular inflammation (18%) (Kent et al. 2004).

Pediatric cases have been estimated to account for less than 5% of all cases of RPC (Belot et al. 2010) but the frequency of chondritis and systemic manifestations of RPC in children is very similar to those seen in adults (Zulian et al. 2009).

RPC can affect the following:

Ear
Conductive hearing loss can result from stenosis of the ear canal, chondritis of the Eustachian tube and secretory otitis media (Kent et al. 2004). Inner ear damage is thought to be due to involvement of the internal auditory artery (Clark et al. 1992).

Eye
Involvement of the eye may be in the form of episcleritis, scleritis, keratitis, and uveitis.

Nose

Crusting, rhinorrheoa, and epistaxis can accompany nasal cartilage inflammation. Chronic inflammation can lead to cartilage destruction resulting in a saddle nose deformity.

Large Airway

Involvement of airways is more common in young patients, and may be more severe than in adults (Clark et al. 1992). Symptoms include dysphonia, aphonia, wheezing, dyspnea, and cough. There may be laryngeal and/or tracheobronchial malacia. There may also be subglottic and/or tracheobronchial stenosis (Lahmer et al. 2010).

Joints

Parasternal joint involvement is typical of RPC. Involvement of peripheral joints is also seen in 70% of cases (usually nonerosive and asymmetric) (Lahmer et al. 2010).

Heart

Ten percent have mitral or aortic valve disease (Lahmer et al. 2010).

Skin

Thirty-six percent of patients have skin lesions like aphthous ulcers, purpura, papules, nodules, or ulcerations. None of these are pathognomonic for RPC (Lahmer et al. 2010).

Nervous System

Vasculitis can result in cranial neuropathies and other neurological sequelae including hemiplegia and seizures (Lahmer et al. 2010).

Diagnosis

The diagnostic criteria proposed by McAdam et al. (1976) have been subsequently modified by Michet et al. (1986). Diagnosis is based on chondritis in two of three sites (auricular, nasal, laryngotracheal) or one of these sites and two other manifestations, including, ocular inflammation, audiovestibular dysfunction, or seronegative inflammatory arthritis. A biopsy is unnecessary in most cases (Kent et al. 2004).

Treatment

The treatment of RPC depends on the disease activity and severity. Local disease (e.g., auricular or nasal chondritis) may be treated with nonsteroidal anti-inflammatory drugs (NSAIDs). If these are not effective, then glucocorticoids at 1 mg/kg bodyweight should be commenced (Lahmer et al. 2010). Colchicine has been reported to be of benefit for auricular chondritis (Kent et al. 2004). If there is significantly compromised organ function, a combination of first- and second-line therapy is necessary. Methotrexate and azathioprine may be used as disease-modifying, steroid-sparing agents. Cyclophosphamide is used for organ-threatening disease. Cyclosporin A may also be used in this scenario (Kent et al. 2004). There have been some successful reports of treatment with TNF alpha antagonists (infliximab and etanercept) (Lahmer et al. 2010).

In order to monitor patients with RPC, regular measurements of renal and lung function should be carried out (Clark et al. 1992).

Outcomes

Mortality rates vary from 28% to 50%. Poor prognostic features include laryngotracheal strictures, systemic vasculitis, microhematuria, and anemia. Deaths may be due to airway involvement with resulting respiratory failure or pneumonia, cardiovascular complications, and opportunistic infections (Clark et al. 1992).

Associated Conditions

Up to a third of cases may be associated with other hematologic, connective tissue, vasculitic, dermatologic, or other autoimmune conditions, including rheumatoid arthritis, systemic lupus erythematosus, and polyarteritis nodosa (Kent et al. 2004).

References

Belot A, Duquesne A, Job-Deslandre C, Costedoat-Chalumeau N, Boudjemaa S, Wechsler B, Cochat P, Piette JC, Cimaz R (2010) Pediatric-onset relapsing polychondritis: case series and systematic review. J Pediatr 156:484–489

Clark LJ, Wakeel RA, Ormerod AD (1992) Relapsing polychondritis – 2 cases with tracheal stenosis and inner-ear involvement. J Laryngol Otol 106:841–844

Kent PD, Michet CJ Jr, Luthra HS (2004) Relapsing polychondritis. Curr Opin Rheumatol 16:56–61

Lahmer T, Treiber M, von Werder A, Foerger F, Knopf A, Heemann U, Thuermel K (2010) Relapsing polychondritis: an autoimmune disease with many faces. Autoimmun Rev 9:540–546

McAdam LP, Ohanlan MA, Bluestone R, Pearson CM (1976) Relapsing polychondritis – prospective-study of 23 patients and a review of literature. Medicine 55:193–215

Michet CJ, McKenna CH, Luthra HS, Ofallon WM (1986) Relapsing polychondritis – survival and predictive role of early disease manifestations. Ann Intern Med 104:74–78

O'Connor Reina C, Garcia Iriarte MT, Barron Reyes FJ, Garcia Monge E, Luque Barona R, Gomez Angel D (1999) When is a biopsy justified in a case of relapsing polychondritis? J Laryngol Otol 113:663–665

Zulian F, Sari M, de Filippis C (2009) Otolaryngological manifestations of rheumatic diseases in children. Int J Pediatr Otorhinolaryngol 73:S56–S60

Distraction Osteogenesis

James Seaward and Alex Kane
Department of Plastic Surgery, University of Texas
Southwestern Medical Center, Dallas, TX, USA

Definition

A surgical technique to lengthen bone together with its soft tissue envelope by creating a bony injury and subsequently modifying the restorative response by the controlled application of external force.

Purpose

Distraction Osteogenesis (DO) is a technique with a wide range of applications. It enables surgeons to lengthen bone together with the surrounding soft tissue envelope. The pediatric craniofacial applications include improving the airway of neonates, potentially avoiding tracheostomy, advancing the midface in children with midface hypoplasia in order to improve significant facial deformities, to protect propotic eyes from morbidity due to exposure and to improve jaw occlusion, and to advance the maxilla in cleft patients with maxillary hypoplasia and severe class II jaw occlusion to improve bite and facial profile. DO can also be used in patients with mandibular asymmetry to improve jaw function, in patients with dental alveolar deficiency to develop sufficient bone to enable dental prostheses to be placed, and to increase intracranial volume in order to reduce the risk of raised intracranial pressure in patients with craniosynostosis.

Principles of Distraction Osteogenesis

The process of distraction osteogenesis involves creating a controlled bony injury, to which the body responds by creating callus. Tension is applied to the callus, elongating it. As tension continues to be applied over time, new bone forms and ossification occurs from the edges of the defect toward the center. When the desired length of bone is achieved, tension ceases to be applied, but the distraction device remains in situ as either external or internal fixation of the distraction site until ossification is adequate for the fixation to be removed. As the bone is lengthened in this process, the surrounding soft tissue envelope is also subject to tensile forces and undergoes a process of tissue expansion with cellular hyperplasia, allowing bony lengthening with lower relapse rates than acute osteotomy and advancement, in which soft tissues are restrictive, and enabling bony lengthening of greater magnitude than would be achievable with acute osteotomy alone.

Distraction osteogenesis consists of three clinical phases: The *latency phase* begins at the end of the first surgical procedure, during which a corticotomy or an osteotomy is made and the distraction device is fitted to the bone. During the latency phase, callus begins to form over and between the cut bony surfaces (McCarthy et al. 2001; Yu et al. 2004; McCarthy 2006). This phase typically lasts between 3 and 7 days.

The *distraction phase* begins as the distractor is activated. Activation of the device typically consists of turning a specific part of the device. Rotational motion at this part is converted to a linear motion across the osteotomy site, separating the two pieces of bone and applying a tensile force to the callus in between. Ilizarov studied distraction rate and discovered that too high a rate led to reduced new bone deposition and the risk of fibrous union, and too low a rate led to an increased risk of premature bony union. He determined that, in long bones, a distraction rate of

1 mm/day was optimal. The rate of craniofacial distraction varies between surgeons: some following Ilizarov's figure of 1 mm/day and others increasing this rate up to 2 mm/day in pediatric mandibles due to the increased bone metabolism in young children and the membranous nature of mandibular bone.

The term *rhythm* is used to describe both the frequency of activation and the amount of lengthening at each activation. Ilizarov's work on distraction frequency determined that the risks of mal-union, fibrous union, and early ossification leading to distraction failure reduced as distraction frequency increased. He determined that distraction of 0.25 mm every 6 h was superior to 0.5 mm every 12 h, which in turn was superior to 1 mm every 24 h. He created a device to provide constant progressive distraction using an electric motor. In practice, a frequency of two to four times daily is used as a compromise between distraction failure due to inadequate activation frequency and due to patient noncompliance.

The *consolidation phase* begins when distraction ceases. During this phase, the distraction device remains in place to support the new bone while it undergoes mineralization and develops adequate strength to support jaw loading and to overcome the tension forces of the soft tissue envelope. At the end of the consolidation phase, the distraction device can be removed in a second surgical procedure.

Distraction osteogenesis can be classified into three types:

1. Unifocal – In this type, the bone begins intact, a single osteotomy is made, and a device is attached to provide forces on either side of the osteotomy.
2. Bifocal – In this type, a defect exists in the bone before treatment. A single osteotomy is made and a device is attached to span the entire bone defect and osteotomy site while providing forces to move the *transport segment*.
3. Trifocal – In this type, a defect also exists in the bone before treatment. Osteotomies are made on both sides of the defect and two *transport segments* are used to fill the defect bidirectionally.

History

Distraction Osteogenesis (DO), in concept, was first published in 1869 by Von Langenbeck, but the first documented clinical application was by the Italian surgeon, Codavilla (McCarthy 2006; Pereira et al. 2007; Saulacic et al. 2008). He used a system of weights and pulleys on a calcaneal bone pin to lengthen the lower limb and, in 1905, published a series of using this technique in 26 patients with a combination of congenital and acquired conditions. This early distraction osteogenesis had a high complication rate including infection, tissue necrosis, malunion and unpredictable reossification rates leading to poor acceptance of this technique. It was the work of Ilizarov, starting in the 1950s in Western Siberia, that allowed distraction osteogenesis to be used safely and reliably. His research into timing, speed of distraction, and surgical technique allowed Ilizarov to develop predictable and effective treatment protocols. He developed a device consisting of two metal rings secured to the proximal and distal fragments with tension wires and secured to each other with threaded wires, which could be manipulated to provide controlled distraction; and he demonstrated the effectiveness of his technique, treating over 15,000 patients and gaining worldwide acceptance for distraction osteogenesis.

The history of mandibular distraction osteogenesis dates back to 1930, when Rosenthal reported using this technique to correct malocclusion secondary to mandibular hypoplasia (Honig et al. 2002). The scientific approach to craniofacial distraction osteogenesis developed in the 1970s and 1980s with several teams undertaking canine studies, but it was Karp et al. who performed detailed histological analysis of the ossification process following distraction osteogenesis in the canine model. This work led to the New York University team performing human mandibular distraction in 1989, published by McCarthy et al. in 1992.

Cellular and Biomechanical Mechanisms of DO

Although there are many similarities in bone healing between fracture and distraction osteogenesis, with the start of the activation phase, bone healing takes a different course. Bone healing occurs as a combination of endochondral ossification and intramembranous ossification. Whereas after fracture, bone healing occurs mostly via endochondral ossification, intramembranous ossification, a type of bone healing without a cartilage precursor, predominates in distraction osteogenesis (McCarthy 2006; Ai-Aql et al. 2008).

Distraction Osteogenesis,
Fig. 1 Cross section of the
osteotomy site during
Distraction Osteogenesis
demonstrating *1* central
fibrous zone, *2* transition zone,
3 remodeling zone, and
4 mature bone zone

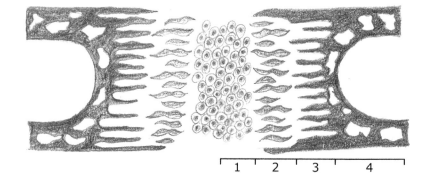

Immediately after the initial bony injury and during the latency phase, the tissue response is as would
be expected during normal fracture healing. Initial
hematoma formation around the cut bone ends leads
to an inflammatory response under the influence of
IL-1 and IL-6, and the recruitment of mesenchymal
stem cells, initiating callus formation influenced
by the TGF-β family (predominantly BMP-2 and
BMP4 early in the latency phase and BMP-6 later
in this phase). Vascular ingrowth from the periosteum and angiogenesis are stimulated by VEGF-C
and VEGF-D.

As the latency phase ends, the space between the
two bone ends is filled with a mix of polymorphonu-
clear leukocytes, endothelial cells, and fibroblasts.
During the start of the distraction phase, as tension
is applied to this mix of cells, Type 1 collagen is
deposited in bundles parallel to the tension line, and
angiogenesis occurs along this collagen matrix. As
the distraction phase develops, a larger gap forms
between the bone ends and, after approximately
14 days, osteoblasts migrate into the bone gap from
the edges and deposit osteoid along the collagen bundles. Later in the distraction phase and subsequently
in the consolidation phase, starting from approximately day 21, mineralization of the osteoid begins.
This new bone is remodeled under the influence of
osteoclasts, eventually becoming mature bone
throughout.

A schematic of a longitudinal section of the bone
gap late into the distraction phase demonstrates all four
of these zones of bone healing from the most immature
in the center of the gap to the most mature at the edges
(Fig. 1).
1. *Central Fibrous Zone* – This is characterized by
   mesenchymal proliferation, angiogenesis, and
   collagen bundle deposition parallel to the vector of
   distraction.
2. *Transition Zone* – Osteoid forms along the collagen
   bundles.
3. *Remodeling Zone* – Osteoclasts remodel the newly
   formed bone.
4. *Mature Bone Zone* – Mature bone similar in structure and appearance to adjacent undistracted bone.

The reason for the 2-week delay before deposition
of osteoid and 3-week delay before the start of mineralization can be explained using the principle of *ultimate tensile strain*. Consider an osteotomized bone
with a bone gap of 1 mm being distracted over the
first day by 1 mm. The tensile strain on the zone
between bone ends is such that 100% lengthening of
the bone gap occurs. On the next day, a further 1 mm
lengthening occurs, but the bone gap on that day is
2 mm, hence the tensile strain required is such that 50%
lengthening occurs. As time progresses and the bone
gap lengthens, the tensile strain across the bone gap
reduces. The *ultimate tensile strain* is the maximum
tensile strain at which bone formation can occur, and is
approximately equivalent to 1–2%. At 2 weeks, the
tensile strain at the bone ends has reduced sufficiently
to allow osteoblast activity and osteoid deposition, and
at 3–4 weeks, the tensile strain at the bone ends has
reduced to a level to allow mineralization and
remodeling.

Indications for Pediatric Craniofacial Distraction Osteogenesis

Distraction Osteogenesis of the Mandible
Distraction osteogenesis of the mandible can be used
to improve vertical deficiencies as seen in hypoplasia

of the ramus, horizontal deficiencies as seen in micrognathia, or a combination of both of these. The direction of distraction is termed the *vector* and is described relative to the maxillary occlusal plane: a vertical vector is at 90° to the maxillary occlusal plane and will lengthen the mandibular ramus, a horizontal vector is parallel to the maxillary occlusal plane and will lengthen the mandibular body, and an oblique vector will lengthen in both of these planes. The desired vector influences choice of osteotomy site as well as direction and placement of the distraction device.

Linear lengthening of one component of a complex structure, such as the mandible, can result in unintended rotational changes in the patient's occlusion. Mandibular DO in a vertical vector has a tendency to produce a posterior open bite whereas DO in a horizontal vector has a tendency to produce an anterior open bite. In neonates and younger children, this is rarely symptomatic as the rapidly growing face readily compensates for these small rotational changes. In older children, however, this can result in malocclusion with speech, feeding, and psychosocial consequences. *Molding the Regenerate* is a process of applying rotational forces late in the activation phase and early in the consolidation phase, while the newly forming bone is still soft. Although previous authors have described manual molding of the soft bone, McCarthy describes using a combination of dental elastics and, for external distraction devices, angulation of the device to achieve optimal occlusion during mandibular DO (McCarthy et al. 2003).

Choice of Device

Distraction devices can be external or semi-buried. The first devices used were external, which consist of multiple pins on either side of the osteotomy, piercing the skin, connected to an external frame. The distraction force is applied at the frame and transmitted through the pins to the bone. Semi-buried devices are inserted through a skin incision and are attached directly to the bone with multiple screws. They span the osteotomy site and the distraction force is applied through the screws to the bone. The activation device exits either through the oral mucosa into the mouth or through a separate skin incision. The advantages of each technique are summarized in the table below.

Advantages of external device	Advantages of semi-buried device

• Can be used in a severely hypoplastic mandible too small for a semi-buried device
• Multivector distraction is possible
• Vector can be altered during distraction
• Device can be removed without further incisions and dissection
	• Improved scarring
	  • Submandibular incision is preferable to skin incisions along the mandibular border, as is necessary with the external device
	  • Non-stretching of skin by distraction pins leads to improved scar outcomes as the length of the scar expected with the external device is the length of the distraction
	• Placing the device in direct contact with the bone confers a mechanical advantage with less torque
	• Less psychosocial morbidity in older children due to a visible device

McCarthy compared complication rates between external and semi-buried devices in more than 200 patients over 20 years and demonstrated that semi-buried devices have a higher rate of minor complications including pain on activation, neuropraxia of the inferior alveolar nerve, device backup and trismus, whereas external devices have a higher incidence of moderate complications including device loosening, improper vector and scarring requiring revision, and a higher incidence of severe complications including fracture, tooth damage, TMJ ankylosis, and scar hypertrophy (Davidson et al. 2010).

Distraction devices are available for use in a wide variety of materials. The senior author's preference for neonatal distraction is for the KLS Martin Micro Zurich device, a semi-buried Titanium device with an integrated ratchet, reducing the risk of the complication of device backup and allowing removal of the activation arm at the end of the activation phase. This device is compact and can be secured to the pediatric mandible with 1 mm screws. A resorbable device, available for neonatal DO is the Biomet Lactosorb® device, which consists of two Lactosorb® plates secured to the mandible with Lactosorb® 1.5 mm screws connected by a steel drive screw, to which the activation arm is attached. At the end of the consolidation phase, the activation arm is withdrawn together with the steel drive screw leaving only the Lactosorb® components, which absorb over 12 months, avoiding a second operation to remove the device. Osteomed has developed a device for neonatal mandibular DO that uses a curvilinear distraction path, varying the vector during distraction in order to prevent the open bite tendency of horizontal vector mandibular DO. It is named the Logic Jr and is a Titanium device fixed to the bone with 1.2 mm screws.

Neonatal Airway Compromise

Neonatal airway obstruction caused by a combination of glossoptosis and micrognathia is seen in a variety of conditions including Stickler Syndrome, Nager Syndrome, Bilateral Hemifacial Microsomia, and Treacher-Collins Syndrome but, most commonly, it is seen in Pierre Robin Sequence. Pierre Robin Sequence is characterized by a combination of micrognathia and glossoptosis in the absence of an underlying recognized syndrome, and is often associated with a wide U-shaped cleft palate. Its incidence is described as between 1 in 2,000 and 1 in 50,000 live births. Frequently, the combination of micrognathia and glossoptosis causes an upper airway compromise. This compromise is compounded because, rather than lying horizontally in the floor of the mouth, the retropositioned tongue frequently lies in more vertical orientation; so when the child attempts to advance the tongue to clear the obstruction, it advances obliquely into the cleft, blocking both the oral and the nasal cavity. In addition to the acute problem, neonatal airway obstruction can cause feeding difficulties and aspiration, failure to thrive due to the increased caloric requirements for breathing and difficulty feeding, and cor pulmonale (Denny and Kalantarian 2002; Denny 2004).

Airway obstruction associated with Pierre Robin Sequence is often successfully managed conservatively by an algorithm starting with prone positioning and progressing to a nasopharyngeal airway and positive pressure respiratory support, as required. If these measures fail to improve the acute obstruction then intubation is required. Neonates who fail to improve with positioning alone are potential surgical candidates and should be investigated with polysomnography, computerized tomography, and, if not intubated, airway endoscopy.

Endoscopy of the airway is important to establish the extent and site of the airway obstruction. Neonates

with obstruction at multiple levels, or with obstruction at a level other than at the base of the tongue are poor candidates for mandibular DO. Polysomnography is important to establish the severity of the obstruction and the pattern of the obstruction, to exclude a central apnea that would not benefit from surgery, and this investigation gives a useful baseline. A preoperative CT scan is helpful in planning the position of osteotomy and the vector of distraction. It also serves to confirm the bony maxillary-mandibular discrepancy at rest.

The main surgical options for neonatal airway obstruction include tongue-lip adhesion, pioneered by Douglas in the 1940s, mandibular DO, and ▶ tracheostomy. Although tracheostomy has been the "gold standard" treatment for children who are born with or who develop airway compromise in the neonatal period, it is not without significant risk and long-term implications. The operation itself can be life saving but it is an operation associated with a mortality of 0.5–5% as well as the continuous risk of accidental decannulation and cannula obstruction (▶ Tracheostomy, Complications). There is the burden of constant close care and maintenance, and patients who have undergone tracheostomy have a higher risk of chronic airway inflammation, airway granulation tissue, impaired speech articulation development, swallowing and feeding difficulty, and psychosocial sequelae.

Mandibular DO, in patients who have not responded to conservative measures, allows resolution of the airway compromise by moving the retropositioned tongue forward but also, by lengthening the mandible, improves the facial contour and brings the anterior jaws into a more anatomically correct position, potentially benefiting mastication and speech development. It can be used as the primary surgery, preventing the need for tracheostomy in both intubated neonates and those who are not intubated but who are dependent on a nasopharyngeal airway or continuous positive airway pressure to manage the obstruction; or as secondary surgery, allowing early decannulation in neonates in whom emergent tracheotomy has been performed.

Assessment of which patients are good candidates for surgery varies between institutions, but a multidisciplinary assessment by at least a craniofacial surgeon, an otolaryngologist, and a neonatologist or pulmonary physician is recommended. Surgical candidates are neonates who are not adequately managed by positioning alone, who have a single level airway obstruction at the level of the base of the tongue, who have no indications of central apnea, and who have a significant overjet. What constitutes a significant overjet varies between surgeons but a minimum discrepancy of 5–8 mm is described. In the well-selected patient group, mandibular DO can achieve a success rate in achieving an adequate, stable airway without the need for tracheostomy of over 90% (Fig. 2).

Mandibular Asymmetry

Asymmetry of the mandible is seen after fractures near growth centers, particularly after condylar fractures (▶ Facial Fractures in Children), and in a variety of congenital conditions, the most common of which is hemifacial microsomia. Hemifacial microsomia occurs in approximately 1 in 5000 births and is usually without any family history. It affects a variety of structures formed from the 1st and 2nd branchial arches and there is a very wide spectrum of severity from mild asymmetry to severe mandibular hypoplasia without a mandibular condyle and temporomandibular joint, macrostomia, anotia, aural atresia, facial nerve dysfunction, orbital dystopia, maxillary deficiency, and facial soft tissue deficiency. DO has an important role in mandibular hypoplasia to lengthen the mandibular body, ramus, or a combination of the two in order to improve bite, facial symmetry, and the function of the temporomandibular joint. The vector for distraction and osteotomy site in these complex deficiencies is chosen depending on the aims of DO on a case-by-case basis (Yu et al. 2004).

Distraction Osteogenesis of the Midface

Applications for DO in the midface include correction of maxillary deficiency such as following cleft lip or palate surgery (▶ Cleft Lip and Palate), to correct a vertical discrepancy in the alveolus or to increase the alveolar thickness prior to dental implant placement, to improve midface hypoplasia as found in Apert and Crouzon Syndromes (▶ Congenital Craniofacial Malformations and Their Surgical Treatment), and to improve facial symmetry in hemifacial microsomia.

In the cleft lip and palate patient, malocclusion caused by maxillary growth restriction is not an uncommon finding. When mild, this can often be treated orthodontically, compensating for the relatively small maxilla, but correction of a discrepancy greater than a few millimeters requires orthognathic surgery. Traditionally the treatment is by maxillary osteotomy at the LeFort I level (Figs. 3 and 4), mobilization of the maxillary segment, repositioning in the desired occlusion, plate fixation with or without bone grafting between the segments, as necessary. While this technique is effective for intermediate discrepancies requiring less than 8 mm of advancement, larger advancements may not be possible due to the soft tissue envelope resisting the forward motion or, if advancement is obtained, then the advanced maxilla may relapse recreating the malocclusion (Yu et al. 2004). Prior to DO, these large discrepancies could be treated with two-jaw surgery: advancing the maxilla as far as the soft tissues would allow and setting the mandible back to give the correct bite occlusion, but the resulting maxillary and mandibular position may not be the optimal site for the overall shape of the face. DO allows these larger maxillary deficiencies to be treated by advancing the maxilla and expanding its soft tissue envelope to bring the upper teeth forward to the correct anatomical position. LeFort I osteotomies are made but the maxilla is not advanced immediately. Instead, the distraction device is attached and, after the latency period, advancement progresses throughout the distraction period until the desired occlusion is achieved. Using DO allows gradual advancement of the maxilla and expansion of the surrounding soft tissue envelope enabling reliable and stable maxillary advancement with lower relapse rates, larger advancements and without the need for bone grafting. The operative time, intraoperative blood loss, and postoperative pain are also reduced, and this technique may have a lower incidence of velopharyngeal dysfunction than LeFort I osteotomy and immediate advancement.

Distraction devices can be internal or external but the most commonly used technique is the hemi-halo type external distractor such as the Rigid External Distraction System. This is an external device anchored to the skull and to either a dental splint or to bone plates. Its advantages are that as the maxillary fixation is often via the teeth, it does not require a second operation to remove the hardware, and it allows a range of distraction vectors including accommodating rotation of the maxillary segment and changing distraction vector during the process (McCarthy et al. 2001). The main disadvantage of this system is psychosocial in that it is readily visible as hardware in

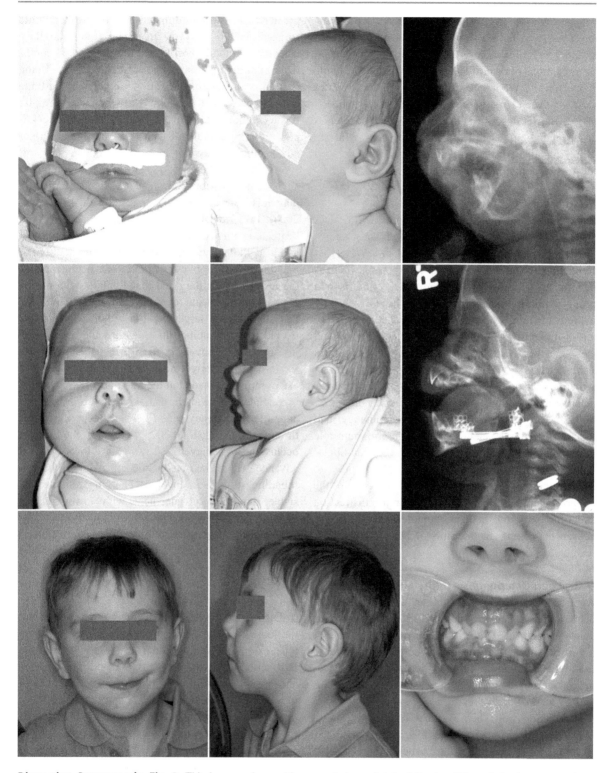

Distraction Osteogenesis, Fig. 2 This boy was born with Pierre Robin Sequence and underwent Mandibular Distraction Osteogenesis as a Neonate. The *top row* demonstrates his clinical and radiographic appearance shortly after birth, the *middle* row is immediately following DO, and the *bottom row* is at 3 years of age and demonstrates a good maintenance of his jaw relationship

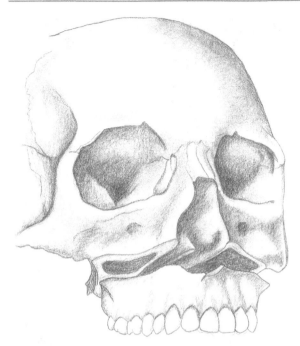

Distraction Osteogenesis, Fig. 3 LeFort I osteotomies

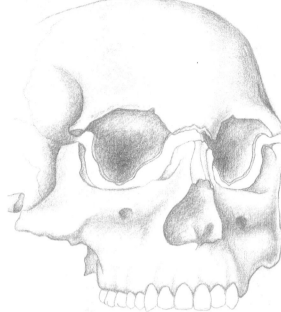

Distraction Osteogenesis, Fig. 4 LeFort III osteotomies

front of the face and it needs to be in place for the entire of the latency, activation, and consolidation phases, which can take several months.

Midface hypoplasia, as seen in craniofacial dysostosis and in syndromic craniosynostoses, such as Crouzon, Apert, and Pfeiffer Syndromes, can result in upper airway obstruction, inadequate protection of the eyes with exposure keratopathy, malocclusion with feeding and speech difficulties, and aesthetic and psychosocial morbidities. Advancement of the entire midface can be used to improve both the patient's function and their facial aesthetics, and this advancement requires either osteotomies at the LeFort III level (Fig. 5) or as a *Monobloc* incorporating midface, orbits, and forehead. Although both internal and external devices can be used, hemi-halo type external devices are most commonly used as they have the ability to vary vector during the distraction process and allow midline traction far from the osteotomy sites. Internal devices distracting via bony fixation laterally have been associated with increased complication rates such as asymmetry of distraction, incorrect vector and fractures of the bony prominences to which the distractors are attached, such as the zygomatic arch.

Calvarial Distraction Osteogenesis

Craniosynostosis, or abnormal fusion of the sutures of the skull, occurs in 1 in 2,500 births and can affect one suture or multiple sutures. Multiple suture involvement is more likely when the craniosynostosis is part of a syndrome, such as Crouzon, Apert, Saethre-Chotzen, or Pfeiffer Syndromes. The suture fusion results in an inability for the skull to grow at that location and so the skull develops an abnormal shape as growth rate increases at other sutures to compensate. In addition to this aesthetic problem, craniosynostosis can result in raised intracranial pressure as skull growth may be inadequate for the underlying growing brain. This is more likely in multiple suture craniosynostosis (Renier et al. 1982). Craniosynostosis tends to be treated surgically addressing the aesthetic deformity and also creating a larger intracranial volume to reduce the risk of raised intracranial pressure. These operations involve removing variable portions of the skull, reshaping and repositioning the bony segments, either in one or multiple stages. These are long operations with relatively high blood loss and the risks of bony necrosis, reabsorption of bone grafts, malunion or nonunion, and bone gaps as well as the risks of meningeal damage or damage, neurological consequences and

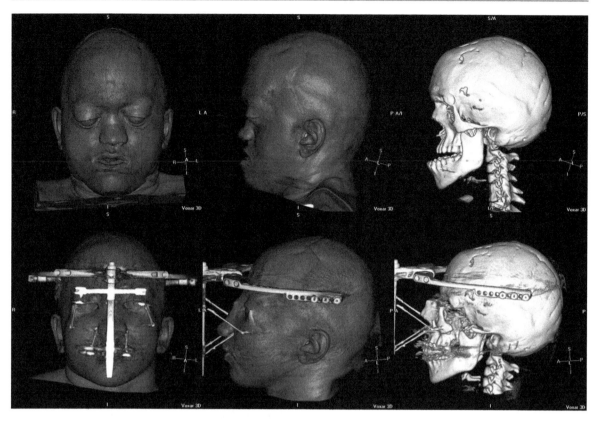

Distraction Osteogenesis, Fig. 5 This girl with Crouzon Syndrome underwent LeFort III osteotomies and DO of her midface. The *top images* are 3D reconstructions of a CT scan before DO and demonstrate her eye proptosis and midface deficiency. The *lower images* are at the end of DO

severe hemorrhage. DO has brought a new dimension to calvarial vault surgery as it allows expansion of the skull without removing, reshaping, and replacing bone, reducing blood loss, surgical time, hospital stay, and morbidity. The devices used for calvarial vault DO can be the same as those used elsewhere on the craniofacial skeleton, but an alternative method of DO using springs was described by Lauritzen in 1998 (Yu et al. 2004). These springs allow for a method of DO, closed to the external environment, and they provide continuous force across the osteotomy rather than patient-controlled activation a few times daily. The force across the osteotomy reduces progressively as DO proceeds, and the springs are custom-made so that when the desired distraction is achieved, the force across the springs reduces to the point at which bony consolidation occurs, following which they can be removed (Fig. 6).

Complications of Distraction Osteogenesis

Although DO is an established and effective method of bone and soft tissue lengthening, complications are encountered. A survey of surgeons undertaking craniofacial distraction around the world identified over 3,000 patients in whom DO had been performed and noted complications in various categories. The most common complication was failure to guide distraction in the correct vector in 8.8% using a single-vector distraction device and 7.2% with multi-vector devices. The next most common complication category was technical failure with a 4.7% rate of noncompliance with distraction protocol, 4.5% rate of hardware failure, 3% rate of device dislodgement, and 1% rate of pain preventing distraction. Premature ossification indicating an inadequate rate of distraction occurred in 1.9% of patients and fibrous nonunion indicating an

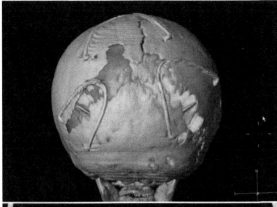

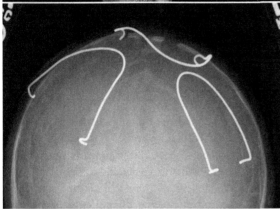

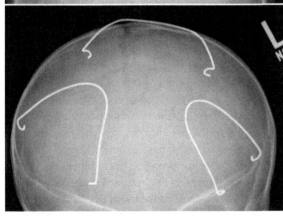

Distraction Osteogenesis, Fig. 6 This girl with Apert syndrome underwent spring cranioplasty of her posterior scalp. The *top image* demonstrates the position of the springs on the skull, the *middle radiograph* is immediately following spring placement, and the *lower radiograph* is 6 months later

excessive rate in 0.5%. The next most common complication was infection. Pin tract infection was noted in 5.2%, infection of the device not requiring removal in 2.9%, infection requiring removal in 0.9% and osteomyelitis in 0.5%. Damage to the inferior alveolar nerve occurred in 3.6% of mandibular distraction, tooth bud injury in 1.9%, and facial nerve injury in 0.4% (Mofid et al. 2001).

Summary

Distraction Osteogenesis has a wide variety of applications throughout the craniofacial skeleton and is used throughout childhood from the neonate with Pierre Robin Sequence through to the skeletally mature teenager to advance the maxilla to correct maxillary hypoplasia. It allows larger movements than osteotomy and immediate advancements, expanding the surrounding soft tissue envelope together with the underlying bony lengthening. Craniofacial DO has been used by surgeons increasingly over the last 20 years and has been proven to be a safe and effective tool for craniofacial reconstruction.

Cross-References

▶ Cleft Lip and Palate
▶ Congenital Craniofacial Malformations and Their Surgical Treatment
▶ Facial Fractures in Children
▶ Hemifacial Microsomia
▶ Tracheostomy
▶ Tracheostomy, Complications

References

Ai-Aql ZS, Alagl AS et al (2008) Molecular mechanisms controlling bone formation during fracture healing and distraction osteogenesis. J Dent Res 87(2):107–118
Davidson EH, Brown D et al (2010) The evolution of mandibular distraction: device selection. Plast Reconstr Surg 126(6):2061–2070
Denny AD (2004) Distraction osteogenesis in Pierre Robin neonates with airway obstruction. Clin Plast Surg 31(2):221–229
Denny A, Kalantarian B (2002) Mandibular distraction in neonates: a strategy to avoid tracheostomy. Plast Reconstr Surg 109(3):896–904; discussion 905–896
Honig JF, Grohmann UA et al (2002) Mandibula distraction osteogenesis for lengthening the mandibula to correct a malocclusion: a more than 70-year-old German concept in craniofacial surgery. J Craniofac Surg 13(1):96–98
McCarthy JG (2006) Principles of craniofacial distraction. In: Thorne C, Grabb WC, Smith JW (eds) Grabb and Smith's

plastic surgery, 6th edn. Wolters Kluwer Health/Lippincott Williams & Wilkins, Philadelphia, pp 96–102

McCarthy JG, Stelnicki EJ et al (2001) Distraction osteogenesis of the craniofacial skeleton. Plast Reconstr Surg 107(7):1812–1827

McCarthy JG, Hopper RA et al (2003) Molding of the regenerate in mandibular distraction: clinical experience. Plast Reconstr Surg 112(5):1239–1246

Mofid MM, Manson PN et al (2001) Craniofacial distraction osteogenesis: a review of 3,278 cases. Plast Reconstr Surg 108(5):1103–1114; discussion 1115–1107

Pereira MA, Luiz de Freitas PH et al (2007) Understanding distraction osteogenesis on the maxillofacial complex: a literature review. J Oral Maxillofac Surg 65(12): 2518–2523

Renier D, Sainte-Rose C et al (1982) Intracranial pressure in craniostenosis. J Neurosurg 57(3):370–377

Saulacic N, Iizuka T et al (2008) Alveolar distraction osteogenesis: a systematic review. Int J Oral Maxillofac Surg 37(1):1–7

Yu JC, Fearon J et al (2004) Distraction osteogenesis of the craniofacial skeleton. Plast Reconstr Surg 114(1):1E–20E

DNI

▶ Pediatric Neck Infections

Donor Site Complications in Free Flap Surgery

Steven B. Cannady[1] and Mark K. Wax[2]
[1]Department of Otolaryngology, SUNY Downstate Medical Center, Brooklyn, NY, USA
[2]Department of Otolaryngology-Head and Neck Surgery, Oregon Health and Science University, Portland, OR, USA

Synonyms

Free flap complications

Definition

Free flap donor site complication = any outcome at the site of flap harvest that results in prolonged recovery, or detrimental effect on patient well-being, or survival.

Introduction

The ultimate goal in the management of head and neck cancer has been to achieve adequate control of the tumor with maximal functional rehabilitation. Achieving this rehabilitation has involved ever increasingly complex reconstructive paradigms.

Treatment of head and neck cancer usually involves multimodality treatment. For some tumors, such as larynx or oropharynx, chemoradiation (CRT) protocols have become the predominant method of treatment. For other tumors in the head and neck, such as in the oral cavity or sino-nasal region, surgery remains the preferred primary method of treatment. Patients who undergo chemoradiation protocols will still occasionally fail treatment and require surgical salvage. Surgical salvage of these patients often times involves transgression into the upper aero-digestive tract. The effects on the soft tissue of the previous treatment, whether it is chemotherapy, radiation therapy, or surgery, along with the usual debilitated state of these patients predisposes them to many local soft tissue and systemic complications. The ability of the local tissues that have already seen a number of treatments to heal in a normal fashion after surgery can be compromised. Furthermore, the normal functions of the head and neck, such as speech, deglutition, and articulation, can all be adversely affected with the removal of the bony or soft tissue components of the head and neck region. Finally, surgical removal of these tissues will lead to a marked cosmetic abnormality that can be devastating to the patient.

Free tissue transfer has become the reconstructive method of choice for complex, three-dimensional composite tissue defects in the head and neck (Wax 2009). Over the last two decades, the use of free tissue to replace the composite tissue that is often times resected during head and neck oncologic procedures has been shown to decrease the postoperative morbidity. Along with this decrease in morbidity, has come an improved ability to both functionally rehabilitate the patient as well as cosmetically and socially optimize their outcomes.

A number of donor sites are available for replacement of the composite tissue losses of the head and neck region. The most common donor site is the radial forearm flap for soft tissue defects. For bony defects, the fibula has become the reconstructive tool of choice. Other soft tissue and bony flaps are described in

Donor Site Complications in Free Flap Surgery, Table 1 The common flaps and their frequency of use from experience with 1,500 free flaps

Type of flap	Frequency of use (%)
Radial/Ulnar	65
Anterolateral thigh	8
Rectus	8
Latissimus dorsi	6
Fibula	20
Others: scapula, jejunum, enteral, and lateral arm	10

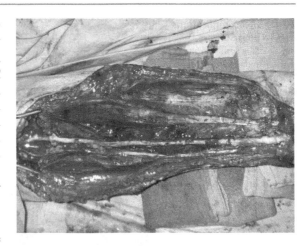

Donor Site Complications in Free Flap Surgery, Fig. 1 This intraoperative photo demonstrates the revascularization of the hand with a saphenous vein graft after sacrifice of the dominant vessel to the hand

Table 1. This entry will discuss the morbidity at the donor site of harvesting the most commonly used free flaps.

Radial/Ulnar Flap

Once the most common free flap used in oral cavity reconstruction, the radial forearm flap is used less today by some surgeons (Avery 2010). Still, the radial forearm, and by extension, the ulnar free flap, are versatile fasciocutaneous free flaps with far reaching applications in head and neck reconstruction. The radial flap harvests both skin and a major blood vessel to the distal forearm. There are two major vascular supplies to the hand: the radial artery and the ulnar artery. In the majority of people, the deep and superficial palmer arches communicate quite well and allow the hand to function well if one of these vascular supplies is compromised. Rarely patients may have a vascular anomaly of the vessels supplying the hand (Fig. 1). Thus, preoperative testing with Allen's test is important in the assessment of whether the flap is appropriate in an individual patient. Vascular anomalies exist with a dominant ulnar blood supply to the hand, or even atrophic or absent ulnar or radial arteries. Without a good Allen's test, these contraindications to forearm flap surgery can elude surgeons until vessel sacrifice and ischemic changes are recognized in the hand (Bell et al. 2011). Flap harvest encroaches upon the nerve supply to the arm, hand, and fingers. The sensory nerves can almost always be preserved to a major degree. Some degree of sensory loss over the wrist is always present. Major motor disability is rare.

Despite the ideal qualities of forearm flaps for some head and neck defects, morbidity from the harvest of a flap can be significant both in the acute and long-term setting (Skoner et al. 2003; de Witt et al. 2007). Early complications tend to be limited to the range of motion and sensory changes. The flap harvest creates a full thickness loss of skin and fascia that exposes underlying muscle and neural tissue responsible for range of motion and sensation to the thumb and hand. Though patients tend to recover function with time, on occasion, branches of the radial nerve are sacrificed to preserve perforators to the radial flap and thus may result in prolonged time periods to nerve regrowth of the anatomical snuffbox and hand. These sensory changes can impact job performance and hobbies related to sensory functions of the hand. Patients that rely on manual dexterity and sensation may become frustrated while waiting for nerve function to return. Most reconstructive surgeons will harvest the flap from the non-dominant arm. The acute management of the arm donor site usually involves some form of immobilization to allow for healing of the split thickness skin graft. Mobilization is then started in a graded manner. As many of these patients also have tracheotomies, the dominant hand is very important to maintain communication. Once the hand is mobilized, a graded physiotherapy regime is instituted to start active mobilization. This program reduces the short-term sequelae.

Once the short-term healing has been completed, one can start to encounter long-term complications as the forearm site is healing. These most often are in the form of delayed healing of the forearm skin site. Long-term

Donor Site Complications in Free Flap Surgery, Fig. 2 This series of photos demonstrates the difference in closure with A meshed split thickness skin graft (**a**) as opposed to a circumferential suture with a non-meshed split thickness skin graft (**b**). Long-term healing demonstrates the differences between the meshed (**c**) and non-meshed split thickness skin grafts (**d**)

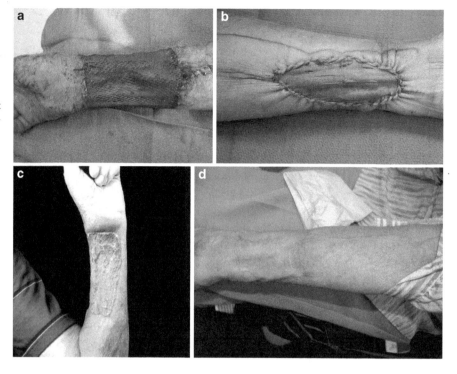

functional deficits of a motor origin are rare. Typically, the harvest site is repaired by split-thickness skin graft, allogenic graft, full-thickness graft, rotational skin flap, purse-string partial closure, or some combination thereof (Winslow et al. 2000) (Fig. 2). Regardless of the method of closure, resultant scar contractures are common, and can result in permanent range of motion limitations. Scarring is considerable after forearm flap harvests, and has led some surgeons to prefer ulnar flaps to hide the scar when a patient stands in the anatomic position. Either scar tends to appear similar to a tissue burn once fully healed, but certainly can be a source of disappointment for patients if not thoroughly discussed preoperatively. The contractures after skin graft can also limit range of motion of the hand or distal forearm, and patients may report difficulty with fine motor function of the thumb and hand. In its most severe form, contractures of the wrist joint can occur and severely limit the use of the affected hand.

Intermediate complications are possible and result most often from partial or full loss of graft repairs of the donor site (Fig. 3). Prolonged wound healing is not uncommon from partial skin graft failure. These complications can typically be managed with wet-to-dry dressings, wound vac, and skin grafting once the wound bed has granulated sufficiently.

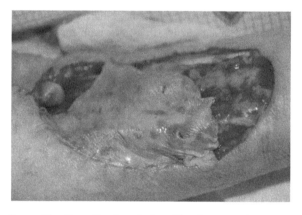

Donor Site Complications in Free Flap Surgery, Fig. 3 The split thickness skin graft has not taken in this example. One hundred percent loss was evident

Osteocutaneous flap harvest adds additional morbidity from possible bony complications associated with future wrist fractures – partial radial bone removal naturally weakens the wrist making fracture more likely after falls (Hartman et al. 2002). Recent experience with prophylactic plating of the radial bone at the time of harvest has decreased the occurrence of fracture to almost zero (Waits et al. 2007). Overall, both in patient perception and functional outcomes, the radial forearm and ulnar flaps appear to have a low-donor-site morbidity profile further preserving it as a versatile reconstructive flap (Werle et al. 2000). Complications are typically low-morbidity, however, patient selection is paramount to good outcome. A patient that requires normal sensation and function of the hand may find even a slight change unacceptable.

Anterolateral Thigh Flap (ALT)

The ALT flap continues to emerge as a replacement for the RFFF with far reaching capabilities (Wong and Wei 2009). Acute and chronic morbidity from harvest of the ALT are typically minor and managed readily. In the authors' experience with over 100 free anterolateral thigh free flaps the most common

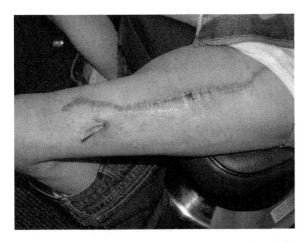

Donor Site Complications in Free Flap Surgery, Fig. 4 The incision for the anterolateral thigh free flap can be long but usually heals well

complications were seroma formation (3%), numbness to lateral thigh (2%), and leg weakness (2%).

Rigorous testing by Kuo et al. (2009) has indicated that the vastus lateralis can be harvested with the flap with minimal morbidity and functional impairment. Infection rates are low following flap harvest. Donor site repair is either via rotation advancement of leg skin, or split thickness grafting, and therefore, wound dehiscence of tense closures are rare (1%), but wound contractures are possible (Fig. 4). Management of seroma may require serial needle drainage or drain replacement, whereas numbness tends to resolve over the year of healing (Fig. 5). Some surgeons recommend quilting sutures to tack skin down to underlying muscle as a measure to prevent seroma formation. The quilting sutures prevent tissue shearing, and reduce potential space at the donor site and in some studies portend a lesser incidence of seroma formation.

Functional outcomes following ALT harvest have been studied closely. Most surgeons sacrifice the nerve to the vastus lateralis when it is closely associated with the flap's blood supply. This creates both skin numbness and muscular strength changes. However, comparisons of patient thigh strength before and after ALT harvest have shown that most patients have very little functional consequence (Hanasono et al. 2010).

Late morbidity from ALT harvest can arise from neuralgias at the incision site or distribution of cutaneous nerves cut during harvest. Some patients report severe pain at the incision, knee, or lateral thigh. These pain syndromes are treated with neurologic medications aimed at blocking aberrant nerve firing.

Overall, the ALT has been lauded for its diversity and lack of morbidity. Patients report few significant morbidities after harvest, making the flap an attractive donor site for use in head and neck reconstructions.

Donor Site Complications in Free Flap Surgery, Fig. 5 When the wound is closed under too much tension it will break down. In these cases, a wound vac will help facilitate granulation tissue (**a**). Once the wound is granulating healing by secondary intention is enough (**b**), although it may take a month or so

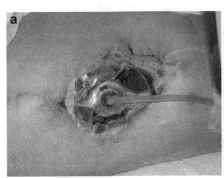
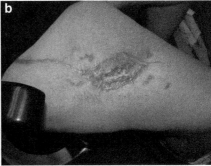

Rectus Flap

Though a good option for large bulky defects, the rectus flap has abdominal morbidities that are not seen with other donor sites. These can be quite significant to the non-general surgeon. However, the variable skin paddle options, and ability to harvest a large muscle, continue to make the musculocutaneous rectus flap (and its variants) a good option for some head and neck defects. In particular, skull base and total glossectomy defects are well suited for the rectus flap. Rectus flap harvest, necessarily, takes muscle and fascia from the abdominal wall pedicled on the inferior epigastric blood supply. Given the anatomy of the abdomen, the flap harvest results in loss of fascial (unless fascia sparing technique is used) and muscular strength, and subsequently, the primary complications of rectus harvest are from anterior wall weakness; Hernia (Fig. 6), abdominal wound dehiscence, infection, and seroma/hematoma are all possible, though rare (Vyas et al. 2008). Abdominal fascial repair with mesh or primary fascial repair seems to prevent long-term risk of hernia. Redundancy of abdominal skin usually allows for primary skin closure. More rare complications such as ileus or small bowel obstruction are possible, but can be avoided with care taken not to inadvertently distract the bowel during closure.

Subscapular System Flaps: Latissimus Dorsi/Serratus/Scapula

The latissimus flap is derived from the largest muscle (in surface area) in the body. It can be harvested alone, or in conjunction with scapula, serratus (+ rib), and skin components. The flexibility of mega-flap options, as well as multiple uses of the latissimus flap itself, makes this system an appealing flap option for multiple head and neck defects. Generally, mega-flap versatility is used when large composite defects are created; for example, a through and through check, mandible, mucosa can be reconstructed with a serratus/rib, latissimus (with multiple paddles), or scapula depending on the individual needs of the patients. The latissimus muscle flap is useful in scalp reconstruction with skin grafting, skull base reconstruction, total glossectomy reconstruction, or large neck defects.

Harvest of the latissimus flap involves elevation of the back skin to expose a large area of muscle

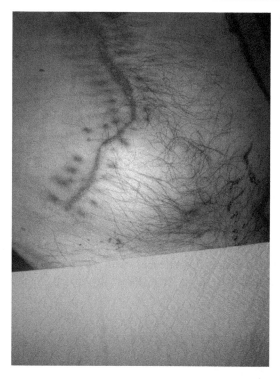

Donor Site Complications in Free Flap Surgery, Fig. 6 This patient developed the acute onset of an incisional hernia 1 month after surgery

extending from the transverse spinal processes to the scapula and posterior-superior illiac crest. The main morbidity/complication associated with this flap harvest is seroma in 5% or more of patients – some role for fibrin sealant has been exposed in recent literature; however, drain placement can be necessary for a mean of 21.5 days following surgery (Bailey et al. 2011).

From a functional standpoint, survey-based studies indicate that patients suffer from weakness (39%), numbness/tightness of skin (50%), and scaring (22%) with a significant number indicating difficulty with vigorous activities of daily life (Adams et al. 2004). Thus, when possible it is best to use the latissimus from a patient's nondominant shoulder to reduce disabilities of the shoulder, arm, and hand (DASH) score changes.

Serratus free flaps can provide additional muscle in conjunction with or independent of latissimus flaps. It can also incorporate a vascularized rib when desirable. Thus, skin elevation morbidity remains similar to the latissimus with resultant tightness, numbness, and seroma formation. Furthermore, rib harvest affords the additional risk of violating the pleural sheath and subsequent pneumothorax, or hemothorax. In addition, atelectasis is common secondary to rib pain after harvest and can create short-term respiratory complications. Muscle dysfunction is usually not significant in serratus flap harvest, with winged-scapula reported rarely, and morbidity affecting return to work nonexistent (Derby et al. 1997).

The harvest of a bony scapula and scapular tip flap are possible in combination with other tissue harvest or alone. It offers considerably diverse options allowing for multiple skin paddles and soft tissue while reliably providing 10 cm of bone, or good bone stock at the scapular tip. Complications directly attributable to the scapula harvest relate to the release of muscular attachments. The aforementioned soft tissue and skin elevation complications are also possible when a scapula is harvest and include seroma, hematoma, and infection. Specific complications of bone removal include weakness and range of motion reduction; yet, patients have reported only minor limitation in activities, strength of shoulder, and overall in DASH scores (Clark et al. 2008; Coleman et al. 2000).

Fibula Free Flap

The fibula free flap, based on the peroneal artery and veins, is a workhorse in bony oromandibular reconstruction. With a long pedicle, and the ability to harvest 20 cm of bone that can harbor dental implants, the fibula is unrivaled in its ability to replace large amounts of bone. A large skin paddle can be harvested with the fibula, and chimeric paddles can allow for reconstruction of intraoral and cheek or neck defects.

The peroneal vessels are one of the three main vascular supplies to the lower extremity. In head and neck cancer patients, coincident peripheral vascular disease can be common, thus, preoperative imaging of the vascular system is pivotal in choosing a leg. If prior existing vessel obstruction is noted on imaging, the leg and foot may become ischemic after peroneal vessel sacrifice. Loss of a foot or lower leg can be a rare but catastrophic complication of fibula harvest. More frequent than total limb loss, significant donor site necrosis can occur due to poor venous return or arterial supply and result in delayed wound healing (Fig. 7). In most cases, wound debridement or vacuum dressing will be sufficient to aid healing, but can prolong this process for months (Fig. 8).

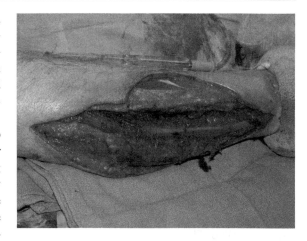

Donor Site Complications in Free Flap Surgery, Fig. 7 This patient developed a severe infection of the lower leg that required debridement. The skin graft was totally lost

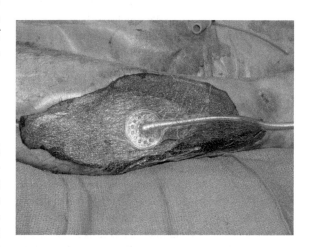

Donor Site Complications in Free Flap Surgery, Fig. 8 A wound VAC has been placed on the lower leg wound to facilitate care

Fibula harvest has traditionally been considered to afford a high rate of short-term complications (31.2%): skin graft loss (15%), cellulitis (10%), wound dehiscence (8%), and abscess (1%). However, long-term morbidity is lower (17%): decreased ankle mobility (12%), great toe contracture (9%), leg weakness (8%), and ankle instability (4%) (Momoh et al. 2011; Ghaheri et al. 2005). A frequently reported vague lower extremity pain without objective clinical findings can be present long after surgery.

In comparing patients that have complications to those without, one study has demonstrated that primary closure resulted in higher complications, and that heavy smokers were more apt to have complications (Shindo et al. 2000).

Clearly, when counseling patients about fibula transfer, the benefits must be weighed against the risks and alternatives. It remains a desirable flap and allows for dual site surgery to be performed, potentially limiting the length of surgery, and consequently, the complications of prolonged anesthetics.

Common Rotational Flaps

Pectoralis Major Flap

The Pectoralis major myocutaneous flap (PMMF) is a common rotational (and sometimes free) flap used in head and neck surgery. Though now more common as a salvage flap (McCarn et al. 2008), it continues to be used reliably when free tissue is not feasible. In settings where internal and external neck reconstruction are necessary, it can both reconstitute the pharynx, and provide muscle for skin grafting as in the case of chemoradiation failure in laryngeal cancer therapy. However, morbidity and cost of free flap reconstruction do not appear to differ from rotation flaps, and thus free tissue has largely supplanted PMMF in their popularity.

PMMF rotates the muscle and skin of the chest wall and its muscular attachments to the ribs, sternum, and humerus. Intercostal perforator vessels traverse the chest wall and have to be meticulously handled to avoid a rare but dreaded complication – hemothorax. More common, but, insidious in presentation is atelectasis secondary to guarding with respirations (Schuller et al. 1994; Seikaly et al. 1990). The pain associated with chest wall surgery can cause patients to breath more shallow and poorly clear the lungs. Hematoma, seroma, infection, and wound dehiscence are also possible, though rare. In women undergoing PMMF, an inframammary incision can help avoid cosmetic morbidity, but puts the breast at risk of necrosis. In most cases, the PMMF is not aesthetically pleasing due to a traversing scar from clavicle to medial areolar skin. In addition, an unsightly muscle bulk can be seen over the clavicle.

Deltopectoral Rotational Flap

The deltopectoral rotational flap is one of the earliest described and employed flaps utilized in head and neck reconstruction. It is based on the intercostals perforators from ribs one to three providing an axial pattern flap with the ability to extend as high as the oropharynx. The large skin defect created is typically covered with split thickness skin grafting. Scar contractures are common, and expected, to a certain extent. The contracture can affect range of motion of the shoulder and chest muscles that it overlies.

Latissimus Rotational Flap

The donor site morbidity of a rotational latissimus mirrors those of the free flap. One additional aspect of rotating involves tunneling the flap through the axilla to the head and neck. As such, the rotated lat flap can add bulk and discomfort to the axilla.

Conclusions

The common free and rotational flaps used in head and neck reconstruction have morbidity to the donor site. The morbidity should be carefully considered in the reconstructive plan, and thoroughly discussed with each patient. The reconstructive surgeon has a plethora of flap choices at his/her disposal, and individual patient characteristics may make one flap choice less morbid than another. Though complications and morbidities are common for some flap donor sites, fortunately most patients recover near normal function. However, without thorough expectations about their surgery, patients can quickly become disappointed in results, despite surgeon satisfaction with outcomes. When faced with a major head and neck resection and reconstruction, it is easy to understand why the overwhelmed patient may not focus on the possible negative outcomes of the donor site choice. Thus, it is incumbent upon the care team to provide concise and understandable descriptions, and goals for both short and long-term recovery. This entry is meant to serve as a summary of the common morbidities at flap donor sites that can be used to help relay this information to patients.

Cross-References

▶ Fibula Free Flap

References

Adams WP Jr, Lipschitz AH, Ansari M, Kenkel JM, Rohrich RJ (2004) Functional donor site morbidity following latissimus dorsi muscle flap transfer. Ann Plast Surg 53:6–11

Avery CM (2010) Review of the radial free flap: is it still evolving, or is it facing extinction? Part one: soft-tissue radial flap. Br J Oral Maxillofac Surg 48:245–252

Bailey SH, Oni G, Guevara R, Wong C, Saint-Cyr M (2011) Latissimus dorsi donor-site morbidity: the combination of quilting sutures and fibrin sealant reduce length of drain placement and seroma rate. Ann Plast Surg [Epub ahead of print]

Bell RA, Schneider DS, Wax MK (2011) Superficial ulnar artery: a contraindication to radial forearm free tissue transfer. Laryngoscope 121(5):933–936. doi:10.1002/lary

Clark JR, Vesely M, Gilbert R (2008) Scapular angle osteomyogenous flap in postmaxillectomy reconstruction: defect, reconstruction, shoulder function, and harvest technique. Head Neck 30:10–20

Coleman SC, Burkey BB, Day TA, Resser JR, Netterville JL, Dauer E, Sutinis E (2000) Increasing use of the scapula osteocutaneous free flap. Laryngoscope 110:1419–1424

de Witt CA, de Bree R, Verdonck-de Leeuw IM, Quak JJ, Leemans CR (2007) Donor site morbidity of the fasciocutaneous radial forearm flap: what does the patient really bother? Eur Arch Otorhinolaryngol 264:929–934

Derby LD, Bartlett SP, Low DW (1997) Serratus anterior free-tissue transfer: harvest-related morbidity in 34 consecutive cases and a review of the literature. Reconstr Microsurg 13(6):397–403

Ghaheri BA, Kim JH, Wax MK (2005) Second osteocutaneous fibular free flaps for head and neck defects. Laryngoscope 115(6):983–986

Hanasono MM, Skoracki RJ, Yu P (2010) A prospective study of donor-site morbidity after anterolateral thigh fasciocutaneous and myocutaneous free flap harvest in 220 patients. Plast Reconstr Surg 125(1):209–214

Hartman EH, Spauwen PH, Jansen JA (2002) Donor-site complications in vascularized bone flap surgery. J Invest Surg 15:185–197

Kuo YR, Yeh MC, Shih HS, Chen CC, Lin PY, Chiang YC, Jeng SF (2009) Versatility of the anterolateral thigh flap with vascularized fascia lata for reconstruction of complex soft-tissue defects: clinical experience and functional assessment of the donor site. Plast Reconstr Surg 124(1):171–180

McCarn KE, Ghanem T, Tartaglia J, Gross N, Andersen P, Wax MK (2008) Second free tissue transfers in head and neck reconstruction. Otolaryngol Head Neck Surg 139:525–529

Momoh AO, Yu P, Skoracki RJ, Liu S, Feng L, Hanasono MM (2011) A prospective cohort study of fibula free flap donor site morbidity in 157 consecutive patients. Plast Reconstr Surg 128(3):714–720

Schuller DE, Daniels RL, King M, Houser S (1994) Analysis of frequency of pulmonary atelectasis in patients undergoing pectoralis major musculocutaneous flap reconstruction. Head Neck 16:25–29

Seikaly H, Kuzon WM Jr, Gullane PJ, Herman SJ (1990) Pulmonary atelectasis after reconstruction with pectoralis major flaps. Arch Otolaryngol Head Neck Surg 116(5):575–577

Shindo M, Fong BP, Funk GF, Karnell LH (2000) The fibula osteocutaneous flap in head and neck reconstruction: a critical evaluation of donor site morbidity. Arch Otolaryngol Head Neck Surg 126:1467–1472

Skoner JM, Bascom DA, Cohen JI, Andersen PE, Wax MK (2003) Short-term functional donor site morbidity after radial forearm fasciocutaneous free flap harvest. Laryngoscope 113:2091–2094

Vyas RM, Dickinson BP, Fastekjian JH, Watson JP, Dalio AL, Crisera CA (2008) Risk factors for abdominal donor-site morbidity in free flap breast reconstruction. Plast Reconstr Surg 121(5):1519–1526

Waits CA, Toby EB, Girod DA, Tsue TT (2007) Osteocutaneous radial forearm free flap: long-term radiographic evaluation of donor site morbidity after prophylactic plating of radius. J Reconstr Microsurg 23(7):367–372

Wax MK (2009) Microvascular reconstructive surgery of the face: preface. Facial Plast Surg Clin North Am 17(2):ix

Werle AH, Tsue TT, Toby EB, Girod DA (2000) Osteocutaneous radial forearm free flap: its use without significant donor site morbidity. Otolaryngol Head Neck Surg 123:711–717

Winslow CP, Hansen J, Mackenzie D, Cohen JI, Wax MK (2000) Pursestring closure of radial forearm fasciocutaneous donor sites. Laryngoscope 110:1815–1818

Wong CH, Wei FC (2009) Anterolateral thigh flap. Head Neck 32:529–540

Doppler Monitoring

▶ Free Flap Monitoring in Head and Neck Reconstruction

Double Transposition Flaps

▶ Z-plasty

Double-Opposing Z-Plasty

▶ Z-plasty

Dribbling

▶ Salivary Gland Disorders, Sialorrhea

Drooling

▶ Salivary Gland Disorders, Sialorrhea

Duplex Theory of Sound Localization

Thomas J. Balkany[1] and Daniel M. Zeitler[1,2]
[1]Department of Otolaryngology-Head and Neck
Surgery, University of Miami Miller School of
Medicine, University of Miami Ear Institute, Miami,
FL, USA
[2]Denver Ear Associates, Denver, CO, USA

Definition

Using both interaural level difference and interaural
time difference together in order to provide binaural
information.

Cross-References

▶ Adult Bilateral Cochlear Implantation

Dupuy's Syndrome

▶ Frey's Syndrome

Dural and Brain Herniation

▶ Temporal Bone Meningocele/Encephalocele

Dural Herniation

▶ Temporal Bone Encephaloceles, Meningoceles, and
CSF Leak, Repair of
▶ Temporal Bone Meningocele/Encephalocele

Dural Sinus Thrombosis

▶ Magnetic Resonance Imaging, Otomastoiditis with
Venous Sinus Thrombosis

Dynamic Facial Nerve Reanimation

Kimberly A. Donnellan[1] and Daniel S. Alam[2]
[1]Department of Facial Plastic and Reconstructive
Surgery, IMC Otolaryngology Facial Plastic and
Reconstructive Surgery, Mobile, AL, USA
[2]Department of Facial Plastic and Reconstructive
Surgery, Head and Neck Institute, Cleveland Clinic
Foundation, Cleveland, OH, USA

Definitions

Epineurium – Layer of connective tissue that
surrounds the entire nerve.
Endoneurium – Layer of connective tissue that
surrounds the individual axons.
House-Brackmann grading scale – Scale between
I and VI is used to grade the function of the facial
nerve.
Neurorrhaphy – Suturing two ends of a nerve together.
Perineurium – Middle layer of connective tissue
encompassing a bundle of nerve fibers.
Wallerian degeneration – Process that occurs after
a nerve is cut or damaged in which the axon degen-
erates distal to the injury.

Introduction

Facial paralysis is a devastating problem that causes
both functional and psychological sequelae. The management is largely based on determining the etiology
and likelihood of spontaneous recovery. While reversible injuries are largely treated with emphasis on
eye care, irreversible injuries require a different
treatment paradigm. Reinnervation of the motor end
plates via dynamic procedures may be capable of
repair when evaluated within an 18–24-month time
frame. Injuries evaluated after 24 months will require
static techniques, muscle transpositions, or free flap
reconstruction.

Analysis of the face at presentation is accomplished
by use of the House-Brackmann grading scale. Additionally, the face is examined by splitting it into vertical thirds: upper face, midface, and lower face. The
primary goal of reanimation is centered around
attaining symmetry and restoring function. Specific

Dynamic Facial Nerve Reanimation, Fig. 1 Split 12 to 7 (Reproduced with permission by D. Alam Curr Opin Otolaryngol Head Neck Surg 18: 232–237)

a   b

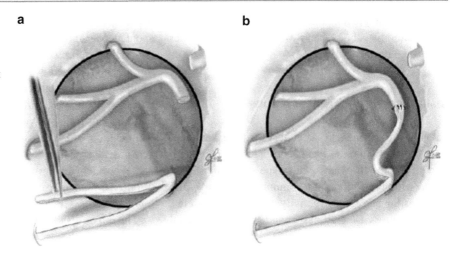

functional goals include the restoration of brow position to assist in visual defects and protecting the globe. Improvement of the nasolabial fold improves external nasal valve stenosis and oral competence. With proper selection of procedures, enhancements in breathing, eating, and speech articulation can be achieved.

Primary Neurorrhaphy

Primary neurorrhaphy can provide the patient with the best prognosis for full recovery in certain injuries. Injuries repaired proximal to the pes anserinus are likely to result in synkinesis. If the individual nerve branches can be identified and repaired distal to the pes anserinus, the outcome is usually without synkinesis. If possible, this coaptation should occur within 72 h prior to Wallerian degeneration. If repair can be completed in a timely fashion, nerve monitors can be utilized to identify the transected ends. Although some authors describe perineurium to perineurium repair, most authors agree that 2 or 3 well-placed 9-0 prolene sutures connecting epineurium to epineurium is sufficient (Fig. 1). These sutures must be placed without tension (Humphrey and Kreit 2008). Despite meticulous, timely repair, the best possible result is similar to House-Brackmann grade III.

Cable Grafting

If primary neurrhaphy is not plausible due to an inability to perform a tensionless primary neurorrhaphy,

cable grafting provides the next best repair. Multiple nerves have been described for use in cable grafting including sensory nerves (great auricular nerve, sural nerve, and medial or lateral antebrachial cutaneous nerves) and motor nerves (ansa cervicalis and nerve to the vastus lateralis). Although all nerves have been shown to have successful outcomes, a randomized double blind placebo rat study indicated that motor nerves had a better recovery than sensory nerves. Motor nerve regeneration was noted to be increased when nerves were approximated using a motor cable graft versus a sensory cable graft (Brenner et al. 2006). A subsequent study suggested that the larger size of typical motor nerve may explain the superior regeneration characteristics (Moradzadeh et al. 2008).

The best outcome following cable grafting, like primary neurorrhaphy, is similar to House-Brackmann grade III. The proximal and distal ends of the nerve need to be identifiable in order to attempt this repair; therefore, this technique is usually only plausible during the acute phase after injury – first 2 weeks. A tensionless repair is essential and is often done with the assistance of a microscope due to the need to use 9-0 prolene sutures (Hazin et al. 2009). Harvest of the donor nerve is largely based on the surgical field, length of nerve needed, and branching patterns. The great auricular nerve can often be harvested in the same operative field but may not be useful in cases of cancer. Harvesting the great auricular and sural nerves can provide lengths up to 10 and 40 cm, respectively. The advantage of the great auricular nerve is the use of one operative site; however, harvesting the sural nerve can be performed via a two-team approach and is easily accessible. The vastus lateralis is most useful when multiple branches need to be reinnervated.

Ipsilateral Nerve Transposition

Patients with permanent facial nerve paralysis without muscle atrophy are the ideal candidates for ipsilateral nerve transfer. In general, this type of repair should occur within the first 18–24 months of injury, and EMG testing can confirm activity of the facial muscles. The hypoglossal-facial nerve and masseteric-facial nerve are most commonly utilized as they do not require a second incision to harvest and have acceptable morbidities. Other nerves that have been reported include the recurrent laryngeal nerve, spinal accessory nerve, phrenic nerve, and ansa cervicalis.

Original harvest of the hypoglossal nerve involves complete transection which often causes problems with articulation and feeding. Modifications to minimize tongue morbidity include harvesting 50% of the superior aspect of the nerve and anastomosing that segment to the distal facial nerve branch via epineural neurorhaphy (Fig. 1) (Shipchandler et al. 2011). Additionally, the facial nerve can be drilled and released at the mastoid process to provide additional length, thus requiring a shorter segment of the hypoglossal nerve. These modifications have been shown to reproduce similar results with respect to facial paralysis while minimizing morbidity. The best results include rest symmetry and a House-Brackmann grade III with non-spontaneous volitional movement (Lin et al. 2009; Venail et al. 2009; Meltzer and Alam 2010). Advantages of using the masseteric nerve include adequate donor length, good size match, and no tongue morbidity. This reanimation was first reported in the 1990s and has gained recent popularity. One study shows that the anastomosis produces excellent results with symmetric voluntary smiles in eight out of ten patients (Faria et al. 2010). Many of these techniques are often used in combination.

Cross-Facial Nerve Grafting (CFNG)

The limitation of ipsilateral nerve transfer is the inability to achieve spontaneous movement. Contralateral nerve transfers, specifically the CFNG, can produce spontaneous movement; however, the literature is conflicting with respect to its efficacy. This procedure must be performed within the 2-year window post-injury while motor end plates are still viable. As stated earlier, it is often used in combination with other techniques. The ipsilateral nerve transfer is often used in combination with a cross-facial nerve graft (CFNG) to act as a "baby-sitter" nerve graft. The "baby-sitter" nerve ensures reinnervation of the affected muscles prior to permanent axonal injury while axons are growing through the CFNG (Terzis and Tzafetta 2009).

The major disadvantage is the unreliability of axon regrowth and the sacrifice of a branch of the facial nerve on the unaffected side in order to anastomosis it to a facial nerve branch on the affected side. The sural nerve is often utilized due to its length to serve as an interposition graft between the two sides (Lee and Hurvitz 2008).

Dynamic Muscle Transposition

After 2 years or more following injury, the native facial muscles can no longer be utilized due to nonviable or absent motor end plates; therefore, alternative muscles may be utilized for reanimation. Patients with congenital facial paralysis or those with large soft tissue defects are also candidates for muscle transposition. The temporalis, masseter, and anterior belly of the diagastric muscles have been described as adequate dynamic slings. The temporalis muscle is by far the most common muscle utilized with multiple modifications described over the years. Traditionally, the muscle belly of the temporalis muscle was transferred over the zygomatic arch to attach to the oral commissure providing volitional, nonspontaneous movement of the lower face. Although the movement was acceptable, the cosmetic outcome was often not ideal given the amount of bulk over the zygomatic arch and the temporal defect. Recent modifications include the orthodromic temporalis tendon transfer (TTT). This technique involves a transfacial or transoral dissection of the coronoid process and temporalis tendon. The temporalis tendon is then suspended at the level of the melolabial fold to address the lower face and to avoid the bulk over the zygomatic arch and the temporal defect. Further modifications include procedures to suspend the lip with fascia lata, palmaris longis tendon, or synthetic materials (Byrne et al. 2007).

Free Tissue Transfer

The use of microvascular free tissue transfer remains a viable option in certain patients. A lot of the variability in success in the literature is most likely secondary to patient selection. Free tissue transfer is most useful for permanent facial paralysis with a large soft tissue defect. The use of a CFNG is often used to innervate the free flap which results in spontaneous, volitional movement; however, innervations with the masseteric nerve have also been described. Frequently used free flaps include the pectoralis minor, latissimus dorsi, and the gracilis muscles with the latter being the most popular (Bae et al. 2006; Rosson and Redett 2008). Manktelow et al. has described spontaneous movement following free flap reconstruction which they attribute to cerebral plasticity, or cortical reorganization (Manktelow et al. 2006). Pediatric patients seem to do particularly well with gracilis free flap reconstruction. One theory is that the cortical reorganization resulting in spontaneous movement is even more efficient than with adult patients.

Cross-References

▶ Static Facial Paralysis Rehabilitation

References

Bae YC, Zucker RM, Manktelow RT et al (2006) A comparison of commissure excursion following gracilis muscle transplantation for facial paralysis using a cross face nerve graft versus the motor nerve to the masseter nerve. Plast Reconstr Surg 117:2407–2413

Brenner MJ, Hess JR, Myckatyn TM et al (2006) Repair of motor nerve gaps with sensory nerve inhibits regeneration in rats. Laryngoscope 116:1685–1692

Byrne PJ, Kim M, Boahene K et al (2007) Temporalis tendon transfer as part of a comprehensive approach to facial nerve reanimation. Arch Facial Plast Surg 9:234–241

Faria JC, Scopel GP, Ferreira MC (2010) Facial reanimation with masseteric nerve: babysitter or permanent procedure? Preliminary results. Ann Plast Surg 64:31–34

Hazin R, Azizzadeh B, Bhatti MT (2009) Medical and surgical management of facial nerve palsy. Curr Opin Ophthalmol 20:440–450

Humphrey CD, Kreit JD (2008) Nerve repair and cable grafting for facial paralysis. Facial Plast Surg 24:170–176

Lee EI, Hurvitz KA (2008) Cross-facial nerve graft: past and present. J Plast Reconstr Aesthet Surg 61:250–256

Lin V, Jacobson M, Dorion J et al (2009) Global assessment of outcomes after varying reinnervation techniques for patients with facial paralysis subsequent to acoustic neuroma excision. Otol Neurotol 30:408–413

Manktelow R, Tomat LR, Zuker RM, Chang M (2006) Smile reconstruction in adults with free muscle transfer innervated by the masseter motor nerve: effectiveness and cerebral adaptation. Plast Reconstr Surg 118:885–899

Meltzer NE, Alam DS (2010) Facial paralysis rehabilitation: state of the art. Curr Opin Otolaryngol Head Neck Surg 18:232–237

Moradzadeh A, Borschel GH, Luciano JP et al (2008) The impact of motor and sensory nerve architecture on nerve regeneration. Exp Neurol 212:370–376

Rosson GD, Redett RJ (2008) Facial palsy: anatomy, etiology, grading, and surgical treatment. J Reconstr Microsurg 24:379–389

Shipchandler T, Seth R, Alam D (2011) Split hypoglossal-facial nerve neurorraphy for treatment of the paralyzed face. Am J Otolaryngol 32(6):511–516

Terzis JK, Tzafetta K (2009) The babysitter procedure: minihypoglossal to facial nerve transfer and cross-facial nerve grafting. Plast Reconstr Surg 123:865–876

Venail F, Sabatier P, Mondain M et al (2009) Outcomes and complications of direct end-to-side facial-hypoglossal nerve anastomosis according to the modified May technique. J Neurosurg 110:786–791

Dysarthria

▶ Speech Development and Disorders

Dysfluency

▶ Fluency Disorders

Dysgeusia

Shelley Segrest Taylor
Department of Otolaryngology and Communicative Sciences, The University of Mississippi Medical Center, Jackson, MS, USA

Definition

The alteration in taste acuity resulting from radiation therapy to the head and neck.

Cross-References

▶ Dental Evaluation in Head and Neck Cancer Patient

Dyslexia

Carol Dinnes and Melissa Ghiringhelli
Massachusetts General Hospital, Revere and Chelsea
Healthcare Centers, Department of Speech-Language,
Swallowing Disorders and Reading Disabilities,
Revere/Chelsea, MA, USA

Synonyms

Literacy disorder; Reading disorder; Written language disorder

Definition

Dyslexia is a neurologically-based, specific learning disability marked by difficulty with acquisition of written language skills. Dyslexia's core deficit is the phonological component of language. Hallmark features are inaccurate and/or nonfluent word recognition, poor decoding, spelling and handwriting. Otherwise, neurologic and cognitive functions are intact. Individuals with Dyslexia present with an unexpected gap between their potential and performance in reading. Secondary consequences may include problems in reading comprehension, vocabulary growth, and background knowledge.

Epidemiology

Dyslexia is the most common form of Learning Disability which may occur in up to 17.4% of school-aged children. In grade 4, 38% of students read below the basic level of proficiency. Incidence is not more prevalent in males or females.

Clinical Features

Individuals with Dyslexia may present with delayed talking and difficulty in following directions, hearing the sound structure of language (phonological awareness), learning letters, phonics (sound/symbol correspondences), and high-frequency sight words. They may also present with varying degrees of deficit in decoding accuracy and rate, reading comprehension, spelling, note-taking, and handwriting. Additional difficulties *may* be seen in learning a foreign language or mathematics, social and organizational skills, and understanding concepts related to time or space. Dyslexia typically occurs in the presence of average intelligence and academic ability outside the realm of reading. Strengths are often apparent in areas of mechanical ability, music, art, drama, sports, or creative writing.

Tests

Dyslexia is diagnosed using standardized testing by a psychologist, neuropsychologist, or neurologist. Characteristics are often identified by reading specialists, speech-language pathologists, or other educators. Standardized test measures assess cognition as it compares to achievement in areas of reading and spelling. Test scores reflect children's performance in comparison to normative data for other children in the same age range. Reports of academic performance and spoken language testing are critical components of the evaluation. If the child is bilingual, testing is ideally completed in both languages.

Differential Diagnosis

Acquired Dyslexia is a disorder of reading following brain damage in individuals who were previously normal readers.

Developmental or congenital language deficits – Hallmark difficulties with comprehension and/or production with vocabulary/semantics, grammar/syntax, and/or social use of language/pragmatics.

Attention Deficit Disorder (ADD; ADHD) – Hallmark difficulties with sustaining attention and/or concentration.

Executive Dysfunction – Hallmark difficulties with organization, self-monitoring, planning, initiating, multitasking, and task completion.

Etiology

There are two main causes for dyslexia: heritable/neurological and environmental

Neurological – There are genetic influences that can cause dyslexia. Specifically, studies have identified certain chromosomes that can be passed down from parents to children. 23–65% of children who are identified with dyslexia also have a parent who was dyslexic. Four central anatomical differences have been identified in the brains of individuals with dyslexia: Planum Temporale Symmetry, Focal Abnormalities in Cerebral Areas, Larger Right Hemisphere, and High Interhemispheric Connectivity.

Environmental – Reading struggles may result from poor reading instruction, a disadvantaged language environment at home, or a combination of both. For these individuals, the neurological system is intact but does not function properly because it was not activated appropriately at an early age.

Treatment

Treatment for dyslexia must include multisensory presentation of specific concepts that are explicitly taught in a highly structured and systematic manner. Instruction must also include regular review of previously presented concepts. Skills to be developed include phonological processing, sound/symbol correspondences as well as rules of syllable structure and spelling. Structural analysis (prefix/stem/suffix), reading fluency, and comprehension are also targets essential to remediation.

Cross-References

▶ Dyslexia
▶ Phonological Awareness
▶ Pragmatics/Social Language Function
▶ Syntax
▶ Vocabulary/Semantics/Content

References

Flynn JM, Rahbar MH (1994) Prevalence of reading failure in boys compared with girls. Psychology in the Schools 31:66–70

Galaburda AM, Sherman GF, Rosen GD, Aboitiz F, Geschwind N (1985) Developmental dyslexia: four consecutive patients with cortical anomalies. Ann Neurol 18(2):222–233

http://www.interdys.org/ewebeditpro5/upload/Definition.pdf

http://www.readingresource.net/causesofdyslexia.html

Kaufman LN, Hook PE (1996) The dyslexia puzzle: putting the pieces together, publication of the New England branch of the international dyslexia association

Lyon GR, Shaywitz SE, Shaywitz BA (2003) A definition of dyslexia. Ann Dyslexia 53:1–14

Shaywitz SE, Shaywitz BA, Fletcher JM, Escobar MD (1990) Prevalence of reading disability in boys and girls: results of the Connecticut longitudinal study. J Am Med Assoc 264:998–1002

Dysphagia

Cathy L. Lazarus
Thyroid Head and Neck Cancer Research Center, Thyroid Head and Neck Cancer Foundation, Department of Otolaryngology, Beth Israel Medical Center, New York, NY, USA

Definition

Dysphagia is a term to describe difficulty in swallowing. It is derived from the Greek *dys*, meaning bad or abnormal, and *phago*, meaning eat. Disorders of swallowing occur in the oropharyngeal and/or the esophageal phases. The oropharyngeal phase can be further divided into the oral preparatory, oral, and pharyngeal phases (Logemann 1998), which overlap in timing, based on the type of bolus of food or liquid being swallowed (Martin-Harris et al. 2005). Dysphagia is typically considered a symptom, as it is the result of disease. But the consequence of dysphagia can often include dehydration, malnutrition, aspiration, and death (Altman et al. 2010). Aspiration is often a symptom and sequela of dysphagia and can occur before, during, and/or after the swallow (Logemann 1988). Aspiration is often silent in is associated with pneumonia (Martin et al. 1994; Lundy et al. 1999).

Epidemiology

Swallowing disorders can occur across the lifespan. Dysphagia can occur in the infant and pediatric populations from a variety of causes, including congenital anatomic abnormalities of the oral cavity, nasopharynx, and larynx, as well as central and peripheral nervous system damage. Respiratory and cardiac problems can also result in dysphagia, resulting in reduced endurance and poor coordination of breathing and swallowing (Arvedson and Lefton-Greif 1996). In the adult population, swallowing impairment has been reported in 23% of the healthy adult primary care population (Wilkins et al. 2007) and 38% in the healthy elderly (Roy et al. 2007). Incidence of dysphagia in the stroke population has been found to be as high as 65% (Daniels et al. 1998). Progressive neurogenic disease such as Parkinson's, multiple sclerosis, amyotrophic lateral sclerosis, myasthenia gravis, and post-polio can cause dysphagia, as well as dystrophies and myopathies, all of which can affect oral, pharyngeal, and esophageal phases. Dysphagia can also occur with systemic disease, such as scleroderma, dermatomyositis, and Sjögren's disease, primarily affecting the pharyngeal phase of swallowing. Esophageal abnormalities within the cervical esophagus can result from such structural/anatomic abnormalities such as cricopharyngeal bar, web, stenosis, and achalasia. In addition, motor disorders within the esophageal body such as dysmotility and achalasia can also result in swallowing impairment. Anatomic/structural disorders of the esophagus can also result in dysphagia, including webs and strictures, as well as tumors and foreign bodies. Esophageal reflux disease can also result in dysphagia.

Dysphagia is often seen in individuals who have become weak and medically debilitated during hospitalization. Normal changes in oropharyngeal swallowing in the healthy elderly can predispose them to dysphagia if medically compromised (Robbins et al. 1992). Increased length of stay has been found in hospitalized patients with a variety of diseases, but most commonly associated with fluid or electrolyte disorder, esophageal disease, stroke, aspiration pneumonia, urinary tract infection, and congestive heart failure (Altman et al. 2010). Treatment of surgery and chemotherapy for head and neck cancer frequently results in dysphagia (Lazarus 2000, 2009).

Clinical Features

Impairment in swallowing can occur during any of the phases of swallowing. Oral preparatory and oral phase impairment can include reduced lip closure, reduced lingual anchoring of the bolus against the palate, reduced ability to manipulate and propel the bolus through the oral cavity, reduced lingual control, strength, speed, and range of motion, as well as reduced lateral motion of the jaw for chewing (Lazarus 2000). Reduced lip closure can result in spillage of material out of the mouth. Reduced lingual functioning can result in impaired pressure generation on the bolus for propulsion through the oral cavity, resulting in oral residue, which can potentially spill into the pharynx and be aspirated after the swallow. Lack of sensory awareness of the bolus within the oral cavity can result in delayed oral initiation of lingual movement. This is often seen with acute and progressive neurogenic impairment, such as dementia, Parkinson's, and traumatic brain injury. However, oral sensory impairment can also be seen after oral cancer surgery and radiotherapy. Motor impairment can also result in lack of or impairment in lingual movement and can be seen in patients with a variety of diagnoses.

Once material is propelled into the pharynx, a pharyngeal motor response is triggered. This motor response is comprised of a series of complex neuromuscular events that include velopharyngeal closure, tongue base retraction to the pharyngeal wall, sequential pharyngeal contraction and pharyngeal shortening, hyolaryngeal elevation and anterior movement, laryngeal vestibule and glottic closure, and upper esophageal sphincter (UES) opening (Logemann 1988). This motor response can be delayed or absent in dysphagic individuals. An absent or delayed triggering of the pharyngeal motor response can result from central or peripheral nervous system damage. In addition, both absent and delayed triggering of the pharyngeal motor response can result in aspiration before the swallow, as the airway is open for breathing and unprotected at this time point. In addition, impairment of lingual function, specifically, reduced lingual range of motion and control, can result in spillage of material into the pharynx before the pharyngeal motor response has triggered, resulting in aspiration before the swallow. Once the pharyngeal motor response occurs, any or all of the various neuromuscular events can be impaired. These can include weakness or reduction in range of motion of the palate, tongue base, pharyngeal constrictors, hyoid, larynx, floor of mouth musculature, and cricopharyngeus muscle, all of which contribute to reduced bolus pressures and reduced clearance through the pharynx and residue which can be aspirated after the swallow. Resection of tissue following treatment for head and neck cancer can also result in reduced valving, and pressure generation within the oral cavity and pharynx and can also result in pharyngeal residue, which can potentially be aspirated after the swallow (Lazarus 2000). Aspiration during the swallow occurs with impairment of glottic and supraglottic (i.e., laryngeal vestibule) closure (Lundy et al. 1999).

Tests

Oropharyngeal swallowing is typically assessed utilizing videofluoroscopy, the modified barium swallow (MBS) (Logemann 1988) or flexible endoscopic evaluation of swallowing (FEES) with or without sensory testing (Leder and Murray 2008). The MBS study examines oropharyngeal swallow physiology, including oral and pharyngeal phase and triggering of the pharyngeal motor response, and can screen the esophageal phase functioning in the lateral, anterior-posterior, and oblique planes. For this exam, the patient is initially seated upright in the lateral plane in order to identify the physiologic swallow disorders and bolus flow during the swallow. Once the physiologic swallow disorders are identified, therapeutic strategies are introduced during the exam to improve swallow safety and/or efficiency, i.e., eliminate aspiration and reduce residue, respectively. Presence, location, amount, and symmetry of oral and pharyngeal residue can be observed in the anterior-posterior plane, as can vocal fold functioning during phonation. Screening of the esophagus is typically accomplished in the upright anterior-posterior and oblique planes. The FEES examination provides excellent visualization of the pharynx and larynx for identification of any structural abnormalities and impairment in laryngeal functioning for breathing and phonation. A flexible laryngoscope is passed transnasally into the upper pharynx in order to view structures and function during swallowing of color-tinged liquids and foods. The FEES procedure examines pharyngeal phase swallow functioning and can also assess triggering of the pharyngeal motor response. Both instrumental assessment techniques utilize various bolus volumes and viscosities to allow for identification of abnormal swallow physiology, results of impaired swallow functioning, including residue and aspiration, as well as utility of therapeutic strategies (Lazarus 2000; Leder and Murray 2008). Manometry can also be utilized to assess oral, pharyngeal, and esophageal pressures generated during swallowing (McConnel 1988). This technique can be utilized alone or paired with fluoroscopy to correlate pressure generation with bolus clearance during the swallow (McConnel 1988).

Evaluation of swallowing should include a thorough history, including symptoms and their onset, frequency, and occurrence, type of oral intake, past medical and surgical history, medications, prior assessment of and treatment for dysphagia, and any medical sequela, such as pneumonia or dehydration. An oral mechanism exam, which assesses the speed, range, precision, coordination, timing, and strength of vocal tract musculature during isolated and rapidly repeated/alternated nonspeech and speech tasks (Lazarus 2000), should be included in the evaluation to provide information on cranial nerve functioning. A bedside or clinical swallow assessment should include an oral mechanism exam and should provide accurate information about the oral preparatory and oral phases of swallowing. In addition, an approximation of the overall timing of the oropharyngeal swallow should be determined, as should an approximation of laryngeal motion during the swallow. Symptoms of dysphagia, such as aspiration, can be observed if they are overt, such as coughing, throat-clearing, and wet gurgly voice. However, aspiration may not be identified on clinical exam since it is often silent both in the neurogenic and treated head and neck cancer populations (Daniels et al. 1998; Lundy et al. 1999; Lazarus 2000). Presence of residue, another symptom of dysphagia, can be inferred from the occurrence of repeat dry swallows. A palpably sluggish laryngeal ascent and descent during the swallow can indicate a weak pharyngeal motor response and resultant reduced bolus clearance through the pharynx. Abnormal volitional cough, abnormal gag reflex, presence of dysarthria and dysphonia, cough after trial swallows, and voice change after trial swallows have been found to be factors associated with aspiration on clinical examination (Daniels et al. 1998).

Treatment

Behavioral treatment for dysphagia should address the physiologic swallow abnormalities identified with instrumental assessment (Lazarus 2000). Some treatment strategies are compensatory in nature, such as modifying posture or bolus type. Others are nonswallow exercises designed to improve range, rate, strength, precision, and coordination of the muscles involved in swallowing. Other behavioral treatments include swallow maneuvers, which are designed to alter swallow physiology.

Nonswallow exercises target the lips, tongue, jaw, palate, and larynx. Exercises to improve range and strength for lip closure are indicated with impairment in lip function. Jaw range of motion exercises can improve jaw range and function for chewing. For lingual impairment, exercises focus on improving lingual control, strength, rate, and range of movement, including range of motion of the tongue base. In addition, swallow maneuvers designed to improve tongue base posterior motion and pharyngeal constrictor motion include the tongue-hold and the effortful swallow, the former of which is designed to improve anterior motion of the pharyngeal constrictors and the latter of which is designed to improve tongue base retraction during swallowing (Lazarus 2000). The tongue-hold maneuver involves anchoring the tongue tip between the teeth or gum while swallowing. This maneuver situates the tongue base more anteriorly, resulting in a compensatory anterior movement of the pharyngeal constrictors during the swallow. The effortful swallow is a maneuver that is designed to improve tongue base posterior motion during swallowing. Patients are instructed to swallow hard, squeezing hard with the throat muscles (Lazarus et al. 2002). This maneuver has been found to improve pharyngeal pressure generation within the upper pharynx for improved bolus clearance within this region (Lazarus et al. 2002). In addition, a pharyngeal squeeze maneuver is also designed to improve pharyngeal contraction for swallowing (Fuller et al. 2009). In this maneuver, the patient says a forceful "eee" in order to effect increased pharyngeal muscle contraction. The supraglottic

swallow is a maneuver designed to improve glottic closure before and during swallowing. This maneuver requires a breath hold before and during the swallow. The super supraglottic swallow maneuver is indicated for those individuals with impaired airway entrance closure, as this maneuver should result in anterior motion of the arytenoids for contact with the epiglottic base before the swallow triggers, in order to provide additional airway protection for those individuals who are penetrating material into the laryngeal vestibule (Lazarus 2000). The super supraglottic swallow requires a tighter breath hold in order to establish laryngeal vestibule closure before the swallow. The Mendelsohn maneuver is designed to improve width and duration of upper esophageal sphincter opening by improving extent and duration of hyolaryngeal motion during the swallow (Lazarus 2000). This maneuver is helpful for those individuals with dysphagia who demonstrate reduced hyolaryngeal motion and reduced opening within the UES region. The Mendelsohn maneuver can also improve overall coordination of the pharyngeal motor response. To perform this maneuver, individuals are instructed to swallow and prolong the swallow at the maximum laryngeal height, thereby increasing the duration and extent of laryngeal motion and width and duration of UES opening. The Shaker exercise is also designed to improve laryngeal motion and UES opening (Lazarus 2000). This exercise involves a head lift which is a suprahyoid muscle strengthening exercise. Other nonswallow treatment strategies found to improve hyolaryngeal motion for swallowing include use of voice (i.e., Lee Silverman Voice Treatment [LSVT]) and respiratory strength training (i.e., expiratory muscle strength training) techniques (El Sharkawi et al. 2002; Sapienza 2008). The LSVT voice exercise program has also been found to improve oral phase swallow functioning (El Sharkawi et al. 2002).

Behavioral strategies to improve swallowing also include techniques to heighten sensory awareness and improve lingual initiation and triggering of the pharyngeal motor response (Lazarus 2000). These strategies include introducing boluses of varying tastes, textures, and temperatures as a preswallow sensory stimulus. Cold, sour, and carbonation have been found to improve initiation of lingual activity and triggering of the pharyngeal motor response, as well as improve the temporal and durational aspects of the swallow (Lazarus 2000). Thermal-tactile stimulation is a technique that has been found to improve triggering of the pharyngeal motor response in those patients with delayed or absent triggering. This technique involves icing a size 00 laryngeal mirror and stroking the base of the faucial arches (Lazarus 2000). Bolus modification, such as altering bolus volume and viscosity, can also heighten sensory awareness and improve lingual initiation and triggering of the pharyngeal swallowing, with slightly larger volumes and more viscous boluses often improving safety and efficiency. This is because the oropharyngeal swallow can accommodate to volume and viscosity, with systematic shifts in airway closure, velopharyngeal closure, and cricopharyngeal opening during the pharyngeal motor response (Lazarus 2000).

Neuromuscular electrical stimulation (NMES) is a technique that has recently been employed to improve swallowing, particularly in those individuals with severe swallow impairment, including reduced pharyngeal motor response and impaired laryngeal motion during swallowing. This technique involves the delivery of therapeutic electrical stimulation to facilitate muscle contraction through surface electrode placement in the region of the submental or thyrohyoid muscles (Ludlow 2010). NMES has been found to lower the hyolaryngeal complex during swallowing, placing the airway entrance at greater risk of penetration of material, particularly in dysphagic patients (Ludlow 2010).

Use of postures can compensate for a physiologic swallow impairment by changing bolus flow during the swallow (Lazarus 2000). Gravity often assists with bolus flow when postures are used. Head back posture is useful for improving transit and clearance of the bolus through the oral cavity. This posture is particularly useful for those patients with reduced lingual functioning, as in dysarthric patients and surgically treated oral cancer patients. Chin tuck posture is useful for those patients with delayed triggering of the pharyngeal motor response, as well as those with airway closure problems, as this posture results in a more posterior tongue base position, a wider vallecular space and a narrowed airway entrance (i.e., arytenoids situated closer to the epiglottic base), all of which assist with providing extra airway protection during the swallow (Lazarus 2000). In addition, chin tuck posture situates the tongue base closer to the pharyngeal wall and can improve bolus clearance through this region on thicker consistencies.

Head rotation posture is useful for unilateral pharyngeal weakness, as it can improve pressure generation within the pharynx and also channel the bolus through the unaffected side of the pharynx (Lazarus 2000). This posture is also useful for those patients with reduced airway closure due to a unilateral vocal fold paralysis or paresis, as well as vertical laryngectomy. In both cases, patients are instructed to turn the head to the paralyzed or operated side to close off and protect the airway, as well as to channel the flow of material through the undamaged/nonsurgical side of the larynx and pharynx (Lazarus 2000). Head tilt posture is useful for unilateral tongue weakness or resection (Lazarus 2000). The patient tilts the head towards the undamaged/nonsurgical side of the tongue so that the tongue can better control the bolus. Lying down posture is reserved for those patients in whom pharyngeal residue cannot be eliminated with other postures and/or maneuvers and who are chronically aspirating after the swallow. In this posture, which can be assessed with a MBS study, utilizing the fluoroscopy table in the horizontal position, the residue sits on the lateral pharyngeal wall and is reswallowed and cleared prior to the patient sitting upright (Lazarus 2000).

Postures are often combined to maximize bolus flow and safety (Lazarus 2000). The head rotation and chin tuck posture are often combined, with the combination improving bolus flow and airway protection. Head tilt and head back posture can often improve bolus transit and clearance through the oral cavity. In addition, postures and maneuvers can also maximize swallow efficiency and safety (Lazarus 2000). The chin tuck and super supraglottic swallow often afford the greatest degree of airway protection. The effortful swallow and chin tuck posture can maximize tongue base to pharyngeal wall contact with a resultant improved bolus clearance through the upper pharynx.

Palatal prosthetics can improve oral and pharyngeal phase swallowing functioning. Three types of palatal prostheses include palatal lift, palatal obturator, and palatal lowering/augmentation (Lazarus 2000). A palatal lift is designed to assist with velar elevation and velopharyngeal closure with neurologic impairment of the palate. A palatal obturator is designed to occlude the velopharyngeal port when there is inadequate velar tissue, as in a palatal resection for treatment of cancer, or in a congenital abnormality as in cleft palate. Both the lift and obturator prostheses are designed to improve velopharyngeal closure to reduce the risk of nasopharyngeal reflux during swallowing, as well as improve bolus clearance through the upper pharynx. A palatal lowering/augmentation prosthesis effectively lowers the palatal vault to improve tongue to palate contact for those with partial or total glossectomy or those with dysarthria severe enough to restrict lingual vertical range of motion. This type of prosthesis can improve bolus control and propulsion of material through the oral cavity (Lazarus 2000).

Compensatory strategies during meals can include modifying bolus volume, such as use of smaller boluses, and modifying bolus consistency, such as softening the diet when pharyngeal clearance issues are present. For those patients who have airway protection problems or have delayed triggering of the pharyngeal swallow and are aspirating on thin liquids, thickening liquids can eliminate aspiration while treatment focuses on addressing the underlying physiologic swallow impairment. Slowing the pace of eating/feeding can also improve swallow safety by allowing time to reswallow and clear oral and pharyngeal residue. Use of a liquid wash can also clear residue from the oral cavity and pharynx. Patients who are using swallow maneuvers when eating and drinking may fatigue from the effort required to perform these maneuvers. Thus, they may benefit from eating smaller, more frequent meals to improve intake and nutrition.

Some patients cannot manage an oral diet due to the severity of their dysphagia. Non-oral nutritional means can include nasogastric tube placement, gastrostomy, jejunostomy, or hyperalimentation. Some patients may be able to receive primary nutrition via non-oral means but may also be eating or drinking for pleasure or with swallow therapy. Not all patients are candidates for direct swallow treatment, such as those with severe cognitive impairment. For these patients, management decisions should be based on clinical and instrumental assessment results, and compensatory strategies are typically utilized, as described above.

Medical/surgical management of dysphagia can include vocal fold medialization, arytenoid adduction, and thyroplasty to improve airway protection by improving glottic closure (Eibling and Boyd 1997). Management of upper esophageal sphincter dysfunction can include dilation, cricopharyngeal myotomy, or botulinum toxin therapy (Eibling and Boyd 1997).

In cases of severe and intractable aspiration, laryngotracheal separation or total laryngectomy can be performed (Eibling and Boyd 1997).

Conclusion

Dysphagia can be a life-threatening problem that can result in malnutrition, dehydration, and medical consequences, including death. A swallowing evaluation should incorporate an instrumental examination of oropharyngeal and esophageal functioning to identify the physiologic swallow impairment. Overall medical status must be incorporated into the treatment plan. A multidisciplinary team should be involved in the management of dysphagia. The overall goal of dysphagia therapy is to maximize swallow efficiency and safety. An additional goal is for the patient to achieve adequate nutrition and hydration by mouth with the safest and highest level diet tolerated.

References

Altman KW, Yu GP et al (2010) Consequence of dysphagia in the hospitalized patient: impact on prognosis and hospital resources. Arch Otolaryngol Head Neck Surg 136(8): 784–789

Arvedson JC, Lefton-Greif MA (1996) Anatomy, physiology, and development of feeding. Semin Speech Lang 17(4): 261–268

Daniels SK, Brailey K et al (1998) Aspiration in patients with acute stroke. Arch Phys Med Rehabil 79(1):14–19

Eibling DE, Boyd EM (1997) Rehabilitation of lower cranial nerve deficits. Otolaryngol Clin North Am 30(5):865–875

El Sharkawi A, Ramig L et al (2002) Swallowing and voice effects of Lee Silverman Voice Treatment (LSVT): a pilot study. J Neurol Neurosurg Psychiatry 72(1):31–36

Fuller SC, Leonard R et al (2009) Validation of the pharyngeal squeeze maneuver. Otolaryngol Head Neck Surg 140(3): 391–394

Lazarus CL (2000) Management of swallowing disorders in head and neck cancer patients: optimal patterns of care. Semin Speech Lang 21(4):293–309

Lazarus CL (2009) Effects of chemoradiotherapy on voice and swallowing. Curr Opin Otolaryngol Head Neck Surg 17(3):172–178

Lazarus C, Logemann JA et al (2002) Effects of voluntary maneuvers on tongue base function for swallowing. Folia Phoniatr Logop 54(4):171–176

Leder SB, Murray JT (2008) Fiberoptic endoscopic evaluation of swallowing. Phys Med Rehabil Clin N Am 19(4):787–801, viii–ix

Logemann JA (1988) Swallowing physiology and pathophysiology. Otolaryngol Clin North Am 21:613–623

Logemann JA (1998) Evaluation and treatment of swallowing disorders, 2nd edn. Austin, TX: Pro-Ed

Ludlow CL (2010) Electrical neuromuscular stimulation in dysphagia: current status. Curr Opin Otolaryngol Head Neck Surg 18(3):159–164

Lundy DS, Smith C et al (1999) Aspiration: cause and implications. Otolaryngol Head Neck Surg 120(4):474–478

Martin BJ, Corlew MM et al (1994) The association of swallowing dysfunction and aspiration pneumonia. Dysphagia 9(1):1–6

Martin-Harris B, Michel Y et al (2005) Physiologic model of oropharyngeal swallowing revisited. Otolaryngol Head Neck Surg 133(2):234–240

McConnel FM (1988) Analysis of pressure generation and bolus transit during pharyngeal swallowing. Laryngoscope 98(1):71–78

Robbins J, Hamilton JW et al (1992) Oropharyngeal swallowing in normal adults of different ages. Gastroenterology 103(3):823–829

Roy N, Stemple J et al (2007) Dysphagia in the elderly: preliminary evidence of prevalence, risk factors, and socioemotional effects. Ann Otol Rhinol Laryngol 116(11): 858–865

Sapienza CM (2008) Respiratory muscle strength training applications. Curr Opin Otolaryngol Head Neck Surg 16(3): 216–220

Wilkins T, Gillies RA et al (2007) The prevalence of dysphagia in primary care patients: a HamesNet Research Network study. J Am Board Fam Med 20(2):144–150

Dysphonia

▶ Hoarseness and Pediatric Voice Disorders
▶ Larynx, Neurological Disorders

Dysplasia

Steven J. Frampton and Emma V. King
Poole Hospital NHS Foundation Trust, Poole, Dorset, UK
Cancer Sciences Division, University of Southampton, Southampton, Hampshire, UK

Definition

Dysplasia is a pathological term used to describe the microscopic appearance of a maturation abnormality.

Cross-References

▶ Field Cancerization

Dysport

▶ Botulinum Toxin

E

Ear Atresia

▶ Congenital Aural Atresia

Ear Canal Wall Replacement/ Reconstruction

John T. McElveen Jr. and Calhoun D. Cunningham III
Carolina Ear & Hearing Clinic, P.C., Raleigh,
NC, USA

Synonyms

Canal wall reconstruction; Mastoid obliteration;
Reversible canal wall down mastoidectomy

Definitions

Cholesteatoma: Skin-lined cyst involving the middle
   ear and mastoid.
Tympanomastoidectomy: Surgical technique to
   remove cholesteatoma and repair the ear drum.
Intact canal wall surgery: Surgical procedure that
   maintains the integrity of the posterior external
   auditory canal.
Canal wall down: Surgical procedure that removes the
   posterior canal wall and connects the mastoid cavity
   to the external auditory canal.
Mastoid obliteration: Surgical technique that fills in
   the mastoid cavity.

Introduction

Canal wall down mastoidectomy is an effective treatment option in the management of cholesteatoma.
Controversy remains, however, regarding how to
address the posterior canal wall. Removing the canal
wall greatly improves successful elimination of middle
ear and mastoid disease, but is not without disadvantages. Canal wall down surgery results in an exteriorized mastoid cavity that tends to accumulate moisture
and debris and can predispose to otorrhea. This
necessitates periodic cleaning of the mastoid cavity
and possibly water restrictions on the part of the
patient. These patients may also experience a "caloric
effect" causing dizziness and vertigo when the ear is
cleaned due to stimulation of the exposed lateral
semicircular canal.

Preserving the posterior canal wall, such as with
intact canal wall surgery, preserves the normal anatomic dimensions of the middle ear thereby improving
hearing results with ossicular reconstruction. The need
for periodic cleaning of the mastoid cavity is eliminated as is the need for water precautions, which is
especially important for pediatric patients. Preservation of the posterior canal wall, however, may impair
direct visualization of some areas within the middle ear
and epitympanum during surgery, potentially leaving
residual disease.

Over the years, a variety of techniques have been
developed to either temporarily displace the posterior
canal wall during cholesteatoma surgery, or to reconstruct it following disease removal.

S.E. Kountakis (ed.), *Encyclopedia of Otolaryngology, Head and Neck Surgery*, DOI 10.1007/978-3-642-23499-6,
© Springer-Verlag Berlin Heidelberg 2013

Canal Wall Reconstruction/Displacement Techniques

In 1963, Schnee first reported on his experience with temporarily displacing the posterior canal wall to facilitate exposure for tympanic membrane grafting.

Lapidot and Brandow (1966) used a small cutting burr to create perforations in the posterior canal wall. The superior osteotomy was made at the level of the superior buttress, and the inferior osteotomy was made at the bottom of the ear canal. A horizontal osteotomy connecting the two vertical cuts was made 1–2 mm lateral to the mastoid segment of the facial nerve. The posterior canal wall with its intact ear canal skin was displaced anteriorly, exposing the ossicular chain and posterior tympanic cavity.

The technique of Richards (1972) differed only slightly from that of Lapidot and Brandow (1966) in that placement of his superior osteotomy started anterior to the head of the malleus; otherwise, the procedure was essentially the same.

In 1969, Gerlach temporarily removed the bony ear canal wall in cases of extensive cholesteatoma. Using small cutting burrs to create his osteotomies, the superior osteotomy was anterior to the head of the malleus and the inferior osteotomy was toward the floor of the ear canal. The bony ear canal was replaced and fixed with Histoacryl glue, and a superiorly based fascia–muscle flap was placed behind the canal wall.

Wullstein (1972) developed the osteoplastic epitympanotomy approach using a 0.3–0.4-mm diamond burr to create a groove in the anterior tympanic spine (Wullstein 1972). Her inferior cut appeared to be in the region of the incudal fossa. The bone was replaced and covered with bone pate and fibrin glue. Fascia was used to cover the bone flap.

Feldmann (1978) used an oscillating saw to create four angled cuts, the superior cuts were above the short process of the malleus and the inferior cuts were along the inferior aspect of the facial recess. By angling the cuts, he was able to create grooves in the posterior canal wall, allowing him to replace the canal wall without other means of fixation.

Mercke (1987) had combined Feldmann's (1978) technique with a musculoperiosteal Palva flap and obliterated the epitympanic space with bone chips. Babighian's (1993) approach involved making canal cuts with a Feldmann saw to temporarily remove the posterior canal wall. The superior cut was made anterior to the head of the malleus and the inferior cut along the inferior aspect of the facial recess. The bone was removed, replaced orthotopically, and fixed using ionomeric cement.

In contradistinction to the Babighian technique, the reversible canal wall down technique developed by McElveen beveled the canal cuts in such a manner that the posterior surface of the canal segment was wider than the anterior segment, minimizing the likelihood of the segment becoming displaced anteriorly into the external auditory canal. In addition, in suitable cases, the reversible canal wall down approach was combined with attempts to preserve the ossicular chain when the cholesteatoma had not engulfed the ossicles.

In 2005, Gantz et al. reported on canal wall reconstruction tympanomastoidectomy with mastoid obliteration. They described their technique of posterior canal wall removal using a microsagittal saw in order to increase intraoperative exposure for cholesteatoma removal as well as removal of any diseased and/or nitrogen-absorbing mastoid epithelium. Using their technique, the canal wall was then replaced and the attic and mastoid were isolated from the middle ear space using a combination of bone chips and bone pâté to obliterate the mastoid. This technique was felt to improve the outcomes of chronic ear surgeries for cholesteatoma by enhancing the surgeon's ability to remove cholesteatoma through improved exposure, as well as preventing the development of postoperative retraction pockets by obliterating the mastoid and epitympanum and removing the nitrogen-absorbing mastoid epithelium. In long-term follow-up of their patients, 98.5% of ears remained safe without evidence of recurrence.

In addition to reversible canal wall reconstruction and mastoid obliteration, various reports describe the use of cartilage to reconstruct the posterior canal wall (Weber and Gantz 1998; Dornhoffer 2004; Barbara 2008; Pennings and Cremers 2009). For large defects or total canal wall reconstruction, cymba cartilage can be successfully employed to reconstruct the canal wall due to its rigidity and natural curvature. Cartilage is readily available, has excellent biocompatibility, and is versatile and easily shaped.

Mastoid Obliteration Techniques

A variety of methods, both medical and surgical, have been suggested for the management of the chronically discharging mastoid cavity. The surgical alternatives have included: (1) lining the mastoid with skin grafts (Kerrison 1930; Lempert 1949; House 1949); (2) filling the cavity with various materials such as bone (Schiller 1963; Shea and Gardner 1970), cartilage (Wullstein 1962), fat (Kuhweide and van Deninse 1960), acrylic (Mahoney 1962), and recently hydroxylapatite (Hartwein and Hoermann 1990); (3) lining or obliterating the mastoid cavity with pedicled soft tissue flaps, either at the time of mastoidectomy or during revision. We focus on the development of soft tissue ablation of the mastoid cavity.

The first use of a pedicled tissue flap after mastoidectomy was reported by Passow in 1908, who used a temporalis musculoperiosteal flap to control persistent fistulae in two patients. In 1910, Gabe reported his experience with this procedure in 28 patients. Mosher (1911) independently described a superiorly based musculoperiosteal flap derived from postauricular soft tissue that he used in an attempt to "shorten the healing, to prevent deformity, and to lessen the frequency of secondary operations." Mastoid obliteration was later advanced by Kisch (1928) who presented three cases with conservative mastoid surgery and a temporalis muscle flap to the Royal Society of Medicine in 1928. Despite successful reports of Kisch's technique in both England and the United States (Almour 1930; Mill 1930), the otologic community was reluctant to adopt this new procedure. In 1935, Popper introduced a periosteal flap with a broad base directed toward the auricle in an effort to provide a viable lining for the mastoid cavity. Meurman and Ojala (1949) incorporated the muscle with the periosteum in an inferiorly pedicled flap designed to obliterate the mastoid tip. In spite of these independent reports of soft tissue mastoid ablation as an alternative to a large open cavity, these methods were not generally accepted at the time.

Interest in mastoid obliteration was revived in 1958, when Rambo described the use of a temporalis muscle flap followed by fenestration of the lateral semicircular canal. Thorburn (1960) suggested that Rambo's obliterative technique might be combined with a Wullstein tympanoplasty procedure, but this idea was rejected by Rambo. Richtnér (1960) later combined mastoid obliteration using skin and muscle flaps with a Wullstein type IV tympanoplasty and Austin (1962) further advanced middle ear reconstruction in combination with mastoid obliteration using a temporalis muscle flap. In 1961, Guilford proposed combining a musculoperiosteal flap as described by Meurman and Ojala with Rambo's temporalis muscle flap to provide a more complete obliteration of the cavity. During this same period, Tauno Palva (1962a) began using a postauricular flap for complete mastoid obliteration in children and later for the reconstruction of the ear canal and middle ear in adults (1962b, 1963). Palva developed an anteriorly pedicled musculoperiosteal flap with a broad base toward the meatus. This flap was similar to that described by Popper (1935), except that Palva included all of the subcutaneous soft tissues with the periosteum. The anterior broad base of this flap provided a rich vascular supply and preserved the innervation to the muscle. These design advantages have made the Palva flap particularly useful in obliterating the mastoid cavity.

One of the problems with soft tissue mastoid obliteration techniques was the potential for atrophy of the soft tissue over time. As a result, interest developed in using bone to obliterate mastoid cavities. Several authors have described techniques for harvesting autogenous bone chips or bone pate to obliterate or reconstruct the canal wall following primary or revision canal wall down mastoid surgeries (Shea and Gardner 1970; Palva 1975; Mills 1987). These techniques require the harvesting of cortical bone posterior to the mastoid cavity using a bone pâté collector. After complete exoneration of any diseased mastoid air cells, the bone pate is compressed into the mastoid defect to obliterate the cavity and reconstruct the canal wall. It is important that the bone pate be covered with either fascia or a local soft tissue flap at the time of reconstruction. Although there is a risk of reabsorption, with proper technique, Roberson and colleagues (2003) reported a take rate of 95%. Bone pate is an excellent resource for mastoid obliteration as it is readily available and has excellent biocompatibility resulting in osteoinduction and osteoneogenesis.

Interest has also been expressed in the use of synthetic materials such as hydroxyapatite cement (Grote 1998). Although readily available and easy to work with, these materials demonstrate a higher rate of extrusion or tissue breakdown over time and may require coverage with a vascularized tissue flap.

Conclusion

Maintenance of the posterior canal wall facilitates normal water activities for the patient and avoids the need for periodic cleansing of the mastoid cavity. A variety of techniques have proven successful in temporarily displacing the posterior canal wall during chronic ear surgery. In addition, other techniques have been developed to reconstruct the posterior canal wall in patients with an exteriorized mastoid cavity. The use of foreign bodies to reconstruct the canal wall may result in tissue breakdown over the implant with time. In light of this, soft tissue or autogenous cartilage or bone techniques are preferable and have proven to be effective with long-term follow-up.

References

Almour R (1930) A method for the repair of persisting postauricular openings. Laryngoscope 40:799

Austin DF, Sanabria F (1962) Mastoidplasty. Arch Otolaryngol Head Neck Surg 76:414–421

Babighian G (1993) Posterior and attic wall 'en bloc' osteoplasty in combined approach tympanoplasty. In: Nakano Y (ed) Cholesteatoma and mastoid surgery. Kugler, Amsterdam, pp 649–653

Barbara M (2008) Lateral attic reconstruction technique: preventive surgery for epitympanic retraction pockets. Otol Neurotol 29(4):522–525

Dornhoffer JL (2004) Retrograde mastoidectomy with canal wall reconstruction: a follow-up report. Otol Neurotol 25(5):653–660

Feldmann H (1978) Osteoplastic approach in chronic otitis media by means of a microsurgical reciprocating saw. Clin Otolaryngol 3:515–520

Gabe E (1910–1911) Über den plastischen Verschluss persistierender retroaurikularer Öffnungen nach Antrumoperationen. Beitr Anat Physiol Path Therap Ohres 18:354–375

Gerlach H (1969) Die hintere Gehorgangswand bei der tympanoplastik. Monatsschr Laryngol Rhinol Otol 48:214–218

Grote JJ (1998) Results of cavity reconstruction with hydroxyapatite implants after 15 years. Am J Otol 19:551–557

Guilford FR (1961) Obliteration of the cavity and reconstruction of the auditory canal in temporal bone surgery. Trans Am Acad Ophthalmol Otolaryngol 65:114–122

Hartwein J, Hoermann K (1990) A technique for the reconstruction of the posterior canal wall and mastoid obliteration in radical cavity surgery. Am J Otol 11(3):169–173

House H (1949) Surgery for the chronically discharging ear. Arch Otolaryngol Head Neck Surg 49:135–150

Kerrison P (1930) Diseases of the ear. JB Lippincott, Philadelphia

Kisch H (1928) Temporal muscle grafts in the radical mastoid operation (with illustrative cases). J Laryngol Otol 43:735–736

Kuhweide W, van Deninse JB (1960) Surgical treatment of chronic otitis media. Acta Otolaryngol 52:143

Lapidot A, Brandow E (1966) A method for preserving the posterior canal wall and bridge in the surgery for cholesteatoma. Acta Otolaryngol 62:88–92

Lempert J (1949) Lempert endaural subcortical mastoidectomy for the cure of chronic persistent suppurative otitis media. Arch Otolaryngol Head Neck Surg 49:20–35

Mahoney JL (1962) Tympanoacryloplasty. Arch Otolaryngol Head Neck Surg 75:519

McElveen JT, Chung ATA (2003) Reversible canal wall down mastoidectomy for acquired cholesteatomas: preliminary results. Laryngoscope 113:1027–1033

Mercke U (1987) The cholesteatomatous ear one year after surgery with obliteration technique. Am J Otol 8:534–536

Meurman Y, Ojala L (1949) Primary reduction of a large operation cavity in radical mastoidectomy with a muscle-periosteal flap. Acta Otolaryngol 37:245–251

Mill WA (1930) Three cases of conservative mastoid operation with temporal muscle graft. J Laryngol Otol 45(11):129–130

Mills RP (1987) Surgical management of the discharging mastoid cavity. Clin Otolaryngol 12:327–329

Mosher HP (1911) A method of filling the excavated mastoid with a flap from the back of the auricle. Laryngoscope 21:1158–1163

Palva T (1962a) Mastoiditis in children. Laryngoscope 72:353–360

Palva T (1962b) Reconstruction of ear canal in surgery for chronic ear. Arch Otolaryngol Head Neck Surg 75:329–334

Palva T (1963) Surgery of chronic ear without cavity. Arch Otolaryngol Head Neck Surg 77:570–580

Palva T (1975) Mastoid obliteration. Arch Otolaryngol 101:271–273

Passow A (1908) Über den Verschluss der Knochenwunden nach Antrumoperationen. Beitr Anat Physiol Path Therap Ohres 1:67–75

Pennings RJE, Cremers CWRJ (2009) Postauricular approach atticotomy: a modified closed technique with reconstruction of the scutum with cymbal cartilage. Ann Otol Rhinol Laryngol 118(3):199–204

Popper O (1935) Periosteal flap grafts in mastoid operations. S Afr Med J 9:77–78

Rambo JHT (1958) Musculoplasty: a new operation for suppurative middle ear deafness. Trans Am Acad Ophthalmol Otolaryngol 62:166–177

Richards S (1972) Tympanoplasty results following the mobilebridge technique. Trans Am Acad Ophthalmol Otol 76:153–159

Richtnér NG (1960) Reconstructive micro surgery of the ear, especially with the cavum minor technique. Laryngoscope 70:1179–1197

Roberson JB, Mason TP, Stidham KR (2003) Mastoid obliteration autogenous cranial bone pÂte reconstruction. Otol Neurotol 24(2):132–140

Saunders JE, Shoemaker DL, McElveen JT (1992) Reconstruction of the radical mastoid. Am J Otol 13(5):465–469

Schiller A (1963) Mastoid osteoplasty. Arch Otolargyngol Head Neck Surg 77:475–483

Schnee I (1963) Tympanoplasty: a modification in technique. Arch Otolaryngol 77:87–91

Shea MC, Gardner G (1970) Mastoid obliteration using homograft bone. Arch Otolaryngol Head Neck Surg 92:358–365

Shea MC Jr, Gardner G Jr, Simpson ME (1970) Mastoid obliteration using homogenous bone chips and autogenous bone paste. Arch Otolaryngol 92:413

Sheehy JL, Crabtree JA (1974) Tympanoplasty: staging the operation. Laryngoscope 83:1594–1621

Sheehy JL, Brackmann DE, Graham MD (1977) Cholesteatoma surgery: residual and recurrent disease. A review of 1024 cases. Ann Otol Rhinol Laryngol 86:451–462

Thorburn IB (1960) A critical review of tympanoplastic surgery. J Laryngol Otol 74:453–474

Weber PC, Gantz BJ (1998) Cartilage reconstruction of the scutum defects in canal wall up mastoidectomies. Am J Otolaryngol 19(3):178–182

Wullstein A (1962) Tympanoplasty today. Arch Otolaryngol Head Neck Surg 76:295

Wullstein S (1972) Die osteoplastische epitympanotomie und ihre resultate. Arch Ohren Nasen Kehlkopfheilkd 202:655–658

Ear Drum Repair

▶ Tympanoplasty, Underlay and Overlay Techniques

Ear Popping

▶ Barotrauma and Decompression Sickness

Ear Reconstruction

▶ Microtia and Atresia

Ear, Nose, Throat Surgery: Anesthetic Management

▶ Anesthetic Techniques for Otolaryngologic Patient

Early/Fast Response

▶ Hearing Testing, Auditory Brainstem Response (ABR)

Ecchordosis Physaliphora

▶ Chordoma

Ectatic Carotid Artery

▶ Imaging for Parapharyngeal Space Masses, Ectatic Internal Carotid Artery

Ectropion

Michael M. Kim
Division of Facial Plastic & Reconstructive Surgery, Department of Otolaryngology-Head and Neck Surgery, Oregon Health & Science University, Portland, OR, USA

Introduction

Ectropion is the outward turning or eversion of the lower lid margin where the mucosal surface of the lid is no longer in apposition to the globe. Untreated, this condition may result in conjunctivitis or exposure keratophy. There are several types of ectropion including involutional (age-related laxity), cicatricial (scar), paralytic, and congenital. The appropriate medical or surgical treatment for this condition is largely determined by the etiology of the disease.

Patient Presentation and Evaluation

Patients with ectropion may present with complaints related to conjunctival and corneal exposure such as epiphora (tearing), irritation, mattering, and edema (Frueh and Schengarth 1982). The practitioner should note the position of the lid margin and the position of the puncta compared to normal anatomy. In the normal lower eyelid, the lower lid rests at the limbus in apposition to the globe with no sclera visible between the lower lid margin and the limbus.

Patients with ectropion may present with concomitant lid retraction. Consequently, the margin reflex distance 2 (MRD2) should be recorded. In patients with epiphora, the patency of the puncta and lacrimal drainage system can be evaluated by irrigation. In these cases of ectropion with punctal eversion, the lack of apposition of the punctum can cause epiphora despite a functional tear drainage system.

"Snap" and "distraction" testing are used to evaluate the horizontal laxity of the lower lid. The "snap" test is performed by manual distraction of the lower lid. Normal support is indicated by a return of eyelid to globe apposition after the lid is released either immediately or at most after one blink. If the lid does not return to the globe after one blink, it is said to exhibit poor support. The "distraction" test also measures horizontal laxity. This is performed by distracting the lid in a caudal direction while measuring the change in position from normal. Distances of greater than 6 mm indicate laxity.

Should there be any concern regarding corneal abnormalities, referral to an ophthalmologist who can perform a more detailed examination through the use of a slit lamp apparatus may be warranted. An examination of the cornea, as well as the quantity and quality of tears can be evaluated through fluorescein administration.

Classification

Ectropion is classified depending on its etiology. First, ectropion is grouped into the rare congenital types or the more common acquired varieties. Primary congenital ectropion results from a primary anomaly of the tarsus while secondary congenital ectropion includes cases caused by birth trauma, skin retraction, and eversion from orbital tumors.

Acquired ectropion occurs with much greater frequency than congenital ectropion, and involutional ectropion is the most common acquired cause. Involutional ectropion results from a progressive laxity of the lid support system with age or with extrinsic factors such as eyelid retraction for ophthalmic surgery (Shore 1985). Factors such as medial or lateral canthal tendon laxity (Ousterhout and Weil 1982), attenuation of the lower lid retractors (capsulopalpebral fascia, Müller's muscle; Putterman 1978), diminishment of orbicularis oculi function, and weakening of the tarsus and septum can all contribute to cause involutional ectropion.

Cicatricial ectropion results from a vertical shortening of the anterior lamella of the lower lid (orbicularis oculi and skin). Causes of anterior lamellar shortening include scarring after trauma, burns, skin conditions, blepharoplasty complications, and after skin cancer defect repair.

Paralytic ectropion is caused by a loss of orbicularis oculi function related to facial nerve paresis. There are myriad causes of facial nerve palsy including neoplastic (cerebellopontine angle or parotid tumors), trauma, iatrogenic (neurosurgery, otologic surgery, parotid surgery), infectious (herpes zoster oticus), and Bell's palsy. Problems related to paralytic ectropion exhibit additional complexity to that of the cicatricial and involutional varieties due to the contribution of concomitant upper eyelid dysfunction (Seiff 1998).

Treatment

Although massage and taping technique can be used with some success in temporary post-procedure ectropion, the treatment of long-term, stable ectropion is primarily surgical. Additional conservative measures such as lubrication and moisturization may be used to prevent corneal complications related to exposure.

Many different techniques have been described for the correction of ectropion. Appropriate selection of specific surgical strategies is largely based on the etiology and severity of ectropion. Although technically possible to perform under local anesthesia, these procedures are frequently done under Monitored Anesthesia Care (MAC) or General Anesthesia (GA) for patient comfort.

The lateral tarsal strip is widely considered the most useful procedure in surgical ectropion treatment because it is often utilized in all of the three major types of acquired ectropion (involutional, cicatricial, and paralytic). The procedure provides support to the lower lid through horizontal shortening of the tarsal plate followed by fixation (Anderson and Gordy 1979). After a lateral canthotomy and inferior lateral cantholysis, the lateral portion of the tarsus is isolated and de-epithelialized. It is then tailored to the appropriate length and then fixated inside the lateral orbital rim at the approximate location of Whitnall's tubercle.

If the patient presents with epiphora due to punctal eversion, the medial spindle procedure is utilized (Nowinski and Anderson 1985). A diamond-shaped excision of conjunctiva and lower lid retractor musculature is resected. This is then followed by suture techniques to invert the lid to a position whereby the medial lid and puncta are in apposition to the globe so that the lacrimal system can drain normally.

Since cicatricial ectropion results from a shortage of anterior lamella, full thickness skin grafts can be used as anterior lamellar replacement tissue. A subciliary incision is made and the lower lid margin is released to expose the posterior lamellar tissue. This is often done in conjunction with a lateral tarsal strip procedure for horizontal support. A full thickness skin graft is then placed between the two sides of the subciliary incision as a spacer in an overcorrected position. Bolstering techniques in addition to the use of a Frost suture to resist the contractile forces of healing are commonly used.

Paralytic ectropion is more difficult to correct since the dynamic nature of the orbicularis oculi muscle is lost. In addition, the concomitant manifestations of upper lid paralysis typically require treatment of the upper and lower lid in order to achieve full eye closure. The lower lid can be treated with the aforementioned lateral tarsal strip procedure. A gold weight will often need to be placed in the upper lid in order to provide a mechanical load for closure.

Complications

Complications related to ectropion include dry eye, lagophthalmos, corneal ulceration, exposure keratopathies, and even blindness. Surgery to correct ectropion may result in complications such as corneal abrasions, inadequate correction, contour abnormalities, and need for additional procedures. Care must be taken when performing lower lid tightening procedures on those with the "negative vector" anatomic configuration. The "negative vector" is characterized by relative proptosis of the globe in relation to the midface. This can be present due to any combination of proptosis and/or malar or orbital rim hypoplasia.

Postsurgical hemorrhage should also be recognized and treated early. Patients should be warned to look for increased swelling, bleeding, pain, and vision changes. If the patient has impending visual loss, the surgeon may need to release sutures and possibly perform lateral canthotomy and cantholysis to decompress the orbit.

Cross-References

▶ Bell's Palsy
▶ Canthal Positions
▶ Canthoplasty
▶ Facial Paralysis
▶ Static Facial Paralysis Rehabilitation

References

Anderson R, Gordy D (1979) The lateral tarsal strip procedure. Arch Ophthalmol 97:2192–2196

Frueh B, Schengarth L (1982) Evaluation and treatment of the patient with ectropion. Ophthalmology 89:1049–1052

Nowinski T, Anderson R (1985) The medial spindle procedure for involutional medial ectropion. Arch Ophthalmol 103:1750–1753

Ousterhout D, Weil R (1982) The role of the lateral canthal tendon in lower eyelid laxity. Plast Reconstr Surg 69:620–622

Putterman A (1978) Ectropion of the lower eyelid, secondary to Mueller's muscle-capsulopalpebral fascia detachment. Am J Ophthalmol 85:814–817

Seiff S, Chang J (1992) Management of ophthalmic complications of facial nerve palsy. Otolaryngol Clin North Am 25:669–690

Shore J (1985) Changes in lower eyelid resting position, movement, and tone with age. Am J Ophthalmol 99:415–423

Eighth Nerve Schwannoma

▶ Cochlear Schwannoma

Electroacoustic Stimulation (EAS)/Hybrid Implants

▶ Implantable Hearing Devices

Electrodiagnostic Test

▶ Electromyogram

Electromyogram

Kofi Derek O. Boahene
Department of Otolaryngology-Head and Neck
Surgery, Johns Hopkins University School of
Medicine, Baltimore, MD, USA

Synonyms

Electrodiagnostic test; EMG

Definition

Electromyogram (EMG) is electrodiagnostic recording of electric potentials or voltage detected by a needle electrode inserted into skeletal muscle. EMG records the variation in electrical potential of insertion, spontaneous, and voluntary activity of muscles with a recording needle electrode. The American Association of Electrodiagnostic Medicine Glossary of Terms provides a uniform agreed-upon framework for expressing electric phenomena encountered in studying patients with EMG.

EMG of the facial muscles is used as an adjunct to neurologic examination of the face to determine the state and function of the facial muscles following facial nerve injury.

Fibrillation Potential
This is the action potential of a single muscle fiber occurring spontaneously or after movement of a needle electrode. Fibrillation potentials usually fire at a constant rate and are indicative of muscle denervation. In the early stage following facial nerve injury, fibrillation potentials are large in size but continue to decrease in amplitude over time. At 6 months the mean amplitude drops by 50–300 µV, and at 1 year 100 µV or smaller. As a rule, larger amplitudes suggest nerve injury within the past few months, whereas smaller amplitudes suggest that injury occurred at least 6 months to a year ago. The presence of fibrillation potentials and their amplitude can be used as an indication of a physiologically responsive muscle that may respond to reinnervation from various nerve grafting techniques.

Polyphasic Potentials
Electrophysiologically, a normal motor unit has a di- or triphasic configuration. One of the earliest signs of muscle reinnervation is the increase in phases of the motor units. Polyphasic potentials are abnormal action potential configurations of a motor unit with five or more phases and indicate neurological recovery and also establish the fact that there is axonal continuity.

Cross-References

▸ Facial Paralysis
▸ Nerve Grafting

References

Anonymous (2001) American Association of Electrodiagnostic Medicine glossary of terms in electrodiagnostic medicine. Muscle Nerve Suppl 10:S1–S50
Dale AJD, Kokmen E, Swanson JW et al (1991) Clinical examinations in neurology, 6th edn. Mosby–Year Book, St. Louis, pp 395–396

Electromyography

J. Edward Hartmann
Georgia Health Sciences, University/Medical College of Georgia, Augusta, GA, USA

Synonyms

Electroneuromyography; Laryngeal electroneuromyography; Needle electromyography

Definition

Electrodes are electrical devices that translate voltage changes into electrical signals for analysis. The *active electrode* is the electrode that records the voltages at the point of interest. Since voltage is a measurement of the electrical potential difference between two points, a second electrode is needed for measurements. This second electrode is the *reference electrode*. A *ground electrode* is placed on the patient for electrical safety.

Electromyography (EMG) is the neurodiagnostic test which samples the electrical activity of a muscle. The electromyographer places a needle intramuscularly for recording for evaluation of its insertional activity at rest and its voluntary motor units during contraction.

Insertional activity is the electrical signal generated when the recording needle is moved within the muscle. Normal muscle will show a short period of electrical changes. Abnormal insertional activity most commonly is increased.

Interference pattern is the appearance of voluntary motor units on the display screen during contraction of a muscle. With submaximal contraction, individual motor units may be analyzed visually or quantitatively for parameters such as amplitude, duration, firing frequency, and recruitment. With full muscle contraction of a normal muscle, the screen is filled with electrical activity and individual motor units cannot be distinguished. Nerve and muscle diseases cause change in these patterns.

EMG utilizes one of two types of needles for testing. A *monopolar needle* consists of a needle that is coated with a material shielding it from electrical activity except at its tip which serves as the active electrode. A reference electrode is placed on nearby skin. A *concentric needle* consists of a needle housing both the active and reference electrodes. The needle tip is beveled exposing a small wire which runs through the center of the needle and acts as the active electrode. The wire within the needle is surrounded by an insulating material, with the outer surface of the needle serving as the reference electrode. Advantages and disadvantages for each are discussed later in this entry.

Recruitment is the orderly fashion in which a muscle increases its power. As a muscle begins to contract, only one motor unit fires. As the muscle needs more power, this single motor unit fires more frequently. At a certain level of increasing force, a second motor unit begins firing (i.e., is recruited), and more motor units activate as the contractile forces increase. With nerve injury, recruitment is delayed, and with muscle injury, recruitment is early.

Purpose

EMG has several purposes. EMG can show injury of the muscle due to muscle or nerve diseases. EMG can demonstrate whether a nerve based lesion is purely demyelinating (no increase in insertional activity) versus wholly or partially involving the axon (when increased insertional activity is seen). Axonal lesions typically reflect more severe injury compared to demyelinating lesions. Also, EMG can demonstrate if the lesion is incomplete by the presence of voluntary motor units versus complete in which no motor units are seen when a patient is asked to contract the muscle of interest. EMG can help with prognosis, especially when it is performed serially, since the motor units' morphology and recruitment patterns change over time in a reinnervated muscle. In addition, specialized hypodermic EMG needles guide the precise delivery of chemodenervation agents such as botulinum toxin (BT). Common disorders in which these purposes are applied in Otolarygologic conditions include Bell's Palsy, Acoustic Neuromas, Hemifacial Spasm, and Spasmodic Dysphonia.

EMG in Bell's Palsy has been reported by several authors. Eighty-one patients with Bell's Palsy who presented over a 4-year period were studied prospectively with several electrodiagnostic studies performed on days 5, 20, and 90 after the clinical onset of symptoms (Ozgur et al. 2010). EMG of the orbicularis oculus was performed, and results were reported as abnormal when insertional activity was increased. Patients whose House-Brackman score was 3 or higher were considered to have a poor prognosis. All EMGs were normal on day 5, reflecting a sample time too early to detect denervation. All seven patients having a poor prognosis on day 90 showed increased insertional activity on day 20 (100% sensitivity). Fifty-two of fifty-eight patients with a good prognosis on day 90 showed normal results on day 20 (90% specificity). Their conclusion was EMG performed on day 20 provided statistically significant information for predicting prognosis. Another publication evaluated 197 patients with four diagnostic tests performed, to include EMG (Hyden et al. 1982). EMGs were performed 7 days after the onset of symptoms. The authors categorized the EMG results into five interference patterns (no motor units, one motor unit, discrete activity, reduced and full interference pattern). If the EMG was showing no motor units, their data showed 13/13 patients demonstrated a bad (severe or moderate weakness) outcome (100% sensitivity). Alternatively, if the EMG showed zero or one motor unit, then 32/41 patients had a bad outcome (78% sensitivity).

Specificity with a "normal" EMG was not as strong – only 50% predictive of a good outcome if any motor units were seen on the interference pattern (and 54% if >1 motor units were seen). An EMG examination of the frontalis, mentalis, and orbicularis oculus (OO) on day 30 of symptoms on patients with Bell's Palsy also was published (Kokotis et al. 2006). Of the 54 patients, only 11 (20%) showed increased insertional activity in the OO, compared to 32 (59%) in the mentalis and 29 (54%) in the frontalis. Patients with increased insertional activity of the OO showed small amplitude responses after facial nerve stimulation and poorer recovery. In summary, an abnormal EMG within 1 month of the onset of Bell's Palsy is helpful in determining which patients have a poor prognosis.

Forty-five preoperative patients with Acoustic Neuromas were studied with EMG to determine prognostic factors (Normand and Daube 1994). The following groups showed abnormalities on EMG: Three of seven patients with facial weakness and 13/38 without facial weakness. Four of nine patients with facial sensation changes showed EMG abnormalities of the masseter muscle (i.e., assessment of the Trigeminal nerve). Among their conclusions, they noted that increased insertional activity was infrequent and less sensitive than the Blink Reflex and Electroneuronography.

Hemifacial Spasm (HS) is the condition in which muscles of facial expression involuntarily contract in a twitching-like movement. HS is a form of segmental myoclonus involving the facial nerve and most commonly affects the orbicularis oculus and zygomaticus muscles. Various causes have been described and can be idiopathic or due to any insult to the facial nerve (such as compression from a nearby vascular structure, trauma, or demyelination from Bell's Palsy). Although a number of medical and surgical therapies have been reported, BT has become the treatment of choice for HS. The available literature was recently reviewed (Kenney and Jankovic 2008). They cited eight articles as being randomized and double-blind studies in support of BT use for HS, although acknowledged that only one of these papers met the Cochrane's review criteria for recommended therapy. Injection sites and doses vary considerably, presumably due to which muscles are involved with HS. Generally, the duration of benefits lasted between 3 and 10 months. Many use EMG guidance for injections as this can direct the delivery of BT to the most active areas of involved muscles. No one has studied if EMG guidance

significantly improves the BT therapy in relieving the myoclonic movements of HS.

Patients with Spasmodic Dysphonia (SD) undergo EMG for two reasons – diagnostic testing and therapeutic injections. EMG can sample laryngeal muscles used for phonation to assess for neuropathic changes. In addition chemodenervation agents are injected through a hypodermic EMG needle into the thyroarytenoid, lateral cricothyroid, and posterior cricothyroid muscles for treatment of SD. The etiology of SD remains unknown, but current theories attribute its pathophysiology to the extrapyramidal pathways similar to other movement disorders. Adductor SD is more common and produces a strained or "strangled" voice due to forced glottal closure. Abductor SD produces a breathy whisper due to forced glottal opening, and patients have trouble with the "voiceless" consonants – d, f, h, k, p, s, and t. Many agree that BT is the "gold standard" of treatment for SD, compared to other treatments such as muscle relaxants, anxiolytics, anticholinergic agents, beta-blockers, and recurrent laryngeal nerve resection (Meyer and Blitzer 2007). Unfortunately, no publications have met the stringent standards of evidenced based recommendations to prove that EMG guidance for injections is the best method for chemodenervation agent delivery. In 2003, the American Association of Electrodiagnostic Medicine (with other organizations) reviewed the published data on laryngeal EMG (LEMG). The article's recommendation was that LEMG was *possibly* (Level C) equally effective for directing BT for the treatment of SD when compared to injection guided by endoscopic techniques based on Class III or IV articles (i.e., most often retrospective articles; but even if prospective, not blinded, randomized, or with a control group). The task force recommended a prospective, randomized, and controlled study to compare BT delivery via laryngoscope versus LEMG. Among several articles published on LEMG guided BT injections, the largest and longest followed group of patients with SD were reported by Blitzer on 901 patients receiving 6,300 injections over the 14 years (Blitzer et al. 1998). Eight-two percent of the cohort had Adductor SD. For Adductor SD, the averages for onset effect was 2–3 days, reaching a peak effect was 9 days, and lasted 15 weeks. The typical dosing of BT for Adductor SD was 1.0 unit to each thyroarytenoid. For Abductor SD, typical dosing was 3.75 units to one posterior cricoarytenoid, administered unilaterally to avoid stridor or even airway obstruction. Its averages for onset effect was 4 days, to peak effect was 10 days, and lasted 10–11 weeks. Only one article has been published with a double-blind, placebo-controlled design for the study of BT for SD (Truong et al. 1991). In it, 13 patients with Adductor SD underwent speech analysis prior to and 4 days following bilateral injections of either 5.0 units of BT or saline. Voices analysis showed significant improvement with BT.

Principle

EMG Equipment

EMGs are performed with an Electromyographic/Nerve Conduction Study (EMG/NCS) machine equipped with a screen to visualize the waveforms and a speaker to listen to them. Newer models have the capability to record short portions of the exam. Several reputable companies manufacture such machines. EMG needles can be monopolar or concentric as described in the definitions section above. Electrodes for the reference and ground leads are most commonly disposable and self-adhesive, although reusable electrodes can be applied with a conductive gel and secured with tape. Exam rooms with EMG capabilities should be electrically shielded in order to minimize radiofrequency interference.

EMG Technique

With the EMG needle properly connected to the EMG machine, the needle is inserted into the muscle of interest. Low- and high-frequency filter settings are usually preset, but one should insure that their settings are 10 Hz and 20 KHz, respectively. Muscles that are typically used for EMG recording or injecting BT are listed in Table 1 and diagramed in Fig. 1.

Possible EMG Results

EMG has two stages – assessment of the insertional activity with the muscle at rest and analysis of voluntary motor units during contraction. Insertional activity can be normal, indicated by a short burst of electrical activity only during needle movements. An increase of insertional activity is the most common abnormality in which abnormal waveforms either are present without needle movement or persist for a prolonged time after needle movement stops. It is due to either muscle disease or injury in the muscle's nerve supply. Rarely,

Electromyography, Table 1

Muscle	Needle insertion point	Use
Orbicularis oculus	Superior and inferior to orbit	BP, HS
Orbicularis oris	Lateral to mouth	BP, HS
Frontalis	Above lateral eyebrow	BP
Thyroarytenoid	Through cricothyroid membrane in an antero-lateral direction	SD
Posterior cricoarytenoid	Posterior to posterior edge of thyroid cartilage, advanced almost to circoid cartilage	SD
Zygomaticus major	Half way between corner of mouth and midpoint of zygomatic arch	BP, HS
Zygomaticus minor	Half way between outer ¼ of mouth and outer corner of eye	BP, HS

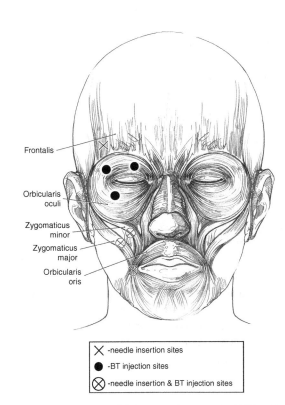

Electromyography, Fig. 1 Locations of needle insertion sites or botulinum toxin injection sites (or both) for muscles of the face (Illustration by Colon Polonsky)

insertional activity is reduced due to fibrotic replacement of the muscle. For assessment of voluntary motor units, the electromyographer visually analyzes the morphologic characteristics of the waveforms.

Parameters evaluated include the motor unit's amplitude, duration, and complexity. Neurogenic lesions usually cause an increase in these variables. Also, neurogenic lesions cause late (or delayed) recruitment of other motor units when resistance against the tested muscle is increased.

Indication

EMG can be performed in any clinical situation in which one suspects a lesion of the muscle or nerve of interest. It can also assist in the delivery of chemodenervating agents for therapy. For otolaryngologic purposes, one performs EMG of the facial or laryngeal muscles when patients present with Bell's Palsy, Spasmodic Dysphonia, Hemifacial Spasm, or having an Acoustic Neuroma. Other conditions may warrant EMG testing based on the physical exam, as the strength of EMG is to extend the exam ability to localize the lesion as well as to assist with prognosis.

Contraindication

EMG should not be performed on a patient who is unwilling to have the procedure performed. Also, postoperative wounds or bandages may obstruct typical insertion sites. The electromyographer should ask if a patient is taking anticoagulants. The electromyographer should account for the patient's level of anticoagulation, the compressibility of the site tested, and the size of the needle used in determining if it is safe to perform an EMG. Guidelines for patients taking anticoagulation have been published by the American Association of Neuromuscular and Electrodiagnostic Medicine.

Advantages/Disadvantages

Monopolar needles are typically smaller, and thus less painful, but it generates a greater amount of electrical interference with the signal output. Monopolar needles can be inserted into smaller muscles more reliably. In addition, monopolar needles can be hypodermic to allow for the delivery of medications such as BT. Concentric needles minimize external electrical interference. Thus, electrical activity from a reference electrode which is relatively distant from the muscle of interest is negated. However, concentric needles usually are larger in diameter, and thus can be more painful.

EMG will not distinguish the etiology of an abnormality, but it can give important clinical information regarding localization and severity of injury. Thus any injury, whether from trauma, Bell's Palsy, a tumor, or other reason, will result in similar abnormalities. Some EMG findings can help with prognosis. Abnormalities on EMG evolve over time, reflecting different stages of denervation and reinnervation of a muscle. Insertional activity usually is not increased until $\sim$10 days after a nerve lesion develops.

Cross-References

▶ Bell's Palsy
▶ Electroneurography
▶ Facial Nerve
▶ Hemifacial Microsomia
▶ Intraoperative Neurophysiologic Monitoring of the Facial Nerve (VII)
▶ Spasmodic Dysphonia

References

AAEM Laryngeal EMG Task Force (2003) Laryngeal electromyography: an evidence-based review. Muscle Nerve 28:767–772

Blitzer A et al (1998) Botulinum toxin management of spasmodic dysphonia (laryngeal dystonia): a 12 year experience in more than 900 patients. Laryngoscope 108(10):1435–1441

Hyden D et al (1982) Prognosis in Bell's Palsy based on symptoms, signs and laboratory data. Acta Otolaryngol 93:407–414

Kenney C, Jankovic J (2008) Botulinum toxin in the treatment of blepharospasm and hemifacial spasm. J Neural Transm 115:585–591

Kimura J (2001) Electrodiagnosis in diseases of nerve and muscle: principles and practice. Oxford University Press, New York

Kokotis P et al (2006) Denervation pattern of three mimic muscles in Bell's Palsy. Neurophysiol Clin 36:255–259

Meyer TK, Blitzer A (2007) Spasmodic dysphonia. In: Stacy MA (ed) Handbook of dystonia. Informa Healthcare USA, New York

Normand MM, Daube JR (1994) Cranial nerve conduction and needle electromyography on patients with acoustic neuromas: a model of compression neuropathy. Muscle Nerve 17:1401–1406

Ozgur A et al (2010) Which electrophysiological measure is appropriate in predicting prognosis of facial paralysis? Clin Neurol Neurosurg 112:844–848

Truong D et al (1991) Double-blind controlled study of botulinum toxin in adductor spasmodic dysphonia. Laryngoscope 101(6):630–634

Electroneurography

▶ Evoked EMG

Electroneuromyography

▶ Electromyography

Electronystagmography

▶ ENG/VNG

Elevated Upper Airway Resistance

▶ Snoring Without Apnea, Evaluation

ELISA

Johnathan Sataloff and Robert T. Sataloff
Department of Otolaryngology-Head and Neck Surgery, Drexel University College of Medicine, Philadelphia, PA, USA

Definition

A method of serologic testing. It is used to screen for Lyme disease but produces false-positive and false-negative results. It is commonly ordered as a "Lyme titer." Western blot provides more definitive testing.

Cross-References

▶ Otologic Manifestations of Lyme Disease

Elite

▶ Surgical Approaches and Anatomy of the Lateral Skull Base

Embryology

▶ Embryology of Ear (General)

Embryology of Ear (General)

Eric R. Oliver[1] and Bradley W. Kesser[2]
[1]Department of Otolaryngology-Head and Neck Surgery, Wake Forest University School of Medicine, Winston-Salem, NC, USA
[2]Department of Otolaryngology-Head and Neck Surgery, University of Virginia Health System, Charlottesville, VA, USA

Synonyms

Developmental anatomy; Embryology; Ontogeny

Definition

Embryologic development from the primitive fetus to a fully functioning organ system

Basic Characteristics

Introduction

The ear is composed of three anatomic divisions, each with unique embryologic origins: (1) the external ear, which consists of the auricle (pinna), the external acoustic meatus and canal, and the external layer of the tympanic membrane; (2) the middle ear, an air-containing space lined by respiratory epithelium housing the three ossicles and containing the internal layer of the tympanic membrane; and (3) the inner ear, which includes the bony and membranous labyrinth

Embryology of Ear (General), Fig. 1 Transverse sections through the rhombencephalon demonstrating formation of the otic vesicles. (**a**) 24 days (**b**) 27 days (**c**) 4.5 weeks (Sadler 2000)

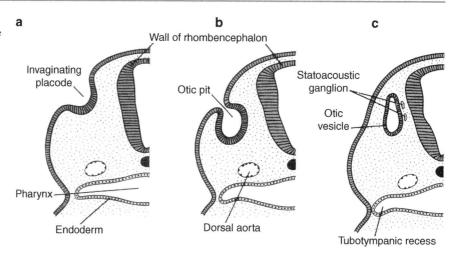

and cochlea. Because inner ear development occurs independent of that of the middle and external ears, congenital sensorineural hearing loss typically occurs in the presence of a normal outer and middle ear, while congenital defects of the middle and/or external ear most often occur in the setting of a structurally and functionally normal cochlea and vestibular system.

Inner Ear

In the auditory system, the inner ear develops earliest. A thickening of the surface ectoderm on each side of the rhombencephalic region (the caudal part of the hindbrain) of each neural fold on embryonic *day 22 or 23* heralds the development of the ear. Formation of this ectodermal thickening, the **otic placode**, is induced by signaling from the paraxial mesoderm and notochord. Head growth translocates the **otic placode** caudally to the level of the second branchial arch region. During the *fourth week*, the **otic placode** invaginates deep to the surface ectoderm into the underlying mesenchyme, forming the **otic pit**. The margins of each **otic pit** subsequently fuse to form the **otic vesicle (otocyst)**, the primordium of the membranous labyrinth. Two regions of the **otic vesicle** become distinguishable: A ventral portion that gives rise to the **saccule** and the **cochlear duct** (pars inferior), and a dorsal portion that forms the **utricle and semicircular canals (pars superior)**, and **endolymphatic duct** (Fig. 1).

Saccule, Cochlea, and Organ of Corti

By *day 26 in the fourth week*, the ventral **otic vesicle** differentiates into the **saccule**. During the *fifth week*, the lower pole of the **saccule** starts to lengthen and coil. This projection, the **cochlear duct**, penetrates the surrounding mesenchyme in a spiral fashion. By completion of the *eighth week*, the duct has made 2.5 turns. The developing membranous cochlea and saccule maintain their connection via the **ductus reuniens**.

During the *seventh week*, cochlear duct epithelial cells differentiate to form the **Organ of Corti**. Initially, these epithelial cells are similar, but with further development, they form two ridges: an **inner** (the future **spiral limbus**) and **outer ridge**. The outer ridge forms one row of **inner** auditory sensory cells (**hair cells**) and 3–4 rows of **outer** hair cells. The stereocilia of the hair cells are contacted by the **tectorial membrane**, which attaches to the spiral limbus. The hair cells, their supporting cells, and the tectorial membrane together constitute the **Organ of Corti**. **Spiral ganglion cells** also differentiate from cells in the wall of the cochlear duct, which migrate along the coiled membranous cochlea to form the ganglion. Neuronal projections extend from the spiral ganglion to the Organ of Corti, terminating at the calyx adjacent to individual hair cells. The cells of the spiral ganglion retain their embryonic bipolar character.

Mesenchyme surrounding the cochlear duct soon differentiates into cartilage. During the *tenth week*, this cartilaginous tissue undergoes vacuolization

Embryology of Ear (General),
Fig. 2 Development of the scala tympani and scala vestibuli. (**a**) The cochlear duct is surrounded by a cartilaginous shell (**b**) During the 10th week, large vacuoles appear in the cartilaginous shell (**c**) The cochlear duct (scala media) is separated from the scala tympani and the scala vestibuli by the basilar and vestibular membranes, respectively (Sadler 2000)

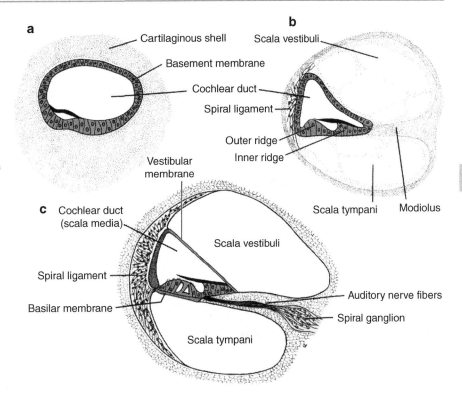

and forms the two perilymphatic spaces: the **scala vestibuli** and **scala tympani**. The **vestibular (Reissner's) membrane** separates the cochlear duct from the scala vestibuli, and the **basilar membrane** separates the cochlear duct from the scala tympani. The lateral wall of the cochlear duct remains attached to the surrounding cartilage by the **spiral ligament**, whereas its medial aspect is supported by the cartilaginous **modiolus**, which later serves as the bony cochlea's axis. The cochlea is structurally developed by the 26th week (Fig. 2).

Utricle, Endolymphatic Sac, and Semicircular Canals
The dorsal region of the otic vesicle begins to elongate by embryonic *day 26*, forming an endolymphatic appendage. Concurrently, the remaining **otic vesicle** begins to differentiate into the **utricle**. The endolymphatic appendage elongates over the next week, and its distal portion expands to form the **endolymphatic sac**. Its connection to the utricle is maintained by a narrow **endolymphatic duct**.

During the *sixth week* of development, **semicircular canals** appear as flattened diverticulae from the utricular portion of the otic vesicle. The central region of the walls of these projections appose each other, fuse, and disappear, giving rise to the three membranous **semicircular canals**. One end of each canal dilates to form the **ampulla**. Since two non-ampullated ends fuse, only five total crura enter the utricle. The **cristae ampullares**, containing hair cells, form as crests within the ampullae of the membranous semicircular canals. Similar specialized receptor areas, the **maculae acousticae** develop in the walls of the utricle and saccule.

Otic Capsule and Perilymphatic Space
In the *ninth week*, the **otic vesicle** stimulates the mesenchyme around the otic vesicle to condense and differentiate into a cartilaginous **otic capsule**. Vacuoles develop within this cartilaginous otic capsule as the membranous labyrinth enlarges. These vacuoles coalesce to form the **perilymphatic space**, which suspends the membranous labyrinth in **perilymph**. The cartilaginous otic capsule ossifies by periosteal and endochondral ossification between *16 and 23 weeks* to form the bony enclosure that houses the

Embryology of Ear (General), Fig. 3 (a) Transverse section of a 7 week embryo in the region of the rhombencephalon, showing the tubotympanic recess, the first branchial cleft, and mesenchymal condensation, preceding development of the ossicles (b)Middle ear showing the cartilaginous precursors of the ossicles (Sadler 2000)

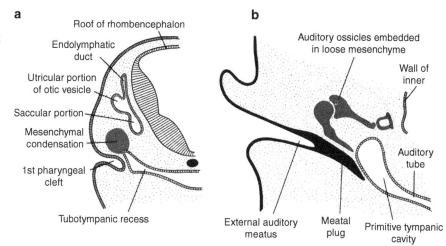

membranous labyrinth and the perilymph, the **bony labyrinth**. The inner ear reaches its adult size and morphology by the midpoint of the fetal period *(20–22 weeks)*.

Middle Ear

Tympanic Cavity and Eustachian Tube

Outpouchings within the endoderm of the embryo form the pharyngeal pouches. The distal part of the first pharyngeal pouch endoderm elongates to form the **tubotympanic recess** and widens further distally to give rise to the **tympanic cavity** (middle ear space). The proximal part remains narrow and forms the **Eustachian (pharyngotympanic or auditory) tube**, through which the tympanic cavity communicates with the nasopharynx. During the *ninth month*, the tympanic cavity expands into the mastoid portion of the temporal bone to form the **mastoid antrum**. The mastoid antrum is close to its adult size at birth. However, no mastoid air cells are typically present in newborns. After birth, the epithelium of the tympanic cavity extends to the bone of the developing mastoid process, and respiratory epithelium-lined air cells are formed (pneumatization).

Ossicles

On the lateral, cranial aspect of the embryo swellings arise from the surface ectoderm – the branchial arches. During the *seventh week*, the cartilaginous precursors of the three **ossicles** condense in the mesenchyme of the first and second branchial arches near the tympanic cavity. The malleus head and neck, incus body and short process, and anterior malleal ligament are derived from cartilage of the first branchial arch (Meckel's cartilage). The second branchial arch (Reichert's cartilage) gives rise to the manubrium of the malleus, long process of the incus, and the stapes (except the vestibular portion of the footplate which arises from the otocyst).

The ossicles remain enveloped in mesenchyme until the *eighth month*, when the surrounding tissue involutes. The endodermal epithelial lining of the tympanic cavity extends along the middle ear space and connects the ossicles in a mesentery-like fashion to the wall of the cavity. The supporting ligaments of the ossicles develop within these mesenteries. During the *ninth month*, the suspended ossicles assume their definitive locations and relationships to adjacent structures. Because the malleus develops from the first branchial arch, its associated muscle, the **tensor tympani**, is innervated by the mandibular branch of the trigeminal nerve. Similarly, the **stapedius muscle** is innervated by the nerve to the second arch, the facial nerve (Fig. 3).

External Ear

External Auditory Canal

Between the branchial arches, the surface ectoderm grows medially, pinching in to form clefts. The external auditory canal precursor develops through

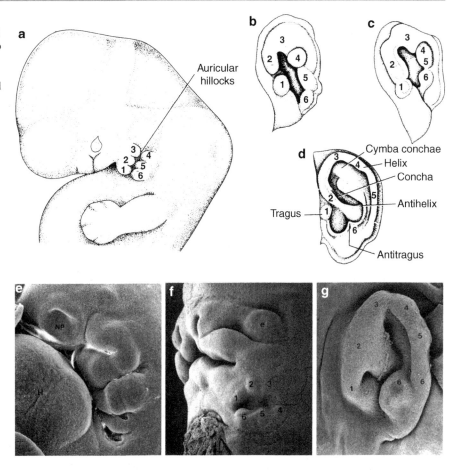

Embryology of Ear (General), Fig. 4 (a) Lateral view of the head of the embryo showing the six auricular hillocks surrounding the dorsal end of the first branchial cleft (b-g) Fusion and progressive development of the hillocks into the adult auricle (Sadler 2000)

a deepening of the distal portion of the first branchial cleft during the *sixth week*. At the beginning of the *third month*, epithelial cells lining the deep portion of the canal proliferate to form a solid epithelial core, the **meatal plug**. The meatal plug completely fills the medial end of the external auditory canal by *week 26*. In the *seventh month* the epithelial cells recanalize by apoptosis in a medial to lateral direction, and the epithelial lining of the floor participates in the formation of the definitive tympanic membrane. The external acoustic canal, relatively short at birth, reaches its final length by approximately the ninth year.

Tympanic Membrane

The primordium of the tympanic membrane is the pharyngeal membrane, which separates the first branchial cleft (ectoderm) from the first pharyngeal pouch (endoderm). As development proceeds, mesenchyme intervenes between the two portions of this membrane. Thus, the tympanic membrane is comprised of an outer lining of ectoderm, an inner lining of endoderm, and an intermediate mesodermal layer (the fibrous stratum).

Auricle

Around the *sixth week* of gestation, the auricle arises from three pairs of mesenchymal proliferations at the dorsal ends of the first and second branchial arches, surrounding the first branchial cleft. These swellings (**auricular hillocks, Hillocks of His**), three on each side of the external auditory canal, begin to enlarge, differentiate, and fuse to produce the definitive form of the auricle during the *seventh week*. The first branchial arch gives rise to Hillocks of His 1–3 (1. tragus; 2. helical crus; 3. helix), and

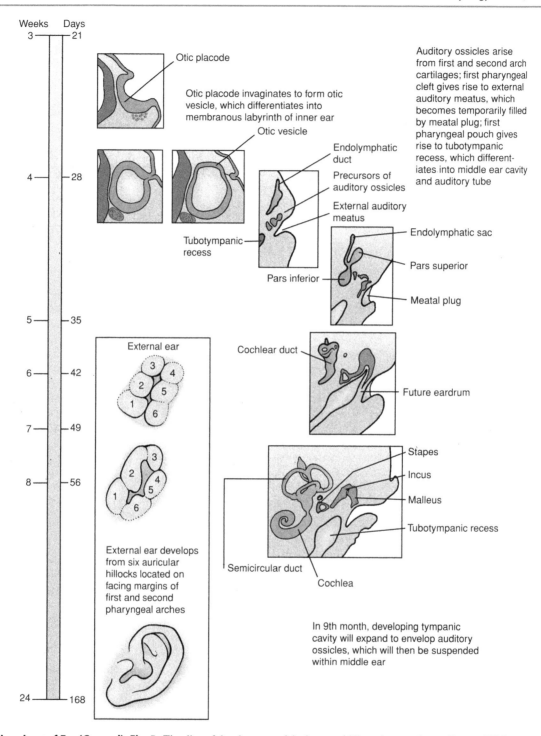

Embryology of Ear (General), Fig. 5   Timeline of development of the inner, middle and external ears (Larsen 2001)

the second branchial arch gives rise to Hillock of His 4–6 (4. antihelical crus; 5. antihelix; 6. lobule and antitragus). As the face and mandible develop, the auricle gradually ascends from its original location in the lower neck region to the side of the head at the level of the eyes (Fig. 4).

For an illustrated overview of the developmental timeline of the ear, see Fig. 5.

Cross-References

▶ Balance (Anatomy: Embryology)
▶ Balance (Anatomy: Vestibular Nerve)
▶ Cochlea, Anatomy
▶ Congenital Aural Atresia
▶ Microtia and atresia

References

Larsen WJ (2001) Human embryology. Churchill Livingstone, Philadelphia, pp 392–398
Moore KL, Persaud T (2008) The developing human. WB Saunders, Philadelphia, pp 431–434
Sadler TW (2000) Langman's medical embryology. Lippincott Williams & Wilkins, Baltimore, pp 382–392

Emergency Airway

▶ Emergent Airway

Emergency Airways

David Furgiuele and Michael Wajda
Department of Anesthesiology, NYU Langone
Medical Center, New York University, New York,
NY, USA

Synonyms

Airway Management; Difficult Airway

Introduction

The emergency airway can be approached in the same way as the difficult airway. In the emergency airway, because of the risk of compromise, there is an inherent urgency in securing the airway. No two situations can be approached the same way. Whether there is structural pathology or traumatic injury, clear understandings of airway anatomy and airway skills are necessary in order to be successful. There is no absolute technique that will guarantee successful intubation in any

airway. Therefore, before managing the emergency airway, it is necessary to be competent with routine airway situations and all intubating techniques.

Characteristics

Evaluation of the Emergency Airway

Airway evaluations are necessary in preparing for an emergency airway. Assessment of the patient will help formulate a coherent and succinct plan to approach securing the airway. This may be the most vital and crucial part, and will ensure the most success. This initial assessment will help in determining whether there will be potential difficulty with intubation and possibly mask ventilation. Many predictors of the difficult airway have been established, which include the Mallampati score, thyromental distance, mouth opening, dentition, and head extension. Used individually, these predictors are of relatively limited value, but when used together, provide better correlation (Miller et al. 2009). The strongest predictor of the difficult airway is a history of previous difficult airway. Especially in the ENT patient, emergency airways tend to have underlying airway pathology such as a tumor, infection, congenital abnormality, stenosis, edema, traumatic injury, and foreign object. Therefore, a very cautious approach must be taken in every situation.

Preparation in the Emergency Airway

In an emergency airway, preparedness is always critical. Even though time is of the essence, a well-prepared environment will aid in securing an airway. In all airways, a well-thought-out plan is needed, as is certain equipment. At every airway there should be an ambu bag connected to oxygen, a mask, and working suction with a yankauer tip. Additionally, all devices that are to be used in the airway should be prepped so that they are readily available when needed. It is also advised that there be someone available when securing the airway to aid in any way possible.

The Difficult Airway Algorithm

"The difficult airway represents a complex interaction between patient factors, the clinical setting and the skills of the practitioner" (American Society of Anesthesiologists [ASA] 2003). The American Society of Anesthesiologists (ASA) developed a difficult airway algorithm in 1993, which was updated in 2003, in which they defined the difficult airway as the "clinical situation in which a conventionally trained anesthesiologist experiences difficulty with face mask ventilation of the upper airway, difficulty with tracheal intubation, or both" (ASA 2003). The algorithm is used as a model for the approach to the emergency and difficult airways, and was created to decrease the rate of adverse outcomes with the more complex airway. When approaching any airway, a clear plan of action is necessary in case any difficulty is encountered. The algorithm provides a clear stepwise approach to the various considerations in attempting to secure an airway. The algorithm also considers awake versus asleep approaches, and noninvasive versus invasive techniques.

Approaches to the Emergency Airway

Asleep Intubation

The determination of whether to manage a patient's airway asleep rather than awake is a critical decision. In emergency airway situations, if the decision has been made to intubate the patient asleep, predictors of a difficult intubation should be relatively small. In these cases, patient's status should be evaluated to assess the risk for regurgitation and pulmonary aspiration. High-risk patients include those that have a full stomach, intra-abdominal processes, or gastroparesis. These patients would necessitate a rapid sequence intubation (RSI), in which a secured airway is established in the shortest amount of time to minimize the chance of aspiration of gastric contents. The essential principles of RSI include preoxygenation, induction of anesthesia, rapid neuromuscular blockade, and intubation, while maintaining cricoid pressure (Barash et al. 2009). Cricoid pressure, also known as the Sellick maneuver, is thought to compress the esophagus against the vertebra in order to prevent pulmonary aspiration (Miller et al. 2009). Once the airway is secured and confirmed, cricoid pressure can be released. Rapid neuromuscular blockade can be achieved with either succinylcholine or double the standard dose of rocuronium, a fast non-depolarizing muscle relaxant. The onset of succinylcholine, a depolarizing muscle relaxant, is about 30 s and duration is between 5 and 10 min. This gives the ability to awaken a patient if a difficulty arises, and proceed with an awake approach if needed. In situations where there is no increased risk of aspiration, a straightforward

anesthetic induction can be followed. If there is any concern that the patient may be a difficult intubation, then an awake approach should be taken.

Awake Intubation

The awake intubation is a technique that allows for the maintenance of spontaneous respirations accompanied with a patent airway. In difficult airways, especially those with significant pathology, the awake intubation may be the only option for a successful and safe intubation. When approaching this technique, there are many points to consider, including the route of anesthetizing the airway, patient positioning to maintain patent airway, the extent of patient cooperation, and whether or not any sedation is feasible. To provide an optimized environment for the awake intubation, 0.2 mg of glycopyrrolate may be given. Glycopyrrolate inhibits salivation and the production of respiratory tract secretions (Morgan et al. 2006).

Techniques for anesthetizing the airway include nebulizers, topical spray, transtracheal injection, and nerve blocks. Usually a combination of these techniques provides the most successful results. Nebulized 2% or 4% lidocaine can be use to anesthetize the entire airway; however, results often vary, and it can take 20 min to completely anesthetize the airway, which can be an issue in the emergent airway. Aerosolized and viscous lidocaine are other approaches to anesthetizing the airway and, when done in a sequential manner, can successfully result in an anesthetized upper airway (Miller et al. 2009). Cocaine is a common local anesthetic used by otolaryngologists when anesthetizing the upper airway because of local anesthetic property and vasoconstrictor ability (Barash et al. 2009). It is possible to increase the extent of topicalization by spraying lidocaine into the trachea while doing an initial laryngoscopy. The transtracheal approach is accomplished by injecting 4ml of 4% lidocaine through the cricothyroid membrane. After the needle makes contact with the skin, constant aspiration of the syringe should be performed until aspiration of air occurs. At this point, the local anesthetic should be injected and needle removed. The patient will typically cough, which aids in the spread of the anesthetic and blockade of the sensory nerve endings of the recurrent laryngeal nerve (Hadzic 2006). Another common nerve block used in awake intubations is the superior laryngeal nerve block. This requires a bilateral nerve block, which anesthetizes the area between epiglottis and vocal cords. This block is accomplished by locating greater cornu of the hyoid bone with a 25G needle, then retracting slightly, and injecting 3 ml of 2% lidocaine after aspiration for air and blood. This will effectively block the internal and external portions of the superior laryngeal nerve (Hadzic 2006).

When dealing with the airway, patient positioning is critical to successful intubations. The sniffing position is the traditional position for successful intubations, and should be used when the emergency airway is encountered. A problem that may occur is when the awake patient cannot tolerate lying flat, and the awake intubation is necessary. In these cases, optimizing the position most tolerated by the patient is necessary. Patient positioning may also dictate which techniques of intubations can be used.

During awake airways, patient cooperation is necessary. Without it, awake intubations are impossible. Patients should be informed of what an awake intubation entails, and should be sure that they are able to cooperate during the procedure. Sedation, especially in the emergency airway, can be very dangerous. Even the smallest amount of sedation may cause airway to be compromised and can make the situation a critical one.

Techniques for Intubation
Careful planning must occur when considering the emergency airway. A logical and succinct plan must be established to have the highest probability for success. The difficult airway algorithm is not only a great example of planning when dealing with the difficult airway, but is a useful tool when dealing with any airway, especially the emergency airway. The ASA difficult airway algorithm dictates a clear and structured way to deal with the difficult airway and can act as a guide in any situation.

Blind Intubation
The blind intubation technique requires no equipment other than an endotracheal tube. It is usually performed through the nasal route in a spontaneously breathing patient. In emergency situations, sedation should be avoided. The nose and upper airway should be adequately anesthetized, after which an endotracheal tube should be slowly advanced while listening to the breath sounds coming from the tube. If breath sounds are no longer heard, it means that the tube has entered into the esophagus and should be pulled back until breath

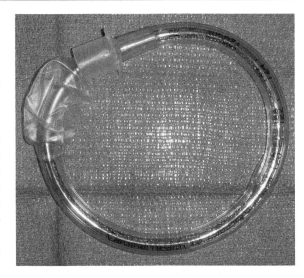

Emergency Airways, Fig. 1 An endotracheal tube connected end to end in preparation for a blind intubation

sounds are heard again. To aid in a blind intubation, prior to placing the tube, connect the tube end to end (Fig. 1). This will give the tube a curve, which makes it more likely to pass anteriorly and end up in the trachea (Morgan et al. 2006). Inflation of the cuff of the tube while in the oropharynx and head flexion are other maneuvers that can be done to aid the placement of the tube (Miller et al. 2009).

Laryngoscopy
The most standard and commonly used way to intubate is by using direct laryngoscopy. This can be accomplished by using a laryngoscope with an appropriately sized blade attached, most commonly the Macintosh or Miller. Direct laryngoscopy can be done in either an asleep or awake patient, if given adequate anesthetic to the airway. Another form of laryngoscopy is done by video laryngoscopy, for example, using the Glidescope (Fig. 2). This involves a specialized laryngoscope and blade that has an optical lens at the end. This is especially useful in patients for whom intubation with direct laryngoscopy is not successful due to limited view. The technique of use is similar to that of direct laryngoscopy, and competence can be achieved rapidly (Miller et al. 2009). Another example of a portable version of an optical laryngoscope is the Airtraq. The Airtraq is a single use laryngoscope with an endotracheal tube–guiding channel that can be used in difficult airways (Barash et al. 2009).

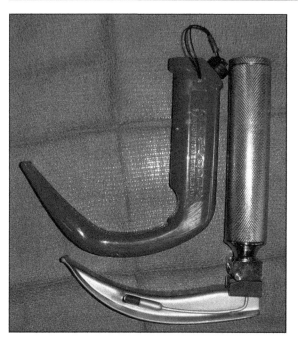

Emergency Airways, Fig. 2 The Glidescope handle and a laryngoscope with a Macintosh blade for comparison

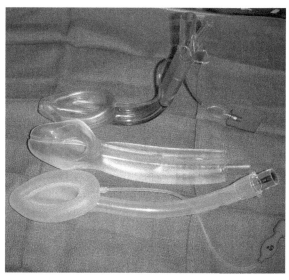

Emergency Airways, Fig. 3 Examples of three LMAs, (*bottom to top*) Laryngeal Mask Airway, i-gel Supraglottic Airway, and LMA Supreme. Both i-gel and LMA Supreme have distal suction ports

Laryngeal Mask Airway Intubation

The laryngeal mask airway (LMA) is a very useful tool in the difficult airway especially when an unanticipated difficulty is encountered. The LMA (Fig. 3) is considered a periglottic device that forms a seal around the larynx when inflated (Miller et al. 2009). The LMA is traditionally used in place of the facemask in anesthetics that do not require intubation but involve general anesthesia. The LMA can be used for ventilation, but it is certainly not a secure airway, and does not protect against aspiration. Some LMAs have distal suction ports that can be used to pass a suction catheter into the stomach. The LMA has become such a useful tool in difficult airways, where the patient cannot be intubated or ventilated, that it has been included in the ASA difficult airway algorithm. In emergency situations, the LMA can also be used to facilitate intubations (Fig. 4) when other techniques have failed. Tubes can either be passed blindly through the LMA, or via fiber-optic, which has a much greater success rate (Miller et al. 2009). A reusable intubating LMA (Fig. 5) has also been created. It has been designed specifically for intubations and has a high success rate, but it is still a blind technique.

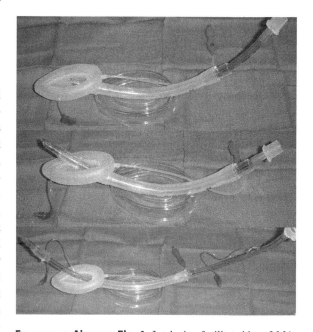

Emergency Airways, Fig. 4 Intubation facilitated by a LMA. (*Top to bottom*) #5 LMA loaded with a well-lubricated #7.0 endotracheal tube (ETT). ETT advanced. Further advancement and removal of LMA facilitated by another #7.0 ETT

Fiber-optic Bronchoscope

Similar to the idea of the video laryngoscope, the fiber-optic scope is an extremely useful tool especially in emergency and difficult airways. It is useful in

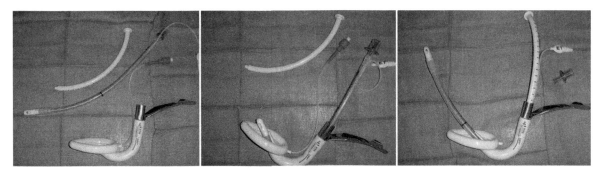

Emergency Airways, Fig. 5 A non-disposable version of an intubating LMA, the LMA Fasttrach

situations with very small mouth openings or severely limited neck mobility, where other laryngoscopes cannot be used (Miller et al. 2009). It is a very safe way to secure an airway in emergency situations. The fiber-optic can be used either via the oral or nasal route. In an awake patient, it can be tolerated and used in any patient position. When using a fiber-optic scope, prior to intubation, glycopyrrolate can be given to reduce secretions and improve the view, and the appropriate tracheal tube should be loaded. While advancing the fiber-optic, the scope can be manipulated in different directions by either hand controls or rotation of the actual scope. In emergency situations, the aspiration channel on the scope can be used both to suction secretions and to provide oxygen (Morgan et al. 2006). After passing the vocal cords with the fiber-optic scope, tracheal rings should be visualized, then the carina, at which point the tracheal tube should be carefully passed. If there is difficulty passing the tracheal tube, twisting of the tube in a counterclockwise manner will sometimes help the advancement. After securing the endotracheal tube, placement should be confirmed by fiber-optic bronchoscopy. If there is difficulty obtaining any view with the fiber-optic bronchoscope, a jaw thrust, Ovassapian oral airway, or direct laryngoscopy can help (Miller et al. 2009).

Retrograde Intubation

Retrograde intubation is a technique that is typically used in difficult or emergency airways. This technique can be used when other techniques of intubation have failed or if it is believed that intubation will be impossible. The most common reasons to perform a retrograde intubation are secretions, blood, airway malignancy, jaw fractures, and an unstable cervical spine (Barash et al. 2009). Retrograde intubations can

also be performed in emergency situations when other equipment is not available for use. Adequate local anesthetic should be given to the airway so that the patient is comfortable during this procedure. This technique involves locating the cricothyroid membrane and puncturing it with an angiocath needle. Before passing the needle, local anesthetic should be given to the skin. If there is difficulty locating the cricothyroid membrane, neck extension can help (Miller et al. 2009). Once the needle enters the trachea, as confirmed by aspiration of air, the angiocath can be advanced while removing the needle. Next a guidewire is passed in the direction of the upper airway until it comes out of the nose or mouth. Once the wire is obtained, the endotracheal tube can be guided into correct position in several ways. The tube can be passed directly over the wire, pulled into the trachea with the wire tied to the Murphy eye of the tube, placing a tube exchanger via the wire, then passing the tube over the exchanger, or by placing a fiber-optic loaded with a tube into the trachea over the wire, then passing the tube to name a few (Barash et al. 2009).

Cricothyrotomy

Cricothyrotomy is a percutaneous airway that is made through the cricothyroid membrane. There are two forms of cricothyrotomy, cannula and surgical. Cannula cricothyrotomy is typically used in the emergency "cannot intubate and cannot ventilate" situations. The procedure is similar to the transtracheal block and the initial steps of the retrograde intubation. Typically, the largest angiocath is placed through the cricothyroid membrane into the trachea. Confirmation of the placement of the cannula is achieved by aspiration of air and should always be done. Ventilation can be achieved thought jet ventilation. There is always a risk of

Emergency Airways,
Fig. 6 Cricothyrotomy
catheter assembly with a 16G
catheter, 3cc syringe, and
tube connector from a
#7.5 endotracheal tube

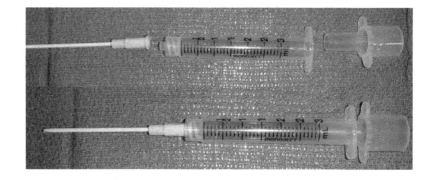

Emergency Airways,
Fig. 7 Connections of the
cricothyrotomy catheter to an
ambu bag and oxygen tubing

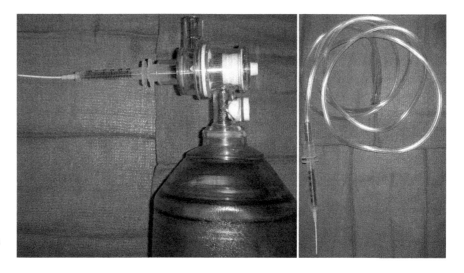

barotrauma to the lungs when using jet ventilation; therefore, considerations should be made when using a jet ventilator. Since deflation of the lungs is through the upper airway during jet ventilation, if there is an upper airway obstruction, the jet ventilator should be disconnected from the cannula to allow for deflation. If a jet ventilator is not available, the cannula can be attached to an ambu bag. To accomplish this, a 3cc syringe with its plunger removed can be fitted with a snugly fitted connector that goes between an endotracheal tube and an ambu bag (Fig. 6). Then it can be attached to the cannula and ambu bag, providing an alternate means of oxygenation and ventilation (Fig. 7).

The surgical cricothyrotomy is a simple procedure that can be done rapidly to secure an airway in emergency situations. This involves identifying the cricothyroid membrane while extending the head and neck, making a horizontal stab with a scalpel through the skin and membrane, and placing the tube trough the

incision. If locating the cricothyroid membrane is difficult, an initial vertical incision can be made to aid in finding the correct location (Miller et al. 2009). Once the tube is secured, ventilation should be confirmed in both lungs. When dealing with the difficult airway in non-emergent situations, the patient should be prepped and anesthetized for surgical cricothyrotomy if the initial plans for securing the airway fail.

Tracheotomy
The tracheotomy is a much more complex and involved procedure compared to the cricothyrotomy. It is a procedure that only an experienced surgeon can perform in a short amount of time, in comparison to the cricothyrotomy, which can be done by anyone with knowledge of the airway anatomy in a few seconds. In anticipated difficult airways, such as laryngeal tumors, an elective tracheotomy can be done when there is a very high likelihood that the airway will be lost during intubation (Miller et al. 2009).

Other Techniques

There are many other intubation techniques and devices that exist, especially for the difficult intubation. The airway bougie and the lighted stylets are two devices that can be used in emergency situations to aid in successful intubations. The bougie is a long, semi-malleable stylet with an angled tip that can be used to help intubate when the vocal cords are unable to be visualized. After direct laryngoscopy, the bougie can be passed under the epiglottis, with its tip aimed anteriorly toward the trachea. Once in the trachea and when the angled tip encounters the tracheal rings, a distinctive clicking will be felt, and the endotracheal tube can then be passed over the bougie to secure the airway (Barash et al. 2009). This technique is considered a blind technique and does not guarantee successful intubation with every use. The lighted stylet is a device that uses a bright light to help guide intubation. This technique is similar to that of the bougie. When in the trachea, the lighted stylet will emit a distinct light in the midline seen through the skin; however, when it is in the esophagus, there will either be no light or a very diffuse glow of light (Miller et al. 2009).

Cross-References

▶ Anesthesia Considerations in Head and Neck Surgery
▶ Anesthetic Techniques for Otolaryngologic Patient
▶ Emergent Airway
▶ Tracheotomy

References

American Society of Anesthesiologists Task Force on Management of the Difficult Airway (2003) Practice guidelines for the management of the difficult airway: an updated report by the American Society of Anesthesiologists Task Force on Management of the Difficult Airway. Anesthesiology 98:1269–1277
Barash PG, Cullen BF, Stoelting RK, Cahalan MK, Stock MC (2009) Clinical anesthesia, 6th edn. Lippincott Williams & Wilkins, Philadelphia
Hadzic A (2006) Textbook of regional anesthesia and acute pain management. McGraw-Hill, New York
Miller RD, Eriksson LI, Fleisher LA, Wiener-Kronish JP, Young WL (2009) Miller's anesthesia, 7th edn. Churchill Livingstone, Orlando
Morgan G, Mikhail M, Murray M (2006) Clinical anesthesiology, 4th edn. McGraw-Hill, New York

Emergent Airway

Eric P. Wilkens
Department of Anesthesiology, Albert Einstein Medical College, New York, NY, USA

Synonyms

Difficult airway; Difficult intubation; Difficult ventilation; Emergency airway

Definition

Difficult Ventilation: The inability of an experienced provider to maintain oxygen saturation greater than 90% in a patient who had normal oxygen saturation prior to induction of anesthesia.

Difficult Laryngoscopy: The inability of an experienced provider to visualize the vocal cords in a patient in multiple attempts at standard laryngoscopy.

Difficult Intubation: The inability of an experienced provider to place an endotracheal tube in a patient's trachea.

Emergent Airway: The transition point at which a patient's oxygen saturation becomes difficult or impossible to maintain above 90% during an intubation or procedure.

Basic Characteristics

Each time a patient endures a trauma, develops respiratory distress, or undergoes an anesthetic for a surgical procedure, there is a very real, yet generally small chance that the process of securing a tube in the patient's trachea becomes "emergent." From the American Society of Anesthesiologists guidelines (ASA 2003), an emergent airway occurs any time a patient's oxygen saturation is unable to be maintained above 90% in the instance that the patient had normal oxygen saturation prior to the event or induction of the anesthetic. The emergent airway is an event for which contingencies must be in place, regardless of whether the patient is considered to have a normal, or "easy" airway, or a predictably more "difficult" airway. The most important thing to remember in treating an emergency airway is situational awareness: that the intubation has diverged from normal and has become "emergent." The primary goal of management of the emergent airway is to reestablish oxygenation. This does not necessarily mean that tracheal intubation need be achieved, as in the case that mask ventilation becomes adequate.

The American Society of Anesthesiologists (ASA) guidelines (ASA 2003) have in their published guidelines for a difficult airway to consider always the value and possibility of allowing the patient to wake up. In an emergency airway event, however, there is simply not enough time for medications to redistribute or to process. An emergency airway is an uncommon enough event that providers who have not had recent simulation training may fixate on "waking up" a patient, or upon using airway techniques that had repeatedly failed in the preceding minutes. Proper management of an emergency airway means that steps have been taken to avoid or mitigate circumstances that foster an emergency event and that a provider thinks of alternate means of ventilating a patient's lungs in an efficient manner. Quite often in these situations, a patient will be in a potentially dangerous middle ground of anesthetic inadequate for the intubation procedure (in hope that they "wake up"), yet too much to have regained spontaneous ventilation. This combined with a low saturation and an increased chance of airway edema associated with multiple attempts at laryngoscopy usually serves to make marginal or emergent airway events worse.

Basic Emergency Airway Management

The more emergent and grave the situation, the smaller the decision tree becomes. In the case of the emergency airway, step one is to recognize that mask ventilation is inadequate and that the emergency is developing and for the provider to request help as soon as possible. The next step, according to the ASA guidelines, is to attempt placement of a laryngeal mask airway (LMA). If this is successful, the provider now has time to consider definitive airway procedures or awakening the patient. If the LMA placement is unsuccessful, the provider may perform one more attempt at direct laryngoscopy (keeping in mind that this is likely already proven unsuccessful) or go to another means of securing the airway, usually but not limited to a subglottic approach such as needle cricothyrotomy,

emergent cricothyrotomy with an endotracheal tube, or emergency tracheostomy. Other methods, described in brief below, include blind intubation, use of hollow tube exchangers, use of lighted stylets, and the like. In extreme circumstances, cardiopulmonary bypass, partial or complete, can provide oxygenation and ventilation.

Airway and Oxygenation Concerns

The preoperative evaluation of a patient's airway from the anesthesiology perspective tries to assess three things: (1) Is it safe to ablate spontaneous ventilation? (2) Is it possible to place a tube in the patient's trachea with ease or in a standard fashion? (3) Is it possible to mask ventilate or deliver oxygen to the patient's lungs if a problem occurs?

Anesthesiology assessment of the airway helps predict the ease of mask ventilation and endotracheal tube placement (Rose and Cohen 1994). The following characteristics represent a predictably "easy" intubation and thus a low risk of developing into an emergency airway:

1. Normal body habitus
2. Free range of motion of the neck (good neck extension)
3. A proportionate thyromental distance (absence of micro- or macrognathia)
4. Palpable cricoid cartilage (absence of goiter, possibility of cricothyrotomy)
5. Normal temporomandibular joint range of motion (greater than 3 cm in an adult)
6. Normal dentition (dentures, condition of teeth, prominence of upper incisors, particularly teeth #8 and #9)
7. Mallampati score of 1 or 2 (visualize all or most of the uvula with extension of tongue and without phonation)
8. No signs/symptoms of sleep apnea

The Mallampati score is a system used to estimate the ease of visualizing the vocal cords during laryngoscopy. It combines the ability of a patient to open and sublux the mandible, the prominence of the teeth, and the size of the tongue, into a simple system. A score of 1 indicates that the palate, faucial pillars, and entire uvula can be visualized with the patient opening their mouth, extending the tongue, and not vocalizing. Mallampati 2 indicates that only the palate, faucial pillars, and base of the uvula may be seen.

Mallampati 3 indicates only some of the faucial pillars and palate are visualized, and Mallampati 4 signifies that only the palate alone or less may be visualized. The Mallampati system estimates the ease of performing laryngoscopy, not necessarily the ability to ventilate the patient's lungs after induction of anesthesia (Mallampati et al. 1985).

As examples, patient may be slender, yet have severe temporomandibular joint dysfunction or have been in a trauma necessitating the use of a cervical spine stabilizing collar, limiting the use of standard laryngoscopy. In these instances, the team could consider inducing the anesthetic and intubating the trachea without direct laryngoscopy with confidence that ventilation will occur easily throughout the intubation process. In contrast, an obese patient with documented sleep apnea, an nonpalpable cricoid cartilage (secondary to adipose tissue), and a Mallampati class 4 mouth opening will be at high risk of emergency airway issues with a standard anesthetic induction due to their pulmonary disease and predicted difficulty with ventilation and intubation.

Otolaryngology procedures commonly present the patient's anesthesiologist with two additional advantages in avoiding and treating emergency airway issues. The otolaryngologist's skill set requires familiarly with the airway, providing the anesthesiologist an additional set of skilled hands when manipulating the patient's airway, and secondly, the surgeon may have specific knowledge of the patient's airway from preoperative scans, preoperative nasopharyngoscopy, or previous procedures. This knowledge would allow the surgeon to communicate that the patient is likely to be difficult to intubate. For example, the care team may opt to begin a partial laryngectomy and modified radical neck dissection by conducting an awake tracheostomy at the beginning of the case, minimizing potentially dangerous airway situations immediately. A more extreme example would be preparing for cardiopulmonary bypass (to guarantee oxygenation) prior to examination and dilatation, an extreme subglottic stenosis.

Common comorbidities associated with otolaryngology patients, particularly those being treated for head and neck malignancies, such as obesity, smoking, and alcohol use, can shorten the time that a provider has to acquire safely a tube in the patient's trachea. Obesity increases oxygen demand and consumption on a systemic level, as well as impairs pulmonary mechanics by restricting chest wall excursion and reducing functional residual capacity in an exaggerated fashion in the supine position. Chronic alcohol use leads to the development of arteriolar-venous vascular malformations, creating left-to-right shunts that efficiently divert oxygenated blood from tissues just prior to reaching capillary beds. Smoking decreases oxygen diffusion capacity and the efficiency of the lungs in many ways.

Time and the Pitfalls of Pulse Oximetry and End-Tidal Carbon Dioxide Detection

The emergent airway is defined as a failure to maintain *oxygenation*, usually monitored by pulse oximetry, but the gold standard for the confirmation that an airway appliance is allowing for *ventilation* is end-tidal carbon dioxide detection.

Standard pulse oximeters measure the oxygenation of the blood by comparing two wavelengths of light absorbed differentially by oxygenated and deoxygenated hemoglobin (Szocik et al. 2000). The most accurate reading is obtained when the following conditions are met:

- A regular heart rate and rhythm
- An adequate blood pressure and cardiac output
- Absence of methemoglobinemia or carbon monoxide
- Adequate blood flow in the extremity with the monitor
- The removal of blue or metallic finger nail polishes if a finger is the monitoring site

The other major consideration with pulse oximetry is the lag time involved between a desaturation event and the monitor registering the correction. Despite a provider seeing that the chest wall is rising and breath sounds are present, the pulse oximeter will continue to decrease and display desaturation because the oxygenated blood must travel through the pulmonary venous system and back out through left heart into the systemic circulation and reach the monitor. In patients with a low cardiac output (heart failure, etc.), it may be 30 s or more before the patient's pulse oximetry reading stops declining.

The gold standard of confirmation for any endotracheal device, supraglottic devices (laryngeal mask airways), or mask ventilation is the monitoring of carbon dioxide (Knill 1993). From the waveform obtained, the carbon dioxide monitor can be used to determine effectiveness of muscle relaxation, demonstrate the presence of restrictive lung disease, and be a rough indicator of cardiac output (low or no cardiac output results in low or no end-tidal carbon dioxide). In most operating rooms, carbon dioxide is measured with other gases in the anesthesia machine gas analyzer. Outside the operating room setting, in "code" situations, the emergency department, or in the field with emergency medical services, the detection relies on an appliance, temporarily placed on the endotracheal tube and in which is a piece of litmus paper that changes color from reaction with the carbon dioxide. It is important to note that end-tidal carbon dioxide may be positive for the first 2–3 breaths, even if the endotracheal tube is in the esophagus, because of air that may be in the stomach. The end-tidal carbon dioxide should rapidly become zero or some low value. Conversely, end-tidal carbon dioxide may read near zero despite a properly placed endotracheal tube.

Treatment Tools and Techniques

The tools and techniques used to manage an emergency airway event fall into three categories: (1) supraglottic, (2) subglottic, and (3) uncommon. Of these categories, the supraglottic techniques are by far the most common and most familiar practiced by providers. These advantages and disadvantages will be discussed briefly. The most common disadvantage of many devices is that they must be removed in order to secure definitively an airway. Supraglottic devices used in treating emergent airway events include (Fig. 1):

- Repositioning patient and jaw thrust
- Nasal airways
- Oral airways
- Laryngeal mask airways
- Direct laryngoscopy
- Video laryngoscopy
- Fiber-optic bronchoscopy
- Eschmann stylet
- Blind intubation
- Lighted stylets
- Intubation stylet
- Tube exchange bougies

In an emergency airway event, it is unlikely that position changes such as flexion or extension of the head, elevating the back and head, performing jaw thrust will allow suddenly for adequate ventilation, but in practiced hands, the bulk of these maneuvers

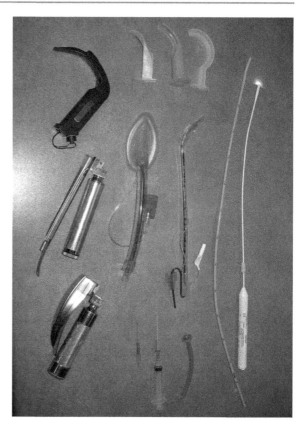

Emergent Airway, Fig. 1 A variety of airway devices commonly used. At the *top*, a lighted stylet and an Eschmann stylet. Below that, from *left* to *right*, oral airways, a styletted endotracheal tube, a nasal airway, needles for cricothyrotomy and jet ventilation, a video laryngoscope blade, a Miller laryngoscope blade, and a Macintosh laryngoscope blade

can be performed in under 3 s and allow for a better view of the glottis using another technique.

Nasal airways hold a distinct advantage over many supraglottic devices because they can be left in place while performing other techniques such as laryngoscopy or placement of a laryngeal mask airway. Nasal airways are simple, pliable tubular devices, are placed into a nostril, and slide behind the tongue. Nasal airways are well tolerated and can be placed easily in awake patients, and when properly sized, prevent obstruction by the tongue and other soft tissues in the neck. Caution must be taken when placing these airways because of their tendency to initiate bleeding from the nasal mucosa. Many providers coat the airways with local anesthetics which can also dilate this friable tissue, increasing the chance that bleeding occurs in the airway.

Emergent Airway, Fig. 2 Three oral airways. At the *top*, a standard oral airway with ventilation channels. In the *middle*, an oral airway with a center channel. At the *bottom*, an oral airway with an open center channel designed to be used to facilitate fiber-optic bronchoscopy

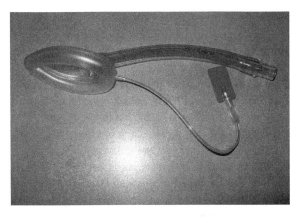

Emergent Airway, Fig. 3 An example of a supraglottic airway device or laryngeal mask airway. The tube portion is thicker than a standard endotracheal tube. The inflatable ring allows for a seal at the larynx

Oral airways are solid plastic devices that are generally have a center channel or two side channels to provide air flow. Oral airways, properly sized, are designed to rest in the mouth cavity on the hard and soft palates. The tip of an oral airway rests in the vicinity of the vallecula and performs a similar function to that of a vigorous jaw thrust maneuver – anteriorly locating soft tissues. Some oral airways even include an inflatable balloon for seating in the pharynx. Gently placed oral airways; create little trauma and bleeding in the airway (Fig. 2). Oral airways are poorly tolerated in conscious patients and can cause coughing, choking, and increase the chance of laryngospasm in a patient emerging from anesthesia. Except in performing fiber-optic bronchoscopy, an oral airway's primary disadvantage is that it must be removed prior to performing other airway techniques.

The most recent and largest change in the American Society of Anesthesiologists difficult airway algorithm is the prominence of the laryngeal mask airway (LMA) (Hung and Murphy 2004). A laryngeal mask airway is a device with a 13 mm adapter to attach to an anesthesia machine circuit or ambu bag. The adapter is at the end of a variably pliable or stiff tube that ends in an oblong, inflatable ring-shaped cup. These devices have variable ability through which to place a bronchoscope, intubating stylet, or endotracheal tube, based on their design. LMAs are bulky items that fully occupy the hypopharynx and much of the oral cavity and pharynx (Fig. 3). LMAs are placed in a blind fashion and a superb for emergency airway situations because of this feature. However, an LMA is not a definitive airway device; it simply facilitates getting air to the level of the glottis. Since an LMA is not a definitive device, it is not sufficient for long-term use, but instead, should be considered a bridge to either emergence from the anesthetic or definitive airway security. There is a tendency to apply much higher airway ventilation pressures than normal during an emergency airway event, and LMAs prevent neither insufflation of the stomach nor reflux of stomach contents into the lungs. The lowest adequate pressure required to ventilate a patient's lungs should be used when ventilating via an LMA. Another caution with LMA use is that the devices themselves are bulky and can cause swelling and increase the chance of bleeding in the pharynx and hypopharynx.

Direct and indirect laryngoscopies are the most practiced of the airway techniques. In anesthesia practice, laryngoscope blades have a light source close to the tip, a blunt-tipped blade, and a flange on the left side (an exception to this rule is the Bizarri California blade which has no flange). Laryngoscope blades are either curved or straight, to varying degrees, with the primary design goal being whether or not to lift the epiglottis out of the way directly or indirectly. The "easiest" and most common technique is to use a curved blade, usually a Macintosh, guide the blunt tip into the vallecula, and elevate the epiglottis indirectly with an anterior and inferior movement.

A straight blade, such as a Miller blade, is designed to be placed just under the epiglottis and elevate it directly, providing a view of the vocal cords (Mulcaster et al. 2003). A recent development gaining popularity is indirect laryngoscopy via the video laryngoscope (White and Elvir-Lazo 2011). Shaped similarly to Macintosh blades, video laryngoscopes provide not only a light source at the tip of the blade, but also a fiber-optic lens and video display, allowing for visualization of the vocal cords with less effort or for patients in whom traditional laryngoscopy provided a poor view. Direct or indirect laryngoscopy has the advantage of actually visualizing the vocal cords the majority of the time and allowing the provider to watch the endotracheal tube pass through the glottis. Considered the gold standard, these techniques have few disadvantages when performed with experienced hands, but must be cautioned that repeated attempts at laryngoscopy lead to airway soft tissue trauma, bleeding, and potential problems with mask ventilation. In an emergency airway situation, it is allowable to try a different blade (straight instead of curved) and to allow a second provider one more attempt prior to other techniques. However, one more attempt with a laryngoscope must be just that, only one more attempt. A common error in emergency airway management is the repeated use of laryngoscopy despite multiple prior failed attempts.

Fiber-optic bronchoscopy is an indirect form of visualizing the vocal cords, trachea, and bronchial tree. It is the gold standard for intubation in the awake patient and an excellent technique for patients who have had or potentially have a difficult laryngoscopy. Bronchoscopes used to intubate patients often have small ports and are not good devices for removing liquids and other materials from the airway. Usually, oxygen is insufflated through the port during its use for this purpose. The fiber-optic technique is susceptible to saliva, blood, and other material in the airway and is often most successful as one of the first techniques in an intubation attempt. As airway swelling and trauma increases from previous attempts at instrumentation, the likelihood of success with a fiber-optic bronchoscope decreases as well.

Other techniques are less reliable and are mentioned here for completeness. Blind intubation, usually with an endotracheal tube with a wire stylet, is unreliable even for an experienced practitioner. Replacing the wire stylet with a "lighted" stylet,

a light at the end of the stylet is marginally more effective, but requires that the room lights be turned down or off to visualize the light at the tip of the endotracheal tube through the skin of the neck. Another disadvantage to this technique is the thickness of the soft tissue of the neck. A thick neck will impede visualization of the light, reducing the success of the procedure. Use of these blind techniques will also irritate tissues that are likely to have been traumatized by prior attempts, worsening the situation. Bougies and the Eschmann stylet, over which endotracheal tubes can be slid, are also poor devices when placed in a blind fashion (Van Zundert et al. 2009). Usually, these supplement a poor video or direct view of the glottis and can render a laryngoscopy with little or no view of the vocal cords into a successful intubation by placement of the smaller stylet. Also, transmission of the vibration of the stylet rubbing on the tracheal rings can confirm correct placement of the stylet despite not seeing it pass through the vocal cords.

The major subglottic techniques include needle cricothyrotomy with jet ventilation, cricothyrotomy with an endotracheal tube, and emergency tracheostomy. These techniques are performed rarely by anesiologists. This author would discourage an anesthesiologist or surgeon with little or no experience with the surgical techniques of cricothyrotomy or tracheostomy from performing them in an emergency situation and promoting the use of needle cricothyrotomy and jet ventilation (Fig. 4). Extreme caution must be used with this technique as well. Placement of a larger bore (20G or 18G) intravenous catheter needle should be performed with the needle on a syringe that is partially filled with saline. The needle should be angled caudad toward the sternum and aimed at the cricothyroid membrane, not into the tracheal rings themselves. Aspiration resulting in bubbles in the syringe signifying that the tip of the needle is in the trachea is a must! After deployment of the catheter into the trachea, aspiration of air must be confirmed again prior to initiation of jet ventilation. The catheter must be held in place for the entirety of the ventilation procedure. Jet ventilators insufflate oxygen directly from wall pipelines and are released at pressures upward of 50 psig. This massive pressure can easily cause pneumothorax or tracheal rupture. The pressure should be administered briefly, and each breath stopped immediately as the chest is seen to start rising

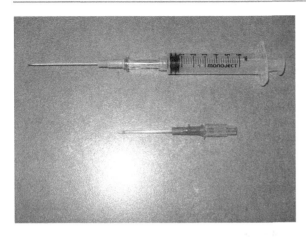

Emergent Airway, Fig. 4 A 20G IV catheter loaded on to a syringe. In an emergency, the provider must partially fill the syringe with saline to effect proper aspiration and confirmation of placement in the trachea. Below this, is an example of a 14G IV catheter, also acceptable for use in jet ventilation

(Nunn et al. 2007). Allowing sufficient time for the lungs to deflate is required to prevent barotrauma from breath stacking, keeping in mind that the glottis and pharynx may be edematous and slow exhalation. If the catheter is dislodged or in the incorrect spot during jet ventilation, air can be insufflated into the neck, head, and mediastinum, causing irreparable harm. Properly placed and performed, jet ventilation can be used for even several hours while definitive airway acquisition is performed. The other surgical techniques have the advantage of using less traumatic, normal insufflation pressures, but all associated problems with these surgical techniques (bleeding, infection, scarring, tracheal stenosis) must be considered.

Finally, there are more rare techniques available in many sites, but not necessarily the most practicable. Cardiopulmonary bypass, partial or complete, can utilize and extracorporeal oxygenator for a short period of time, but the time required to find a bypass machine, perfusionist, and surgeon to place the cannulae required is often far too long to be practical for the patient. Helium-oxygen mixtures for ventilation again may facilitate oxygenation, but not all facilities have this gas mixture readily available.

Summary

Emergency airways arise from unforeseen events. Proper airway assessment and communication between the surgical and anesthesia staff are critical in avoiding and managing emergent airway events. In summary, the emergent airway can arise any time a patient is in the process of being intubated, or has an endotracheal or tracheostomy tube in place to maintain their oxygenation. The emergent airway exists at the time that adequate saturation cannot be maintained by either mask ventilation or standard intubation techniques. Of most importance is (1) recognizing that an emergency condition has arisen, (2) that the time available to correct the situation and prevent permanent injury to the patient is very limited (1–2 min), and (3) the practitioner is familiar with a reasonable set of alternative techniques to secure the airway and guarantee oxygenation.

Cross-References

▶ Adult Glottic Stenosis
▶ Subglottic and Tracheal Stenosis in Adults
▶ Tracheostomy
▶ Vocal Cord Surgery

References

American Society of Anesthesiologists (2003) Practice guidelines for management of the difficult airway: an updated report by the american society of anesthesiologists task force on the management of the difficult airway. Anesthesiology 98:1269–1277

Hung O, Murphy M (2004) Unanticipated difficult intubation. Curr Opin Anaesthesiol 17(6):479–481

Knill RL (1993) Practical CO_2 monitoring in anaesthesia. Can J Anaesth 40:R40

Mallampati SR, Gatt SP, Gugino LD (1985) A clinical sign to predict difficult tracheal intubation: a prospective study. Can Anaesth Soc J 32:429–434

Mulcaster JT, Mills J, Hung OR (2003) Laryngoscopic intubation: learning and performance. Anesthesiology 98(1):23–27

Nunn C, Uffman J, Bhananker SM (2007) Bilateral tension pneumothoraces following jet ventilation via an airway exchange catheter. J Anesth 21(1):76–79

Rose DK, Cohen MM (1994) The airway: problems and predictions in 18,500 patients. Can J Anaesth 41(5 pt 1):372–383

Szocik JF, Barker SJ, Tremper KK (2000) Fundamental principles of monitoring instrumentation. In: Miller RD (ed) Anesthesia, 5th edn. Churchill Livingstone, Philadelphia, pp 1053–1077

Van Zundert A, Maassen R, Lee R (2009) A macintosh laryngoscope blade for viedoe laryngoscopy reduces stylet use in patients with normal airways. Anesth Analg 109(3):825–831

White P, Elvir-Lazo OL (2011) Video-laryngoscopy: great glottic view, but does it really make a difference clinically in routine practice?. Anesth News Guide to Airway Management, pp 34–35

EMG

▶ Electromyogram

EMG Bursts

Amir Ahmadian, Angela E. Downes and A. Samy
Youssef
Department of Neurosurgery, University of South
Florida, Tampa, FL, USA

Definition

Spontaneous EMG muscular discharges occurring in
close relation to surgical manipulations.

Cross-References

▶ Cranial Nerve Monitoring – *VIII, IX, X, XI*

Encephalocele

▶ Temporal Bone Encephaloceles, Meningoceles, and
CSF Leak, Repair of

Encephalopathy

Johnathan Sataloff and Robert T. Sataloff
Department of Otolaryngology-Head and Neck
Surgery, Drexel University College of Medicine,
Philadelphia, PA, USA

Definition

A disorder of the brain. Encephalopathy occurs in
a substantial number of patients with Lyme disease.

Cross-References

▶ Otologic Manifestations of Lyme Disease

End-of-Life Care

▶ Palliative Care and Head and Neck Cancer

Endolaryngeal Surgery

▶ Vocal Cord Surgery

Endolymph

Gerald T. Kangelaris and Lawrence R. Lustig
Department of Otolaryngology-Head and Neck
Surgery, University of California, San Francisco, San
Francisco, CA, USA

Definition

The potassium-rich fluid of the scala media. Its highly
positive charge generates an electrical gradient
(dubbed "endocochlear potential") allowing for the
highly metabolic neuronal activity of the cochlea.

Cross-References

▶ Sensorineural Hearing Loss

Endolymphatic Hydrops

Johnathan Sataloff and Robert T. Sataloff
Department of Otolaryngology-Head and Neck
Surgery, Drexel University College of Medicine,
Philadelphia, PA, USA

Definition

Distention of the scala media of the cochlea, associated
with fluctuating hearing loss, episodic vertigo, aural
fullness, and tinnitus (often of a seashell character).

Cross-References

▶ Otologic Manifestations of Lyme Disease
▶ Vestibular Dysfunction, Meniere's Disease

Endolymphatic Sac Tumors

Badr Eldin Mostafa
Department of Otorhinolaryngology-Head and Neck
Surgery, Faculty of Medicine, Ain-Shams University,
Nasr City, Cairo, Egypt

Synonyms

Aggressive papillary middle ear tumors (APMET)

Definition

Aggressive tumors arising from the endolymphatic sac. They are slow growing locally aggressive adenocarcinomas.

Etiology

Endolymphatic sac tumors have been identified as a manifestation of von Hippel-Lindau disease (VHL). VHL is an autosomal dominant disorder associated with a defect on chromosome 3p25-26. The disease manifests itself as multiple hemangioblastomas of the retina and central nervous system accompanied by renal cysts, renal carcinoma, pheochromocytoma, pancreatic cysts, papillary cystadenomas of the epididymis, and endolymphatic sac tumor. The incidence of endolymphatic sac tumor is higher in patients with von Hippel-Lindau disease, and there are more bilateral tumors. Approximately 11% of patients with von Hippel-Lindau disease have endolymphatic sac tumor. However, as many as 60% of patients with von Hippel-Lindau disease who also have hearing loss may eventually develop an endolymphatic sac tumor (Eby et al. 1983; Horiguchi et al. 2001; Choo et al. 2004).

Clinical Presentation

These are tumors of middle aged patients. Some studies report a female predominance (Gaffey et al. 1988; Li et al. 1993). Average duration of symptoms varies from 9.3 to 10.6 years. Unilateral hearing loss is the most common symptom, and can often be of sudden onset. Other common presentations include tinnitus and vertigo. As the tumor spreads along the endolymphatic sac and duct, the posterior labyrinth and facial canal are eroded and eventually the middle ear and external canal are invaded. Many have a bluish-red discoloration seen through an intact tympanic membrane, or a vascular mass protrude through it into the external auditory canal. Extension along the petrous ridge may lead to involvement of the IAM, CPA, and trigeminal nerve (Roche et al. 1998; Russell et al. 2007).

Diagnosis

Radiology
On CT, the tumor bone margins are geographic or "moth-eaten," and the intratumoral bone appears reticular or spiculated. All papillary endolymphatic sac tumors had a thin peripheral rim of calcification, representing the expanded cortex of the petrous bone. Sparing of the jugular foramen helps distinguish the endolymphatic sac tumors from jugular or jugulotympanic glomic tumors. On MR imaging, the small tumors show heterogeneous signal with a peripheral rim of increased signal intensity, and on T1-weighted images, these tumors show heterogeneous intratumoral contrast enhancement (Fig. 1). The presence of intratumoral scattered areas of increased signal intensity on T1-weighted images is related to the presence of breakdown products of subacute hemorrhage, cholesterol clefts, and proteinaceous cysts in the large tumors. On angiography, the tumor displays a high degree of vascularity, with blood supply from the ascending pharyngeal and stylomastoid arteries (Mukherji et al. 1997; Mafee and Shah 2003).

Pathology
Microscopically, the tumor is composed of nonciliated columnar or cuboidal cells lining one layer

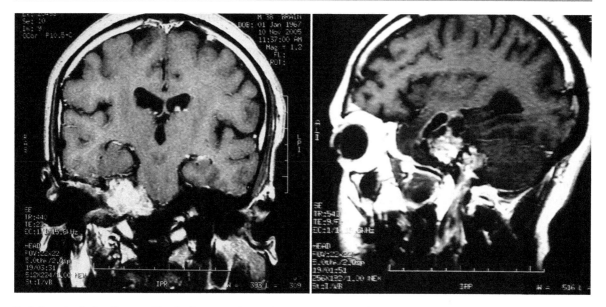

Endolymphatic Sac Tumors, Fig. 1 Contrast-enhanced MRI of an invasive ELST

and mainly showed a papillary. Glandular structures may be noted, with colloid-like fluid. Tumor cells are eosinophilic and occasionally clear cytoplasm and a round to oval nucleus without atypia. There is a fine granular chromatin pattern. Neither nuclear inclusion nor mitosis is present (Fig. 2). The stroma consists of thick fibrous connective tissue and numerous microvessels. Hemorrhage and hemosiderin deposits may be seen. The lumen of the cystic component of the tumor contains a proteinaceous material. This material may be indistinguishable from thyroid colloid. Consequently, it is important to use thyroglobulin staining to distinguish metastatic papillary thyroid carcinoma from endolymphatic sac tumor. Immunohistochemical expression of cytokeratins (CKs) and VEGF has been noted in ELST (Lonser et al. 2004).

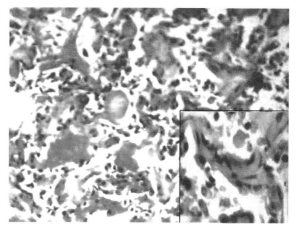

Endolymphatic Sac Tumors, Fig. 2 Histopathology of an ELST (Hx and E. X150, inset ×400)

Differential Diagnosis

Adenocarcinoma of the middle ear, Metastatic thyroid papillary carcinoma

Therapy

The treatment of choice is total surgical removal after preoperative embolization. However, as many of these tumors present late, extensive surgery is usually required. Partial removal results in massive recurrences. Radiation therapy and chemotherapy are used almost exclusively as palliative treatments for endolymphatic sac tumors that cannot be resected completely but do not control tumor growth (Roche et al. 1998; Russell et al. 2007).

Prognosis

Prognosis is poor with multiple recurrences and a protracted course and eventual intracranial invasion.

Cross-References

▶ Langerhans Cell Histiocytosis of Temporal Bone
▶ Middle Ear Adenoma
▶ Radiologic Evaluation of Central Skull Base
▶ Skull Base Neoplasms
▶ Temporal Bone Resection

References

Choo D, Shotland L, Mastroianni M et al (2004) Endolymphatic sac tumors in von Hippel-Lindau disease. J Neurosurg 100:480–487
Eby T, Makek M, Fisch U (1988) Adenomas of the temporal bone. Ann Otol Rhinol Laryngol 97:605–612
Gaffey MJ, Mills SE, Fechner RE et al (1988) Aggressive papillary middle ear tumor: a clinicopathologic entity distinct from middle-ear adenoma. Am J Surg Pathol 12:790
Horiguchi H, Sano T, Toi H, Kageji T, Hirokawa M, Nagahiro S (2001) Endolymphatic Sac Tumor Associated with a Von Hippel-Lindau disease patient: an immunohistochemical study. Mod Pathol 14(7):727–732
Li JC, Brackman DE, Lo WWM (1993) The reclassification of aggressive adenomatous mastoid neoplasm endolymphatic sac tumors. Laryngoscope 103:1342
Lonser RR, Kim HJ, Butman JA et al (2004) Tumors of the endolymphatic sac in von Hippel-Lindau disease. N Engl J Med 350:2481–2486
Mafee M, Shah H (2003) Endolymphatic sac tumors and papillary adenocarcinoma of the temporal bone: role of CT and MRI, Iran. J Radiol 53–59
Mukherji SK, Albernaz VS, Lo WM et al (1997) Papillary endolymphatic sac tumors: CT, MR imaging and angiographic findings in 20 patients. Radiology 202:801–808
Roche PH, Dufour H, Figarella P et al (1998) Endolymphatic sac tumors: report of three cases. Neurosurgery 42:927–932
Russell R, Lonser MD, Jeffrey Kim H (2007) Microsurgical resection of endolymphatic sac tumors. Oper Techn Otolaryngol 18:65–70

Endonasal Skull Base Surgery

▶ Endoscopic Surgery of Skull Base

Endoneurium

Wojciech K. Mydlarz and Kofi Derek O. Boahene
Department of Otolaryngology-Head and Neck Surgery, Johns Hopkins University School of Medicine, Baltimore, MD, USA

Definition

Layer of delicate protective sheath composed of connective tissue that encloses the myelin sheath of a single nerve fiber.

Cross-References

▶ Sunderland Classification of Nerve Injury

Endoscopic Cranial Base Surgery

▶ Endoscopic Surgery of Skull Base

Endonasal Endoscopic Sinus Surgery

▶ Endoscopic Sinus Surgery in Children

Endonasal Sinus Surgery

▶ Endoscopic Sinus Surgery in Children

Endoscopic Laser Surgery

▶ Transoral Laser Resection of Larynx

Endoscopic Parathyroidectomy

▶ Minimally Invasive Parathyroid Surgery

Endoscopic Pituitary Surgery

Mitchell Gore and Brent A. Senior
Department of Otolaryngology-Head and Neck
Surgery, University of North Carolina at Chapel Hill,
Chapel Hill, NC, USA

Synonyms

Endoscopic transphenoidal pituitary surgery; Minimally invasive pituitary surgery

Definition

Transnasal, transsphenoidal minimally invasive surgery for removal of pathology of the pituitary gland and parasellar area.

Purpose

Pituitary and Sellar Masses

Pituitary and sellar masses may present with neurologic symptoms, visual field deficits, diplopia, or headache. These masses may also present with hormonal aberrations such as inappropriate lactation or low testosterone levels. They are also frequently discovered as an incidental finding on magnetic resonance imaging (MRI) performed for some other reason, such as workup of headache or in cases of head trauma.

Pituitary adenomas are the most common cause of sellar masses in adults and may account for 10% of all intracranial neoplasms (Gsponer et al. 1999; Freda and Post 1999; Saeger et al. 2007). Pituitary adenomas are benign tumors, typically of the anterior pituitary gland, with prolactin secreting tumors most common.

The development of certain types of pituitary tumors may be associated with genetic causes, such as loss of the MEN1 tumor suppressor gene (associated with multiple endocrine neoplasia type 1 syndrome involving parathyroid, pancreatic islet, and pituitary gland tumors), an activating mutation of the guanine nucleotide stimulatory protein (Gs-alpha) gene in somatotroph adenomas (Landis et al. 1989; Vallar et al. 1987), or PTTG – The pituitary tumor transforming gene, which is overexpressed in most human pituitary adenomas (Zhang et al. 1999; Vlotides et al. 2007).

Pituitary adenomas are classified according to size. Microadenoma describes lesions <1 cm, while macroadenoma describes lesions >1 cm. Pituitary adenomas are also grouped by cell of origin, with adenoma types including gonadotrophic, thyrotrophic, corticotrophic (causing Cushing's disease), lactotrophic (prolactin-secreting), somatotrophic (causing acromegaly), and mixed adenomas such as lactotrophic/somatotraphic mixed adenomas. Any lesion can cause decreased levels of other hormones from gland compression.

Other Sellar Lesions

Pituitary hyperplasia and other benign tumors such as craniopharyngiomas (solid or mixed solid-cystic benign tumors that arise from remnants of Rathke's pouch along a line from the nasopharynx to the diencephalon) may also present as sellar masses. They may present as growth retardation in children and abnormal vision in adults, and pituitary hormonal deficiencies such as diabetes insipidus.

A meningioma is a usually benign tumor arising from the meninges anywhere within the head. Some arise near the sella, causing visual impairment and hormonal deficiencies.

Pituicytoma is an uncommon, low-grade glioma arising from the pituicytes of the posterior pituitary. It presents as a sellar mass, which is usually mistaken for a pituitary adenoma, and has no known hormonal secretory function.

Malignant Tumors

Primary malignancies that arise in the parasellar region are relatively rare compared to benign adenomas. These malignancies include germ cell tumors, sarcomas, chordomas, and lymphomas. Germ cell tumors usually occur through the third decade of life and may present with headache and signs and symptoms of increased intracranial pressure, diplopia, and hypopituitarism. Serum concentrations of human chorionic gonadotropin-beta, and alpha fetoprotein may be elevated. Although these lesions are highly malignant and metastasize readily, they are also highly radiosensitive. Chordomas are locally aggressive tumors that are thought to arise from a remnant of the embryologic notochord and can metastasize. They often arise in the clivus and present with headaches, visual impairment, and anterior pituitary hormonal deficiencies. Primary central nervous system (CNS) lymphoma may sometimes involve the pituitary, and is a rare sellar lesion.

Other Sellar Masses

Metastases to the hypothalamus and pituitary gland account for 1–2% of sellar masses (Gsponer et al. 1999; Fassett and Couldwell 2004) and occur most commonly with breast cancer in women and lung cancer in men, but can be seen with other cancers (Schubiger and Haller 1992; Sansur and Oldfield 2010). Symptoms are similar to those of large primary sellar lesions including visual disturbances and hypopituitarism. Cystic masses such as Rathke's cleft, arachnoid, and dermoid cysts can present as sellar masses, again resulting in visual impairment, diabetes insipidus, anterior pituitary hormonal deficiencies, and hydrocephalus. Pituitary abscesses are rare but can occur in a normal or diseased pituitary gland.

Evolution of Surgical Approaches to the Pituitary

In 1897, Davide Giordano, chief of surgery at the University of Venice, proposed a transsphenoidal approach to the pituitary. This consisted of a transglabelar approach where the anterior wall of the frontal sinus and ethmoid bone were removed. While Giordano never performed his procedure, it laid the foundation for Hermann Schloffer of Austria, who in 1907 performed the first transsphenoidal approach to the pituitary. Performed in three stages under local cocaine anesthesia, the first stage involved a left-sided lateral rhinotomy incision reflecting the nose to the right and removing the inferior turbinates, middle turbinates, and septum. In the second stage, he removed the vomer and the sphenoid rostrum, and in the third stage he chiseled off face of the sella after removal of the sphenoid mucosa (Lindholm 2007; Senior et al. 2008).

In 1909, Theodore Kocher, professor of surgery in Berne, Switzerland, performed a transnasal hypophysectomy by resecting the septum via a midline incision over the nasal dorsum, sparing the frontal, ethmoid, and maxillary sinuses. This midline approach was believed to result in improved visualization of the

sella without violating the sinuses, thereby reducing infection risk (Lanzino and Laws 2001).

Harvey Cushing performed his first transsphenoidal procedure in 1909 on an acromegalic. He performed a modification of the Schloffer technique by making an omega shaped incision over the forehead, fashioning a frontal osteoplastic flap. Under headlight illumination, ethmoidectomy was followed by placement of a 2 cm window in the sphenoid and removal of the thinned, enlarged sellar floor with a chisel. Using a curette, partial removal of the tumor was then accomplished. Cushing eventually modified the technique by incorporating features introduced by others such as a sublabial incision described by Halstead and the submucosal resection of the septum reported by Kocher. He thus developed and performed the first sublabial-transseptal transsphenoidal approach on June 4, 1910. Using a modified Sewell mouth gag, he made a sublabial incision elevating mucosal flaps off the septum allowing for the placement of lateral retractors. Cartilage, perpendicular plate of the ethmoid, and vomer were removed, and a self-retaining speculum was placed. Under headlight visualization, this then allowed the sphenoid to be entered and the sella opened.

Cushing presented these improvements in his 1912 work, "The Pituitary Body and its Disorders." Cushing later reported on his early experience with the transsphenoidal approach involving 74 operations on 68 patients in 1914 (Schubiger and Haller 1992). Twenty-two patients experienced a slight visual improvement or stabilization of vision over months to years after the operation, whereas another 22 experienced a sudden significant visual improvement. Seven deaths occurred with a mortality rate of 9.5% in that report. Cushing eventually reduced the mortality rate to 5.6% for surgical treatment of pituitary tumors later in his career (Cushing 1912, 1914).

By 1929 though, Cushing had abandoned the sublabial-transseptal transsphenoidal approach in favor of transcranial approaches due to a perception of better visualization and decompression of the optic apparatus with improved vision recovery and lower recurrence rate (Welbourn 1986). Because of Cushing's influence as the father of modern Neurosurgery, a majority of neurosurgeons converted to transcranial approaches for the next three decades. During this period, the endonasal transsphenoidal approach was maintained by Oskar Hirsch, a rhinologist from Vienna. He championed the endonasal transseptal transsphenoidal technique using a method similar to Hajek's for the management of empyema of the sphenoid. Hirsch used a head mirror for lighting with a nasal speculum and a suctioning device to enhance visualization (Senior et al. 2008). Hirsch performed his first endonasal approach to a pituitary tumor in 1910 in Vienna, several weeks ahead of Cushing performing his first sublabial transsphenoidal approach. Hirsch performed a five stage procedure over a 5-week period utilizing local cocaine anesthesia on a 35-year-old woman with headaches and visual loss. The procedure resolved the patient's headaches and improved her vision. Soon after, Hirsch modified his technique into a single stage with incorporation of Kocher's submucous resection of the septum. By 1937, Hirsch reported a mortality rate of 5.4% in 277 patients.

Norman Dott, a neurosurgeon from Edinburgh, learned the transsphenoidal technique while visiting Cushing in 1923. To improve visualization, he pioneered novel illumination techniques by developing a lighted speculum. In 1956, Dott demonstrated the endonasal transsphenoidal approach to a French neurosurgeon, Gerard Guiot, who ultimately performed more than 1,000 cases while also introducing intraoperative fluoroscopy to help define the anatomy of the nasal passages. A student of Guiot, Jules Hardy revolutionized the transsphenoidal pituitary approach when he introduced the use of the operating microscope and microsurgical instrumentation in 1967 (Liu et al. 2001). The microscope with increased illumination and magnification permitted a more thorough and safer resection without deaths or major morbidities (Liu et al. 2001). Hardy's contributions led to a paradigm shift in pituitary tumor surgery, with microsurgical techniques allowing for complete resection and surgical cure of hormonal disease in microadenomas. The procedure described by Hardy underwent numerous modifications and was the main procedure performed by neurosurgeons for removal of pituitary tumors from the 1960s through the early 1990s.

Principle

Endoscopic Pituitary Surgery

Introduction of Endoscopic Pituitary Surgery
The use of the endoscope by otolaryngologists to treat inflammatory sinus disease as pioneered by Kennedy, Stammberger, and others grew in popularity in the early 1990s. The visual clarity and brightness of the endoscope led to the rapid application of the endoscope for transsphenoidal pituitary surgery (Liu et al. 2001). Guiot initially reported the use of the endoscope as a complementary tool to improve visualization during conventional microscopic sublabial-transseptal surgery many years earlier but its use did not catch on. With the exception of Bushe and Halves, no other descriptions of endoscopic transsphenoidal pituitary surgery appeared until 1992 when Jankowski reported on endoscopic transsphenoidal pituitary surgery in three patients (Liu et al. 2001). The landmark 1997 article by Jho and Carrau presented a 46 patient series that demonstrated the safety, efficacy, and advantages of endoscopic transsphenoidal pituitary surgery (Senior et al. 2008), and marked the initiation of the modern era of minimally invasive pituitary surgery (MIPS).

High resolution computed tomography (CT) and magnetic resonance imaging (MRI) scans have significantly improved assessment of sellar masses, allowing for improved detection of microadenomas. Stereotactic navigational guidance systems have become the standard of care, providing improved intraoperative localization and safety (Senior et al. 2008).

The endoscope has provided improved visualization and lighting, allowing for multiple visual angulations when using angled scopes, reduced operative time, and improved differentiation between normal glandular tissue and tumor. The MIPS approach essentially eliminates the risk of tooth numbness, deprojection of the nose and denture difficulties seen with the sublabial approach, and decreases the risk of septal perforation and nasal obstruction seen after the transnasal transseptal approach.

Disadvantages of the MIPS approach include the loss of binocular visualization provided by the microscope, while neurosurgeons not trained in the use of the endoscope nor in the intricacies of sinonasal anatomy experience a certain learning curve (Senior et al. 2008). Many neurosurgical curricula do not include this training, while otolaryngologists have extensive endoscopic training and are typically comfortable with the anatomy of the sphenoid and sinonasal cavities. For this reason, a joint effort by the otolaryngologist and the neurosurgeon for resection of pituitary tumors allows for a safe and rapid approach in which each surgeon performs that part with which he is the most comfortable.

Surgical Indications

Indications for excision of hormonally inactive adenomas include compressive symptoms such as hypopituitarism and visual changes, pituitary apoplexy (hemorrhage into the tumor), or severe headaches. Patients with hormonally active prolactinomas are referred for surgery after failure of medical management. Patients with acromegaly, hypothyroidism, Cushing's disease, Rathke's cleft cysts (RCCs), chordomas, and arachnoid cysts are offered surgery as a primary therapy.

Preoperative Evaluation

Patients with pituitary adenomas are best evaluated by a multidisciplinary team including an endocrinologist, a neurosurgeon, an otolaryngologist, an ophthalmologist, and a radiation oncologist. Flexible endoscopy is essential for evaluating the sinonasal anatomy and ruling out any concurrent infectious process that may mandate a delay in surgery. Image guidance fine-cut CT scan without contrast is reviewed for further anatomic details such as the presence of Onodi cells as well as sphenoid pneumatization (sellar, presellar or conchal), asymmetry, and septations. Possible dehiscence of the carotid arteries in the sphenoid, which may be present in 20% of sphenoids is also assessed. Preoperative MRI with and without gadolinium is also obtained, allowing differentiation of normal pituitary from tumor, cystic lesions from solid lesions, and assessment of suprachiasmatic or intracavernous extention. The position of the carotid artery with regard to the tumor and the sella is also assessed, a feature particularly important in the setting of revision surgery. The risks and benefits of the procedure are discussed at length and all questions are answered. The expected postoperative course and potential complications are also explained to the patient and family.

Preoperative evaluation by an ophthalmologist is recommended. This includes visual acuity and visual fields as well as a retinal exam, all serving as a baseline for postoperative comparisons to determine improvement, or possibly, degeneration in vision.

A significant number of patients with pituitary tumors will present to the surgical team referred by an endocrinologist, after unsuccessful conservative medical management. These preoperative medications are usually continued; hypothyroidism is ideally well-controlled, and stress doses of steroids are given preoperatively and postoperatively as necessary.

Surgical Technique

The patient is positioned in the "beach-chair" position with the torso elevated at approximately 30° and the knees slightly bent for comfort. The head is rotated approximately 15° toward the surgeon. A computer-guided navigation system is routinely used, preferably with CT and MRI fused; this facilitates identification of sellar landmarks and orientation in relation to the tumor.

The patient's face is left nonsterile since the instruments will be passing through the contaminated nasal cavity. The abdomen is prepared in sterile fashion in case a fat graft is required at the end of the procedure, e.g., for cerebrospinal fluid (CSF) leak repair. Care is taken to maintain sterility of the abdominal region with the nasal field being kept distinct throughout the procedure.

Hemostasis is aided by performing greater palatine blocks by injecting approximately 1.5 mL of a solution of 1% lidocaine with 1/100,000 epinephrine transorally into each greater palatine canal. The nasal cavities are decongested with pledgets soaked in 0.05% oxymetazoline hydrochloride. Under endoscopic guidance, lidocaine with epinephrine is injected at the junction of the horizontal portion of the basal lamella and lateral nasal wall in the region of the sphenopalatine foramen to obtain a sphenopalatine artery block.

For smaller pituitary lesions that are parasagittal, and for larger tumors extending laterally into the cavernous sinus, the contralateral nasal cavity presents a better angle of approach. Generally, however, a binarial approach is utilized allowing for use of multiple simultaneous surgical instruments in addition to the endoscope.

The approach to the anterior face of the sphenoid utilizes the transnasal corridor, medial to the middle turbinate. This approach allows the remaining sinuses lateral to the middle turbinate to be left undisturbed, minimizing the risk of postoperative sinusitis. When necessary, gentle lateralization of the middle turbinate is performed.

Key to the identification of the sphenoid sinus ostium is the identification of the superior turbinate and the region of the sphenoethmoid recess. The recess is bounded by the skull base superiorly, the superior turbinate laterally, and the septum medially and nearly always contains the ostium of the sphenoid sinus. The ostium can be well seen after decongesting the superior turbinate with local anesthesia and displacing it laterally or occasionally conservatively resecting its posterior-inferior third using a powered shaver/microdebrider. Located medial to the turbinate, the ostium is just posterior to its inferior edge in the sphenoethmoid recess. Additionally, Jho has described using the inferior edge of the middle turbinate as a landmark for orientation to the floor of the sella, with this landmark specifically leading to the clival indentation, about 1 cm below the level of the sellar floor (Senior et al. 2008).

The posterior septal branch of the sphenopalatine artery crosses the inferior aspect of the sphenoethmoidal recess on its way to supply the mucosa of the septum. Transection of this artery while performing the sphenoidotomy can lead to annoying intraoperative bleeding but can usually be well-controlled with bipolar cautery. Vasoconstriction may be further obtained by injection of lidocaine or epinephrine solution along the posterior septum, before any incision in the face of the sphenoid. Alternatively, this posterior septal branch, serving as the primary blood supply and pedicle for nasoseptal flaps, should be meticulously preserved in cases where a nasoseptal flap for skull base reconstruction is planned.

Once the sphenoid sinus ostium is identified, the sinus is entered and the ostium enlarged in an inferior and medial direction, away from structures along the lateral wall of the sinus until the ostium has been enlarged to a point where the endoscope can be inserted into the sinus to visualize the lateral extent of the sinus. The bone of the sphenoid rostrum is resected using a combination of Kerrison rongeurs and punches until the nasal septum is encountered; the coarse diamond burr on a high-speed drill can also be used for resection of this relatively thick bone. A partial posterior septectomy is then performed using backbiting forceps, allowing for exposure of the contralateral face of the sphenoid. The intersinus septum is resected, exposing the sellar face. Great care is taken in resection of the intersinus septum, which often attaches posteriorly over the carotid artery or optic nerve or both.

The tuberculum sella is found rostrally, with the clival recess located caudal to the sella. The optic nerves are seen at 11 and 1 o'clock, with the C-shaped carotid arteries laterally and the cavernous portions of the internal carotid arteries located at 5 and 7 o'clock. Caution must be exercised when dissecting or drilling near the carotid arteries, as these can be dehiscent in up to 22% of sphenoids (Kennedy et al. 1990).

Once the sella is identified, the surgical team typically moves to a four-handed, two surgeons, two-sided technique. One surgeon maintains visualization with the endoscope whereas the other uses both hands introducing instruments on the same side or opposite side or both. The mucosa on the posterior wall of the sphenoid sinus is removed and the sella is entered with a high-speed drill in order to expose the dura of the sella. The dural exposure is enlarged with a Kerrison rongeur or a currette. The dura is then cauterized and opened with a sickle knife and rotating scissors. The tumor mass typically bulges through the dural opening and at this point specimen is obtained for frozen section and permanent pathology before any suction is used, especially when dealing with microadenomas and smaller lesions. The tumor is then removed with a combination of suction and neurosurgical ring curettes with different angulations. Tumor tissue is usually easily differentiated from normal yellow pituitary tissue.

Once the bulk of the tumor is removed, straight and angled scopes may be inserted into the sella to facilitate more detailed exploration for residual tumor. The diaphragm of the sella and normal pituitary tissue will tend to descend into the defect. Hydroscopy, or inspection of the interior of the sella under gentle irrigation under low, continuous water pressure, will expand the soft tissue boundaries of the sella including the diaphragm while also washing away small amounts of blood and clot. With improved visualization, this technique allows inspection of the cavity and ensures as complete a removal of tumor tissue as possible (Senior et al. 2005).

At the end of the procedure, hemostasis is obtained using a hemostatic substance such as microfibrillar collagen in thrombin. This is allowed to sit for a few minutes in the sella and is then irrigated out.

Reconstruction of the sella is frequently unnecessary. However, reconstruction is necessary, in the presence of intraoperative CSF leak. Skull base/sellar reconstruction may be performed with a small fat plug placed in the sellar opening and bolstered by resorbable packing. High flow leaks or very large defects may also be reconstructed with a pedicled nasoseptal flap if necessary.

Postoperative Management

Postoperatively, the patient is admitted for routine neurologic monitoring, monitoring for CSF leak, and measurement of hormone levels if indicated. An MRI is obtained on the first postoperative day to evaluate completeness of resection and to serve as a post-resection baseline. Patients are generally discharged home on antibiotics, and hormonal replacement and steroid replacement as necessary. Patients are instructed to avoid nose blowing or sneezing through the nose to avoid displacement of mucus into the open sellar cavity.

At the first postoperative visit approximately 3–4 weeks later, sinonasal endoscopy is performed to confirm appropriate healing; typically, the sellar opening is usually covered by a healthy mucosal layer and patients may resume gentle nose blowing. Patients are closely followed by the neurosurgery and the endocrinology teams; visits to the otolaryngologist beyond that are on an as-needed-basis only.

Cross-References

▶ Endoscopic Surgery of Skull Base

References

Cushing H (1912) The pituitary body and its disorders: clinical states produced by disorders of the hypophysis cerebri. JB Lippincott, Philadelphia

Cushing H (1914) The Weir Mitchell lecture. Surgical experiences with pituitary disorders. J Am Med Assoc 63:1515–1525

Fassett DR, Couldwell WT (2004) Metastases to the pituitary gland. Neurosurg Focus 16(4):E8

Freda PU, Post KD (1999) Differential diagnosis of sellar masses. Endocrinol Metab Clin North Am 28:81

Gsponer J, De Tribolet N, Déruaz JP et al (1999) Diagnosis, treatment, and outcome of pituitary tumors and other abnormal intrasellar masses. Retrospective analysis of 353 patients. Medicine (Baltim) 78:236

Kennedy D, Zinreich SJ, Hassab M (1990) The internal carotid artery as it relates to endonasal sphenoethmoidectomy. Am J Rhinol 4:7–12

Landis CA, Masters SB, Spada A, Pace AM, Bourne HR (1989) Vallar L GTPase inhibiting mutations activate the alpha chain of Gs and stimulate adenylyl cyclase in human pituitary tumours. Nature 340(6236):692

Lanzino G, Laws ER Jr (2001) Pioneers in the development of transsphenoidal surgery: Theodor Kocher, Oskar Hirsch, and Norman Dott. J Neurosurg 95:1097–1103

Lindholm J (2007) A century of pituitary surgery: Schloffer's legacy. Neurosurgery 61(4):865–867

Liu JK, Das K, Weiss MH, Laws ER Jr, Couldwell WT (2001) The history and evolution of transsphenoidal surgery. J Neurosurg 95:1083–1096

Saeger W, Lüdecke DK, Buchfelder M et al (2007) Pathohistological classification of pituitary tumors: 10 years of experience with the German pituitary tumor registry. Eur J Endocrinol 156:203

Sansur CA, Oldfield EH (2010) Pituitary carcinoma. Semin Oncol 37(6):591–593

Schubiger O, Haller D (1992) Metastases to the pituitary – hypothalamic axis. An MR study of 7 symptomatic patients. Neuroradiology 34(2):131

Senior BA, Dubin MG, Sonnenburg RE, Melroy CT, Ewend MG (2005) Increased role of the otolaryngologist in endoscopic pituitary surgery: endoscopic hydroscopy of the sella. Am J Rhinol 19(2):181–184

Senior BA, Ebert CS, Bednarski KK, Bassim MK, Younes M, Sigounas D, Ewend MG (2008) Minimally invasive pituitary surgery. Laryngoscope 118(10):1842–1855

Vallar L, Spada A, Giannattasio G (1987) Altered Gs and adenylate cyclase activity in human GH-secreting pituitary adenomas. Nature 330(6148):566

Vlotides G, Eigler T, Melmed S (2007) Pituitary tumor-transforming gene: physiology and implications for tumorigenesis. Endocr Rev 28(2):165

Welbourn RB (1986) The evolution of transsphenoidal pituitary microsurgery. Surgery 100:1185–1190

Zhang X, Horwitz GA, Heaney AP, Nakashima M, Prezant TR, Bronstein MD, Melmed S (1999) Pituitary tumor transforming gene (PTTG) expression in pituitary adenomas. J Clin Endocrinol Metab 84(2):761

Endoscopic Sinus Surgery (ESS)

▶ Endoscopic Sinus Surgery in Children
▶ Primary Sinus Surgery

Endoscopic Sinus Surgery in Children

Sancak Yuksel[1] and Samer Fakhri[1,2]
[1]Department of Otorhinolaryngology-Head and Neck Surgery, University of Texas Medical School at Houston, Houston, TX, USA
[2]Texas Skull Base Physicians and Texas Sinus Institute, Houston, TX, USA

Synonyms

Endonasal endoscopic sinus surgery; Endonasal sinus surgery; Endoscopic sinus surgery (ESS); Functional endonasal sinus surgery; Functional endoscopic sinus surgery (FESS); Pediatric endoscopic sinus surgery (PESS); Pediatric functional endoscopic sinus surgery; Sinus surgery; Transnasal endoscopic surgery

Definition

Functional endoscopic sinus surgery (FESS) is a minimally invasive surgical technique in which diseased mucosa and bone are removed from sinus air cells and sinus ostia under endoscopic visualization.

Purpose

The rationale for performing FESS in the pediatric population has traditionally followed that of its adult counterpart. As such, the primary purpose of FESS is to restore normal function of the paranasal sinuses in patients with chronic rhinosinusitis (CRS) or to manage acute rhinosinusitis complicated with orbital or intracranial involvement.

Principle

Historical Perspective

Before the era of proper understanding of paranasal sinus physiology and mucociliary function, aggressive and nonfunctional surgical interventions were performed on patients with sinonasal disease. Messerklinger and Stammbergerin Europe used their studies on paranasal sinus physiology and developed the concept of functional endoscopic sinus surgery in the 1970s. In the United States, FESS was further defined and popularized by Kennedy in the mid-1980s.Since then, it has become a well-established and commonly performed procedure in adults with CRS. In children, the trend followed a similar pattern. FESS in children was initially explored in Europe, but it was not until 1989 that the initial results appeared in the literature (Gross et al. 1989). The role of FESS in the pediatric population is still evolving and despite ongoing debates about timing, indications, and potential negative effects on the facial development of the child, the current literature supports FESS as a safe and effective treatment for refractory pediatric sinus disease.

Patient Evaluation and Imaging

The diagnostic approach to children with CRS is largely similar to that in adults. It starts with a thorough history and includes physical examination, nasal endoscopy, allergy testing, and immune workup as needed. The diagnosis of rhinosinusitis in children is more challenging than in adults because of the difficulty of eliciting and communicating historical factors such as nature, chronicity, and severity of symptoms. In addition, the symptoms of viral upper respiratory tract infections and adenotonsillar hypertrophy may overlap with the symptoms of chronic rhinosinusitis. Nasal endoscopy in the office setting is not easily tolerated especially in the younger patient population. Therefore, greater weight needs to be placed on radiographic imaging in the assessment of CRS. A consensus report by the American College of Radiology provided appropriateness criteria of various radiographic imaging modalities in evaluating pediatric sinus disease (McAlister et al. 2000). They recommended coronal CT as the diagnostic imaging modality of choice in the evaluation of sinus disease in any age category. It is fast, allows accurate assessment of soft tissue and bony changes, and can be performed in children without the need for sedation. The American Academy of Pediatrics (AAP) recommends sinus CT scan when rhinosinusitis has been refractory to medical treatment especially if surgery is considered. Plain sinus radiographs, while widely available, are not optimal for the accurate assessment of paranasal sinus disease.

Patient Selection and Surgical Decision Making

In children with CRS, surgery may be considered when symptoms and objective findings fail to improve following appropriate trials of medical therapy, typically consisting of 3–6 weeks of broad-spectrum or culture-directed antibiotics and adjunctive therapy (Felisati and Ramadan 2007).

Current surgical options for the treatment of recalcitrant CRS are adenoidectomy, FESS, or combination of both. Some investigators suggested a stepwise protocol including adenoidectomy alone with intravenous antibiotic as an alternative to FESS (Don et al. 2001). Common consensus is that adenoidectomy should be offered first especially in children younger than 6 years of age (Felisati and Ramadan 2007).This procedure removes the reservoir of pathogenic bacteria, relieves nasal obstruction, and allows better drainage of sinonasal secretions. Middle meatal culture and maxillary sinus aspiration with irrigation may be performed during adenoidectomy, therefore directing postoperative antimicrobial therapy.

Preoperative Planning

Careful preoperative review of the CT scan in both the coronal and axial planes is imperative, and provides a road map for the safe execution of the surgical procedure. Computer-aided surgery with preoperative planning and intraoperative navigation is often used in revision cases where the anatomy is distorted, or when more comprehensive FESS is indicated (Lusk 2002; Postec et al. 2002). Preoperative review of triplanar images enables the surgeon to build a three-dimensional mental appreciation of the surgical field. Surgical navigation allows the preoperative images to be directly correlated to the operative field, helping the surgeon effectively execute the surgical plan and avoid injury to surrounding structures.

Technique and Scope of Surgery

The key concept that is critical to the success of FESS is to remove sources of sinus obstruction and restore ventilation and normal mucociliary function. In children with CRS, inflammation typically affects the ostiomeatal complex with involvement of the anterior ethmoid and maxillary sinuses. Intervention should be tailored to the disease configuration. In most children, surgical objectives are achieved by performing an uncinectomy, widening of the maxillary sinus natural ostium, and anterior ethmoidectomy (Lusk 2002). Surgical management of the sphenoid and frontal sinuses is rarely needed. Comprehensive FESS is used in cystic fibrosis and ▶ allergic fungal rhinosinusitis patients to improve quality of life and optimize the sinonasal cavity for subsequent topical therapy.

The technique of the surgery is similar to its adult counterpart. The operation is performed under general anesthesia with orotracheal intubation. The patient is placed on the operating table supine or in a slight reverse Trendelenburg position. The anesthesia team is requested to maintain the lowest mean arterial pressure and pulse that is safe for the patient. The eyes should be left uncovered but corneal exposure should be avoided. The nose is decongested with 1%

oxymetazoline hydrochloride on cotton pledgets placed in the nasal cavity. This should be done in the least traumatic way to avoid mucosal lacerations and unnecessary bleeding. A sphenopalatine block is performed with 1% lidocaine with 1:100,000 units of epinephrine. The mucosa of the lateral nasal wall is also injected with the same solution. Multiple mucosal stabs should be avoided considering the bleeding potential of inflamed mucosa.

Frequent and sequential decongestion is often required to achieve optimal visualization as the surgeon proceeds deeper into the sinonasal cavity. Additional measures to improve hemostasis and/or enhance visualization may be considered but are often unnecessary. Lens-cleaning devices such as Endo-Scrub (Medtronic Xomed, Jacksonville, FL) are helpful but they add to the diameter of the telescope and their use may therefore become problematic in pediatric noses. Microdebriders with their concurrent suction and fast tissue removal are useful tools to enhance visualization and expedite the surgical procedure. They should be used cautiously to avoid complications and mucosal injury.

Four millimeter telescopes are used in the majority of pediatric cases but 2.7 mm and newer 3 mm scopes should be given consideration in pediatric patients with relatively small nasal passages. The 0° telescope is used to perform the uncinectomy, ethmoidectomy, and sphenoidotomy if the latter is indicated. The 30° telescope is used to perform the maxillary antrostomy and frontal recess dissection if indicated. If frontal sinusotomy is necessary, optimal visualization may require 70° telescopes. Angled telescopes afford significant surgical advantages, but they also add to visual distortion and their use should be reserved for experienced surgeons.

At the beginning of the procedure, any purulence in the middle meatus should be collected in a sterile fashion and the specimen sent for cultures. The results are used to guide postoperative antimicrobial therapy. The initial maneuver is to remove the uncinate process and identify the ethmoidal infundibulum and the natural ostium of the maxillary sinus. The natural ostium is enlarged and included in the final surgical antrostomy. The bulla ethmoidalis is then penetrated and removed with through-cutting instruments or with a microdebrider. Care should be taken to avoid injury to the middle turbinate and medial orbital wall especially when using powered instrumentation. The blade of the microdebrider should be pointing perpendicular to the medial orbital wall. At the end of the procedure, a dissolvable middle meatal spacer may be placed.

A second-look procedure under general anesthesia (GA) has been traditionally performed 2–3 weeks after FESS because of the difficulty of performing meaningful postoperative care in the office setting in children. This approach, however, has not resulted in superior surgical outcomes (Fakhri et al. 2001). In fact, 72% of surveyed pediatric otolaryngologists do not routinely perform a second-look endoscopy under GA (Cable and Mair 2006).

Outcome of Pediatric FESS

The safety and efficacy of pediatric FESS has been largely assessed based on collection of data through satisfaction surveys. A meta-analysis using data from 882 patients in eight published studies as well as the authors' own data showed a beneficial outcome in 89% of children undergoing FESS (Hebert and Bent 1998). The complication rate was 0.6%. The study concluded that pediatric FESS is a safe and effective treatment for refractory CRS in children. Other studies in the literature have supported this notion. One particular study looked at the long-term outcome of FESS in children (Lusk et al. 2006). The study reported that parents of young children with chronic rhinosinusitis appear to be more satisfied with the outcome of surgical management compared to medical management when assessed 10 years later.

A prospective non-randomized study over 10 years with follow-up assessment at 12 months evaluated the effect of FESS, adenoidectomy, and age at the time of surgery on the outcome of surgical intervention. The author showed that success rates of FESS with adenoidectomy, FESS alone, and adenoidectomy alone were 87%, 75%, and 52%, respectively (Ramadan 2004). When the results were stratified according to the age of the child at the time of surgery, children aged over 6 years had better overall success rate when compared to children 6 years and younger. In the latter group there was no statistical difference between FESS with adenoidectomy, FESS alone, and adenoidectomy alone. Other variables such as asthma, smoke exposure, and Lund-McKay CT score were also analyzed. The results of this study support a stepwise surgical management algorithm

whereby adenoidectomy alone may be performed in children 6 year of age or younger who have failed medical therapy, have no asthma, and a low burden of disease on sinus CT scan.

As the pool of patients who have undergone FESS has increased over the years, revision FESS is more commonly performed and outcome data on these revision procedures have become available. Ramadan reported that 13% of 243 children required ▶ revision sinus surgery. The most common finding was adhesions (57%), maxillary sinus ostium stenosis, or missed maxillary sinus ostium at the time of the initial procedure (52%), recurrent disease (39%), sinus disease in non-operated site (26%), deviated septum (17%), and mucocele (13%). Presence of asthma and younger age were risk factors for undergoing a revision procedure (Ramadan 2009).

Extended Endoscopic Approaches for Noninflammatory Disease

Building on improved understanding of the endoscopic regional anatomy of the sinonasal cavity, endoscopic techniques were applied to increasingly complex sinonasal, orbital, and skull base pathology such as ▶ cerebrospinal fluid (CSF) leaks, encephaloceles, nasolacrimal duct obstruction, choanal atresia, dysthyroid orbitopathy, and optic neuropathy (Castelnuovo et al. 2010). More recently, endoscopic skull base surgery with resection of selected tumors, including inverted papilloma, angiofibroma, and hypophyseal tumors, has become common. Further developments in sophisticated surgical instrumentation and computer-aided surgery have facilitated the resection of skull base malignancies using minimally invasive endoscopic techniques.

Indication

The role of endoscopic surgery in the treatment of pediatric sinusitis is still in evolution and there is no clear consensus regarding timing of FESS for CRS in children. An ideal FESS candidate was described by Clary as a child with normal immune function who has failed to respond to maximal medical therapy and adenoidectomy and meets criteria for CRS by history and CT findings (Clary 2003). In an international consensus meeting that took place in Belgium in 1996, the indications for ESS in children were identified as follows: (1) complete nasal obstruction in cystic fibrosis due to massive polyposis or closure of the nose by medialization of the lateral nasal wall, (2) antrochoanal polyp, (3) intracranial complications, (4) mucocoeles or mucopyocoeles, (5) orbital abscess, (6) traumatic injury in the optic canal, (7) dacryocystorhinitis due to sinusitis and resistant to appropriate medical treatment, (8) fungal sinusitis, (9) some meningoencephaloceles, and (10) some neoplasms (Clement et al. 1998). Possible indications for FESS include persistent symptoms of chronic rhinosinusitis despite optimal medical management and after exclusion of any systemic disease. In these patients, endoscopic sinus surgery is a reasonable alternative to continuous medical treatment. In general, optimal medical management is defined as 2–6 weeks of adequate antibiotics (intravenous or oral) and treatment of concomitant diseases. The participants of the Consensus Panel stressed that children who are eligible for sinus surgery represent only a small fraction of all children suffering from chronic rhinosinusitis.

The above indications continue to hold until today with a trend toward more conservative approach especially in children less than 6 years of age, as many of these patients outgrow their sinus disease with time.

Contraindications

There are probably no absolute contraindications to FESS. Intracranial or orbital complications of frontal sinusitis may represent relative contraindications to endoscopic techniques but may be considered depending on surgeon experience and available instrumentation. Other contraindications include medical conditions precluding general anesthesia.

Advantage/Disadvantage

Advantages
Endoscopic sinus surgery allows for excellent illumination and magnification and the ability to see around corners with angled telescopes and high-definition monitors. This facilitates precise tissue removal and visualization of sinus drainage pathways, as well as preservation of uninvolved structures. There is improved access and exposure to the sphenoid sinus and frontal recess. The endoscopic approach avoids facial incisions and allows for more rapid recovery, and fewer overall complications. Another advantage of this technique is its effectiveness in managing complicated acute rhinosinusitis by addressing both the offending sinus and the extrasinus complication (Fakhri and Pereira 2006).

Disadvantages
FESS requires specialized and expensive technology (video endoscopy), specialized instrumentation (especially for the frontal recess and sinus), and a thorough knowledge of endoscopic anatomy. The main limitation relates to the bleeding potential of inflamed tissue that may compromise the endoscopic visualization of the surgical field.

Other non-proven disadvantages include risks to the normal development of the maxillofacial skeleton of the young child. These concerns stem from studies demonstrating such an effect in piglets. However, prospective studies indicated that midfacial growth is not significantly affected by ESS in humans (Lieser and Derkay 2005).

Another limitation relates to postoperative care in children which is difficult to perform in the office setting, and may in select cases require a second-look surgery in the operating room.

Finally, inexperienced endoscopists may be challenged during endoscopic sinus surgery to generate movements in a three-dimensional space based on feedback provided by two-dimensional display monitors. Compromised depth perception may lead to complications such as injury to the orbit, optic nerve, or skull base.

Cross-References

▶ Rhinosinusitis, Pathophysiology and Medical
  Management
▶ Sinusitis
▶ Temporal Bone Meningocele/Encephalocele

References

Cable BB, Mair EA (2006) Pediatric functional endoscopic sinus surgery:frequently asked questions. Ann Otol Rhinol Laryngol 115(9):643–657

Clary R (2003) Is there a future for pediatric sinus surgery? An American perspective. Int J Pediatr Otorhinolaryngol 67:213–216

Clement PA, Bluestone CD, Gordts F, Lusk RP, Otten FW, Goossens H et al (1998) Management of rhinosinusitis in children: consensus meeting, Brussels, Belgium, September 13, 1996. Arch Otolaryngol Head Neck Surg 124:31–34

Don DM, Yellon RF, Casselbrant ML, Bluestone CD (2001) Efficacy of stepwise protocol that includes intravenous antibiotic therapy for the management of chronic rhinosinusitis in children and adolescents. Arch Otolaryngol Head Neck Surg 127(9):1093–1098

Fakhri S, Pereira K (2006) Endoscopic management of orbital abscesses. Otolaryngol Clin North Am 39(5):1037–1047

Fakhri S, Manoukian JJ, Souaid JP (2001) Functional endoscopic sinus surgery in the paediatric population: outcome of a conservative approach to postoperative care. J Otolaryngol 30(1):15–18

Felisati G, Ramadan H (2007) Rhinosinusitis in children: the role of surgery. Pediatr Allergy Immunol 18(Suppl 18): 68–70

Gross CW, Gurucharri MJ, Lazar RH, Long TE (1989) Functional endoscopic sinus surgery (FESS) in the pediatric age group. Laryngoscope 99(3):272–275

Hebert R, Bent J (1998) Meta-analysis of outcomes of pediatric functional endoscopic sinus surgery. Laryngoscope 108:796–799

Lieser JD, Derkay CS (2005) Pediatric sinusitis: when do we operate? Curr Opin Otolaryngol Head Neck Surg 13: 60–66

Lusk RP (2002) Pediatric endoscopic sinus surgery. Op Tech Otolaryngol Head Neck Surg 13(1):36–40

Lusk RP, Bothwell MR, Piccirillo J (2006) Long-term follow-up for children treated with surgical intervention for chronic rhinosinusitis. Laryngoscope 116(12):2099–2107

McAlister WH, Parker BR, Kushner DC, Babcock DS, Cohen HL, Gelfand MJ, Hernandez RJ et al (2000) Sinusitis in the pediatric population. American College of Radiology. ACR Appropriateness Criteria. Radiology 215(Suppl): 811–818

Postec F, Bossard D, Disant F, Froehlich P (2002) Computer-assisted navigation system in pediatric intranasal surgery. Arch Otolaryngol Head Neck Surg 128:797–800

Ramadan HH (2004) Surgical management of chronic sinusitis in children. Laryngoscope 114(12):2103–2109

Ramadan HH (2009) Revision endoscopic sinus surgery in children: surgical causes of failure. Laryngoscope 119(6): 1214–1217

Endoscopic Surgery of Skull Base

Li-Xing Man[1], Amber Luong[2,3], Martin J. Citardi[2,3] and Samer Fakhri[2,3]
[1]Department of Otolaryngology-Head and Neck Surgery, University of Rochester School of Medicine and Dentistry, University of Rochester Medical Center, Rochester, NY, USA
[2]Department of Otorhinolaryngology-Head and Neck Surgery, University of Texas Medical School at Houston, Houston, TX, USA
[3]Texas Skull Base Physicians and Texas Sinus Institute, Houston, TX, USA

Synonyms

Endonasal skull base surgery; Endoscopic cranial base surgery; Exclusively endoscopic approach (EEA); Expanded endonasal approach (EEA); Minimally invasive endoscopic resection (MIER); Transnasal endoscopic resection (TER)

Definition

Endoscopic skull base surgery is a surgical approach to the ventral skull base using telescopes through the nose.

Purpose

The advent of endoscopic technology has revolutionized the management of sinonasal disorders. Nasal endoscopy has been used for the diagnosis and treatment of inflammatory disease in the paranasal sinuses since the 1970s. Building on improved understanding of the endoscopic regional anatomy of the sinonasal cavity, endoscopic techniques were then applied to increasingly complex sinonasal, orbital, and skull base pathology such as ▶ cerebrospinal fluid (CSF) leaks, encephaloceles, nasolacrimal duct obstruction, dysthyroid orbitopathy, and optic neuropathy (Castelnuovo et al. 2010). More recently, endoscopic resection of selected tumors, including inverted papilloma, angiofibroma, and hypophyseal tumors, has become common. Further developments in sophisticated surgical instrumentation and computer-aided surgery have facilitated the consideration of resection of skull base malignancies using minimally invasive endoscopic techniques. Endoscopic resection of skull base malignant tumors has emerged as an alternative to traditional craniofacial resection (tCFR).

Principle

Multidisciplinary Evaluation and Treatment

Management of skull base neoplasms requires a multidisciplinary approach. The rhinologic skull base surgeon often plays a primary role in facilitating patient care when the endoscopic approach is considered. It is essential to involve neurosurgery and ophthalmology to address intracranial and orbital disease, respectively. The head and neck surgeon may be recruited to address regional neck disease via neck dissection. Radiation and medical oncology should be consulted if induction or adjuvant radiotherapy or chemotherapy is contemplated. All patients with malignancies should be discussed at a multidisciplinary tumor board if the treating institution sponsors such a forum. The consensus that arises from the discussion leads to a comprehensive treatment strategy for each patient. Patients should actively participate throughout the process to understand the implications of their diagnosis and its treatment. If endoscopic resection is recommended, patients should have the option to undergo consultation to consider alternative surgical approaches, including "open" tCFR.

The multidisciplinary team approach is extended to the surgical suite, especially when tumors transgress the dura. Endoscopic skull base surgery involves the otolaryngologist and neurosurgeon operating in concert rather than sequentially. One surgeon directs the field of view with the endoscope while the other dissects with both hands. The potential benefits of this collaborative approach to surgery include improved visualization, increased surgical efficiency, enhanced decision making, and augmentation of each surgeon's energy and enthusiasm (Snyderman et al. 2008; Nogueira et al. 2010). Moreover, the experience and technical skills of both surgeons enhances the ability to manage a crisis such as a vascular injury.

Principles of Resection

The most frequently cited reservation regarding endoscopic skull base surgery is the inability to achieve the classical en bloc resection. Additional concerns include the ability to visualize tumor margins, manage bleeding, and reconstruct skull base defects. These criticisms must be addressed to affirm the endoscopic approach as an alternative to traditional craniofacial resection.

Surgical Oncology

The tenets of surgical oncology remain paramount in endoscopic resection of skull base malignancy. The primary objective is complete tumor extirpation. This must be achieved while taking into account important functional and quality of life considerations, including preservation of neurologic function, vision, swallowing, voice, and physical appearance (Batra and Citardi 2006). Traditional craniofacial resection has been touted as the only means to achieve en bloc resection of ventral skull base malignancies with negative margins. In reality, en bloc resection of bulky, easily fragmented tumors filling the nasal cavity and paranasal sinuses is rarely achieved even with traditional "open" techniques (McCutcheon et al. 1996). Generous margins are impossible given the close proximity to critical neurovascular structures. In a multicenter series of 1,307 patients undergoing traditional craniofacial resection, negative margins were accomplished in only 54.3% of patients (Patel et al. 2003).

Endoscopic resection of skull base malignancy often requires tumor debulking to gain access to the area of attachment or invasion. This approach has been criticized as having a theoretically higher risk for local recurrence or tumor seeding. Such concerns have not been borne out clinically (Snyderman et al. 2008; Eloy et al. 2009). Ultimately, en bloc resection of the neoplasm is less important than achieving sound oncologic resection with clear surgical margins (Batra et al. 2010; Ong et al. 2010). Indeed, local recurrence and both disease-specific and overall mortality are associated with positive surgical margins (Patel et al. 2003). The paradigm of piecemeal resection without compromising complete tumor extirpation is analogous to situations such as laser excision of laryngeal squamous cell carcinoma and Mohs micrographic surgery for skin cancer.

Technological Advances

The advent of high-definition videoendoscopy and angled telescopes has enhanced our ability to visualize

Endoscopic Surgery of Skull Base, Fig. 1 CT-MR fusion images may be combined with surgical navigation. This still image capture was obtained during computer-aided endoscopic resection. The lower right image is the standard endoscopic view, and the remaining quadrants show fused CT-MR images

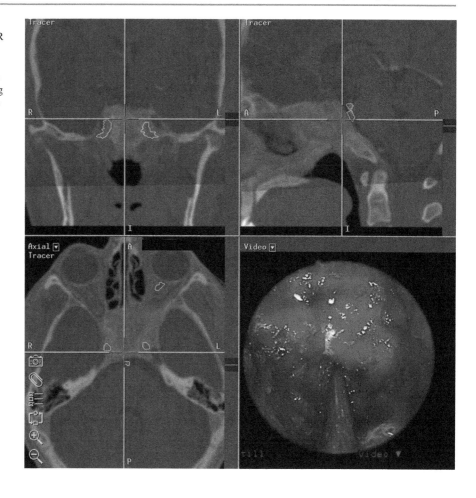

the surgical field and to discern tumor boundaries and their interface with normal tissue. Computer-aided surgery with preoperative planning and intraoperative navigation is often instrumental in facilitating precise endoscopic resection of skull base malignancy (Knott et al. 2006). Preoperative review of triplanar images enables the surgeon to determine tumor margins in relationship to associated critical structures and build a three-dimensional mental appreciation of tumor location and extent. Surgical navigation allows the preoperative images to be directly correlated to the operative field, helping the surgeon effectively execute the surgical plan and avoid neurovascular injury. Both CT and MRI are essential and complementary in the evaluation of skull base lesions. CT-MR fusion technology (Fig. 1) merges the two imaging modalities and generates a hybrid image that can be adjusted and viewed on a continuous spectrum between CT (bone) and MRI (soft tissue) windows. This improves the delineation of tumor extent along the skull base and

help the surgeon maximize tumor resection while minimizing collateral injury (Leong et al. 2006).

The main limitation of endoscopic techniques probably relate to the bleeding potential of malignant and vascular lesions. Even for the most experienced endoscopists, significant bleeding impairs intraoperative visualization and may seriously compromise the safety and completeness of the resection. Advances in technology and refinement in surgical strategies have allowed the endoscopic surgeon to successfully address large vascular tumors such as hemangiopericytomas with relatively less blood loss compared with external approaches for similar tumors (Gomez-Rivera et al. 2010). A number of specialized intranasal bipolar devices currently on the market allow for hemostasis and minimize bloody contamination of the surgical field. A wide assortment of topical hemostatic agents is also available. Preoperative embolization may be considered in large vascular tumors that draw some of their blood supply from the

Endoscopic Surgery of Skull Base,
Fig. 2 Endoscopic view of a large skull base defect from orbit to orbit and crista galli to planum sphenoidale after endoscopic resection of a T4 adenocarcinoma (**a**). Multilayered reconstruction with an intradural collagen dural substitute and bone with additional collagen dural substitute in the epidural space (**b**), to be followed by a mucosal graft

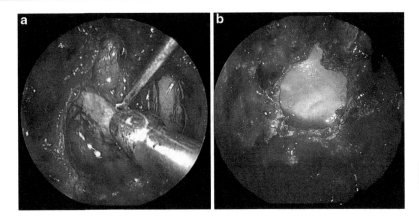

external carotid system. Radiofrequency coblation technology may decrease blood loss during tumor removal (Kostrzewa et al. 2010).

Skull Base Reconstruction

After traditional craniofacial resection, almost any skull base defect can be repaired using various techniques including vascularized pericranial flaps, split thickness bone flaps, temporalis muscle flaps, and dural substitutes (Zimmer and Theodosopoulos 2009). The ability to reconstruct the skull base following resection was initially a significant obstacle to endoscopic skull base surgery. A number of techniques have evolved. Smaller defects are repaired using free tissue autografts. Ideally, grafts should be placed on the intracranial side of the defect with use of an underlay technique. Larger defects may require a multilayered reconstruction including solid support from cartilage or bone grafts placed in the epidural or intradural space (Citardi and Fakhri 2010) (Fig. 2). Large ventral skull base defects may also be managed with vascularized mucosal pedicled flaps, especially when adjuvant radiation therapy is anticipated. The nasoseptal flap, pedicled on the posterior septal branch of the sphenopalatine artery, provides coverage for dural defects extending from frontal sinus to sella and orbit to orbit (Hadad et al. 2006). Various other pedicled mucosal flaps and a minimally invasive, anteriorly based pericranial flap harvested without a craniotomy have also been described (Ong et al. 2010). These techniques have lowered the postoperative CSF leak rate to approximately 4% (Zimmer and Theodosopoulos 2009; Ong et al. 2010). Moreover, endoscopic techniques may be used to address residual

or recurrent CSF leaks seen after previous external skull base reconstruction with pericranial or other flaps (Clark et al. 2010).

Outcomes

Direct comparisons between endoscopic resection of skull base malignancy and traditional craniofacial resection through "open" techniques are difficult due to the rarity of disease and heterogeneity of histology. Making meaningful comparisons of survival rates is also hindered by differences in tumor stage and length of follow-up between studies. Nevertheless, evidence suggests that short-term endoscopic outcomes are at least equivalent to those obtained through traditional techniques.

Eloy et al. compared 18 patients treated with endoscopic resection to 48 patients who underwent craniofacial resection for anterior skull base malignancy (Eloy et al. 2009). There was no significant difference in perioperative complication rates. The endoscopic group had a significantly decreased length of hospital stay. There was a trend toward a higher recurrence rate in the craniofacial resection group, but this may be attributed to differences in the distribution of tumor stage and histology.

In a larger series, 93 patients with sinonasal malignancy resected endoscopically were compared to 27 patients who received a combined endoscopic and craniotomy approach (Hanna et al. 2009). The 5- and 10-year disease-specific survival rates for the entire cohort were 87% and 80%, respectively. There were no significant differences in disease recurrence and survival between the purely endoscopic and combined approach groups. However, patients with higher tumor stage or skull base involvement were more likely to be treated with the combined approach.

Nicolai et al. published the largest series to date of sinonasal and skull base malignancies treated with purely endoscopic ($n = 134$) and combined cranioendoscopic ($n = 50$) techniques with a mean follow-up time of 34.1 months (Nicolai et al. 2008). The 5-year disease-specific survival rate for the purely endoscopic group was 94.4% for adenocarcinoma, 60.7% for squamous cell carcinoma, and 100% for ▶ esthesioneuroblastoma and adenoid cystic carcinoma. The 5-year disease-free survival for the purely endoscopic group was 91.4% compared to 58.8% for the combined cranioendoscopic group. This disparity is not surprising given that 65% of the patients who underwent a purely endoscopic approach had only T1 or T2 disease while 92% of those who had a combined approach had T3 or T4 disease.

Batra et al. reported on 25 patients with T3 or T4 skull base malignancies treated with minimally invasive endoscopic resection (Batra et al. 2010). The most common histopathologies were squamous cell carcinoma ($n = 6$), ▶ esthesioneuroblastoma ($n = 5$), mucosal melanoma ($n = 5$), and sinonasal undifferentiated carcinoma ($n = 4$). The calculated 5-year overall and disease-free survival rates were 58.6% and 51.7%, respectively. These rates compare favorably to the estimated rates in large craniofacial resection series: 5-year overall and disease-free survival rates were 48.3% and 45.8%, respectively, in a 17-institution series of 334 patients who underwent craniofacial resection (Ganley et al. 2005).

In sum, these studies and other reports provide strong evidence for the utility of endoscopic surgery of the skull base. Endoscopic resection may be an emerging standard for select tumors of the ventral skull base. The endoscopic approach, however, will not supplant craniofacial resection. Rather, the skull base surgeon should be well versed in both endoscopic and "open" techniques and select the approach – endoscopic, "open," or combined – based on the individual patient and characteristics of the tumor.

Indication

The indications for endoscopic surgery of the skull base continue to evolve with technological advances and advancements in surgical technique and experience. The entire ventral skull base may be accessed endoscopically. In the midline, this extends from the frontal sinus to the body of C2. The anterior, middle, and posterior cranial fossae may be accessed in the coronal plane (Snyderman et al. 2008). Based on a 10-year experience, Nicolai et al. concluded that candidates for an endoscopic approach include patients with minimal dural involvement and tumor not invading the orbit, nasolacrimal canal, anterior face of the maxillary sinus, massive intracranial extension, or dural extension lateral to the orbit (Nicolai et al. 2008).

Contraindication

Limitations to endoscopic surgery of the skull base include anatomical restrictions on surgical access, technical challenges of dural reconstruction and hemostasis, and lack of technological and human resources (Solares et al. 2010). Skull base malignancies deemed inoperable by traditional methods are not candidates for curative resection endoscopically, although there may be a role for palliative resection in selected cases. Endoscopic treatment of tumor infiltrating the cavernous sinus or infratemporal fossa is a relative contraindication but may be considered depending on surgeon experience (Luong et al. 2010). Patients with facial soft tissue invasion may be better treated with a craniofacial resection approach. Other contraindications include lack of surgeon expertise and specialized instrumentation.

Advantage/Disadvantage

Advantages
Endoscopic surgery of the skull base allows for excellent illumination and magnification and the ability to see around corners with angled telescopes and high-definition monitors. This facilitates precise tissue removal with improved judgment of tumor origin and boundaries as well as preservation of uninvolved vital structures. There is improved access and exposure to the sphenoid sinus, orbital apex, and frontal recess. The endoscopic approach avoids facial incisions and allows for more rapid recovery, decreased hospitalization and cost, and fewer overall complications (Eloy et al. 2009; Neal et al. 2007).

Disadvantages

The endoscopic approach to the skull base requires specialized technology (image guidance, intraoperative imaging), specialized instrumentation (long drills, long bipolar forceps, hand dissection instruments), and a thorough knowledge of endoscopic anatomy. Technological limitations continue to shrink; current and future developments include three-dimensional videoendoscopy, flexible or malleable instruments and telescopes, and robotic skull base surgery (Nogueira et al. 2010). The team approach requires a relatively long learning curve. Early on, the otolaryngologist may be inexperienced with neuroanatomy while the neurosurgeon may be unfamiliar with sinonasal anatomy. Both must integrate existing anatomic knowledge with the field of view provided by the endoscope. Finally, patients undergoing an endoscopic approach may have higher rates of sinonasal bleeding, crusting, synechiae, septal perforations, and nasal obstruction compared to those undergoing craniofacial resection.

Cross-References

▶ Computer Assistance in Sinus Surgery
▶ CSF Leak
▶ Endoscopic Pituitary Surgery
▶ Esthesioneuroblastoma
▶ Juvenile Nasopharyngeal Angiofibroma
▶ Radiologic Evaluation of Central Skull Base
▶ Sinonasal Neoplasms
▶ Skull Base Metastases
▶ Skull Base Neoplasms
▶ Skull Base Reconstruction
▶ Temporal Bone Meningocele/Encephalocele

References

Batra PS, Citardi MJ (2006) Endoscopic management of sinonasal malignancy. Otolaryngol Clin N Am 39:619–637

Batra PS, Luong AL, Kanowitz SJ, Sade B, Lee J, Lanza DC et al (2010) Outcomes of minimally invasive endoscopic resection of anterior skull base neoplasms. Laryngoscope 120:9–16

Castelnuovo P, Dallan I, Battaglia P, Bignami M (2010) Endoscopic endonasal skull base surgery: past, present and future. Eur Arch Otorhinolaryngol 267:649–663

Citardi MJ, Fakhri S (2010) Cerebrospinal fluid rhinorrhea. In: Flint PW et al (eds) Cummings otolaryngology-head & neck surgery, 5th edn. Mosby Elsevier, Philadelphia

Clark DW, Citardi MJ, Fakhri S (2010) Endoscopic management of skull base defects associated with persistent pneumocephalus following previous open repair: a preliminary report. Otolaryngol Head Neck Surg 142(6): 820–826

Eloy JA, Vivero RJ, Hoang K, Civantos FJ, Weed DT, Morcos JJ et al (2009) Comparison of transnasal endoscopic and open craniofacial resection for malignant tumors of the anterior skull base. Laryngoscope 119(5):834–840

Ganley I, Patel SG, Singh B, Kraus DH, Bridger PG, Cantu G et al (2005) Craniofacial resection for malignant paranasal sinus tumors: report of an international collaborative study. Head Neck 27(7):575–584

Gomez-Rivera F, Fakhri S, Williams MD, Hanna EY, Kupferman ME (2010) Surgical management of sinonasal hemangiopericytomas: a case series. In: Paper presented at AHNS 2010 research workshop on the biology, prevention and treatment of head and neck cancer, October 28–30, Arlington, VA

Hadad G, Bassagasteguy L, Carrau RL, Mataza JC, Kassam A, Snyderman CH et al (2006) A novel reconstructive technique after endoscopic expanded endonasal approaches: vascular pedicle nasoseptal flap. Laryngoscope 116: 1882–1886

Hanna E, DeMonte F, Ibrahim S, Roberts D, Levine N, Kupferman M (2009) Endoscopic resection of sinonasal cancers with and without craniotomy: oncologic results. Arch Otolaryngol Head Neck Surg 135(12):1219–1224

Knott PD, Batra PS, Citardi MJ (2006) Computer aided surgery: concepts and applications in rhinology. Otolaryngol Clin North Am 39:503–522

Kostrzewa JP, Sunde J, Riley KO, Woodworth BA (2010) Radiofrequency coblation decreases blood loss during endoscopic sinonasal and skull base tumor removal. ORL J Otorhinolaryngol Relat Spec 72(1):38–43

Leong JL, Batra PS, Citardi MJ (2006) CT-MR image fusion for the management of skull base lesions. Otolaryngol Head Neck Surg 134(5):868–876

Luong A, Citardi MJ, Batra PS (2010) Management of sinonasal malignant neoplasms: defining the role of endoscopy. Am J Rhinol 24(2):150–155

McCutcheon IE, Blacklock JB, Weber RS, DeMonte F, Moser RP, Byers M et al (1996) Anterior transcranial (craniofacial) resection of tumors of the paranasal sinuses: surgical technique and results. Neurosurgery 38(3):471–479

Neal JG, Patel SJ, Kulbersh JS, Osguthorpe JD, Schlosser RJ (2007) Comparison of techniques for transsphenoidal pituitary surgery. Am J Rhinol 21(2):203–206

Nicolai P, Battaglia P, Bignami M, Bolzoni Villaret A, Delù G et al (2008) Endoscopic surgery for malignant tumors of the sinonasal tract and adjacent skull base: a 10-year experience. Am J Rhinol 22(3):308–316

Nogueira JF, Stamm A, Vellutini E (2010) Evolution of - endoscopic skull base surgery, current concepts, and future perspectives. Otolaryngol Clin North Am 43: 639–652

Ong YK, Solares CA, Carrau RL, Snyderman CH (2010) New developments in transnasal endoscopic surgery for malignancies of the sinonasal tract and adjacent skull base. Curr Opin Otolaryngol Head Neck Surg 18(2): 107–113

Patel SG, Singh B, Polluri A, Bridger PG, Cantu G, Cheesman AD et al (2003) Craniofacial surgery for malignant skull base tumors: report of an international collaborative study. Cancer 98(6):1179–1187

Snyderman CH, Carrau RL, Kassam AB, Zanation A, Prevedello D, Gardner P et al (2008) Endoscopic skull base surgery: principles of endonasal oncologic surgery. J Surg Oncol 97(8):658–664

Solares CA, Ong YK, Snyderman CH (2010) Transnasal endoscopic skull base surgery: what are the limits? Curr Opin Otolaryngol Head Neck Surg 18(1):1–7

Zimmer LA, Theodosopoulos PV (2009) Anterior skull base surgery: open versus endoscopic. Curr Opin Otolaryngol Head Neck Surg 17(2):75–78

Endoscopic Thyroidectomy

Melanie W. Seybt and David J. Terris
Department of Otolaryngology, Medical College of Georgia, Georgia Health Sciences University, Augusta, GA, USA

Synonyms

Minimally invasive thyroidectomy; MIVAT; Video-assisted thyroidectomy

Definition

Basic Characteristics

Origins of Minimally Invasive and Endoscopic Neck Surgery

Over the past decade, minimally invasive and endoscopic endocrine neck surgery has evolved significantly. The first endoscopic parathyroidectomy was performed by Michel Gagner 1996 at the Cleveland Clinic (Gagner 1996). Surgery lasted over 5 h and the patient developed massive subcutaneous emphysema. Concerns were subsequently raised regarding sustained intravascular absorption and subcutaneous emphysema from long duration of exposure to CO_2 insufflation (Gottlieb et al. 1997). In 1998, Miccoli and his team in Pisa pioneered an endoscopic technique which used a 15 mm central neck incision and only 3–4 min of CO_2 insufflation in order to create an operative pocket (Miccoli et al. 1998). Once the working space was created, visualization was maintained using external retractors. The procedure continued to develop and eventually involved no use of CO_2 insufflation. The operative pocket was created by minimal dissection through a 15 mm anterior neck incision, and visualization of the operative field was obtained using a 5-mm 30° high-resolution endoscope.

Endoscopic thyroid surgery evolved from these early investigations in parathyroid surgery. Drs. Paolo Miccoli in Pisa (Miccoli et al. 1999), and Rocco Bellantone in Rome (Bellantone et al. 1999) essentially simultaneously developed similar minimally invasive video-assisted approaches to performing thyroid surgery. The technique consists of a small single central incision, use of advanced energy devices to maintain hemostasis in a small space, and endoscopic guidance primarily for the management of the vasculature of the thyroid gland, and the identification and preservation of the recurrent laryngeal nerves and parathyroid glands. These procedures are accomplished without the need for drainage, and are routinely performed on an outpatient basis in the USA (Terris et al. 2007a).

Endoscopic Thyroid Surgery Technique

Endoscopic thyroidectomy is actually a three-part procedure starting with an open technique, which is followed by the endoscopic component and then completed in an open fashion.

Patients are positioned with the neck only mildly extended and a 15–20-mm horizontal cervical incision was made. After exposure the thyroid gland, and careful placement of retractors, a 5-mm 30° laparoscopic telescope was properly positioned and used to facilitate ligation of the superior pole vessels utilizing an ultrasonic energy device (Fig. 1). Once the vessels are safely ligated (Fig. 2), the superior pole can be freed up from its remaining attachments and mobilized inferiorly. The superior parathyroid gland is usually readily identified at this point, and is dissected gently away from the thyroid gland.

The field of view is repositioned to the inferior pole, and the 30° telescope is angled downward. The inferior pole is mobilized to facilitate identification of the recurrent laryngeal nerve. With the thyroid gland retracted medially, the nerve is identified inferiorly. Once the nerve is identified, the inferior parathyroid gland is located, and gently mobilized away from the

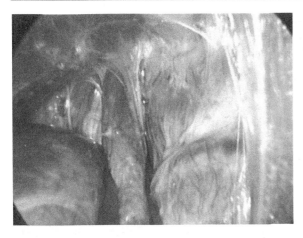

Endoscopic Thyroidectomy, Fig. 1 Endoscopic visualization of the superior pole

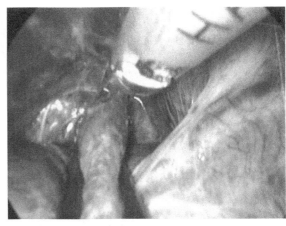

Endoscopic Thyroidectomy, Fig. 2 Ligation of the superior pole vessels using an ultrasonic energy device

gland. The inferior thyroid artery and vein are sealed and divided with the ultrasonic shears.

The thyroid isthmus can be divided at this point with either electrocautery or the ultrasonic shears. The thyroid gland is delivered through the wound, and remains attached primarily by the ligament of Berry. Once the gland has been delivered through the incision (Fig. 3a, b), it is grasped with a sponge, and the recurrent laryngeal nerve is traced to its entry in the region of the cricothyroid joint. The connective tissue attachments between the gland and the trachea are divided using the ultrasonic shears, with care taken to orient the active blade away from the nerve at all times.

After liberal irrigation and careful inspection of the wound, and assurance of hemostasis, surgicel is placed in the thyroid bed, and the strap muscles reapproximated with a simple figure of eight suture of 3-O Vicryl. Two interrupted sutures of 4-O Vicryl are used to approximate the subcutaneous tissues, and Dermabond is used to seal the wound. No external sutures or drains are required.

Evolution of Endoscopic Thyroid Surgery

The Miccoli technique is the most widely practiced variation of endoscopic thyroid surgery, likely due to the relative ease of performance in addition to the substantial patient advantages. More importantly, a number of publications have appeared that clarify the oncologic safety of the procedure (Miccoli et al. 2002), demonstrate the profound cosmetic

(Miccoli et al. 2001) and even functional superiority relative to conventional surgery (Lombardi et al. 2008), and confirm the compatibility with other technologies such as nerve monitoring or the use of ultrasonic energy (Terris et al. 2007b).

Miccoli accomplished a very convincing prospective randomized trial comparing minimally invasive video-assisted thyroidectomy with conventional thyroidectomy for the management of thyroid cancer (Miccoli et al. 2002), which served to alleviate concerns regarding the thoroughness of resection in thyroid malignancy. Postoperative measures of serum thyroglobulin and radioactive iodine uptake confirmed that the endoscopic technique yielded a thorough thyroid removal when compared with conventional thyroidectomy. Additionally, prospective trials were conducted by the Miccoli (Miccoli et al. 2001) and Bellantone (Lombardi et al. 2008) groups in which the cosmetic and functional advantages of the endoscopic technique were validated. In a comparison between minimally invasive video-assisted thyroidectomy and conventional surgery, patients described greater satisfaction with their scar outcome and reduced pain with the minimally invasive technique (Miccoli et al. 2001). Finally, after describing a large North American multi-institutional application of this technique (Terris et al. 2008), Terris et al. subsequently highlighted the complementary application of endoscopic surgery and laryngeal nerve monitoring (Terris et al. 2007b), which helps to compensate for the inherently reduced surgical aperture

Endoscopic Thyroidectomy, Fig. 3 Delivery of the gland

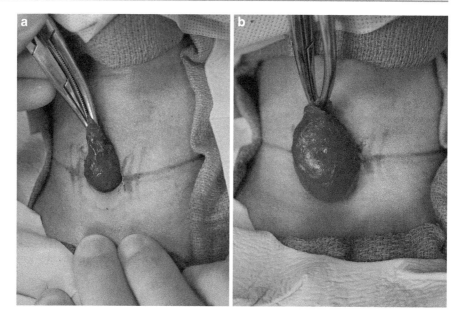

associated with minimally invasive surgery. Excellent functional outcomes were achieved with a very low rate of transient nerve dysfunction, likely due to the magnified visualization of the recurrent laryngeal nerves.

The Future of Endoscopic Thyroid Surgery

With improvements in technology, there seems to be little doubt that endoscopic thyroid surgery will continue to evolve with three possible directions of this evolution. These include expanded indications for the endoscopic thyroidectomy, the further development of remote access surgery via several different routes, and the application of robotics to further assist the surgeon in accomplishing these techniques (as discussed in another entry).

There are already early reports of the expansion of indications for endoscopic surgery. Miccoli has described the use of this procedure for carriers of the ret proto-oncogene (Miccoli et al. 2004) and for bilateral neck exploration (Miccoli et al. 2008). Bellantone has published on endoscopic lymph node dissection, both in the central compartment (Bellantone et al. 2002) and in the lateral compartment (Lombardi et al. 2007). As instrumentation improves, and as retrieval of the gland is facilitated, ever larger glands and lesions may be removed through ever smaller incisions.

Summary

After nearly a century of performing thyroidectomy essentially the way it was described by Theodore Kocher in the nineteenth century, the technique has rapidly evolved. Endoscopic thyroidectomy can now be performed in many patients who benefit from the reduced dissection and smaller incisions associated with this approach. While many of the cosmetic, quality of life, and functional improvements have been proven, a better understanding of the procedure and the appropriate indications for its application will continue to develop even as the technique itself evolves, and as new approaches emerge.

Cross-References

▶ Follicular Thyroid Cancer
▶ Medullary Thyroid Cancer
▶ Minimally Invasive Parathyroid Surgery
▶ Papillary Thyroid Cancer
▶ Parathyroidectomy
▶ Thyroidectomy
▶ Thyroidectomy, Complications
▶ Thyroid Nodules, Evaluation
▶ Well-Differentiated Thyroid Cancer

References

Bellantone R, Lombardi CP, Raffaelli M, Rubino F, Boscherini M, Perilli W (1999) Minimally invasive, totally gasless video-assisted thyroid lobectomy. Am J Surg 177(4):342–343

Bellantone R, Lombardi CP, Raffaelli M, Boscherini M, Alesina PF, Princi P (2002) Central neck lymph node removal during minimally invasive video-assisted thyroidectomy for thyroid carcinoma: a feasible and safe procedure. J Laparoendosc Adv Surg Tech A 12(3):181–185

Gagner M (1996) Endoscopic subtotal parathyroidectomy in patients with primary hyperparathyroidism. Br J Surg 83(6):875

Gottlieb A, Sprung J, Zheng XM, Gagner M (1997) Massive subcutaneous emphysema and severe hypercarbia in a patient during endoscopic transcervical parathyroidectomy using carbon dioxide insufflation. Anesth Analg 84:1154–1156

Lombardi CP, Raffaelli M, Princi P, De Crea C, Bellantone R (2007) Minimally invasive video-assisted functional lateral neck dissection for metastatic papillary thyroid carcinoma. Am J Surg 193(1):114–118

Lombardi CP, Raffaelli M, D'alatri L, De Crea C, Marchese MR, Maccora D, Paludetti G, Bellantone R (2008) Video-assisted thyroidectomy significantly reduces the risk of early postthyroidectomy voice and swallowing symptoms. World J Surg 32(5):693–700

Miccoli P, Bendinelli C, Conte M et al (1998) Endoscopic parathyroidectomy by a gasless approach. Jnl Lap Adv Surg Tech 8(4):189–194

Miccoli P, Berti P, Conte M, Bendinelli C, Marcocci C (1999) Minimally invasive surgery for thyroid small nodules: preliminary report. J Endocrinol Invest 22:849–851

Miccoli P, Berti P, Raffaelli M, Materazzi G, Baldacci S, Rossi G (2001) Comparison between minimally invasive video-assisted thyroidectomy and conventional thyroidectomy: a prospective randomized study. Surgery 130:1039–1043

Miccoli P, Elisei R, Materazzi G, Capezzone M, Galleri D, Pacini F, Berti P, Pinchera A (2002) Minimally invasive video-assisted thyroidectomy for papillary carcinoma: a prospective study of its completeness. Surgery 132:1070–1073

Miccoli P, Elisei R, Berti P, Materazzi G, Agate L, Castagna MG, Cosci B, Faviana P, Ugolini C, Pinchera A (2004) Video assisted prophylactic thyroidectomy and central compartment nodes clearance in two RET gene mutation adult carriers. J Endocrinol Invest 27(6):557–561

Miccoli P, Berti P, Materazzi G et al (2008) Endoscopic bilateral neck exploration versus quick intraoperative parathormone assay (qPTHa) during endoscopic parathyroidectomy: a prospective randomized trial. Surg Endo 22(2):398–400

Terris DJ, Moister B, Seybt MW, Gourin CG, Chin E (2007a) Outpatient thyroid surgery is safe and desirable. Otolaryngol Head Neck Surg 136(4):556–559

Terris DJ, Anderson SK, Watts TL, Chin E (2007b) Laryngeal nerve monitoring and minimally invasive thyroid surgery: complementary technologies. Arch Otolaryngol Head Neck Surg 133(12):1254–1257

Terris DJ, Angelos P, Steward DL, Simental AA (2008) Minimally invasive video-assisted thyroidectomy: a multi-institutional North American experience. Arch Otolaryngol Head Neck Surg 134(1):81–84

Endoscopic Transphenoidal Pituitary Surgery

▶ Endoscopic Pituitary Surgery

ENG/VNG

Jorge E. González[1] and Alexander Kiderman[2]
[1]Bloomsburg University of Pennsylvania, Bloomsburg, PA, USA
[2]Neuro-Kinetics, Inc., Pittsburgh, PA, USA

Synonyms

Electronystagmography; Videonystagmography

Definition

Electronystagmography (ENG) is the use of electrodes for collecting and analyzing nystagmic eye movements, while videonystagmography (VNG) uses video recording methods to collect and analyze nystagmus. ENG takes advantage of the corneoretinal potential (CRP), the biological dipole between the cornea (positively charged) and the retina (negatively charged), to detect eye position. ENG and VNG are types of oculography, the recording of eye movements using electrodes (EOG) or video (VOG). ENG and VNG are frequently used to describe a test battery using the ENG/VNG recording to assess vestibular and/or balance disorders. The ENG/VNG battery includes ocular motility, positioning (Dix-Hallpike), positional, and caloric tests.

Purpose

The ENG/VNG test battery is a common diagnostic tool for the evaluation of vestibular or balance disorder patients. The different components of the battery provide information on ocular motor, central vestibular, and peripheral vestibular function. The Dix-Hallpike test is performed to determine the presence of Benign Paroxysmal Positional Vertigo (BPPV) of the posterior semicircular canal. Caloric testing provides information regarding the functioning of the individual horizontal semicircular canals.

Principle

Equipment and Preparation

The equipment needed for ENG and VNG is similar. For both methods of testing, a means of providing a visual stimulus for ocular motility testing is needed. The means of stimulus production typically involve light emitting diodes (LED) in a light bar, video projector, or laser presentation techniques.

In order to utilize electrodes to record eye movements, a differential amplifier capable of recording DC from the corneoretinal potential is needed. Commercially available Ag/AgCl electrodes and electrode leads are used. To record eye movements through VOG technique an infrared camera system capable of capturing at least 60 frames per second is needed. The VNG systems require a means by which the infrared cameras can be affixed to the patient's head. This is typically done through the use of modified goggles or headbands.

A means of graphing the eye movements is required in order to analyze the test results. Traditionally this was done for ENG through the use of graphed strips of paper, or strip charts. However, modern ENG systems use computers to acquire and store eye and stimulus data for analysis. The method of data collection also must allow for analysis of the resultant eye movements. For computerized testing, the software should allow examination of horizontal and vertical (for EOG) and horizontal, vertical, and torsional (for VOG) components of the eye movements.

Caloric testing requires a water or air irrigator. The standard water irrigation system, called open-loop irrigation, involves the direct application of water into the ear canal. An alternative to open-loop water is the air irrigation. Air irrigators provide direct application of air to the ear canal/ear drum. Generally, air irrigators require more diligence from the operator since air, as a poor conductor of temperature, must be directed at the ear drum in order to deliver the full thermal effect. In cases where ice water caloric testing is required, a thermometer is needed to determine that the temperature of the water is appropriate.

Patient medication should also be taken into account prior to the ENG/VNG testing. It is known that a significant number of medications have vestibular side effects. These can generally be divided into those that act upon the peripheral vestibular system and those that act upon the central nervous system (CNS) or central vestibular system (Bhansali 2001). The medications acting on the peripheral vestibular system include aminoglycosides, loop diuretics, antineoplastics, and ototoxic medications. ENG/VNG test results can also be influenced by antihypertensive, antidepressant and vestibulosuppressants or CNS acting medications.

Nystagmus

The main type of eye movement that is observed during the ENG/VNG examination is nystagmus. The presence of nystagmus is a normal response in some test conditions (e.g., optokinetic and caloric testing), while abnormal in other conditions (pursuit and positional testing). Nystagmus is an involuntary rhythmic motion of the eyes that consists of a "slow" component in one direction and a "fast" correction of the eye in the other direction. A graphic representation of nystagmus as obtained via ENG/VNG techniques is shown in Fig. 1. Slow component eye movements are the sloped portion of the nystagmus trace (black solid line) while the fast components are vertical. Direction of the nystagmus is defined by the fast phase, while velocity of the nystagmus is defined by the slow phase. Slow component eye velocity (SCEV) is the number of degrees of eye movement for single nystagmus beat over the time for that particular nystagmus beat (change in eye position for one nystagmus beat in degrees/time of this nystagmus beat in seconds). In this example, the SCEV of the highlighted nystagmus beat is approximately 20°/s.

Analysis of nystagmus is based upon two characteristics; velocity and direction. The velocity of the nystagmus is defined by the slow component (sloped traces), while the direction is defined by the fast component (vertical traces). Nystagmus is displayed graphically with degrees of eye movement vertically and time graphed horizontally. The calculation of SCEV is performed by determining the degrees of movement that occur over 1 s of time. Rightward movements of the eyes are graphed upwards, while leftward movements are graphed downwards. Further discussion of nystagmus can be found in the section on ▶ Nystagmus.

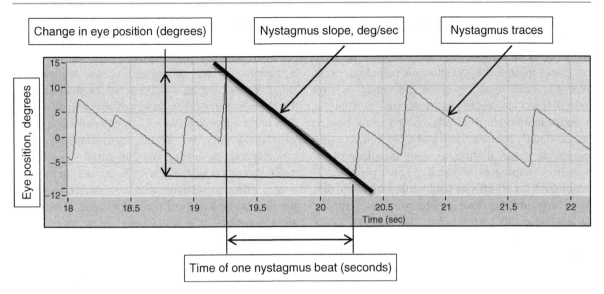

ENG/VNG, Fig. 1 Graphic display of right-beating horizontal nystagmus. Note the characteristic saw-tooth pattern representing the slow and fast components of the nystagmus. The slow component (black diagonal line) plots the amount of deviation of the eye over the course of 1 s. The fast component (vertical tracing) indicates the direction of the corrective saccade. Upward movements of the tracings are right beating saccades, while downward movements represent left beating saccades. Time is represented on the abscissa and degrees are displayed on the ordinate. Left beating nystagmus would be shown as a horizontal inversion of this image

Technique

ENG testing requires proper placement of the electrodes on the patient's skin. Minimally, two channels: horizontal and vertical, should be used. Skin preparation for electrodes occurs on the high forehead as a ground, above and below one eye for the vertical channel, and at the outer canthus of each eye for the horizontal channel. The preparation sites should be placed such that the electrode placement will nearly bifurcate the eye position across the electrodes. When using VNG, the goggles/headband should be placed on the patient such that the video camera(s) are positioned to maximize the viewing of the eye. The use of four electrode channels for ENG or binocular cameras for VNG allow for the precise examination of both eyes and should be considered in circumstances where the eyes do not move conjugately. In order to prevent the suppression of vestibular nystagmus by visual fixation, the Dix-Hallpike, positional, and caloric tests are performed in the absence of visual fixation for VNG and with the eyes closed for ENG.

The ocular motor test battery includes tests of spontaneous nystagmus, horizontal and vertical gaze evoked nystagmus, saccades, smooth pursuit, and optokinetics. Once the ocular recording method (ENG or VNG) has been properly selected, the patient is positioned in front of the stimulus that will be used for the ocular motility test battery. Spontaneous nystagmus testing requires the patient to maintain focus in the primary position (in front) in the presence and in the absence of a visual target. During horizontal and vertical gaze evoked nystagmus tests, the patient is asked to look at a target that is offset from the primary position in the respective planes. The patient is asked to quickly and accurately follow a rapidly moving target during the saccade test. During the smooth pursuit test, the patient must follow a visual target that moves smoothly back and forth. Smooth pursuit testing can be performed in the horizontal and the vertical planes. Optokinetic testing requires that the patient follow a series of visual targets as they move in one direction and then in the other. Further description of the test techniques can be found in other sources (Leigh and Zee 2006).

The Dix-Hallpike or positioning test requires motion of the patient as well as observation of the eyes. The visualization of the patient's eyes is done with VNG or Frenzel lenses. As a test of posterior semicircular canal BPPV, proper placement is important. Prior to the movement, the patient is seated with his/her head turned approximately 45° from the sagittal plane toward the symptomatic/pathologic side. With the head in this position the patient is then moved from a seated to a supine position at a reasonable speed. Typically, the patient's head is placed slightly below the horizontal plane, in an effort to provide maximal stimulus along the plane of the posterior semicircular canal. This position is maintained for 30–60 s or until vertigo subsides, during which time the clinician observes or records the patient's eye movements. Once the time or vertigo expires, the patient is then assisted to the seated position while maintaining the position of the head. The clinician observes the eyes as before. The rate of movement does not need to be aggressive, and movements at a normal pace for the individual are usually sufficient to elicit symptoms. Modifications to the Dix-Hallpike test, such as the side lying technique or roll test, can be performed in order to accommodate restricted patient motion or suspicion of involvement of the horizontal or anterior semicircular canals.

Positional testing involves searching for the presence of nystagmus while the patient is oriented in different static positions. The positional test battery includes different head positions and body positions. The head positions include supine, head left, and head right, while the body positions include body right, body left, and the caloric position. Patients are engaged with mental alerting tasks within all head and body positions. Fixation suppression, where the patient is asked to focus on a visual target, should be included in all the different head positions; especially if any nystagmus is found during the testing. Head hanging positions are often included to examine for vertigo of cervical origin.

The main underlying principle behind how the caloric test works, first postulated by Bárány, is that of convection. By warming or cooling the endolymph of the canals, a convective flow is created causing stimulation of the cristae. The convective theory is supplemented by neural warming/cooling, as caloric responses have been found in space experiments in the absence of gravity (Baloh and Honrubia 2001). During the caloric test, the patient is placed in the supine position approximately 30° off of the horizontal (aka caloric position). This arrangement places the horizontal semicircular canals in a plane that is nearly perpendicular to earth, in order to maximize the convective effect.

When an ear is irrigated with warm water a warming of the endolymph of the semicircular canal occurs creating a decrease in the fluid density. This decrease in density causes an upward convective flow of the endolymph which causes a deflection of the cupula toward the utricle (utriculopetal). The utriculopetal deflection of the cupula results in a depolarization of the hair cells and an increase in neural firing. Irrigations with cool water cause an increase in the density of the endolymph, thereby creating cupular deflection away from the utricle (utriculofugal). Utriculofugal movement causes a hyperpolarization of the hair cells and a decrease in neural firing. The increased neural firing causes the patient to sense motion toward the irrigated ear, while decreases in neural firing will cause a sense of motion away from the irrigated ear. The acronym COWS, (Cold – Opposite, Warm – Same) indicates the direction of the fast component of the nystagmus that results from the different temperatures of irrigation. The cool irrigation of the left ear (LC) and warm irrigation of the right ear (RW) elicit right-beating nystagmus, while cool irrigations of the right ear (RC) and warm irrigations of the left ear (LW) elicit left-beating nystagmus.

The standard procedure for the caloric test was initially developed by Fitzgerald and Hallpike in 1942. The process of Alternating Binaural Bithermal (ABB) calorics involves irrigating each ear with both warm and cool stimuli. The temperatures of the irrigations are 30°C and 44°C for the cool and warm water irrigations, respectively. The duration of the water irrigation is usually 30 s. The poor thermal conductivity of air requires a greater temperature differential and duration of irrigation when using air stimuli. The cool and warm air irrigations (24°C and 50°C) are maintained for approximately 60 s. The durations of irrigations may vary among clinics; however, the duration of the irrigations should remain consistent within each patient. The irrigations are administered to the ear canal and eye movements are recorded for a period of 2–3 min after the irrigations ceases. Upon completion of the caloric irrigation, a waiting time of 3–5 min is recommended to allow the temperature effect on the endolymph to reduce. The order of the irrigations does not seem to have a significant effect on the responses elicited by the caloric test (Barin 2008a). A monothermal warm screening test (MWST) has been shown to be a viable alternative to the ABB when time constraints or patient discomfort are concerns (Murnane et al. 2009).

The main analyses of ABB caloric test results look at both peripheral and central aspects of vestibular function. Unilateral Weakness (UW) or Unilateral Vestibular Weakness (UVW) compares the strength of the average peak SCEV for the warm and cool irrigations of each ear. The UW gives information to lateralize weaknesses in vestibular function in one ear or the other. The formula for UW calculation is:

$$UW\% = \frac{(RW + RC) - (LW + LC)}{(RW + RC + LW + LC)} \times 100$$

Using this formula when the right ear responses are stronger than the left ear responses, the UW percentage will be positive. Stronger responses in the left ear will result in negative percentages. These calculations will be described as left unilateral weakness (LUW) and right unilateral weakness (RUW), respectively.

Bilateral weakness (BW) or Bilateral Vestibular Weakness (BVW) quantifies the overall function of both peripheral vestibular systems based upon the sum of the SCEV in all conditions. The formula for BW calculation is:

$$BW = RW + RC + LW + LC$$

Directional Preponderance (DP) compares the strength of the average peak SCEV for the right-beating versus the left-beating responses. The formula for UW calculation is:

$$DP\% = \frac{(RW + LC) - (LW + RC)}{(RW + RC + LW + LC)} \times 100$$

Similar to calculations for UW, the directional preponderances are described based upon the percentages. Right directional preponderances (RDP) are found when the SCEV of the right beating responses (RW + LC) are stronger than those of the left beating responses (LW + RC). Left directional preponderances (LDP) occur when the opposite is true. Using this formula, the RDP will exhibit a positive percentage, while LDP will be negative.

The measurement of the central vestibular function is based upon the Fixation Index (FI). The FI compares the peak average SCEV of the nystagmus during the fixation condition and compares it to the peak average SCEV prior to fixation. This calculation is done for each direction of the fast component. Since caloric responses do not usually differ significantly between directions FI can be calculated off of only one caloric per direction; although it is typically calculated for all irrigations tests.

$$RB\ FI\% = \frac{(RB\ Fixation)}{(RB\ No\ Fixation)} \times 100$$

$$LB\ FI\% = \frac{(LB\ Fixation)}{(LB\ No\ Fixation)} \times 100$$

The ice water caloric method requires some modification of the test technique compared to the standard temperature protocol, and are primarily used to confirm absent or reduced nystagmus SCEV. First, the temperature of the irrigation should be approximately 2–4°C. This provides maximal thermal stimulation to the vestibular organ being tested and can be monitored through the use of a thermometer. Typically, the duration of the ice water caloric test is shorter (10–30 s) than that of the ABB stimuli. The patient is placed in the supine position and the head is turned to orient the test ear superiorly. The ear canal and concha of the pinna are filled with the ice water. After the predetermined irrigation time the patient's head is centered. In some clinical settings, the patient is then moved to the caloric position to allow for maximal convective effect along the plane of the horizontal semicircular canal. Analysis of function via ice calorics looks specifically at the difference between the right and left ear ice water responses SCEV (RI and LI, respectively) relative to the total responses. The formula is:

$$Ice\ water\ UW\% = \frac{RI - LI}{RI + LI} \times 100$$

Mental alerting tasks are performed during each caloric test, and the patient is asked to visually focus on a target near the maximal response. The purpose of the mental alerting tasks is to minimize central suppression of the vestibular response, while the fixation provides information regarding the integrity of the central vestibular pathways.

Findings and Interpretation

The types of eye movements found during the ocular motility tests and the manner in which they are analyzed differ based upon the test. Spontaneous and gaze evoked nystagmus testing looks for the presence of nystagmus in those different test conditions. Positive findings for spontaneous nystagmus testing could be in the fixation present or the fixation absent conditions. Nystagmus found in the fixation absent condition alone is indicative of a peripheral vestibular dysfunction, while nystagmus present in the fixation present condition is indicative of central involvement. During the saccade testing, measurements of saccadic latency, accuracy, and velocity are performed. These values represent the time delay between the patient's eye movement after the target movement, the amplitude of eye movement relative to target movement, and the time required for the patient's eye to travel from its initial position to the final target position, respectively. Smooth pursuit eye movements are often examined in terms of the amplitude gain. The velocity gain examines the velocity of the eye relative to the velocity of the target (Shepard and Schubert 2008). Additional examination of phase differences between the target and the eyes and asymmetry of velocity gain in one direction versus the other can be performed. Qualitative analysis of smooth pursuit morphology and calculation of percentage of saccadation may also be performed. The optokinetic test results are analyzed respective to the velocity gain of the eye movements. Specifically, the velocity of the eye movements should approximate that of the visual target motion.

In cases of posterior semicircular canal BPPV, the characteristic eye movement observed in a Dix-Hallpike test is rotatory or torsional nystagmus. Torsional nystagmus cannot be recorded by traditional ENG testing and few commercially available VNG systems can properly analyze torsion. Involvement of the right posterior canal typically elicits a counter clockwise torsional nystagmus, while left posterior canal involvement elicits a clockwise torsional nystagmus. Horizontal canal BPPV will elicit horizontal nystagmus, although lateralization of the pathologic ear is often difficult based solely upon examination of the fast component. Further discussion of nystagmus can be found in the entry on Examination (Vestibular Dysfunction-Benign Paroxysmal Positional Vertigo).

The presence of nystagmus during positional testing is suggestive of either peripheral or central involvement regardless of the position in which it is elicited. Nystagmus of peripheral vestibular origin will be suppressible in the presence of a fixation stimulus and often beats in the direction of the intact labyrinth. In addition, peripheral nystagmus will be direction-fixed within a particular head position, horizontal or torsional in nature, and may diminish over time within a particular position. Two principal characteristics of positional nystagmus of central origin are that it is not suppressible with fixation and it may change direction within one position. Central nystagmus also is most often vertical in nature, does not diminish within a position, and may be secondary to medications (El-Kashlan and Handelsman 2008; Roberts and Gans 2008).

The caloric test is widely regarded as the most sensitive test of the ENG/VNG test battery (Baloh and Honrubia 2001; Barin 2008b). Caloric nystagmus has a latency of approximately 15 s, gradually increases over approximately 1 min and then decreases back to its baseline. By calculating the UW, BW, DP, and FI the integrity of the horizontal semicircular canals can be determined. The normal percentage for UW varies slightly among clinics, but typically ranges between 20% and 25% (Baloh and Honrubia 2001; Barin 2008b). Any UW values above the normative values are indicative of peripheral vestibular pathology in the weaker ear. While the SCEV values differ among individuals, larger UW percentages are suggestive of lesser function in the weaker ear. When performing the MWST, interaural differences of less than 10% can be interpreted as symmetric function (Murnane et al. 2009). Cool water irrigations should be performed to complete the ABB protocol when MWST differences are larger than the 10% cutoff. Numerous pathologies can result in a unilateral weakness including labyrinthitis, Ménière's Disease, vestibular schwannoma, ischemic disorders affecting the labyrinth, and multiple sclerosis.

Along with determining if there is an asymmetry in vestibular response, the overall function, BW must be calculated. The sum of the caloric responses (BW) for all irrigations should be above 20–25°/s (Baloh and Honrubia 2001; Barin 2008b). A positive finding of BW can indicate that both vestibular labyrinths are dysfunctional. Common causes for BW include bilateral meningitis, chronic otitis media, ototoxicity, bilateral Ménière's Disease, cerebellar degeneration, and autoimmune inner ear disorders.

Nystagmus exhibited during caloric stimulation should exhibit suppressibility if it is purely peripheral in origin. In light of this, suppression of caloric nystagmus as measured by FI, should be suppressed by between 50% and 70% (Barin 2008b, El-Kashlan and Handelsman 2008). Using the formula to calculate FI, complete suppression of the nystagmus with fixation will yield an FI of 0%. A failure of fixation suppression is an indicator of central pathology which is often associated with the cerebellar flocculus.

Directional preponderance is the standard calculation of caloric responses that has limited clinical utility (Barin 2008a). Abnormal DP has been found in patients with central involvement as well as individuals with normal vestibular function. DP is often interpreted as an asymmetric peripheral disorder (Shepard 2001). There are other rare abnormalities of caloric testing including caloric inversion and caloric perversion. Since these abnormalities will rarely be encountered by clinicians, the reader is referred to other sources.

Indication

ENG/VNG is indicated in patients with complaints of vertigo or balance disorders. In particular, these diagnostic procedures may be helpful in diagnosing individuals who present with complaints that suggest vestibular disorders, Ménière's Disease, instability, light-headedness, or abnormalities of gait. Ocular motility testing should be included in every initial ENG/VNG test. Dix-Hallpike testing is indicated in cases where BPPV is suspected.

Contraindication

There are relatively few contraindications to ENG/VNG. Since the evaluation of the results of all of the subtests are based upon calibrated eye movements, a patient's inability to see a target or to voluntarily move the eyes to acquire the target make the data difficult to collect and interpret. In addition, some retinal pathology can impact the integrity of the CRP tracings (Jacobson et al. 2008). Dix-Hallpike/positional testing may be contraindicated by restricted mobility or disorders of the lower back. Patient cooperation is needed for all of the different test components of the ENG/VNG battery.

Caloric testing may be contraindicated by several factors. Open-loop water calorics should not be performed in ears with perforated tympanic membranes or tympanostomy tubes, as the introduction of water to the middle ear space could promote otitis media. In cases of perforated eardrums, air caloric testing should be performed. Typically, caloric testing can be performed on ears that have undergone mastoidectomy; however, interpretation of the data from that ear is questionable. In the cases of perforated tympanic membranes and mastoidectomy the consistency of the thermal transfer compared to the intact ears is unclear.

Advantage/Disadvantage

The main advantage of ENG/VNG testing is that it provides reliable information on the function of the vestibular system. The caloric component of the ENG/VNG provides stimulation of the horizontal semicircular canals independent of the other and it can be easily performed (Baloh and Honrubia 2001). The ocular motor battery provides information on the integrity of the ocular motor pathways. One of the disadvantages of the ENG/VNG test is that the results of the test do not always reflect the patient's reported symptoms or disability (Shepard 2001). A patient may yield normal results despite symptoms typically associated with vestibular disorders. Because of this, interpretation of test findings may be challenging. Additionally, the caloric stimulus may cause nausea and vomiting in some patients which may create patient discomfort, obscure the results or necessitate stopping the test battery before completion.

Cross-References

▶ Auditory System Exam
▶ Balance (Anatomy: Embryology)
▶ Balance (Anatomy: Labyrinth and Otoliths)
▶ Balance (Anatomy: Vestibular Nerve)
▶ Mastoidectomy

▶ Nystagmus
▶ Rotary Chair
▶ Superior Canal Dehiscence
▶ Testing, Posturography
▶ Unilateral Vestibular Weakness
▶ Vestibular and Central Nervous System, Anatomy
▶ Vestibular Dysfunction, Meniere's Disease
▶ Vestibular Rehabilitation

References

Baloh RW, Honrubia V (2001) Clinical neurophysiology of the vestibular system, 3rd edn. Oxford University Press, New York

Barin K (2008a) Background and technique of caloric testing. In: Jacobson GP, Shepard NT (eds) Balance function assessment and management. Plural, San Diego, pp 197–228

Barin K (2008b) Interpretation and usefulness of caloric testing. In: Jacobson GP, Shepard NT (eds) Balance function assessment and management. Plural, San Diego, pp 229–252

Bhansali SA (2001) Medication side effects. In: Goebel JA (ed) Practical management of the dizzy patient. Lippincott, Williams and Wilkins, Philadelphia, pp 45–60

El-Kashlan HK, Handelsman JA (2008) Computerized vestibular testing. In: Weber PC (ed) Vertigo and disequilibrium. Thieme, New York, pp 4–14

Jacobson GP, Shepart NT, Dundas JA, McCaslin DL, Piker EG (2008) Eye movement recording techniques. In: Jacobson GP, Shepard NT (eds) Balance function assessment and management. Plural, San Diego, pp 27–44

Leigh RJ, Zee DS (2006) The neurology of eye movements, 4th edn. Oxford University Press, New York

Murnane OD, Akin FW, Lynn SG, Cyr DG (2009) Monothermal caloric screening test performance: A relative operating characteristic curve analysis. Ear Hear 30:1–7

Roberts RA, Gans RE (2008) Background, technique, interpretation, and usefulness of positional/positioning testing. In: Jacobson GP, Shepard NT (eds) Balance function assessment and management. Plural, San Diego, pp 171–196

Shepard NT (2001) Electronystagmography (ENG) testing. In: Goebel JA (ed) Practical management of the dizzy patient. Lippincott, Williams and Wilkins, Philadelphia, pp 113–127

Shepard NT, Schubert M (2008) Background and technique of ocular motor testing. In: Jacobson GP, Shepard NT (eds) Balance function assessment and management. Plural, San Diego, pp 133–146

ENoG

▶ Evoked EMG

Epicanthal Folds

Michael M. Kim
Division of Facial Plastic & Reconstructive Surgery, Department of Otolaryngology-Head and Neck Surgery, Oregon Health & Science University, Portland, OR, USA

Definition

The epicanthal fold is a skin fold of the upper eyelid that obscures the medial canthus. This feature is often present in patients with Down's Syndrome and may also be seen in individuals of Eastern Asian descent. The epicanthal fold may be reduced through the use of various z-plasty techniques in conjunction with the double-eyelid fold procedure.

Cross-References

▶ Z-plasty

Epicranial Aponeurosis

Derek Robinson and Bradley W. Kesser
Department of Otolaryngology-Head and Neck Surgery, University of Virginia Health System, Charlottesville, VA, USA

Synonyms

Galea aponeurotica

Definition

Fibrous membrane that covers the cranium between the occipital and frontal muscles of the scalp. Also called the galea aponeurotica.

Cross-References

▶ Pinna and External Auditory Canal, Anatomy

Epidermoid

▶ Cholesteatoma, Acquired
▶ Cholesteatoma of Childhood

Epidermoid Cyst

▶ Cholesteatoma, Acquired
▶ Lateral Skull Base Epidermoids

Epidural Abscess

▶ Sinusitis in Children, Complications

Epineurium

Wojciech K. Mydlarz and Kofi Derek O. Boahene
Department of Otolaryngology-Head and Neck
Surgery, Johns Hopkins University School of
Medicine, Baltimore, MD, USA

Definition

It is the outermost layer of connective tissue surrounding a peripheral nerve. It is made of dense irregular connective tissue that contains multiple nerve fascicles as well as the blood supply to the nerve.

Cross-References

▶ Sunderland Classification of Nerve Injury

Epiphora

▶ Sinus Surgery, Complications

Epiphora and Dacryocystorhinostomy

Richard N. Palu
Section of Ophthalmic Plastic and Reconstructive
Surgery, New York University Medical Center,
New York, NY, USA

Synonyms

Nasolacrimal duct surgery; Tear duct surgery; Tearing

Definitions

Epiphora/Tearing – Overflow of tears (tearing) from the surface of the eye. It may be due to abnormal tear production (excess or decreased), abnormal tear distribution, or abnormalities in tear drainage.

Nasolacrimal Drainage System/Tear Drainage System – Composed of the punctum (puncti), canaliculus (canaliculi), nasolacrimal (tear) sac, and nasolacrimal (tear) duct. Tear flow is from the ocular surface, into the puncti, through the canaliculi, into the tear sac, down the tear duct, and into the nose. The tear drainage system on the right side is the mirror image of the system on the left side.

Punctum – The small opening at the eyelid margin in the medial aspect of each of the four eyelids. The punctum is the beginning of the tear drainage system. Each punctum is approximately 0.25–0.33 mm^2 in diameter with the lower puncti being larger. The punctum leads to the canaliculus.

Canaliculus – The microtubular pathway in the nasal-most aspect of the eyelid. It is the conduit of tear flow from the punctum to the nasolacrimal sac.

Nasolacrimal Sac/Tear Sac – A mucosal-lined structure in the medial canthus residing in a bony fossa made up of the thick ascending process of the maxillary bone anteriorly and the thin lacrimal bone posteriorly. Tears pass into the tear sac from the upper and the lower canaliculi. The upper and lower canaliculi join to form a common canaliculus before entering the tear sac. The opening of the common canaliculus into the lateral wall of the tear sac is an important anatomic landmark in nasolacrimal surgery.

Nasolacrimal Duct/Tear Duct – A canal-like structure in the lateral wall of the nose/medial maxillary wall. Tears drain from the tear sac down the tear duct and into the nose. The tear duct enters the nose at an opening in the inferior meatus approximately 1.0 cm from the opening of the nostril.

Dry Eye Syndrome/DES/Dry Eyes – Ocular symptoms and ophthalmologic findings on the ocular surface resulting from decreased tear production.

Dacryocystorhinostomy/DCR/Tear Duct Surgery – Surgical anastomosis between the nasolacrimal sac of the tear drainage system and the nose.

Clinical Features

Epiphora (Tearing)

Epiphora is the overflow of tears (tearing) from the surface of the eye.

It may be due to abnormal tear production (excess or decreased), abnormal tear distribution, or abnormalities in tear drainage. Tearing is a "final common pathway" in many ophthalmologic conditions, including intraocular diseases. A formal work-up of the tearing patient is a necessary evaluation in every patient with symptomatic tearing. (Holds 2012).

Note: Epiphora in the newborn or infant is most often due to delayed opening of the nasolacrimal duct as it enters the nose. Rarely, intranasal pathology or more severe ophthalmologic conditions can cause tearing in this age group. The tear duct opens spontaneously in the vast majority of patients by 1 year of age. In those that do not open spontaneously, probing or balloon dacryoplasty of the nasolacrimal duct is indicated.

Tests

The Epiphora Work Up

The work up of the adult tearing patient includes:

1. A complete ophthalmologic evaluation to rule out intraocular disease (anterior segment inflammation, glaucoma, cataract, vitritis, retinitis, retinal diseases, intraocular tumor, etc.) and ocular surface disease (DES, conjunctivitis, conjunctival tumors, blepharitis, meibomian gland dysfunction, etc.) (Holds 2012).
2. A directed examination of:
   A. Tear production
   B. Tear distribution
   C. Tear drainage

Abnormalities of tear production, tear distribution, and tear drainage all may cause tearing. Tearing may be multifactorial.

A. *Examination of Tear Production* – This is an evaluation of the quantity and the quality of tear production.

   Many clinical tests are available for qualitative and quantitative assessment of tear production. No one test alone will suffice. Most commonly used tests include a combination of the Basic Tear Secretion Test, Schirmer Tests (Type I and II), and qualitative and quantitative evaluation of the tear film at the slit lamp (tear breakup time, fluorescein staining, Rose Bengal staining).

   Abnormalities of Tear Production – Tear Production abnormalities most commonly include low tear production (DES) and a qualitatitively poor tear film from meibomian gland dysfunction.

B. *Examination of Tear Distribution* – This is an evaluation of eyelid position and function. This is a visual and manual evaluation involving the static position and the dynamic activity (function) of the eyelids.

   Abnormalities of Tear Distribution – Abnormalities involving the static position of the eyelids include upper eyelid malpositions (ptosis, entropion, ectropion, and retraction) and lower eyelid malpositions (entropion, ectropion, and retraction). Disorders of eyelid function include facial paralysis, facial synkinesis, facial mass movement, blepharospasm, and hemifacial spasm.

C. *Examination of Tear Drainage* – This is an evaluation of the nasolacrimal drainage system. It begins and ends as a direct examination but for the most part it is an indirect examination of the complex drainage system that begins in the eyelid and ends in the nose. The examination begins at the puncti, with direct examination at the slit lamp. The canaliculi are examined indirectly via probing. The nasolacrimal sac and duct are also evaluated indirectly by means of irrigation. An intranasal examination is then performed to examine the lateral wall of the inferior meatus, where the nasolacrimal duct enters the nose. The opening of the nasolacrimal duct into the nose is not visible without endoscopy.

Abnormalities of Tear Drainage – Abnormalities include:

Punctal abnormalities including malposition, stenosis, occlusion from conjunctivalchalasis, etc.

Canalicular abnormalities including stenosis and canaliculitis.

Nasolacrimal sac disorders include dacryolyth and tumors (benign and malignant).

Nasolacrimal duct abnormalities include partial and complete obstruction on an involutional basis, obstruction secondary to tumor (endogenous via extension from the canaliculi or sac, or exogenous via compression from tumors of the nose or paranasal sinuses), and obstruction secondary to a foreign body (advanced punctal plug).

Treatment

Abnormalities of tear production, tear distribution, and tear drainage which cause symptomatic tearing must be addressed individually. Some can be treated simultaneously (Linberg 1988) (Black et al. 2012).

The work up itself may improve tearing by clearing partial, non-fixed obstructions of the punctum, canaliculus, or tear duct or by dilating a narrow punctum or canaliculus to facilitate nasolacrimal irrigation.

In addition, partial or incomplete obstructions of the puncti, canaliculi, and tear duct can sometimes be successfully treated by dilation and stenting the stenotic anatomy.

Dacryocystorhinostomy is indicated:

1. In the patient with symptomatic tearing and a clinically proven nasolacrimal duct obstruction (NLDO) where:
   A. Tearing is NOT due to dry eye syndrome (DES) or other abnormalities of tear production.
   B. Other causes of tearing, described above, have been ruled out or will be treated simultaneously.
2. In the patient with chronic dacryocystitis:
   A. *Dacryocystorhinostomy SHOULD NOT be performed when tearing is due to Dry Eye Syndrome (DES) or other abnormalities of tear production.* DES can cause tearing on a reflex basis, mimicking nasolacrimal drainage obstruction including nasolacrimal duct obstruction (NLDO). It the case of nasolacrimal drainage obstruction and DES, treatment of the

DES is necessary. If the DES is not addressed, nasolacrimal surgery may worsen the DES as a result of improved tear drainage. In fact, occlusion of the nasolacrimal drainage system, in the form of punctal plugs or surgical canalicular occlusion, is sometimes used to treat severe DES.

   B. *Dacryocystorhinostomy may be performed if NLDO is found and if other causes of tearing, described above, have been ruled out or will be treated simultaneously.* If NLDO is among the findings, then DCR can be performed along with other surgery to treat conditions causing tearing. For example, ectropion repair and DCR or punctalplasty and DCR are commonly performed. An exception would be any treatment aimed at DES, where, except in unusual circumstances, DCR is contraindicated. This is because the improved drainage resulting from DCR may make an already compromised (i.e., dry) ocular surface, even more compromised (drier) and put the eye at serious risk for vision threatening disease such as corneal ulcer and perforation.

3. *Dacryocystorhinostomy is also indicated in the patient with dacryocystitis.* Dacryocystitis is an infection of the nasolacrimal sac due to nasolacrimal duct obstruction. The obstruction, most commonly at the junction of the sac and the upper duct, blocks tear flow, creates tear stasis, and can lead to an infection in the sac. In most cases, the patient will give a history of chronic tearing prior to the onset of infection. Initial treatment is systemic antibiotics. Usual organisms are staph and strep. Once resolved, DCR is indicated to treat the underlying anatomic abnormality creating the milieu for infection. The patient is at risk for recurrent dacryocystitis unless the obstruction is treated. It is the procedure of choice after medical management of acute dacryocystitis and in chronic dacryocystitis. It can be used to treat severe acute dacryocystitis in extreme cases.

Dacryocystorhinostomy: The Procedure

The traditional, external transcutaneous approach is via an incision in the medial canthus on the lateral wall of the nose. Success rate is described at 96%.

Endoscopic DCR and laser-assisted trancanalicular DCR have been described. Their advantage is the avoidance of a cutaneous incision. The success rate varies with these techniques. Some studies show results that may approach but do not exceed traditional transcutaneous DCR. In addition, some of these approaches do not allow the option of obtaining surgical specimens of the sac and/or nasal mucosa should pathology be suspected or examination warranted (Linberg 1988; Black et al. 2012).

In external DCR, many incision types and locations have been described. General details of DRC are described here. After injecting the medial canthal skin with lidocaine and epinephrine, a skin incision is made. Dissection is carried down through skin, muscle, and periostium, which are reflected medially toward the nasal bridge and laterally over the anterior lacrimal crest. At the anterior lacrimal crest, the anterior aspect of the nasolacrimal sac is encountered. Subperiosteal dissection then allows for reflection of the sac out of its fossa. Direct visualization of the bony fossa is then possible. The anterior part of the fossa is the sturdy frontal process of the maxillary bone. The posterior part of the fossa is thin lacrimal bone. Using a curved hemostat or Kerrison punch, the thin posterior wall of the fossa is infractured and an osteotomy is created using an up biting rongeur. Care is taken to preserve the nasal mucosa internal to this osteotomy. Meticulous hemostasis is also required. A lacrimal probe is then passed into the punctum, through the canaliculus, and into the sac. The probe is seen to tent up the periosteum overlying the medial aspect of the reflected sac adjacent to the osteotomy, the former site of its fossa. A vertical incision is made into the sac and, depending on the type of flaps planned (if any), horizontal incisions are also made. I prefer a U-shaped incision. This allows me to create anterior flaps and to amputate the smaller posterior flap. Success rate is not dependent on the type of flap created. Once the sac is opened, the lacrimal probe is directly visible entering the sac via the common canaliculus. A mirror-image incision/flap(s) is created in the nasal mucosa through the osteotomy. The middle turbinate and nasal septum are directly observed through this mucosa opening into the nose. Microtubular intubation is often done to "stent" the system during healing. Once the tubes are in place, anterior flaps are sutured to one another. The skin wound is then closed. Post-op care includes steroid-antibiotic drops and nasal

hygiene. Patients should be instructed to avoid blowing their nose and valsalva maneuvers for about 1 month.

Endoscopic examination shows that osteotomy heals an opening of 2–4 mm in diameter by about 6 weeks.

Endoscopic DCR also centers around creation of a mucosal-lined anastomosis between the nasolacrimal sac and the nasal mucosa. In this technique, the intranasal region is approached first. After injecting the mucosa of the lateral nasal wall and the middle turbinate with lidocaine and epinephrine, a posterior-based mucosal flap of nasal mucosa is created. The vertical anterior incision of the flap is placed just anterior to the middle turbinate. The parallel horizontal incisions continue posteriorly to the groove between the uncinate process and the lacrimal bone. (The middle turbinate can be mobilized medially and the uncinate process can be removed if needed, for better access to the lateral nasal wall). The intranasal aspect of the lacrimal sac fossa is now directly visualized in the surgical field. Next, a light source (fiber optic light pipe) is then placed intra-canalicularly and advanced into the nasolacrimal sac to illuminate the nasolacrimal sac fossa from within the sac. This is simultaneously visualized endoscopically on the lateral nasal wall. Using the trans-oseal illumination as a guide, an osteotomy is made in the lateral nasal wall revealing the periosteum overlying the medial aspect of the nasolacrimal sac. At this point, dye can be irrigated into the sac via the punctum. The sac is then opened through the intranasal osteotomy by creating a posteriorly based mirror image (to the nasal mucosal flap) flap. The visualization of the dye in the sac upon opening it further confirms the correct surgical anatomy. Microtubular intubation is then performed. The flaps are approximated but not sutured. Post-op care is the same as for external DCR.

Transcanalicular laser-assisted DCR is a newer technique which is well described elsewhere.

Cross-References

References

Black EH, Nesi FA, Gladstone GJ, Levine MR, Calvano CJ (eds) (2012) Smith and Nesi's ophthalmic plastic and reconstructive surgery, 3rd edn. Springer

Holds J (ed) (2012) 2011–2012 Basic and clinical science course, section 7: Orbit, eyelids, and lacrimal system. American Academy of Ophthalmology

Linberg J (ed) (1988) Lacrimal surgery. Churchill Livingstone, New York

---

Epistaxis

Adam M. Becker
Division of Otolaryngology-Head and Neck Surgery, Department of Surgery, Duke University School of Medicine, Durham, NC, USA

Synonyms

Nose bleed

Definition

Anterior epistaxis – This generally refers to bleeding from the anterior nasal septum in Kiesselbach's plexus or Little's area or, less commonly, the anterior-inferior turbinate

Kiesselbach's plexus – This is also known as Kiesselbach's triangle or Little's area. It is the area on the anterior septum that is the most common site of epistaxis. A number of vessels contribute to the vascular supply of this region

Posterior epistaxis – This generally refers to bleeding from a source posterior to the anterior nasal septum or anterior-inferior turbinate

Woodruff's plexus – This is located in the posterior nasal cavity in the inferior meatus

Basic Characteristics

Epistaxis is an extremely common condition, although only a fraction of cases will require the care of an otolaryngologist. Although the true incidence is difficult to calculate, roughly 60% of persons will experience epistaxis in their lifetime (Gifford and Orlandi 2008).

Of those, approximately 10% will seek emergency care, making epistaxis the most common otolaryngic emergency (Gifford and Orlandi 2008). Though usually only a nuisance, nosebleeds may be associated with systemic disorders and can, rarely, be life threatening. Epistaxis can be categorized into minor epistaxis and major epistaxis, though other classifications have been described. The most common causes include nose picking, desiccation of the nasal mucosa with resultant epithelial disruption, superficial vasculature, benign and malignant neoplasms, granulomatous diseases, and trauma. Factors that have been related to exacerbations of epistaxis include hypertension, coagulopathy, and antiplatelet medications. Associated conditions that often present with epistaxis include hereditary hemorrhagic telangiectasia (HHT) and juvenile nasoangiofibroma (JNA). The diagnosis is made based on history and/or evidence of bleeding on examination with diagnostic testing in select cases. The treatment of epistaxis can range from conservative measures such as nasal moisturizing agents, to invasive, including packing, cauterization, angiography with embolization, and surgical vessel ligation.

Anatomy

A thorough understanding of sinonasal anatomy is critical to successfully diagnose and treat the causes of epistaxis. The vascular supply of the nasal cavity can be divided into the external carotid artery (ECA) distribution and the internal carotid artery (ICA) distribution.

External Carotid Distribution

The majority of the nasal blood supply originates from the internal maxillary artery (IMA). The IMA arborizes within the infratemporal and pterygomaxillary fossa. The nasal cavity is supplied by a number of these branches: the sphenopalatine artery, the greater palatine artery, and the pharyngeal artery. The sphenopalatine artery provides the majority of the arterial supply via its lateral and medial branches. The lateral branches supply the inferior, middle, and superior turbinates. The medial branch, or posterior septal artery, supplies the nasal septum. The greater palatine artery enters through the greater palatine foramen and supplies the palate. The terminal branch of the greater palatine artery then reenters the nasal cavity via the incisive foramen to contribute to the blood supply of the anterior-inferior nasal septum. The pharyngeal artery, also known as the vidian artery, generally originates as a small branch of the pterygopalatine portion of the IMA that runs with the vidian nerve through the vidian canal and provides some distribution to the upper part of the nasopharynx and torus tubarius. It is worth noting that this artery can originate as a branch of the petrous portion of the internal carotid artery or exist as a significant anastomosis between the internal carotid artery and the sphenopalatine artery. The superior labial artery, a branch of the facial artery, contributes blood supply to the nasal vestibule and anterior nasal cavity. Kiesselbach's plexus, also known as Little's area, is a region of mucosa located on the anterior, inferior nasal septum. It is a highly collateralized region supplied by branches of the sphenopalatine, greater palatine, and facial arteries and is the site of most anterior epistaxis.

Internal Carotid Distribution

The internal carotid artery supplies the nasal cavity through terminal branches of the ophthalmic artery, namely, the anterior and posterior ethmoidal arteries. The anterior ethmoid artery accompanies the nasociliary nerve through the anterior ethmoidal canal to supply the anterior and middle ethmoid air cells, frontal sinus, and anterosuperior aspect of the lateral nasal wall. Anatomic studies have shown that the anterior ethmoid artery is dehiscencent in the nasal cavity between 16% and 30% of cases (Yang et al. 2009; Floreani et al. 2006). The posterior ethmoid artery usually runs tangentially along the skull base within a bony cavity or intracranially. The posterior ethmoid artery is typically found anterior to anterior face of the sphenoid sinus but can occasionally be found posterior to this. It exits into the nasal cavity to supply posterior ethmoid air cells and nasal septum.

Venous

Woodruff's plexus can be found as a prominent venous plexus in the posterior part of the inferior meatus. It is a rare source of posterior epistaxis.

Assessment

Evaluation of the epistaxis patient includes a detailed history with particular attention to volume of blood loss, timing and frequency of prior episodes, any medical comorbidities, anticoagulant medications, surgery or trauma, and any recreational drug use. Patients should be assessed for signs of hypovolemia, including pallor, diaphoresis, cool skin, or tachycardia. IV access should be obtained, and laboratory evaluation to assess for coagulopathy, anemia, and crossmatching should be considered. In general, routine clotting studies only add to the management when patients have a history of a bleeding disorder or are undergoing anticoagulant therapy. Fresh frozen plasma may be considered for an INR greater than 4 (Choudhry et al. 2004). Other medications associated with bleeding include aspirin, clopidogrel, alcohol, and nonsteroidal anti-inflammatory drugs.

Hypertension is commonly identified during the initial evaluation of the epistaxis patient. However, the association between hypertension and epistaxis is controversial (Jackson and Jackson 1988; Theodosis et al. 2009). In one study, patients with hypertension upon presenting to the emergency room with nosebleeds are more likely to require admission (Jackson and Jackson 1988).

The causes of epistaxis can be divided into local and systemic disease states (Table 1). Local factors include vascular abnormalities, infectious or inflammatory states, traumatic (including iatrogenic injuries), neoplasm, desiccation, and foreign bodies. Systemic factors include hypertension, atherosclerosis, infectious/inflammatory diseases, blood dyscrasias, platelet abnormalities, coagulopathies, as well as kidney and liver disease (Simmen and Jones 2010; Wormald 2006).

Treatment

A number of options exist in the treatment of epistaxis, ranging from conservative to invasive. Universal precautions, including eye protection, to protect from blood-borne illness cannot be overemphasized regardless of the treatment option utilized. Since about 90% of nosebleeds occur from the anterior nasal septum, conservative measures are successful at stopping most nosebleeds. These include pinching the lower portion of the nose to apply pressure to the anterior nasal septum. Patients often need to be informed that pinching the nose along the bony dorsum is not helpful, and pressure needs to be applied along the alae to

Epistaxis, Table 1 Causes of Epistaxis

Local factors	Systemic factors
Anatomic abnormalities	Alcohol
Septal deviation	Altitude
Septal perforation	Blood dyscrasias
Septal spur	Hematologic malignancies
Environmental	Liver failure
Chemical irritants	Platelet dysfunction
Coagulopathies	Warfarin
Iatrogenic	Von Willebrand's disease
Nasal oxygen	Hereditary hemorrhagic
Nasal surgery	telangiectasia
Idiopathic	Hypertension
Inflammatory/Infectious	Malnutrition
Allergic rhinitis	Vascular abnormalities (Fig. 2)
Granulomatous diseases	
Rhinosinusitis (viral and	
bacterial)	
Drugs	
Cocaine	
Nasal sprays	
Neoplasms	
Angiofibroma	
Hemangioma	
Hemangiopericytoma	
Juvenile nasoangiofibroma	
(Fig. 1)	
Malignancy	
Papilloma	
Pyogenic granuloma	
Trauma	
Foreign body	
Fracture	
Nasal cannula	
Nose picking	

(Simmen and Jones 2010; Wormald 2006)

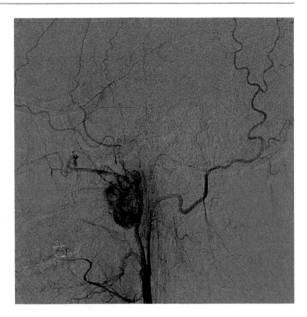

Epistaxis, Fig. 1 Angiography demonstrating the appearance of a juvenile nasoangiofibroma

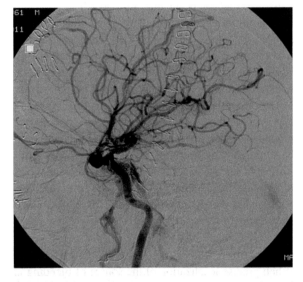

Epistaxis, Fig. 2 Angiography demonstrating an internal carotid aneurysm that presented with massive epistaxis

compress the site of bleeding. Topical vasoconstrictors can be useful in stopping nosebleeds in the emergency setting.

Children

Recurring epistaxis is commonly seen in children. As with adults, initial treatment consists of conservative measures, such as nasal creams and saline spray. Kubba and colleagues reported that topical antiseptic cream was more effective than ointment in reducing the frequency of epistaxis (Kubba et al. 2001). If old enough, silver nitrate cauterization in the office can be attempted; however, many children may require operative endoscopy under general anesthesia or sedation. Bipolar or suction monopolar cauterization may be used. It is advisable to minimize cautery in overlapping areas of septal mucosa in cases of bilateral epistaxis to avoid septal cartilage necrosis and perforation.

Nasal Packing

Packing has been a long time mainstay in the treatment of epistaxis. A number of commercially available products exist to aid the clinician, ranging from absorbable materials to nasal sponges or inflatable balloon devices. The guiding principle is to localize the source of epistaxis and apply the packing material of choice to tamponade the site of bleeding.

In the event that a well-placed anterior pack is unsuccessful, posterior packing may be utilized. This method employs a pack placed to obstruct the choanae, thus allowing for more vigorous packing to be applied without this material extending into the oropharynx. Generally, this is achieved with either tonsil packs that are sewn together and retrieved through the oral cavity with a red rubber catheter placed through the nasal cavity. Alternatively, a Foley catheter or commercially available balloon can be inflated in the nasopharynx and pulled anteriorly to obstruct the choanae. The anterior pack is placed and the posterior pack held in position with a device, such as an umbilical clamp, to clip over the posterior pack as it emerges through the anterior pack, thus providing stabilization. Particular care is taken to avoid pressure on the columella or alae from the packing or clip to avoid necrosis of these structures that can occur in as little as 4 h.

It is important to recognize the potential for toxic shock syndrome, hemodynamic changes, apnea, necrosis, and discomfort that nasal packing of any sort can induce. Patients are often placed on antistaphylococcal antibiotics to avoid toxic shock syndrome, although the exact incidence is unknown and there is not sufficient evidence to support this practice. Any patient receiving a posterior pack should be admitted to the hospital, and cardiopulmonary monitoring in an intensive care unit is recommended for older patients, children, and those with comorbidities. Packing has a reported failure rate of 10–52% (Pollice and Yoder 1997; Schaitkin et al. 1987).

Cauterization

When precise localization of the source of bleeding is possible, cauterization can be used to provide hemostasis. In the emergency setting, silver nitrate can be used, though bleeding may often be too brisk to allow adequate chemical cauterization. Temporary packing with topical vasoconstrictors can be utilized first to improve the results of silver nitrate cautery. If silver nitrate cautery fails, electrocautery may prove more effective. If bilateral cauterization is necessary, the procedures are generally performed 4–6 weeks apart to avoid the risk of septal necrosis. The failure rate of cauterization has been reported to be around 17–33%

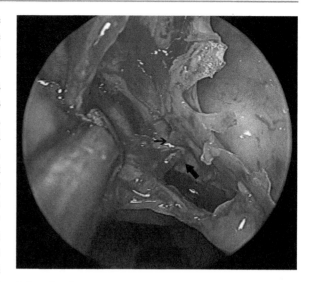

Epistaxis, Fig. 3 Intraoperative photograph demonstrating the sphenopalatine artery emerging from its foramen (*large arrow*). A relatively small crista ethmoidalis is also seen (*small arrow*)

(Schwartzbauer et al. 2003). Complications are uncommon but include pain, eschar, rhinitis, acute sinusitis, injury to neural structures, and damage to the lacrimal duct (Pollice and Yoder 1997; Schwartzbauer et al. 2003).

Arterial Ligation

No consensus exists regarding the surgical management of epistaxis. In general, arterial ligation can be considered for failure of medical treatment, nasal anatomy that precludes local treatments, patient refusal of packing, the need for blood transfusion, and as initial treatment of posterior epistaxis. Local nasal care after surgical treatment of epistaxis may include antibiotic ointments as well as saline irrigations or sprays.

Sphenopalatine artery ligation is now the preferred method for surgical management of persistent posterior epistaxis (Schwartzbauer et al. 2003) (Fig. 3). The morbidity associated with endoscopic ligation of the sphenopalatine artery is low compared with that for ligation of the maxillary or external carotid artery with success rates reported at 98% (Kumar et al. 2003). It should be noted that upon entering the nasal cavity, the sphenopalatine artery may be present as two or more branches. Schwartzbauer et al. have described the possible variation. In their series, 16% of arteries branched within the foramen, allowing the two arteries to exit together; in 42%, the branches exited much more posteriorly; and in the remaining 42%, the septal branch

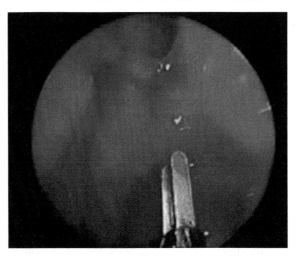

Epistaxis, Fig. 4 Photograph of the right orbit. The frontoethmoid suture line has been enhanced to show its location *(small arrow)*. The lacrimal fossa can be seen anteriorly. The anterior ethmoid artery foramen (labeled 1) is located approximately 24 mm beyond the lacrimal crest. The posterior ethmoid artery foramen (labeled 2) is located approximately 12 mm beyond the anterior ethmoid artery foramen

Epistaxis, Video 1 Intraoperative video demonstrating coagulation of the left anterior ethmoid artery with bipolar artery. The lamina papyracea had been carefully removed and bone over the artery carefully thinned with a fine diamond burr to adequately expose the artery

exited through a separate foramen posterior to the sphenopalatine foramen. Failure to address all branches may lead to treatment failure.

Anterior and posterior ethmoid artery ligation may be performed in conjunction with ligation of the sphenopalatine artery. Traditionally, this is performed through a lynch incision. The lacrimal fossa and crest are identified, and the location of the anterior ethmoid artery is expected to be approximately 24 mm posterior to the lacrimal crest within the frontoethmoid suture line (Fig. 4). After isolating the artery, which can be facilitated using a nasal endoscope through the incision, the vessel is either clipped or cauterized with bipolar cautery. Complications of this approach include telecanthus, ectropion, and permanent epiphora, although a z-plasty modification may reduce the risk of these (Esclamado and Cummings 1989). Transnasal endoscopic approaches for ligation of the anterior ethmoid artery have been described, but may require removal of the lamina papyracea to expose the vessel within the orbit (Video 1). In addition, occasionally, the artery can be difficult to reach via this approach with only 20% of arteries being accessible in one cadaver study (Floreani et al. 2006). The advantage of the endoscopic endonasal approach is the avoidance of a noticeable skin incision and associated risk of lid contracture. Finally, Morera et al.

demonstrated the feasibility of a transcaruncular approach to the anterior ethmoid artery (Morera et al. 2011). The authors report on their experience with eight patients who underwent the approach, which was combined with sphenopalatine artery ligation. In their series, there was one incident of transient epiphora and no other complications. The scar was inconspicuous in all cases after 1 month.

Another technique to control posterior epistaxis is ligation of the internal maxillary artery in the pterygopalatine fossa. It has a reported success rate of approximately 90% (Strong et al. 1995). Treatment failures are due to the difficulty in finding the artery and all its branches. Because this procedure is done through a Caldwell-Luc approach, complications include sinusitis, facial pain, oroantral fistula, as well as facial and dental paresthesia can occur (Morgan and Aldren 1997). There are also reports of blindness, ophthalmoplegia, and decreased lacrimation from dissection within the pterygomaxillary fossa (Johnson and Parkin 1976). The overall complication rate has been reported at 28% (Strong et al. 1995).

External carotid artery ligation has been described as a means of controlling epistaxis. Treatment failures are more frequent due to extensive collateralization in the external carotid system. With advances in endoscopic endonasal techniques, this procedure would appear to be essentially obsolete with regard to epistaxis.

Embolization

As an alternative to surgical ligation, embolization has been shown to be successful in the management of refractory epistaxis. Overall, embolization has a long-term success rate of 93–100% (Fukutsuji et al. 2008). Major complications include ischemic stroke, hemiplegia, facial paralysis soft tissue necrosis, and blindness (Ntomouchtsis et al. 2010; Cullen and Tami 1998). Minor complications include headache, jaw pain, and facial edema. In addition, facial pain and numbness may be seen in around 54% of patients and appear to be more likely in patients in whom embolization of more than one artery is necessary (Fukutsuji et al. 2008).

Although success rates of embolization and surgical ligation may be similar, there are several differences that should be considered. In a retrospective comparison, Cullen et al. noted greater success with surgical ligation compared to embolization (Cullen and Tami 1998). They found embolization to be more cost-effective than ligation by $1,639.70 per patient, primarily because of operating room costs. Internal maxillary artery (IMA) ligation was associated with a higher minor complication rate and is associated with a major complication rate similar to that for IMA embolization. It is important to consider, however, that the types of major complications associated with IMA embolization are more serious than those for surgical ligation and include internal carotid artery injury, facial paralysis, and hemiplegia. They noted that the cost savings with embolization are offset by the higher failure rate and increased risks.

Hot Water Irrigation

A technique for hot water irrigation has been described for the treatment of epistaxis (Stangerup et al. 1999). They describe utilizing a balloon pack to obstruct the choanae, followed by copious irrigation with 50°C tap water for approximately 3 min. It is speculated that thermal changes due to the hot water result in tissue edema and compression of the vasculature, thereby slowing or stopping bleeding. Subsequent analysis has shown a success rate of 82% for hot water irrigation alone, with no complications. Hot water irrigations have also been utilized in expanded endonasal approaches to the skull base to improve the surgical field (Kassam et al. 2005). Hot water irrigation has the advantages of avoiding packing, hospitalization, and

immediate surgery while also allowing for normal nasal breathing after treatment.

Hereditary Hemorrhagic Telangiectasia

Hereditary hemorrhagic telangiectasia (HHT) deserves special mention in the discussion of epistaxis. Also known as Osler-Weber-Rendu syndrome, HHT is an autosomal dominant disorder with a prevalence of approximately 1 in 10,000 (Guttmacher et al. 1995). The disorder is characterized by vascular dysplasia and hemorrhage. Although the exact pathophysiology is still being elucidated, two distinct genes have been identified: the endoglin gene and the activin receptor–like kinase type I (ALK-1) gene. Endoglin and ALK-1 are type III and type I transforming growth factor-beta (TGF-B) receptors, and both are found exclusively on vascular endothelial cells (Shovlin et al. 1997). Mutations of endoglin genes and ALK-1 genes are involved in the genetic pathogenesis of HHT type 1 and HHT type 2, respectively. The precise mechanisms of by which these mutations elicit the vascular abnormalities in patients with HHT remain uncertain. Angiodysplasia, which is the hallmark feature of HHT, is thought to be caused by a number of factors including a lack of elastin fibers in the smooth muscle layer of vessels, endothelial cell degeneration, and endothelial cell junction defects (Karapantzos et al. 2005). Increased tissue plasminogen activator has also been demonstrated in HHT, leading to hyperfibrinolysis manifest by epistaxis (Kwaan and Silverman 1973).

Telangiectasias most often present in the nasal cavity, followed by the lungs, gastrointestinal tract and brain (Haitjema et al. 1997). Fifty to eighty percent of patients experience recurrent epistaxis, and in half of the patients, this becomes more serious with age. Blood transfusions are required in roughly 25% of patients (Hoag et al. 2010).

Along with bleeding from the aerodigestive tract, patients are at risk for developing pulmonary and cerebrovascular arteriovenous malformations later in life (Byahatti et al. 1997).

There are a number of management options in the management of epistaxis in HHT. Cauterization of the telangiectasias is the most common management practice. A variety of lasers including CO_2, KTP, pulsed dye, and Nd:YAG lasers as well as argon plasma coagulation have been used to control epistaxis. The greatest volume of data exists for Nd:YAG and KTP lasers. The Nd:YAG laser has the advantage of greater depth of penetration compared with KTP. KTP has an intermediate wavelength, falling in between CO_2 and Nd:YAG. This allows the KTP laser to cut, coagulate, and vaporize (Vickery and Kuhn 1996). Karapantoz and colleagues have shown improvement in physical and mental health dimension after laser treatment (Karapantzos et al. 2005). They also highlighted the importance of preparation of the nose, including gentle cleaning of clots, application of topical vasoconstrictor, and moisturization to reduce coagulation necrosis of superficial tissues and allow deeper penetration. Ghaheri et al. reported their experience with bipolar electrocautery in the treatment of HHT. They showed excellent improvement in epistaxis rates, without new perforations or new synechia formation (Ghaheri et al. 2006). Bipolar cautery has the advantage of ready availability at most institutions without the need for specialized training, a dedicated laser nurse, and additional setup or precautions. Cautery techniques are best suited for mild to moderate cases of HHT epistaxis.

In HHT requiring frequent transfusions or parenteral iron supplementation, more aggressive surgical intervention such as septodermoplasty or nasal closure may require (Levine et al. 2008). Septodermoplasty involves removal of a portion of the nasal septal mucosa, while preserving the mucoperichondrium and periosteum. The denuded surface is relined with a split-thickness skin graft, which is better able to resist formation of telangiectasias (Harvey et al. 2008). One study showed that patients undergoing septodermoplasty experienced a 57% reduction in the need for subsequent laser treatments within their study period (Harvey et al. 2008). The need for septodermoplasty must be weighed against the risks including septal perforation, increased crusting, and decreased sensation of airflow, anosmia, and atrophic rhinitis. In a review of the complications of septodermoplasty, Levin et al. found that the main complication was nasal odor, which occurred in 78% of cases, followed by nasal crusting in 72%, hyposmia in 58%, and increased sinusitis in 30% (Levine et al. 2008). Nasal closure has shown success in the literature; however, this comes at the expense of nasal breathing and olfaction (Lund and Howard 1997).

Medical therapy for HHT-related epistaxis is typically reserved for persistence after surgery. There are multiple agents that have been reported to improve bleeding rates in HHT including aminocaproic acid, tranexamic acid, bevacizumab, as well as hormonal and antihormonal therapy. Aminocaproic acid is a potent inhibitor of the fibrinolytic system. In low doses, it blocks the conversion of plasminogen to the powerful fibrinolytic enzyme plasmin. By stabilizing blood clots, HHT patients could, in theory, experience a reduction in epistaxis. Though there are some anecdotal reports showing benefit when aminocaproic acid was administered, other reports have shown poor results, likely reflecting the multifactorial nature of the bleeding diathesis. Tranexamic acid, another antifibrinolytic agent, also has conflicting reports (Klepfish et al. 2001).

There is little consensus regarding the use of hormonal and antihormonal therapy in HHT. Based on Jameson and Cave's review of the literature, oral contraceptives containing estrogen and progesterone could be considered as initial therapy in fertile women with HHT-related epistaxis (Jameson and Cave 2004). They also described dramatic improvement with the use of tamoxifen in two cases.

Bevacizumab is a humanized monoclonal antibody that binds to vascular endothelial growth factor, thus blocking angiogenesis. Recognizing that the genetic alterations associated with HHT are members of the vascular endothelial growth factor (VEGF) signaling cascade, Davidson and colleagues sought to assess the efficacy and safety of intranasal bevacizumab in the treatment of HHT-related epistaxis (Karnezis and Davidson 2011; Chen et al. 2011). Thirty-two patients with recurrent HHT epistaxis were treated with 25–100 mg of intranasal bevacizumab, either as a submucosal injection or as a topical spray (Karnezis and Davidson 2011). Twelve patients were treated concurrently with KTP laser photocoagulation. Patients receiving combined therapy had a reduction of epistaxis severity score from 7 to 2.9, a result that was statistically significant. When the cohort receiving only topical bevacizumab were examined, they noted a reduction in epistaxis severity score from 6.6 to 3.6, also statistically significant. In a follow-up report, septal perforation was the most common complication noted (Chen et al. 2011). They pointed out that all patients who experienced septal perforation were treated with submucosal injection of bevacizumab in addition to KTP laser along the bilateral cartilaginous septum. Since observing these findings, their protocol was modified, and no further perforations were identified.

Cross-References

▶ Acute and Chronic Rhinosinusitis
▶ Allergic Rhinitis
▶ Arteriovenous Malformations
▶ Benign Sinonasal Neoplasms
▶ Granulomatous Disorders
▶ Juvenile Nasopharyngeal Angiofibroma
▶ Nasal and Sinus Trauma
▶ Septal Perforation
▶ Sinonasal Neoplasms
▶ Sinus Surgery, Complications
▶ Vascular Anomalies of Head and Neck

References

Byahatti SV, Rebeiz EE, Shapshay SM (1997) Hereditary hemorrhagic telangiectasia: what the otolaryngologist should know. Am J Rhinol 11(1):55–62

Chen S, Karnezis T, Davidson TM (2011) Safety of intranasal Bevacizumab (Avastin) treatment in patients with hereditary hemorrhagic telangiectasia-associated epistaxis. Laryngoscope 121(3):644–646

Choudhry N, Sharp HR, Mir N, Salama NY (2004) Epistaxis and oral anticoagulant therapy. Rhinology 42(2):92–97

Cullen MM, Tami TA (1998) Comparison of internal maxillary artery ligation versus embolization for refractory posterior epistaxis. Otolaryngol Head Neck Surg 118(5):636–642

Esclamado RM, Cummings CW (1989) Z-plasty modification of the Lynch incision. Laryngoscope 99(9):986–987

Floreani SR, Nair SB, Switajewski MC, Wormald PJ (2006) Endoscopic anterior ethmoidal artery ligation: a cadaver study. Laryngoscope 116(7):1263–1267

Fukutsuji K, Nishiike S, Aihara T, Uno M, Harada T, Gyoten M, Imai S (2008) Superselective angiographic embolization for intractable epistaxis. Acta Otolaryngol 128(5):556–560

Ghaheri BA, Fong KJ, Hwang PH (2006) The utility of bipolar electrocautery in hereditary hemorrhagic telangiectasia. Otolaryngol Head Neck Surg 134(6):1006–1009

Gifford TO, Orlandi RR (2008) Epistaxis. Otolaryngol Clin North Am 41(3):525–536

Guttmacher AE, Marchuk DA, White RI (1995) Hereditary hemorrhagic telangiectasia. N Engl J Med 333:918–924

Haitjema T, Westermann C, Overtoom T, Timmer R, Disch F, Mauser H, Lammers J (1997) Hereditary hemorrhagic telangiectasia (Osler-Weber-Rendu Disease): new insights in pathogenesis, complications, and treatment. Arch Intern Med 156:714–719

Harvey RJ, Kanagalingam J, Lund VJ (2008) The impact of septodermoplasty and potassium-titanyl-phosphate (KTP)

laser therapy in the treatment of hereditary hemorrhagic telangiectasia-related epistaxis. Am J Rhinol 22(2):182–187

Hoag JB, Terry P, Mitchell S, Reh D, Merlo CA (2010) An epistaxis severity score for hereditary hemorrhagic telangiectasia. Laryngoscope 120(4):838–843

Jackson KR, Jackson RT (1988) Factors associated with active, refractory epistaxis. Arch Otolaryngol Head Neck Surg 114:862–865

Jameson JJ, Cave DR (2004) Hormonal and antihormonal therapy for epistaxis in hereditary hemorrhagic telangiectasia. Laryngoscope 114(4):705–709

Johnson LP, Parkin JL (1976) Blindness and total ophthalmoplegia. A complication of transantral ligation of the internal maxillary artery for epistaxis. Arch Otolaryngol 102(8):501–504

Karapantzos I, Tsimpiris N, Goulis DG, Van Hoecke H, Van Cauwenberge P, Danielides V (2005) Management of epistaxis in hereditary hemorrhagic telangiectasia by Nd:YAG laser and quality of life assessment using the HR-QoL questionnaire. Eur Arch Otorhinolaryngol 262(10):830–833

Karnezis TT, Davidson TM (2011) Efficacy of intranasal Bevacizumab (Avastin) treatment in patients with hereditary hemorrhagic telangiectasia-associated epistaxis. Laryngoscope 121(3):636–638

Kassam A, Snyderman CH, Carrau RL, Gardner P, Mintz A (2005) Endoneurosurgical hemostasis techniques: lessons learned from 400 cases. Neurosurg Focus 19(1):E7

Klepfish A, Berrebi A, Schattner A (2001) Intranasal tranexamic acid treatment for severe epistaxis in hereditary hemorrhagic telangiectasia. Arch Intern Med 161(5):767

Kubba H, MacAndie C, Botma M, Robison J, O'Donnell M, Robertson G, Geddes N (2001) A prospective, single-blind, randomized controlled trial of antiseptic cream for recurrent epistaxis in childhood. Clin Otolaryngol Allied Sci 26(6):465–468

Kumar S, Shetty A, Rockey J, Nissen E (2003) Contemporary surgical treatment of epistaxis: what is the evidence for sphenopalatine artery ligation? Clin Otolaryngol Allied Sci 28:360–363

Kwaan HC, Silverman S (1973) Fibrinolytic activity in lesions of hereditary hemorrhagic telangiectasia. Arch Dermatol 107:571–573

Levine CG, Ross DA, Henderson KJ, Leder SB, White RI Jr (2008) Long-term complications of septal dermoplasty in patients with hereditary hemorrhagic telangiectasia. Otolaryngol Head Neck Surg 138(6):721–724

Lund VJ, Howard DJ (1997) Closure of the nasal cavities in the treatment of refractory hereditary haemorrhagic telangiectasia. J Laryngol Otol 111(1):30–33

Morera E, Artigas C, Trobat F, Ferrén L, Tomás M (2011) Transcaruncular electrocoagulation of anterior ethmoidal artery for the treatment of severe epistaxis. Laryngoscope 121(2):446–450

Morgan MK, Alden CP (1997) Oroantral fistula: a complication of transantral ligation of the internal maxillary artery for epistaxis. J Laryngol Otol 111(5):468–470

Ntomouchtsis A, Venetis G, Zouloumis L, Lazaridis N (2010) Ischemic necrosis of nose and palate after embolization for epistaxis. A case report. Oral Maxillofac Surg 14(2):123–127

Pollice PA, Yoder MG (1997) Epistaxis: a retrospective review of hospitalized patients. Otolaryngol Head Neck Surg 117(1):49–53

Schaitkin B, Strauss M, Houck JR (1987) Epistaxis: medical versus surgical therapy – a comparison of efficacy, complications, and economic considerations. Laryngoscope 97:1392–1396

Schwartzbauer HR, Shete M, Tami TA (2003) Endoscopic anatomy of the sphenopalatine and posterior nasal arteries: implications for the endoscopic management of epistaxis. Am J Rhinol 17(1):63–66

Shovlin CL, Hughes JM, Scott J, Seidman CE, Seidman JG (1997) Characterization of endoglin and identification of novel mutations in hereditary hemorrhagic telangiectasia. Am J Hum Genet 61(1):68–79

Simmen DB, Jones NS (2010) Epistaxis. In: Flint PW, Haughey BH, Lund VJ, Niparko JK, Richardson MA, Robbins KT, Thomas JR (eds) Cummings otolaryngology: head and neck surgery, 5th edn. Mosby, Philadelphia, pp 682–693

Stangerup SE, Dommerby H, Siim C, Kemp L, Stage J (1999) New modification of hot water irrigation in the treatment of posterior epistaxis. Arch Otolaryngol Head Neck 125:686–690

Strong EB, Bell DA, Johnson LP, Jacobs JM (1995) Intractable epistaxis: transantral ligation vs embolisation: efficacy review and cost analysis. Otolaryngol Head Neck Surg 113(6):674–678

Theodosis P, Mouktaroudi M, Papadogiannis D, Ladas S, Papaspyrou S (2009) Epistaxis of patients admitted in the emergency department is not indicative of underlying arterial hypertension. Rhinology 47(3):260–263

Vickery CL, Kuhn FA (1996) Using the KTP/532 laser to control epistaxis in patients with hereditary hemorrhagic telangiectasia. South Med J 89(1):78–80

Wormald PJ (2006) Epistaxis. In: Bailey BJ, Johnson JJ, Newlands SD (eds) Head and neck surgery – otolaryngology, 4th edn. Lippincott Williams and Wilkins, Philadelphia, pp 505–514

Yang YX, Lu QK, Liao JC, Dang RS (2009) Morphological characteristics of the anterior ethmoidal artery in ethmoid roof and endoscopic localization. Skull Base 19(5):311–317

Epistaxis in Pediatric Patient

J. Brett Chafin[1], Cindy Gauger[2] and Gary D. Josephson[1]
[1]Division of Pediatric Otolaryngology-HNS, Nemours Children's Clinic, Jacksonville, FL, USA
[2]Division of Pediatric Hematology-Oncology, Nemours Children's Clinic, Jacksonville, FL, USA

Synonyms

Nasal hemorrhage; Nose bleed

Introduction

Epistaxis in the pediatric population is common and can become a nuisance for the child, the parent or caretaker, and even the caring clinician. Oftentimes the events occur sporadically leaving the treating physician a difficult task of identifying the occult source, as well as offering a definitive treatment expeditiously. Fortunately, most cases of epistaxis in children are benign in etiology and self-limiting with or without therapy. This entry presents a broad overview of the problem, evaluation, and treatment options.

Thirty percent of children 0–5 years, 56% of those 6–10, and 64% of those 11–15 have had at least one episode of epistaxis (Middleton 2004). Infantile epistaxis is overall much rarer at <1:5,000. A retrospective review of infants hospitalized for epistaxis revealed no identifiable cause in almost one third of the population. Identifiable causes in decreasing prevalence included acute rhinitis, trauma, coagulation disorder, congenital anomaly, and one smothering attempt. The vast majority of the patients required no treatment (Paranjothy et al. 2009).

Most episodes of epistaxis are minor in nature and do not require any intervention or medical attention. Epistaxis seems to lessen as children enter puberty, although up to 9% of teenagers suffer from the problem. The condition can account for up to 9% of outpatient referrals to the otolaryngologist (Whymark et al. 2008). Unfortunately, surveys have revealed a surprisingly poor understanding of proper treatment from the general public as well as from treating emergency department clinicians (Robertson et al. 2010). An interesting Australian study evaluated the characteristics of children admitted to the hospital with a primary diagnosis of epistaxis. They found a male predominance, most requiring a short stay with minimal intervention, and the initial control of bleeding was managed in the emergency department. Most of these children had a previous history of epistaxis. Approximately one third required some type of packing, while an additional one third eventually required surgical intervention. In these patients no underlying bleeding disorder was discovered (Brown and Berkowitz 2004).

Despite the relative frequency of this condition, the current literature is sparse on the best workup and management strategy to care for this common and often frustrating condition. Two algorithms are

Active Bleeding

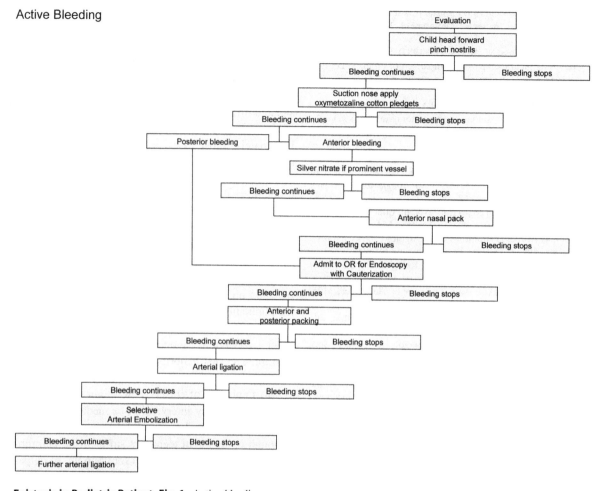

Epistaxis in Pediatric Patient, Fig. 1   Active bleeding

suggested below to the approach of treating the child with either active bleeding on presentation (Fig. 1) or with the presentation of recurrent epistaxis with no active bleeding (Fig. 2). This will offer the clinician an easy reference guide on how to approach the child with epistaxis.

Etiology

Epistaxis can be categorized in several different ways. It has been described in terms of local versus systemic, anterior versus posterior, environmental, traumatic, and iatrogenic to name a few. We like to think of this disease in regard to where it is occurring first, that is, anterior or posterior, and use this nomenclature in addressing the problem. This is then

followed by the search for the underlying etiology to determine the best definitive treatment plan.

The blood supply to the nose is extensive and the astute clinician must have a keen understanding of this blood supply if he or she is requested to definitively address the patient with epistaxis. The nose is supplied indirectly by feeding vessels off the internal and external carotid artery. The internal carotid's contribution is through its branching anterior and posterior ethmoid arteries. These vessels enter the nose superiorly and join a confluence of vessel on the anterior nasal septum known as Kiesselbach's plexus (KP). The external carotid artery offers blood supply to the nose from two of its branches; the facial artery and the internal maxillary artery(IMA). The facial artery contributes to KP as it comes up the anterior nasal spine. The IMA also supplies the anterior nose by joining KP via the

Evaluation of Child Without Active Bleeding

Epistaxis in Pediatric Patient, Fig. 2 Evaluation of child without active and bleeding

greater palatine artery which runs forward in the hard palate. The sphenopalatine artery, also a branch off the IMA, divides into several terminal branches supplying the posterior nasal wall (Middleton 2004).

The most common site of epistaxis in children arises anteriorly as the terminal branches of the descending palatine artery joins the terminal branches of the ethmoid, sphenopalatine, and facial arteries to form a vascular triangle (KP) across the anterior surface of the septal cartilage, which is referred to as Little's area (Gifford et al. 2008). This vascular nasal mucosa is readily damaged in children by their well-intentioned fingers. It is an area prone to drying, irritation, and crusting. Accidental and self-inflicted trauma (nose picking) due to this crusting and associated nasal vestibulitis is the most commonly suspected etiology for epistaxis (Gifford et al. 2008). Recurrent traumatization of the mucosa with devitalization of the perichondrium can eventually lead to septal cartilage exposure and perforation. Further, mucosal disruption can lead to disturbance of laminar airflow, increased turbulence, and further drying leading to scab formation and bleeding. Other inflammatory predisposing conditions including acute upper respiratory infection, allergic rhinitis, or even a nasal foreign body can exacerbate the problem. Blunt and penetrating trauma, anatomic variations, septal deviation, benign and malignant tumors, and bleeding disorders must also be in the differential diagnosis and be explored as potential etiologies.

Crusting on the mucosa of the anterior septum is the most common finding on physical exam, present in nearly two thirds of children with epistaxis. In addition, visible vessels on the anterior septum can be seen in up to 40–50% of patients (Middleton 2004). Bleeding that occurs posteriorly is much more severe in nature and more commonly seen in the adult population. The incidence of epistaxis peaks in the winter months especially in Northern climates. Frequent changes from cold outside air to warm heated dry indoor temperatures alter the normal nasal cycle leading to increased nasal congestion, nasal dryness, crusting, and irritation.There is also an increase in upper respiratory infections during this time of year, which further leads to more friable inflamed mucosa7. It has been demonstrated in comparison to controls, children with nosebleeds are more likely to have nasal colonization of *Staphylococcus aureus*. The organism may replace the normal flora and increase crusting,

inflammation, and vessel formation (Whymark et al. 2008). This may be an explanation as to the effectiveness of antibiotic creams/ointments over lubricating jellies alone.

Facial trauma in children can be the cause of epistaxis, however less common than in adults. This is because the midface of a child is relatively compact and dense, it is smaller in size, has lack of developed sinuses, and undescended teeth. Therefore, the cranium bares the brunt of head trauma in children sparing the midface (Middleton 2004; Gifford et al. 2008). When it does occur however, blunt trauma to the nose or orbit can lead to arterial injury and even the development of pseudoaneurysms. The event may disrupt one or both ethmoid arteries exiting the orbit and traversing the roof of the ethmoid labyrinth. The history may be significant for recurrent episodes of severe bleeding followed by temporary spontaneous resolution. In contrast, bleeding associated with foreign body is usually accompanied with purulent rhinorrhea, a distinctively foul odor, and friable mucosa.

Aneurysms and benign tumors such as nasal papilloma, hemangioma, juvenile nasopharyngeal angiofibroma are relatively uncommon causes of epistaxis, but must be considered in the differential diagnosis. Malignant causes such as esthesioneuroblastoma, melanoma, squamous cell, and adenocarcinoma are even rarer in the pediatric population. These tumors generally present with unilateral bleeding from the affected side, often with a history of nasal obstruction on the ipsilateral side. Epistaxis in the postsurgical patient recovering from sinus or nasal surgery is also a recognized possible complication of this type of surgery. Depending on the type of procedure and the severity of the bleeding, the surgeon can decide on the degree of intervention necessary.

Overview of Hemostasis

The clinician may be faced with the child having no apparent etiology, yet the episodes of nasal bleeding continue. If the physical examination is unrevealing and there is a strong history of excessive bleeding or easy bruising either in the family or the child, an evaluation for an underlying bleeding disorder may be warranted. Understanding hemostasis is essential in diagnosing and treating this group of patients as well as knowing which tests to order that will offer the greatest value. It will also give the clinician confidence in deciding when it is necessary to obtain consultation from the hematologist.

Hemostasis is a delicately balanced system designed to maintain blood in a fluid state within the vasculature, yet rapidly promote clot formation following endothelial injury. Hemostasis is generally thought of in three phases, intricately linked: primary hemostasis, secondary hemostasis, and fibrinolysis. Abnormalities in any phase of hemostasis may lead to a clinical bleeding disorder.

Primary hemostasis describes the formation of a platelet plug, which involves the interaction between platelets, vonWillebrand factor (vWF), and the vessel wall at the site of vascular injury. These interactions lead to platelet adhesion, secretion of platelet granules, platelet aggregation, and finally the platelet plug that is effective in arresting immediate bleeding, although is unstable. The platelet plug must be reinforced by the formation of an organized fibrin clot through activation of secondary hemostasis (blood coagulation system).

Secondary hemostasis involves a cascade of activation reactions converting zymogens to their respective serine proteases in the presence of calcium and a phospholipid surface provided by the platelet or damaged endothelium. In vivo, secondary hemostasis is initiated through the "extrinsic pathway" when tissue factor is exposed on the damaged endothelium and binds to factor VII. Ultimately, a small amount of thrombin is generated. The "intrinsic pathway" is responsible for the subsequent propagation and amplification of a thrombin burst. One of thrombin's primary roles is conversion of soluble fibrinogen into insoluble fibrin, further strengthened through crosslinking by factor XIII (Lichtman et al. 2006).

Following tissue repair and healing, the blood clot is dissolved and eliminated by the fibrinolytic system. Physiologically specific inhibitors regulate each step of the coagulation and fibrinolytic processes.

Clinical Evaluation of a Child with a Bleeding Disorder

Epistaxis is a common childhood bleeding symptom that often prompts referral to a pediatric hematologist. While severe bleeding disorders often present in the first year of life, less severe bleeding disorders, such as von Willebrand disease (vWD), may be clinically silent for years until a hemostatic challenge occurs.

The bleeding history, with a focus on the child's personal history of excessive bleeding through their lifetime, as well as the family history, is critical in the evaluation of a child with a bleeding disorder. The history of bleeding should identify the severity, the site, the spontaneity, duration, and ease with which hemostasis was achieved. Care should be taken in documenting concurrent medications, as several may exacerbate bleeding. The clinical evaluation of bleeding symptoms is often a challenge because mild bleeding symptoms are commonly reported by healthy individuals. Epistaxis is a common childhood complaint; among patients referred to pediatric hematology for evaluation of recurrent epistaxis, 25–33% are diagnosed as having a bleeding disorder (Lichtman et al. 2006; Sharathkumar and Pipe 2008). A retrospective review of 178 children with recurrent epistaxis in a single institution found that only a family history of bleeding was predictive of diagnosing a coagulopathy. However, some studies in literature have found that children with severe epistaxis, epistaxis occurring in association with other bleeding signs, identification of family members with an established bleeding disorder, anemia, and those patients that have undergone nasal cauterization were more likely to have a diagnosable coagulopathy (Lippi et al. 2007).

Mucosal bleeding, in addition to recurrent epistaxis, is characterized by: easy bruising, menorrhagia, petechiae, oral bleeding, genitourinary or rectal bleeding, prolonged bleeding from trivial wounds/abrasions, and prolonged bleeding after surgery including dental extractions. Mucosal bleeding is highly suggestive of a defect in primary hemostatsis, such as platelet defects and vWD. While ecchymoses have been reported in up to 50% of surveyed healthy controls, bruises associated with a defect in primary hemostasis are usually located over bony protuberances of the extremities and the spinous processes along the back, are larger than a quarter, and may be associated with palpable hematomas. The bruising generally appears to be out of proportion to the mechanism of injury (Sharathkumar and Pipe 2008).

Deep tissue bleeding such as hematomas, muscle and joint bleeding, and "delayed" surgical bleeding, especially when there is a need for transfusion, is more suggestive of a coagulation factor deficiency associated with secondary hemostasis.

A detailed history of medications and underlying medical disorders is also very important in the evaluation of a child with a bleeding disorder. Several medications have well-known antiplatelet adverse effects (aspirin, NSAIDs, Plavix, Coumadin, heparins) which may exacerbate bleeding.

Laboratory Evaluation of a Child with a Bleeding Disorder

Coagulation testing in patients with suspected bleeding disorders can be divided into first-line (screening) and second-line (specific test) testing. First-line screening for patients with a significant bleeding history should include a complete blood count (CBC), consideration for the PFA100, PT/INR, APTT, and fibrinogen.

First-line screening for evaluation of primary hemostasis must include the CBC and evaluation of blood smear morphology. The PFA100 is also a screen for abnormalities in primary hemostasis, but cannot be relied upon to identify all patients who have vWD or platelet function defects. Routine use of the PFA100 remains controversial. Therefore, when disorders of primary hemostasis are strongly suspected based on the clinical bleeding history, initial von Willebrand disease testing should be considered: vWF:Ag, vWF:RCo, and FVIII activity. vWF:Ag measures the amount of vWF protein present in the plasma, vWF:RCo is a measure of the function of the protein, and FVIII activity is a measure of the ability of the vWF to serve as a carrier protein to maintain normal FVIII survival. If any of these tests are abnormal the patient should be referred to a hematologist. Additionally, if clinical symptoms or a family history is strongly suggestive of vWD, a single set of vWD assays does not rule out the diagnosis. This patient should also be referred to the hematologist for further evaluation and consideration of repeated laboratory measurements, including RIPA and multimeric analysis (Lichtman et al. 2006; Sandoval et al. 2002).

The combination of the Prothrombin Time (PT)/International Normalized Ratio (INR), Activated Prothrombin Time (APTT), and fibrinogen assay provides an overview of the global function of blood coagulation – secondary hemostasis. The PT is commonly reported along with the INR to adjust for different reagent sensitivities. The PT is a measure of the extrinsic (VII) pathway and the common pathway (V, X, prothrombin, and fibrinogen) clotting factors. The APTT is a measure of the intrinsic (XII, XI, IX, VIII) and common pathway clotting factors. Neither test measures the activity of FXIII. Interpretation of these screening assays will guide the physician to additional specific factor assays, if necessary, as second-line

coagulation testing. Additional second-line testing may include the thrombin time, reptilase time, functional assays of the fibrinolytic system, and FXIII activity (Sandoval et al. 2002). Hematologists should be consulted to perform and interpret the more specific second-line coagulation evaluations.

Inherited Bleeding Disorders

Primary Hemostasis. Disorders of primary hemostasis include vWD and quantitative and qualitative platelet disorders. vWD is the most common genetic bleeding disorder with a prevalence of 1–2%. vWD is classified into three major categories and must be distinguished as therapy may vary: Type 1 (70–80% of all cases) is a partial quantitative deficiency of the von Willebrand protein, Type 2 is a qualitative defect in vWF function and is divided further into four variants (2A, 2B, 2M, 2N), and Type 3, a near total deficiency of vWF.

Bleeding is typically of mild-moderate severity reflecting the predominance of type 1 vWD and usually involves mucous membrane and skin sites. Epistaxis if often the most common bleeding symptom reported in up to 60% of all patients. However, life-threatening bleeding (CNS/GI) can occur in type 3 vWD. Therapeutic choice is dependent on the type and severity of vWD and the severity of the hemostatic challenge (Sharathkumar and Pipe 2008). This is best managed by referral to a hematologist.

Three strategies are generally employed: First, one may chose to increase the plasma concentration of vWF by releasing endogenous vWF stores through stimulation of endothelial cells with DDAVP (nasal, subcutaneous, or IV routes of administration). A second approach is to replace vWF with human plasma-derived viral-inactivated concentrate. The third strategy promotes hemostasis without altering the concentration of vWF, such as the use of Amicar or Tranexamic acid, to inhibit fibrinolysis.

Thrombocytopenia is another common cause of bleeding manifestations. Acquired disorders are more common and may be secondary to medications, underlying systemic disorders, or immune thrombocytopenic purpura (ITP). Inherited platelet disorders are less common and may involve any of the steps in primary hemostasis. Examples include: Bernard-Soulier syndrome, Glanzmann's thrombasthenia, and May-Hegglin syndrome. Other inherited platelet disorders include those involving platelet storage granules: Hermansky-Pudlak, Chediak-Higashi, Wiskott-Aldrich syndrome, Gray Platelet Syndrome, and Quebec syndrome. Finally, platelet-type vWD is characterized by mild thrombocytopenia and increased affinity of the platelet for vWF (Streif et al. 2010).

Secondary Hemostasis

The most common and most important congenital coagulation disorders are: Hemophilia A (deficiency Factor VIII) and Hemophilia B (deficiency Factor IX). As the genes for hemophilia are located on the X chromosome, hemophilia primarily affects males, although females may be symptomatic carriers. Three severities of hemophilia are generally defined: mild disease (6–30%), moderate (1–5%), and severe (less than 1%) depending on the activity of Factor VIII or Factor IX. All hemophilia patients may experience severe bleeding after surgical procedures or trauma. Patients with severe hemophilia may experience severe spontaneous bleeding in any tissue; joint, muscle, or soft tissue bleeding is common. Patients with hemophilia can be treated with infusion of factor concentrates.

Additional rare congenital coagulation disorders have autosomal recessive inheritance and include deficiencies of Factors V, VII, X, XI, XIII and fibrinogen. Inherited abnormalities of the fibrinolytic system while uncommon often present with recurrent episodes of epistaxis, easy bruising and prolonged abnormal bleeding after surgery and dental procedures. Acquired bleeding disorders may also be encountered due to systemic disorders such as liver disease, acquired vitamin K deficiency, uremia, and DIC.

Medical Management

Optimal treatment of recurrent idiopathic epistaxis is unknown, with no proven advantage of observation versus various forms of intervention. Nor is there consensus on how frequent or severe epistaxis needs to be to warrant consultation. Fortunately, 90–95% episodes of epistaxis will stop spontaneously or with simple first aid including digital compression to the anterior nose for 10–15 min, ice to the nasion, and/or nape of the neck, which is believed to promote a reflexive constriction of nasal vessels (Middleton 2004).

When brought to medical attention, care should be taken to examine the body for petechiae, purpura, and lymphadenopathy, cautioning one to a systemic cause. When examining the bleeding nose, universal precautions should be taken and clots should be gently suctioned to achieve better visualization. Vasoconstriction can be achieved with epinephrine 1:1,000 or 0.05% oxymetazoline. Anesthetizing with topical lidocaine allows for better tolerance should further intervention be necessary. These simple measures alone have been reported to stop anterior epistaxis in up to 65% of patients (Middleton 2004).

Cauterization is a commonly employed technique if an accessible site is found. Silver nitrate sticks are a frequent means for cauterization. The silver precipitates and is reduced to a neutral silver. This process releases oxygen to coagulate tissue. Utilization is thought to sclerose vessels and thickens mucosa. However, in the presence of flowing blood, the reaction will not occur and the agent will simply be washed away in the stream of blood. Application should be focused to small areas applying in a peripheral to central manner for no more than 4–5 s. A gray/black eschar residue will be noted and excess should be removed to reduce penetration through the perichondrium. Use of laser has proven of little benefit, and there is no clear advantage using electrocautery though it is likely more helpful in the face of aggressive bleeding. Unfortunately, cautery is often a painful event that can cause mucosal atrophy, and delay healing. In addition, use of cautery, especially when applied bilaterally, raises a theoretical concern regarding possible septal perforation. However, a recent investigation has found no such evidence (Link et al. 2006). This treatment is associated with a high failure rate.

Application of petroleum jelly to cover the dried mucosa and exposed vessels have been found to be no more effective than observation alone (Loughran et al. 2004). However, use of antibiotic cream/ointment has been found to have an advantageous effect. Studies investigating the use of neomycin impregnated ointment have shown better results than petroleum jelly, and likely better results than observation (McGarry 2006). It also appears to be equal in effectiveness to silver nitrate cauterization, without the associated pain (Ruddy et al. 1991). Proper application involves placing the open tube in the anterior nares and squeezing enough to coat the vestibule, anterior septum when the nostrils are pinched. This can be a challenge with many children and compliance can be an issue.

When local measures fail, packing may be necessary. Anterior packing applies direct pressure to the bleeding site. Whereas posterior packing provides a buttress with which an anterior pack can tamponade the entire nasal cavity. There are several anterior packs available and include absorbable and nonabsorbable forms. Ribbon packing has long been used in conjunction with petroleum, to minimize pain with removal, and an antibiotic cream to prevent bacterial infections such as toxic shock syndrome (though there is poor evidence to support this). Packing should start horizontally along the floor from the posterior-inferior area of the nasal cavity to the apex.

Merocel packs are dehydrated polyvinyl polymer sponges that are 8 or 10 cm in length. They are inserted into the bleeding nares and hydrated with water, saline, or blood. They expand threefold and fill the nasal cavity. They can be coated with ointment prior to application for less painful removal and are technically easier to place than the traditional ribbon/gauze pack. Overall control rate has been found to be 92%, with most failures noted as posterior in nature (Middleton 2004).

Balloon packs have variations of anterior, posterior (which can be used in conjunction with an anterior pack, such as a Merocel), or combined. They tamponade the nasal cavity and control bleeding but often struggle to remain secured in its desired placement. However, applied pressure can be modulated based upon the amount of fluid used to distend the balloon/s.

Less than 5% of epistaxis is primarily posterior in nature and tend to result from complications of hypertension and arterial degeneration, which are uncommon in children (Middleton 2004). The posterior nasal space is cylindrical and packs have a tendency to fall back and down. The utilized pack must conform to the nasopharynx and occlude the posterior choanae and provide a buttress for the anterior pack. This pack may take the form of ribbon, rolled gauze pad, or double balloon 12–14 French foley catheter (filled with water or saline, not air). The packs are notoriously painful and associated with cardiopulmonary strain causing hypoxia and arrhythmias. This may be due to intrapulmonary shunting through stimulation of the nasopulmonary "diving" reflex (Gifford et al. 2008). These associated issues may also be due to aspirated blood or sedation from pain medication. Nevertheless, these patients require a monitored environment, oxygen support, and antibiotics.

In general, nonabsorbable packs are difficult to place in the conscious child, quite painful on insertion, in positioning, and upon removal. Furthermore, concern exists that removal will induce further bleeding. The packs should stay in place for 48–72 h, and antibiotics, such as a penicillin or first generation cephalosporin, should be used to prevent toxic shock syndrome and reduce acute rhinosinusitis. Nonabsorbable pack complications include mucosal ulceration, septal perforation, synechiae, platelet sequestration, bacterial colonization, and tissue necrosis (Middleton 2004; Gifford et al. 2008).

Absorbable packs tend to promote platelet aggregation, tamponade and protect the mucosa from further dissection or trauma, and promote healing. Surgicel, regenerated oxidized cellulose, and Avitene are common examples of microfibrillar collagen dressings that promote platelet adhesion. Rather than packed into the nose, they are inserted/applied to the nasal mucosa where they adhere, maintain nasal airflow, and dissolve in 2–3 weeks.

Floseal is a slurry combination of thrombin and gelatin that is easily applied and painless, but less useful in high-flow bleeding. In a controlled field, its results are comparable to silver nitrate and electrocautery. Like many absorbable options, it may prove ideal in the coagulopathic patient. Unfortunately, absorbable packs are not able to provide a great deal of pressure to tamponade and are not ideal in the face of aggressive bleeding.

Rapid Rhino (Arthrocare) is a balloon pack with a hydrocolloid fabric coating. It has several advantages of both absorbable and nonabsorbable pack. They include ease of insertion, balloon-assisted tamponade, and a colloid gel-like coating to allow a less painful removal and reduced sticking to nasal mucosa and clots, theoretically reducing further induction of bleeding upon removal. The product comes in varying lengths so that a most appropriate size for the patient can be chosen.

Surgical Management

When bleeding is severe and/or unable to be controlled with conservative measures or packing attempts, surgical options must be considered. More traditional techniques focus on open attempts at arterial ligation. Internal maxillary ligation requires a Caldwell Luc approach with access to pterygomaxillary fossa through the posterior maxillary sinus wall. The vessels are identified and ligated. The failure rate is reported to be up to 40%, often due to bleeding distal to ligation (Gifford et al. 2008). It is also a technically difficult approach, especially in children with a smaller field and thicker posterior wall. Inability to find the vessel and/or terminal branches has been reported. Complications with the approach and procedure include tissue ischemia, fistulas, opthalmoplegia, and dental and/or infraorbital nerve injury.

Ethmoid artery ligation, anterior and possibly posterior, may be necessary in the face of uncontrollable bleeding. This is usually approached with a Lynch incision and the anterior ethmoid artery is generally found 24 mm posterior to the lacrimal crest with the posterior vessel about 10 mm behind. The optic nerve is 6–8 mm further posterior. These anatomic relationships are fairly constant posteriorly during growth, but the anterior orbit tends to expand to greater degree and the distance from the anterior vessel to the lacrimal crest can be variable depending on age. In addition, some patients do not have a posterior vessel, adding to the surgical challenge. Its close proximity to the optic nerve is also a concern and risk of accidental ligation exists. As these vessels abut thin dura near the cribriform plate, they are not candidates for intranasal ligation or cauterization due to risk of intracranial injury or cerebrospinal leak (Isaacson and Monge 2003).

Embolization for epistaxis was first described by Sokoloff in 1974. Targets of this procedure are mainly the internal maxillary artery and the facial artery. Agents such as cyanoacrylate glue, polyvinyl alcohol sponges, and metal coils have been used. Overall success rate is quoted between 76% and 94% (Sadri et al. 2006). Complications of embolization include rebleeding, stroke, blindness, facial numbness, and tissue necrosis. The ethmoid vessels are not candidates as they branch from the ophthalmic artery, a branch of the internal carotid artery, and are associated with higher risk of stroke and blindness. This approach is approximately twice as expensive as other surgical options. Embolization is frequently used in the treatment of juvenile nasopharyngeal angiofibromas. Classically described as the pubescent male with unilateral nasal obstruction and episodic severe primarily unilateral nasal bleeding, these patients tend to experience less intraoperative blood loss and shorter hospital stay when undergoing embolization of the feeding vasculature preoperatively.

Endoscopic sphenopalatine artery ligation has shown encouraging results (Peloquin and Bissada 2007). This end branch of the internal maxillary artery supplies the major portion of the posterior nasal cavity.

The procedure was first described in 1992 and has a success rate over 90% (Isaacson and Monge 2003). The first successful utilization in a child was reported in 2007 (Peloquin and Bissada 2007). After endoscopic visualization of the attachment of the posterior middle turbinate to the lateral nasal wall (near the face of the sphenoid sinus), a 10–20 mm vertical incision is made 5 mm anterior to the site. A mucosal flap is elevated to the crista ethmoidalis. The artery is just posterior and dissected free. It is then clipped and cauterized close to the lateral nasal wall. Effectiveness stems from disruption of the nasal vasculature at a point distal enough to avoid all retrograde and anastamotic blood flow, and relatively consistent anatomic relationships. Complications include palatal numbness, sinusitis, intranasal adhesions, and decreased lacrimation. This technique appears to be faster and less invasive than IMA ligation (Isaacson and Monge 2003).

Summary

Epistaxis in children is a common phenomenon, fortunately usually self-limiting and benign in etiology. In the child with active bleeding at the time of visit, the clinician must be prepared to identify the area of the nose that is bleeding and offer prompt treatment. Once the acute bleeding is stopped, or in the child that presents with intermittent but not current bleeding, the clinician can obtain the appropriate history and clinical information, and perform a thorough physical examination to determine the etiology of the epistaxis. Less frequent, a laboratory evaluation or consultation with a hematologist may be deemed necessary to determine if the cause of the bleeding is from an underlying bleeding disorder. Having a developed protocol as described above, on how to approach these patients, offers the clinician a time-efficient, cost-considerate opportunity that will be rewarding in treating this disorder successfully with high patient and physician satisfaction in an otherwise often frustrating clinical problem.

Cross-References

► Allergic Rhinitis
► Angiography
► Arteriovenous Malformations
► Deviated Nasal Septum

▶ Endoscopic Sinus Surgery in Children
▶ Epistaxis
▶ Juvenile Nasopharyngeal Angiofibroma
▶ Nasal and Sinus Trauma
▶ Nasal Polyps
▶ Nasal Washes
▶ Sinonasal Malignancies
▶ Sinusitis in Children, Complications

References

Brown N, Berkowitz R (2004) Epistaxis in healthy children requiring hospital admission. Int J Pediatr Otorhinolaryngol 68(9):1181–1184

Burton M, Doree C (2004) Interventions for recurrent idiopathic epistaxis (nosebleeds) in children. Cochrane Database Syst Rev 1:CDO04461

Gifford T et al (2008) Epistaxis. Otolaryngol Clin N Am 41:525–536

Isaacson G, Monge J (2003) Arterial ligation for pediatric epistaxis: developmental anatomy. Am J Rhinol 17(2):75–81

Lichtman MA et al (2006) Williams hematology, 7th edn. McGraw-Hill Medical, New York, pp 1741–1747, 1929–1946

Link T et al (2006) Bilateral epistaxis in children: efficacy of bilateral septal cauterization with silve nitrate. Int J Pediatr Otorhinolaryngol 70(8):1439–1442

Lippi G et al (2007) Diagnostic approach to inherited bleeding disorders. Clin Chem Lab Med 45:2–12

Loughran S et al (2004) A single-blind, randomized controlled trial of petroleum jelly/Vaseline for recurrent pediatric epistaxis. Clin Otolaryngol Allies Sci 29(3):266–269

McGarry G (2006) Nosebleeds in children. Clin Evid 31(3):496–499

Middleton PM (2004) Epistaxis. Emer Med Aust 16:428–440

Paranjothy S et al (2009) The incidence and aetilolgy of epistaxis in infants: a population-based study. Arch Dis Child 94(6):421–424

Peloquin L, Bissada E (2007) Endoscopic transnasal sphenopalatine arterial ligation for intractable posterior epistaxis in a young child. J Otolaryngol 36(4):E57–E59

Robertson A et al (2010) Frequency and management of epistaxis in schools. J Laryngol Otol 124:302–305

Ruddy J et al (1991) Management of epistaxis in children. Int J Pediatr Otorhinolaryngol 21:139–142

Sadri M et al (2006) Assessment of safety and efficacy of arterial embolisation in the management of intractable epistaxis. Eur Arch Otorhinolaryngol 263:560–566

Sandoval C et al (2002) Clinical and laboratory features of 178 children with epistaxis. J Pediatr Hem Onc 24:47–49

Sharathkumar A, Pipe S (2008) Bleeding disorders. Pediatr Rev 29:121–130

Streif W et al (2010) Inherited disorders of platelet function in pediatric clinical practice: a diagnostic challenge. Klin Pediatr 222:203–208

Whymark A et al (2008) Childhood epistaxis and nasal colonization with Stapylococcis aureus. Otolaryngol Head Neck Surg 138(3):307–310

Epithelial Inclusion Cyst

▶ Lateral Skull Base Epidermoids
▶ Magnetic Resonance Imaging, Epidermoid

Epithelial Papilloma

▶ Benign Sinonasal Neoplasms

Epithelial Tumor

▶ Magnetic Resonance Imaging, Epidermoid

Epitympanum

Sébastien Schmerber[1,2,3], Arnaud Attye[1,2,4], Ihab Atallah[5], Cédric Mendoza[1,2,4] and Alexandre Karkas[1,4,6]

[1]Department of Otolaryngology-Head and Neck Surgery, Otology/Neurotology Unit, University Hospital of Grenoble, Grenoble, France
[2]Service ORL. Hôpital A. Michallon, Grenoble, France
[3]Otology, Neurotology and Auditory Implants Department, University Hospital of Grenoble CHU A. Michallon, Grenoble, France
[4]Department of Neuroradiology, University Hospital of Grenoble, Grenoble, France
[5]Department of Otolaryngology-Head and Neck Surgery, University Hospital of Grenoble, Grenoble, France
[6]Clinique Universitaire Oto–Rhino–Laryngologie, Centre Hospitalier Universitaire A. Michallon, Grenoble, France

Definition

The upper portion of the middle ear (i.e., space above tympanic membrane annulus).

Erosive Otitis Externa

▶ Benign Osteonecrosis of Temporal Bone

Erythema Migrans

Johnathan Sataloff and Robert T. Sataloff
Department of Otolaryngology-Head and Neck
Surgery, Drexel University College of Medicine,
Philadelphia, PA, USA

Definition

A target-like rash associated with Lyme disease, but absent or unrecognized in approximately 25% of patients diagnosed with Lyme disease.

Cross-References

▶ Otologic Manifestations of Lyme Disease

Erythroplakia

Steven J. Frampton and Emma V. King
Poole Hospital NHS Foundation Trust, Poole,
Dorset, UK
Cancer Sciences Division, University of Southampton,
Southampton, Hampshire, UK

Definition

Erythroplakia is a clinical term used to describe a flat red patch or lesion on the mucosal surface that cannot be attributed to any other pathology.

Cross-References

▶ Field Cancerization

Esophagus

▶ Upper Digestive Anatomy and Function

Esteem®: Totally Implantable Hearing System

Jack A. Shohet
Shohet Ear Associates Medical Group, Inc., Newport
Beach, CA, USA

Synonyms

Active middle ear implant; IMEHD; Implantable middle ear hearing device; Totally implantable hearing device

Definition

The Esteem® by Envoy Medical is a totally implantable middle ear hearing device which senses vibrations from the incus body and drives the stapes capitulum using piezoelectric transduction.

Purpose

Implantable middle ear hearing devices (IMEHD) were devised to address the shortcomings of conventional hearing aids. They facilitate improved hearing by allowing direct transmission of sound to the inner ear. In addition, IMEHDs improve comfort by allowing the ear canal to stay open and avoid feedback by decoupling the receiver from the microphone.

The totally implantable Esteem® is invisible when implanted, which mitigates cosmetic considerations and allows the user to bathe, swim, and exercise while enjoying the benefits of their device.

Principle

Conventional digital hearing aids work by digitizing and processing the sound received by an external microphone. The signal is filtered, compressed, amplified, and eventually processed back into sound waves. This sound energy is then directed toward the middle ear transduction mechanism via the ear canal. The conversion of sound into digital signal and then back into sound introduces distortion to the system.

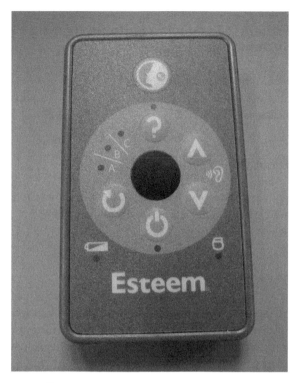

Fig. 1 Esteem Transducers and Sound Processor

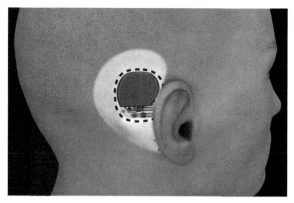

Fig. 2 Esteem implanted postauricularly

Implantable middle ear devices work by a direct drive mechanism whereby the sound is picked up through a microphone, processed, and then delivered directly to the middle ear as energy in the form of ossicular vibration. The distortion inherent in converting the signal back to sound energy is thus eliminated.

The Esteem's direct drive system consists of two piezoelectric transducers, a sound processor and a battery (Fig. 1). A piezoelectric sensor, which is cemented to the body of the incus, picks up the ossicular vibrations in response to sound hitting the tympanic membrane. The piezoelectric transducer converts these mechanical vibrations into an electric signal, which is relayed to the sound processor. The sound processor (SP) and battery are housed in a unit resembling a pacemaker. It is implanted in a drilled recess over the mastoid and parietal bones (Fig. 2). The SP filters, compresses, and amplifies the electric signal and then delivers it to the driver, which is cemented to the stapes capitulum. The piezoelectric driver transducer converts the electrical signal into mechanical vibrations, which stimulate the inner ear via the stapes (Chen et al. 2004) (Fig. 3).

The surgical procedure is initiated as a postauricular incision, through which all the components are implanted. A well is drilled over the posterior mastoid and parietal bones to accommodate the SP. A mastoidectomy is performed, which includes exposure of the head of the malleus and incus body in the epitympanum as well as an extended facial recess exposure of the long crus of the incus and posterior crus of the stapes. In order to avoid feedback through the ossicular chain, the lenticular process and a portion of the long crus of the incus are resected and removed through the facial recess. The bodies of the sensor and driver transducers are cemented into the mastoid cavity. The piezoelectric projection of the sensor is cemented to the body of the incus in the epitympanic exposure and the driver projects through the facial recess into the middle ear where it is cemented to the stapes capitulum. The transducer cables are plugged into the SP, the wound is closed, and the SP is turned off.

Intraoperative testing of the system is done at several steps using laser Doppler interferometry and a speaker positioned in the ear canal. Intact ossicular chain measurements are made at the body of the incus and posterior stapes crus to ensure sufficient ossicular movement. Additional testing is performed after the sensor and driver are implanted to measure displacement of the ossicles in response to sound stimuli. Feedback tests investigate whether there are gross sources of feedback in the implanted system. Finally,

Esteem®: Totally Implantable Hearing System, Fig. 3 Sound pathway with Esteem. Vibrations of tympanic membrane are sensed by the piezoelectric transducer cemented to the incus. The electrical current generated by the piezoelectric movement is relayed to the sound processor which processes the sound and delivers it to the driver which is implanted on the stapes

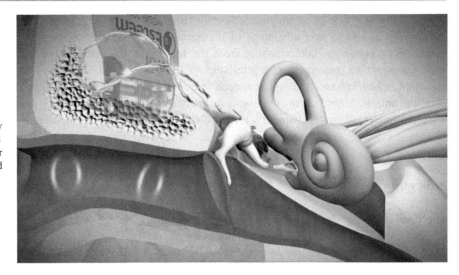

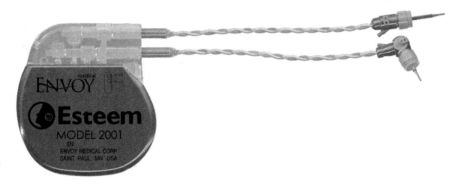

Esteem®: Totally Implantable Hearing System, Fig. 4 Personal Programmer which control power to the device, volume control and selection of preset programs

the displacement of the stapes in response to a sound stimulus in the ear canal is measured when the entire system is in place and activated.

The postoperative course involves routine wound care for the first several days after surgery followed by several weeks until the implant is activated. Blood and eventually a serous effusion occupy the middle ear for several weeks after the surgery and impair device performance if activated too early.

Once the effusion has resolved, the device is programmed and activated in the office with specialized software and hardware. The implant can be interrogated and information about the individual components can be obtained. Soundbooth testing is performed to determine efficacy and ensure that sensorineural hearing has not been affected. Periodic

adjustments to the programming are performed as needed. A wireless personal programmer (Fig. 4), which allows for volume control and selection of 3 preset programs, is dispensed at the time of device activation.

The current battery life is expected to be between 5 and 9 years depending on how long it is used during the day and how much power is required for the individual's settings. An operation to remove the battery is done under local anesthetic through the postauricular incision. The transducer leads are unplugged from the SP and remain in place. Only the SP is changed out. In this way, the Esteem is retrograde compatible. The patient can benefit from advances in battery and sound processing technology when the battery is replaced.

A microphone that picks up sound directly from the ossicles is able to take advantage of the normal human ear physiology. Directionality from the forward-facing pinna, resonance characteristics of the ear canal, which enhance the higher speech frequencies, and amplification via the ossicular lever mechanism are leveraged by the Esteem's sensor (Maurer and Savvas 2004).

Indication

The Food and Drug Administration (US Department of Health and Human Services) lists the indications as:
(a) Moderate to severe hearing loss as defined by the Pure Tone Average (PTA) at 500, 1,000, and 2,000 Hz
(b) Eighteen years old and above
(c) Stable hearing loss
(d) Speech discrimination test score greater than or equal to 40%
(e) Normal function of the middle ear (Eustachian) tube
(f) Normal middle ear anatomy
(g) Normal tympanic membrane
(h) Adequate space to house the transducers as determined through a high resolution Computed Tomography (CT) scan
(i) Minimum of 30 days experience with appropriately fitted hearing aids

In addition, it is important that the patient has reasonable expectations regarding the potential extent of hearing rehabilitation.

Contraindication

Conversely, the FDA lists a history of the following as contraindications:
(a) Post-adolescent chronic middle ear infections
(b) Inner ear disorders or recurring vertigo requiring treatment
(c) Chronic mastoid infections
(d) Swelling in the inner ear (hydrops)
(e) Meniere's disease
(f) Disabling tinnitus which requires treatment
(g) Fluctuating air and/or bone conduction hearing loss over the past 1 year period of 15 decibels (dB)

in either direction at two or more hearing frequencies (from 500 to 4,000 Hz)
(h) Otitis externa or eczema of the external auditory canal
(i) Destructive middle ear disease (cholesteatoma)
(j) Central auditory disorders (retrocochlear)
(k) Keloid formation in other wounds
(l) Excessive sensitivity to silicone rubber, polyurethane, stainless steel, titanium, and/or gold

Advanced age is not a contraindication as long as the patient's health status permits a 3–5 h operation under general anesthetic.

Advantage/Disadvantage

There are many IMEHD hearing device advantages that are realized using Esteem's technology. The direct drive system improves fidelity of the sound. The closest measure of sound fidelity used in the Esteem FDA clinical trial was the Abbreviated Profile of Hearing Aid Benefit (APHAB). This questionnaire assesses four different categories including Ease of Communication, Reverberation, Background Noise, and Aversiveness of Sounds and was used to compare the subjects' hearing aid experience with their Esteem implant. In the clinical trial, APHAB scores improved in all categories with the greatest improvement found in the Ease of Communication category.

A totally implanted hearing system facilitates many other advantages: comfort is optimized as there are no external components to irritate the skin, or create hygiene issues; cosmetic concerns are obviated as it is invisible; being able to hear while swimming, bathing, and exercising is always possible; the occlusion effect is not an issue; and, feedback is minimized since the microphone and speaker of the system are decoupled.

During the pivotal phase 2 clinical trial, which included 57 subjects implanted in three centers in the USA, the subjects' hearing with their hearing aid in the same ear before surgery and with the Esteem 12 months after surgery were compared. On average, the Speech Reception Threshold (SRT) improved from 41.2 to 29.4 dB. The Word Recognition Score (WRS) at 50 dB HL improved from 46.3% to 68.9%. Furthermore, the Pure Tone Average (PTA) scores improved by 27 +/− 1 dB (Kraus et al. 2011)

A five-patient subgroup of the original 57 patients had a profound high-frequency sensorineural hearing loss. SRT was improved from 48 to 26 dB and WRS at 50 dB improved from 23% to 78%. WRS at the most comfortable level (MCL) improved from 69% to 88% (Shohet et al. 2011).

The primary disadvantage of implantable middle ear hearing devices is that they require surgery with the attendant risks of the primary procedure and anesthetic. The most common side effect was temporary taste disturbance, which was experienced by 42% of the trial subjects. Nineteen percent (19%) reported imbalance/vertigo/dizziness which resolved in 82% by the end of the 12-month follow-up period. Eighteen percent (18%) experienced tinnitus, which resolved in 70% by the end of the trial follow-up period. Five percent (5%) experienced a delayed facial paralysis, which completely resolved with steroid treatment (Kraus et al. 2011).

Explantation of the Esteem requires reconstruction of the incus defect. A partial ossicular reconstruction prosthesis (PORP) was designed by one of the primary investigators to address this specific defect. Called the K-Helix Crown prosthesis (Grace Medical, Memphis, Tennessee), the prosthesis spans the defect and is optimally stabilized with glass ionomer cement.

Other disadvantages includes the fact that, as with other implantable hearing devices, the Esteem is MRI-incompatible. In addition, the cost of the implant, procedure, and intensive postoperative programming may hamper accessibility to the device. Finally, the Esteem implantation surgery is a complex procedure requiring many steps that build upon each other. The operation utilizes surgical cements and intricate 3-dimensional positioning of the components, which are new to most otologic surgeons. Suboptimal completion of an earlier step can compound into a much more difficult issue to confront later in the surgery. This has led to a steep surgical learning curve and a need to complete a considerable number of procedures before proficiency is attained.

Cross-References

▶ Hearing Aid
▶ Implantable Hearing Devices
▶ Ossiculoplasty

References

Chen DA, Backous DD, Arriaga MA (2004) Phase 1 clinical trial results of the envoy system: a totally implantable middle ear device for sensorineural hearing loss. Otolaryngol Head Neck Surg 131(6):904–916

Kraus EM, Shohet JA, Catalano PJ (2011) envoy esteem totally implantable hearing system: phase 2 trial, 1-year hearing results. Otolaryngol Head Neck Surg 145(1):100–109

Maurer J, Savvas E (2010) The esteem system: a totally implantable hearing device. Adv Otorhinolaryngol 69:59–71

Shohet JA, Kraus EM, Catalano PJ (2011) Profound high-frequency sensorineural hearing loss treatment with a totally implantable hearing system. Otol Neurotol 32(9):1428–1431

Esthesioneuroblastoma

Adrienne M. Laury[1] and Sarah K. Wise[1,2]
[1]Department of Otolaryngology-Head and Neck Surgery, Emory University School of Medicine, Atlanta, GA, USA
[2]Department of Otolaryngology, Emory University, Atlanta, GA, USA

Synonyms

Blue cell tumor; Neuroepithelial tumor; Olfactory neuroblastoma

Definition

A sinonasal malignancy of neuroectodermal origin that arises from the olfactory system within the nasal cavity.

Epidemiology

Esthesioneuroblastoma (ENB) is a relatively rare malignancy accounting for only 6% of nasal cavity and paranasal sinus cancers (McLean et al. 2007). Approximately 1,000 cases have been reported since its initial discovery in 1924 (Gabory et al. 2010). ENB is typically identified at an advanced stage, primarily because of its typical presentation with benign and nonspecific symptoms. In a cohort of 311 patients diagnosed with ENB, approximately 17% of patients presented with a Kadish A stage tumor, 50% presented with Kadish stage B, and 34% with more advanced stage Kadish C or D tumors (Jethanamest et al. 2007). ENB has a bimodal age distribution between 10–20 years and 50–60 years. It also appears to have no predilection based on sex. No identifiable genetic or environmental causes or risk factors have been identified for ENB.

History

As stated above, patients frequently present with a relatively benign history secondary to the anatomic origin of the tumor high in the nasal vault. Tumor growth in this location often prevents early detection until there is a significant increase in the size of the tumor and subsequent mass effect. Symptoms usually include nasal obstruction, epistaxis, anosmia, and headache (Flint et al. 2010). Five percent of patients also concurrently present with a palpable neck mass, concerning for nodal metastasis (Zanation et al. 2010). Additionally, another 1.5% initially present with coexisting distant metastases (Jethanamest et al. 2007). Due to this relatively small percentage of distant metastasis and the overall rarity of ENB, the primary locations for the ENB distant metastases have not been extensively studied.

Clinical Features

On physical examination, rigid nasal endoscopy commonly reveals a unilateral nasal mass, which may appear consistent with a benign polyp or, occasionally, a firm mass. The nasal cavity mass is often vascular in appearance. If the mass has significantly expanded by the time of initial presentation, ocular symptoms, such as proptosis or paretic extraocular movements, may also exist. The discovery of neck disease may also be a significant part of the initial clinical exam. Most metastatic cervical nodes are located ipsilateral to the primary disease. However, more rarely, bilateral nodes and even retropharyngeal nodes can occur. Throughout the course of the disease, level II is the most common area of presentation for neck metastasis, with approximately 93% of patients with cervical disease having at least one positive node in this region. However, additional nodes can be often be identified in levels I (57% of patients with neck disease) and III (50% of

N + patients), and retropharyngeal nodes have been found in up to 43% of patients (Howell et al. 2011).

Diagnostics

When the diagnosis of ENB is suspected, an MRI with gadolinium should be immediately obtained. Typically, when compared to gray matter, ENBs appear hypointense on a T1-weighted noncontrast image. On a T2-weighted MRI image, ENBs often appear hyperintense. Gadolinium contrast enhancement is intense and of variable uniformity on MRI scans (Figs. 1a and 2a). Gadolinium helps to distinguish the mass from obstructed secretions in the paranasal sinuses, as well as determine meningeal and extradural spread and detect perineural invasion (Derdeyn et al. 1994). CT imaging is also useful for defining bony destruction as well as skull base defects that may require repair following resection (Figs. 1b and 2b). No large-scale studies have been performed to evaluate the utility of PET scanning in the initial workup of esthesioneuroblastoma. However, work is currently underway examining the role of PET in the posttherapeutic patient and their long-term monitoring for recurrence (Fig. 1c).

After imaging studies have been performed, a biopsy must be obtained for diagnosis and pathologic staging. Many surgeons will choose to perform biopsies of suspected ENB in the operating room due to its highly vascular nature. Workup for potential metastases includes laboratory evaluation including CBC and complete chemistry profile with liver function tests. Imaging of the neck and lungs for diagnosis of regional and distant metastases is also essential.

Staging

The original and most commonly utilized staging system was first put forth by Kadish in the 1970s and subsequently revised by Morita (Jethanamest et al. 2007). Table 1 displays the modified version of the staging system.

Although the Kadish staging system is the most commonly utilized staging system for ENB, several downfalls must be noted. The discrimination between stages A and B represents little clinical difference and, therefore, is of low prognostic significance.

Esthesioneuroblastoma,
Fig. 1 (**a–c**) These images are
from a 25-year-old patient
with Kadish stage D
esthesioneuroblastoma.
(**a**) Coronal T1-weighted MRI
scan shows a right-sided nasal
cavity mass. This mass effaces
the right medial orbit and
medial rectus muscle.
Intracranial extension is also
noted. (**b**) Coronal CT scan
image in bone window
algorithm from the same
patient. Erosion of the medial
aspect of the bony skull base
and crista galli can be
visualized. (**c**) Axial PET-CT-
fused images reveal bilateral
lymph node metastases in the
neck with notable tracer
uptake

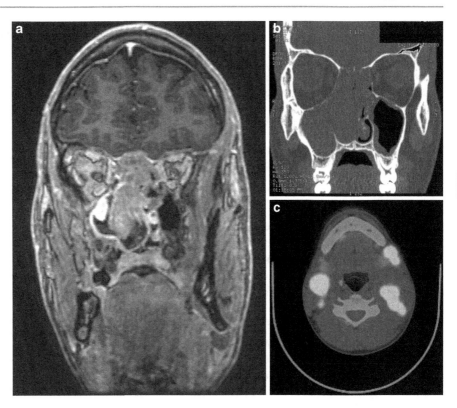

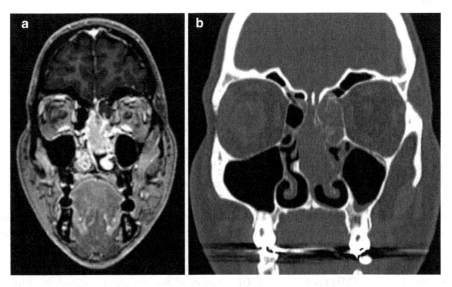

Esthesioneuroblastoma, Fig. 2 (**a–b**) These images are from
a 33-year-old patient with Kadish stage A esthesioneuroblastoma. (**a**) Coronal T1-weighted MRI scan with gadolinium
contrast enhancement reveals a left-sided nasal cavity mass
arising from the region of the olfactory cleft, without significant
intracranial or intraorbital extension. Gadolinium contrast in this
image reveals heterogeneous tumor enhancement. (**b**)
Corresponding CT scan image in coronal bone windows also
demonstrates the left nasal cavity mass with pressure effect on
the nasal septum, causing bowing of the nasal septum to the
right. There is no significant erosion of the bony skull base

Esthesioneuroblastoma, Table 1 Revised Kadish staging system for esthesioneuroblastoma

Staging	Tumor extension
Kadish A	Mass is limited to the nasal cavity
Kadish B	Mass involves the nasal cavity and paranasal sinuses
Kadish C	Mass extends beyond the nasal cavity and sinuses
Kadish D	Mass additionally has regional (cervical lymph nodes) or distant metastases

Esthesioneuroblastoma, Table 2 Hyams pathologic grading system for esthesioneuroblastoma

Feature	Grade I	Grade II	Grade III	Grade IV
Architecture	Lobular	Lobular	± Lobular	± Lobular
Mitotic activity	Absent	Present	Prominent	Ubiquitous
Nuclear pleomorphism	Absent	Moderate	Prominent	Ubiquitous
Fibrillary matrix	Prominent	Present	Minimal	Absent
Rosettes	± Homer Wright	± Homer Wright	Flexner	Absent
Necrosis	Absent	Absent	± Present	Frequent

Stage A is exceedingly rare, due to the nature and location of the disease. Finally, no differentiation is made regarding tumors which have intracranial or intraorbital extension. Because of these numerous deficiencies, a myriad of other staging systems have been proposed. However, in a comparative study between the Kadish staging system versus the Biller and Dulguerov staging systems (two systems based on a more classic TNM staging), the Kadish staging system was the only classification that yielded a statistically significant discrimination between stages (Dias et al. 2003).

Pathologic Features

The pathologic grading of ENB has also been shown to be an important predictor of clinical outcome. There are several findings which assist in diagnosing ENB. Common features are mitotically active, small, round neuroepithelial cells (blue cells) arranged in rosette or pseudorosette patterns, separated by fibrous elements. True rosettes, known as Flexner rosettes, consist of an empty central space ringed by columnar cells with radially oriented nuclei. Alternatively, pseudorosettes, or Homer-Wright rosettes, present with the same ring of columnar cells, but the central space is filled with a meshwork of fibrin. Hyams described a pathologic grading system based on the presence or absence of distinct microscopic features. Grade I tumors have an excellent prognosis, while grade IV tumors are associated with a very high mortality (Miyamoto et al. 2000). Table 2 displays Hyams grading system which is still used today (Bluestone et al. 2001).

Some controversy still exists regarding poorly differentiated tumors and whether these should be classified as a Hyams grade IV or sinonasal undifferentiated carcinoma (SNUC). This is important given that the overall prognosis for ENB is significantly better than SNUC (Flint et al. 2010).

Differential Diagnosis

Sinonasal Undifferentiated Carcinoma (SNUC), Squamous Cell Carcinoma, Inverted Papilloma, Adenocarcinoma, or Sinonasal Melanoma.

Sinonasal undifferentiated carcinoma – SNUC is a rare (less than 100 literature-reported cases to date) and highly aggressive neoplasm arising from the nasal cavity and paranasal sinuses that was first described in 1986. Prior to its "discovery," SNUC tumors were typically classified as ENB and, to date, are still commonly misdiagnosed. The tumor is composed of small- to medium-sized undifferentiated cells arranged in nests, frequently accompanied by extensive necrosis. Generally, the tumor is extensive at presentation and involves multiple sinonasal structures. Invasion into the orbit and intracranial cavity is frequent. Although presentation, and at times, pathology is very similar to ENB, the prognosis is significantly worse. Overall survival was 22% at 5 years, and the estimated 5-year distant metastasis-free survival was 35% (Lin et al. 2010).

Squamous cell carcinoma – Squamous cell carcinoma of the paranasal sinuses is considerably more common than ENB, accounting for over 80% of all malignancies that present in the nasal cavity and sinuses. Paranasal sinus squamous cell carcinoma encompasses several variants including, verrucous carcinoma, basaloid squamous cell carcinoma, spindle cell carcinoma, and transitional or cylindrical cell carcinoma. The presenting symptoms are similar to ENB – nasal obstruction, rhinorrhea, epistaxis, cranial neuropathies, or pain. However, neck and distant metastases are significantly less common. Histologic examination reveals sheets, ribbons, and individual squamous, polyhedral, or round-to-ovoid cells with various degrees of keratinization. Prognosis is relatively similar to ENB, with the overall 5-year survival rate being 60–64% and the recurrence rate estimated at 31% (Klem and Thaler 2009).

Inverted papilloma – Inverted papilloma (IP) is a benign lesion with a locally aggressive nature. It initially presents as a red-tan mass in the nasal cavity and, like ENB, is frequently unilateral. Approximately 10% of IP harbor squamous cell carcinoma is making histologic evaluation essential. Pathology typically demonstrates hyperplastic multilayered squamous-to-columnar epithelium with or without atypia. Prognosis is good, as the lesion is most often benign, but recurrence rates range between 13% and 34% depending on resection technique utilized (Mirza et al. 2007).

Adenocarcinoma – Adenocarcinoma of the nasal cavity and paranasal sinuses is historically important and is associated with specific risk factors including exposure to wood dust, lacquers, and other organic compounds. Presenting signs are again similar to those for ENB, primarily obstructive symptoms, rhinorrhea, or epistaxis. Additionally, local destruction of the orbits and skull base is frequently seen. Distant metastases and cervical lymph node spread are both rare. Treatment is surgical excision with wide margins and postoperative radiotherapy for advanced disease or positive margins. The prognosis for low-grade adenocarcinoma is far better than that for high-grade tumors of the sinonasal area – with a 5-year survival of 80%. High-grade adenocarcinomas have a reported survival rate of less than 35% at 3 years (Klem and Thaler 2009).

Malignant melanoma of the paranasal sinuses – Melanoma is a relatively rare disorder of the nasal cavity accounting for less than 4% of the sinonasal malignancies. Melanomas rarely metastasize to this location but more often originate here as the primary site of disease. Presentation is again similar to ENB with the finding of a firm, gray-white, or pink-to-black ulcerated mass. However, on presentation, the concurrent finding of cervical metastases is much higher at nearly 26%. Immunohistochemistry is extremely important in diagnosis and is positive for S-100, HMB-45, melan-A, or pigment epithelium-derived factor. Surgery plus radiation for advanced disease is the primary therapeutic modality. However, despite optimal treatment, prognosis is significantly worse than ENB, with median survival being less than 2 years (Klem and Thaler 2009).

Treatment

The treatment of ENB is still a widely debated topic. The use of combined modality treatment with surgery, radiation therapy (RT), and chemotherapy in various combinations has been applied more frequently over the past few years. Recently, it was shown that the combined use of surgery and radiation therapy resulted in a better survival rate (65%) than surgery alone (48%), chemoradiotherapy (51%), or radiotherapy alone (37%) (Dulguerov et al. 2001). This was based upon all grades of ENB, regardless or Kadish or Hyams staging.

However, when analyzing treatment based upon Kadish tumor staging, the extent of therapy for the rare cases of solely nasal cavity disease (Kadish A) is debatable. While some studies advocate for surgical resection as the sole form of treatment, others still support a concomitant modality incorporating both surgery and RT (Zafereo et al. 2008; Gabory et al. 2010, respectively).

Additionally, for more severe cases with extranasal extension (Kadish C), the role of chemotherapy, given concomitantly with surgery and RT, has been supported. The addition of platinum-based chemotherapy resulted in significantly better event-free survival (65% vs. 20%) (Eich et al. 2005).

The type of surgical resection is also a topic of contention in the treatment of ENB. Open en bloc craniofacial resection versus endoscopic removal has recently incited controversy. As endoscopic skull base tumor resections are performed more frequently and data on long-term follow-up becomes available, many have increasingly advocated for endoscopic resection of ENB. Meta-analyses show significantly improved survival rates, reaching nearly 100%, when the mass is resected entirely endoscopically (Devaiah and Andreoli 2009). However, it must be taken into account that open resections have overall longer follow-up data and are utilized for more extensive

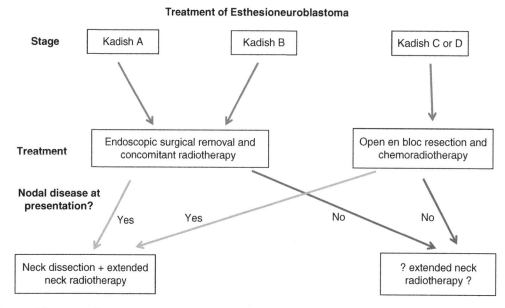

Esthesioneuroblastoma, Fig. 3 Treatment of esthesioneuroblastoma

disease, while endoscopic resections are more commonly reserved for less severe tumor spread (Kadish A and B). This selection bias, in turn, may over amplify the success rates of endoscopic resection. Yet, these early data showing good survival with endoscopic resection are promising.

Radiation therapy is commonly administered postoperatively in the treatment of ENB. However, some studies have also applied radiation as a neoadjuvant therapy. Most patients receive approximately 5,000–6,000 cGy using standard fractionation techniques. Of note, studies have shown that the use of radiotherapy as a single modality treatment results in high local recurrence rates (Flint et al. 2010).

The treatment of cervical nodal disease in ENB must also be considered. Although only 5% of patients initially present with concurrent nodal metastases, approximately 20–25% will develop neck disease over time (Zanation et al. 2010). In patients initially presenting with cervical disease, 5-year survival rates drop to only 29% compared to 64% in those with N0 disease. Given this significant decrease, the addition of a neck dissection(s) along with elective neck irradiation to traditional treatment regimens has been increasingly advocated for (Zanation et al. 2010).

Finally, the prophylactic treatment of the neck in patients initially presenting with N0 disease is

undetermined. Some studies have shown promising results with prophylactic neck irradiation but nothing which reaches statistical significance in preventing regional recurrence. To date, no study has examined prophylactic neck dissections in patients presenting with N0 disease, yet this could pose a promising option in minimizing cervical recurrence. Figure 3 is a treatment flowchart based on statistically significant clinical data for the management of patients presenting with ENB.

Prognosis

Overall, the prognosis of ENB is relatively good with a 5-year disease free survival rate of between 60% and 71% (McLean et al. 2007). Recently, the University of Virginia Health System updated a series of 50 cases (the largest cohort to date) and reported higher disease-free survival rates of 86.5% and 82.6% at 5 and 15 years; all patients received multimodality treatment including craniofacial resection, radiotherapy, and chemotherapy for stage C disease (Jethanamest et al. 2007).

Unfortunately, treatment failures may also occur immediately after completion of therapy in as many as 10% of patients. Additionally, local recurrence as well as regional and distant metastases has been shown to occur in up to 38% of patients and for up to 12 years posttreatment. Specifically, during the first decade after treatment, regional nodal recurrence was shown to be the most common, as opposed to in the second decade where local or distant metastases occurred more frequently (Gabory et al. 2010).

Hyams grading has also been proven to be an important prognostic factor with studies showing patient's with Hyams grade I disease having a 100% 5-year survival versus grades II and III having a 75% and 57% 5-year survival, respectively (McLean et al. 2007).

Overall, despite the relatively good prognosis, especially for ENB with a low Hyams score and low Kadish grade, long-term follow-up is required to allow for early identification of any recurrence.

References

Bluestone CD, Stool SE, Alper CM, Arjmand EM (2001) Pediatric otolaryngology. Elsevier Health Sciences, Philadelphia

Derdeyn CP, Moran CJ, Wippold FJ et al (1994) MRI of esthesioneuroblastoma. J Comput Assist Tomogr 18:16–21

Devaiah AK, Andreoli MT (2009) Treatment of esthesioneuroblastoma: a 16-year meta analysis of 361 patients. Laryngoscope 119:1412–1416

Dias FL, Sa GM, Lima RA et al (2003) Patterns of failure and outcome in esthesioneuroblastoma. Arch Otolaryngol Head Neck Surg 129:1186–1192

Dulguerov P, Allal AS, Calcaterra TC (2001) Esthesioneuroblastoma: a meta-analysis and review. Lancet Oncol 2:683–690

Eich HT, Muller RP, Micke O et al (2005) Esthesioneuroblastoma in childhood and adolescence: better prognosis with multimodal treatment? Strahlenther Onkol 181: 378–384

Flint PW, Haughey BH, Lund VJ et al (2010) Cummings otolaryngology – head and neck surgery, 5th edn. Mosby, St Louis

Gabory L, Abdulkhaleq HM, Darrouzet V et al (2010) Long-term results of 28 esthesioneuroblastomas managed over 35 years. Head Neck 33(1):82–86

Howell MC, Branstetter Iv BF, Snyderman CH (2011) Patterns of regional spread for esthesioneuroblastoma. AJNR Am J Neuroradiol 32(5):929–933

Jethanamest D, Morris LG, Sikora AG, Kutler DI (2007) Esthesioneuroblastoma: a population-based analysis of survival and prognostic factors. Arch Otolaryngol Head Neck Surg 133:276–280

Klem C, Thaler J (2009) Malignant tumors of the sinuses. Emedicine. http://emedicine.medscape.com/article/847189-overview. Accessed March 3, 2009

Levine PA, Gallagher R, Cantrell RW (1999) Esthesioneuroblastoma: reflections of a 21 year experience. Laryngoscope 109:1539–1543

Lin EM, Sparano A, Spalding A et al (2010) Sinonasal undifferentiated carcinoma: a 13-year experience at a single institution. Skull Base 20:61–67

McLean JN, Nunley SR, Klass C et al (2007) Combined modality therapy of esthesioneuroblastoma. Otolaryngol Head Neck Surg 136:998–1002

Mirza S, Bradley PJ, Acharya A et al (2007) Sinonasal inverted papillomas: recurrence, and synchronous and metachronous malignancy. J Laryngol Otol 121:857–864

Miyamoto RC, Gleich LL, Biddinger PW et al (2000) Esthesioneuroblastoma and sinonasal undifferentiated carcinoma: impact of histological grading and clinical staging on survival and prognosis. Laryngoscope 110:1262–1265

Zafereo ME, Fakhri S, Prayson R et al (2008) Esthesioneuroblastoma: 25-year experience at a single institution. Otolaryngol Head Neck Surg 138:452–458

Zanation AM, Ferlito A, Rinaldo A et al (2010) When, how and why to treat the neck in patients with esthesioneuroblastoma: A review. Eur Arch Otorhinolaryngol 267:1667–1671

Estlander Flap

Eric J. Dobratz
Department of Otolaryngology, Eastern Virginia Medical School, Norfolk, VA, USA

Synonyms

Cross-lip flap; Lip-switch flap

Definition

One-staged cross-lip flap for lip reconstruction involving the oral commissure. The medial-based pedicle from the lip opposite the defect remains intact and is incorporated into the reconstructed commissure.

Basic Characteristics

Lip reconstruction using a cross-lip flap was first described more than 250 years ago by Johann Hierzel (Vrebos et al. 1994). This account of the first cross-lip flap described an almost V-shaped full-thickness flap of the corner of the lower lip based on the lower labial artery that was rotated into the upper lip. Nearly 100 years later, in 1872, Estlander described

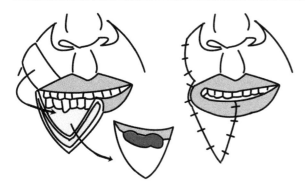

Estlander Flap, Fig. 1 Estlander cross-lip flap. A full-thickness wedge of tissue is rotated to repair a defect, that includes the commissure, in the opposite lip. The donor site is closed primarily. A new medialized commissure is created at the site of the pedicle

a single-stage cross-lip flap used to reconstruct a lateral defect that involved the oral commissure that was similar to that originally described by Hierzel (Tommaso 2009). The flap that Estlander described involved the transfer of a full-thickness flap that used a point of rotation at the commissure and a pedicle that remained attached and was incorporated into the reconstructed commissure (Fig. 1).

In 1837, prior to Estlander's description of a cross-lip flap, Sabittini detailed a lip reconstruction using a two-staged cross-lip flap to repair more central lip defects. Abbe was the first to describe a two-staged cross-lip flap in the English literature in 1898 and now has his name linked to this type of lip reconstruction. The Sabattini and Abbe cross-lip flaps were used for defects that did not involve the oral commissure, and therefore required a second stage to divide the pedicle and release the attached upper and lower lip.

Cross-lip flaps are pedicled flaps based off of the labial artery that are used to transfer composite labial tissues from the opposite lip. This allows for reconstruction of lip defects with the "like" tissue contained in the opposite lip. Cross-lip flaps may be used to reconstruct defects of the upper or lower lip. The cross-lip flap that was described by Hiertzel was a V-shaped full-thickness flap of the corner of the lower lip that was rotated into the upper lip. The flap described by Estlander involved the transfer of a triangular-shaped full-thickness segment of lip tissue from the upper lip to a full-thickness defect of the lower lip. In fact, there is more often a need to transfer a flap from the upper lip to reconstruct a defect of the lower lip,

where cancer occurs with greater frequency. Using the upper lip as a donor site is generally more challenging due to greater complexity of the upper lip anatomy. The effects on the complex upper lip anatomy should taken into account while planning for lower lip reconstruction with a cross-lip flap. This is less of a concern for laterally based Estlander-type cross-lip flaps since the anatomy of the lateral subunit of the upper lip is less complex than the medial subunit. However, it is important to note that the lateral subunit of the upper lip will be shortened as compared to the contralateral subunit when the upper lip is used as a donor site.

Whichever lip contains the defect, the donor flap is pedicled off of the labial artery of the opposite lip from the defect. The donor flap is pedicled medially off of supply from the contralateral labial artery. The newly created oral commissure starts at the pedicle on the lip opposite from the repaired defect. The anatomical basis of the Abbe-type cross-lip flap was studied by Schulte et al. (Schulte et al. 2001). The arterial anatomy that is discussed in this entry is important for Estlander flaps as well. Schulte described the location of the superior and inferior labial arteries as they course from lateral to medial. Laterally, near the oral commissure, the vessel may be as far as 1.5–2.5 cm from the free margin of the lip. Two other points were measured between the oral commissure and the midline, the area of the pedicle of most Estlander flaps, and the artery was noted to be as far as 1.5 cm from the free margin of the lip. At these points, the superior labial artery was within the vermilion 44% and 75% of the time. The inferior labial artery was within the vermilion 80% and 87% of the time. This data illustrates the importance of searching for the artery prior to reaching the vermilion as the vessel may lie outside of the vermilion. Careful dissection may then be continued to reduce the bulk of the pedicle allowing for greater rotation and closure of the donor site on the side of the pedicle. One must be careful to leave enough tissue around the pedicle to allow for adequate drainage through the small veins that parallel the course of the artery.

The donor flap may be designed as a triangular or "V"-shaped flap as originally described by Estlander, or may be modified to be shaped as a W, rectangle or other configurations depending on the shape of the defect. In general, the width of the donor flap is half the width of the recipient site. This allows for the two lips to remain proportionally similar in size after flap

Estlander Flap, Fig. 2 A representation of Buck's two flap closure of a central lower lip defect. A transposition flap is created from the lateral lower lip to close the central lower lip defect. The donor defect from the transposition flap is closed with an Estlander flap

transfer. When estimating the size of the defect, one should take into account the pull of the orbicularis oris on the wound edges, which will widen the appearance of the defect (McCarn and Park 2005). The height of the donor flap is generally the same height as the defect.

Baker (Renner 2007) described a modification of the triangular flap originally described by Estlander, which places the donor site scar within the melolabial crease (as shown in Fig. 1). This provides better scar camouflage of the donor site while still allowing for an easy pivot of the flap into the lower lip defect.

Techniques have also been described to incorporate an Estlander flap with other types of flaps to repair lip defects. Buck (Renner 2007) described a two flap reconstruction involving an Estlander cross-lip flap and a transposition flap to reconstruct a full-thickness defect of the central lower lip (Fig. 2). This type of reconstruction involved the transfer of the remaining lateral segment of the lower lip to reconstruct the central defect. The donor site from the transposition flap was then closed with an Estlander cross-lip flap from the upper lip.

One of the major drawbacks of the Estlander flap is the resultant microstomia and blunting of the oral commissure. A new commissure is created at the point of rotation, which is at the medially located pedicle on the lip opposite from the defect. The modiolus and the corresponding muscles that are lateral to the defect are rotated medially with the new commissure resulting in microstomia and rounding of the commissure. Although the Estlander flap allows for a one-stage reconstruction, patients will often require a secondary **commissuroplasty** in an attempt to

restore a more normal appearance of the blunted commissure. In fact, Hierzel (Vrebos et al. 1994) described performing "a final revision at the corner of the mouth."

Cross-lip flaps involve the transfer of full-thickness lip tissue, which includes the transfer of muscle that has been separated from its innervation from the donor lip. This results in a temporary denervation of the muscle and loss of the orbicularis oris sphincter function over the reconstructed portion of the lip. The function of the orbicularis sphincter generally returns to a near-normal with time. The first signs of motor reinnervation of the cross-lip flap begin to appear a few months after flap transfer and are demonstrated by irregular low-amplitude motor unit potentials (Renner 2007). By 1 year, the amplitude increases to a near-normal level. The quality of movement may vary from near-normal function to some degree of persistent weakness. Rarely patients may experience oral incompetence due to this weakness.

Cross-lip flaps will also sustain a temporary loss of sensation as well. In a study of denervated cross-lip flaps (Smith 1960), sensation returned in a few months, starting with pain sensation at 2 months, tactile sensation at 3 months, cold at 6 months, and warmth at 9 months.

Techniques

The full-thickness defect involving one third to two thirds of the upper or lower lip and also involving the oral commissure is assessed and determined to be amenable to a one-staged cross-lip reconstruction. Some defects may result in significant destruction of the orbicularis oris muscle, but portions of the muscle and mucosa remain. In these cases, the sphincter function has already been compromised and it is generally best to excise the remaining tissue and create a full-thickness defect. The lip can then be reconstructed with a full-thickness flap.

The defect is analyzed and flap size and shape is determined based on the defect. The defect template is created and then transferred to the opposing lip. In many cases, the defect will be a wedge, which will require a V-shaped flap. This flap is created to be half the width of the defect, which allows for equalization of the lip proportions after flap transfer. The donor flap for rectangular-shaped defects may be created as a "W" to minimize the length of the burrow triangle required to close the donor defect.

A full-thickness incision is created through the cutaneous portion of the lip on the nonpedicled side of the flap. The incision is carried through the vermilion and will meet up with the vermilion at the edge of the defect that is nearest to the flap. Next, a full-thickness incision is created on the pedicle side through the cutaneous portion of the lip, starting at the point away from the vermilion. The full-thickness incision is created toward the vermilion and it is stopped approximately 5 mm from the vermilion. A partial thickness incision through the skin is created to the vermilion at this point and careful, blunt dissection is carried through the muscle to the vermilion. If the artery is encountered, dissection is stopped and the flap is rotated into place. If the artery is not encountered and the vermilion is reached, the flap is rotated into place. The tissues surrounding the donor site may need to be undermined to close the defect.

The recipient site is closed in layers through the vermilion on the nonpedicle side. All layers are reapproximated including the mucosa, the muscle, and subcutaneous/cutaneous tissues. The donor site is closed upon itself and sutured in layers as well. The skin of the cheek lateral to the new commissure is then sutured to the vermilion at the new medialized commissure.

Conclusion

The Estlander flap describes a one-staged cross-lip flap that is used for reconstruction of full-thickness defects of the upper or lower lip measuring one third to two thirds the width of the lip. This pedicled flap is used for defects that involve the oral commissure. Although this is a single-staged reconstruction, the newly created commissure is medialized and often blunted, requiring a secondary commissuroplasty. The flap will usually regain motor and sensory innervation allowing for competent oral sphincter function.

Cross-References

▶ Abbe Flap
▶ Commissuroplasty
▶ Lip Reconstruction

References

McCarn KE, Park SS (2005) Lip reconstruction. Facial Plast Surg Clin North Am 13:301–314

Renner G (2007) Reconstruction of the lip. In: Baker S (ed) Local flaps in facial reconstruction. Elsevier, Philadelphia, pp 498–505

Schulte DL, Sherris DA, Kasperbauer JL (2001) The anatomical basis of the Abbe flap. Laryngoscope 111(3):382–386

Smith JW (1960) The anatomical and physiologic acclimatization of tissue transplanted by the lip switch technique. Plast Reconstr Surg 26:40

Tommaso A (2009) Reply to "the cross-lip flap from 1756 to 1898. Reply to 'the Sabattini-Abbe flap: a historical note'". Plast Reconstr Surg 124(2):666–667

Vrebos J, Dupuis C, Hierzel JG (1994) A lip-switch flap in 1756. Plast Reconstr Surg 93:201–204

Eustachian Tube Dysfunction

▶ Barotrauma and Decompression Sickness

Eustachian Tube, Anatomy and Physiology

Ojas A. Shah and Ravindhra G. Elluru
Department of Otolaryngology, Cincinnati Children's Hospital and University of Cincinnati College of Medicine, Cincinnati, OH, USA

Definitions

Eustachian tube – connects the middle ear and the nasopharynx and serves to equalize pressure, clear secretions, and protect the middle ear.

Introduction

The physiological status of the Eustachian tube (ET) is critical to the proper functioning of the middle ear and normal hearing. Therefore, it is essential to understand the factors that give rise to normal function of the ET: the anatomy and physiology of the Eustachian tube.

The ET is not just "a tube," but instead is a sophisticated organ whose function is intimately connected to surrounding structures. In general, the ET consists of a lumen with a mucosal surface, surrounding soft tissue, osseous and cartilaginous components, and associated musculature which will be described below.

Eustachius was the first known individual to attempt to describe the function of the Eustachian tube in the late fifteenth century. In the eighteenth century, Antonio Valsalva also attempted to categorize the function of the Eustachian tube while describing an insufflation technique of the middle ear. He is credited with giving the ET its name. In the nineteenth century, Carus and Rathke both published separate reports that the development of the Eustachian tube was related to the respiratory tract from the study of gills in fish and pig embryos, respectively. In the same century, Adam Politzer further advanced the technique of middle ear insufflation and developed a primitive middle ear ventilation tube.

Anatomy

The ET is located in the skull base and connects the middle ear cleft to the nasopharynx. The tube has an osseous component, located in the temporal bone, and a cartilaginous component, located in the nasopharynx. The ratio of the osseous to cartilaginous components of the ET varies with age. In adults, the osseous component is less than one third the total length of the tube.

The torus tubarius is a projection along the lateral wall of the nasopharynx which serves as the orifice of the ET. It is composed of cartilage with overlying soft tissue. The ET also abuts several different spaces and structures. Adenoid tissue, which is lymphoid tissue, is found just posterior and medial to the ET. The pharyngeal recess, otherwise known as the fossa of Rosenmuller, lies directly posterior and superior to the torus tubarius. Lymph nodes found in this region can be implicated in certain head and neck cancers, notably nasopharyngeal carcinoma.

The osseous ET originates in the tympanic mesotympanum just above the floor of the middle ear. At this location, the tube varies from 3 to 5 mm in diameter. The osseous ET then continues anteromedially in the petrous portion of the temporal bone where it is associated with several important structures. The carotid artery abuts the medial wall, the middle fossa dura the superior wall, and the glenoid fossa (containing the temporomandibular joint) the lateral wall. The osseous portion of the ET progressively narrows as it approaches the cartilaginous portion of the tube. At this point, the diameter of the tube is less than a millimeter in diameter.

The Eustachian tube reveals some differences from infancy to adulthood, which helps explain the increased incidence of otitis media in the pediatric population. The tube is longer in an adult compared to an infant, typically ranging from 31 to 38 mm in adulthood. The spatial orientation also changes from infancy to adulthood, transitioning from 10° to 45° in relation to the horizontal plane. It does appear that the ET reaches its adult length and orientation by 7 years of age.

Four muscles are in close association with the ET, assisting in its function. These muscles are the (1) tensor veli palatini, (2) levator veli palatini, (3) tensor tympani, and (4) salpingopharyngeus. The tensor veli palatini is a thin muscle that serves as the only dilator of the ET. It arises from three different locations and inserts via a tendon at the pterygoid hamulus. The origin sites for the muscle are the base of the medial pterygoid plate, the spina angularis of the sphenoid, and the lateral wall of the cartilaginous ET. The levator veli palatini is a thicker muscle in comparison to the tensor veli palatini. It also has multiple sites of origin, arising from the petrous portion of the temporal bone and the medial lamina of the cartilage of the ET. Laterally, each muscle arises above the superior pharyngeal constrictor muscle and then meets with the opposite muscle at the midline. The salpingopharyngeus muscle originates from the ET and extends inferiorly. Its role is unclear, and it may be involved in the opening of the ET with deglutination or yawning. The tensor tympani is located in a bony canal above the osseous ET. It originates from three different locations and inserts onto the manubrium of the malleus. The sites of origin of the tensor tympani are the cartilaginous portion of the ET, the greater wing of the sphenoid, and the attachments in the bony canal.

The arterial blood supply to the ET is different for the cartilaginous and osseous components. The internal maxillary artery, the ascending pharyngeal, and the ascending palatine artery supply the cartilaginous tube. The caroticotympanic artery from the internal carotid artery and a branch of the accessory meningeal artery supply the osseous portion of the tube. The venous drainage parallels the arterial supply. Sensory innervation of the ET similarly arises from multiple sources, including contributions from the otic ganglion, sphenopalatine nerve, and glossopharyngeal nerve.

Physiology

The ET is normally found to be closed, but opens during both voluntary and involuntary actions like swallowing and sneezing. The opening of the ET then permits the equalization of pressure in the nasopharynx (i.e., atmospheric pressure) and the pressure in the middle ear. The proper functioning of the Eustachian tube is critical to the health of the ear. It has three main physiologic functions: (1) pressure equalization, (2) drainage of secretions from the middle ear into the nasopharynx, and (3) protection from the nasopharyngeal environment.

1. *Pressure equalization.* The ET serves a critical function in equilibrating the ambient pressure in the nasopharynx and the middle ear. While at rest, the normal ET is collapsed and the ambient middle ear has a slightly negative pressure. Intermittent opening of the ET allows for bidirectional gas exchange that continues equilibration of the pressure. The pressure equalization function of the ET can be best illustrated by the example of flying on an aircraft. During takeoff and while ascending, a relatively positive pressure develops in the middle ear due to the decreasing atmospheric pressure. For most people, airflow proceeds through the tube causing an equilibration of pressure. However, during the descent the opposite pressure differential develops with a negative pressure in the middle ear and an increasing positive atmospheric pressure. The negative pressure keeps the ET orifice closed and leads to a blocked sensation in the ears. Most individuals with normal ET function are able to re-equilibrate the pressure by actions that dilate the tube by yawning, swallowing, or popping the ears. Defective functioning of the ET can lead to excessive negative pressure in the middle ear

causing a retraction of the tympanic membrane. In addition, excessively high negative pressure in the middle ear may lead to a buildup of fluid, which can become secondarily infected, leading to otitis media.

2. *Clearance of secretions.* The ET plays a vital role in the clearance of secretions from the middle ear to the nasopharynx. The movement of secretions through the tube requires coordination of the cilia that line the surface of the tube. Movement of secretions into the tympanic segment of the ET is an active process as the ET orifice lies above the floor of the hypotympanum. Viral and bacterial infections are suspected to disrupt mucociliary clearance by affecting the function of the cilia. Although the mechanisms of viral and bacterial pathogenesis are different, normal return to function can take up to a month after the clearance of an infection.

3. *Middle ear protection.* The ET serves as a barrier protecting the middle ear from microorganisms and the relatively insterile environment of the nasopharynx. The tubal mucosa secretes various antimicrobial substances including lactoferrin and lysozyme that serve as intrinsic defenses against microbial migration. In addition, the lymphoid tissue associated with the tube serves another immunologic function. Surfactant proteins may also play in role in protecting the middle ear. Besides helping keep the ET open, the surfactant proteins are believed to be 'anti-inflammatory and promote phagocytosis. The ET also plays a role in the protection of the middle and inner ear from sound generated from the larynx and the pharynx. The coordinated contraction of the tube seals the transmission of this sound. In addition, the opening of the ET dissipates sound entering the external auditory canal from complete transmission to the middle and inner ear. The ET also serves the function of protecting the middle ear from the nasopharyngeal airflow. Excessively patulous ETs are unable to prevent this airflow, which causes movement of the tympanic membrane with every breath. The middle ear protection function of the ET has been well illustrated in "the flask model" by Bluestone. In this model, the orifice and the neck represent the nasopharyngeal opening and the ET, and the bulbous portion

represents the mastoid and the middle ear. Bluestone used this model to demonstrate that a shorter ET or a hole in the tympanic membrane predisposes toward reflux of nasopharyngeal secretions into the middle ear.

Evaluation of the ET

Assessment of ET function always starts with a thorough history and physical. The most common complaints related to the ET are fullness or pain in the ears, which may be associated with dizziness, tinnitus, and/or hearing loss. These symptoms are frequently not relieved by actions that dilate the ET like swallowing or yawning.

On physical examination, a noncompliant tympanic membrane on pneumatic otoscopy is concerning for ET dysfunction. Further evaluation of the ET orifice in the nasopharynx can be performed with rigid or flexible fiber-optic endoscopy. Pathologic states such as edema secondary to infection, or obstruction secondary to adenoid hypertrophy or tumor can be seen. It is to be noted that a new unilateral concern for ET dysfunction is an indication for nasal endoscopy to rule out malignancy. Recently smaller sub-centimeter endoscopes have also been used to evaluate the ET itself.

Along with pneumatic otoscopy, the Valsalva and Toynbee maneuver can be used to qualitatively assess ET function. Both of these tests require pinching the nose; the Valsalva requires blowing out with a closed mouth while the Toynbee requires a swallow. Normally, these tests demonstrate an alteration in the middle ear pressure that stabilizes to ambient pressure indicative of normal ET function.

Sonotubometry is another method to assess the function of the ET. In this test, a sound is applied to the nostril and a microphone is placed in the external auditory canal. The sound pressure in the canal can be used to assess the patency of the ET. Audiometric evaluation can also be used to evaluate the function of the ET. A tympanogram can be obtained separately or as a part of an audiogram. It provides a quantitative assessment of the compliance of the tympanic membrane, and can thereby indirectly assess the function of the ET. A type A tympanogram is consistent with normal compliance of the tympanic membrane.

A type B tympanogram reveals a flat tracing and is consistent with a noncompliant tympanic membrane. A type C tympanogram demonstrates a negative pressure in the middle ear.

Conclusion

The Eustachian tube is an anatomic entity that is critical in the functioning of the middle ear. An understanding of the ET requires an understanding of the surrounding structures and the underlying physiologic considerations that affect its functioning. Anatomically, the ET is composed of an osseous and cartilaginous component, and is intimately associated with the middle ear, the nasopharynx, and associated muscles that play a role in its opening. Age also plays a role in the length and orientation of the tube. The ET has the functions of pressure equalization, clearance of secretions, and middle ear protection.

References

Bluestone CD (2004) Studies in otitis media: children's hospital of Pittsburgh – University of Pittsburgh progress report. Laryngoscope 114:1–26

Bluestone CD (2006) Anatomy and physiology of the eustachian tube system. In: Bailey BJ (ed) Baileys head and neck surgery – otolaryngology, 4th edn. Lippincott Williams & Wilkins, Philadelphia, pp 1253–1264

Bluestone CD, Doyle WJ (1998) Anatomy and physiology of eustachian tube and middle ear related to otitis media. J Allergy Clin Immunol 81:997–1003

Hughes GB, Pensak ML (2007) Clinical otology, 3rd edn. Thieme, New York

Northrop C, Piza J, Eavey RD (1996) Histological observations of amniotic fluid cellular content in the ear of neonates and infants. Int J Pediatr Otolaryngol 11:113–127

Persaud R, Hajioff D, Trinidade A et al (2007) Evidence-based review of aetiopathogenic theories of congenital and acquired cholesteatoma. J Laryngol Otol 121:1013–1019

Proctor B (1967) Embryology and anatomy of the eustachian tube. Arch Otolaryngol 86:51–62

Reilly RC, Sando I (2010) The eustachian tube. In: Flint PW (ed) Cummings otolaryngology: head and neck surgery, 5th edn. Mosby, Philadelphia, pp 1866–1875

Seibert JW, Danner CJ (2006) Eustachian tube function and the middle ear. Otolaryngol Clin North Am 39:1221–1235

Takasaki K, Takahashi H, Miyamoto I et al (2007) Measurement of angle and length of the eustachian tube on computed tomography using multiplanar reconstruction technique. Laryngoscope 117:1251–1254

Evidence-Based Medicine and Clinical Outcomes Research

Zachary M. Soler[1] and Timothy L. Smith[2]
[1]Department of Otolaryngology-Head and Neck Surgery, Medical University of South Carolina, Charleston, SC, USA
[2]Oregon Sinus Center, Department of Otolaryngology-Head and Neck Surgery, Oregon Health and Science University, Portland, OR, USA

Definition

Evidence-Based Medicine

Evidence-based medicine (EBM) is a set of principles and methods intended to ensure that to the greatest extent possible, medical decisions, guidelines, and policies are based on and consistent with good evidence of effectiveness and benefit (Eddy 2005).

Overview

The definition of EBM given above encompasses both clinical decisions for the individual patient and decision-making on a broader group level. The former has been referred to as evidence-based individual decision-making (EBID) and has been defined by Sackett et al. as the "conscientious, explicit, and judicious use of current best evidence in making decisions about the care of individual patients" (Sackett et al. 2000). In practice, this involves integrating the physician's clinical appreciation of the current medical problem, the specific patient's treatment preferences, and the best available evidence. EBM also involves decisions that occur on a broader, group level, as might occur with public health practices or policy coverage decisions. Group level guidelines and policies are by necessity generic but nonetheless are often informative for individual decision-making, as they represent rich sources of aggregated evidence. Regardless of its setting, the defining feature of EBM is a focus on rigorous, scientific research as the foundation of medical decision-making.

Brief History

"Evidence-based. . ." became a catch phrase in the 1990s, and the focus on evidence in medicine persists to the present. The introduction of EBM was spurred by important research findings which questioned the manner by which medical decisions were being made. Traditional medical decision-making was considered an art form, which arose from the rigors of medical training, journal readership, and clinical experience. This view assumes that the physician is able to appropriately synthesize individual pieces of information into a cohesive and logical framework for decision-making. However, research in the 1970s and 1980s began to call into question the validity of this practice. Studies showed that physician' practice patterns diverged in significant ways, without appropriate justification (Geyman et al. 2000). The origin of common practices was often traced back to expert opinion that had been forged over many years without any substantive evidentiary basis. Additionally, the volume and complexity of existing information surpassed that which could be readily acquired and organized by any individual physician. These issues, in concert with the exponential rise in medical costs, drew widespread attention to a heretofore underappreciated problem (Manchikanti 2008).

At the same time as traditional medical practices were called into question, new methodological techniques were developed to acquire, analyze, and organize medical research findings. These methods included an emphasis on randomized clinical trials, the development of meta-analytic techniques, and advances in technologically driven data management and access (McGovern et al. 2001). A 25-part series, entitled "Users Guide to the Medical Literature," was published by JAMA between 1993 and 2000, helping to highlight these issues and catalyze the transformation toward EBM (Guyatt 1993). Since this time, many influential programs have been established, including the Cochrane Collaboration, the Agency for Healthcare Research and Quality (AHRQ), and formal incorporation of EBM into existing medical curricula. The result has been the general acceptance that clinical experience, pathophysiologic rationale, and tradition alone are not sufficient for medical decision-making. Instead, the principals of EBM explicitly mandate that rigorous clinical evidence serve as the foundation for all decisions, in concert with individual circumstances and patient values (Hamer 2005).

Evidence-Based Individual Decision-Making (EBID)

Every patient encountered by a physician is unique with regard to history, presenting signs/symptoms, and individual preferences. Therefore, a strict "cookbook" application of rules or guidelines is unlikely to optimize outcomes and represents a mischaracterization of EBM (Sackett et al. 1996). Instead, the principals of EBM can be utilized to arrive at an individually informed decision that maximizes available research evidence, clinical expertise, and individual patient preferences (Gray 2001).

The practice of EBID within the clinical setting consists of four steps which can be explicitly outlined (Sackett et al. 2000). The initial step involves developing a clinically relevant question, whose answer provides the information which is unknown and/or critical to the problem at hand. The question may pertain to treatment of a specific disease, prevention strategies, or diagnostic considerations. Although this step may seem straightforward, considerable general knowledge, experience, and acumen contribute to proper formulation of the relevant question. In many ways, the traditional concept of the "art of medicine" applies to this step, in that the expert physicians are able to separate signal from noise and focus on the relevant issue(s) at hand.

The second step involves searching for and identifying the available research which pertains to the question of interest. In the third step, the evidence must be critically evaluated, with greater importance given to those studies adhering to methodologies which allow the strongest conclusions. The quality of evidence can be graded with respect to internal and external validity and overall effect size. Internal validity represents the likelihood that the study findings reflect actual truth. Criteria for internal validity vary by study design, but principles such as control groups, randomization, blinding, and intention-to-treat minimize the risk of systematic biases (McGovern et al. 2001). Only after internal validity is ensured can one consider the study's external validity. External validity refers to the extent to which the study findings are generalizable to the

individual patient or circumstance of interest. If a study's inclusion/exclusion criteria are such that the study population differs substantially from the patient of clinical interest, then the study may not be applicable regardless of its internal validity.

The final step involves integrating the best available evidence with the patient's unique circumstance and preferences to arrive at the optimal decision. Although evidence from research studies serves as the foundation, the final decision should be customized to each encounter. A paradigm is thus formed whereby the clinician and patient together arrive at a decision which best optimizes the clinical outcomes of interest.

Identification of Evidence

Technological advancements have greatly simplified the search for and retrieval of medical information. In the past, a literature review for a pressing clinical question might consist of thumbing through a previously purchased textbook or archive of medical journals. Today, a vast quantity of information is readily retrievable from electronic databases. Abstracts of original research are available from PubMed and EMBASE via straightforward search strategies, with full-length articles available electronically in many instances. Given the abundance of primary research, it may prove inefficient to review all available studies for each and every question that arises. In these instances, secondary review databases are available, including the Cochrane Database of Systemic Reviews, the York Database of Abstracts of Reviews of Effectiveness (DARE), the American College of Physicians Physicians' Information and Education Resource (ACP PIER), and Dynamed. Evidence-based guidelines can also be found online at sites such as the National Guidelines Clearinghouse, which is maintained by the AHRQ.

Ranking of Evidence

Quite often, a primary literature search will return numerous sources of information directly or indirectly related to the topic of interest. A principle component of EBM is the rigorous evaluation and grading of the available evidence (Geyman et al. 2000). This is

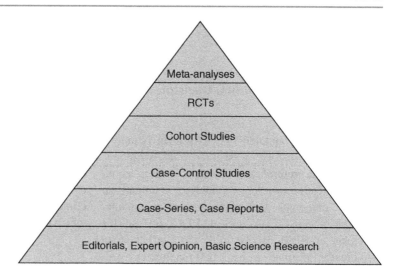

Evidence-Based Medicine and Clinical Outcomes Research, Fig. 1 Hierarchy of evidence provided by individual study designs. *RCT* randomized controlled trial

especially important when findings qualitatively disagree among studies. The underlying concept is that all study designs are not created equal. Instead, a hierarchy of evidence exists, and the evidence inherent in any given study must be weighted by its overall quality (Fig. 1).

Several different methodologies exist for ranking or grading the quality of a study. Some of the most widely utilized algorithms include the Center for Evidence-Based Medicine (CEBM) Levels of Evidence (Table 1), the United States Preventive Service Task Force (USPSTF) Levels of Evidence (Table 2), and the Grading of Recommendations Assessment, Development and Evaluation (GRADE) approach (Guyatt et al. 2008). The rank or grade of a study is usually closely associated with the overall study design, with specific study designs felt to confer a greater likelihood of validity than others. Although overall study design is important, additional factors contribute to the quality of a study, such as the rigor with which the study was actually carried out and the generalizability of the study to the patient of immediate clinical interest.

Study Design

In Vitro Experiments, Animal Research

Although considered "low-level" evidence, basic science experimentation is a fundamental component of medical research. These experiments often establish the underlying pathophysiologic and therapeutic

mechanisms and provide the initial proof of concept needed to begin human experimentation. However, extrapolating in vitro or animal findings to humans is rarely straightforward and often misleading without additional confirmatory research.

Editorial, Expert Opinion

The opinion of medical experts and consensus panels continues to be influential in shaping medical practice. Ideally, expert opinion would be grounded within the available evidence. However, situations arise where there is a lack of available evidence, such as during outbreaks of new infectious diseases. In circumstances where evidence does not exist, is flawed, or entirely conflicting, the opinion of clinicians experienced in the field may serve as the best available evidence.

Case Reports, Case Series

Reports of individual cases or series of cases continue to represent a rich source of medical information, especially when a disease process is rare or a novel therapeutic option is described. In these situations, larger more rigorous study methodologies are not yet feasible and may never be done. Case series might then provide the only source of information, and in cases of new diseases, the impetus for further research and exploration.

Case–Control Studies

Case–control studies are ideally suited to study rare disease outcomes. When a disease has a low incidence,

Evidence-Based Medicine and Clinical Outcomes Research, Table 1 Oxford centre for evidence-based medicine levels of evidence

Level	Therapy/prevention, aetiology/harm	Prognosis	Diagnosis	Differential diagnosis/ symptom prevalence study	Economic and decision analyses
1a	SR (with homogeneity*) of RCT	SR (with homogeneity*) of inception cohort studies; CDR† validated in different populations	SR (with homogeneity*) of Level 1 diagnostic studies; CDR† with 1b studies from different clinical centres	SR (with homogeneity*) of prospective cohort studies	SR (with homogeneity*) of Level 1 economic studies
1b	Individual RCT (with narrow Confidence Interval‡)	Individual inception cohort study with >80% follow-up; CDR† validated in a single population	Validating** cohort study with good††† reference standards; or CDR† tested within one clinical centre	Prospective cohort study with good follow-up****	Analysis based on clinically sensible costs or alternatives; systematic review(s) of the evidence; and including multi-way sensitivity analyses
1c	All or none§	All or none case-series	Absolute SpPins and SnNouts††	All or none case-series	Absolute better-value or worse-value analyses†††††
2a	SR (with homogeneity*) of cohort studies	SR (with homogeneity*) of either retrospective cohort studies or untreated control groups in RCTs	SR (with homogeneity*) of Level >2 diagnostic studies	SR (with homogeneity*) of 2b and better studies	SR (with homogeneity*) of Level >2 economic studies
2b	Individual cohort study (including low quality RCT; e.g., <80% follow-up)	Retrospective cohort study or follow-up of untreated control patients in an RCT; Derivation of CDR† or validated on split-samples§§§ only	Exploratory** cohort study with good††† reference standards; CDR† after derivation, or validated only on split-sample§§§ or databases	Retrospective cohort study, or poor follow-up	Analysis based on clinically sensible costs or alternatives; limited review(s) of the evidence, or single studies; and including multi-way sensitivity analyses
2c	"Outcomes" research; Ecological studies	"Outcomes" research		Ecological studies	Audit or outcomes research
3a	SR (with homogeneity*) of case–control studies		SR (with homogeneity*) of 3b and better studies	SR (with homogeneity*) of 3b and better studies	SR (with homogeneity*) of 3b and better studies
3b	Individual case–control study		Non-consecutive study; or without consistently applied reference standards	Non-consecutive cohort study, or very limited population	Analysis based on limited alternatives or costs, poor quality estimates of data, but including sensitivity analyses incorporating clinically sensible variations
4	Case-series (and poor quality cohort and case–control studies§§)	Case-series (and poor quality prognostic cohort studies***)	Case–control study, poor or non-independent reference standard	Case-series or superseded reference standards	Analysis with no sensitivity analysis
5	Expert opinion without explicit critical appraisal, or based on physiology, bench research or "first principles"	Expert opinion without explicit critical appraisal, or based on physiology, bench research or "first principles"	Expert opinion without explicit critical appraisal, or based on physiology, bench research or "first principles"	Expert opinion without explicit critical appraisal, or based on physiology, bench research or "first principles"	Expert opinion without explicit critical appraisal, or based on economic theory or "first principles"

Produced by Bob Phillips, Chris Ball, Dave Sackett, Doug Badenoch, Sharon Straus, Brian Haynes, and Martin Dawes since November 1998. Updated by Jeremy Howick March 2009 (For definitions of terms used, see glossary at http://www.cebm.net/?o=1116)

Evidence-Based Medicine and Clinical Outcomes Research, Table 2 United States Preventive Services Task Force Levels of Evidence

Level of evidence	Study design
I	Properly powered and conducted randomized controlled trial (RCT); well-conducted systematic review or meta-analysis of homogeneous RCTs
II-1	Well-designed controlled trial without randomization
II-2	Well-designed cohort or case–control analytic study
II-3	Multiple time series with or without the intervention; dramatic results from uncontrolled experiments
III	Opinions of respected authorities, based on clinical experience; descriptive studies or case reports; reports of expert committees

prospectively enrolling and following a nondiseased cohort in hopes of observing cases is inefficient. Instead, cases can be identified after they present and then analyzed in comparison to a control group without the disease of interest. The prevalence of exposure can then be compared, allowing some inference regarding the exposure-disease relationship. The main drawback of case–control studies is that exposure history is most often obtained in a retrospective fashion. Retrospective assessment of exposure status (and other covariates) can introduce bias which can significantly affect the study's validity. Furthermore, directly controlling for unidentified confounding factors is not possible.

Cohort Studies

Cohort studies involve enrolling a group of patients and following their progress over time. Exposure status and relevant covariates can be assessed at baseline, before disease status or outcome is known, eliminating an important source of bias possibly present in case–control studies. Covariates that might cause confounding can also be assessed and controlled for in subsequent data analysis, although unmeasured confounding might still exist.

Randomized Clinical Trials

Clinical trials which employ randomization are considered the highest quality individual study design. The process of assigning treatment by a random

process ensures that factors which might confound the treatment-outcome relationship are equally allocated to each group. Although many possible confounders are still measured, it is the random allocation of unmeasured confounders (that may not have been appreciated) that separates RCTs from lower level studies. In most situations, evidence from a well-conducted, large RCT will supersede evidence from expert opinion, case series, and observational studies (Hamer 2005).

Systematic Review +/− Meta-Analysis

A systematic review brings together the available evidence on a topic in a methodical and transparent fashion. The search algorithm, inclusion/exclusion criteria, and critical assessment strategy are explicitly prespecified to guard against author bias and allow reproducibility (Crowther et al. 2010). The formalized structure of a systematic review contrasts with the narrative review style used historically. Narrative reviews lack formal methodology and can easily be shaped by the authors' opinion and agenda. The reader is often unable to appreciate why some studies are discussed and others unmentioned.

The pinnacle of evidence is thought to be systematic reviews of multiple, large RCTs (Geyman et al. 2000). If the RCTs are sufficiently homogenous, then the estimated effects of individual studies can be pooled via meta-analytic techniques to arrive at an overall effect estimate with great precision (Fig. 2). The most informative systematic reviews often include both RCTs and observational study designs. Sensitivity analysis can then be done such that the reader can appreciate the effect of inclusion/exclusion of specific studies and/or study designs.

Study Quality

The quality of a study is not determined solely by its overall design. The largest RCT may be substantially flawed in its design and execution such that its results carry little or no validity. The critical components of a valid RCT include but are not limited to randomization, blinding (patients, physicians/assessors), and intention-to-treat analysis (Sibbald 1998). As previously mentioned, randomization assures that confounding factors are equally allocated between treatment groups, eliminating an important source of

Evidence-Based Medicine and Clinical Outcomes Research, Fig. 2 Forest plot describing meta-analysis of six RCTs comparing budesonide to placebo for nasal polyposis
Figure reprinted with permission from Joe et al. (2008)

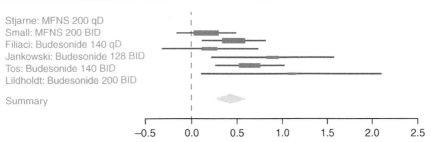

Difference in Mean Changes in Polyp Size Score between Treatment and Placebo Groups

bias. Blinding also assures that knowledge of treatment group does not systematically influence the results. An intention-to-treat analysis protocol ensures that all patients are analyzed with the group to which they were initially allocated, regardless of whether they switched protocols (drop-out /drop-in). The Consolidated Standards of Reporting Trials (CONSORT) 2010 statement is a 25-item checklist designed to ensure the proper reporting of parallel-group RCTs (Schulz et al. 2010). Trials which report results in accordance with CONSORT will have sufficient detail such that their quality can be readily ascertained.

Just as RCTs can vary in quality, systematic reviews can be performed with varying degrees of rigor. The pooling of data can result in impressively precise results, but the validity of these estimates is only as good as the soundness of the underlying data and rigor in which it was synthesized. In some situations, the data may not be of sufficient quality or homogeneity to pool via meta-analysis. Similar to the CONSORT, standards exist for reporting systematic reviews. The PRIMSA statement is an evidence-based minimum set of items for reporting in systematic reviews and meta-analyses (Moher et al. 2010). Although it is not a quality assessment instrument, the items required by PRIMSA will allow the quality of the analyses to be readily determined.

Study Quality in Otolaryngology

The adoption of EBM techniques has led to steady improvements in the quality of available medical research, including evidence in the field of otolaryngology. A longitudinal analysis of published studies in leading otolaryngology journals between 1993 and 2003 was performed by Rosenfeld (Wasserman et al. 2006). This study showed a steady increase in the quality of studies, including increased sample sizes, use of control groups, and reporting of p-values and confidence intervals. Although the quality of evidence increased with time, the majority of studies were still of low quality (level 4). This was especially true for studies evaluating therapeutic interventions. A similar study by the same author indicated that 80% of the therapeutic recommendations in otolaryngology journals were based on descriptive case series and only 7% utilized randomized controlled trials (Bentsianov et al. 2002). Although this data is now dated, the need for high-level evidence within otolaryngology remains.

Evidence-Based Guidelines

Clinical practice guidelines are systematically developed statements which evaluate the available medical evidence related to a specific topic and provide summary recommendations based upon that evidence. These instruments are most often developed and supported by the governing bodies such as the AHRQ or specialty bodies such as the American Academy of Otolaryngology-Head and Neck Surgery (AAO-HNS). Evidence-based guidelines are unique in that they developed via an explicit, multidisciplinary process which stresses transparency and flexibility. The available evidence is appraised for its quality based upon the above schema and evaluated with regard to its applicability to the clinical population of interest. Recommendations based upon the evidence are then suggested, with value judgments clearly articulated. Inherent within guidelines are the assumption that individual patients and clinical situations may not

Evidence-Based Medicine and Clinical Outcomes Research, Table 3 AAO-HNS levels of recommendation for clinical practice guidelines

Aggregate evidence quality	Preponderance of benefit or harm	Balance of benefit and harm
A. Well-designed RCTs or diagnostic studies on relevant populations with minor limitations; highly consistent evidence from observational studies	Strong recommendation	Option
B. RCTs or diagnostic studies with minor limitations; highly consistent evidence from observational studies	Recommendation	Option
C. Observational studies, case control and cohort design	Recommendation	Option
D. Expert opinion, case reports, reasoning from first principles	Option	No recommendation
X. Exceptional situations where validating studies cannot be performed and there is a clear preponderance of benefit or harm	Recommendation or strong recommendation	

Source: Rosenfeld and Shiffman (2009)

precisely fit into the framework of the guideline, and thus, a guideline is not a substitute for sound clinical judgment.

The AAO-HNS has been endorsing clinical practice guidelines since 2006 using a formal development process. These guidelines are typically published in the academy's journal and also are available publicly at www.entnet.org. In addition to specific guidelines, a manual is provided to direct guideline development as well as an e-mail address where topics can be suggested for consideration by the Guideline Development Task Force (Rosenfeld 2009). Guidelines pertaining to head and neck cancer can also be found at the National Comprehensive Cancer Network. Perhaps, the largest collection of otolaryngology-related guidelines can be found at the National Guideline Clearinghouse, a database maintained by the AHRQ.

Grades of Recommendation

Guidelines are useful not only as a source of evidence but as a critical synthesis of that evidence toward a therapeutic recommendation. Just as several systems exist to evaluate levels of evidence, different methods exist to grade the strength of recommendations. Perhaps, the most popular is an A-I format suggested by the USPSTF (Guirquis-Blake et al. 2007). The strength of recommendations endorsed by the AAO-HNS includes "strong recommendation," "recommendation," "option," "recommend against," and "strongly recommend against" (Table 3). A strong recommendation means the benefits of the recommended approach clearly exceed the harms

(or, in the case of a strong negative recommendation, that the harms clearly exceed the benefits) and that the quality of the supporting evidence is excellent (Grade A or B). Therefore, recommendations incorporate not only the soundness of the underlying evidence but also a balance between risk and benefits. Although judgment is required during the course of guideline development, these judgments should be made in a transparent fashion so that the reader can easily understand the value trade-offs involved.

Definition

Clinical Outcomes Research

Outcomes research has been defined as a multidisciplinary field of inquiry, both basic and applied, that examines the use, costs, quality, accessibility, delivery, organization, financing, and outcomes of health-care services to increase the knowledge and understanding of health services for individuals and populations (Institute of Medicine 1990).

Overview

Clinical outcomes research seeks to formally measure, understand, and improve the impact of health-care interventions on the health outcomes of individual patients and patient populations. Outcomes research focuses on those endpoints which patients are most likely to experience and care about. For chronic illnesses in particular, quality of life (QOL) and mortality are often the primary endpoints which capture the benefits most important to patients with regard to any particular intervention. By incorporating rigorous scientific methodologies, outcomes research serves as an important source of evidence useful in clinical decision-making.

The definition given above highlights the comprehensive nature of outcomes research. For clinicians and patients, outcomes research provides evidence regarding risks, benefits, and results of treatment. However, outcomes research encompasses more than just evidence of health benefit for a particular intervention. Outcomes research also examines associated costs and logistical realities that influence accessibility and utilization. In this regard, outcomes research can include pragmatic trials which emphasize real-world outcomes of medical interventions. This source of evidence is highly informative for physicians, payers, and policymakers who must make decisions regarding not only individual patients but entire populations of patients.

Endpoints of Outcomes Research

Primary Clinical Endpoints

All research endeavors measure and evaluate specific endpoints in order to make inference regarding the effectiveness of an intervention. A traditional efficacy study of an antihypertensive medication might utilize change in systolic blood pressure in millimeters of mercury as an endpoint. However, outcomes research would focus instead on an endpoint that is felt to be "clinically relevant." A clinically important endpoint would be an outcome measure considered important by the patient receiving the treatment. In the case of an antihypertensive, change in systolic blood pressure is of little importance to an individual patient. Instead, they are much more likely to care about changes in the risk of stroke, vision changes, or death irrespective of its effect on blood pressure (Fleming 1996). Additionally, a patient would care if the drug of interest affects their overall QOL, which might encompass side effects of the drug, costs, and overall inconvenience.

The appropriate clinical endpoint for an outcomes study will by necessity vary based on the disease of interest and the overall goal of the study. Taking chronic rhinosinusitis (CRS) as an example, there are numerous endpoints that one could consider to measure outcomes after an intervention. An endpoint such as mortality would be of considerable interest to the patient but makes little sense since CRS is rarely a life-threatening condition. One might consider using changes in computed tomography (CT) scans as a primary endpoint; however, one could argue that change in CT findings are not of particular concern to the individual patient. The same argument could be made against a molecular endpoint, such as change in expression of a mucosal inflammatory marker. Currently, most outcomes of CRS focus on QOL changes after an intervention such as medical therapy or endoscopic sinus surgery (Soler 2010). Evaluating changes in overall QOL, such as with the Short-Form 36 instrument, allows global evaluation using a metric which captures health changes relevant to the individual patient. Disease-specific QOL instruments have also been developed, including the Rhinosinusitis Disability Index (RSDI), the Chronic Sinusitis Survey (CSS), and the Sinonasal Outcomes Test-22 (SNOT-22). The CRS-specific instruments capture QOL aspects most likely to be affected by those with CRS. These instruments have been formally designed such that they validly and reliably measure the QOL of patients with CRS (Linder 2004). In many cases, researchers have identified values which indicate the minimal clinically important difference (MCID) for each scale (Beaton et al. 2002). Outcomes studies after sinus surgery have shown that patients demonstrate statistically significant and clinically relevant improvements in general and CRS-specific QOL.

Surrogate Endpoints

In many diseases, measuring the clinical endpoints most important to patients can be time-consuming, expensive, and require significant sample sizes. This is especially true for diseases that have rare but critically important outcomes, such as mortality, stroke, or myocardial infarction. In these circumstances, researcher would prefer to measure surrogate endpoints rather than the actual clinical endpoint. An example would be assessing the presence/absence of rash as a surrogate for antitumor activity of epidermal growth factor receptor (EGFR) inhibitors in head and neck cancer. If rash was a true surrogate, than patients responding to EGFR inhibitors could be identified quickly and easily as compared to those not responding. The surrogate marker would thus allow rapid decision-making, as opposed to following a patient for many years to assess the ultimate outcome of interest (mortality). To justify use of surrogate markers in outcome studies (whose focus is on clinically relevant endpoints), a specific set of criteria must be satisfied, as outlined by Prentice (1989). In short, (1) the experimental treatment must have a significant impact on the true clinical endpoint, (2) the experimental treatment must have a significant impact on the proposed surrogate endpoint, (3) the surrogate endpoint must have a significant impact on the true endpoint, and (4) the full effect of the intervention on the true endpoint must be captured by the surrogate endpoint. The reality is that this set of criteria is very hard to satisfy, and thus, it is rare that surrogate markers are valid substitutes for true clinical endpoints in outcomes research.

Using CRS as an example again, CT scan findings might serve as a surrogate for long-term QOL changes after surgical intervention. Studies have shown that patients with CRS have worse CT scores and that CT scores do improve after surgery (Smith et al. 2010). However, the correlation between QOL and CT scores is low (Hopkins et al. 2007). Thus, some patients with significant QOL impairment have relatively little disease on CT scan and vice versa. The result is that CT scan findings after treatment are a poor proxy for QOL changes and thus not an excellent surrogate marker.

Study Designs in Outcomes Research

The same basic study designs utilized in traditional medical research are applicable to outcomes research, with specific emphasis on clinically relevant endpoints as described above. The basic construct of an RCT can still be employed, but these are often done in a pragmatic fashion. Pragmatic trials seek to evaluate the efficacy of a treatment as it exists in real-world applications (Roland 1998). Whereas a traditional RCT would strictly control inclusion/exclusion criteria to optimize homogeneity, a pragmatic trial would seek to enroll all patients that typically utilize the treatment of interest. Pragmatic trials often have simple designs with fewer variables but make up for these deficiencies with large sample sizes.

Many outcomes studies are primarily concerned with the cost-effectiveness of a given diagnostic strategy or therapeutic regimen. With health-care expenditures increasing in the United States, the US Congress passed the Health Care and Education

Reconciliation Act of 2010. This law established a nonprofit corporation known as the Patient-Centered Outcome Research Institute, whose purpose is to "assist patients, clinicians, purchasers, and policymakers in making informed health decisions" (Clancy 2010). This emphasis on comparative effectiveness is likely to continue for the foreseeable future given the rising costs of health care and limited resources available.

Conclusion

EBM has become an entrenched philosophy within the fabric of Western medicine. Although initially resisted by some, EBM is now embraced as a methodology that adds additional validity and efficacy to the art of medicine. The current emphasis on outcomes research has also placed renewed focus on clinically relevant outcomes of primary importance to patients. As health-care dollars are forced to stretch further and further, it will remain imperative that medical practice be based on solid evidence with proven comparative effectiveness.

References

Beaton D, Boers M, Wells G (2002) Many faces of the minimal clinically important difference (MCID): a literature review and directions for future research. Curr Opin Rheumatol 14:109–114

Bentsianov B, Boruk M, Rosenfeld R (2002) Evidence-based medicine in otolaryngology journals. Otolaryngol Head Neck Surg 126:371–376

Clancy C, Collins F (2010) Patient-centered outcomes research institute: the intersection of science and health care. Sci Transl Med 37:37

Crowther M, Lim W, Crowther M (2010) Systematic review and meta-analysis methodology. Blood 116:3140–3146

Eddy D (2005) Evidence-based medicine: a unified approach. Health Aff 24:9–17

Fleming T, Demets D (1996) Surrogate end points in clinical trials: are we being misled? Ann Intern Med 125:605–613

Geyman J, Deyo R, Ramsey S (2000) Evidence-based clinical practice: concepts and approaches. Butterworth Heinemann, Woburn

Gray J (2001) Evidence-based healthcare: how to make health policy and management decisions. Churchill Livingstone, London

Guirquis-Blake J, Calonge N, Miller T, Siu A, Teutsch S, Whitlock E (2007) Current processes of the US Preventive Services Task Force: refining evidence-based recommendation development. Ann Intern Med 147:117–122

Guyatt G, Rennie D (1993) Users' guides to the medical literature. JAMA 270:2096–2097

Guyatt G, Oxman A, Vist G, Kunz R, Falck-Ytter Y,
Schunemann H (2008) Grade: what is "quality of evidence"
and why is it important to clinicians? BMJ 336:995–998

Hamer S, Collinson G (2005) Achieving evidence-based practice: a handbook for practitioners. Bailliere Tindall,
Endinburgh

Hopkins C, Browne J, Slack R, Lund V, Brown P (2007) The
Lund-Mackay staging system for chronic rhinosinusitis: how
is it used and what does it predict? Otolaryngol Head Neck
Surg 137:555–561

Institute of Medicine committee to design a strategy for quality
review and assurance in Medicare (1990) Medicare:
a strategy for quality assurance. National Academy Press,
Washington, DC

Joe SA, Thambi R, Huang J (2008) A systematic review of the
use of intranasal steroids in the treatment of chronic
rhinosinusitis. Otolaryngol Head Neck Surg 139:340–347

Linder J, Atlas S (2004) Health-related quality of life in patients
with sinusitis. Curr Allergy Asthma Rep 4:490–495

Manchikanti L (2008) Evidence-based medicine, systematic
reviews, and guidelines in interventional pain management,
part 1: introduction and general considerations. Pain Physician 11:161–186

McGovern D, Valori R, Summerskill W, Levi M (2001) Key
topics in evidence-based medicine. Bios Scientific, Oxford

Moher D, Liberati A, Tetzlaff J, Altman D, The PRISMA Group
(2010) Preferred reporting items for systematic reviews and
meta-analyses: The PRISMA statement. Int J Surg 8:
336–341, DOI:dx.doi.org

Prentice R (1989) Surrogate endpoints in clinical trials: definition and operational criteria. Stat Med 8:431–440

Roland M, Torgerson D (1998) Understanding controlled trials:
what are pragmatic trials? BMJ 316:285

Rosenfeld R, Shiffman R (2009) Clinical practice guideline
development manual: a quality-driven approach for translating evidence into action. Otolaryngol Head Neck Surg 140:
S1–S43

Sackett D, Rosenberg W, Gray J, Haynes R, Richardson W
(1996) Evidence based medicine: what it is and what it
isn't. BMJ 312:71

Sackett D, Straus S, Richardson W, Rosenberg W, Haynes R
(2000) Evidence based medicine: how to practice and teach
EBM. Churchill Livingstone, London

Schulz F, Altman D, Moher D, CONSORT Group (2010) CON-
SORT 2010 statement: updated guidelines for reporting parallel group randomised trials. Ann Intern Med 152:726–732

Sibbald B, Roland M (1998) Understanding controlled trials:
why are randomized controlled trials important? BMJ
316:201

Smith T, Litvack J, Hwang P, Loehrl T, Mace J, Fong K, James K
(2010) Determinants of outcomes of sinus surgery: a multi-
institutional prospective cohort study. Otolaryngol Head
Neck Surg 142:55–63

Soler Z, Smith T (2010) Quality of life outcomes after functional
endoscopic sinus surgery. Otolaryngol Clin North Am
43:605–612

Wasserman J, Wynn R, Bash T, Rosenfeld R (2006) Levels of
evidence in otolaryngology journals. Otolaryngol Head Neck
Surg 134:717–723

Evoked EMG

Michael H. Rivner
Department of Neurology, Georgia Health Sciences
University, Augusta, GA, USA

Synonyms

Electroneurography; ENoG; Facial nerve conductions

Definition

The facial nerve is stimulated at the angle of the jaw
and a response is recorded from muscles of the face.
Many muscles have been studied but most commonly the nasalis muscle is recorded at the
nasolabial fold either with a bar electrode
containing an active electrode that is usually angled
upward with the active electrode located proximal
to the reference or with paired electrodes on either
side of the nose (Fig. 1) (Dumitru et al. 1988).
Following stimulation, a response is recorded with
an electromyography machine. The size of the
response and the latency of the response are
recorded (Fig. 2). The amplitude of the response
may be recorded between baseline and negative
peak or from positive peak to negative peak
depending on the technique used. The latency of
the response is the time from the onset of the stimulus to the initial negative deflection from the
baseline. Typically, waveforms are displayed
with negative displayed upward, so the upward
peak is usually negative. In the case of the facial
nerve, the amplitude of the abnormal side is compared to the normal side. An electroneurographic
quotient is calculated by dividing the difference in
amplitudes between the normal and the abnormal
side, by the amplitude of the normal side, to
give a percent reduction in amplitude.
$elect\,quot = \left(\frac{(amp2-amp1)}{amp2}\right) \times 100$ Where amp1 is
the amplitude of the abnormal side and amp2 is
the amplitude of the normal side. If this index is
less than 90%, the likelihood of a favorable result is
80–100% (Fisch 1984). If this index is greater than
95% than the likelihood of a favorable result is 60–

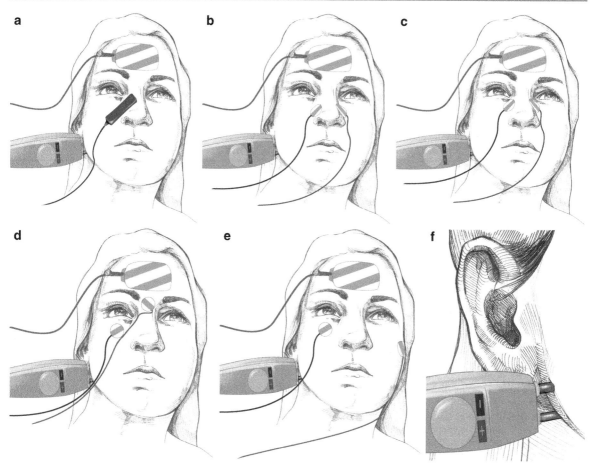

Evoked EMG, Fig. 1 The electrode placement for various methods of facial nerve electroneurography. The stimulator is viewed at stylomastoid foramen. (**a**) A bar electrode is used to record a response at the nasal labial fold. (**b**) Bi-nasal electrodes. (**c**) Bi-nasal electrodes. (**d**) Recording from the orbicularis oculi with a reference at the top of the nose. (**e**) Recording from the orbicularis oculi with a reference at the contralateral cheek. (**f**) Location of the stimulating electrode (Illustrations by Colby Polonsky)

70%. If between 90–95% the likelihood of a favorable result is 70%. A favorable result is considered to be a House-Brackmann score of I or II after 6–12 month recovery time. Figure 3 shows an example of a patient with a facial nerve lesion on the left. In this case, the electroneurographic quotient is 57.7% indicating that this patient has a good prognosis.

Purpose

This test is used to evaluate facial nerve lesions. It is also used to determine the prognosis of unilateral facial nerve lesions such as Bell's palsy.

Principle

The distal portion of the facial nerve is stimulated electrically at the angle of the jaw with the cathode on the trunk of the facial nerve and the anode in the stylomastoid foramen (Fig. 1f). Responses may be recorded from many muscles in face. Usually either the nasalis or orbicularis oculi muscles are recorded (Fig. 1). This test is quantitative as the muscle response is recorded and the amplitude and latency of the responses can be measured. Normal values for this test have been established so unlike the ▶ NET or ▶ MST, bilateral facial nerve lesions may be detected using this test. If the latency of the response is delayed initially after a lesion, suspicion for a distal facial

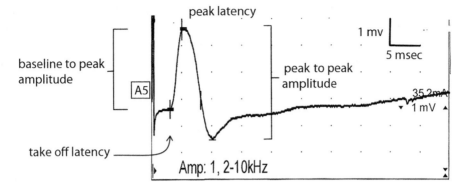

Evoked EMG, Fig. 2 This is an example of a facial nerve waveform recorded using the method demonstrated in Fig. 1d. Negative is displayed upward. The gain and sweep speed are displayed on the figure. The take-off latency represents the time between the stimulus onset and the initial negative deviation from the baseline. The peak latency represents the time between the stimulus onset and the peak of the negative waveform. Baseline to peak amplitude represents the amplitude between the baseline and negative peak. Peak to peak amplitude represents the amplitude between the negative and positive peaks (Illustrated by Colby Polonsky)

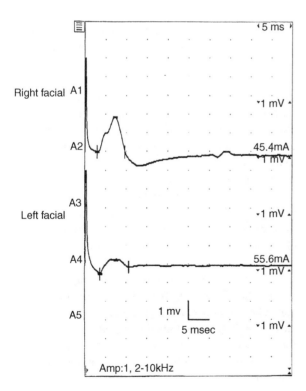

Evoked EMG, Fig. 3 This is an example of electroneurography in a patient with a Bell's Palsy. The top trace is the normal right side. The bottom trace is the abnormal left side. The amplitude of the abnormal side is lower and the facial waveform differs from that of the normal side. Its amplitude is 58% that of the normal side which is indicative of a good prognosis (Illustrated by Colby Polonsky)

nerve lesion or a neuropathy such as Guillain-Barre syndrome should be entertained. Even though some authors have felt that a prolonged distal latency may occur following a proximal nerve lesion.

Since the most common cause of facial nerve damage is from a proximal lesion in the fallopian canal, such as in ▶ Bell's palsy, most often the site of damage is proximal to the stimulation site. In the case of neuropraxia at that site, electroneurography will remain normal. In the case of a Bell's palsy this would indicate a favorable prognosis. If axonotmesis or neurotmesis has occurred, after 5–10 days, there will be Wallerian degeneration of the distal facial nerve and the amplitude of the facial nerve will be reduced. It is believed that no noticeable reduction in facial strength will be noticed with up to a 50% reduction in amplitude. While classically it was believed that the prognosis will be good if the response of the abnormal side is greater than 10% of normal (Fisch 1984; Linder et al. 2010), several studies have used a higher value of 25–30% as their cutoff value (May et al. 1983; Engstrom et al. 2000; Chow et al. 2002; Grosheva et al. 2008). Most authors believe that electroneurography is the best predictor of facial nerve prognosis but others believe that the variability of electroneurography makes other tests more reliable (Adour et al. 1980; Sittel et al. 1998). Others believe that the inter-trial variability is low enough to detect severe lesions (Di Bella et al. 1997; Engstrom et al. 2000). Some authors feel that electroneurography by itself is not adequate to determine prognosis but ▶ needle electromyography is needed for adequate prognosis (Grosheva et al. 2008; Sittel and Stennert 2001). Interestingly, the response recorded on the normal side with ▶ Bell's palsy also changes with time (Psillas and Daniilidis 2002). At 3 weeks following the onset of weakness, the amplitude of the contralateral side increases. The amplitude progressively increases until 1–2 months when it plateaus and may gradually increase up to the 4th month. At 6 months the response amplitude is lower than at 4 months but higher than baseline. This may affect the electroneurographic quotient.

Since facial nerve conductions test only the distal portion of the facial nerve, it is not the best test for localization of the lesion, since most facial nerve lesions are proximal to the stimulation point at the angle of the jaw. ▶ Transcranial magnetic stimulation, blink reflexes, and f-waves will allow for localization of the lesion proximal to the jaw. The former two topics will be discussed elsewhere. F-waves are long latency responses that are produced by the antidromic conduction of the nerve impulse to the cell body in the facial nerve nucleus. The cell body of the facial nerve is depolarized and if still depolarized at the end of the refractory period it will generate an impulse that will travel back down the nerve producing a small late response occurring around 10–12 msec after the initial stimulus. Usually only one cell body will be sufficiently depolarized by this antidromic volley so the f-wave will represent the firing of a single motor unit and be of much smaller amplitude than the compound muscle action potential seen in the standard orthodromic response. The latency of the f-wave will vary since different facial nerve motor neurons are activated with each volley. A prolonged facial f-wave may indicate a proximal lesion (Wedekind and Klug 2000).

Nakatani described a method for antidromically recording a facial nerve response from the posterio-superior part of the annulus tympanicus and the entrance to the external auditory canal (Nakatani et al. 2002). They stimulated the facial nerve at Stensen's duct with a catheter electrode. They subtracted the response from the external auditory canal from the annulus tympanicus to eliminate muscle responses. They related prognosis of ▶ Bell's palsy to the shape and presence of the antidromically recorded response. In a normal subject, the response was triphasic. In ▶ Bell's palsy it was biphasic. If the shape remains biphasic and does not become monophasic or absent it was associated with a good prognosis. They recommended using this technique with standard electroneurography. It is this author's opinion that this technique appears too invasive and difficult to use on a routine basis.

Many different recording sites have been used to record responses in electroneurography which complicates comparing studies. Classically Esslen described using a bar with two electrodes angled superiorly to record the nasalis muscle (Esslen 1977; Coker et al. 1992). Other authors have used bilateral nasal electrodes and nasal reference to the tip of the nose to record the response from the nasalis muscle (May et al. 1983; Di Bella et al. 1997; Engstrom et al. 2000). Other recording sites used have been the orbicularis oculi, orbicularis oris, mentalis, and frontalis muscles (Engstrom et al. 2000). Coker found that nasolabial fold recordings correlated best with with NET and using an amplitude difference of 3.5 millamps was equivalent to 90% degeneration using electroneurography recording from the nasolabial folds. They also found less variance using nasolabial recordings (Coker et al. 1992). Forehead and chin recordings were not recommended by these authors. Engstrom felt that while recording from a single muscle had high predictive value, recording from multiple muscles increased the prognostic value of electroneurography (Engstrom et al. 2000). They found that the best prediction was obtained using the nasalis and mentalis muscles using electroneurography quotients of less than or equal to 75% and 78%, respectively; recording from the frontalis and orbicularis oris muscles were less useful. The results obtained from electroneurography depend somewhat on which muscles are tested but if the same muscles are used to compare responses on both sides this comparison will be of value. Recording from the frontalis muscles is generally not as useful as recordings from other muscles. The highest amplitude responses are usually found recording from the orbicularis oculi with a reference at the top of the nose or contralateral cheek bone (Fig. 1d, e).

Indications

Bell's Palsy, Facial Nerve Trauma, Facial Nerve Palsy, Neuropathy.

Contraindications

None

Advantages/Disadvantages

The main advantage of electroneurography is that it is an objective test that does not require grading by the evaluator. The results are quantitative and less subject to interpretation. There are still many technical issues such as which muscles to record responses from. As mentioned above there is no uniform agreement about the muscles to record from. This makes comparing the results from one study to another more difficult. It does appear that valid results can be obtained using many different methods. It is recommended that the best results are obtained from the nasalis, mentalis, or lower orbicularis oculi muscles (Engstrom et al. 2000). Orbicularis oris and frontalis muscles are more prone to error. The method of stimulation is important as well. It is important to supramaximally stimulate the nerve at its most sensitive point. It is important not to activate the muscles of the mandibular branch of the trigeminal nerve as this may give spurious values for the amplitude of the test (Adour et al. 1980; Hughes 1989; Engstrom et al. 2000). Most of the studies use peak to peak amplitudes to study the amplitude of responses even though this is different than the way most motor response amplitudes are recorded. Usually baseline to negative peak is used. It is important to pay attention to the location of the reference electrode as this may interfere with one's ability to properly measure the amplitude of the response. With modern equipment the measurement of area is now possible rather than amplitude which might give a more accurate measurement of the response. Data on this has not been studied. As mentioned above there may be some inter-test variability but this may be minimized if the person doing electrodiagnostic studies is compulsive and makes sure that they use the same technique each time they do the study. Despite these problems, electroneurography is believed by most workers to be the most reliable study in predicting outcome in facial nerve palsy (Fisch 1980).

Electroneurography allows the response latency to be measured. This can be useful to determine if the facial nerve lesion is distal to the stimulation point and might indicate an otherwise overlooked generalized nerve disturbance. The response waveform may be examined which may give additional information. An irregular response waveform might give additional information about the nerve lesion.

The major disadvantage of electroneurography is that it may take 5–10 days for abnormalities from axonal damage proximally to be seen using this technique. Other techniques including ▶ NET and ▶ MST have this same limitation. With electroneurography, the initial waveform obtained before this time might give one an idea about the preexisting health of the nerve. Also the progression of the changes with time may be studied in a more quantitative manner than with ▶ NET and ▶ MST. The equipment needed to do this testing is not generally available to the ENT physician and trained personnel must perform this test. However, most communities have well-trained physicians in electrodiagnostic medicine who can perform this test.

Cross-References

▶ Bell's Palsy
▶ Blink Reflex
▶ Electromyography
▶ Nerve Excitability Test
▶ Transcranial Magnetic Stimulation of Facial Nerve

References

Adour KK, Sheldon MI, Kahn ZM (1980) Maximal nerve excitability testing versus neuromyography: prognostic value in patients with facial paralysis. Laryngoscope 90:1540–1547

Chow LCK, Tam RCN, Li MF (2002) Use of electroneurography as a prognostic indicator of Bell's palsy in Chinese patients. Otol Neurotol 23:598–601

Coker N, Fordice JO, Moore S (1992) Correlation of the nerve excitability test and electroneurography in acute facial paralysis. Am J Otol 13:127–133

Di Bella P, Logullo F, Lagalla G, Sirolla C, Provinciali L (1997) Neurophysiol Clin 27:300–308

Dumitru D, Walsh NE, Porter LD (1988) Electrophysiological evaluation of the facial nerve in Bell's palsy. Am J Phys Med Rehabil 67:137–144

Engstrom M, Jonsson L, Grindlund M, Stalberg E (2000) Electroneurographic facial muscle pattern in Bell's palsy. Otolaryngol Head Neck Surg 122:290–297

Esslen E (1977) Electromyography and electroneurography. In: Fisch U (ed) Facial nerve surgery: proceedings of the third international symposium on facial nerve surgery, 9–12 August, 1976. Aesculapius Publishing Co/, Zurich/Birmingham, pp 93–100

Fisch U (1980) Maximal nerve excitability testing vs electroneurography. Arch Otolaryngol 106:352–357

Fisch U (1984) Prognostic value of electrical tests in acute facial paralysis. Am J Otol 5:494–498

Grosheva M, Wittekindt C, Guntinas-Lichius O (2008) Prognostic value of electroneurography and electromyography in facial palsy. Laryngoscope 118:394–397

Hughes GB (1989) Prognostic tests in acute facial palsy. Am J Otol 4:304–311

Linder TE, Abdelkafy W, Cavero-Vanek S (2010) The management of peripheral facial nerve palsy: "paresis" versus "paralysis" and sources of ambiguity in study designs. Otol Neurotol 31:319–327

May M, Blumenthal F, Klein SR (1983) Acute Bell's palsy: prognostic value of evoked electromyography, maximal stimulation, and other electrical tests. Am J Otol 5:1–7

Nakatani H, Iwai M, Takeda T, Hamada M, Kakigi A, Nakahira M (2002) Waveform changes in antidromic facial nerve responses in patients with Bell's palsy. Ann Otol Rhinol Laryngol 111:128–134

Psillas G, Daniilidis J (2002) Facial electroneurography on the contralateral side in unilateral Bell's palsy. Eur Arch Otorhinolaryngol 259:339–342

Sittel C, Guntinas-Lichius O, Streppel M, Stennert E (1998) Variability of repeated facial nerve electroneurography in healthy subjects. Laryngoscope 108:1177–1180

Sittel C, Stennert E (2001) Prognostic value of electromyography in acute peripheral facial nerve palsy. Otol Neurotol 22:100–104

Wedekind C, Klug N (2000) Assessment of facial nerve function in acoustic tumor disease by nasal muscle f waves and transcranial magnetic stimulation. Muscle Nerve 23:58–62

Exclusively Endoscopic Approach (EEA)

▶ Endoscopic Surgery of Skull Base

Exon

Gerald T. Kangelaris and Lawrence R. Lustig
Department of Otolaryngology-Head and Neck Surgery, University of California, San Francisco, San Francisco, CA, USA

Definition

A sequence of DNA transcribed to messenger RNA that encodes information for protein synthesis.

Cross-References

▶ Sensorineural Hearing Loss

Exostoses

Ted A. Meyer
Department of Otolaryngology-Head and Neck Surgery, Medical University of South Carolina, Charleston, SC, USA

Definition

Exostoses are benign bony lesions of the external auditory canal. Many patients have multiple exostoses. Exostoses are thought to develop in response to repeated cold water exposures. The majority of exostoses are asymptomatic, but if cerumen, water, squamous debris, or other material becomes trapped medially to the exostosis, the patient can present with ▶ otorrhea, otalgia, or ▶ conductive hearing loss. If this occurs, most often, once the debris is removed, and any minor infection is treated, no further treatment is necessary. If the patient has recurrent problems, exostoses are removed surgically, typically with an otologic drill. Surgery can be performed either through a transcanal approach or with a postauricular incision depending on exposure needs and surgeon preference.

Cross-References

▶ Osteoma

Exostoses and Osteomas of External Auditory Canal

Brendan P. O'Connell and Paul R. Lambert
Department of Otolaryngology-Head and Neck Surgery, College of Medicine, Medical University of South Carolina, Charleston, SC, USA

Definitions

1. *Exostosis* – Non-neoplastic bony outgrowth that projects from the surface of a bone or root of a tooth.
2. *Osteoma* – Benign, slow growing bony tumor often originating from skull or facial bones.

3. *Periosteum* – Dense connective tissue membrane that closely invests the surface of bones except at articular surfaces. Its outer layer consists of blood vessels and nerves that nourish and innervate the underlying bone. The inner layer contains osteoblasts which play a role in bone formation and remodeling.
4. *Otitis externa* – Inflammation of the skin of the external auditory canal, most commonly due to bacterial infection.
5. *Canalplasty* – Surgical procedure performed to restore the normal width and bony contour of the external auditory canal.
6. *Tympanic membrane* – Thin membrane which transmits vibrations produced by sound waves from the outer ear to the ossicular chain in the middle ear. It is also known as the eardrum.

Introduction

External auditory canal exostoses and osteomas (▶ Osteoma) are benign, hyperplastic bony growths that present with similar clinical signs and symptoms. Historically grouped together, they represent distinct clinical entities.

Exostoses

Exostoses are hyperostotic outgrowths that usually develop as multiple, bilateral, bony swellings in the medial portion of the external auditory canal (Graham 1979; Fenton et al. 1996). Graham noted that exostoses invariably originate along the anterior, inferior, and posterior surfaces of the bony external auditory canal, however no definitive predilection for a specific canal wall site has been established (Graham 1979). An overall incidence of 0.6% has been demonstrated in general otolaryngology patients (House and Wilkinson 2008). Exostoses have been shown to occur with much greater frequency in males than females. In a recent retrospective review of 327 patients undergoing canalplasty for external auditory canal exostoses, 98% of the patients were men (House and Wilkinson 2008).

While the exact etiology remains unclear, it is generally accepted that multiple cold water immersions trigger a periosteal reaction that results in temporal bone growth (Fenton et al. 1996). Van Gilse was the first to propose a relationship between cold water exposure and exostosis formation. He observed that warm water swimmers did not develop aural exostoses whereas those bathing in the cold, North Sea did (Van Gilse 1938). Prevalence amongst surfers ranges from 70% to 80%, with similar patterns of affliction described in underwater breath-hold divers. Further, severity of external ear canal obstruction has been shown to increase as a function of the number of years surfed and the number of surfing sessions per year (Deleyiannis et al. 1996).

Van Gilse demonstrated that irrigation of the human external auditory canal with cold water resulted in prolonged hyperemia of the canal's epidermal lining (Van Gilse 1938). Harrison performed similar studies in guinea pigs and showed that repeated irrigation of the external auditory canal resulted in localized production of new bone. Histological sectioning of these bone specimens revealed underlying bone vasodilation (Harrison 1951). Given these findings, it is possible that cold water exposure initiates a vasodilatory response in canal epithelium. Resultant increased vascular flow may be sufficient to cause proliferation of the underlying periosteum.

Osteoma

Osteomas are fibro-osseous bony tumors of unknown etiologic origin. Compared to exostoses, osteomas are relatively rare. Benign in nature, osteomas are neoplastic bone tumors characterized by slow, progressive growth. They are the most common bony neoplasm of the temporal bone (▶ Temporal bone tumors) and are most frequently found in the external auditory canal (Fenton et al. 1996; Tran et al. 1996). These lesions usually present as solitary, unilateral, pedunculated growths originating from the tympanosquamous or tympanomastoid suture lines (Fenton et al. 1996). Similar to exostoses, osteomas have no malignant potential.

Histology

Exostoses are sessile lesions consisting of dense, stratified lamellar bone. The newly formed bone is arranged in layers suggestive of a periodic growth pattern. Subperiosteal bone comes in direct contact with the surface of the native canal bone (Graham 1979).

Osteomas are more often pedunculated masses characterized by abundant fibrovascular channels surrounded by irregularly oriented lamellar bone (Graham 1979). Osteomas typically lack the laminated growth pattern of exostoses (Schuknecht 1993). Both lesions are covered by the squamous epithelium of the external auditory canal.

Controversy exists, however, as to whether these lesions can be differentiated entirely on histological features. While Graham stresses that exostoses are uniformly devoid of intervening fibrovascular channels, Fenton argues that the presence of fibrovascular channels should not be considered an absolute differentiating factor (Graham 1979; Fenton et al. 1996). Fenton studied the histological features of osteomas and exostoses excised from 13 patients and found that fibrovascular channels were present in all pathological specimens. In this group of patients, two clinically diagnosed exostoses were misdiagnosed as osteomas on a histological basis as they were single, rounded specimens with large fibrovascular channels (Fenton et al. 1996). Further studies with larger sample sizes are needed to definitively characterize the histological differences between exostoses and osteomas.

Clinical Presentation

Most exostoses and osteomas do not cause clinical symptoms and the majority of affected patients will never present for medical care. Primary care physicians discover these lesions, particularly pedunculated osteomas, incidentally on routine otoscopic examination in asymptomatic patients. This subset of patients is frequently referred to otolaryngologists for further management. As such, it is important for otolaryngologists to be familiar with the diagnosis and management of these bony lesions.

When symptomatic, exostoses and osteomas manifest similarly. Patients often begin to experience symptoms when bony stenosis becomes severe enough to cause disruption of the normal physiologic clearance of desquamated epithelium from the external auditory canal. Resultant obstruction leads to buildup of debris and moisture proximal to the site of obstruction

creating a nidus for infection. Affected patients frequently present with otitis externa or otorrhea. Accumulation of cerumen, exfoliated epithelium, and other debris can also manifest as ▶ otalgia in the absence of active infection.

The association of osteoma with cholesteatoma (▶ Cholesteatoma, Acquired) is exceedingly rare, however there have been a few reports of postobstructive cholesteatoma formation (Tran et al. 1996). In such cases, surgical resection of osteoma should be considered to prevent cholesteatoma extension posteriorly into the mastoid. Osteoma presenting with unilateral headache and external auditory canal polyp has also been described in case reports.

In both exostoses and osteomas, trapped debris can impede tympanic membrane movement resulting in a conductive hearing loss (Tran et al. 1996). In rare cases, canal narrowing can be so severe that passage of sound waves is impaired. Canal apertures of 3 mm or less can result in loss of high-frequency sounds, with lower frequency loss arising as disease progression further compromises canal diameter (Brackmann et al. 2001).

Recurrent otitis externa is the most common presenting complaint in patients undergoing surgery for either exostoses or osteomas, followed by the sensation of ear blockage and hearing loss. Data from a large, retrospective review of patients undergoing canalplasty for exostoses demonstrated that 41.9% of patients presented initially with otitis externa or otorrhea. Plugged sensation was the second most common complaint on presentation (29.4%), followed by hearing loss (25.4%), pain (7.3%), and tinnitus (2.4%) (House and Wilkinson 2008).

Diagnosis

Exostoses and osteomas of the external auditory can be diagnosed clinically with otoscopic examination. Exostoses manifest as broad-based lesions, often multiple and bilateral, which protrude into the external auditory canal causing narrowing. Conversely, osteomas are typically solitary, unilateral, and more pedunculated than sessile in configuration.

When gross morphology is difficult to appreciate during office examination or surgical intervention is planned, high-resolution ▶ CT imaging of the

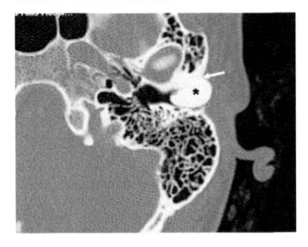

Exostoses and Osteomas of External Auditory Canal,
Fig. 1 High-resolution axial CT scan of the left temporal bone demonstrating osteoma (*asterisk*) arising from the anterolateral portion of the external auditory canal (*arrow*). Note the pedunculated configuration of the lesion (Reprinted with permission from *Otology and Neurotology*, 2008; 29:875. External Auditory Canal Osteoma. Yuen HW, Chen JM)

temporal bone should be considered for further evaluation of these lesions (Figs. 1 and 2).

Medical Management

Medical management is the mainstay of treatment. Cerumen disimpaction and debridement should be performed periodically. Patients who suffer from recurrent episodes of otitis externa should be prescribed appropriate topical antibiotics. If an exostosis is suspected, patients are cautioned against further water exposure as this could accelerate disease progression. Surfers or divers who choose to continue to participate in aquatic activities are advised to wear ear plugs or occlusive hoods to minimize water exposure.

Surgical Management

Surgical removal of osteomas and exostoses is occasionally necessary. Surgery is generally indicated for patients who have chronic/recurrent otitis externa refractory to medical management or a documented conductive hearing loss on audiometric examination. Surgery may also be indicated if the region medial to the site of canal stenosis needs to be

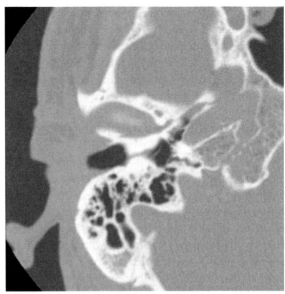

Exostoses and Osteomas of External Auditory Canal,
Fig. 2 High-resolution axial CT scan of the right temporal bone demonstrating broad-based osseous outgrowths consistent with exostoses. Note the significant narrowing of the external auditory canal (Reprinted with permission from *Cummings Otolaryngology Head and Neck Surgery*, 2010; 5th edition: 1918. Part 7: Otology, Neuro-otology, and Skull base Surgery. Flint, PW et al)

accessed for other otologic procedures such as stapedectomy (▶ Stapedectomy and Stapedotomy) or tympanoplasty. Surgery is not necessary in patients with significant canal stenosis who demonstrate no evidence of recurrent infection or hearing impairment (Brackmann et al. 2001).

Timing of surgical intervention, particularly in patients with otitis externa, must be taken into consideration when planning operative intervention. Active infection may delay wound healing and compromise the ability of canal wall skin to reepithelialize postoperatively. Clinicians should attempt to establish a pattern of recurrence and ideally schedule surgery at a time when active infection is not present. Adequate microscopic cleaning and topical therapy is essential during the preoperative period.

As previously mentioned, osteomas usually present as discrete, pedunculated lesions. In some of these cases, the osteoma can be removed under local anesthesia with a curette via a transcanal approach. Alternatively, osteomas can be removed with a drill.

Depending on surgeon preference, exostoses can be removed with either a transcanal or postauricular approach. The postauricular approach is generally considered safer as it allows for easier identification of landmarks and provides greater access to the medial portion of the canal. Ability to lateralize and preserve meatal skin is also maximized with this approach.

Canalplasty Via the Postauricular Approach

The ear is injected with local anesthestic and a postauricular incision is made. The canal skin overlying the exostosis is incised as far medially as possible. At 12 and 6 o'clock radial incisions are then made to create anterior and posterior skin flaps pedicled laterally. These flaps are elevated with a round knife to expose the exostoses, which are drilled out in a 360° fashion. Once the level of the remaining canal skin is reached, that skin is reflected medially toward or onto the tympanic membrane. This deeper portion of the exostosis is removed with a diamond burr. A thin piece of Silastic or foil from a suture pack can be placed over the reflected skin and tympanic membrane to minimize inadvertent injury to the structures.

Once drilling is complete, the medially and laterally pedicled skin flaps are repositioned onto the new contour of the canal wall. Depending on the degree of canal narrowing, it may not be possible to maintain all the deep canal skin intact. If there are significant areas of exposed bone, these can be covered by a split thickness skin graft from the postauricular area or from the posterior surface of the auricle.

Many surgeons feel that anterior exostoses should be addressed before posterior ones (Brackmann et al. 2001). By drilling the anterior exostosis first, the temporomandibular joint can be identified, which safely directs the surgeon toward the tympanic membrane. Verification of the tympanic membrane position allows for safe dissection of the posterior exostosis in the area lateral to the annulus. The surgeon must always be cognizant of the mastoid segment of the facial nerve, particularly given the distorted canal anatomy secondary to new bone growth. For this reason, facial nerve monitoring is recommended.

The degree of surgical difficulty in drilling exostoses should not be underestimated. Major complications of canalplasty include prolonged healing, ▶ facial paralysis, tympanic membrane perforation, canal stenosis, infection, ▶ temporomandibular joint symptoms, and hearing loss (Brackmann et al. 2001).

A study examining iatrogenic facial nerve paralysis following otologic surgery at a single institution (excluding neurotologic procedures) revealed that a surprisingly high number (14%) of patients sustained facial nerve injury during removal of exostoses (Green et al. 1994). It is important to keep in mind that the distal mastoid segment of the facial nerve courses lateral to the tympanic annulus. Care should also be taken when drilling the medial extent of posterior canal exostoses as the chorda tympani runs beneath the bone near this field of dissection. If an injury to the tympanic membrane occurs, it should be addressed with a fascia graft.

Patients are usually seen 2–4 weeks postoperatively; if any granulation tissue is present, a steroid-antibiotic eardrop is recommended. Additional absorbable or nonabsorbable packing may also be required. Strict dry ear precautions are recommended until complete healing has occurred.

Conclusion

Exostoses and osteomas are distinct, benign bony growths of the external auditory canal. Exostoses occur bilaterally and may be secondary to a periosteal reaction triggered by repeated cold water exposure. Osteomas typically arise unilaterally and are true bony neoplasms. Conservative medical management is the first line treatment for all asymptomatic patients. When symptomatic, patients most commonly present with otitis externa or conductive hearing loss likely resulting from canal obstruction and accumulation of debris. In most cases, surgery should be reserved for symptomatic patients who have failed medical management. The postauricular approach should be strongly considered in any patient undergoing removal of exostosis or advanced osteoma.

References

Brackmann DE, Shelton C, Arriaga MA et al (2001) Otologic surgery, 2nd edn. W.B. Saunders, Philadelphia, p xxii, 680 p
Deleyiannis FW, Cockcroft BD, Pinczower EF (1996) Exostoses of the external auditory canal in Oregon surfers. Am J Otolaryngol 17:303–307
Fenton JE, Turner J, Fagan PA (1996) A histopathologic review of temporal bone exostoses and osteomata. Laryngoscope 106:624–628
Graham MD (1979) Osteomas and exostoses of the external auditory canal. A clinical, histopathologic and scanning electron microscopic study. Ann Otol Rhinol Laryngol 88:566–572

Green JD Jr, Shelton C, Brackmann DE (1994) Iatrogenic facial nerve injury during otologic surgery. Laryngoscope 104:922–926

Harrison DF (1951) Exostosis of the external auditory meatus. J Laryngol Otol 65:704–714

House JW, Wilkinson EP (2008) External auditory exostoses: evaluation and treatment. Otolaryngol Head Neck Surg 138:672–678

Schuknecht HF (1993) Pathology of the ear, 2nd edn. Lea & Febiger, Philadelphia, p. xv, 672 p

Tran LP, Grundfast KM, Selesnick SH (1996) Benign lesions of the external auditory canal. Otolaryngol Clin North Am 29:807–825

Van Gilse P (1938) Des observations ulterieures sur la genese exostoses du conduitexterne par l'iritatio d'eau froid. Acta Otolaryngol 26:343–352

Expanded Endonasal Approach (EEA)

▶ Endoscopic Surgery of Skull Base

Explantation of Cochlear Implant

▶ Cochlear Implantation, Revision – Adult
▶ Surgical Devices (Cochlear Implantation, Revision – Pediatric)

Expressivity

Matthew Ng[1] and Drew M. Horlbeck[2]
[1]Department of Surgery, Division of Otolaryngology, University of Nevada School of Medicine, Las Vegas, NV, USA
[2]Department of Surgery, Division of Pediatric Otolaryngology, Nemours Children's Clinic, Jacksonville, FL, USA

Definition

Presenting with different manifestations of an affected gene.

Cross-References

▶ Sensorineural Hearing Loss-Congenital-Genetics

Extended Lateral Temporal Bone Resection

▶ Lateral Temporal Bone Resection

Extended Retrolabyrinthine Transtentorial Approach

▶ Surgical Approaches and Anatomy of the Lateral Skull Base

Extended Transcochlear Approach

▶ Surgical Approaches and Anatomy of the Lateral Skull Base

External Auditory Canal (EAC)

▶ Pinna and External Auditory Canal, Anatomy

External Auditory Meatus

▶ Pinna and External Auditory Canal, Anatomy

Extracapsular Spread

Jonathan R. Clark[1] and Douglas Shaw[2]
[1]Sydney Head and Neck Cancer Institute, Royal Prince Alfred Hospital, Camperdown, Sydney, NSW, Australia
[2]Sydney Head and Neck Cancer Institute, Camperdown, NSW, Australia

Definition

Extension of tumor from within a nodal deposit through the capsule of the lymph node. ECS may be macroscopic or microscopic, with macroscopic ECS portending the worse prognosis.

Cross-References

▶ Lymphatic Spread from Cutaneous Neoplasms of Head and Neck

Extraesophageal Reflux

▶ Reflux Disease and LPR

Extranodal Deposit

Jonathan R. Clark[1] and Douglas Shaw[2]
[1]Sydney Head and Neck Cancer Institute, Royal Prince Alfred Hospita, Camperdown, Sydney, NSW, Australia
[2]Sydney Head and Neck Cancer Institute, Camperdown, NSW, Australia

Synonyms

Extranodal spread; Soft tissue deposit

Definition

Also known as extranodal spread (ENS) or a soft tissue deposit of metastatic cancer; ENS is the presence of tumor within defined nodal basins without any evidence of lymph node. This may represent a lymph node metastasis that has completely destroyed the lymph node or a "true" extranodal deposit of tumor. This may occur via lymphatic or hematogenous spread, and in cutaneous squamous cell carcinoma, ENS is probably associated with a worse prognosis than extracapsular spread.

Cross-References

▶ Extracapsular Spread
▶ Lymphatic Spread from Cutaneous Neoplasms of Head and Neck

Extranodal Spread

▶ Extranodal Deposit

Exudative Tracheitis

▶ Pediatric Inflammatory Airway Disorders

F

Facial Fractures in Children

Todd M. Brickman and Anita Jeyakumar
Department of Otolaryngology-Head and Neck
Surgery, Louisiana State University School of
Medicine-Health Science Center, New Orleans,
LA, USA

Definitions

Displaced fracture – Separation of bone fragments, usually causes form and function disturbances due to loss of anatomical alignment.

Greenstick fracture – A crack or partial break of a bone, typically does not cause form or function disturbances as anatomical alignment is retained.

Lefort I fracture – A horizontal fracture of the lower maxilla just above the tooth roots which usually allows the upper jaw to float freely. Fracture goes through pterygoids, lower maxilla, and into piriform aperture.

Lefort II fracture – A transverse fracture of the mid-maxilla that looks pyramidal when fracture occurs bilaterally. Fracture extends from the pterygoids through maxillary sinus, infraorbital rim, orbital floor, and through the nasal bones.

Lefort III fracture – This is also called craniofacial disjunction as maxilla is separated from skull base. Fracture extends from frontozygomatic suture through the lateral, floor and medial wall of the orbit to the nasal bones.

Maxillo-mandibular fixation (MMF) – Attaching the mandible to the maxilla with wires, appliances, screws, or arch bars to prevent movement. Also known as wiring jaw shut.

Orbital blowout fracture – Fracture that occurs from force to orbital rim or globe itself. The forces are dispersed from the orbital rim to the globe and then to the thin, elastic orbital floor that cracks as it expands.

Trapdoor fracture – As the hydraulic forces from an orbital blowout fracture cause the orbital floor to expand, the orbital fat and muscle push through this crack; but due to the elasticity of the bone, the bone quickly retracts back to its original position entrapping fat and muscle.

White-eyed fracture – A type of isolated trapdoor fracture from a low-velocity blunt trauma that can sometimes present without any visible signs of trauma (periorbital echymosis, edema, or subconjunctival hemorrhage). Due to a strong oculocardiac reflex in children, hypotension, bradycardia, nausea, and vomiting may accompany this type of trapdoor fracture and possibly be the only presenting symptoms.

Zymaticomalar complex (ZMC) fracture – Fracture of the zygomatic arch, lateral orbital wall (frontalzygomatic suture), and the inferior orbital rim. Also known as a tripod fracture.

History

Historically, facial trauma was related to interpersonal violence in adults. Evolving patterns of presentation changed as the use of motorized transportation was introduced to the masses in the 1940s and the 1950s. Advances in speed and size of vehicles outpaced safety measures, so the presentation of pan facial fractures and life-threatening injuries dominated the early rise of the automobile-related crashes. Implementation of safety measures such as the

S.E. Kountakis (ed.), *Encyclopedia of Otolaryngology, Head and Neck Surgery*, DOI 10.1007/978-3-642-23499-6,
© Springer-Verlag Berlin Heidelberg 2013

National Traffic and Motor Vehicle Act of 1966 requiring cars to have seat belts and the US government decreasing highway speeds in the mid-1970s led to a decrease in mortality-related crashes. Additional measures of air bags, child safety seats, and reduction of alcohol-impaired driving in the 1990s continued the downward trend in automobile-related morbidity and mortality until leveling off in the early part of this century. However, these measures not only decreased incidence rates of facial fractures but introduced new types of trauma patients – those with extensive isolated injuries and those with traditionally non-survivable injuries. Technological advances in the provision and speed of hospital care in tertiary medical hospitals and intensive care units (ICU) have allowed patients with traditionally mortal injuries to survive. Evolving technology has also changed the prevention, presentation, and treatment of facial fractures for both the adult and pediatric population.

Epidemiology

The medical school pediatric rotation teaching that children are not small adults also holds true for pediatric facial trauma. There are many contributing factors to these differences. Anatomy, facial growth patterns, societal and psychosocial issues all impart their own influence on the differences between adult and pediatric facial trauma. However, the facial trauma mantra – achievement of pre-injury form and function while minimizing intervention and impairment – holds true for both adult and pediatric populations.

Since the mid-twentieth century, injury has been the leading cause of death for infants and children. More specifically for the years 1999–2008, unintentional injury was the leading cause of death from age 1 to age 45 with motor vehicle collisions being the number one cause of mortal injury. Unintentional fall is the leading cause of non-fatal trauma treated in pediatric hospital emergency rooms (CDC - 2010).

There exists wide variability in the incidence of pediatric facial fractures reported in the literature over the years. The reason for this variability is multi-factorial. One of the reasons may be a real change in the incidence rate from mid- to late-twentieth century. However, the rates may be influenced by reporting bias from analyses of academic versus private institutions, local versus regional

hospitals, and single versus multi-institutional studies. Vyas et al. analyzed a large national database and reported pediatric facial fractures as 14.7% of all facial fractures. Less than 1% of all facial fractures occurred in children less than 5 years of age (Vyas et al. 2008). It is generally accepted that facial fractures in children younger than 5 is rare (5% of all pediatric facial fractures) with an increasing incidence at every age range until the rate in the later teenage years mimics the adult rate. Most reports demonstrate a similar or slight increased male-to-female fracture ratio in children younger than 5 with the ratio increasing with aging to reach the adult ratio of approximately 3:1. Many reports list nasal and mandible fractures as the most common facial bone fractures. Nasal fractures are more common as these are not likely to be admitted to the hospital and hence underreported. Mandible fractures account for about 30% of facial fractures. The mandibular condyle is most prone to fracture in children with rates equaling out between the condyle, body and arch in the adolescence years. Orbital fractures are the most common midface fracture and account for approximately 25% of all facial fractures. The incidence of pediatric complex midfacial fractures is less than 10%. Pediatric panfacial fractures are infrequent.

Anatomy

Some of the differences in adult versus pediatric facial trauma can be explained by anatomical differences. The pediatric facial skeleton has more cartilage than adults, and children obviously have more growth centers than adults. Pediatric bone has a higher percentage of cancellous to cortical bone ratio thereby providing more elasticity and resistance to fracture. Bone is less mineralized and more elastic in children with a thicker facial soft tissue envelope to provide additional padding from traumatic forces compared to adults.

Dentition also influences pediatric facial trauma. Deciduous teeth predominate until 6 years of age with a mixed dentition from 6 to12 years of age. These unerupted permanent teeth provide additional support to the mandible and maxilla until the permanent teeth fully erupt during adolescence. The combination of a dense mandible and maxilla connected with flexible cartilaginous joints and growth centers renders facial bones solid but elastic and hence less resistant to fractures.

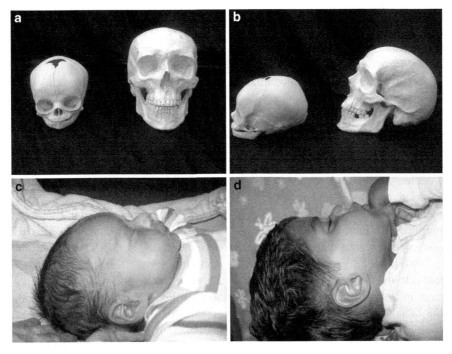

Facial Fractures in Children, Fig. 1 Comparison of skull sizes demonstrating differences in the contribution of the mandible and maxilla to the craniofacial ratio. (**a**) Frontal view of neonate and adult skull models. Note the contribution of the mandible and maxilla in the facial region, and significant vertical height difference between the neonate and adult. (**b**) Lateral view of neonate and adult skull models. Note the contribution of the mandible and maxilla bone accounting for the differences in facial projection between the neonate and adult. Photos of (**c**) newborn and (**d**) 6-year-old, demonstrating the evolving differences in facial projection, height, and craniofacial ratio. Note the increased mandibular projection and thinning of the soft tissues in the cheek during these few years of development

Facial Growth

The ratio of cranium to face at birth is 8:1. In the first 2 years of life, 80% of cranial growth occurs with the head size doubling from birth to age 5. Cranial growth is complete by age 7 but facial growth continues, thus accounting for the shrinking craniofacial ratio to 4:1 at 5 years of age. As the face continues to grow, the craniofacial ratio reaches 2–2.5:1 at adulthood (see Fig. 1).

Facial growth is broken down into the midface and mandibular components. Midface growth is inferiorly (downward) and laterally (sideways). The maxillary sinus growth starts around 5 months and continues to 16 years of age. The ethmoid sinus starts at 1 year of age and the frontal sinus starts around 6 years with both continuing growth into adulthood.

Mandibular growth is anteriorly (forward) and laterally (sideways). There are multiple growth centers in the mandible. The growth center consists of a fibrous cap with an inner chondrogenic layer, a layer of cartilage, and a layer of ossifying cartilage. With the increase in both the vertical and horizontal facial components, the soft tissue envelope is stretched and thinned thereby providing less cushioning and a greater chance for fracture.

As the cranium and facial structures take shape and change growth patterns, the incidence of fractures concomitantly changes. With the growth of the midface and mandible, they become more prominent on the facial profile and are more inclined to be injured. The infant's mandible and midface are relatively retruded and so are protected, whereas the frontal area is prominent and prone to injury. In adults and older children, the zygomaticomaxillary complex (ZMC), nasal, and Le Fort fractures become more common.

Psychosocial

Just as the growth of the midface influences fracture patterns, the pediatric patient undergoes social evolution which influences fracture patterns and incidence.

Infants are swaddled and cared for with close observation preventing many of the occurrences which would cause facial trauma. As toddlers gain independence with walking, caregivers still keep a watchful eye and can redirect toddlers away from potentially fracture-causing situations. As the child enters kindergarten and elementary school there is more independence and an increase in higher risk behaviors. Children are more likely to climb jungle gyms and playgrounds as well as now participating in sporting activities. Into adolescence as independence grows and adult supervision decreases, higher speed and force generating sports as well as driving and interpersonal relationships will increase the opportunity for facial trauma. As adolescents mature into the late teenage years, lifestyle development of increased driving for school activities and employment in addition to an increase in interpersonal violence bridges the gap into the facial trauma presentation that is typically seen with adulthood.

Clinical Features

Management

Regarding the facial trauma patient, treatment starts with the ABCs. Initial evaluation and resuscitation follows Advanced Trauma Life Support (ATLS) protocols. While facial fracture diagnosis, management, and treatment are important, it must be completed within the context of the overall patient well-being. The pediatric airway is smaller with a retruded tongue. This larger tongue to mouth ratio at baseline can make for airway distress and a difficult airway in mandible fractures. Infants are obligate nasal breathers so midface and nasal fractures along with blood and vomitus can impede the airway. If positioning techniques and airway appliances are inadequate to secure the airway, orotracheal intubation may be required with tracheotomy reserved as a last effort.

The secondary exam can be more difficult due to swelling, ecchymosis, asymmetry, lacerations, crepitus, paresthesias, and bleeding. A complete systematic examination of the head and neck is performed. Overall assessment is evaluated with visual inspection looking for facial asymmetry, ecchymosis, lacerations, and malocclusion as these can be predictors for facial fractures. Palpation of the bony architecture is performed assessing for asymmetry,

step-offs, fractures, and bony deformities. Midface mobility is assessed by rocking the premaxilla while the head is held steady. Dental occlusion is assessed as malocclusion is highly suggestive of a mandible fracture. Trismus and deviation on opening the mouth should also alert the clinician to a possible mandible fracture. Anterior rhinoscopy evaluates for septal/nasal fractures and a septal hematoma. Ocular exam checking pupillary reflexes, motility, and gross vision is performed. A comprehensive ophthalmologic evaluation in pediatric patients with midface and orbital fractures should be considered.

Due to the force needed in causing facial fractures, over 50% of facial trauma patients will have injury outside of the head and neck region. The rule of one/thirds for facial fractures is that a third will have a brain injury, a third will present with a skull fracture, and a third will have other organ injuries (Imadara et al. 2008). Cervical spine injury presents in less than 10% of pediatric facial fracture patients, which is lower than adults, but must be ruled out with proper imaging and examination. Coordination of care for all injuries must be performed in a systematic fashion with the overall well-being of the patient as the first priority, even if this means delaying treatment or less than optimal outcome for the repair of the facial fractures.

Diagnosis

Taking a history and diagnosing facial trauma is more difficult in the pediatric population. Children generally communicate less effectively and have decreased recall when compared to adults. They may have distracting injuries, or more life-threatening injuries and not be able to respond (Ryan et al. 2011).

Plain films provide limited information for midface and mandibular fractures. Towne, Caldwell, lateral oblique and intraoral projections can provide additional information but are not all encompassing. A panoramic X-ray provides more information regarding mandible fractures, especially those in the body. However, these require a patient to sit upright in occlusion and cannot be performed in an intubated patient or uncooperative child.

Ultrasound has been described to evaluate facial fractures. Skull, orbital floor, and zygomatico-orbital complex fractures have shown some promise being evaluated with ultrasound. However, midface and mandibular fracture diagnosis has shown poor sensitivity and specificity with ultrasonography. A major limitation of ultrasound is the inability to diagnose non-displaced or greenstick fractures and fractures of the mandibular ramus and condyle (Friedrich et al. 2003).

Multi-slice axial computed tomography (CT) with coronal, sagittal, and three-dimensional reconstructions is the gold standard for diagnosing facial fractures (Alcala-Galiano et al. 2008). It provides improvement in diagnostic accuracy and mapping the extent of fractures. Recently, appropriate concerns regarding high-dose radiation exposure in children has led to the development of low-dose radiation protocols, which has not been fully evaluated and established but is being practiced in numerous pediatric facilities.

Treatment

Overall the approach and treatment of pediatric facial fractures is more conservative than adult interventions. Children heal faster so the time to treatment and duration of intervention will be reduced compared to adults. The goals of treatment are similar – reduction and stabilization of the horizontal and vertical buttresses to re-establish occlusion, normal facial proportions, and symmetry.

Future growth and development of the child must also be considered when deciding treatment. An invasive approach that acutely restores stability and aesthetics but compromises future growth leading to deformities is not ideal. The trauma itself can affect future normal growth and bone remodeling, predisposing patients to form and functional alterations with advancing age. Injuries to growth centers (mandibular condyle, ramus, body) can lead to future growth concerns. Crush injuries have shown a higher propensity for growth disturbances and may indicate a need for a more aggressive intervention. However, a younger-aged child is more adaptable to an injury. Children are more capable of remodeling and the increased time for growth and compensation allows for correction of the deformity and return to more normal form and function. In addition, the approach and intervention itself can be traumatic thereby causing additional growth deformities leading to aesthetic and functional issues.

An injury that may be surgically treated in an adult could be managed non-operatively in a pediatric patient. Clinical acumen must be used on a case-by-case basis to determine whether intervention is needed to produce a better long-term outcome. Untreated displaced fractures and over treating fractures with excessive periosteal elevation, soft tissue manipulation, and plating may result in growth disturbance. However, stability and accurate reduction supersede the effect of facial growth alteration as a consequence of periosteal elevation needed for the reconstruction (Bailey and Johnson 2006). It is recommended to fixate unstable, displaced fragments with the fewest number and smallest-size plates through a small opening with minimal intervention and dissection. Additionally, interval removal of hardware may help avoid future growth disturbances.

Due to the relatively low incidence of pediatric facial fractures, data are limited regarding long-term outcomes for a large pediatric population. Adverse outcomes have been reported to range from 5% to 30% with isolated fractures resulting in fewer complications. Patients treated operatively have also shown higher complication rates (Rottgers et al. 2011). However, data are lacking to sufficiently determine whether the cause of the poor outcomes is a consequence of the initial trauma, the intervention, the compromised growth, or a combination of these factors. Those patients with multiple injuries and fractures requiring surgical intervention should be followed with longitudinal evaluations and counseled that form and functional abnormalities are likely. Future interventions such as surgery or orthodontia may be necessary.

ORIF

There has been a revolution in treatment over the last 20 years for both adult and pediatric facial fractures. The advancement of titanium plate and screw technology in the 1990s has provided a more reliable system of fixation with improved outcomes over traditional measures. However, implementation of the titanium technology into the pediatric population still has not resolved the conundrum of whether the benefits of rigidly fixating unstable fractures outweigh the drawbacks of the surgical intervention upon future facial growth. One drawback of titanium plates is that they are permanent. It is believed that the plates and screws may impede growth, especially if placed across suture lines. A single plate should not be placed across more than one suture line as this can tether growth. One solution to this disadvantage is interval removal of the hardware. This approach alleviates the potential of limiting future growth from the plates and screws but it also requires a second surgery.

Another technological advancement that has shown some promise is resorbable plates and screws. A combination of biodegradable copolymers with differing strengths, degradation times, and reactivity quotients comprise resorbable plates which undergo a two-step degradation process. The first step is hydrolysis, which breaks the long chains into shorter ones and markedly reduces the strength of the substance. The second step is phagocytosis of the shorter chains by macrophages which decreases the mass of the substance. Most current resorbable systems are made of a combination of polyglycolic acid (PGA), which is subject to rapid hydrolysis and poly L-lactic acid (PLA), which is more slowly resorbed. There are a handful of commercially available resorbable systems with different ratios of the copolymers which provide an array of strengths and degradation times. The stronger a resorbable plate is, the longer it will take to degrade, with most clinicians preferring the degradation time to be within 9–12 months. The load-bearing forces needed for the specific fracture repair has to be evaluated and the system that provides the best strength that will resorb in an acceptable time frame determined.

There has been individual retrospective evidence provided for and against both titanium and resorbable plating systems throughout the years. However, no prospective, randomized trial has evaluated the outcomes using these systems for facial fractures. In a review by The Cochrane Collaboration, there was insufficient evidence to demonstrate the effectiveness of resorbable compared to titanium systems for facial fractures (Dorri et al. 2009).

Frontal Bone Fracture

Frontal bone fractures are seen more commonly in children under 6 years of age due to the prominence of the forehead and a higher craniofacial ratio. In this age range, frontal fractures are more likely to extend to include skull and orbital roof fractures. This association decreases with age as the frontal sinus pneumatizes and is better able to absorb and disperse impact forces. There is a greater association with neurocranial injury due to increased force needed for frontal bone fractures. Non-displaced fractures can be watched and anterior table frontal sinus fractures can also be conservatively treated unless cosmetic depressions or injury to the nasofrontal duct exist/exists. If displacement of the posterior table by more than the thickness of the table exists, cranialization or obliteration of the frontal sinus with debridement of the mucous membranes and occlusion of the nasofrontal duct is warranted. Frontal bone fractures may also be associated with skull fractures and the orbital roof. This fracture pattern is more likely to cause brain injury and cerebral spinal fluid leak. Neurosurgical evaluation is needed and management is coordinated among services based upon severity of injury and the child's status.

Orbital Fracture

The fracture pattern for superior orbital fractures is similar to frontal bone fractures. The orbital roof is most likely to fracture in patients under 7 years of age due to the increased craniofacial ratio and a direct bony connection to the frontal bone from a less pneumatized frontal sinus. As the frontal sinus and midface develop, the forces are dispersed within the now more prominent midface and orbit, resulting in an increasing incidence of floor and medial orbital wall fractures.

The patient should be examined for rim step-offs, paresthesias, diplopia, and gaze restriction and treated if fracture segments are grossly displaced, decreased extraocular muscle movements with positive forced duction testing are noticed, or significant alteration of orbital volume exists. Ocular injuries, such as retrobulbar hematoma, pupillary defects, vision changes, globe injury, etc., prompt an urgent ophthalmologic evaluation. Children with isolated blowout fractures can be conservatively watched for 7–10 days. If enopthalmos, diplopia, or ophthalmodynia persists, exploration is performed. CT scans should be reviewed for muscle entrapment, especially the inferior rectus muscle in isolated orbital floor fractures. Since children's bones are very elastic, they are more likely to have muscle entrapment. As the trauma forces are dispersed from the orbital rim to the globe to the thin, elastic floor, the floor cracks as it expands. The orbital fat and muscle push through this crack; but due to the elasticity of the bone, the bone quickly retracts back to its original position possibly entrapping fat and muscle. This trapdoor fracture requires early intervention with correction within 24 h providing the best results. Isolated trapdoor fractures from low-velocity blunt trauma can sometimes present without any visible signs of trauma (periorbital echymosis, edema, or subconjunctival hemorrhage) and are called white-eyed fractures. Due to a strong oculocardiac reflex in children, hypotension, bradycardia, nausea, and vomiting may accompany trapdoor fractures and should prompt ophthalmologic evaluation as the diagnosis may be subtle.

Midface Fracture

Midface fractures are rare in preschool-aged children due to a high craniofacial ratio, but as the mandible and midface grow, incidence increases with age reaching its peak in late teen years. The traditional zymaticomalar complex (ZMC) or tripod fracture seen in adults also becomes more likely as the patient's age increases. Maxillary fractures are mainly caused by high-velocity injury from motor vehicle collisions or interpersonal violence, both of which also increase with age. Fractures like these in young children have concomitant neurocranial injury and may preclude timely intervention. Unerupted dentition provides strength to the alveolus, and a cushioning thick adipose layer over a soft spongy maxilla also protects children and leads to more greenstick than displaced fractures. Non-displaced fractures can be managed with soft diet and activity restrictions. Palpable step-offs, paresthesias, malocclusion, and excessive pain can all be indications for treatment with closed or open reduction. Moderately displaced, comminuted, and/or unstable fractures warrant intervention to reduce and stabilize the fractures. Isolated fractures, such as zygomatic arch fractures, may be treated with a closed or minimal exposure approach. However, extensive midface fractures, such as comminuted ZMC or Lefort II or III fractures, require more exposure and open surgical intervention.

Nasal Fracture

Nasal and septal fractures are more commonly encountered throughout the whole pediatric population. An increasingly prominent nasal profile with aging along with thinner bones than elsewhere in the head that more easily fracture from less traumatic forces cause this consistent fracture incidence from childhood to teenage years. Nasal trauma usually presents with significant external edema making initial fracture diagnosis difficult. Plain films are usually taken in the emergency room and should be reviewed for nasal and septal fractures. Photographs and plain films should always be completed for documentation as future surgery may be needed and insurance companies are more commonly requiring evidence of previous trauma. Nasal deviation, palpable step-offs, depressed fragments, nasal obstruction, and soft tissue edema are all potential signs of a nasal fracture. Treatment includes closed or open reduction with internal or external splint stabilization. Isolated nasal fractures can be treated with a closed technique. Extensive damage or fractures that have a delay in diagnosis most likely will require an open approach. All reduced fractures should be stabilized with external splints not only to help decrease edema but also prevent any secondary displacement caused by unintentional patient manipulation. Internal splints may be needed for septal stabilization from fractures of the septum itself or dislocation from the maxillary crest. Rhinoscopy should be performed in all patients evaluating for a septal hematoma and incised and drained if present. Septal hematomas can occur independently of fractures. As the tight septal perichondrial covering is separated from the cartilage, a space is created into which bleeding occurs. The result is a purplish bulging mucosa that is compressible but not shrinkable with decongestant spray. Untreated septal hematomas may lead to loss of the quadrilateral cartilage, saddle-nose deformity, and possible midface growth restrictions.

Nasal Orbital Ethmoid (NOE) Fracture

NOE fractures are very rare in children and usually accompany other facial fractures. Symptoms include a depressed and flattened nasal root, telecanthus, subconjunctival hemorrhage, and mobility of the medial canthal tendon on bimanual palpation. Additional clinical features include rounding of the medial canthus, horizontal shortening of the palpebral fissure, and an intercanthal distance greater than the palpebral fissure width. CT scan is used for diagnosis and treatment planning. The surgical approach is tailored to the extent of fractures, and fixation can be accomplished with mini-plates, wiring, or suture techniques. Special attention is given to the medial canthus and determining its attachment to the central fragment and status of the nasomaxillary buttress. Undercorrection of the intercanthal distance is common and therefore, overcorrection of both the intercanthal distance and nasal projection should be attempted.

Mandible Fracture

Mandibular fractures are more common in children than adults but a larger percentage of these fractures are non-displaced, greenstick fractures and therefore, would only need a soft diet for treatment. Malocclusion, open lacerations, open bite deformity or deviation are all indications of a mandible fracture. Teenage patients can be treated as adults because their dentition is fully erupted and will not be injured with screw placement from internal fixation or maxillo-mandibular fixation (MMF). The goal of restoring occlusion is the same for both adults and children. However, treatment of a younger pediatric mandible fracture, especially less than 6 years old is controversial. Greenstick fractures and slightly displaced fractures that cause mild malocclusion can be conservatively managed as the pediatric mandible will compensate with bone remodeling. Unstable, displaced, or comminuted fractures need repair. Deciduous teeth do not tolerate maxillo-mandibular fixation with wire techniques very well as these teeth lack a cingulum for the wire to snug the bar down to the gingiva. Bicortical screw placement in mixed and deciduous dentition run the risk of injury to permanent unerupted teeth. Some advocate maxillo-mandibular fixation with wires passing around the mandible and through the piriform aperture or the use of an acrylic mandibular splint. Others advocate monocortical screw placement for internal fixation. However, some believe that this interferes with mandibular growth and recommend these internal fixation plates be removed after healing. In an attempt to avoid this second surgery from plate and screw removal, absorbable plates have been introduced but are only for midface and upper face treatment and not FDA approved for mandibular fractures. However, some have used absorbable systems off label for mandible fractures in the younger pediatric population as the mandibular bite forces created are not as substantial as adults and can withstand the plate fracture force. Research is continuing which may lead to the development of an absorbable plating system that is appropriate for mandibular fractures, but until then monocortical plates and screws placed at the inferior

mandibular border provide for excellent stabilization in those patients whose fractures warrant surgical intervention.

Special attention is paid to mandibular condyle fractures as this is a major growth center. Intracapsular fractures are managed nonsurgically with a soft diet and sometimes immobilization with MMF. If normal range of motion and occlusion exists for high condylar neck and subcondylar fractures, a soft diet is sufficient treatment. If normal occlusion but deviation upon mouth opening exists, arch bars with guiding elastics may be considered. For more displaced fractures that cause occlusal and deviation disturbances, controversy exists whether open surgical treatment is needed or MMF is sufficient. A remarkable remodeling capacity of the pediatric mandible allows for significant compensation over time and must be considered when determining the intensity of intervention, especially in the younger pediatric population.

Conclusion

The pediatric population has different incidence, presentation, and treatment patterns than adults. The incidence of fractures is influenced by anatomy, psychosocial aspects, and facial development. There is a significant change around 6 years of age, as the infants' solid but elastic facial frame transitions to a more rigid adult structure, and psychosocial interactions account for more high-risk behaviors.

The coupling of changes in facial growth patterns with psychosocial evolution explains the changes seen in facial fracture patterns from infancy to adulthood. The largest transition is seen in these elementary school years and then slowly evolves through adolescent and teenage years to adult levels. Trauma in early childhood tends to cause greenstick fractures which can be managed conservatively. With aging, more severe fractures and anatomical changes call for surgical intervention. Attention to disruption of anatomy and future growth must be appreciated with any considered intervention. The goals of facial fracture treatment are anatomic reduction and stabilization to re-establish occlusion, normal facial proportions, and symmetry. Clinical acumen is used to balance the need for intervention with the extent of the intervention needed. Stability and reduction take precedence over an anticipated alteration of facial growth.

More invasive techniques like rigid fixation are reserved when more conservative, closed techniques will not provide adequate results.

References

Alcala-Galiano A, Arribas-Garcia IJ, Martin-Perez MA, Romance A, Montalvo-Moreno JJ, Millan Juncos JM (2008) Pediatric facial fractures: children are not just small adults. Radiographics 28:441–461

Bailey B, Johnson J (2006) Head & neck surgery – Otolaryngology, vol 4. Lippincott Williams & Wilkins, Philadelphia

Centers for Disease Control (CDC) and Prevention (2010). Office of Statistics and Programming, National Center for Injury Prevention and Control. Data Source: National Center for Health Statistics (NCHS), National Vital Statistics System. http://www.cdc.gov/injury/wisqars/index.html

Dorri M, Nasser M, Oliver R (2009) Resorbable versus titanium plates for facial fractures. Cochrane Database Syst Rev 1: CD007158

Friedrich RE, Heiland M, Bartel-Friedrich S (2003) Potentials of ultrasound in the diagnosis of midfacial fractures. Clin Oral Investig 7:226–229

Imadara SD, Hopper RA, Wang J, Rivara F, Klein MB (2008) Patterns and outcomes of pediatric facial fractures in the United States: a survey of the National Trauma Data Bank. J Am Coll Surg 207(5):710–716

Rottgers SA, Decesare G, Chao M, Smith DM, Cray JJ, Naran S, Vecchione L, Grunwaldt L, Losee JE (2011) Outcomes in pediatric facial fractures: early follow-up in 177 children and classification scheme. J Craniofac Surg 22(4): 1260–1265

Ryan ML, Thorson CM, Otero CA, Ogilvie MP, Cheung MC, Saigal GM, Thaller SR (2011) Pediatric facial trauma: a review of guidelines for assessment, evaluation, and management in the emergency department. J Craniofac Surg 22:1183–1189

Vyas RM, Dickinson BP, Wasson KL, Roostaeian J, Bradley JP (2008) Pediatric facial fractures: current national incidence, distribution, and health care resource use. J Craniofac Surg 19(2):339–349

Facial Hemiatrophy

▶ Parry-Romberg Syndrome

Facial Nerve

▶ Facial Nerve Imaging, CT and MRI
▶ Intraoperative Neurophysiologic Monitoring of the Facial Nerve (VII)

Facial Nerve Conductions

▶ Evoked EMG

Facial Nerve Function, Examination

Shelby Topp[1] and Michael E. Hoffer[2]
[1]Department of Otolaryngology, Naval Medical Center San Diego, San Diego, CA, USA
[2]Department of Otolaryngology, Spatial Orientation Center, Naval Medical Center, San Diego, CA, USA

Assessment of Facial Nerve Function: History and Physical

When an individual presents with complaints of altered facial nerve function a thorough history should be obtained. Pertinent questions include time since onset, rate of progression of paralysis, and associated symptoms to include facial twitching, facial numbness, changes in hearing, dizziness, mental status changes, or loss of function of other nerves (Schaitkin et al. 2001). Once the examiner has a good idea of the status of the history surrounding the paralysis, background information must be collected. Pertinent background information includes history of facial trauma (blunt or penetrating), history of facial paralysis in the past, history of recent upper respiratory infections, history of exposure to ticks, and history of foreign travel. Other questions may be pertinent depending on the patient population and site of the clinic. A complete past medical and surgical history should be performed.

Physical examination should include a complete head and neck examination with particular attention paid to the external auditory canal (EAC), skin around the EAC, and all cranial nerves (especially cranial nerves 8 – hearing/balance and 5 – facial sensation). In order to test the facial function, the patient is asked to move muscles covering all segments of the facial nerve (with the exception of the cervical) on each side. For the temporalis branch, an eyebrow or forehead raise is used; for the zygomatic branch, nasal motion is observed; for the buccal branch, upper lip motion is observed; and for the mandibular branch, lower lip motion is observed. Some examiners use a hand especially in the temporal region to prevent cross-pulling of fibers. Once a complete examination is done, the examiner needs to classify the facial nerve paralysis.

Most examiners currently use a modified House-Brackmann scale (House and Brackmann 1985). The scale is enclosed in the text below.

Grade	Characteristics
I. Normal	Normal facial function in all areas
II. Mild dysfunction	Gross • Slight weakness noticeable on close inspection • May have slight synkinesis • At rest, normal symmetry and tone Motion • Forehead – Moderate-to-good function • Eye – Complete closure with minimal effort • Mouth – Slight asymmetry
III. Moderate dysfunction	Gross • Obvious but not disfiguring difference between the two sides • Noticeable but not severe synkinesis, contracture, or hemifacial spasm • At rest, normal symmetry and tone Motion • Forehead – Slight-to-moderate movement • Eye – Complete closure with effort • Mouth – Slightly weak with maximum effort
IV. Moderately severe Dysfunction	Gross • Obvious weakness and/or disfiguring asymmetry • At rest, normal symmetry and tone Motion • Forehead – None • Eye – Incomplete closure • Mouth – Asymmetric with maximum effort
V. Severe dysfunction	Gross • Only barely perceptible motion • At rest, asymmetry Motion • Forehead – None • Eye – Incomplete closure • Mouth – Slight movement
VI. Total paralysis	No movement

The scale was originally developed to describe outcomes of individuals who had suffered a facial nerve paralysis at an earlier date but has now become a fairly common nomenclature and a standard way of communicating the facial function between medical care team members.

Radiological Studies

In cases where a known etiology is causing the facial paralysis (parotid mass, SCCA of the temporal bone, etc.) appropriate imaging (MRI, CT, or nuclear medicine) should be ordered for the primary disorder. The facial nerve will best be visualized in its intratemporal portion by thin cut CT or MRI whereas MRI is best for all other portions of the nerve. For individuals with idiopathic facial paralysis, the need for radiologic study and the study of choice is more difficult. If there is a suspicion that a tumor could be present in the brainstem (hearing changes, slow progression of paralysis, unsteadiness, or mental status changes) an MRI scan should be obtained. Sequencing required to examine the brainstem varies between institutions. In the absence of such signs, idiopathic facial paresis or paralysis does not, initially, require imaging. Nevertheless, in a recent study of the management of such lesions, just over two thirds of experienced providers obtained an MRI at the time of presentation (Smouha et al. 2011). Prior to the findings of this study, the standard practice had been not to obtain imaging unless the lesion progresses for too long a period of time or surgery is contemplated. Once again, CT scan will prove more effective at delineating the course of the nerve through the temporal bone and the relationship of this bone to the nerve, whereas MRI will be better for other portions of the nerve. The decision of which scan to do and when to do the scan varies by institution (Kefalidis et al. 2010; Quesnel et al. 2010).

Electrical Tests

There are three electrical tests of facial nerve function – the nerve excitability test (NET), electroneurography (ENoG), and electromyography (EMG). The utility and timing of these testes has been an issue of significant debate over the years (Fisch 1984; May et al. 1983). Some individuals argue aggressive testing and early intervention whereas others argue for more conservative measures. However, it is important to note that in the same survey quoted above 97% of respondents said they would obtain an ENoG and only 17% ordered EMGs.

This entry briefly describes the two most commonly used tests: ENoG and EMG. It is important to remember that these tests are only used in individuals with a total paralysis (HB 6/6). Individuals with any function are observed. ENoG is only valuable when performed within the first 10 days of paralysis. This test compares the amplitude of facial muscle contractions of the affected side to the normal side using suprathreshold electrical stimulation at the stylomastoid foramen. Those patients that have more than 90% loss of amplitude on the paralyzed side have a poorer prognosis (Fisch 1984).

EMG testing is often used in conjunction with ENoG; either to confirm the results or in cases when surgery is contemplated. The test will not be useful in the first 72 h because even in muscles whose motor nerve is severed, normal latency and normal muscle action potentials can persist for 2–3 days. The test can be helpful at the 5–8 day mark but fibrillation potentials may not appear until 2–3 weeks after injury/onset of paralysis. In EMG testing a needle electrode is placed in the muscle of interest and patients are asked to attempt to contract the muscle. Lack of spontaneous motor unit action potentials implies no innervation or reinnervation and the presence of fibrillation potentials suggests a poor prognosis. On the other hand, voluntary action potentials imply that the muscle is innervated and polyphasic reinnervation potentials suggest a good prognosis.

Summary

Analysis of facial nerve function begins with a thorough history and physical examination. The findings on this initial evaluation guide future diagnostic steps. Radiologic imaging can be helpful but may not be necessary in uncomplicated idiopathic palsy. Whereas there are many electrodiagnostic tests, most individuals only utilize ENoG for patients with total paralysis with EMG reserved to confirm the results of ENoG and as a presurgical test.

Disclaimer

The views expressed in this article are those of the author(s) and do not necessarily reflect the official policy or position of the Department of the Navy, Department of Defense, or the U.S. Government.

Cross-References

▶ Evoked EMG
▶ Facial Nerve Paralysis Due to Bacterial Etiology
▶ Facial Nerve Paralysis Due to Viral Etiology
▶ Facial Paralysis
▶ Nerve Excitability Test

References

Fisch U (1984) Prognostic value of electrical tests in acute facial paralysis. Am J Otol 5(6):494–498
House JW, Brackmann DE (1985) Facial nerve grading system. Otolaryngol Head Neck Surg 93:146–147
Kefalidis G, Riga M, Argyropoulou P, Katotomichelakis M, Gouveris C, Prassopoulos P, Danielides V (2010) Is the width of the labyrinthine portion of the fallopian tube implicated in the pathophysiology of Bell's palsy?: a prospective clinical study using computed tomography. Laryngoscope 120(6):1203–1207
May M, Blumenthal F, Klein SR (1983) Acute Bell's palsy: prognostic value of evoked electromyography, maximal stimulation, and other electrical tests. Am J Otol 5(1):1–7
Quesnel AM, Lindsay RW, Hadlock TA (2010) When the bell tolls on Bell's palsy: finding occult malignancy in acute-onset facial paralysis. Am J Otolaryngol 31(5):339–342
Schaitkin BM, May M, Klein SR (2001) Office evaluation of the patient with facial palsy: differential diagnosis and prognosis. In: May M, Schaitkin BM (eds) The facial nerve, 2nd edn. Thieme, New York
Smouha E, Toh E, Schaitkin BM (2011) Surgical treatment of bells palsy: current attitudes. Laryngoscope 121(9):1965–1970

Facial Nerve Imaging, CT and MRI

Ramón E. Figueroa
Department of Radiology, Georgia Health Sciences University, Augusta, GA, USA

Synonyms

CN 7; CN VII; Cranial nerve 7; Facial nerve

Definition

The facial nerve, also known as the cranial nerve VII, is a mixed function cranial nerve with dominant motor function, but also parasympathetic and gustatory functions. Its motor fibers control the muscles of facial expression, while its parasympathetic efferent fibers control secretory functions of the lacrimal, submandibular and sublingual glands. Its afferent fibers receive the taste sensation from the anterior two thirds of the tongue.

Purpose

The appropriate imaging evaluation of the facial nerve depends on which segment of the facial nerve is being explored, which must be deducted from the clinical signs and symptoms of the affected nerve. Computed tomography (CT) is most useful for evaluation of the facial nerve segments contained within the temporal bone, while magnetic resonance imaging (MRI) is most appropriate for the evaluation of the intra-axial, cisternal, and extracranial segments.

Principles

The facial nerve is a mixed function nerve that controls the muscles of facial expression; the secretory innervation to the lacrimal, submandibular, and sublingual glands; and the taste sensation for the anterior two thirds of the tongue. Its motor division, comprising about 70% of the total volume of nerve fibers, supplies somatic motor innervation to the muscles of the face, scalp, and auricle; the buccinators and platysma; the stapedius; stylohyoideus; and the posterior belly of the digastric muscle (Harnsberger et al. 2006). It is subdivided into four main anatomic segments: the intra-axial segment, cisternal, intratemporal, and extracranial segments. The facial nerve is anatomically comprised of two roots, the larger size motor root made up of heavily myelinated fibers, and the sensory root that carries the parasympathetic and gustatory fibers. This sensory root, of smaller caliber, is known as the nerve of Wrisberg, or by its more common name, nervus intermedius, since it arises in intermediate position between the motor root of the facial nerve and the vestibulocochlear nerve (cranial nerve VIII) at the lateral pontomedullary junction (Curtin et al. 2003).

The intra-axial pathways of the facial nerve start from pyramidal neurons at the precentral frontal motor cortex, where the eloquent cortex controlling facial expression is topographically represented by the complexity of motor tasks, with more complex function

having a larger number of neurons. The facial motor cortical representation along the precentral gyrus and somatosensory representation along the post-central gyrus are sequentially organized from top to bottom in frontal, periorbital, midface, perioral, and tongue cortical zones. The facial motor pathways continue through the posterior genu of the internal capsule as the corticobulbar tracts. Upon reaching the pons, most of the frontal motor fibers decussate to the contralateral facial nerve nucleus, while some remain ipsilateral, resulting in bilateral supranuclear innervation to the muscles of the upper face. The supranuclear fibers for the lower face decussate completely to the contralateral facial nucleus. This anatomic asymmetry is responsible for the clinical subdivision of facial palsy into central (facial palsy with sparing of frontal expression) and peripheral (palsy involving the entire hemiface) (May 2000).

The intra-axial pontine facial nerve is comprised of three nuclei: the motor nucleus, the parasympathetic superior salivatory nucleus, and the gustatory nucleus of the tractus solitarius, arranged sequentially from medial to lateral within the ventral-lateral pons (Raghavan et al. 2009). The larger of these nuclei, the motor nucleus of the facial nerve, is divided into an upper and lower half, with the upper half receiving ipsilateral and contralateral cortical innervation for the upper face, while the lower half receive only contralateral innervation for the lower face. Central lesions affecting the intra-axial facial nerve pathways (supranuclear) will thus express facial paralysis with sparing of upper frontal facial expression (due to bilateral cortical innervation to the upper division). Peripheral lesions (distal to the facial nerve motor nucleus or infra-nuclear) will have complete (upper and lower) facial paralysis ipsilateral to the lesion. The motor nucleus of the facial nerve lies within the reticular formation of the lower third of the pons, ventral to the sixth cranial nerve nucleus. Its efferent fibers run around the dorsal margin of the abducens nerve nucleus, forming a contour elevation on the floor of the fourth ventricle, known as the facial colliculus, easily recognizable by MRI (Fig. 1). This loop around the abducens nucleus is known as the facial nerve internal genu. Facial nerve motor fibers continue anterolaterally to emerge from the brainstem at the lateral pontomedullary junction.

The superior salivatory nucleus, the second nucleus of the facial nerve, lies lateral to the facial motor

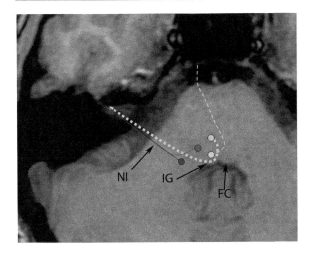

Facial Nerve Imaging, CT and MRI, Fig. 1 Axial T1-weighted image at the level of the pontine tegmentum shows the facial colliculus at the floor of the fourth ventricle. Overlaid diagram shows the motor nucleus of the facial nerve (*yellow circle*) and the motor root of the facial nerve (*intermittent yellow line*) forming the internal genu (*IG*) around the abducens nucleus (*light blue circle*). Notice also the tractus solitarius nucleus (*dark blue circle*) and the superior salivatory nucleus (*red circle*), both of which contribute to the formation of the nervus intermedius (*NI*)

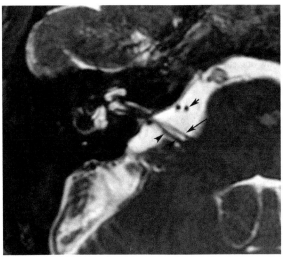

Facial Nerve Imaging, CT and MRI, Fig. 2 Axial T2-weighted image at the level of the cerebellopontine angle shows the cisternal portion of the facial nerve (*long arrow*) just anterior to the vestibulocochlear nerve (*double arrowheads*), both extending toward the internal auditory canal. Notice a prominent anterior inferior cerebellar artery (*short arrow*)

nucleus. Its efferent parasympathetic fibers emerge from the brainstem posterolateral to the motor root, as the nervus intermedius, running together next to the motor root through the cisternal segment into the internal auditory canal. This nucleus controls the secretory function of the lacrimal, submandibular, and sublingual glands.

The nucleus of the tractus solitarius is lateral to the superior salivatory nucleus. It receives the afferent taste input from the anterior two thirds of the tongue through fibers that travel from the tongue through the chorda tympani nerve to synapse at the geniculate ganglion, and from there through the nervus intermedius to the nucleus of the tractus solitarius. The intra-axial segment of the facial nerve is best evaluated by MRI.

The cisternal segment of the facial nerve is made up of the larger motor root running anterior to the smaller sensory nervus intermedius along the cerebellopontine angle cistern to enter the internal auditory canal (IAC). Both emerge from the brainstem at the lateral pontomedullary sulcus, just anterior to the vestibulocochlear nerve. This facial nerve segment is also best evaluated by MRI (Fig. 2).

The intratemporal segment of the facial nerve can be subdivided into IAC, labyrinthine, tympanic, and mastoid segments, all enclosed by bone, best evaluated by high-resolution CT. The IAC segment runs from the porus acusticus to the superior anterior quadrant of the apex of the IAC, where the entrance to the fallopian canal is found (Fig. 3a, b). The motor root and the nervus intermedius form a common trunk at the IAC, still with the nervus intermedius fibers remaining posterior to the motor fibers. The fallopian canal of the facial nerve starts at the apex of the IAC superior to the falciform crest and anterior to Bill's bar, running for a length of approximately 14 mm to end at the stylomastoid foramen. The facial nerve through the fallopian canal is subdivided into labyrinthine, tympanic, and mastoid segments. The labyrinthine segment crosses the otic capsule at the superior medial border of the cochlea, extending from the apex of the IAC to the fossa of the geniculate ganglion (Fig. 4a, b, c, d). The facial nerve does a hairpin turn at the geniculate ganglion, to continue along the medial tympanic wall as the tympanic segment (Fig. 5a, b). This turn at the geniculate ganglion is known as the anterior genu. The greater superficial petrosal nerve arises from the geniculate ganglion, extending anterior-medially to contribute to the formation of the vidian nerve,

Facial Nerve Imaging, CT and MRI, Fig. 3 Axial CT and axial T2-weighted images at the internal auditory canal show otic capsule contour on CT (**a**) matching membranous labyrinth and IAC segment of the facial nerve on MRI (**b**). Notice vestibule (*V*), basal turn of the cochlea (*C*), and tympanic segment (*TS*) of the facial nerve on each image. IAC segment shows best on MRI (*arrowheads*)

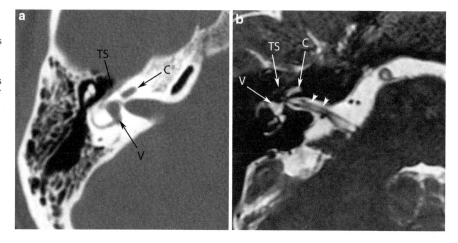

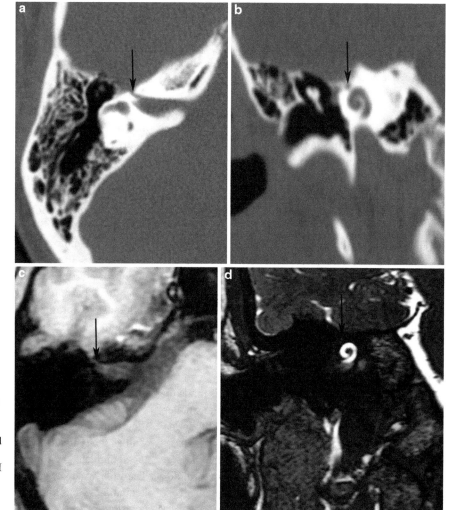

Facial Nerve Imaging, CT and MRI,
Fig. 4 Labyrinthine segment of the Facial Nerve: Top row axial CT (**a**) and coronal CT (**b**) with anatomically matched axial T1-weighted MRI (**c**) and coronal T2-weighted MRI (**d**) show the labyrinthine segment (*vertical arrow*) of the facial nerve

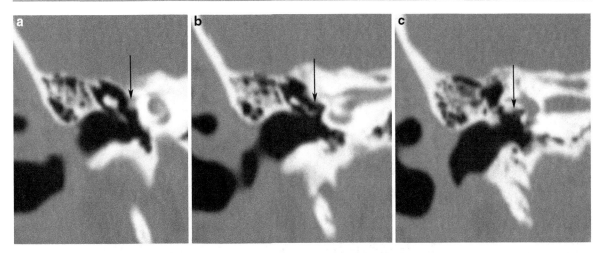

Facial Nerve Imaging, CT and MRI, Fig. 5 a–c: Tympanic segment of the facial nerve is shown best on sequential coronal CT images in bone detail (*vertical arrows*), extending between the geniculate ganglion and the posterior genu along the medial wall of the tympanic space

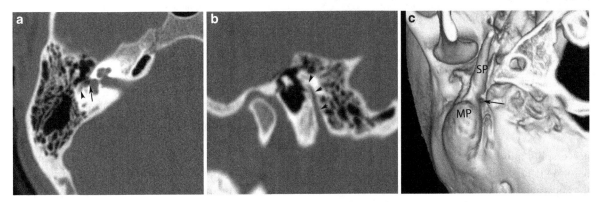

Facial Nerve Imaging, CT and MRI, Fig. 6 a–c: Mastoid segment of the facial nerve is vertically oriented, between the posterior genu and the stylomastoid foramen. **a:** axial CT shows the tympanic segment of the facial nerve ending at the posterior genu (*arrowhead*). Notice the oval window (*arrow*). **b:** Sagittal CT reformatted image shows the posterior genu and the mastoid segment to best advantage (*arrowheads*). **c:** 3D Volume rendered CT image shows the mastoid process (*MP*) and styloid process (*SP*) framing the aperture of the stylomastoid foramen (*arrow*)

transmitting parasympathetic innervation to the lacrimal gland. The tympanic segment runs horizontally along the medial wall of the tympanic space just above the oval window, continuing right under the lateral semicircular canal to the roof of the sinus tympani, where the nerve turns 90° downward (posterior genu) to constitute the mastoid segment, finally to exit through the stylomastoid foramen (Fig. 6a, b, c).

The stapedius nerve arises from the mastoid segment of the facial nerve just below the posterior genu, innervating the stapedius muscle within the pyramidal eminence, to control and modulate the sound transmission dampening effects of the stapedius muscle upon the ossicular chain. The chorda tympani is the next branch of the facial nerve, usually at the inferior mastoid segment above the stylomastoid foramen. The afferent gustatory fibers from the anterior two thirds of the tongue travel with the lingual branch of the trigeminal nerve mandibular division to form the chorda tympani, which crosses the middle ear and joins the facial nerve at the inferior mastoid segment.

The facial nerve beyond the stylomastoid foramen comprises the extracranial segment of the facial nerve, crossing lateral to the styloid process to enter the substance of the parotid gland. The intraparotid facial

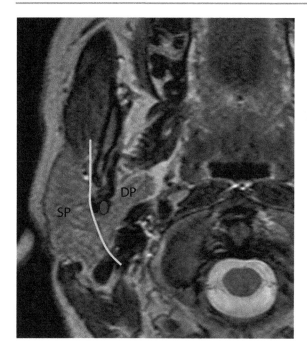

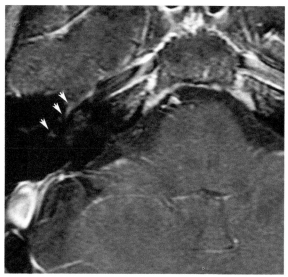

Facial Nerve Imaging, CT and MRI, Fig. 7 Axial T2-weighted MRI at the parotid space level shows the course of the intraparotid facial nerve (*yellow line*) immediately lateral to the retromandibular vein (*blue circle*) separating the parotid substance into a superficial parotid (*SP*) and deep parotid (*DP*) components

Facial Nerve Imaging, CT and MRI, Fig. 8 Axial Gadolinium-enhanced T1-weighted MR with fat suppression technique shows the discrete pattern of normal enhancement from circumneural vascular plexus along the tympanic segment (*arrowheads*)

nerve splits into its major branches as it crosses the parotid gland, establishing a virtual plane that defines the superficial and deep portions of the parotid gland. The intraparotid facial nerve runs lateral to the retromandibular vein, where it separates into five major branches: the temporal (frontal), zygomatic, buccal, marginal mandibular, and cervical branches (Fig. 7). The facial nerve vascular supply within the fallopian canal is provided by a circumneural arterial and venous plexus, supplied by vascular pedicles from the anterior inferior cerebellar artery at the IAC end of the fallopian canal and by external carotid artery branches at the stylomastoid foramen. This slow-flowing vascular arcade may provide mild enhancement of the facial nerve within the fallopian canal on Gadolinium-enhanced MRI studies (Fig. 8).

Indication

The determination of which study to use for imaging of a facial nerve palsy is dictated by the type of clinical defect found. If a central facial nerve lesion is suspected by the presence of a paralysis of muscles of facial expression with forehead sparing, MRI of the brain is indicated, looking for ischemic, demyelinating or tumoral lesions in the intra-axial facial nerve pathways above the facial nerve nuclei. MRI imaging protocol includes pre- and post-Gadolinium axial and coronal T1-weighted 3 mm images, diffusion-weighted images for detection of ischemic lesions, and a heavy T2-weighted 3D volume acquisition partitioned at 1 mm. If on the other hand, a peripheral facial nerve injury is suspected, expressed as paralysis of ipsilateral muscles of facial expression, with variable impairment of lacrimation, sound dampening and taste, a temporal bone lesion should be excluded, best screened by high-resolution temporal bone CT. CT images are acquired with a multidetector CT scanner in axial plane parallel to the hard palate with 0.625 mm slices at 0.3 mm intervals in edge enhancement bone detail, with targeted small field of view processed for each temporal bone independently. The resulting isotropic voxel data can be reviewed with high-resolution detail in any plane at the imaging workstation, allowing for a thorough evaluation of the entire intratemporal course of the facial nerve.

Contraindication

MRI may be contraindicated in patients with cardiac pacemakers, old aneurysm clips, or neural stimulator implanted devices, such as vagus nerve stimulators, deep brain stimulators, or cochlear implants. In such cases, high-resolution temporal bone CT remains the main diagnostic modality.

Cross-References

The pathology of the facial nerve varies from inflammatory **Bell's palsy**, to **facial nerve congenital anomalies**, **hemifacial spasm** from vascular compression, facial nerve tumors such as **schwannomas**, **intratemporal benign vascular tumors** and malignant lesions, especially **perineural spread** from malignancies such as adenoid cystic carcinoma, squamous cell carcinoma, melanoma, and lymphoma. For more information on specific entries of facial nerve pathology, please see also: Facial nerve paralysis due to Bacterial Etiology, Facial nerve paralysis due to Viral Etiology, Facial Nerve Anatomy and Physiology-Embryology, Facial Nerve Anatomy and Physiology-Examination, Facial Neuroma, hemangioma and other neoplasms, Facial paralysis in children.

References

Curtin H, Sanelli P, Som P (2003) Temporal bone: embryology and anatomy. In: Som PM, Curtin HD (eds) Head and neck imaging, 4th edn. Mosby, St. Louis, pp 1057–1092

Harnsberger H, Osborn AG, Macdonald AJ et al (2006) Diagnostic and surgical imaging anatomy: brain, head and neck, spine. Amyrsis, Inc, Salt Lake City, Utah, pp 224–231

May M (2000) Anatomy of the facial nerve for the clinician. In: May M, Schaitkin B (eds) The facial nerve. Thieme Medical, New York, pp 19–56

Raghavan P, Mukherjee S, Phillips CD (2009) Imaging of the facial nerve. Neuroimag Clin N Am 19:407–425

Facial Nerve Palsy

▶ Post-parotidectomy Facial Nerve Paralysis

Facial Nerve Paralysis due to Bacterial Etiology

George S. Conley
Department of Otolaryngology-Head and Neck Surgery, University of Pittsburgh, Pittsburgh, PA, USA

Definitions

Neuropraxia: A temporary loss of motor and sensory neural function due to blockage of nerve conduction, usually lasting weeks to months before a full recovery is observed.

Petrous apicitis: An infection involving the apex of the petrous portion of the temporal bone. It is usually superimposed on a middle ear infection and may clinically present with an abducens nerve palsy and deep facial pain associated with inflammation of the trigeminal nerve.

Subperiosteal abscess: A collection of purulent fluid lateral to the mastoid cortex that may be associated with a mastoiditis and coalescence of the mastoid air cell system.

Tympanosclerosis: A condition where chronic ear disease may elicit the production of dense connective tissue and calcification of various middle ear structures to include the tympanic membrane, middle ear bones, and mucosa of the middle ear and mastoid cavity.

Cholesteatoma: A skin cyst in the middle ear and/or mastoid. This cyst consists of keratinizing squamous epithelium that may enlarge and erode the middle ear bones or other structures within the temporal bone.

Introduction

Management of patients who present with acute facial paralysis can be a challenging task. The clinician must have a thorough understanding of the anatomy and physiology of the facial nerve and must be aware of the numerous disease processes that elicit facial nerve disorders. Although most cases of acute facial paralysis are mediated by an idiopathic or viral etiology, the initial evaluation should focus on identifying other common causes such as trauma, neoplasm, or bacterial infection.

The identification of a bacterial-related facial palsy is very important since early treatment of infection has a profound impact on improving long-term clinical outcomes. The most common bacterial diseases associated with facial paralysis are acute otitis media, chronic otitis media, malignant otitis externa, and Lyme disease. Each presents with characteristic clinical features that may be discovered through a detailed history and comprehensive clinical exam. Identification of the specific bacterial disease will lead to an appropriate treatment plan that prevents additional morbidity and improves facial nerve recovery.

Acute Otitis Media

Acute suppurative otitis media (ASOM) is a bacterial infection of the middle ear lasting less than 3 weeks in duration. Typically, it is identified in young children who present with fever, otalgia, decreased hearing, and otoscopic findings suggestive of a middle ear mucopurulent infection. *Streptococcus pneumoniae*, *Haemophilus influenzae*, and *Moraxella catarrhalis* are common pathogens associated with ASOM (Agrawal et al. 2005). Oral antibiotics are highly successful in resolving the infection with minimal adverse effects but in rare instances, a progressive facial weakness may occur with ASOM.

The overall incidence of facial palsy associated with ASOM is estimated at 0.005% (Vrabec and Coker 2006). It is commonly believed to arise from the various bacterial and inflammatory substrates that exist within a suppurative effusion. These substrates produce neural inflammation that eventually leads to facial nerve edema and neuropraxia (Kitsko and Dohar 2007). Congenital dehiscences of the fallopian canal commonly found in the tympanic segment are sites where infection may directly contact the facial nerve to induce an inflammatory effect (Mattox 2010). Other potential pathways are through the small bony canaliculi that transmit the chorda tympani and stapedial nerves from the mastoid segment of the fallopian canal to the middle ear (Yetiser et al. 2002).

If facial nerve palsy is observed with ASOM, a computed tomography (CT) scan of the temporal bone should be obtained to determine the extent of disease. Using intravenous antibiotics and a wide myringotomy, initial treatment is directed at eradicating the ear infection and its toxic metabolites from the temporal bone. Middle ear fluid obtained during the myringotomy should be cultured for bacterial sensitivities that may further direct antibiotic therapy. If the patient is known to have a significant history of recurrent otitis media, a myringotomy tube may also be placed for prolonged ventilation of the middle ear. These measures typically lead to the prompt resolution of ASOM and an excellent prognosis. A complete facial nerve recovery can be expected in greater than 95% of patients with ASOM associated facial palsy (Agrawal et al. 2005).

However, if the fever and otalgia do not respond to appropriate therapy or if facial paralysis persists for longer than a week, a cortical mastoidectomy should be performed to debride recalcitrant areas of infection. A mastoidectomy is also advocated if other complications of ASOM such as a coalescent mastoiditis, petrous apicitis, or subperiosteal abscess are identified (Agrawal et al. 2005). When completing a mastoidectomy for ASOM, facial nerve decompression is not recommended (Kitsko and Dohar 2007). This may further expose the nerve to toxic metabolites and it increases the possibility of an iatrogenic injury to an already inflamed nerve.

Chronic Otitis Media

Chronic Suppurative Otitis Media/Cholesteatoma

Chronic suppurative otitis media (CSOM) is defined as an active bacterial infection of the middle ear or mastoid that is associated with chronic ear disease and a history of past or present tympanic membrane perforation. CSOM is mainly found in adults and typically presents with chronic ear drainage, hearing loss, and signs of chronic infection such as eardrum perforation, atelectasis, tympanosclerosis, or cholesteatoma. Common pathogens of CSOM include *Pseudomonas aeruginosa*, *Proteus mirabilis*, and *Staphylococcus aureus* (Agrawal et al. 2005). The long-term inflammatory effect of these pathogens on the mucosa of the middle ear and mastoid commonly leads to fibrosis, granulation tissue, and sometimes cholesteatoma.

Uncomplicated CSOM is initially treated in a similar fashion as ASOM. Systemic antibiotics are directed at clearing active infection from the middle ear and mastoid. If the eardrum is intact, a myringotomy is completed and the middle ear fluid is cultured for bacterial sensitivity. However, when CSOM is complicated by facial palsy, the role of cholesteatoma and granulation tissue must be considered. Both are capable of eroding the fallopian canal and producing an enlarged area of facial nerve exposure that is susceptible to toxic or compressive elements. Any development of facial weakness associated with CSOM should be evaluated with a CT scan of the temporal bone. This will determine the status of the fallopian canal and the presence of cholesteatoma or additional intratemporal complications. Patients with facial nerve palsy and cholesteatoma have a worse prognosis for functional facial recovery than those with CSOM alone (Toh and Lee 2008).

When CSOM is complicated by facial dysfunction, surgical debridement of the mastoid and middle ear is necessary to provide the patient with a safe ear. During a tympanomastoidectomy, the facial nerve should be inspected and carefully decompressed of any diseased tissue without opening the epineurium (Vrabec and Coker 2006). Surgery should be performed early since higher rates of facial nerve recovery are associated with earlier intervention (Makeham et al. 2007). If facial paralysis is present for longer than 3 weeks, functional facial improvement is rarely observed (Vrabec and Coker 2006). Overall, the prognosis of complete facial nerve recovery in CSOM is reported to be between 58% and 70% (Agrawal et al. 2005).

Tuberculous Otitis Media

Tuberculous otitis media (TOM) is caused by *Mycobacterium tuberculosis* and accounts for 0.05–0.9% of chronic infections of the middle ear (Vaamonde et al. 2004). In developed countries, it is commonly associated with immigrants, lower socioeconomic status, patients suffering from human immunodeficiency virus, and those with a personal or family history of tuberculosis. The classic description of TOM includes painless otorrhea, multiple tympanic membrane perforations, and facial palsy. However, most patients do not demonstrate this triad and instead manifest a presentation that can be easily confused with CSOM.

Clinical findings suggestive of TOM include chronic otorrhea, tympanic membrane perforation, abundant pale granulation tissue, polypoid mucosal inflammation, the formation of bony sequestra, and cervical lymphadenopathy. A mixed hearing loss is usually identified and may be attributed to ossicular erosion and an inner ear labyrinthitis. Facial palsy develops in approximately 10% of adults and 35% of children with TOM (Schleuning et al. 2006). CT scans of the temporal bone typically show soft tissue opacification of the middle ear and mastoid that is typically indistinguishable from CSOM.

Since TOM is a rare cause of bacterial mediated facial paralysis, it is imperative that this disease be identified early so that proper medical treatment can be administered. A key finding suggestive of TOM is chronic otorrhea refractory to medical management. Once TOM is suspected, testing should be directed toward identifying a mycobacterial source. Although not highly sensitive, aural exudate should be cultured for mycobacteria. A positive PPD (tuberculosis skin test) or evidence of pulmonary tuberculosis on chest X-ray or CT scan may also lend support for the diagnosis of TOM. If still uncertain, histologic and microbiologic analysis of biopsied middle ear tissue is the gold standard for identifying TOM. It is important that any biopsies meant for culture be sent as fresh specimens without using formalin. Once diagnosed, TOM is treated with a standard antituberculosis multidrug chemotherapy regimen. This commonly includes isoniazid, rifampin, and pyrazinamide. Most studies show that medical management with appropriate antibiotics results in good facial recovery, resolution of otorrhea, and spontaneous closure of eardrum perforations (Vaamonde et al. 2004). If antibiotic treatment of aural tuberculosis does not improve clinically, some advocate surgery to eradicate recalcitrant disease (Schleuning et al. 2006).

Malignant Otitis Externa

Malignant otitis externa (MOE) is a severe infection of the external auditory canal (EAC) that gradually progresses into an osteomyelitis of the temporal bone and skull base. In the majority of cases, MOE is associated with immunocompromised individuals and the gram-negative aerobe, *Pseudomonas aeruginosa* (Hirsch 2005). The diagnosis of MOE is based on its clinical presentation along with supportive radiographic imaging and laboratory findings. MOE is commonly found in the elderly diabetic who describes severe otalgia (usually worse at night), aural fullness, hearing loss, and otorrhea. Otoscopy typically demonstrates purulent otorrhea and granulation tissue localized at the bony-cartilaginous junction of the EAC floor. There is usually an absence of any middle ear pathology.

The external ear infection travels to the skull base through small perforations in the cartilaginous portion of the EAC known as the fissures of Santorini. An ensuing osteomyelitis will spread medially to the various skull base foramina and this may result in multiple cranial neuropathies. Since, the stylomastoid foramen is in close proximity to the EAC, facial nerve paralysis is commonly observed in up to 25% of MOE patients (Carfrae and Kesser 2008).

Laboratory evaluation of MOE focuses on the analysis of biopsied granulation tissue from the EAC. Biopsies are primarily used to rule out malignancy of the EAC since carcinoma has a similar clinical presentation as MOE. Although pseudomonas is identified in up to 98% of cases of MOE, tissue cultures are routinely grown to identify the specific bacteria involved and its antibiotic sensitivities. Rarely, a fungal pathogen such as an *Aspergillus* species may be identified. Leukocytosis and other laboratory signs of systemic infection are not commonly identified, but an elevated erythrocyte sedimentation rate (ESR) is a typical finding in cases of MOE (Carfrae and Kesser 2008).

A variety of radiographic modalities are used in the diagnosis and management of MOE. CT scans of the temporal bone are routinely obtained early in the diagnostic stage to determine if erosive bony changes of the EAC and skull base are consistent with MOE. Nuclear imaging studies using technetium and gallium may also support a diagnosis of MOE. Technetium concentrates in areas of high osteoblastic activity and serves as an early indicator of osteomyelitis (Hirsch 2005). Gallium concentrates in areas of high inflammation and will identify both bony and soft tissue involvement of infection.

Appropriate treatment of MOE is accomplished using long courses of high dose antibiotic therapy and occasional selective surgical debridement. Although symptoms may resolve quickly, antipseudomonal antibiotics such as ciprofloxacin are advocated for at least 6–8 weeks (Carfrae and Kesser 2008). With a focus on early medical management, past mortality rates of up to 50% have been reduced to less than 15%. Still, recurrence rates of up to 20% have been reported (Carfrae and Kesser 2008). The

overall prognosis of MOE with facial paralysis is not significantly different than MOE without facial dysfunction. However, in contrast to lower cranial nerve recovery, patients who experience facial nerve paralysis rarely recover normal facial function (Carfrae and Kesser 2008). As indicators of inflammation, gallium scans and the ESR are commonly used to confirm resolution of MOE and may serve as an endpoint for medical therapy.

Lyme Disease

Lyme disease is a systemic illness that occurs when the spirochete *Borrelia burgdorferi* is transmitted to humans through the bite of an *Ixodes* tick. It occurs throughout the United States, Europe, and Asia, and is endemic in various regions. After the initial tick bite, the symptoms of Lyme disease typically develop in stages but the clinical manifestations are highly variable. Early findings may include a characteristic rash at the site of the tick bite known as erythema migrans and generalized flu-like symptoms such as headache, myalgias, fevers, chills, and profound fatigue (Schleuning et al. 2006). Late findings occur months after the initial bite and may include the development of cardiac inflammation (specifically A-V block), meningitis, multiple neuropathies, encephalopathy, and arthritis (Marques 2010). The facial nerve is the most common cranial nerve affected and facial nerve paralysis can occur in up to 11% of patients with a 3:1 ratio of unilateral to bilateral involvement (Limb and Niparko 2005). In certain endemic regions, Lyme disease may be responsible for up to 50% of facial paralysis seen in children (Mattox 2010).

A diagnosis of Lyme disease is based primarily on a history of possible tick exposure and the characteristic progression of systemic, cutaneous, and neurologic symptoms throughout the varied stages. Early detection can be difficult because many patients will not remember an insect bite. In the late stages, serologic testing with an enzyme-linked immunosorbent assay (ELISA) followed by the more reliable western blot testing is recommended (Marques 2010). These tests can corroborate a diagnosis of Lyme disease but they do not distinguish between an active and inactive infection.

Most manifestations of Lyme disease spontaneously resolve. However, antibiotic therapy is recommended to enhance recovery and prevent long-term sequelae. Lyme disease is commonly treated with 14–28 day regimens of doxycycline, amoxicillin, cefuroxime axetil, or penicillin (Marques 2010). The prognosis for facial nerve recovery is excellent. Most patients achieve complete recovery and the few affected patients usually experience mild residual impairment or synkinesis.

Conclusion

In the management of acute facial palsy, current evidence suggests that infectious etiologies are implicated in the majority of cases. Although viruses comprise the largest source, various bacteria are associated with facial nerve paralysis. In all cases of facial nerve palsy, a careful investigation should determine if an underlying bacterial process is present. If bacterial pathology is recognized, prompt antibiotic and selective surgical treatment should be initiated to resolve the infection, prevent further morbidity, and improve long-term facial function.

Disclaimer

The views expressed in this presentation are those of the author and do not necessarily reflect the official policy or position of the Department of the Navy, Department of Defense, or the United States government.

Cross-References

▶ Cholesteatoma, Acquired
▶ Facial Paralysis
▶ Facial Paralysis in Children
▶ Otologic Manifestations of Lyme Disease
▶ Otitis Media with Effusion
▶ Otitis Media, Complications

References

Agrawal S, Husein M, MacRae D (2005) Complications of otitis media: an evolving state. J Otolaryngol 34(Suppl 1):S33–S39
Carfrae MJ, Kesser BW (2008) Malignant otitis externa. Otolaryngol Clin North Am 41(3):537–549, viii–ix
Hirsch B (2005) Otogenic skull base osteomyelitis. In: Jackler R (ed) Neurotology. Elsevier, Philadelphia, pp 1096–1106
Kitsko DJ, Dohar JE (2007) Inner ear and facial nerve complications of acute otitis media, including vertigo. Curr Allergy Asthma Rep 7(6):444–450
Limb C, Niparko J (2005) The acute facial palsies. In: Jackler R (ed) Neurotology. Elsevier, Philadelphia, pp 1231–1247
Makeham TP, Croxson GR, Coulson S (2007) Infective causes of facial nerve paralysis. Otol Neurotol 28(1):100–103
Marques A (2010) Lyme disease: a review. Curr Allergy Asthma Rep 10:13–20
Mattox D (2010) Clinical disorders of the facial nerve. In: Niparko J (ed) Cummings otolaryngology – head and neck surgery. Elsevier, Philadelphia, pp 2391–2402
Schleuning A et al (2006) Otologic manifestations of systemic disease. In: Hirsch B, Gadre A (eds) Head & neck surgery-otolaryngology. Lippincott Williams & Wilkins, Philadelphia, pp 2155–2168
Toh E, Lee K (2008) Facial nerve paralysis. In: Lee K (ed) Essential otolaryngology head & neck surgery. McGraw Medical, New York, pp 198–223
Vaamonde P et al (2004) Tuberculous otitis media: a significant diagnostic challenge. Otolaryngol Head Neck Surg 130(6):759–766
Vrabec J, Coker N (2006) Acute paralysis of the facial nerve. In: Hirsch B, Gadre A (eds) Head & neck surgery-otolaryngology. Lippincott Williams & Wilkins, Philadelphia, pp 2139–2154
Yetiser S, Tosun F, Kazkayasi M (2002) Facial nerve paralysis due to chronic otitis media. Otol Neurotol 23(4):580–588

Facial Nerve Paralysis due to Viral Etiology

George S. Conley
Department of Otolaryngology-Head and Neck Surgery, University of Pittsburgh, Pittsburgh, PA, USA

Definitions

1. Bell's palsy: A form of facial paralysis that is idiopathic, sudden in onset, predominantly unilateral, and typically self-limiting. It is commonly referred to as a diagnosis of exclusion and reserved for facial nerve dysfunction that has no known etiologies.
2. Ramsay Hunt Syndrome: A form of acute facial paralysis that is associated with the varicella zoster virus. It is typically characterized as a unilateral facial paralysis that is accompanied by a specific vesicular rash that is commonly localized to the

ear. It is typically more severe than Bell's palsy and is frequently associated with vestibulocochlear symptoms such as hearing loss, tinnitus, and vertigo.

3. EMG: Electromyography is an electrophysiologic test that determines the activity of a muscle. It measures spontaneous and voluntarily initiated postsynaptic membrane potentials. After a specific nerve injury, it reflects degeneration in the form of fibrillation potentials. If reinnervation of the muscle and recovery occur, it will demonstrate high frequency polyphasic potentials prior to actual voluntary muscle movement.

4. ENOG: Electroneuronography or evoked EMG is an electrophysiologic test that determines facial motor response to a supramaximal electrical stimulus of the facial nerve. The elicited response is a compound muscle action potential and its amplitude forms a quantitative assessment of nerve integrity. This response is compared to the normal side of the face.

5. Facial Synkinesis: Involuntary movements of some facial muscles when attempting to make purposeful voluntary movement of other facial muscles.

Introduction

Management of patients presenting with acute facial paralysis can be a challenging task. The clinician must have a thorough understanding of the anatomy and physiology of the facial nerve and must be aware of the numerous disease processes that elicit facial nerve disorders. Common causes of acute facial paralysis include Bell's palsy, trauma, Ramsay Hunt syndrome, neoplasm, infection, congenital anomalies, and systemic processes.

Many of these common causes of facial paralysis are well defined and have specific evaluation and treatment protocols. However, Bell's palsy, accounting for up to two third of acute facial paralysis has been an idiopathic disorder of unknown etiology and its management has been controversial. Historically, mechanisms such as microcirculatory failure, autoimmune reaction, and viral inflammation were leading etiologies proposed for this disorder. Now after much investigation, the type 1 herpes simplex virus (HSV-1) has gained the strongest

support for causing most cases of Bell's palsy (Toh and Lee 2008). Ramsay Hunt syndrome, another common cause of acute facial paralysis has long been associated with the varicella zoster virus (VZV). Together, these viruses strengthen the concept of viral-mediated inflammation as a predominant etiology for acute facial paralysis.

Both HSV-1 and VZV are derived from the herpes family of viruses, and as such, they share many common characteristics. Most importantly, they demonstrate an affinity for the peripheral nervous system and the ability to establish a dormant site of infection within various sensory cranial nerve ganglia (Sweeney 2001; Simmons 2002). Periodically, these viruses will reactivate from the latent state and manifest characteristic mucosal or skin lesions in a dermatomal pattern. This is most commonly seen with reactivation of HSV-1 in the trigeminal ganglion and its subsequent production of recurrent mucocutaneous lesions (Simmons 2002). It is hypothesized that these viruses will reactivate in the geniculate ganglion and trigger an inflammatory response that causes the facial nerve paralysis seen in Bell's palsy and Ramsay Hunt syndrome.

Pathophysiology

To formulate a theory for the pathogenesis of Bell's palsy and to further define Ramsay Hunt syndrome, investigators correlated clinical observations with anatomic, physiologic, and histopathologic studies. Through these studies, HSV-1 and VZV were implicated as the likely etiologic agents for Bell's palsy and Ramsay Hunt syndrome, respectively. Also, the meatal foramen was identified as the most likely intratemporal location for initiating a viral-mediated facial nerve injury.

Viral-Mediated Pathogenesis

Clinical support for a viral-mediated mechanism of acute facial palsy originated from the fact that acute facial paralysis was observed in many viral illnesses including measles, mumps, herpes simplex infection, infectious mononucleosis, and HIV infections. However, some discounted these observations as circumstantial since viral serology markers and clinical signs of active viral infection were inconsistently identified in many cases of Bell's palsy or Ramsay Hunt syndrome. Others suggest that these inconsistencies are best explained by the fact that HSV-1 and VZV produce their effect as latent reactivations of sensory ganglia (Mattox 2010). Therefore, the clinical signs or serologic markers commonly seen in an initial infection may not be present in viral-mediated facial paralysis.

The most significant evidence relating HSV-1 with Bell's palsy and VZV with Ramsay Hunt syndrome was determined through studies of the geniculate ganglion by Murakami and associates (Murakami et al. 1996). They used polymerase chain reaction (PCR) techniques confirmed by Southern blot analysis to detect HSV-1 and VZV DNA in the endoneural fluid and postauricular muscle of subjects undergoing facial nerve decompression for paralysis. Eleven of fourteen patients with Bell's palsy were positive for HSV-1 and eight of nine patients with Ramsay Hunt syndrome were positive for VZV. All the control subjects who had facial paralysis for other known causes such as trauma or neoplasm were negative for any viral pathology.

Additional support for the role of HSV-1 in Bell's palsy was suggested from an animal model experiment performed by Sugita and coworkers (Sugita et al. 1995). They were able to replicate the clinical course of Bell's palsy after inoculating the auricle or lateral tongue of mice with HSV-1. The resultant facial paralysis developed in 6–9 days, persisted for up to a week and spontaneously resolved in all cases. Through these studies and others, it has been postulated that the initiating event for the facial paralysis of Bell's palsy and Ramsay Hunt syndrome is the reactivation of latent HSV-1 or VZV from the geniculate ganglion of the facial nerve.

Although early studies on Bell's palsy and Ramsay Hunt syndrome demonstrated abnormal facial nerve conduction within the intratemporal segment, a specific mechanism for how viruses mediate their pathogenic affect on the facial nerve was unknown. Anatomically, the facial nerve arises from the pontine portion of the brainstem and travels across the cerebellopontine angle to enter the temporal bone. From proximal to distal, the intratemporal course of the facial nerve is divided into four segments: meatal, labyrinthine, tympanic, and mastoid. The meatal segment is approximately 8–10 mm long and spans the internal auditory canal (IAC) from the porus acousticus medially to the fundus laterally. In this meatal segment, the facial nerve is accompanied by the vestibulocochlear nerve. At the fundus, the facial nerve proceeds on its own through the fallopian canal. The first portion of the fallopian canal is the labyrinthine segment. It is approximately 2.5 mm in length and extends from the meatal foramen (opening of fundus) to the geniculate ganglion. At the geniculate ganglion, the facial nerve makes a posterior turn and travels through the tympanic cavity toward the pyramidal eminence. This 8–11 mm segment is known as the tympanic or horizontal segment. Finally, the facial nerve will make an inferior turn at the second genu to extend vertically from the pyramidal eminence to the stylomastoid foramen. This final 10–14 mm segment is known as the mastoid segment.

Fisch analyzed the intratemporal course of the facial nerve in detail and he found that the meatal foramen had a mean diameter of 0.68 mm (Fisch 1972). This marked the narrowest location for the facial nerve to transgress as it coursed through the temporal bone. The narrowest segment was the labyrinthine segment that begins at the meatal foramen and ends at the geniculate ganglion. Building on these anatomic findings, other investigators completed electrophysiologic studies on Bell's palsy and Ramsay Hunt patients who underwent surgical decompression of the facial nerve. The decompressed facial nerve was electrically stimulated at various locations along its intratemporal course and a conduction differential was identified across the meatal foramen (Limb and Niparko 2005). Adding to the evidence that the meatal foramen was the major site of viral-mediated facial nerve injury, many histopathology studies demonstrated diffuse inflammatory infiltrates and demyelination of the facial nerve, with the most severe changes affecting the meatal foramen and labyrinthine segment (Mattox 2010).

Accounting for the intrinsic properties of HSV-1 and VZV, the intratemporal anatomy of the facial nerve, and the various studies described above; a viral-mediated etiology for facial nerve injury is likely. A postulated sequence of events includes a viral reactivation within the geniculate ganglion, subsequent diffuse inflammation throughout the facial nerve, and a compression facial neuropathy originating in the labyrinthine segment.

Management of Viral-Mediated Facial Palsy

The initial evaluation of the patient with acute facial paralysis should focus on excluding nonviral etiologies. Each evaluation should include a detailed history, an extensive review of systems, a complete physical exam, and a routine audiology exam. The onset and progression of facial paralysis (sudden or gradual), any associated neurologic or sensory findings, and the degree of facial paralysis (complete or incomplete), are key clinical elements that must be addressed.

In the history, a key factor is the onset and progression of the paralysis. Viral mediated causes such as Bell's palsy or Ramsay Hunt syndrome will typically demonstrate facial paralysis that develops within 2–3 weeks and will demonstrate some recovery in facial movement within 3–4 months. However, if a carefully observed facial paralysis continues to progress after the initial 3 weeks or if no improvement is noticed after 4–6 months, other pathology such as neoplasm must be investigated (Toh and Lee 2008).

On physical exam, it is critical to accurately assess the level of facial motor dysfunction in terms of completeness. The clinician should remember that upper eyelid movement derived from the levator palpebral muscle is innervated by the oculomotor nerve and not the facial nerve. Therefore, subtle upper eyelid movement in the context of a complete facial paralysis should not be misinterpreted as a partial paralysis. Furthermore, a standardized facial nerve grading system such as the House-Brackmann scale should be used to document the status of facial movement. This serves as a consistent scale for comparative assessment of facial nerve dysfunction in both the diagnostic and recovery phases.

While excluding common nonviral causes of facial paralysis, the clinical presentations of Bell's palsy and Ramsay Hunt syndrome should be considered.

Bell's Palsy – HSV1: Although categorized as a diagnosis of exclusion, Bell's palsy has a specific set of clinical findings that are characteristic of this disease. It is typically described as an acute unilateral palsy of the face that occurs with rapid onset and limited duration. The facial dysfunction typically develops within 48–72 h and it may commonly be associated with other symptoms such as pain or numbness in the face or postauricular area, taste disturbance, hyperacusis, and decreased lacrimation. Some level of spontaneous facial nerve recovery should be identified within 4–6 months, however up to 85% will occur in less than 3 weeks (Vrabec and Coker 2006). Overall, there is no age or sex predilection and it rarely affects children. It has a slight female predominance in the early adult years and this changes to a slight male predominance in older adults (Mattox 2010). Bell's palsy is known to recur in approximately 10% of patients. Known risk factors for Bell's palsy include pregnancy and HIV infection but the risk level of diabetes mellitus is controversial (Limb and Niparko 2005).

Ramsay Hunt – VZV: Ramsay Hunt syndrome develops from the reactivation of the VZV in the geniculate ganglion. It clinically manifests with an acute facial palsy, ear pain, and herpetic vesicular eruptions appearing in a dermatomal fashion along sensory areas innervated by the facial nerve such as the external auditory canal and concha. The vesicular eruptions usually appear at the same time as the facial paralysis but 25% may appear earlier and these patients will have an improved prognosis (Mattox 2010). Some eruptions appear later and require careful repetitive examination to ensure proper identification of Ramsay Hunt syndrome. The pain usually precedes the palsy and rash by a few days. Facial nerve degeneration is noted to be more severe than in Bell's palsy and there is a higher degree of associated symptoms such as sensorineural hearing loss, vertigo, tinnitus, hyperacusis, dysgeusia, and decreased lacrimation (Sweeney 2002). Although more severe than Bell's palsy, the initial progression of facial paralysis in Ramsay Hunt syndrome is slower, many times lasting up to 3 weeks. Like Bell's palsy, there is no sex predilection however unlike Bell's, it is commonly found in the elderly population with increased incidence after age 60 (Mattox 2010). Recurrence is uncommon.

A variant of Ramsay Hunt syndrome is the diagnosis of Ramsay Hunt syndrome zoster sine herpete. This syndrome is characterized by a peripheral facial paralysis and radicular pain but without the dermatomal rash normally affecting the ear or mouth. In the absence of a rash, zoster sine herpete may be clinically confused with Bell's palsy (Sweeney 2001). Correct identification of this variant is found when a fourfold rise in serum antibody titers to VZV or positive evidence of VZV DNA on PCR is obtained (Sweeney 2001).

Diagnostic Testing

A comprehensive clinical approach to facial nerve palsy will narrow the differential diagnosis and determine if additional diagnostic testing needs to be performed. If the pathognomonic characteristics of Bell's palsy or Ramsay Hunt syndrome are identified, no further diagnostic testing is necessary. However, if the diagnosis is uncertain or if common pathologies such as trauma, bacterial infection, or neoplasm are suspected; radiographic imaging is used for further evaluation.

High resolution computed tomography (CT) and magnetic resonance imaging (MRI) are commonly used to evaluate head and neck disorders. In facial nerve disorders, the primary role of radiographic imaging is to identify or further define nonviral pathology. Excellent at evaluating bony anatomy, CT imaging of the temporal bone is particularly useful for cases of trauma, infection, and for identifying facial nerve injury along the course of the bony fallopian canal.

MRI is sensitive for evaluating soft tissue densities and therefore it is useful in examining the intrinsic facial nerve throughout its entire intra- and extracranial course. Specifically, contrast enhanced MRI is highly sensitive for identifying neuronal enhancement that is due to inflammation or neoplasm (Vrabec and Coker 2010). Investigators found that Bell's palsy and Ramsay Hunt syndrome demonstrate a diffuse enhancement of the facial nerve as compared to the focal enhancement seen with neoplasm (Limb and Niparko 2005). This may be particularly helpful when early neoplastic processes mimic Bell's palsy. The fact that the diffuse enhancement is mainly identified at the distal meatus and labyrinthine segment, lends further support to the theory of a viral-mediated pathogenesis for Bell's palsy and Ramsay Hunt syndrome, (Mattox 2010). Unfortunately this is nondiagnostic, since a similar enhancement of the facial nerve has been seen in MRI evaluations of normal patients (Limb and Niparko 2005).

Prognosis and Electrophysiologic Testing

The prognosis for most patients with Bell's palsy is very good. Approximately one third of the patients will only suffer a partial paralysis and if so, they have a high likelihood of obtaining an excellent recovery with only a few experiencing mild residual deficits. Of the two third of patients who develop a complete paralysis, all will experience some recovery but the extent of recovery is variable. In multiple studies on the natural progression of Bell's palsy, approximately 15–40% of the patients who experience a complete paralysis will go on to suffer long-term major sequelae (Limb and Niparko 2005). The primary indicator for determining the level of recovery is the amount of time elapsed before some recovery is evident. If the time delay is longer than 6–8 weeks, major sequelae such as synkinesis, residual weakness, and muscle spasms are more likely to occur. The prognosis for Ramsay Hunt syndrome is much worse than Bell's palsy. Several studies show poor rates of complete recovery ranging from 16% to 22% and of those who have incomplete recovery, approximately 50% will suffer major sequelae such as synkinesis, weakness, and spasm (Vrabec and Coker 2006; Mattox 2010).

The role of electrophysiologic testing in facial nerve paralysis is to determine which patients are likely to recover from those who will suffer long-term disability and might benefit from medical or surgical intervention. In patients with a partial paralysis, electrical testing is not helpful since almost all of these patients experience an excellent prognosis for complete recovery. However, in complete paralysis with its varied recovery rates, certain electrophysiologic tests such as electroneuronography (ENoG) and electromyography (EMG) have been useful in determining prognosis. When using ENoG, if the measured amplitude of the compound muscle action potential (CMAP) from the impaired side of the face decreases to 10% or less than the normal side (especially within the first 14 days of onset), the patient is likely to experience a poor clinical outcome (Limb and Niparko 2005). A worse prognosis can be expected if the 10% threshold is met early within the first few days after onset of facial paralysis. EMG testing of the facial nerve is commonly used in coordination with ENoG to confirm absence of voluntary muscle activity. It is also useful in documenting nerve degeneration in the form of fibrillation potentials and it can predict an eventual recovery when polyphasic potentials are observed.

Treatment

The various treatment options for Bell's palsy and Ramsay Hunt syndrome have been controversial. Medical treatment of facial paralysis from a presumed viral-mediated inflammatory reaction would suggest a significant role for corticosteroid and antiviral therapy. However, numerous clinical trials and meta-analyses have explored these options and only steroid therapy has proven to be effective in improving facial function for both Bell's palsy and Ramsay Hunt syndrome (Limb and Niparko 2005; Lockhart et al. 2009). Although consensus is lacking on the dosage and duration of steroid therapy, early use is advocated and many studies show a marginal improvement in complete facial nerve recovery as compared to placebo. Recent investigations on the role of antiviral therapy in Bell's palsy have shown no significant benefit for facial nerve recovery and its use is not currently advocated (Lockhart et al. 2009). In Ramsay Hunt syndrome, antiviral agents have shown significant benefit in improving postherpetic neuralgia and for resolving vesicular skin lesions, but its affect on facial nerve outcomes has been controversial (Sweeney 2002; Uscategui 2008). Combination therapy with steroids and antiviral agents are commonly advocated for Ramsay Hunt syndrome but no high quality evidence has proven its efficacy (Sweeney 2002).

Surgical decompression of the facial nerve for Bell's palsy remains controversial. In a well-controlled multicenter trial, Gantz and colleagues clearly showed improvement in facial nerve outcomes for patients with severe facial paralysis who demonstrated greater than 90% degeneration on ENoG and no voluntary EMG potentials within the first 2 weeks of facial paralysis (Gantz et al. 1999). However, using the same criteria, clinical trials have shown that up to 50% of these patients treated conservatively will achieve adequate recovery with minimal weakness. In consideration of the fact that a middle fossa decompression surgery is not without risk for iatrogenic injury and current electrophysiologic testing is not able to conclusively predict which patients will go on to suffer major sequelae, many clinicians do not routinely operate on viral-mediated facial paralysis. Yet it still remains a valid option for those patients with severe degeneration who meet ENoG and EMG criteria.

Conclusion

In the management of acute facial nerve palsy, current evidence suggests that a viral pathogen may be implicated in the majority of cases. Certain clinical findings are characteristic of a presumed viral etiology and a plausible pathophysiologic mechanism has been proposed. However, a consensus on the specific evaluation and treatment of viral-mediated facial nerve palsy is still evolving. A comprehensive approach that explores other etiologies for facial nerve paralysis is still of primary importance. If a viral etiology is ultimately suspected and a complete paralysis is evident, electrophysiologic testing may be used to predict long-term outcomes and to possibly direct further medical or surgical management. Although anti-inflammatory and antiviral pharmacologic agents are well tolerated by most patients, further investigation will be necessary to determine their specific roles in the overall management of viral-mediated facial paralysis. Corticosteroids have shown some benefit in the treatment algorithm for acute facial palsy and its early use is advocated. Antiviral therapy alone has not been found to be clinically significant. However, in severe facial paralysis, combined early antiviral and corticosteroid therapy is supported. In regard to surgery, a middle fossa decompression of the labyrinthine segment of the facial nerve has proven to be effective in certain clinical circumstances and it remains a viable treatment option for severe complete facial paralysis.

Disclaimer

Cross-References

- ▶ Bell's Palsy
- ▶ EMG
- ▶ Facial Paralysis
- ▶ Idiopathic Facial Nerve Paralysis
- ▶ Synkinesis

References

Fisch U, Esslen E (1972) Total intratemporal exposure of the facial nerve. Pathologic findings in Bell's palsy. Arch Otolaryngol 95(4):335–341

Gantz BJ et al (1999) Surgical management of Bell's palsy. Laryngoscope 109(8):1177–1188

Limb C, Niparko J (2005) The acute facial palsies. In: Jackler R (ed) Neurotology. Elsevier, Philadelphia, pp 1231–1247

Lockhart P et al (2009) Antiviral treatment for Bell's palsy (idiopathic facial paralysis). Cochrane Database Syst Rev (4):CD001869

Mattox D (2010) Clinical disorders of the facial nerve. In: Niparko J (ed) Cummings otolaryngology – head and neck surgery. Elsevier, Philadelphia, pp 2391–2402

Murakami S et al (1996) Bell palsy and herpes simplex virus: identification of viral DNA in endoneurial fluid and muscle. Ann Intern Med 124(1 Pt 1):27–30

Simmons A (2002) Clinical manifestations and treatment considerations of herpes simplex virus infection. J Infect Dis 186(Suppl 1):S71–S77

Sugita T et al (1995) Facial nerve paralysis induced by herpes simplex virus in mice: an animal model of acute and transient facial paralysis. Ann Otol Rhinol Laryngol 104(7):574–581

Sweeney CJ, Gilden DH (2001) Ramsay Hunt syndrome. J Neurol Neurosurg Psychiatry 71(2):149–154

Toh E, Lee K (2008) Facial nerve paralysis. In: Lee K (ed) Essential otolaryngology head & neck surgery. McGraw Medical, New York, pp 198–223

Uscategui T et al (2008) Antiviral therapy for Ramsay Hunt syndrome (herpes zoster oticus with facial palsy) in adults. Cochrane Database Syst Rev (4):CD006851

Vrabec J, Coker N (2006) Acute paralysis of the facial nerve. In: Hirsch B, Gadre A (eds) Head & neck surgery-otolaryngology. Lippincott Williams & Wilkins, Philadelphia, pp 2139–2154

Facial Nerve Paresis

▶ Post-parotidectomy Facial Nerve Paralysis

Facial Nerve Schwannoma

▶ Facial Neuroma, Hemangioma, and Other Neoplasms

Facial Nerve Transposition

▶ Jugular Foramen, Approaches

Facial Nerve, Embryology

Christopher M. Johnson and Michael E. Hoffer
Department of Otolaryngology, Spatial Orientation center, Naval Medical Center, San Diego, CA, USA

Basic Characteristics

The complex anatomy of the facial nerve can best be appreciated with an awareness of its embryologic development. This awareness allows the surgeon to understand and often anticipate anatomic variations. In this entry, the developmental anatomy of the facial nerve is outlined from roughly the third week of gestation through birth, although the majority of its development takes place within the first 3–4 months of fetal life. It concludes with a comment on the clinical implications of aberrant development of the facial nerve. The content was summarized primarily from two sources, so the reader is referred to publications by Gasser and May as well as Sataloff and Selber for more detailed discussion.

It would be difficult to discuss facial nerve embryology without an understanding of facial nerve anatomy, therefore a brief overview is provided here for reference. The motor nucleus of the adult facial nerve is located in the caudal portion of the pons. As the axons exit the motor nucleus medially, they bend around the abducens nucleus and exit laterally between the olive and the inferior cerebellar peduncle. The nervus intermedius consists of sensory neurons from the geniculate ganglion as well as parasympathetic axons from the superior salivatory nucleus. This sensory root of the facial nerve enters the central nervous system at the pontocerebellar groove. The facial nerve and the nervus intermedius travel with the eighth cranial nerve into the internal auditory canal. Through its course, the facial nerve gives rise to three major intratemporal branches and seven extratemporal branches terminating primarily to innervate the facial musculature (Sataloff and Selber 1993).

The developing brain and brainstem are derived from three primary vesicles or dilations of the neural tube: the prosencephalon (forebrain), mesencephalon (midbrain), and rhombencephalon (hindbrain). The rhombencephalon divides into the myencephalon and metencephalon, the latter eventually forms the pons

and cerebellum. At the end of the third week of gestation, a cluster of neural crest cells becomes apparent
rostral to the otic placode attached to the metencephalon. This collection of cells gives rise to both the
seventh and eighth cranial nerves and is therefore
named the facioacoustic (or acousticofacial) primordium. By the end of the fourth week, the facial and
acoustic portions become better defined. The facial
portion forms a cell column terminating near
a thickened area of surface ectoderm called an
epibranchial placode on the surface of the second
branchial arch. The acoustic portion terminates on the
otocyst, which is formed at roughly the same time by
invagination of the otic placode.

In the early part of the fifth week, the distal segment
begins to separate into two parts. The caudal portion,
which represents the main trunk, terminates in the
mesenchyme of the second arch. The rostral portion
courses into the first (mandibular) arch to become the
chorda tympani nerve. Where the nerve approaches
the epibranchial placode, large dark nuclei indicate
the location of the developing geniculate ganglion.
At the end of the fifth week, the facial motor nucleus
can be recognized in the region of the metencephalon
that will become the pons.

Near the end of the seventh week, the facial nerve
roots are evident and the geniculate ganglion is more
distinct. The nervus intermedius extends from the ganglion to enter the brainstem and comprises the sensory
portion of the nerve. The motor fibers of the facial
nerve develop independently from the sensory pathway, which allows individuals with congenital facial
paralysis to taste and produce tears normally.

As stated earlier, the facial nerve gives rise to three
major intratemporal branches. The chorda tympani
nerve and the greater superficial petrosal nerve
(GSPN) are the first to form. The chorda tympani is
identifiable during the fifth week coursing into the
mandibular arch terminating near the mandibular
branch of the trigeminal nerve. By the end of the
seventh week it joins with the lingual nerve just proximal to the developing submandibular ganglion. The
GSPN forms rostral to the geniculate ganglion shortly
after the chorda tympani nerve is evident. By the eigth
week, the GSPN is well developed and joins with the
deep petrosal nerve near the developing internal
carotid artery to form the nerve of the pterygoid
canal. It then terminates into a group of cells that will
become the pterygopalatine ganglion. The stapedius

muscle is innervated from the time it is formed during
the seventh week; however, a distinct branch (nerve to
the stapedius) is not evident until the eigth week of
gestation.

The intratemporal segment, which forms before the
extratemporal segment, initially travels in a vertical
direction straight into the second pharyngeal arch. By
the end of the fifth week, the developing nerve takes
a slight caudal bend at the site of the developing
geniculate ganglion. This horizontal segment becomes
more apparent as the region expands during the sixth
and seventh week of development. Gasser and May
(2000) states that the formation of the horizontal segment is due to a caudal shift of second arch structures,
which draws the distal portions of the nerve caudally.
The geniculate ganglion and nerve segments proximal
to it may remain essentially stationary due to tethering
from the developing GSPN. The region immediately
distal to this horizontal segment turns vertically at the
pyramidal process to run through the mastoid and exit
at the stylomastoid foramen. This caudal shift progresses throughout fetal life and the vertical segment
tends to lie in a more anterior position in relation to the
middle and external ear until it rests essentially in its
adult position at birth.

By the eigth week of gestation, the membranous
labyrinth reaches its adult configuration and the cartilaginous otic capsule forms around it. At this point, the
relationships of the intratemporal segment are predominantly established. Shortly after this, the nerve can be
observed lying in a sulcus within the cartilaginous
capsule which will eventually ossify and begin to
enclose the nerve forming the fallopian canal.

Initially, the terminal fibers of the facial nerve end
blindly in the mesenchyme of the second branchial
arch. The extratemporal branches tend to develop
from proximal to distal, when the cervicomandibular
region begins to enlarge. The posterior auricular
branch is the first to appear followed by the branch to
the posterior belly of the digastric muscle, both of
which are identifiable by the sixth week of gestation.
The upper and lower divisions separate early in the
eigth week. By the end of the eigth week, the temporal,
zygomatic, buccal, mandibular, and cervical branches
are apparent, although it should be noted that the
temporal portions are the last to appear.

The development of muscles and their innervating
branches are temporally related. The second branchial
arch gives rise to distinct collections of myoblasts

around the seventh and eigth week that correspond to the newly formed extratemporal facial nerve branches. Analogous to the development of the facial nerve branches, the more proximally innervated muscle groups (cervicomandibular and occipital) develop first. The superficial layer of the second arch mesenchyme separates to form laminae, from which facial muscle groups evolve. The occipital, cervical, temporal, and mandibular laminae are formed first, with the infraorbital lamina developing in the latter part of the eigth week. These laminae rapidly differentiate over the following weeks, such that all facial muscles are identifiable in their respective positions by 12 weeks gestational age.

The facial nerve forms more communications with other nerves than any other cranial nerve. Around the eigth week, a small branch arises from the geniculate ganglion to join the glossopharyngeal nerve forming a communication to the tympanic plexus. At the same time, the auricular branch of the vagus nerve communicates with both the glossopharyngeal and facial nerves. Branches of these three cranial nerves provide sensory innervation to the external auditory canal. The cutaneous branches of the second and third cervical ganglia are the first to establish communication with the extratemporal segments. The great auricular and transverse cervical nerves communicate with the posterior auricular and cervical branches of the facial nerve in the seventh week. Following that, communications become apparent with the mental, infraorbital, buccal, and auriculotemporal branches of the trigeminal nerve. The majority of interconnections are made by 12 weeks; however, several communications to the trigeminal nerve in the periorbital region are made around 4.5 months gestation.

Early in the eigth week, the parotid primordium, which is unbranched, grows dorsally as an outgrowth of the lateral oral cavity region. At this point, a small branch overlies the developing parotid in the buccal region. By the end of the eigth week, the gland enlarges and rapidly divides into second- and third-order ductules to reach the preauricular region. During this period of expansion, the gland lies superficial to the lower buccal, marginal mandibular, and cervical branches of the facial nerve. Fourth-order ductules are formed at 10 weeks. At this time, branches of the upper division of the nerve lie superficial to the gland, while branches of the lower division are deep to it. By the 12th week, the branching patterns of the developing gland become increasingly

complex and the ductules begin to connect the superficial and deep portions of the gland by growing between the branches of the facial nerve. This establishes the complex relationship between the parotid gland and the extratemporal facial nerve.

Ossification of the cartilaginous otic capsule begins at 16 weeks and bone begins to enclose the nerve at around 5 months. Dehiscences of the fallopian canal are most commonly located adjacent to the oval window (Beddard and Saunders, 1962) and are not necessarily an uncommon finding. Specter and Ge (1993) examined the ossification patterns in the tympanic segment in fetal and neonatal temporal bones and concluded that fallopian canal dehiscence should be regarded as a variant of normal development rather than a congenital anomaly.

At roughly 14 weeks, the geniculate ganglion is fully developed. By 16 weeks, all definitive communications of the facial nerve have been made. At birth, the facial nerve exits a very superficially located stylomastoid foramen leaving it more vulnerable to injury due to absence of the mastoid process. Between ages2 and 4, the mastoid process forms and the nerve occupies its more protected adult position.

The external and middle ear develop at roughly the same time as the facial nerve, which explains the frequent coexistence of intratemporal anomalies of the facial nerve with deformities of the external and middle ear. In patients with congenital malformations, the fetal age at which disruption occurred can often be determined with knowledge of normal embryologic development. If the course of the facial nerve is aberrant, its development was likely disrupted at the same time as the development of the ear. Also, malformations in other systems, most notably the renal system, can suggest the presence of otologic malformations because the two systems evolve concurrently. Because of this, the otologic surgeon can often predict the location of an aberrant facial nerve in the presence of other malformations.

Sataloff (1990) emphasizes that knowledge of facial nerve embryology must be integrated with the embryologic development of other otologic structures. To illustrate this point, the stapes begins to form at the time of development of the horizontal segment of the facial nerve. The time at which the stapes begins to form and the position of the developing facial nerve at that particular time determine whether the nerve will pass above, below, or even through the stapes. Sataloff

(2003) also describes a case of a 6-year-old boy with microtia and atresia to illustrate the importance of knowledge of facial nerve embryology. He reports that the appearance of the auricle placed the time of disruption of normal development at around the eigth week. Computed tomography revealed a hypoplastic middle ear space and an absent external auditory canal. Based on this information, the surgeon surmised that the vertical portion of the facial nerve would course more anterior, inferior, and superficial. His suspicions were confirmed intraoperatively, and if adult relationships had been utilized for surgical planning, the facial nerve would have been at risk for injury during the course of creating an external auditory canal and removing the atresia plate. The nerve may bifurcate, trifurcate, or take any number of different aberrant routes through the temporal bone. Although rare, the possibility of an aberrant facial nerve is always present. Knowledge of facial nerve embryology can provide the otologic surgeon the information to accurately predict the course of the nerve before surgery is undertaken.

Cross-References

▶ Balance (Anatomy: Embryology)
▶ Embryology of Ear (General)
▶ Hemifacial Microsomia
▶ Microtia and Atresia

References

Beddard D, Saunders WH (1962) Congenital defects in the fallopian canal. Laryngoscope 72:112–115
Gasser RF, May M (2000) Embryonic development. In: May M, Schaitkin BM (eds) The facial nerve, 2nd edn. Thieme Medical, New York, pp 1–17
Sataloff RT (1990) Embryology of the facial nerve and its clinical applications. Laryngoscope 100:969–984
Sataloff RT, Selber JC (2003) Phylogeny and embryology of the facial nerve and related structures. Part 2: embryology. Ear Nose Throat J 82:704–724
Spector GJ, Ge X (1993) Ossification patterns of the tympanic facial canal in the human fetus and neonate. Laryngoscope 103:1052–1065

Facial Neurilemmomas

▶ Facial Neuroma, Hemangioma, and Other Neoplasms

Facial Neurilemoma

▶ Magnetic Resonance Imaging, Facial Nerve Schwannoma

Facial Neurinoma

▶ Facial Neuroma, Hemangioma, and Other Neoplasms

Facial Neuroma

▶ Facial Neuroma, Hemangioma, and Other Neoplasms
▶ Magnetic Resonance Imaging, Facial Nerve Schwannoma

Facial Neuroma, Hemangioma, and Other Neoplasms

Ilka C. Naumann and Jack M. Kartush
Michigan Ear Institute, Farmington Hills, MI, USA

Synonyms

Facial nerve schwannoma; Facial neurilemmomas; Facial neurinoma; Facial neuroma

Definition

Facial neuromas are rare benign tumors arising from Schwann cells. They occur throughout the length of the facial nerve from the cerebellopontine angle to its distal branches but are most commonly found in the perigeniculate area. Facial weakness is the most common clinical symptom.

Classification

Facial neuromas can be classified into intracranial, intratemporal, extratemporal, or a combination of these. Less than 10% of facial neuromas occur extratemporal (Forton et al. 1994). Most common location of facial neuromas is along the perigeniculate region (Dort 1991).

Clinical Presentation

Due to the close proximity of the facial nerve (CN VII) to cochlear and vestibular nerves, the clinical picture will largely depend on the location of the facial nerve tumor and its compression of surrounding structures. Facial neuromas limited to the cerebellopontine angle and internal auditory canal (IAC) frequently mimic acoustic neuromas (vestibular schwannomas) and may be very difficult to distinguish clinically or radiographically (Sherman et al. 2002).

Facial nerve dysfunction is the most common presenting symptom, with facial nerve weakness occurring in 75% of the patients (Lipkin 1984). Facial twitching or spasms also occur frequently. Normal facial nerve function as well as a sudden onset of a facial paralysis has a reported incidence of up to 25% each. Facial nerve paralysis is much more often seen in intratemporal facial neuroma due to earlier compression of the nerve fibers within the narrow fallopian canal. A facial neuroma should be considered in the differential diagnosis in patients with "Bells palsy" who do not show any signs of recovery within 6 months or if the paralysis recurs (O'Donoghue et al. 1989).

Auditory-vestibular symptoms develop from compression of the tumor along CN VIII or from involvement of the middle or inner ear. Conductive or sensorineural hearing loss, tinnitus, and dizziness have been found as chief complaints in decreasing incidence. Pain, otorrhea or masses in the ear canal are more rare symptoms of neuromas involving the intratemporal facial nerve (Lipkin et al. 1987).

Extratemporal facial neuromas usually present as a painless parotid mass with normal facial function (Balle 1984) (Fig. 1).

Clinical symptoms are seen early in tumors along the meatal foramen due to its extremely narrow diameter at the start of the fallopian canal.

Other tumors of the facial nerve, including benign vascular tumors (hemangiomas and vascular malformations), cholesteatomas, paragangliomas, choristomas, metastatic lesions along the nerve

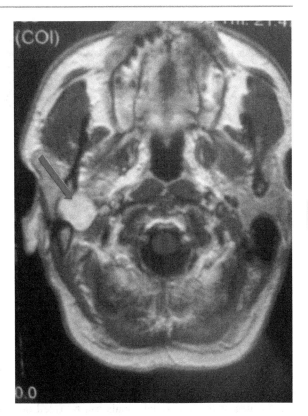

Facial Neuroma, Hemangioma, and Other Neoplasms, Fig. 1 MRI of extratemporal facial neuroma, right parotid

may lead to recurrent facial nerve paresis, often with incomplete recovery between recurrences.

Radiological Findings

Intratemporal facial neuromas when diagnosed preoperatively should be imaged with Magnetic resonance imaging (MRI) of the IAC and a high resolution computer tomography.

MRI and HRCT scans each have their own strengths in imaging facial neuromas based on their location, i.e., within soft tissue versus bone. Due to the lack of specific symptoms, the "optimal" scan may not always available prior to surgery. An MRI scan will likely be the only imaging modality available to a surgeon for facial neuromas of the cerebellopontine angle. Exclusively extratemporal facial neuromas are likely imaged with either a contrasted CT of the parotid region or an MRI. A fusiform mass along the course of the nerve in the absence of other masses should raise the suspicion for a facial neuroma.

Facial Neuroma, Hemangioma, and Other Neoplasms, Fig. 2 Coronal HRCT of intratemporal facial neuroma, left perigeniculate area

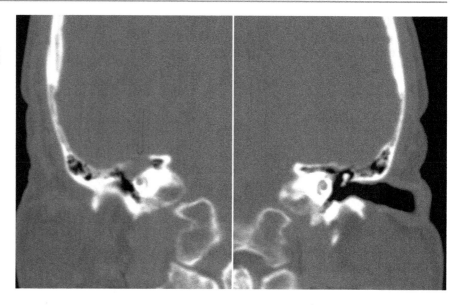

The HRCT scan is optimal for lesions originating in or extending into the temporal bone. As these tumors enlarge, involvement of the otic capsule along the cochlea or the horizontal canals can be ruled out preoperatively (Fig. 2). Facial neuromas within the IAC may result in widening of the bony IAC. A widened meatal foramen may be the only differentiation compared to a vestibular schwannoma. Intratemporal facial neuromas will enlarge the fallopian canal as a smooth expansile mass. Tumor involvement along the tympanic segment can lead to opacification of the mastoid secondary to an attic block as well as a conductive hearing loss. Poor aeration can lead to chronic otitis media.

An MRI scan may help in these cases differentiating this tumor from a cholesteatoma, which is hypointense on T1, isointense on T2, and diffusion restriction on DWI weighted images. The T1-weighted MRI scan shows a smooth, well delineated, usually isointense (ranging from mildly hypo- to hyperintense) lesion that enhances strongly with contrast. Smaller lesions will frequently be more homogenous whereas larger lesion can develop cystic areas leading to heterogeneity with contrast enhancement. Careful evaluation of an IAC lesion should include an assessment of the labyrinthine segment of the facial nerve. Enhancement along the meatal foramen may be the only hint leading to the diagnosis of a facial neuroma over a vestibular schwannoma. Parasagittal reformatted images of the

IAC may assist localizing a facial neuroma in the anterior superior quadrant.

Hemangiomas of the facial nerve may appear hyperintense on T2 or FLAIR (Veillon et al. 2008) and will markedly enhance with contrast. The fusiform expansion may also suggest an intratemporal benign vascular lesion rather than a schwannoma (Raghavan et al. 2009).

When reviewing images in patients with a facial neuroma one should note:
- Intracranial extension
- Most proximal and distal involved segments of the facial nerve
- Intratemporal involvement
  - Ossicles
  - Otic capsule (cochlea, vestibule, semicircular canals)

Histology

Facial neuromas are slow growing benign, encapsulated tumors which typically originate from the outer sheath, the epineurium. The tumor may grow longitudinally along the fallopian canal and may involve more than one segment of the nerve (Schuknecht) and clinically present as multicentric. Facial nerve dysfunction frequently will be caused by compression rather than actual invasion. Histologically, they are identical to its much more common counterpart the vestibular schwannoma with Antoni A or Antoni B cells.

Facial nerve hemangiomas are rare tumors, most commonly located along the geniculate ganglion and are thought to arise from a perigeniculate plexus (Balkany et al. 1991). They are more likely to infiltrate the facial nerve.

Electrophysiologic Testing

There is a redundancy of facial nerve fibers such that the slow loss of axons over time may result in little to no weakness until nearly 50% of fibers are affected. Facial electroneurography (ENoG) can sometimes detect subclinical levels of facial nerve involvement preoperatively or if used to follow patients serially over time (Kartush et al. 1986). ENoG is performed by transcutaneous stimulation of the facial nerve near the stylomastoid foramen with recording of the compound muscle action potential (CMAP) responses near orbicularis oris using surface electrodes. The amplitude of the evoked CMAP is compared to the contralateral side to obtain a percent difference. Obesity and large parotid glands can affect the accuracy of testing as does clinical experience. Therefore, up to 30% interside differences are considered within normal limits. Consequently, when ENoG reveals marked amplitude reduction, e.g., 40–50%, it may indicate subclinical neural degeneration. Patients with marked preoperative ENoG abnormalities can be counseled that they may have a higher chance of facial palsy and be made aware of options including subtotal resection dependent upon actual intraoperative findings.

ENoG can also be used to follow the course of patients who either choose to defer treatment or do not have their tumor resected at the time of surgical exploration. In these cases, ENoG can be an adjunct to observing growth on scans as well as clinical symptoms.

Treatment

The treatment of benign facial nerve tumors remains controversial. Twenty years ago some authors recommended total resection of tumor including sacrifice of the nerve with grafting even for minimally symptomatic patients (Dort 1991). The logic was that nerve grafting of normally functioning nerves has the best chance of recovery. Today, however, a more conservative approach is frequently taken with decompression, subtotal resections, stereotactic radiosurgery, or watchful waiting.

Treatment of facial neuromas depends on location, size, hearing, and the patient's age as well as timing of diagnosis, e.g., unexpected finding during surgery for "chronic ear disease" or a "parotid tumor." The surgeon has a wide range of treatment options to consider and, if the diagnosis is suspected preoperatively, to discuss with the patient:
- Resection with attempted nerve preservation
- Resection with nerve grafting
- Subtotal resection
- Decompression
- Diagnose, stop, and observe
- Diagnose and treat with stereotactic radiosurgery, e.g., Gamma Knife

We classify facial neuromas as either "eccentric" or "intrinsic" facial neuromas depending on the ability of the surgeon to fully resect the tumor without transecting the nerve itself. An intrinsic tumor will grow inside the fascicles and is tightly adherent to the nerve, making it impossible for the surgeon to remove the tumor without losing facial nerve function. In these cases, even a small "biopsy" may result in complete facial paralysis. In contrast, eccentric tumors grow peripherally along the nerve and have a much higher chance of being separated from the majority of nerve fibers. Neither the size nor any currently available imaging modality allows prediction of the type of the tumor in its relation to the nerve. Preoperative signs of facial weakness or spasms increase the likelihood of an intrinsic tumor if they are seen with small tumors in the CPA or parotid area. Conversely, tumors originating in the fallopian canal often cause early facial nerve symptoms due to compression – regardless of whether the tumor is eccentric. They may also cause conductive hearing loss, dizziness, and SNHL.

Clearly, patients with preoperative facial weakness have a higher chance of postoperative paralysis. However, as noted above, slow tumor growth may result in progressive subclinical degeneration of fibers that predispose the nerve to injury at the time of resection even when using gentle microdissection techniques that would not ordinarily traumatize a normal nerve. Consequently, intraoperative facial nerve monitoring using intramuscular needle electrodes to detect small amplitude responses is critical in resecting these neuromas in order to detect the earliest signs of neural trauma.

Facial neuromas that occur in the IAC and CPA may look identical to acoustic neuromas on MRI scans. There are two telltale signs, however, that may alert the surgeon to the possibility that the tumor is actually of facial nerve origin: (1) facial neuromas tend to be much more sensitive to even slight mechanical trauma resulting in high frequency, sustained runs of EMG "trains" and (2) "intrinsic" type neuromas typically spread normal facial nerve fibers diffusely around the tumor – thus, electric stimulation often results in responses over a broad area of the tumor.

While intraoperative monitoring has become accepted as a standard for acoustic tumor resection (Acoustic Neuroma, NIH Consensus Statement 1991), unfortunately, most residency training programs do not have a formal curriculum for the technical and interpretive fundamentals of intraoperative neurophysiologic testing. Many centers perform only "passive" monitoring – i.e., rely only on listening for EMG evidence of trauma (e.g., train and burst potentials). Conversely, "active" monitoring entails frequent, nearly continuous use of electrically triggered EMG responses during tumor dissection that alert the surgeon not just to injury but to nerve proximity and nerve conductivity. Kartush Stimulating Instruments (KSI) – allow *simultaneous* surgical dissection with ongoing electrical stimulation (Kartush 1989) (Fig. 3).

Surgical treatment depends on the location of the tumor and has to be tailored individually for each case. Proper preoperative imaging (MRI and CT) allows for accurate planning of the procedure especially with large tumors. If intraoperatively an unexpected facial neuroma is diagnosed, the risks versus benefits of a biopsy should be carefully weighed. Even a small biopsy might lead to a complete facial paralysis in a clinically intact nerve, if subclinical degeneration is present – the reduced number of functioning nerve fibers may lie on the surface in the area of the biopsy.

The approaches for tumors in the cerebellopontine angle and the internal auditory canal will depend on the patient's preoperative hearing, age, health, and tumor size. For hearing preservation, a retrosigmoid approach or a middle cranial fossa approach (for smaller tumors in the IAC) can be used. If hearing preservation is of no concern a transtemporal

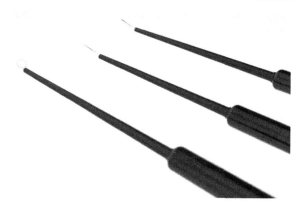

Facial Neuroma, Hemangioma, and Other Neoplasms, Fig. 3 Kartush Stimulating Instruments (KSI) – allow *simultaneous* surgical dissection with ongoing electrical stimulation (Neurosign – Wales, UK)

translabyrinthine route will allow for good exposure with minimal brain retraction. Such an approach also increases exposure should nerve grafting in the CPA be needed. Resection and if possible grafting is indicated for large tumors compressing the brain stem. Early reanimation is recommended if grafting is impossible.

For tumors along the tympanic or vertical segment, a transmastoid approach with opening of the facial recess is used. Even with normal hearing, the incus may need to be removed to increase exposure, followed by ossicular chain reconstruction. If the tumor appears to be eccentric a resection may be attempted; conversely, intrinsic tumors may be widely decompressed if facial function is normal. They are then followed with scans, ENoG, and observance of new symptoms. Tumor progression may prompt subsequent surgical resection with grafting or radiosurgery

Tumors of the parotid gland exclusively in the soft tissue can frequently be followed for many years because of the absence of constricting bone. The diagnosis is typically established by exploration for a presumed benign tumor of the parotid gland – however, if facial nerve monitoring is used with frequent electric stimulation, the surgeon may be alerted to the possibility of a facial neuroma by obtaining responses when the stimulator is placed on the tumor as well as encountering hypersensitivity to mechanical manipulation.

There has been controversy about timing and indications for surgery when a facial neuroma is known or suspected – rather than encountered unexpectedly. For

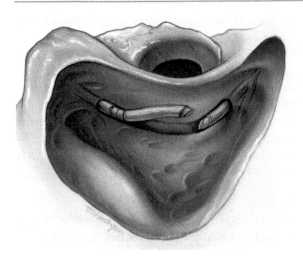

Facial Neuroma, Hemangioma, and Other Neoplasms, Fig. 4 Placement of a great auricular nerve graft in the mastoid

most patients with normal facial function, preserving this function is paramount unless the tumor may be life threatening, e.g., large CPA tumors – or eroding into the labyrinth.

Due to the slow growth of these tumors, wide decompression of an intratemporal tumor can allow years or decades of normal facial function, as has been the experience of the senior author over the last 25 years. If surgery is eventually needed and performed before function worsens to a House Brackmann Grade IV, resection and grafting typically result in long-term Grade III function – nearly the same as if resection were performed for a clinically intact nerve (Fig. 4). Numerous factors can impact the final outcome including age, diabetes, radiation, etc.

In contrast to conventional surgical treatment options, stereotactic radiosurgery has been used on some tumors with excellent facial function (HB1 and 2). In a review of a small series with six patients who underwent Gamma Knife treatment in a single dose of 12 Gy, there was 100% tumor control. Pre and posttreatment facial nerve function did not change within the 26 months of median follow-up (Lunsford 2009). Long-term follow-up of patients treated with radiosurgery is needed. There are rare reported cases of other benign tumors undergoing radiosurgery that have undergone malignant transformation.

Follow-up should include annual clinical exams, and ENoG 6 after the diagnosis is made and if stable yearly. In the early phase biyearly MRI scans for known residual tumors or during times of observation should be obtained. Any new onset of symptoms, such as weakness or spasms should trigger an exam, repeat ENoG and MRI. If facial nerve functions or symptoms worsen the patient should be re-counseled about the above stated options.

Facial reanimation procedures should be considered if the facial nerve function did not return or a re-anastomosis of the nerve at the time of the surgery was not feasible. In all cases of facial palsy, assuring corneal protection is crucial. Early gold weight eyelid implantation should be considered for any patient in whom lubrication is inadequate (Kartush et al. 1990). Such a concern is increased when the facial nerve has been involved proximal to the geniculate ganglion due to lost greater superficial petrosal function with attendant drying of the cornea.

References

Acoustic Neuroma, NIH Consensus Statement (1991) 9(4):1–24.

Balkany T, Fradis M et al (1991) Hemangioma of the facial nerve: role of the geniculate capillary plexus. Skull Base Surg 1(1):59–63

Balle VH, Greisen O (1984) Neurilemmomas of the facial nerve presenting as parotid tumors. Ann Otol Rhinol Laryngol 93(1 Pt 1):70–72

Dort JC, Fisch U (1991) Facial nerve schwannomas. Skull Base Surg 1(1):51–56

Forton GE, Moeneclaey LL et al (1994) Facial nerve neuroma. Report of two cases including histological and radiological imaging studies. Eur Arch Otorhinolaryngol 251(1):17–22

Kartush JM (1989) Electroneurography and intraoperative facial monitoring in contemporary neurotology. Otolaryngol Head Neck Surg 101(4):496–503

Kartush JM, Graham MD, Kemink JL (1986) Electroneurography: preoperative facial nerve assessment in acoustic neuroma surgery: a preliminary study. Am J Otol 7(5):322–338

Kartush JM, Linstrom CJ, McCann PM, Graham MD (1990) Early gold weight eyelid implantation for facial paralysis. Otolaryngol Head Neck Surg 103(6):1016–1023

Lipkin AF, Coker NJ et al (1987) Intracranial and intratemporal facial neuroma. Otolaryngol Head Neck Surg 96(1):71–79

Lunsford LD, Sheehan JP (2009) Stereotactic radiosurgery for nonvestibular schwannomas. In: Dade Lunsford L, Sheehan JP (eds) Intracranial stereotactic radiosurgery. Thieme, New York

O'Donoghue GM, Brackmann DE et al (1989) Neuromas of the facial nerve. Am J Otol 10(1):49–54

Raghavan P, Mukherjee S et al (2009) Imaging of the facial nerve. Neuroimaging Clin N Am 19(3):407–425

Sherman JD, Dagnew E et al (2002) Facial nerve neuromas: report of 10 cases and review of the literature. Neurosurgery 50(3):450–456

Veillon F, Taboada LR et al (2008) Pathology of the facial nerve. Neuroimaging Clin N Am 18(2):309–320

Facial Paralysis

▶ Bell's Palsy
▶ Congenital Unilateral Lower Lip Paralysis
▶ Cross-Facial Nerve Grafting (CFNG), Procedure
▶ Idiopathic Facial Nerve Paralysis, Medical and Surgical Management

Facial Paralysis in Children

Kenneth H. Lee
Department of Otolaryngology-Head and Neck
Surgery, University of Texas Southwestern Medical
Center at Dallas, Dallas, TX, USA

Synonyms

Palsy; Paresis

Definition

1. Paralysis: A general term most often used to describe severe or complete loss of muscle strength due to motor system disease anywhere along the path from the cerebral cortex to the muscle fiber. This term may also occasionally refer to a loss of sensory function.
2. Paresis: A general term referring to a mild to moderate degree of muscular weakness, occasionally used as a synonym for paralysis (severe or complete loss of motor function).

Basic Characteristics

Epidemiology

Facial paralysis overall is a rare clinical problem affecting 20–32 per 100,000 in the general population annually (Peitersen 2002; Rowlands et al. 2002). In children, it is even more rare as it is found 2–10 times less frequently in the pediatric population (Rowlands et al. 2002; El-Hawrani et al. 2005). Facial paralysis in the pediatric population appears to have a bimodal distribution with infectious etiologies accounting for

the palsy in younger children aged 1–3 years and trauma in older patients aged 8–12 years (Evans et al. 2005). While Bell's palsy, or idiopathic facial nerve paralysis, is the most common diagnosis in adults, in a majority of children presenting with a paralyzed face, the palsy is secondary to an identifiable diagnosis. Thus, prompt evaluation to identify the underlying etiology to provide treatment when appropriate is critical when caring for children with facial paralysis (Shargorodsky et al. 2010).

Anatomy

The facial nerve is the VIIth cranial nerve (CN) and provides both sensory and motor function to the areas of the face, head, and neck. The facial nerve is particularly at risk of injury secondary to head trauma and infection as it has the longest intraosseous course of any cranial nerve. Upon exiting the brainstem at the cerebellopontine angle anterior to the vestibulocochlear nerve (the VIIIth CN), it is joined by the nervus intermedius (nerve of Wrisberg). The fibers originating from the nervus intermedius provide the secretomotor function to the lacrimal and salivary glands as well as the gustatory function to the oral tongue.

The intraosseous course of CN VII has four segments within the temporal bone: meatal, labyrinthine, tympanic (horizontal), and mastoid (vertical) (Fig. 1, reprinted with permission from KK Adour). CN VII enters the porus acousticus and travels with CN VIII and nervus intermedius in the internal auditory canal (IAC) to comprise the meatal segment. Laterally in the IAC near the fundus, CN VII incorporates nervus intermedius within its sheath. Subsequently, they diverge from the cochlear and vestibular nerves to enter the Fallopian canal at the meatal foramen marking the beginning of the labyrinthine segment. The meatal foramen is the narrowest portion of the Fallopian canal measuring 0.61–0.68 mm and is accepted to be the site of nerve compression accounting for facial palsy secondary to inflammatory conditions (Ge and Spector 1981; Eicher et al. 1990). Near the midpoint of the short labyrinthine segment, the nerve takes a sharp 75° turn backward at the geniculate ganglion. At this first intratemporal genu, the greater superficial petrosal nerve exits anteriorly to travel to and supply secretomotor function to the lacrimal gland. Following the first genu, the nerve then travels posteriorly and horizontally along the medial wall of

Facial Paralysis in Children,
Fig. 1 Schematic diagram of
intratemporal course of facial
nerve (Reprinted with
permission from Dr. Kedar K.
Adour)

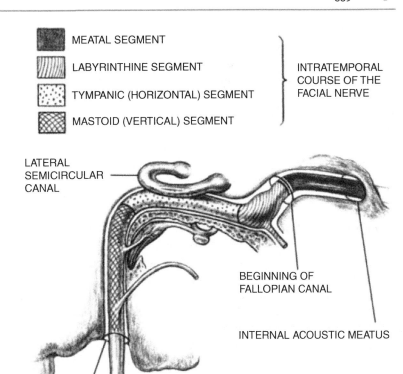

- MEATAL SEGMENT
- LABYRINTHINE SEGMENT
- TYMPANIC (HORIZONTAL) SEGMENT
- MASTOID (VERTICAL) SEGMENT

INTRATEMPORAL COURSE OF THE FACIAL NERVE

LATERAL SEMICIRCULAR CANAL

BEGINNING OF FALLOPIAN CANAL

INTERNAL ACOUSTIC MEATUS

STYLOMASTOID FORAMEN

the mesotympanum in the tympanic segment until it makes its second intratemporal genu to the vertical mastoid segment. From the mastoid segment, a branch emerges from the main trunk to supply motor innervation to the stapedius muscle and inferior to this, the chorda tympani nerve arises to course through the middle ear space and provides secretomotor function to the submandibular and sublingual salivary glands as well a taste to the anterior two thirds of the tongue. The mastoid segment terminates at the stylomastoid foramen where it exits its intraosseous course and goes on to innervate the facial musculature.

Due to the functions of the three intratemporal branches of facial nerve, in some cases the location of injury can be determined or narrowed down by the patients' symptoms and/or results of stapedial reflex testing. Thus, the care provider should assess for decreased lacrimal, salivary, and gustatory function as well as hyperacusis when evaluating a patient with facial nerve palsy. In addition, based on the manner in which the motor fibers of the facial nerve cross in at the level of the brainstem, the lower half of the face is

controlled solely by the contralateral motor cortex while the upper half receives input from both sides. Therefore, a unilateral palsy that spares the forehead suggests a contralateral central lesion and should be evaluated with intracranial imaging of the central nervous system.

Clinical Presentation

Facial nerve dysfunction in children most commonly presents with rapid onset of partial or complete paralysis of the face and is most easily noted by decreased forehead movement, incomplete eye closure, or pulling of the oral commissure on the affected side to the unaffected side. As infants cannot respond to display these findings on command, observation of grimacing while crying provides an opportunity to determine facial nerve function in the extreme young patient. In most cases, the facial paralysis with or without associated lacrimal, salivary, or gustatory dysfunction or hyperacusis as noted above are the only symptoms. However, patients can also present with facial numbness, fever, headache, sore throat, and neck stiffness (Jäämaa et al. 2003). Also in most cases, the palsy presents only on one side. Cases of acquired bilateral facial nerve palsy would most likely suggest Lyme disease (Cook et al. 1997). However, sarcoidosis can also present with bilateral facial paralysis (Teller and Murphy 1992). When evaluating children with congenital facial paralysis, careful observation should be made to note general dysmorphic features and/or other cranial nerve neuropathies as these children may have an associated syndrome (Carr et al. 1997; Gorlin et al. 1990).

Diagnostics and Tests

As with other conditions that brings a patient to see an otolaryngologist, a key to making the correct diagnosis is obtaining a good history and performing an accurate physical examination. As mentioned earlier in this entry, because a majority of children presenting with facial paralysis have an underlying diagnosis that has led to the symptom of palsy, prompt evaluation and treatment of the underlying etiology is critical in the pediatric population.

Review of the history should be directed at the timing of onset, duration of symptoms, rate of progression, previous occurrences, and presence of other symptoms or systemic illnesses. Particular note should be made of any history of tick bites or risk of bites based on recent activity and travel. It should be determined if the patient is immunocompromised due to HIV infection or immunosuppression, or has diabetes mellitus. If the patient is a newborn or if the symptoms were present at birth, one should elicit a birth history to determine if there was prolonged labor, birth weight greater than 3,500 g, use of forceps, or if any facial ecchymosis was noted after delivery (Harris et al. 1983).

The physical exam should include a detailed evaluation of lower and upper facial motion, complete otological examination including the attention to the concha, external ear canal, mastoid, tympanic membrane, middle ear, as well as pneumatic otoscopy and tuning fork exam if the patient is able to comply. A complete cranial nerve exam should be performed. The exam should also include inspection of the oral cavity, specifically for a fissured tongue suggesting Melkersson-Rosenthal syndrome, as well as palpation of the parotid gland and neck for masses. In addition, the skin of the extremities should be evaluated for rashes suggestive of Lyme disease.

All children presenting with facial paralysis should receive an audiogram and tympanogram. Patients with a history of chronic otitis media, cholesteatoma, previous otologic surgery, temporal bone trauma, or physical exam findings revealing a middle ear mass, acute otitis media, or acute mastoiditis should undergo imaging with a temporal bone computed tomogram (CT). All other patients, especially those who demonstrate other cranial nerve neuropathies, other neurological symptoms, and lower facial paralysis with normal forehead motion or a parotid mass should undergo imaging with a Magnetic Resonance Imaging (MRI) with and without contrast (Shargorodsky et al. 2010).

While mild leukocytosis can be noted due to associated viral infection, this does not provide specific diagnostic information, and the value of laboratory testing in children with facial palsy is limited mainly to patients at risk or suspected to have Lyme disease. In patients who live in or have recently traveled to Lyme disease endemic areas, or those who present with a rash, serological testing for B. burgdorferi should be performed (Nigrovic et al. 2008). The added value of lumbar puncture (LP) with evaluation of cerebrospinal fluid for elevated mononuclear cells and antibodies to B. burgdorferi is controversial. The current recommendations by the American Academy of Pediatrics is that LP is not routinely performed in children with Lyme-associated facial paralysis unless they have overt clinical symptoms of meningitis (Pickering et al. 2009).

As with adults, the severity of facial nerve palsy is most commonly determined using the House Brackmann (HB) facial nerve grading scale (Table 1, adapted from House and Brackmann 1985). For patients with complete paralysis (House Brackmann grade VI), electroneuronography (ENoG) should be performed after sufficient time is allowed for Wallerian degeneration (3–5 days). The diagnostic value of ENoG diminishes with prolonged paralysis. Based on this, ENoG is most useful as a prognostic indicator when obtained 6–14 days after the onset of complete paralysis (Gantz et al. 1999). The results of the ENoG are coupled with electromyography (EMG). Based on outcomes of facial nerve recovery, patients who demonstrate >90% degeneration on ENoG with no motor potential units on EMG are recommended to undergo surgical decompression of the nerve to achieve improved functional recovery (Gantz et al. 1999).

Facial Paralysis in Children, Table 1 House Brackmann facial nerve grading scale (Adapted from House and Brackmann 1985)

Grade	Degree of dysfunction	Characteristics
I	Normal	Normal function all areas
II	Slight	Appearance: slight weakness noticeable close inspection; my have very slight synkinesis At rest: normal symmetry and tone Forehead motion: moderate to good Eyelid closure: complete with minimal effort Mouth motion: slight asymmetry
III	Moderate	Appearance: obvious but not disfiguring weakness between the 2 sides; noticeable but not severe synkinesis, contracture and/or hemifacial spasm At rest: normal symmetry and tone Forehead motion: slight to moderate movement Eyelid closure: complete with effort Mouth motion: slightly weak with maximal effort
IV	Moderately severe	Appearance: obvious weakness and/or disfiguring asymmetry At rest: normal symmetry and tone Forehead motion: none Eyelid closure: incomplete Mouth motion: asymmetric with maximal effort
V	Severe	Appearance: only barely perceptible motion At rest: asymmetric Forehead motion: none Eyelid closure: incomplete Mouth motion: slight movement
VI	Total	No facial function

Differential Diagnosis

Congenital Facial Nerve Paralysis

Congenital facial nerve paralysis occurs in 2.1 per 1,000 children and in most cases, up to 90%, results from *birth trauma* (Falco and Eriksson 1990). Facial palsy at birth due to trauma is associated with prolonged labor, birthweight greater than 3,500 g, and use of forceps in delivery. When facial paralysis at birth is associated with craniofacial or other anomalies, one must consider that the palsy is part of a genetic syndrome (Lorch and Teach 2010). Intermittent facial paralysis with a fissured tongue is classically associated with *Melkersson-Rosenthal syndrome*, which also includes facial swelling. In patients with this syndrome,

permanent facial paralysis can develop in 30–50% (Greene and Rogers 1989). Patients with *Goldenhar syndrome* have hemifacial microsomia associated with their facial palsy, which in most cases, is unilateral and right sided (Jones 2006). Patients with *Mobius syndrome* have bilateral congenital facial paralysis and often have dysfunction of other cranial nerves. Bilateral facial paralysis can also be seen in *Osteopetrosis* or *Albers-Schonberg* disease. This is a genetic disorder in which the facial palsy is delayed and progressive as bony overgrowth of at the stylomastoid foramen results in impingement of the facial nerve. Other syndromes that can include facial palsy include *DiGeorge syndrome*, *CHARGE association*, and *Poland syndrome*.

Acquired Facial Nerve Paralysis

In children, more than one third of acquired facial nerve paralysis is due to infectious etiologies, of which, *Lyme disease* is the most common in children. Up to 50% of the cases of facial palsy in children living in endemic areas can be attributed to Lyme disease (Cook et al. 1997; Jäämaa et al. 2003). Infection with *Herpes Simplex Virus (HSV)* is another common etiology for acquired facial nerve paralysis in children accounting for the palsy in a majority of children who are seronegative for Lyme disease. While less common than HSV, *Vericella Zoster Virus (VZV)* can cause facial paralysis in an infected child. Infection with VZV leading to facial paralysis is also known as *Ramsay Hunt syndrome* or *Zoster Oticus* and may or may not present with the classic vesicular lesions in the ear canal and concha. In the absence of these lesions, the diagnosis can be confirmed by identifying the virus in serum or the saliva of the patient. Infection from other viruses such as *herpes*, *mumps*, *coxsackie*, and *adenovirus* can also cause facial nerve palsy.

Due to antibiotics, complications of *acute otitis media (AOM)*, including facial paralysis have dramatically decreased in recent decades. Currently, only 0.005% of patients with AOM develop a facial palsy (Ellefsen and Bonding 1996). The exact pathophysiology of AOM leading to facial paralysis is unclear and hypotheses range from retrograde infection via the chorda tympani nerve, contact with bacterial toxins, to erosion of the fallopian canal. A recent case of unilateral facial palsy was presented in a child with acute otitis media and a facial nerve that was dehiscent in the tympanic segment seen on a temporal bone CT (Fig. 2). Regardless of whether there is direct contact

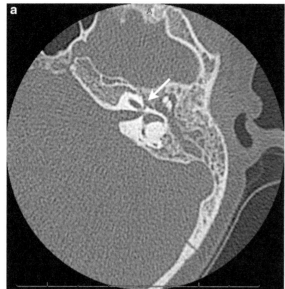

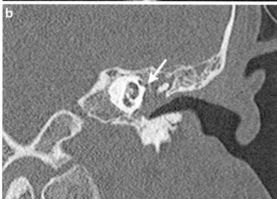

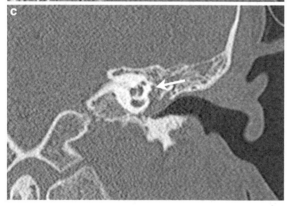

Facial Paralysis in Children, Fig. 2 Axial (**a**) and coronal (**b** and **c**) slices of high-resolution temporal bone CT of patient who presented with acute otitis media and left unilateral HB grade VI facial palsy. *White arrows* point to Fallopian canal and scan shows areas of facial nerve dehiscence

of purulent fluid with the nerve sheath, the underlying cause of the nerve dysfunction secondary to infection is likely due to an inflammatory process.

Facial palsy in children can also result from *trauma* to the face or temporal bone. A recent review of patients presenting with facial palsy at a children's hospital revealed a bimodal distribution in terms of age with peaks at 2.4 years and 8.6 years of age (Evans et al. 2005). Interestingly, in this series, while the overall numbers were small, the number of girls presenting with facial palsy was more than twice the number of boys. The trauma can also be *iatrogenic* during otologic surgery. Fortunately, in a recent review of cases of facial palsy in children, three cases were identified to result after otologic surgery and in all three cases, the patients recovered function (Evans et al. 2005).

When a facial palsy in a child is gradual and progressive, *cholesteatoma* should be considered at the top of the differential diagnosis as it is the most common neoplastic etiology in children (Jackson and Doersten 1999). In children, while neoplasms in general are less common than in adults, when they are present, one must consider malignancies. A review of patients presenting to a children's hospital with idiopathic facial palsy reported that 12% had malignancies such as *leukemia*, *astrocytoma*, and *rhabdomyosarcoma* (Grundfast et al. 1990). In addition, although rare, one must also consider the benign neoplasms that are more often the underlying etiologies for facial palsies in adults: *facial nerve schwannomas, vestibular schwannomas*, and *meningiomas* (Shargorodsky et al. 2010).

While *Bell's palsy* or idiopathic facial nerve palsy is relatively more common in adults, it is rare in children and accounts for as low as 9% of cases in the pediatric population (Evans et al. 2005). Another rare etiology for facial paralysis in children is *hypertension*. A review of cases at a pediatric hospital revealed that 8% of children with acquired facial palsy were attributable to hypertension (Lloyd et al. 1966).

Considering that a majority of cases of facial palsy in children can be attributed to an underlying diagnosis, the physician evaluating these patients must carefully review the history and findings to arrive at the correct or likely diagnosis so that proper treatment can be initiated. An algorithm for diagnosing the etiology of facial nerve palsy in children has been proposed by Lorch and Teach and is shown in Fig. 3.

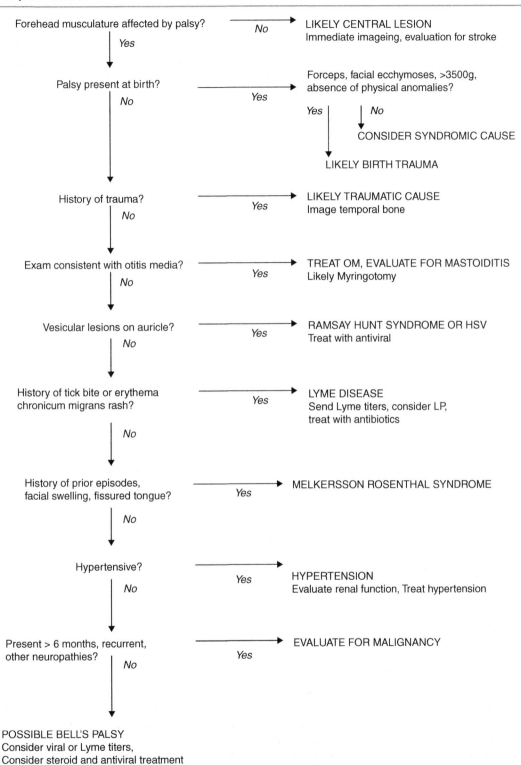

Facial Paralysis in Children, Fig. 3 Algorithm for diagnosis of facial palsy in children (Reprinted with permission from Lorch and Teach 2010)

Treatment

In general, as with adults, eye care is critical in cases where closure is incomplete, in order to prevent keratitis and compromise of vision. This includes the use of saline eye drops during the day and ophthalmic ointment at night while the child sleeps. If an eye patch or taping of the eyelid is used, it must be done with great care to prevent the inadvertent opening of the eyelid under the patch that can lead to corneal injury. In cases of permanent facial nerve dysfunction, a gold weight implant can be considered.

In any case of facial paralysis where the underlying etiology is identified, it obviously should be addressed. When the cause is infectious in nature, antimicrobial or antiviral therapy should be initiated as soon as possible. Any patient with a history of living in or visiting a Lyme endemic area should be started on empiric therapy, particularly during peak season of Lyme disease which is late spring through summer (Nigrovic et al. 2008). Current recommendations are for oral doxycycline or amoxicillin for 21–28 days (Pickering et al. 2009).

Patients with AOM and facial palsy should be initiated on IV antibiotics and surgical management dictated by the finding on temporal bone CT scan. If the child simply has otitis media with or without a dehiscent facial nerve, he should undergo myringotomy and tympanostomy tube placement with postoperative administration of antibiotic ear drops containing a steroid such as Ciprofloxacin/Hydrocortisone. A culture of the middle ear fluid should be obtained to ensure appropriate antibiotic therapy is being administered. If the CT scan shows coalescent mastoiditis or cholesteatoma, the family should be counseled and a mastoidectomy performed.

The treatment for Bell's palsy and Ramsay Hunt disease or zoster oticus with antiviral agents and oral steroids has been a subject of much controversy and varying results from different studies. The results of many of these studies are summarized in two recent reviews (Shargorodsky et al. 2010; Lorch and Teach 2010). Based on review of the current literature, the author recommends the use of oral steroids in any child with a severe facial nerve dysfunction (HB grade V or VI) and the addition of an antiviral agent if herpetic lesions are present in the external ear, face, or oral cavity.

If a child presents or develops complete facial paralysis (HB grade VI), ENoG and EMG can direct the need for surgical management and help determine prognosis. Based on known neuropathology after complete transection, degeneration of the distal axon takes up to 5 days post-injury. Delayed progression to complete paralysis after 14 days of the onset of symptoms has been shown to have good return of function without surgical intervention (Fisch 1984). Thus, the use of ENoG and EMG physiological testing has most prognostic value when performed 6–14 days post-injury. Surgical decompression is recommended when the paralyzed side shows >90% degeneration on ENoG compared to the contralateral normally functioning side and when the EMG shows no motor potential units (Gantz et al. 1999).

Prognosis

The likelihood of recovery from facial nerve paralysis in children overall is very good. However, it can vary depending on the etiology of the palsy. In cases of blunt trauma either due to birth or other causes later in life, prognosis for spontaneous recovery is good with 80–90% of patient having return of function, and often within 1 month of injury (Smith et al. 1981; Guerrissi 1997). Children with acute otitis media and facial paralysis who underwent myringotomy and tympanostomy tube placement with subsequent antibiotic and steroid treatment have excellent recovery. A recent study showed that around 80% recovered to a HB grade I and 100% recovered to a HB grade II or better (Evans et al. 2005). In the case of patients with complete paralysis (HB grade VI) and ENoG showing >90% degeneration and no motor unit potentials on EMG within 2 weeks of onset, greater than 90% of patients who underwent surgical decompression recovered to a HB grade I or II, whereas only 42% of patients achieved the same outcome if treated with steroids alone (Gantz et al. 1999).

Cross-References

References

Carr MM, Ross DA, Zuker RM (1997) Cranial nerve defects in congenital facial palsy. J Otolaryngol 26(2):80–87

Cook SP, Macartney KK, Rose CD, Hunt PG, Eppes SC, Reilly JS (1997) Lyme disease and seventh nerve paralysis in children. Am J Otolaryngol 18(5):320–323

Eicher SA, Coker NJ, Alford BR, Igarashi M, Smith RJ (1990) A comparative study of the fallopian canal at the meatal foramen and labyrinthine segment in young children and adults. Arch Otolaryngol Head Neck Surg 116(9):1030–1035

El-Hawrani AS, Eng CY, Ahmed SK, Clarke J, Dhiwakar M (2005) General practitioners' referral pattern for children with acute facial paralysis. J Laryngol Otol 119(7):540–542

Ellefsen B, Bonding P (1996) Facial palsy in acute otitis media. Clin Otolaryngol Allied Sci 21(5):393–395

Evans AK, Licameli G, Brietzke S, Whittemore K, Kenna M (2005) Pediatric facial nerve paralysis: patients, management and outcomes. Int J Pediatr Otorhinolaryngol 69(11):1521–1528. Epub 2005 Jun 27

Falco NA, Eriksson E (1990) Facial nerve palsy in the newborn: incidence and outcome. Plast Reconstr Surg 85(1):1–4

Fisch U (1984) Prognostic value of electrical tests in acute facial paralysis. Am J Otol 5(6):494–498

Gantz BJ, Rubinstein JT, Gidley P, Woodworth GG (1999) Surgical management of Bell's palsy. Am J Otol 20(6):781–788

Ge XX, Spector GJ (1981) Labyrinthine segment and geniculate ganglion of facial nerve in fetal and adult human temporal bones. Ann Otol Rhinol Laryngol Suppl 90(4 Pt 2):1–12

Gorlin RJ, Cohen MM, Levin LS (1990) Syndromes of the head and neck, 3rd edn. Oxford University Press, New York

Greene RM, Rogers RS 3rd (1989) Melkersson-Rosenthal syndrome: a review of 36 patients. J Am Acad Dermatol 21(6):1263–1270

Grundfast KM, Guarisco JL, Thomsen JR, Koch B (1990) Diverse etiologies of facial paralysis in children. Int J Pediatr Otorhinolaryngol 19(3):223–239

Guerrissi JO (1997) Facial nerve paralysis after intratemporal and extratemporal blunt trauma. J Craniofac Surg 8(5):431–437

Harris JP, Davidson TM, May M, Fria T (1983) Evaluation and treatment of congenital facial paralysis. Arch Otolaryngol 109(3):145–151

House JW, Brackmann DE (1985) Facial nerve grading system. Otolaryngol Head Neck Surg 93(2):146–147

Jäämaa S, Salonen M, Seppälä I, Piiparinen H, Sarna S, Koskiniemi M (2003) Varicella zoster and Borrelia burgdorferi are the main agents associated with facial paresis, especially in children. J Clin Virol 27(2):146–151

Jackson CG, von Doersten PG (1999) The facial nerve. Current trends in diagnosis, treatment, and rehabilitation. Med Clin North Am 83(1):179–195

Jones KL (2006) Oculo-auriculo-vertebral spectrum (first and second branchial arch syndrome, facio-auriculo-vertebral spectrum, hemifacial microsomia, Goldenhar syndrome). In: Smith's recognizable patterns of human malformation, 6th edn. Elsivier Saunders, Philadelphia

Lloyd AV, Jewitt DE, Still JD (1966) Facial paralysis in children with hypertension. Arch Dis Child 41(217):292–294

Lorch M, Teach SJ (2010) Facial nerve palsy: etiology and approach to diagnosis and treatment. Pediatr Emerg Care 26(10):763–769

Nigrovic LE, Thompson AD, Fine AM, Kimia A (2008) Clinical predictors of Lyme disease among children with a peripheral facial palsy at an emergency department in a Lyme disease-endemic area. Pediatrics 122(5):e1080–e1085. Epub 2008 Oct 17

Peitersen E (2002) Bell's palsy: the spontaneous course of 2,500 peripheral facial nerve palsies of different etiologies. Acta Otololaryngol Suppl 549:4–30

Pickering LK, Baker CJ, Kimberlin DW, Long SS (eds) (2009) American Academy of Pediatrics. Lyme disease. In: Report of the committee on infectious diseases, (28th edn), Elk Grove Village, pp 430–435

Rowlands S, Hooper R, Hughes R, Burney P (2002) The epidemiology and treatment of Bell's palsy in the UK. Eur J Neurol 9(1):63–67

Shargorodsky J, Lin HW, Gopen Q (2010) Facial nerve palsy in the pediatric population. Clin Pediatr (Phila) 49(5):411–417. Epub 2010 Feb 4

Smith JD, Crumley RL, Harker LA (1981) Facial paralysis in the newborn. Otolaryngol Head Neck Surg 89(6):1021–1024

Teller DC, Murphy TP (1992) Bilateral facial paralysis: a case presentation and literature review. J Otolaryngol 21(1):44–47

Facial Paresis

▶ Idiopathic Facial Nerve Paralysis, Medical and Surgical Management

Facial Recess

Brian J. McKinnon
Department of Otolaryngology-Head and Neck Surgery, Georgia Health Sciences University, Augusta, GA, USA

Definition

An anatomic area bounded by the facial nerve, chorda tympani nerve, and the incus buttress.

Cross-References

▶ Canal Wall Up Mastoidectomy
▶ Mastoidectomy
▶ Mastoidectomy – Canal Wall-Up Technique, Posterior Tympanotomy (Facial Recess)
▶ Vibrant Soundbridge: Application in Sensorineural Hearing Loss

Facial Recess Approach

► Posterior Tympanotomy

Facioauriculovertebral Dysplasia

► Hemifacial Microsomia

Facioauriculovertebral Malformation Complex

► Hemifacial Microsomia

Failed Extubation in NICU

Sunita Pereira
Division of Newborn Medicine, Department of
Pediatrics, Tufts Medical Center, Boston, MA, USA

Definitions

1. *Extreme Low Birth Weight (ELBW)*: Newborn infants weighing less than 1,000 g at birth
2. *Bronchopulmonary Dysplasia (BPD)*: is a form of chronic lung disease that develops in preterm neonates treated with oxygen and positive pressure ventilation (PPV) and involves a continuum of inflammation and repair.
3. *Patent Ductus Arteriosus (PDA)*: a condition in which there is a persistent communication between the descending thoracic aorta and the pulmonary artery
4. *Ventilator-Associated Pneumonia (VAP)*: is a subtype of hospital-acquired pneumonia which occurs in newborns who are receiving mechanical ventilation
5. *Tracheoesophageal Fistula (TEF)*: is an abnormal connection (fistula) between the esophagus and the trachea
6. *Tracheostomy* is a surgical procedure to create an opening through the neck into the trachea

7. *Spontaneous Breath Test (SBT)*: Extubation Readiness test where the newborn is placed on CPAP through the endotracheal tube and allowed to breathe spontaneously with the help of pressure support for 15–30 min
8. *Continuous Positive Airway Pressure (CPAP)*: A ventilatory treatment that uses mild airway pressure to keep airway open
9. *Noninvasive Intermittent Positive Pressure Ventilation (NIPPV)*: ventilation through the nasal passages without intubation of trachea
10. *Direct Laryngo Bronchscopy (DLB)*: A procedure to visualize the larynx and bronchi done under inhalation anesthesia in a spontaneously breathing infant

Introduction

Extubation failure of is defined as re-intubation within 72 h of an extubation attempt in mechanically ventilated infants and neonates (Kamlin et al. 2006). Limiting the time on the ventilator is one of the primary goals of neonatal intensive care. Early extubation reduces neonatal morbidity and mortality related to barotrauma, volutrauma, oxidant stress, bacterial colonization, sepsis, and bronchopulmonary dysplasia (BPD). Neonates are generally extubated once the underlying causes for intubation and mechanical ventilation have resolved. Extubation failure occurs in 22–40% of premature neonates and 16.3% of infants and children (Kamlin et al. 2006). Although several variables that predict successful extubation in adults have been validated and published, similar data in neonates and children are limited. In this entry, the pathogenesis of extubation failure, current status of knowledge with regards to assessment of readiness for extubation, and strategies to improve successful extubation will be discussed. The role of a pediatric otolaryngologist in cases of extubation failure will be enumerated and illustrated.

The decision to extubate is usually based on clinical assessment, blood gas results, and ventilator settings. However, up to 40% of infants weighing ≤1,000 g who are extubated based on these criteria require re-intubation (Stefanescu et al. 2003). The most common causes of re-intubation are atelectasis, apnea, patent ductus arteriosus (PDA), BPD, subglottic stenosis, ventilator-associated pneumonia (VAP), and muscle atrophy from prolonged ventilation (Greenough and Prendergast 2008). Failure of extubation may be related to the presence of associated comorbidities such as neurologic and musculoskeletal pathology, and chromosomal, craniofacial, aero diges- tive, or cardiac anomalies (Ward et al. 1995). Laryn- geal nerve injury following tracheoesophageal fistula (TEF) repair or Phrenic nerve injury following chest tube placement or cardiac surgery may interfere with a successful extubation in a newborn (Guillemaud et al. 2007). In many cases, a tracheostomy is required for prolonged ventilatory support or for upper airway obstruction. However, with improved NICU care, tracheostomies are less often performed for airway obstruction and more often needed for prolonged ven- tilator assistance due to BPD or other comorbidities (Ward et al. 1995). Failure of extubation is relatively common in the NICU and sometimes avoidable.

Assessment of Readiness to Extubate

Discontinuation of mechanical ventilation is generally successful if the neonate has adequate capacity to sustain spontaneous breathing without undue effort and adequate gas exchange. This is possible if there is normal respiratory drive and respiratory muscle strength, and the absence of excessive load on the respiratory muscles due to underlying lung disease, airway abnormality, or chest wall compliance (Greenough and Prendergast 2008). Clinical assess- ment for readiness to wean off mechanical ventilation is made daily in the NICU. However, as yet there are no reliable objective tools that could enhance this assessment. Measurement of pulmonary function tests (PFT) in neonates is not practical, technically difficult, and less informative than in children and adults (Kamlin et al. 2006). In neonates, breath-to- breath variability in respiratory mechanics and ventila- tor-related issues lead to inconsistent measurements. Calculated total respiratory compliance, spontaneous minute ventilation, and spontaneous expiratory tidal vol- umes show variable results as predictors of extubation failure and need to be validated in larger studies (Greenough and Prendergast 2008). Unlike adults, a trial of spontaneous breathing for 3 min on endotra- cheal CPAP (Spontaneous Breathing trial, SBT) has not proven to be beneficial, may lead to muscle fatigue, and needs to be validated in larger studies.

The graphics on newer ventilators with built-in air flow sensors provide a wealth of information on expiratory tidal volume (V_{TE}), minute ventilation, air flow, airway resistance, airway pressure, and pressure and flow volume loops of spontaneous and supported breaths. These measurements display in real time the infant's spontaneous respiratory drive, change in respi- ratory compliance, and the interplay of the respirator and the infant. Improved understanding and interpre- tation of data from real-time ventilator graphics will be necessary to further decrease extubation failures in the NICU. This tool is underutilized in the NICU.

Etiopathogenesis of Delayed or Failed Extubations in the NICU

The possible etiologies associated with failed extubation attempts is summarized in Table 1 (modi- fied from Prendergast and Greenough) (Greenough and Prendergast 2008). Recurrent extubation failure is most often a problem of extreme prematurity caused by abnormal respiratory load due to underlying lung disease, diminished respiratory drive, inadequate dia- phragmatic muscle strength, and occasionally increased airway resistance. Prolonged intubation, repeated extubation and re-intubation cycles, use of larger endotracheal tubes, and the unique anatomy of the newborn trachea place the baby at risk for subglottic edema, stenosis, or cyst formation (Dankle et al. 1987; da Silva 1996). A pediatric otolaryngolo- gist is consulted when potential airway injury as man- ifest by increased airway resistance is suspected or when prolonged ventilation is required due to lung pathology or neuromuscular issues. Adjuvant therapies are used routinely and sometimes concurrently in the neonatal intensive care nursery to improve pulmonary function and extubation success.

Adjuvant Therapies to Improve Successful Extubation

Timely extubation of the NICU patient decreases respiratory and other related morbidities reduce venti- lator-associated pneumonia (VAP), length of stay, and cost of care. Extubation to noninvasive means of respi- ratory support is essential to reduce morbidity of BPD and associated adverse neurologic outcomes. ELBW infants who fail extubation due to poor pulmonary function may need multiple adjuvant therapies to

Failed Extubation in NICU, Table 1 Etiopathogenesis of failed extubations in the NICU patients

Abnormal respiratory load	Inadequate respiratory drive	Inadequate respiratory muscle strength	Increased airway resistance
Residual lung disease, BPD, atelectasis Gastroesophageal Reflux (GERD) related lung injury	Prematurity	Prematurity; Disuse atrophy from prolonged ventilation	Choanal stenosis/atresia Epignathus Retropharyngeal mass glossoptosis
PDA	Hypercapnia	Hypochloremia, hypokalemia Due to diuretic therapy	Subglottic stenosis Vocal cord paralysis: traumatic, S/P PDA ligation or S/P TEF repair Traumatic avulsion of vocal fold
Pneumonia	Sedation	Prolonged use neuromuscular blocking agents	Vascular rings around trachea Mediastinal mass compressing trachea
Severe edema of chest wall	Intracranial Pathology	Neurolomuscular disorders	laryngeal web: congenital
Pleural effusion		Diaphragmatic dysfunction/ Phrenic nerve palsy	Laryngo/trachea/bronchomalacia Primary or associated with other anomalies including esophageal atresia or cardiac anomalies

Modified from Greenough and Prendergast (2008)

enhance the chances of a successful extubation before a tracheostomy is considered. Strategies to decrease pulmonary load, reduce muscle fatigue, improve muscle strength, and improve respiratory drive (Table 2) should be employed before an otolaryngologist is consulted to evaluate for airway obstruction or need for tracheostomy.

Strategies to Decrease Respiratory Load

• *Ventilation Strategies.* Patient triggered ventilation (PTV) strategies such as assist control ventilation (ACV) that supports every spontaneous breath or synchronized intermittent mandatory ventilation (SIMV) where the mandatory breaths are synchronized to neonatal breathing have increased the success of extubation and decreased duration of ventilation in ELBW infants recovering from respiratory complications. Pressure or volume support added to SIMV or AC, in the recovery phase of respiratory distress syndrome, facilitates weaning to minimal settings before extubation (Greenough and Prendergast 2008) by improving diaphragmatic fitness. In volume targeted (VT) ventilation mode, the ventilator responds to changes in respiratory

Failed Extubation in NICU, Table 2 Adjuvant treatments to improve extubation success

Strategies to decrease respiratory load	
1.	CPAP/SNIPPV
2.	Diuretics/bronchodilators/inhaled steroids (BPD)
3.	Diagnosis and treatment of symptomatic PDA(PDA)
4.	Prevention of ventilator-associated pneumonia (VAP)
5.	Chest physiotherapy
Strategies to improve respiratory drive	
1.	Caffeine
2.	Doxapram
3.	SNIPPV/CPAP
4.	Avoidance/timely Weaning of sedation and paralysis
Strategies to improve respiratory muscle strength	
1.	Patient triggered ventilation
2.	Correction of hypokalemia and hypochloremia due to diuretics
3.	Avoidance of neuromuscular blocking agents
4.	Diagnosis and treatment diaphragmatic paralysis
Strategies to diagnose and treat Upper airway obstruction	
1.	Ventilator graphics
2.	ENT evaluation
3.	Airway Dexamethasone
4.	Others evaluations

Modified from Greenough and Prendergast (2008)

compliance such that the preset targeted volume can be delivered at lower pressures as compliance improves. However, if targeted volume is set lower than 6 ml/kg during the weaning process, excess work of breathing may lead to muscle fatigue. Further work needs to be done to determine which of these modes is superior for weaning off the ventilator and reducing diaphragmatic muscle fatigue while protecting the lung from injury.

- *Optimizing Pulmonary Function.* Intubation and assisted ventilation in premature or term newborns is associated with lung injury, oxidant stress, and resultant inflammatory pulmonary edema which may begin as early as 24 h after intubation. Furthermore, when total body and lung water increases, lung compliance decreases. Fluid restriction, use of diuretics along with aggressive nutrition, abrogates this inflammatory edema. Late, targeted use of systemic steroids in ELBW infants who are ventilator dependent may be considered to improve extubation success, but only if current AAP guidelines are followed (Halliday 2010). Neonates with BPD may have airway hyperreactivity and smooth muscle hypertrophy and may respond to bronchodilators. Beta-agonists and anticholinergics can improve lung function in ventilator-dependent ELBW infants and have been used alone or in combination in such patients with variable results. Bronchodilators improve pulmonary function by reducing reversible airway obstruction and increasing airway conductance in ELBW infants studied at 32–44 weeks post conception. However, 15% of infants demonstrate paradoxical effects and actually increase airway resistance, due to loss of intrinsic smooth muscle tone and dynamic compression of the small airways during expiration. Treatment with bronchodilators therefore should be individualized and clinical outcome measures established. Treatment of gastroesophageal reflux disease (GERD) to reduce recurrent aspirations and lung injury should be instituted after obtaining objective evidence of severe GERD and aspiration. Other factors which may play a role in extubation success or failure are cardiac function, presence or absence of pulmonary hypertension, neurologic disabilities, and nutritional status. Each patient should be assessed systematically for these issues.

Failed Extubation in NICU, Table 3 VAP bundle at Tufts Medical Center NICU

1. Head end of the bed elevated 15–30°
a. Assist with prevention of aspiration of gastric contents
b. Encourage full expansion of lungs
2. Daily assessment of readiness to wean
a. Proven to improve likelihood of weaning off ventilator
3. Sterile intubation, limit number of attempts at intubation and unplanned extubations
a. Reduces chances of introducing pathogens into the respiratory tract
4. Limit hyperoxia
a. Use of 100% oxygen produces oxidative damage that has been linked to endotracheal infection and septicemia
b. Blended oxygen in the delivery room and during transport
c. Strict oxygen policy in the NICU
5. Oral care with sterile water or Colostrum
a. Decrease oral colonization with pathogenic bacteria

- *Diagnosis and Treatment of Hemodynamically Significant PDA.* Hemodynamically significant PDA is an important risk factor in extubation failure in extremely low birth weight (ELBW) infants. The significant left to right shunt leads to pulmonary overcirculation, pulmonary edema, and increased ventilatory load. Indomethacin or Ibuprofen is used to achieve medical closure in such cases. The failure rate of medical treatment in infants with lower gestational ages may be as high as 25–40%. Surgical ligation is associated with increased neurodevelopmental morbidity and risk of recurrent laryngeal nerve palsy.

- *Prevention of Ventilator-Associated Pneumonia (VAP).* Ventilator-associated pneumonia, defined as a pneumonia that develops in a neonate after 48–72 h or more of mechanical ventilatory support, is the second most common hospital-acquired infection. Infants weighing <1,000 g are at greatest risk. VAP increases respiratory load, causes lung injury, increases risk of BPD, and also increases risk of poor neurodevelopmental outcomes. In the NICU, institution of the VAP bundle has significantly decreased the incidence of VAP by encouraging sterile intubations, oral care, elevation of head end of the bed to prevent aspirations, and timely extubations. The essential features of the VAP bundle are shown in Table 3.

Strategies to Improve Respiratory Drive

- *Respiratory Stimulants (Caffeine/Doxapram).* Caffeine, a trimethylated xanthine, reduces the incidence of apnea of prematurity, has broncho-relaxant effect and reduces diaphragmatic muscle fatigue, improves respiratory mechanics, and reduces extubation failure. Starting Caffeine early (less than 3 days of life) results in significant reductions in duration of respiratory support. High-dose (20 mg/kg) compared with low-dose (5 mg/kg) Caffeine appears to be more effective. In infants unresponsive to Caffeine, Doxapram, a respiratory stimulant may be tried; however, its safety profile is poor and currently, this therapy is not recommended for ELBW neonates.
- *Continuous Positive Airway Pressure (CPAP) and Noninvasive Positive Pressure Ventilation (NIPPV).* Post-extubation CPAP or NIPPV help maintain functional residual capacity (FRC) and prevent atelectasis. Nasal CPAP reduces the incidence of adverse effects post extubation including failure of extubation. NIPPV may be superior to nasal CPAP at preventing post-extubation respiratory failure. Nasal CPAP, NIPPV, and methylxanthines are evidence-based treatments to facilitate weaning and extubation of preterm infants. Similarly, synchronized noninvasive intermittent positive pressure ventilation (SNIPPV) is an effective method of augmenting the beneficial effects of nasal CPAP in preterm infants in the post-extubation period.
- *Avoidance of and Weaning from Sedation.* Sedation of ventilated newborns is occurring less frequently in the NICU due to potential associated morbidities. Sedation/analgesia is generally practiced in postoperative surgical patients and occasionally in patients with severe primary pulmonary hypertension. Sedation needs to be weaned to allow infant to have adequate respiratory drive, and prolonged sedation can lead to respiratory muscle weakness and difficulty with extubation.

Strategies to Improve Respiratory Muscle Strength

- *Patient Triggered Ventilation.* Neonates, especially premature neonates, have a paucity of fatigue resistant high oxidative muscle fibers in their diaphragm and intercostal muscles. Synchronized intermittent mandatory ventilation or assist control ventilation along with pressure or volume support during the weaning phase reduces muscle fatigue and atrophy.
- *Correction of Hypokalemia/Hypochloremia/Hypocarbia/Hypercarbia.* Premature infants who are hypocarbic/hypercarbic may not have adequate central respiratory drive to maintain respirations once extubated. Hypercapnic ventilatory response to CO_2 is significantly reduced in preterm infants and improves with advancing gestation. Furthermore, the CO_2 apneic threshold is close to the baseline CO_2 and hyperventilation can lead to apnea. Chronic and acute loop diuretic induced hypokalemia, hypochloremia and contraction alkalosis also causes muscle weakness. These metabolic derangements need to be corrected prior to attempted extubation especially in preterm infants.
- *Avoidance of Neuromuscular Blocking Agents.* Paralysis during ventilation leads to decreased chest wall compliance, fluid overload, impaired pulmonary function, and need for higher ventilator settings which cause barotrauma. Neuromuscular blocking agents are used during anesthesia for surgery and rarely for rapid sequence intubation. Neonates are at greater risk for residual neuromuscular blockade than older children and adults. Immaturity of the neonatal neuromuscular system, reduced level of type I fibers in the ventilatory musculature, greater elimination half-life for neuromuscular blocking agents, and overlap of closing lung volume with tidal volume are some of the causes. This places them at greater risk for failure of extubation after surgery. Non-depolarizing muscle relaxants that competitively antagonize autonomic cholinergic receptors such as Pancuronium and Vecuronium have their neuromuscular blocking effect potentiated by simultaneous use of aminoglycosides, presence of acidosis, and hypokalemia. Residual muscle paralysis during the postoperative period may lead to mildly impaired respirations, pulmonary atelectasis, apnea, hypoxemia, hypercarbia, and acidosis which further potentiate the effect of neuromuscular blockade. Prolonged use of aminoglycosides can have the same effect because of their cholinergic effect.
- *Diagnosis and Management of Phrenic Nerve Injury.* Phrenic nerve injury is a rare complication of chest tube placement, cardiac surgery, tracheoesophageal fistula repair, or as a result of obstetric

trauma. It is difficult to diagnose in a ventilated patient as the positive pressure ventilation may obscure the raised diaphragm in a chest radiograph. An asymmetric or tented diaphragm on a chest radiograph and failure to extubate should raise concern for this complication. Ultrasound may reveal a hypokinetic diaphragm, but may not differentiate between diaphragmatic eventration and Phrenic nerve palsy. Direct percutaneous electromyographic stimulation or noninvasive electromagnetic stimulation of the Phrenic nerve shows prolonged Phrenic nerve latency or an absent signal. Treatment is plication of the hemidiaphragm once it is clear that the nerve injury is irreversible and the infant repeatedly fails extubation (Williams et al. 2003). Once the repair has been performed, the infant is generally able to extubate with 3–5 days of treatment.

Strategies to Diagnose and Treat Upper Airway Obstruction

- *Clinical Exam.* The clinical examination remains a vital part of evaluation of an infant who has difficulty when extubated. The presence of stridor is not always clinically apparent soon after extubation and may appear after a few hours. Stridor may be inspiratory, expiratory, or both. Presence of biphasic stridor along with retractions suggests subglottic stenosis or edema. Knowledge of the size of endotracheal tube used prior to extubation and difficulty experienced with re-intubation may confirm any suspicions (Pereira et al. 2007). Change in the quality of stridor with change in head position is important. Stridor in laryngomalacia is relieved in the prone position with head extended. Stridor of unilateral vocal cord paralysis improves when infant is placed on the side of the paralyzed vocal cord. Severe airway obstruction may present with aphonia, weak or almost no airway stridor but with distress and apnea. Loudness of stridor bears no relation to severity. Unilateral nasal obstruction either dominant or nondominant increases total and inspiratory airway resistance and decreases minute ventilation in premature newborns (Martin et al. 1989). Examination of airflow at both nostrils is essential. Most of the times, the unilateral obstruction is from edema of the nasal passage from a prolonged

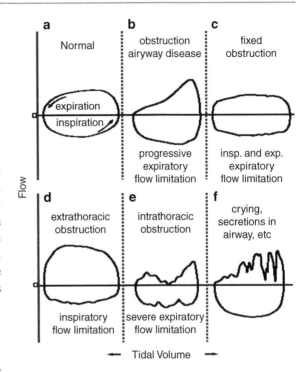

Failed Extubation in NICU, Fig. 1 Ventilator Graphics showing Tidal Flow Volume loops. (**a**): Normal tidal flow volume loop; (**b**): Progressive expiratory flow limitation due to obstructive airway disease such as BPD; (**c**): Inspiratory and expiratory flow limitation due to fixed obstruction such as Subglottic stenosis; (**d**): Inspiratory flow limitation due to extrathoracic obstruction such as Aberrant Subclavian artery; (**e**): Sever expiratory flow limitation due to intrathoracic obstruction such as tracheomalacia; (**f**): A craggy flow volume curve due to airway secretions or crying (Adapted from Goldsmith JP, Karotkin E Assisted ventilation of the neonate 5th edition)

indwelling nasogastric tube. However, unilateral choanal stenosis or obstruction due to epignathus (Maartens et al. 2009) may not be apparent until the infant has been extubated. A Pediatric Otolaryngology evaluation is required to diagnose and treat causes of airway obstruction.

- *Ventilator Graphics in Assessment of Airway Obstruction.* Tidal-flow volume (F-V) loops (Fig. 1) are a graphic expression of airflow at different lung volumes (Graph 1a). The expiratory part of the flow volume loop becomes concave in cases of bronchospasm due to airflow limitation which improves with bronchodilators. A "Ski slope loop" is observed with expiratory airflow limitation as seen in babies with BPD (Graph 1b).

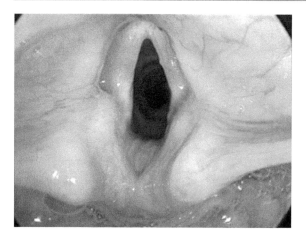

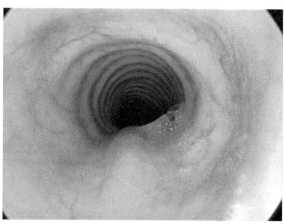

Failed Extubation in NICU, Fig. 2 Normal larynx

Failed Extubation in NICU, Fig. 3 Normal trachea

A cigar shaped loop due to inspiratory and expiratory air flow limitation is seen in subglottic stenosis, tracheal web, or with a narrow endotracheal tube (Graph 1c). A bun shaped loop may be observed in infants with extra-thoracic inspiratory airflow obstruction as in an aberrant vessel compressing the trachea (Graph 1d). A "crumpled loop," or severe expiratory flow obstruction is seen in tracheobronchomalacia where the airway is unstable and air flow is hampered due to airway collapse (Graph 1e). A craggy flow volume loop is seen with secretions or due to crying (Graph 1f). Similarly, pressure volume (P-V) loops can be used to assess lung compliance, presence of air leaks, and airway resistance. Ventilator graphics can be helpful in optimizing conditions for weaning off the ventilator and diagnosing potential risk factors for failure of extubation (Bhutani and Sivieri 2001).

- *Airway Dexamethasone*. The neonatal airway is narrow and relatively rigid (Figs. 2 and 3) at the level of the cricothyroid cartilage and may be more prone to injury and obstruction in the subglottic region. Subglottic edema or stenosis is the most common cause of extubation failure especially in low birth weight population and in postoperative cardiac patients. Subglottic edema occurs following repeated attempts at intubation or after prolonged intubation for ventilation (Dankle et al. 1987). In a meta-analysis, intravenous Dexamethasone given prior to extubation in newborns significantly

reduced the need for re-intubation (Davis and Henderson-Smart 2001). It has been suggested that the use of Dexamethasone be restricted to infants at increased risk for airway edema and obstruction, such as those who have had repeated or prolonged intubations. Dexamethasone is started 24 h prior to a planned extubation and continued for 24 to 48 h after extubation.

Failed Extubation in the NICU: When to Call an Otolaryngologist

An Otolaryngology consult should be obtained in a NICU patient who fails multiple extubation attempts, has stridor post extubation, or when there is concern about anomalies of the aero digestive tract. Abnormal laryngotracheal findings are common in such neonates. Rigid or fiber-optic laryngo-tracheobronchoscopy evaluation of the airway in the operating room under anesthesia is often required to assess airway patency, presence of laryngo-tracheo or bronchomalacia (Figs. 4 and 5a, b), vocal cord paralysis, subglottic stenosis (Fig. 6a, b), laryngeal webs, laryngeal clefts (Fig. 7a, b), hemangiomas (Fig. 8a, b, c), lymphangiomas, papillomas or cysts (Fig. 9a, b), or presence of extrinsic pressure on the airway (Fig. 10). Vocal cord paralysis may follow PDA ligation, cardiac surgery, or tracheoesophageal fistula repair. Neonates who are successfully extubated following PDA ligation are generally asymptomatic despite vocal cord paralysis (Pereira et al. 2006). Congenital laryngeal web is a rare malformation caused by an anomalous embryologic development of the primitive larynx. Most of the reported cases are of the glottic type; the subglottic web is extremely rare. Laryngo-tracheobronchoscopy plays an essential role in the diagnostic workup of this lesion, and endolaryngeal resection is the preferred treatment whenever a structural cartilaginous subglottic stenosis is not present (Anton-Pacheco et al. 2009). Increased airway resistance due to tracheobronchomalacia or laryngomalacia in the presence of poor pulmonary reserve due to BPD can also lead to extubation failure (Downing and Kilbride 1995).

A Systematic Approach to the Problem of Failed Extubation in the NICU

The literature is replete with reviews of complications of prolonged ventilatory support in premature neonates. However, recommendations regarding the management of those who fail extubation are varied and often without consensus. In addition, there exists a fair amount of inter- and intra-institutional variation regarding the optimal number of trials of extubation prior to deciding on alternate airway management strategies (Pereira et al. 2007). Pereira and colleagues retrospectively analyzed the data from records of all premature (gestational age <37 weeks) infants who underwent direct laryngo-bronchoscopy (DLB) in the operating room (OR) for failed extubation between January 1998 and December 2006 at their institution (see Table 4). DLB was performed in 63 neonates to evaluate the cause of failed extubation. Fifty (80%) infants required a tracheostomy and had an average gestational age of 30 weeks, birth weight of 1,457 g, and 2.68 failed extubation attempts. Thirteen patients who did not undergo tracheostomy were older in gestation, weighed more, and had 1.33 failed extubation attempts; 44% of the former and 23% of the latter group had some degree of subglottic stenosis. When compared to their counterparts with similar

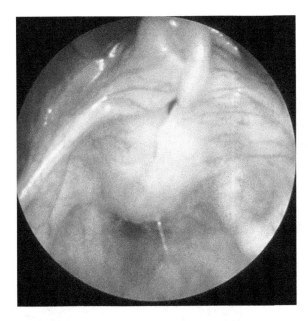

Failed Extubation in NICU, Fig. 4 Laryngomalacia

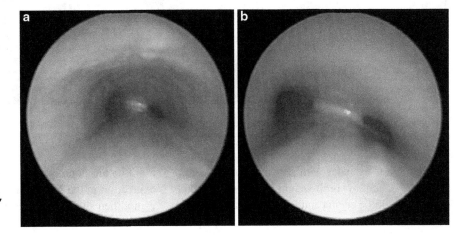

Failed Extubation in NICU, Fig. 5 (a and b): Tracheomalacia

Failed Extubation in NICU,
Fig. 6 (**a** and **b**): Subglottic
scarring due to intubation
injury

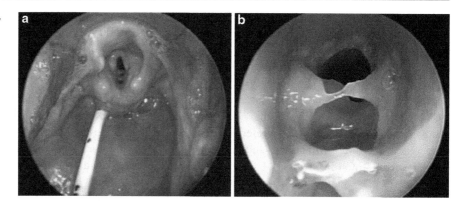

Failed Extubation in NICU,
Fig. 7 (**a** and **b**): Laryngeal
cleft type 3

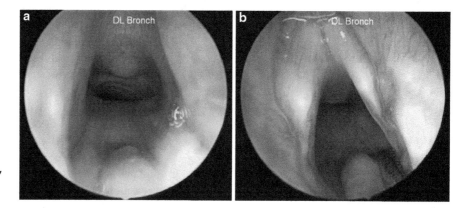

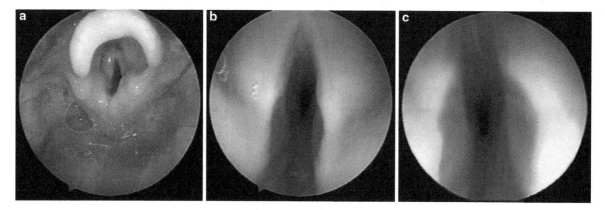

Failed Extubation in NICU, Fig. 8 (**a**, **b**, **c**): Laryngeal hemangioma

comorbidities, neonates with BPD, gestational age of ≤30 weeks, and low birth weight were twice as likely to have subglottic edema and failed extubation(Pereira et al. 2007). Pereira and colleagues have proposed a rational approach to the problem of failed extubation in the NICU based on their findings which is modified slightly to a gestational cutoff of 28 weeks (Fig. 11).

**Failed Extubation in NICU,
Fig. 9** (a and b): Sunglottic
cyst

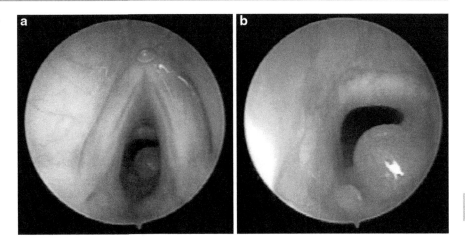

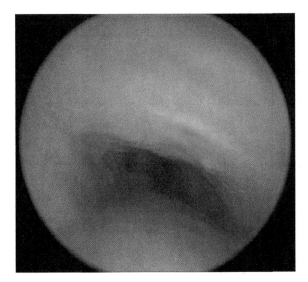

Failed Extubation in NICU, Fig. 10 Aberrant innominate
artery

Failed Extubation in NICU, Table 4 Failed extubation in the
neonatal intensive care unit (Pereira et al. 2007)

Characteristics	Group A (N = 50)	Group B (N = 13)
Average gestational age (weeks)	30	34.5
Average birth weight (g)	1,457	2,309
Average days intubated	88.7	43.2
Average number of failed extubations	2.68	1.33
Average number of endoscopies	1.82	1.17
Chronic lung disease (%)	56	38.5
Laryngopharyngeal reflux (%)	50	61.5
Comorbidities (%)	96	92.3
Abnormal airway (%)	92.7	90.9
Subglottic edema or stenosis (%)	44	23.1

With improved NICU care, especially with shortened period of ventilation, restrictive oxygen policies,
aggressive nutrition, prevention of VAP and central
line–associated sepsis, severe BPD is an increasingly
rare complication in infants born at >28 weeks of
gestation. Failed extubation in this group of premature infants is likely due to either upper airway anomalies or airway injury leading to increased airway
resistance. In these neonates, an Otolaryngology
opinion is warranted when the infant fails extubation.
Extubation failure is rarely due to poor lung
function but due to other causes including airway
abnormalities. An individualized approach is
recommended and individualized treatment plan is
warranted.

In infants <28 weeks, BPD, airway obstruction,
and other comorbidities related to prematurity may
lead to recurrent extubation failures. An Otolaryngology consult is recommended in this group after three
failed extubation attempts (Pereira et al. 2007). An
aero digestive team comprising of an otolaryngologist, pulmonologist, gastroenterologist, neonatologist, and a pediatric surgeon often manage these
patients. The approach consists of optimizing pulmonary function, aggressively treating gastroesophageal

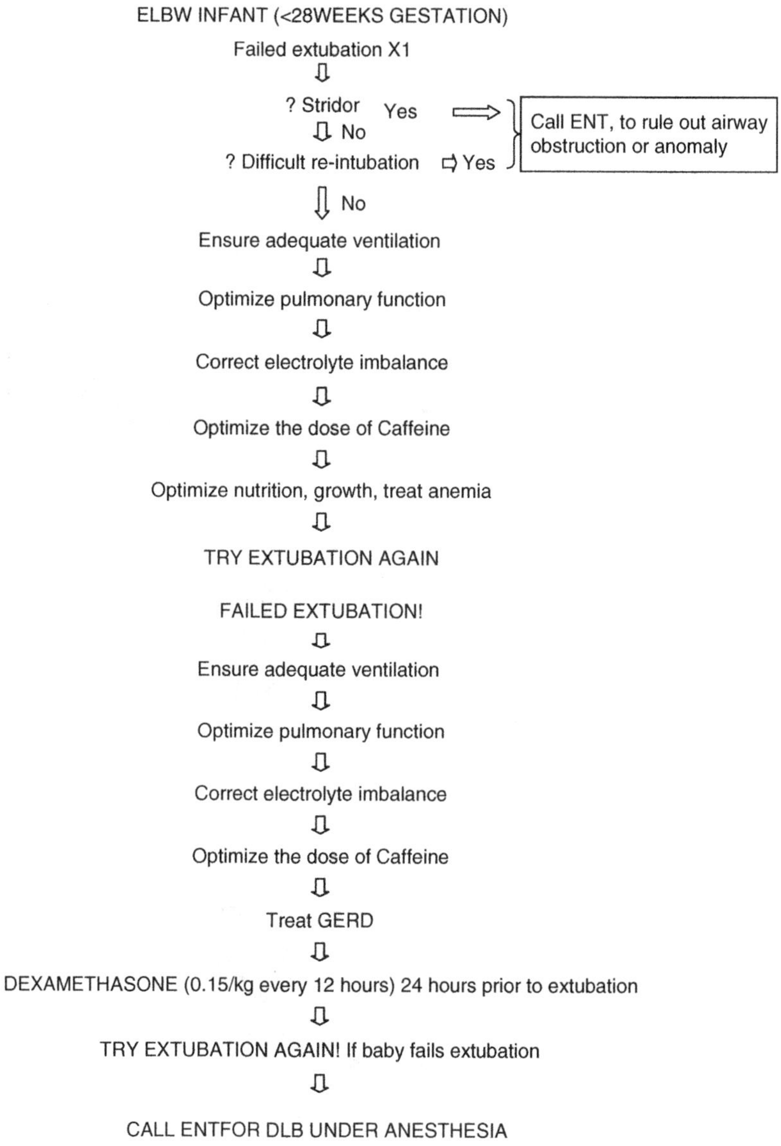

Failed Extubation in NICU,
Fig. 11 A proposed approach
to an ELBW infant who fails
extubation

ELBW INFANT (<28WEEKS GESTATION)

Failed extubation X1

⇩

? Stridor   Yes ⟹ ⎫

⇩ No   ⎬ Call ENT, to rule out airway obstruction or anomaly

? Difficult re-intubation ⇨ Yes ⎭

⇩ No

Ensure adequate ventilation

⇩

Optimize pulmonary function

⇩

Correct electrolyte imbalance

⇩

Optimize the dose of Caffeine

⇩

Optimize nutrition, growth, treat anemia

⇩

TRY EXTUBATION AGAIN

FAILED EXTUBATION!

⇩

Ensure adequate ventilation

⇩

Optimize pulmonary function

⇩

Correct electrolyte imbalance

⇩

Optimize the dose of Caffeine

⇩

Treat GERD

⇩

DEXAMETHASONE (0.15/kg every 12 hours) 24 hours prior to extubation

⇩

TRY EXTUBATION AGAIN! If baby fails extubation

⇩

CALL ENTFOR DLB UNDER ANESTHESIA

reflux, treating nasal stuffiness and optimizing the airway with Dexamethasone 24–48 h before an assessment by rigid or flexible bronchoscopy to look for airway obstruction and other anomalies(Pereira et al. 2007). Those infants who show evidence of ongoing respiratory instability due to recurrent aspirations and GERD may need a gastrostomy tube and fundoplication. A proposed approach to extubation failure is outlined in Fig. 11.

An Otolaryngology consultation includes a thorough evaluation of the airway of the infant in the NICU and then under anesthesia in the operating room. Nasal obstruction due to edema is easily treated with nasal saline drops or with ophthalmic suspension of Dexamethasone with Tobramicin twice a day for 2–3 days. However for nasal obstruction due to other causes, such as unilateral/bilateral choanal atresia/ stenosis or an epignathus, a magnetic resonance imaging (MRI) is required to delineate the extent of the lesion and plan further management. A laryngoscopy may reveal posterior pharyngeal or laryngeal pathology; however, a detailed exam under anesthesia with either a rigid or flexible bronchoscope is generally necessary (Downing and Kilbride 1995; Lim et al. 2003). Dynamic studies such as a cine computerized tomography (CT) (Fig. 12) or a MRI (Fig. 13) of the airway may be necessary to evaluate the extent of tracheobronchomalacia or extrinsic compression. Rarely a contrast bronchogram (Fig. 14) may be necessary to diagnose stenosis of the tracheobronchial tree (Torer et al. 2008). Further diagnostic studies and management are planned depending on the

pathology found. Many of the infants will need to undergo a tracheostomy at the time of the DLB because of severity of the disease process or for prolonged ventilator support. Preparing the parents of these patients about the possibility of this outcome prior to examination under anesthesia is necessary so that they understand that these infants will require extended medical and home care (Schlessel et al. 1993).

Conclusion

In summary, failed extubations are relatively common in the NICU. With earlier extubations to prevent lung and airway injury and a lack of reliable predictors for successful extubation, many infants may need multiple attempts before they are finally extubated. A thorough knowledge of the causes of extubation failure, a good understanding of the anatomy and pathophysiology of the respiratory system, and a systematic approach to examining the infant who fails extubation is needed. Treating the underlying causes of extubation failure such as poor lung compliance, inadequate respiratory drive, and reversible airway pathology (e.g., nasal obstruction, subglottic edema, GERD) is necessary before an otolaryngologist is consulted. Ideally, a multidisciplinary team comprising of the neonatologist, pulmonologist, gastroenterologist, and an

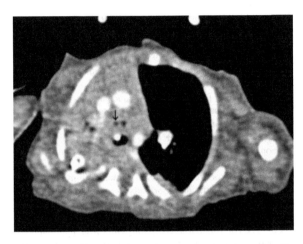

Failed Extubation in NICU, Fig. 12 Computed tomography showing Bronchomalacia with narrowing of both bronchi, more pronounced on the right (*arrow*) and collapse of the right lung

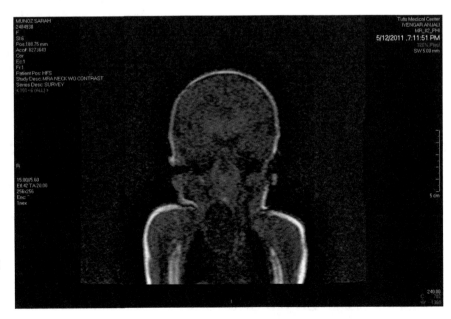

Failed Extubation in NICU, Fig. 13 MRI of the head and neck showing an extrinsic mass compressing and deviating the trachea

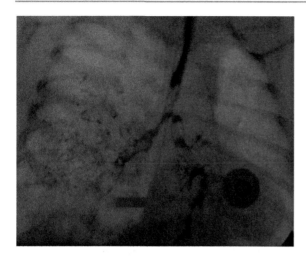

Failed Extubation in NICU, Fig. 14 Bronchography performed during DLB shows the narrowing of the trachea and both bronchi

otolaryngologist should manage these babies in the NICU and follow them post discharge to ensure best outcomes.

Cross-References

▶ Gastroesophageal Reflux in Children
▶ Imaging of Pediatric Neck and Airway
▶ Nasal Obstruction in Newborn
▶ Subglottic and Tracheal Stenosis

References

Anton-Pacheco JL, Villafruela M et al (2009) Congenital subglottic web: a rare cause of neonatal stridor. J Pediatr Surg 44(1):e25–e27
Bhutani VK, Sivieri EM (2001) Clinical use of pulmonary mechanics and waveform graphics. Clin Perinatol 28(3):487–503, v
da Silva OP (1996) Factors influencing acquired upper airway obstruction in newborn infants receiving assisted ventilation because of respiratory failure: an overview. J Perinatol 16(4):272–275
Dankle SK, Schuller DE et al (1987) Prolonged intubation of neonates. Arch Otolaryngol Head Neck Surg 113(8):841–843
Davis PG, Henderson-Smart DJ (2001) Intravenous dexamethasone for extubation of newborn infants. Cochrane Database Syst Rev (4):CD000308
Downing GJ, Kilbride HW (1995) Evaluation of airway complications in high-risk preterm infants: application of flexible fiberoptic airway endoscopy. Pediatrics 95(4):567–572

Greenough A, Prendergast M (2008) Difficult extubation in low birthweight infants. Arch Dis Child Fetal Neonatal Ed 93(3): F242–F245
Guillemaud JP, El-Hakim H et al (2007) Airway pathologic abnormalities in symptomatic children with congenital cardiac and vascular disease. Arch Otolaryngol Head Neck Surg 133(7):672–676
Halliday HL (2010) Postnatal steroids: the way forward. Arch Dis Child Fetal Neonatal Ed 96(3):F158–F159
Kamlin CO, Davis PG et al (2006) Predicting successful extubation of very low birthweight infants. Arch Dis Child Fetal Neonatal Ed 91(3):F180–F183
Lim J, Hellier W et al (2003) Subglottic cysts: the Great Ormond Street experience. Int J Pediatr Otorhinolaryngol 67(5):461–465
Maartens IA, Wassenberg T et al (2009) Neonatal airway obstruction caused by rapidly growing nasopharyngeal teratoma. Acta Paediatr 98(11):1852–1854
Martin RJ, Miller MJ et al (1989) Effects of unilateral nasal occlusion on ventilation and pulmonary resistance in infants. J Appl Physiol 66(6):2522–2526
Pereira KD, Webb BD et al (2006) Sequelae of recurrent laryngeal nerve injury after patent ductus arteriosus ligation. Int J Pediatr Otorhinolaryngol 70(9):1609–1612
Pereira KD, Smith SL et al (2007) Failed extubation in the neonatal intensive care unit. Int J Pediatr Otorhinolaryngol 71(11):1763–1766
Schlessel JS, Harper RG et al (1993) Tracheostomy: acute and long-term mortality and morbidity in very low birth weight premature infants. J Pediatr Surg 28(7):873–876
Stefanescu BM, Murphy WP, Hansell BJ et al. (2003) A randomized controlled trial comparing two different continuous positive airway pressure systems for successful extubation of extremely low birth weight infants. Pediatrics 112(5): 1031–1038
Torer B, Gulcan H et al (2008) Use of balloon-expandable metallic stent in a premature infant with congenital tracheobronchial stenosis. Pediatr Pulmonol 43(4):414–417
Ward RF, Jones J et al (1995) Current trends in pediatric tracheotomy. Int J Pediatr Otorhinolaryngol 32(3): 233–239
Williams O, Greenough A et al (2003) Extubation failure due to phrenic nerve injury. Arch Dis Child Fetal Neonatal Ed 88(1):F72–F73

False Aneursym of Carotid Artery

▶ Imaging for Parapharyngeal Space Masses, Carotid Artery Pseudoaneurysm

False Croup

▶ Pediatric Inflammatory Airway Disorders

Fascial Flaps

▶ Fasciocutaneous Flaps

Fascicle

Wojciech K. Mydlarz and Kofi Derek O. Boahene
Department of Otolaryngology-Head and Neck
Surgery, Johns Hopkins University School of
Medicine, Baltimore, MD, USA

Definition

It is the inner subunit of a peripheral nerve composed
of a number of nerve fibers invested in a sheath of
connective tissue called the perineurium.

Cross-References

▶ Sunderland Classification of Nerve Injury

Fasciocutaneous Flaps

Kal Ansari[1,2], Yaser Alrajhi[1] and Praby Singh[3]
[1]Walter Mackenzie Center, University of Alberta
Hospital, Edmonton, AB, Canada
[2]Department of Otrolaryngology, University of
Alberta, Edmonton, AB, Canada
[3]Division of Otolaryngology-Head and Neck Surgery,
Walter Mackenzie Centre, University of Alberta
Hospital, Edmonton, AB, Canada

Synonyms

Fascial flaps; Locoregional flaps; Microvascular free
flaps; Pedicled flaps

Definition

A fasciocutaneous flap consists of skin, subcutaneous
tissue, and deep muscle fascia and has a defined axial
blood supply, which is the pedicle. Adiposofascial
flaps consist of subcutaneous tissue and fascia while
fascia-only flaps consist only of fascia. Both of these
later flaps also have a definable axial blood supply.

Purpose

The purpose of a fasciocutaneous flap is to resurface
cutaneous or mucosal defects of the head and neck
while having its own independent blood supply.
Adiposofascial flaps bring vascularized subcutaneous
tissue to restore volume to a head and neck defect.
Fascial-only flaps provide a thin layer of vascular
fascia where thin lining is critical to the reconstruction (i.e., coverage of carved costal cartilage to form
an auricle, or provide a thin lining for
a hemilaryngectomy defect).

Principle

A sound knowledge of the vascular anatomy of fascial
flaps allows the surgeon to efficiently harvest these
extremely well-vascularized flaps in predictable and
reliable way. The dermal, subdermal, suprafascial, and
subfascial vascular plexuses of these flaps can be
supplied through perforator vessels from an axial
blood supply (major named vessel) that can either sit
on top of a muscle (direct cutaneous artery) or
underneath a muscle, or between muscles. For
example, if the axial supply originates underneath
a muscle and the perforators going to the flap travel
through the muscle, these perforators are referred to as
the musculocutaneous type. Similarly, if the axial supply resides between two muscles and the perforators
travel through an intermuscular septum, which lies
between the two muscle bellies, to the vascular plexuses of the flap, these perforators are the
septocutaneous type. A single fascial flap can have
multiple perforators and combinations of different
types of perforators (Mathes and Nahai 1982). Mathes
and Nahai have classified fasciocutaneous flaps: Type
A has a direct cutaneous pedicle to the fascia (i.e.,
temporoparietal fascial flap); Type B has
a septocutaneous perforator (i.e., radial forearm free
flap); and Type C has perforators from
a musculocutaneous source (i.e., anterolateral thigh
free flap) (Lamberty and Cormack 1990). Cormack
and Lamberty classified fasciocutaneous flaps based

on the number of definable perforators: no identifiable perforators because flap is supplied by the fascial plexus from a direct cutaneous artery; a flap with single perforator; and flaps with multiple perforators from a segmental artery source. Perforators supply defined areas of skin, subcutaneous tissue, and fascia. These areas are referred to as ▸ angiosomes (Geddes 2003). The concept of "free style" free flap or ▸ perforator flap refers to incising the skin, and then supra- or subfascially elevating the skin till a robust perforator is identified. The perforator is dissected to its parent segment vessel. The area of skin that is reliably supplied by the perforator(s) is incised into an island and the flap is elevated. When the fascial flap can be transferred to the defect site without dividing its parent blood supply, it is referred to as a ▸ pedicled or locoregional flap. On the other hand if the pedicle flap will not reach the defect, its parent blood is divided. The flap is transferred to the defect as a free flap where microvascular anastomosis is performed. The axial blood supply of a free flap will often consist of an artery and its attendant vena comitantes. Occasionally, a superficial venous system can also be identified to drain the flap (i.e., cephalic vein of the radial forearm free flap). The flap is inset into the defect and the flap vessels are microvascularly anastomosed to native recipient vessels of the head and neck.

Indication

For defects in the head and neck, fascial flaps are considered in the reconstructive ladder when simplifier options are not viable such as local flaps (pedicled or random blood supply) and free grafts (i.e., tissue grafts that do not have their own blood supply and rely on the recipient bed for vascularity like skin grafts). In radiated defects, the utilization of free grafts is essentially precluded because of the poor blood supply of the bed from radiation endarteritis. Although this vascular depleted environment can be somewhat remedied with hyperbaric oxygen (HBO) treatments, even with HBO, the reliability and the success of a pedicled fascial flaps still far exceeds that of any free graft. Furthermore, fascial flaps bring with them a rich, independent blood supply that dramatically enhances the healing potential of chronically infected and poorly healing wounds. When considering ▸ local flap, we are referring to flaps that are adjacent to the defect

and have a random blood supply based on the deep dermal and subdermal plexus. An example is a rotation flap. These flaps may not be an option if prior surgical incisions have crossed the area of proposed flap elevation, thus compromising the flap. Even though such flaps maybe successfully raised in a delayed fashion, they will not be as reliable as a regional pedicled or free fasciocutaneous flap. Although local flaps provide better tissue match due to the proximity to the defect, they may not provide an adequate amount of tissue to resurface or fill the defect. Furthermore, if the blood supply of a local flap is random in nature, the vascularity, and therefore reliability, will never exceed that of a pedicled fascial flap. Compared to some fascial flaps which can be harvested with multiple vascularized layers, multiple skin paddles, fascia, and other components such as muscle and bone, a single local flap may simply lack the adequate composition required to reconstruct complex and multilayered defects (i.e., through-and-through defect of the cheek and maxilla into the oral cavity).

Contraindication

If simpler reconstructive options with better functional and aesthetic results, and less donor morbidity are available, they should be exhausted first before turning to a regional or distal fascial flap. If prior surgery or trauma has compromised the pedicled blood supply to the flap, it should not be harvested (i.e., prior axillary node dissection on the side of proposed harvest of a ▸ scapular/parascapular free flap, or recent intra-arterial line in radial artery or intravenous in the cephalic vein at site of a proposed radial forearm free flap harvest). If there is major donor site morbidity predicted with the flap harvest, it should be abandoned as a reconstructive option. For example, if a patient's Allen's test or preoperative Doppler ultrasound fails to demonstrate good collateral flow through the vascular arches of the hand with radial artery occlusion, a radial forearm free flap should not be harvested because of the substantial risk of ischemic injury to the hand.

Advantage/Disadvantage

The advantages of fascial flaps have been asserted in the aforementioned sections: easy and efficient flaps to harvest; a reliable and independent blood supply and, therefore, highly successful reconstructions; enhanced wound healing in the chronically infected and vascular depleted recipient beds; highly versatile flaps in terms of number flap layers, and independent skin paddles; the flaps can be extremely thin fascial-only flaps (temporoparietal fascial flaps) to flaps with thick subcutaneous tissue such as the anterolateral thigh free flap; fascial flaps can also be harvested with other vascularized tissue components such as muscle or bone (these composite flaps will be discussed in the section on ▶ musculocutaneous and ▶ osteocutaneous flaps); and lastly, some of these flaps can also be sensate (lateral antebranchial cutaneous nerve of the radial forearm free flap).

The disadvantages of these flaps are the associated donor site morbidity. This can include poor healing in the donor site including wound break down, and failure of skin grafts to take resulting in tendon exposure such as that might occur when repairing the radial forearm donor site. Furthermore, there is the possibility of seromas and/or hematomas, sensory or motor nerve injury, and muscle injury. Buried adiposofascial flap and fasciocutaneous flaps can be difficult to monitor without an external skin paddle. Implantable Doppler devices are useful in this situation. Of course as with any flap, flap failure is a possibility, resulting in an adverse situation where the patient incurs donor site morbidity without making any progress towards rehabilitating the defect. Fortunately, as one will observe in the subsequent sections, there are multiple fasciocutaneous flap options available as a backup in the event of a flap failure.

Whenever considering fascial type of flaps, one must select a flap where the advantages of the flap reconstruction far outweigh the disadvantages and potential complications.

Commonly Used Fasciocutaneous Flaps

Radial Forearm Free Flap

This is the workhorse free flap of head and neck reconstruction. It provides a relatively thin, pliable, and sensory neurotized flap which makes it ideal for oral cavity reconstruction. As an adiposofascial flap, it is ideal to restore volume in defects such those created by total parotidectomy. A vascularized palmaris tendon can also be included to suspend a total lower lip reconstruction. The pliability of the flap allows it to be tubed for total laryngopharyngectomy defects (Urken et al. 1995), particularly after chemoradiotherapy failures for laryngeal cancer requiring laryngectomy and reconstruction. Multiple independent skin paddles can be used for resurface mucosal and cutaneous defects at the same time (i.e., through-and-through defect of the cheek). The long pedicle length allows it to reconstruct the skull base while the pedicle can easily reach the neck to be anastomosed. To provide even thinner lining, such as that required for the internal nasal mucosa for total rhinectomy defects, the flap can be prelaminated with split thickness skin graft and then can be later harvested for intranasal lining reconstruction. A subcutaneous paddle can also be harvested in continuity with the cutaneous paddle. The subcutaneous paddle can be separated from the pedicle but is deliberately kept attached to the cutaneous paddle, thus maintaining its blood supply through the subdermal plexus in a retrograde fashion. By this way the vascularized subcutaneous paddle can be rolled onto itself to provide the necessary bulk for base of tongue reconstruction.

The flap design extends longitudinally over the forearm while being centered over the radial artery pedicle and cephalic vein. The entire forearm from the flexor crease to the antecubital fossa can be harvested. The radial artery pedicle is located between the brachioradialis and flexor carpi radialis. Between these two muscles, septocutaneous perforators traverse the intermuscular septum to supply the fasciocutaneous paddle. Many of these perforators also supply the radial bone. Therefore, a portion of the radial bone can be harvested to create an osteocutaneous flap. Often the vena comitantes can be dissected to a common bridging vein that connects to the superficial cephalic vein system, although this is not absolutely necessary.

Potential morbidity associated with this flap is wound breakdown resulting in tendon exposure due to poor split thickness skin graft take at the donor site. Elevating the skin paddle in a suprafascial plane minimizes the occurrence of this complication. During flap elevation, care also has to be taken not to injure the radial sensory nerve branches. A preoperative Allen's test is mandatory to ensure good collateral circulation from the ulnar vessels through the superficial and deep palmer arches to the thumb and index finger. Patients with questionable Allen's tests should undergo Doppler ultrasound with radial artery occlusion to quantify collateral flow. Serious morbidity can be incurred with loss of blood supply to the thumb, index finger, and thenar eminence if these preoperative checks are ignored to identify poor collateral blood supply in the hand. Lastly, another disadvantage of the flap is that it transfers hair-bearing skin. Some authors have advocated removing the mid dermis to epithelium portion of the flap with a dermatome prior to transfer. While the partial skin graft that was removed resurfaces the secondary forearm defect, the transferred flap now has a depleted number of pilosebaceous units and subsequent minimal hair growth upon healing. This technique can only be applied if flap is not folded in the defect causing opposing bare surfaces to scar together, and thus compromising the reconstruction. As an aside, if postoperative radiation is planned, during its course, many of the pilosebaceous units will also damaged and hair growth will be minimized. Opposing de-epithelialized segments of the inset flap should not contact each other in order to avoid synechiae. Furthermore, there is a potential risk of injury to radial sensory nerve branches to the thumb.

Temporoparietal Fascial Flap

The temporoparietal fascia (TPF) lies deep to the subcutaneous tissue and hair follicles of the dermis of the temple. TPF is continuous with the galea aponeurotica above the superior temporal line and with the SMAS (superficial musculoaponeurotic system) below the zygomatic arch. Therefore, the galea can be harvested with the flap, creating flaps as large as 17 by 14 cm (Bailey et al. 2006). The flap cannot be harvested below the zygomatic because of the following anatomical considerations. At the zygomatic arch, the TPF is adherent to the periosteum of the zygomatic arch. Along the zygomatic arch, the frontal branch of the facial nerve pass into the TPF through a corridor that is 2 cm in front of the tragus and 2 cm behind the orbital rim. In this corridor along the zygomatic arch, the frontal branches are vulnerable to injury if the dissection is not in a subperiosteal or subcutaneous plane. Above the arch, the frontal branches travel within the TPF anterior to Pitanguy's line. This is a line that connects a point 0.5 cm below the tragus to another point 1.5 cm above the lateral tail of the brow. Therefore, only the TPF that is posterior to this line can be harvested safely without injuring the facial nerve. The

superficial temporal artery and vein typically arise from the parotid to cross the zygomatic arch and enter into the TFP just anterior to the root of the helix and behind the aforementioned danger zone of the facial nerve at the zygomatic arch. The pedicle can be safely dissected further proximally into the parotid as long as one remains superficial to the bony-cartilaginous junction of the external auditory canal in order to avoid the main trunk of the facial nerve. Just above the zygomatic arch, the pedicle sends the middle temporal artery branch which supplies the deep temporal fascia. Therefore, a two layer vascularized fascial flap can be harvested (Bailey et al. 2006). Approximately 3 cm above the root of the helix, the superficial temporal artery divides into a frontal and parietal branch. The frontal branch of the superficial temporal artery is ligated well behind Pitanguy's line to harvest the flap.

As a pedicled flap, it is the preferred method for reconstructing the external lining of the external pinna when it is deficient and local flaps will not suffice (i.e., burn victim with poor overlying skin in auricle region). This thin lining flap is usually draped over the cartilaginous ear reconstruction, and then a skin graft is applied. Because the flap is thin, it easily adapts to the delicate contours of the reconstructed ear, bringing the architecture of the neo-constructed pinna into broad relief. As a free flap, it is also thin enough to reconstruct hemilaryngectomy defects without compromising the airway with an excessively thick flap. The TPF quickly mucosalizes in the airway.

The disadvantages of the flap are its short pedicle length, making it difficult to transfer a large surface area of the flap to the anterior skull base. Because the hair-bearing skin of the temporal area is elevated in the near subdermal plane in order to expose the flap, there is possibility of injury to hair follicles, resulting in temporary or permanent alopecia. There is usually unavoidable sensory numbness in the distribution of the auriculotemporal nerve, although patients rarely complain about this symptom. As discussed, the frontal branch of the facial nerve can be placed in jeopardy during this dissection.

Anterolateral Thigh Free Flap

This flap has been progressively adopted by many centers as a "workhorse flap" like the radial forearm due to its purported thinness in Asian patients, the large surface area of skin that can be transferred while allowing for primary closure of the leg, a long vascular pedicle, and sensory innervation from the lateral femoral cutaneous nerve. However, due to the generous body habitus of many North Americans, the ALT is usually a thick subcutaneous flap in North America (Microsurgeon.org). Different authors have proposed that up to 20–25 cm longitudinally and 8–12 cm of width of skin flap can be harvested with primary closure of the leg. Like the radial forearm free flap, two team simulataneous oncologic ablation and flap elevation can be performed simultaneously. The pedicle of the flap is the descending branch of the lateral femoral circumflex artery (LFCA). This pedicle usually resides between the rectus femoris muscle and the vastus lateralis deep in the lateral intermuscular septal plane. Occasionally the pedicle travels within the substance of the vastus lateralis itself. There are on average two major perforators to the flap. When more than one perforator is present, independent skin paddles can be harvested. These perforators are most often located in the midpoint of the line connecting the lateral patella and the anterior superior iliac spine, and thus the flap should be centered at this point. At least initially, it is important to preserve the consistent tensor fascia lata perforator located more cephalically in the leg, till a more inferior perforator is identified. If one does not identify a reasonable distal perforator, tensor fascia lata (TFL) perforator can serve as the lifeboat of the anterolateral thigh free flap. However, basing the flap on this TFL perforator reduces the overall length of the pedicle. Because most of the perforators identified are more commonly of the musculocutaneous type, traveling through the vastus lateralis, two thirds of the flap width should be located over this muscle. In terms of flap design, this means that two thirds of the width of flap should be located behind the line connecting the lateral patella and anterior superior illiac spine. The musculocutaneous nature of the perforators and their variable location can make the dissection tedious for inexperienced surgeons. On the other hand, vascularized vastus lateralis can be harvested with the flap and can also have motor neurotization via the nerve to the vastus lateralis. Such a flap may have applications in reconstructing the bulk and functional muscle of the tongue or for facial reanimation. As a perforator flap, one can harvest a TFL fascial-only flap or adiposofascial flap.

Potentially donor site morbidities associated with this flap include postoperative hematomas and seromas due to large area of dissection. Rarely, there can be weakness of knee extension resulting in gait alteration. Avoiding damage to proximal perforators coming off the LFCA to the rectus femoris muscle can minimize this. Sensory disturbances can occur to the lateral thigh. Aesthetic issues include abnormal scarring from the conspicuous long lateral leg incision, and contour deformities from resection of subcutaneous tissue.

Scapular/Parascapular Fasciocutaneous Free Flap
The pedicle originates from the subscapular artery whose origin is based on the third part of the axillary artery. The subscapular artery divides into a thoracodorsal branch supplying the latissimus dorsi and serratus anterior muscles (and tip of scapular bone via the angular branch), and a circumflex scapular branch, supplying the scalpular/parascapular fasciocutaneous skin paddles. The circumflex scapular artery (CSA), the main pedicle of the scapular/parascapular fasciocutaneous free flap, emerges through the triangular fossa from dorsal to ventral. The teres minor superiomedially, teres major inferiomedially, and the long head of triceps laterally are the boundaries of the triangular fossa. Prior to emerging from the triangular fossa, a branch from the proximal CSA supplies the lateral border of the scapular bone. The teres major muscle has to be divided in order to expose and dissect out the pedicle. It is prudent to reattach the muscle via drill holes in remainder of the lateral scapular bone so that occurrence of postoperative shoulder dysfunction is reduced. After the CSA emerges from the triangular fossa, the pedicle divides into a transverse branch, supplying the horizontally oriented scapular flap, and a descending branch, supplying the vertically oriented parascapular flap. If all the components (i.e., scapular and parascapular skin paddles, lateral scapular bone, angle of scapular bone, latissmus dorsi, serratus anterior with possible overlying skin paddles) are harvested on the ▶ subscapular system, this is referred to as the "scapular megaflap."

The advantage of this flap is the large surface area of thin, pliable, and hairless skin it provides. The flap can provide multiple skin paddles, bone, and large volume of muscle and therefore it is ideal for three dimensionally reconstructing large, complex, and multilayered tissue defects. Also the flap provides a long pedicle length (Bailey et al. 2006). The pedicle length is 7–10 cm if it is harvested at the CSA, and 11–14 cm if the subscapular artery is harvested.

Fasciocutaneous Flaps, Table 1 Faciocutaneous flap types, transfer method, advantages, disadvantages, indications, & contraindications

Flap	Regional versus Free	Pedicle	Advantages	Disadvantages	Common uses	Contraindications
Radial forearm	Free	• Radial artery and venae comitantes (VCs) and septocutaneous perforators (SCPs) • Cephalic vein	• Workhorse attributes (easy to harvest, long pedicle, large surface area of thin, pliable skin, multiple paddles, adiposal fascial option, sensory innervation), also bone option	• Requires split thickness skin graft for closure of donor site • Pathologic # of radius possible if excessive bone harvested • Hairy flap	• Workhorse for oral cavity, and pharynx reconstruction • Facial recontouring procedure • Ramus of mandible reconstruction when using bone	• Poor preoperative Allen's test • Prior arterial line in radial artery or prior intravenous line in cephalic vein
Ulnar	Free	• Ulnar artery and its VCs and SCPs	• Same as RFFF except somewhat more difficult flap elevation • Possible ulnar nerve injury	• Same as RFFF • Potential injury to the radial sensory nerves causing numbness of thumb	• Same as RFFF	• Same as RFFF
ALT	Free	• Descending branch of lateral circumflex artery and VCs and 80% musculocutaneous perforators and 20% SCP's	• Workhorse attributes, and can also harvest vascularized vastus lateralis with its motor nerve	• Difficult dissection of musculocutaneous perforators	• Same as RFFF and resurfacing large skin defects	• Prior surgery in the region of the pedicle
Temporoparietal fascia	Pedicled or Free	• Superficial temporal artery and vein	• Thin fascial flap • Deep temporal fascia based on middle temporal branch can also be harvested	• Short pedicle as a free flap • Possible morbidity to frontal branch of facial nerve and alopecia	• Soft tissue coverage of neo-reconstructed cartilage pinna as a pedicled flap • Hemilaryngectomy reconstruction as free flap	• Beware of prior parotidectomy damaging pedicle
Scapular/ Parascapular	Free	• Circumflex scapular artery and its VCs giving direct cutaneous arteries (transverse and descending branch)	• Large surface area of thin, hairless, pliable skin • Long pedicle • Multiple skin paddles, muscle, and bone can be harvested in the mega flap	• Lateral decubitus positioning making 2 team surgery difficult, longer operative time • Contralateral brachial plexus injury	• Complex, large, multilayered three-dimensional full thickness defects of head and neck	• Prior axillary node dissection or some form of radical neck dissection on same side
Lateral arm	Free	• Posterior radial collateral artery and VCs giving off SCPs	• If skin paddle width is <8 cm, primary closure of arm is possible • Sensate • Occasionally muscle, bone, and nerve can be included	• Possible injury to the radial nerve • Slightly shorter pedicle than forearm (8 cm) • Possible shoulder dysfunction	• Same as radial forearm	• Prior surgery in area of flap and pedicle

Flap	Type	Vascular supply / Technique	Advantages	Disadvantages / Cautions	Uses	Contraindications
Posterior tibial	Free	• Posterior tibial artery and VCs giving off SCPs	• Thin, supple skin paddle	• Avoid injury to posterior tibial nerve • Do not strip periosteum off tibial bone as split thickness skin graft will not take resulting in chronic wound over tibial bone • Short pedicle	• Same as radial forearm	• Preoperative CT angiogram to ensure good collateral flow through anterior tibial and peroneal vessels to foot
Paramedian forehead flap	Pedicled	• Direct cutaneous artery (supratrocheal or supraorbital) • One staged/interpolated or two stage with subsequent pedicle division	• Good skin match to nasal skin • Easy to harvest usually with frontalis muscle to protect pedicle • Can harvest vascularized pericranium as a separate layer	• Forehead scar, medial eyebrow distortion, forehead numbness	• External skin of nose in nasal reconstruction • Can be folded to provide inner lining of nose as well. • Pericranium can be used for inner nasal lining or frontal sinus obliteration	• Prior surgery in regional of pedicle
Melolabial flap	Pedicled	• Direct cutaneous artery (angular artery) • Can be superiorly or inferiorly based • Can be one stage interpolated or two stage (less blunting of the nasofacial isthmus)	Good match to sebaceous skin of nasal side wall, nasal ala, easy to harvest	• Melolabial scar with resultant flatness of the nasolabial fold • One stage can blunt nasofacial sulcus	• Superiorly based is good for reconstructing alar lobule • Inferiorly based good for reconstructing upper or lower lip external skin	• Prior extensive surgery in medial cheek region in melobial fold
Deltopectoral flap	Pedicled	• Direct cutaneous artery (first two parasternal perforators of the internal thoracic artery)	Provides a large surface of skin. If extending the paddle past the deltopectoral groove, it should be delayed	• Requires a large split thickness skin graft to cover secondary defect	• Often a last option after a pectoralis major flap for carotid artery coverage after ▲ pharyngocutaneous fistula, or large skin reconstruction in lower face	• Prior mastectomy or other chest wall surgery around sternum • Prior harvest of internal mammary for cardiac bypass

The obvious disadvantage is that simultaneous flap harvest and oncologic ablation is very difficult. Therefore, harvesting this flap can lead to protracted operative times. The lateral decubitus positioning can injure the contralateral brachial plexus if one does not use an axillary roll in the contralateral axilla. Winging of the scapular and shoulder dysfunction is aggravated if the teres major muscle is not reattached to the lateral border of the scapula. Furthermore, if the flap is harvested on the same side as radical or modified radical neck dissection, which causes spinal accessory nerve morbidity, shoulder dysfunction can be quite debilitating. Prior axillary node dissection can damage the pedicle vessels, and therefore this is an obvious contraindication for harvesting the scapular systems of flaps (Table 1).

Cross-References

▸ Angiosomes
▸ Classification of Flaps
▸ Delay of Flap
▸ Donor Site Complications in Free Flap Surgery
▸ Free Tissue Transfer in Head and Neck
▸ Local Flaps
▸ Mandible Reconstruction
▸ Musculocutaneous Flap
▸ Nasal Reconstruction
▸ Oropharyngeal Reconstruction
▸ Pedicled Flaps
▸ Perforator Flaps
▸ Pharyngocutaneous Fistula
▸ Regional Flaps
▸ Subscapular System Flaps

References

Bailey BJ et al (2006) Head and neck surgery – otolaryngology. Lippincott Williams & Wilkins, Philadelphia
Geddes C, Morris S, Neligan P (2003) Perforator flaps: evolution, classification and applications. Ann Plast Surg 50:90–99
Lamberty BG, Cormack GC (1990) Fasciocutaneous flaps. Clin Plast Surg 17(4):713–726, Review
Mathes SJ, Nahai F (1982) Clinical applications for muscle and musculocutaneous flaps. Mosby, St. Louis
www.microsurgeon.org. Anterolateral thigh flap anatomy and flap dissection
Urken ML, Cheney ML, Sullivan MJ, Biller HJ (1995) Atlas of regional and free flaps for head and neck reconstruction. Raven, New York

^{18}F-FDG PET

▸ Positron Emission Tomography (PET) and Head and Neck Cancer

FDG PET

▸ Positron Emission Tomography (PET) and Head and Neck Cancer

Feeding Difficulties

▸ Feeding Disorders

Feeding Disorders

Anjali Malkani[1] and Nidhi Rawal[2]
[1]Department of Pediatric Gastroenterology and Nutrition, University of Maryland, School of Medicine, Baltimore, MD, USA
[2]Department of Pediatric Gastroenterology and Nutrition, University of Maryland, Baltimore, MD, USA

Synonyms

Childhood eating disorder; Feeding difficulties; Feeding problems; Food intolerance; Food selectivity; Picky eater

Definition

The term "feeding disorder" refers to a condition when a child is unable or refuses to eat, or has difficulty eating. Feeding problems that persist not only undermine the child's growth and development, but can affect the whole family. This causes stress and a disturbed interaction between caregiver and child. Early identification and appropriate management is essential to avoid these long-term problems.

Epidemiology

The prevalence of feeding disorders in normally developing children is estimated to be between 25% and

45%, with figures soaring to as high as 80% in children with developmental disabilities (Lefton-Greif and Arvedson 2007; Manikam and Perman 2000). However, these estimates represent the tip of the iceberg, as there are not many studies reporting the epidemiological figures for feeding disorders and nor is there a registry or systematic reporting system.

Development of Feeding Skills

Feeding is a complex developmental process and the child eventually acquires self-feeding with socially acceptable skills by the age of 3 years. Evolution of feeding is dependent on the acquisition of oral sensorimotor skills, posture and tone, and psychosocial differentiation as the child matures.

Infant feeding is characterized by suckling in the first 6 months and sucking in the latter 6 months of infancy. Suckling is characterized by liquid drawn into the mouth by rhythmic extension and retraction of the tongue (horizontal movement), the backward phase being more pronounced, combined with opening and closing of the jaw. Tongue protrusion does not extend beyond the border of the lips, and the lips are loosely approximated. In the sucking pattern, there is vertical movement of the tongue due to strong activity of its muscles, which results in vertical excursion of the jaw. The lips are sealed firmly and there is negative pressure in the mouth. The developmental sequence from suckling to sucking is one of the steps in oral preparation for weaning to soft foods and spoon-feeding. Transitional feeding period begins at 4–6 months of age when semisoft textures can be handled. This is accomplished by an increase in the oral cavity due to growth of the mandible and resorption of the sucking pads to accommodate the food, along with lateral movement of the tongue to move the food between the tongue and the buccal wall. Chewing at this stage is by vertical motion of the jaw referred to as "munching." Though teeth may erupt at this time, they are not essential for chewing. Food is effectively chewed even with no teeth, on the "molar tables." As development progresses, the vertical movement of the jaw alternates with lateral movement and finally a mature mastication process evolves: chewing with molars and rotatory motion of the jaw. Concurrent with the evolution of feeding patterns, the child also develops speech to verbalize hunger and food preferences, while posture develops with the ability to control the head, neck, and trunk. As the child acquires new motor skills, feeding skills evolve as well. Self-feeding begins at around 9 months of age when the pincer grasp develops (apposition of thumb and forefinger). This is also a time when the mealtime experience broadens from a one-on-one relationship with the primary feeder to participation in the family meal.

Etiology

Feeding disorder results from interplay of organic and psychosocial factors. Though most feeding disorders can have an organic cause, there is often a concurrent behavioral issue. For successful feeding, there must be an adequate and appropriate nutrition source available. The child must be able to swallow safely with no untoward symptoms after swallowing and the environment (including the cues from the caregiver) must be conducive for feeding.

Both early and late weaning may be associated with feeding problems. It is felt that there is a "critical" period when children should be challenged with solid foods (6–7 months of age) in order to develop appropriate feeding skills. If children miss this solid-food feeding-window, they may resist the challenges imposed by foods requiring chewing and continue to prefer smooth textured foods.

Similarly, if higher textured foods are offered too early when the child has not achieved developmentally appropriate oro-motor skills, the caregiver may misinterpret the refusal or "spitting" out of the food as rejection of the food. This perceived rejection might result in anger by the caregiver or pressure on the child to eat. Together, this may result in maladaptive behavior on both the child and caregivers' part.

Classification

Feeding disorders can be broadly classified into three categories, based on the key etiology:
1. Behavioral
2. Oral sensorimotor dysfunction
3. Inability to accept food due to medical conditions and comorbidities

These discrete categories operate at an interface of the physical and emotional developmental age of the child, as well as on social learning and behavioral adaptation. More often, there is a "mixed" etiology

Feeding Disorders, Table 1 Most common behaviors associated with feeding disorders

Temper tantrums (screaming, running around, hitting food with hands)
Regression behaviors (going back to easier textures like puree and liquid, preferring bottles over cups)
Food selectivity (texture, color, temperature, consistency)
Engaging in playful activities while caregiver is trying to feed
Refusing to swallow a bite
Self-induced emesis
Negative behavior during eating
Exceedingly slow eating
Angry outbursts while eating

for childhood feeding disorders, but the maladaptive behavior resulting from this is uniform.

Behavioral

Food refusal can be complete or partial. Complete food refusal occurs when it is to all foods, irrespective of their physical and chemical properties. Partial food refusal (aka food selectivity) occurs when it applies to specific texture, volume, temperature, type, color, appearance, smell, or brand. Children may refuse food after a negative experience such as pain or discomfort. Such presentations are usually behavior related, but it is also important to rule out any medical condition that could be contributing to the feeding problem. If found and treated, there is a high probability of reverting the child's feeding pattern back to normal and ensuring adequate nutritional status. Some parents would describe their children as "picky" eaters, who only eat a limited number of foods. The child might also indulge in difficult behaviors during mealtimes in order to avoid eating food, such as temper tantrums, spitting out the food, and refusal to open the mouth to take a bite. Often parents attempt to correct this behavior by negative reinforcement, but it appears as positive reinforcement to the child as he is able to hold the parents' attention. This results in persistence of inappropriate mealtime behavior. In such instances, behavioral intervention plays an extremely significant role. Table 1 lists some of the typical behaviors associated with a feeding disorder.

Oral Sensorimotor Dysfunction

Oral sensorimotor dysfunction occurs in normally developing young children as well as children with developmental disabilities and medical conditions. Children often are either hypersensitive to texture/ taste/smell of the food or are unable to initiate or complete different phases of swallowing. Some infants/children might also have impaired suck and swallow reflex, secondary to a previous insult to the nervous system or anatomical malformations. Swallow function may be affected in smaller premature infants with anoxic brain injury, as well as children with acquired brain injury – traumatic, post-infectious, or metabolic. Conditioned dysphagia occurs in children who have had multiple procedures around their mouth (NG tube, suctioning, tracheostomy) who subsequently develop food hypersensitivity. A typical presentation of oral motor dysphagia includes drooling, inability to form a bolus of food during the oral phase of swallowing, packing food inside the cheeks for prolonged periods, or spitting out the bolus of food. Dysfunctional swallow caused by entry of food into the respiratory system manifests as a coughing spell immediately after swallowing food. Children with oromotor problems might also exhibit language delays due to incoordinated oral motor infrastructure. Hence, language delay coupled with feeding problems should prompt a medical as well as an oral motor evaluation. Exhaustive oral sensorimotor evaluation and intensive oral motor therapy is the key to success in these children. Studies have shown that developmentally disabled children with oral motor dysfunction have a more severe course of feeding disorder than those without it (Wilson and Hustad 2009). Language delays have also shown to improve with intensive and consistent therapy.

Inability to Eat Due to Medical Conditions and Comorbidities

Medical disorders can be the initial trigger or a coexisting condition contributing to the feeding problem (Levy et al. 2009) (Table 2). Since such medical disorders can be extremely subtle, every child with a feeding disorder should be medically evaluated to assess if the symptoms have an organic cause to them or are behavioral and/or are environmental in origin. Presence of certain conditions predisposes children to a relatively more complicated course of feeding disorder. Examples of these conditions include children with cerebral palsy (Wilson and Hustad 2009), hemiplegia/diplegia/quadriplegia, autism spectrum disorders (Provost et al. 2010), seizure disorder, special needs children (Gal et al. 2011), extreme prematurity (Samara et al. 2010), ventriculo-peritoneal shunts,

Feeding Disorders, Table 2 Most common medical conditions associated with feeding disorders

Gastrointestinal	Esophagitis
	Gastritis
	Duodenitis
	Inflammatory bowel disease (Crohn's, ulcerative colitis)
	Celiac disease
	Malabsorption syndromes
	Bowel resection
	Short gut syndrome
	Constipation
	Hirschsprung's disease
	Dumping syndrome
	Chronic abdominal pain syndrome
	Chronic pancreatitis
	Chronic hepatitis
	Motility disorders: GERD, antroduodenal dysmotility, colonic hypomotility
	Assisted tube feedings: gastrostomy, gastro-jejunostomy, jejunostomy, naso-gastric
	Stomas: post-ileostomy, cecostomy, colostomy
Neurodevelopmental	Cerebral palsy
	Delayed milestones
	Myopathy syndromes (congenital muscular dystrophy, Duchenne muscular dystrophy)
	Hypoxic-ischemic encephalopathy
	Congenital malformations (Arnold-Chiari)
	Syndromes(Riley-Day, Noonan, Russell-Silver, Pierre Robin sequence, Klippel-Feil, Beckwith-Wiedemann, Trisomy 18, Kabuki, Velocardiofacial, Prader-Willi, Oculo-mandibulo-facial, Smith-Lemli-Opitz, de Lange)
	Post-traumatic brain injury (traumatic encephalopathy, brain stem injuries)
	Polyneuropathies (myasthenia gravis)
	Rett syndrome
Pulmonary	Cystic fibrosis
	Bronchopulmonary dysplasia
Oro-laryngeal	Language disorders
	Acute infectious processes (Otitis media, sinusitis)
	Structural anomalies of the upper respiratory tract (micrognathia, tongue tie, midfacial hypoplasia)
	Vocal cord dysfunction

(continued)

Feeding Disorders, Table 2 (continued)

Cardiovascular	Chronic and complex congenital heart disease
Medications (with mechanism of action)	Anti-epileptic drugs (arousal abnormalities)
	Neuroleptics (arousal abnormalities)
	Benzodiazepines (suppression of brain stem regulation of swallowing)
	Antihistamines (arousal abnormalities)
	Anticholinergics (diminished salivation)
Metabolic	Lysosomal storage diseases
	Peroxisomal disorders
	Purine and pyrimidine disorders
Psychological	Disordered child-caregiver interaction
	Acute or chronic stressors
	Rumination, pica, psychogenic vomiting, purging, depression

delayed milestones, congenital malformations, metabolic disorders, and genetic syndromes. Recent illness, especially if it ran a complicated course requiring hospitalization for a prolonged period, has also found to be an important trigger or precipitating factor for some feeding difficulties.

Symptoms that raise concern for an underlying organic cause for feeding disorder include vomiting, abdominal pain, nausea (esophagitis, gastritis, duodenitis); and feeling of food getting stuck in the throat (eosinophilic esophagitis, reflux or infectious esophagitis, esophageal motility disorders). Failure to thrive is another red flag that needs to be investigated. Recurrent GI symptoms from celiac disease, hirschsprung's disease, dysmotility or POTS can also disrupt a normal eating cycle.

Evaluation of a Child with Feeding Disorder

Clinical Assessment

A highly comprehensive and multidisciplinary assessment is critical to understand the process of any ongoing feeding problem. It involves inquiring about symptoms pertaining to a medical condition, behavioral difficulties, lack of oropharyngeal coordination, parent–child interaction, and assessment of the child's nutritional status. Identification of predisposing, precipitating, and perpetuating factors should be meticulously sought out. Parental responses and coping mechanisms are often intertwined with the existing feeding problem

There are five components to a comprehensive feeding assessment of a child with feeding disorders:

- Medical evaluation
- Nutritional status evaluation
- Behavioral evaluation
- Oral motor and speech evaluation
- Psychosocial

Medical Evaluation

Presence of medical conditions can make the treatment of feeding disorder more challenging as they interact with both behavioral and social factors (Berlin et al. 2011; Zangen et al. 2003). A thorough history and a comprehensive systemic exam form the cornerstone for diagnosis. A detailed neurodevelopmental exam is also important to rule out any organic cause for delayed milestones. GI motility disorders have been found to contribute significantly to feeding difficulties, and a motility expert (Zangen et al. 2003) should evaluate such children. Any red flags such as intellectual disability, recent illness/events, recent surgeries, tone abnormalities, worsening headache, seizures, cardiac rhythm abnormalities, sensory losses, significant weight loss, recurrent abdominal pain, vomiting, blood in stools, melena, bilious emesis, jaundice, steatorrhea, constipation, and recurrent diarrhea should be further investigated. A simultaneous assessment of the child's nutritional status is also very important. It is not uncommon for new symptoms of motility disorder, food allergies, and lactose intolerance to emerge after the child has been taught to consume larger volumes, especially if the child's intake was never substantial to begin with. Children with special needs like cerebral palsy, seizure disorder with delayed milestones, congenital syndromes, and those with chronic diseases like short gut syndrome or cystic fibrosis might need the combined effort of other specialties to work toward improving the oral intake (Table 6).

Nutritional Evaluation

Since feeding disorders can affect the growth and nutritional status, a thorough evaluation of the child's growth parameters and nutritional intake is important. Not only is it important to plot the child's current growth parameters on the CDC growth charts, the growth trend also needs to be evaluated. Detailed history of solid and liquid intake by a dietitian will uncover any possible deficiencies in macro- and micronutrients. Children with extreme food selectivity are more likely to have nutritional deficiencies (Kirby and Danner 2009) like iron deficiency anemia, Vitamin B-12 deficiency anemia, hypocalcemia, and vitamin D deficiency. When found, appropriate treatment should be ensued per the most current guidelines. Before starting feeding therapy, child's food preferences should be noted so appropriate recommendations can be made during therapy.

Behavioral Evaluation

Assessment of behaviors during and outside of meals is an important part of the comprehensive clinical assessment (Kedesky and Budd 1998). Significant deviation from normal feeding behavior affects the caregiver's attitude, just as the caregiver's feeding techniques affect child's feeding pattern. Hence, observation of feeding behaviors and the techniques employed to optimize the feeding time are of tremendous value, as they provide the best insight into the most complicated aspect of this disorder. This can be done by direct observation or viewing previously recorded video tapes. Even though the significance of "in-clinic" observation cannot be undermined, it is often not representative of the "real" events. When parents or caregivers videotape a meal session at home, the child should be unaware of the recording. Feeding disorders in typically developing and healthy children usually manifest as behavioral difficulties. It is also important to assess whether the feeding behaviors are appropriate for the child's age and neurodevelopmental status. Both meal time and out of meals behaviors should be evaluated and compared through a series of questions that can be completed by the child's caregiver. Table 3 lists some of the questions that can be answered by the child's caregivers.

Behavioral assessment of children with special needs has some unique challenges. These children are often predisposed to chronic medical conditions, which can be a significant contributor to the ongoing feeding problem. Their neurodevelopment status, ambulatory status, ability to express their needs and hunger, degree of independence, motor and sensory impairments (whole body as well as oral motor strength), coordinating capability, and social support can affect their feeding. The multivariable nature makes taking care of these children more challenging.

Feeding Disorders, Table 3 Behavioral assessment questionnaire

What are the specific problem behaviors associated with child's feeding?
Which behavior do you think is contributing the most to the feeding problem?
How long have these behaviors been a part of the child's meal routine?
What techniques, if any, have caregivers tried out to resolve these behaviors?
Have any of the past treatment or techniques been helpful?
Is there any particular time of the meal when the behaviors are at their worst, like beginning, mid-meal, or at the end of the meal?
Does any particular food item or texture make them worse?
Are the behaviors in question also depicted outside of home setting, like school, grandparents' house, day care, and restaurants?
What effect does distraction, with either a toy or a TV/video, have on the behaviors?
Does the child display such behaviors toward all the caregivers? Are such behaviors directed toward any specific individual?
Describe a particular meal time at home
If the child expresses any regressive behaviors with meals, are they also seen in-between meal sessions?
What has been the course (getting better or worse) since the beginning of the behaviors?
How does the child interact with other children in the family?
Do you think that eating food with the other children of the family improves or worsens the behaviors?
Was there ever a time that the child was eating normally with other developing children of his age?

However, an interdisciplinary team approach has shown to benefit their feeding and the subsequent quality of life (Laud et al. 2009).

Oral Motor and Speech Evaluation

All children with feeding difficulties should be assessed for oral motor weakness, hypersensitivities, oral motor coordination, and language delays (Kedesky and Budd 1998). Children with such deficits are unable to communicate effectively with their parents or caregivers, which contributes to their feeding difficulties (Fabrizi et al. 2010). Occupational therapists and speech and language therapists assess the overall neurodevelopmental status of the child as well as the strength of muscles involved in the process of mastication. Cranial nerve exam will reveal any abnormalities in the cranial nerves 9, 10, 11, 12 and hence any disordered swallowing. Feeding trials are done to evaluate body positioning, oral motor coordination,

Feeding Disorders, Table 4 Airway assessment

Audible pharyngeal secretions
Stridor
Chest retractions
Anatomic obstruction to airflow
Aspiration while feeding (History: bronchospasm, recurrent pneumonia, chronic lung disease; Exam: tachypnea, diminished breath sounds, inspiratory crepitations)

and self-feeding skills. Since swallowing involves both deglutition and respiration taking place at the same time, upper airway assessment at rest and during feeds becomes important, especially in patients with clinically significant dysphagia. Children with neurodevelopmental abnormalities are more likely to have dysphagia and its complications. Any suspicion of dysfunctional swallow is confirmed by a Modified Barium Swallow study. The child consumes a preferred food item, of the texture that he is known to tolerate (without developing any symptoms suggestive of aspiration). Swallowing is then observed under real-time fluoroscopy, in the presence of an occupational or speech/language therapist, to evaluate if there is penetration or aspiration into the airway.

Table 4 enlists some of the important markers of a compromised airway and/or disordered swallowing.

Psychosocial Evaluation

Psychosocial evaluation involves a pediatric psychologist with expertise in childhood feeding disorders. The psychologist assesses the quality of parent–child interaction during and out of mealtimes and any adjustment problems or psychopathology in the participants in the feeding relationship and evaluates the child for any cognitive or developmental problems. Presence of multiple stressors in the family, even if not directly involving the child, can have significant impact on child's eating patterns (Kedesky and Budd 1998).

Investigations

Once clinically significant medical symptoms are identified in a child with a feeding disorder, they must be completely investigated. Some of the most commonly ordered tests and lab evaluations, with their medical conditions, are listed in Table 5. This is a comprehensive list, but is not uncommon for physicians to order

Feeding Disorders, Table 5 Common symptoms and appropriate tests

Symptom/sign	Differential diagnoses	Possible tests/procedures
Nausea, emesis, abdominal pain	Gastritis, duodenitis, esophagitis, GERD, peptic ulcer disease	Esophagogastroduodenoscopy
		Multiple intraluminal impredance
		pH monitoring
		Upper GI motility studies
Choking on feeds, drooling, recurrent Pneumonias, prolonged feeding time	Dysfunctional swallow	Modified Barium Swallow study (MBS)
Failure to thrive	Malabsorption syndromes	Nutritional assessment with hemoglobin
		Serum calcium
		Vitamin D levels
		Bone density assessment
		Stool tests for malabsorption (fat, protein)
Chronic abdominal pain, dizziness, dyspepsia, weight loss, alternating constipation and diarrhea, s/p resection, positive family history	POTS[a]	CT scan
	Malabsorption	Small bowel biopsy and brushing
	Short gut syndrome	
	Small bowel resection	EGD
	Celiac disease	Antroduodenal manometry study
	Small bowel motility disorder	Celiac Panel
	Irritable Bowel syndrome	
Chronic constipation, abdominal pain, bleeding per rectum, anal fissures, fecal soiling, positive family history for inflammatory bowel disease	Inflammatory bowel disease	CT scan
	Hirschsprung's disease	MRI
	Colonic motility disorders	Genetic and inflammatory markers for IBD
		Colonoscopy with biopsies
		Rectal suction biopsy
		Colonic motility studies
		Anorectal motility studies
Delayed milestones, muscle weakness, fidgety, short attention span in more than one setting	Autism	Detailed neurodevelopmental assessment with ADHD questionnaires
	Cerebral Palsy	
	ADHD	
Staring spells, involuntary movements	Seizure disorder	EEG
	Movement disorder	CT scan
		MRI
		Movement studies

[a]*POTS* postural orthostatic tachycardia syndrome

additional rare and more sophisticated tests and procedures, in order to ensure appropriate diagnosis and management.

Treatment

Due to its team approach and prolonged, persistent intensive management the treatment of feeding disorders is at times referred to as Feeding therapy.

Effective management of feeding disorders in children requires a multidisciplinary team approach. This may be initiated once the child is considered medically stable to undergo therapy after a detailed medical assessment. Such an interdisciplinary team can include a gastroenterologist, nutritionist, otolaryngologist, behavioral psychologist, occupational therapist, and a social worker, with each member having defined roles and responsibilities. This is illustrated in Table 6.

Feeding Disorders, Table 6 Role of feeding team members

Team member	Role
Physician	Developmental assessment
	Management of active medical conditions
	Recommend appropriate diagnostic tests
	Assessment of oral feeding safety with different textures
Occupational therapist/ speech therapist	Assess and treat oromotor, fine motor, and sensory skills
	Increase competencies through skill acquisition
	Assess and modify posture and positioning
	Recommend appropriate utensil usage
Nutritionist	Evaluate nutritional status
	Assessment of current diet
	Monitor daily caloric and fluid intake
	Assist in preparation of meals
	Caregiver education
Behavioral therapist	Assess and treat mental health
	Eliminate interfering behavior and develop appropriate behaviors
	Behavioral and skills training to increase daily functional capacity
	Decrease caregiver stress and increase caregiver functioning
	Conduct parent training
Social worker	Evaluate family functioning and support system
	Evaluate caregiver stress and coping mechanisms
	Provide resources to improve coping skills
	Mediate between team and caregiver
	Secure community services

It is important to remember that children with inadequate oral intake, malnutrition, and failure to thrive might need supplemental enteral feeding via a nasogastric or gastrostomy tube prior to the initiation of therapy.

All meals (3 meals with 1–2 snacks per day) during therapy are conducted in a room, under direct observation of behavioral therapists through one-way mirror. The primary caregiver is asked to conduct the meals for the first 1–2 days, so a baseline is established and initial goals are set. The behavioral therapists make appropriate behavioral recommendations after carefully observing child's behavior and temperament. Such modifications are introduced one at a time and the progress of the child noted with the help of highly sophisticated software, which provides detailed statistical analysis. Numerous studies have shown successful results of applied behavior analysis in children with food selectivity, food refusal, and disruptive meal behaviors (Levine et al. 2011; Woods et al. 2010).

Pediatric nutritionists assess daily calorie and fluid intake; make recommendations about foods with adequate nutritional value, tube feeding management, and food preparation and storage. They also educate the caregiver about appropriate food choices.

Outside of meal times, the child undergoes intensive occupational and speech/language therapy daily, focusing on the areas of weakness. A detailed record is kept for the child's progress over the next 4–8 weeks and modifications made on an as needed basis. The initial goals are revisited depending on the child's progress. Over the course of intensive therapy, individualized attention is given to factors which are found to be the most important barriers to normal feeding.

For children who are unable to handle higher texture foods, occupational and speech therapists slowly introduce small quantities of higher texture foods. Direct and indirect approaches may be used to improve oral sensorimotor function. Direct approaches include "oral exercises" to stimulate cheeks and lips for improved function and encourage oral exploration. This may be aversive for the child and stimulate oral secretions. Indirect approaches include altering the environment so as to reduce distractions, ensuring appropriate positioning and seating so there is better support for feeding, and improving communication signals by using visual or tactile cues. Alterations in the physical properties of the food (texture, taste and temperature), size of bolus and changing the interval for food presentation are other approaches used to improve sensorimotor function.

Once the child accepts a new texture, it is then introduced into the meal sessions, where behavioral therapists work with the behaviors associated with the higher texture food. Reward techniques, distraction, and positive and negative reinforcement techniques are some of the methods utilized by the behavioral therapists to increase desired behaviors or decrease undesired behaviors. Recommendations are made keeping in mind what would be practically feasible at home, to allow for as smooth a transition as possible.

The physician/gastroenterologist also evaluates the child daily and intervenes for any alarming or new signs and symptoms.

The primary caregiver is present during all the therapy sessions, unless certain behaviors are worse in their presence. The team evaluates any problematic interaction between the child and the caregiver. At the same time, out of meal behaviors that interfere with a positive parent–child interaction or contribute to the inside-meal negative behaviors need to be addressed. The caregiver initially observes the therapy, is gradually "faded" into the mealtime, and finally completes the feeding session independently.

Children with significant deviations from normal feeding behavior need Intensive therapy, which could be administered in an inpatient setting or in an outpatient-feeding program. This depends on the resources available. Usually medically fragile children and children with extreme behaviors are admitted to an inpatient unit for feeding therapy. The duration of Intensive therapy is from 4 weeks to 12 weeks. Intensive outpatient therapy requires the child and caregiver to be at the Feeding Clinic 6–8 h daily for 6–12 weeks.

All the team members meet 1–2 times/week to discuss progress and make any necessary changes. The primary caregiver is updated about their child's progress. The decision to terminate the intensive-therapy is based on the success of the child. If the child has achieved the pre-set realistic goals and is able to maintain a healthy oral intake, the intensive therapy is terminated and the child is transitioned to home. It is critical to closely follow up on the child after being discharged, as it is not uncommon to see reversal of behaviors once the child goes back home. Occasionally key members of the team make special home visits to "fine-tune" the meal sessions and make new recommendations, if needed. The team might also decide to have the child and the family come to the clinic for a more prolonged meal session, to re-evaluate the mealtime behaviors.

In summary, therapeutic techniques and modifications are available to treat pediatric feeding disorders effectively. However, the evaluation and management is a complex process and it can be challenging to address social, medical, psychological, and environmental factors. All available resources should be mobilized to treat the multifactorial and complex nature of pediatric feeding disorders. A cohesive team and a multidisciplinary approach is the key to successful outcomes (Miller 2009).

References

Monographs

Arvedson JC, Brodsky L (2002) Pediatric swallowing and feeding: assessment and management, 2nd edn. Singular Publishing Group, Albany

Kedesky JH, Budd K (1998) Childhood feeding disorders: behavioral assessment and intervention. Paul H. Brookes Publishing, Baltimore

Journal Articles

Berlin KS, Lobato DJ, Pinkos B, Cerezo CS, LeLeiko NS (2011) Patterns of medical and developmental comorbidities among children presenting with feeding problems: a latent class analysis. J Dev Behav Pediatr 32(1):41–47

Fabrizi A, Costa A, Lucarelli L, Patruno E (2010) Comorbidity in specific language disorders and early feeding disorders: mother-child interactive patterns. Eat Weight Disord 15(3):e152–e160

Gal E, Hardal-Nasser R, Engel-Yeger B (2011) The relationship between the severity of eating problems and intellectual developmental deficit level. Res Dev Disabil 32(5):1464–1469

Kirby M, Danner E (2009) Nutritional deficiencies in children on restricted diets. Pediatr Clin North Am 56(5):1085–1103

Laud RB, Girolami PA, Boscoe JH, Gulotta CS (2009) Treatment outcomes for severe feeding problems in children with autism spectrum disorder. Behav Modif 33(5):520–536

Lefton-Greif MA, Arvedson JC (2007) Pediatric feeding and swallowing disorders: state of health, population trends, and application of the international classification of functioning, disability, and health. Semin Speech Lang 28:161–165

Levine A, Bachar L, Tsangen Z et al (2011) Screening criteria for diagnosis of infantile feeding disorders as a cause of poor feeding or food refusal. J Pediatr Gastroenterol Nutr 52(5):563–568

Levy Y, Levy A, Zangen T et al (2009) Diagnostic clues for identification of nonorganic vs organic causes of food refusal and poor feeding. J Pediatr Gastroenterol Nutr 48(3):355–362

Luijk MP, Saridjan N, Tharner A et al (2010) Attachment, depression, and cortisol: deviant patterns in insecure-resistant and disorganized infants. Dev Psychobiol 52(5):441–452

Manikam R, Perman J (2000) Pediatric feeding disorders. J Clin Gastroenterol 30:34–46

Miller CK (2009) Updates on pediatric feeding and swallowing problems. Curr Opin Otolaryngol Head Neck Surg 17(3):194–199

Provost B, Crowe TK, Osbourn PL, McClain C, Skipper BJ (2010) Mealtime behaviors of preschool children: comparison of children with autism spectrum disorder and children with typical development. Phys Occup Ther Pediatr 30(3):220–233

Samara M, Johnson S, Lamberts K, Marlow N, Wolke D (2010) Eating problems at age 6 years in a whole population sample of extremely preterm children. Dev Med Child Neurol 52(2): e16–e22

Wilson EM, Hustad KC (2009) Early feeding abilities in children with cerebral palsy: a parental report study. J Med Speech Lang Pathol nihpa57357

Woods JN, Borrero JC, Laud RB, Borrero CS (2010) Descriptive analyses of pediatric food refusal: the structure of parental attention. Behav Modif 34(1):35–56

Zangen T, Ciarla C, Zangen S et al (2003) Gastrointestinal motility and sensory abnormalities may contribute to food refusal in medically fragile toddlers. J Pediatr Gastroenterol Nutr 37(3):287–293

Feeding Problems

▶ Feeding Disorders

Festoons

Michael M. Kim
Division of Facial Plastic & Reconstructive Surgery, Department of Otolaryngology-Head and Neck Surgery, Oregon Health & Science University, Portland, OR, USA

Definition

Redundant folds of lax skin and orbicularis oculi of the lower eyelid and cheek. An age-associated anatomic deformity whose removal can be performed either by direct excision or extended lower blepharoplasty techniques.

Fetal Development

▶ Balance (Anatomy: Embryology)

Fever

▶ Oral Mucosal Lesions

Fibrous Osteoma

▶ Congenital Craniofacial Malformations and Their Surgical Treatment

Fibula Free Flap

Daniel S. Schneider[1] and Mark K. Wax[2]
[1]Microvascular/Facial Plastic Surgery, Oregon Health & Science University, Portland, USA
[2]Department Otolaryngology-Head and Neck Surgery, Oregon Health and Science University, Portland, OR, USA

Introduction

The mandible may need to be resected or removed for many reasons. Reconstruction of these mandibular defects whether they result from benign and malignant oncologic surgery, osteoradionecrosis, or severe ▶ trauma continues to challenge head and neck reconstructive surgeons. The issues surrounding postoperative recovery can be complex and result in significant healing problems. These defects leave the patient with a severe degree of functional and cosmetic disability. Quality of life can be negatively impacted with devastating results. In the past, such composite defects have been reconstructed with nonvascularized bone grafts or soft tissue reconstructions with a bridging reconstructive plate. Historically, soft tissue flaps combined with bridging reconstructive plates had variable success and high rates of plate extrusion, especially for anterior mandibular defects (Head et al. 2003; Wei et al. 2003). The ability to reconstruct composite soft tissue defects with similar composite vascularized soft tissue has revolutionized the postoperative rehabilitation of these patients. Depending on the location and extent of the mandibular defect and the underlying indication for reconstruction, ▶ free tissue transfer with soft tissue alone or combined with bone is now more commonly chosen for mandibular reconstruction.

Recent literature examining head and neck reconstruction confirms that the optimal reconstructive method to improve the function and quality of life of these patients has shifted to free tissue transfer (Smith et al. 2007; Bozec et al. 2008).

Mandibular Reconstruction

The goals of ▶ mandibular reconstruction are similar to the goals of reconstructive surgery in the head and neck: mainly to restore form and function. This includes (1) restoration of mandibular continuity with appropriate projection and width of the lower 1/3 of the face and (2) functional considerations including understandable speech, oral competence, return of sensation, and potential dental restoration while enabling the patient to have adequate mastication and deglutition to allow for oral nutrition. At the present time, no single free flap allows for a comprehensive reconstruction for a segmental mandibular defect that restores complete form and function. The three most common bone flaps that are utilized are the ▶ fibula, the radial forearm, and the ▶ scapula. Other flaps including vascularized serratus with rib have been described. Soft tissue characteristics and amount of bone to be replaced all play into determining which bone flap to use in the particular patient (Table 1).

The focus of this entry is on the vascularized fibular flaps. It is the most common and allows for adequate bone stock to take dental implants. It also comes with an acceptable soft tissue component that allows reconstruction of the soft tissue defect. Lateral segmental defects less than 5 cm and benign mandibular lesions that do not require postoperative radiotherapy and traumatic defects less than 5 cm are often treated with nonvascularized bone grafts. The remainder of this entry will review the use of the vascularized fibula osteoseptocutaneous flap as it remains the most common flap for reconstruction of composite mandibular defects.

Fibula Free Flap

The fibula free flap was first described by Taylor in 1975 with a subsequent series for mandibular reconstruction published in 1989 by Hidalgo (Hidalgo 1989). It remains the most frequently used osseous flap for mandibular reconstruction with multiple advantages compared to other osseous flaps such as the radial forearm or the scapula. Not only does it have

Fibula Free Flap, Table 1 The characteristics of the various bony flaps used for mandibular reconstruction are defined

Flap	Bony characteristics	Soft tissue characteristics	Ability to place dental implants
Fibula	>20 cm	Large	Excellent
	Thick	Tethered by septum	
	Many osteotomies	Thick	
Radial	10 cm	Large	Not possible
	Thin	Very malleable	
	Single osteotomy	Thin	
Scapula	10 cm	Large	Excellent
	Thick	Malleable	
	Single osteotomy	Thick	

better bone for rehabilitation but the overall donor site morbidity is felt to be less than other bony flaps. Other characteristics of this flap are the reliable and consistent vascular anatomy. Finally, the flap allows for a two-team approach with the ablative and reconstruction teams being able to work simultaneously.

The fibular bone has dense cancellous bone quality and can provide up to 25 cm of bone stock thereby providing for multiple osteotomies and total mandibular reconstruction. The dense bone allows for placement of osseointegrated implants for dental rehabilitation with the caveat that these implants tend to be quite costly and are seldom covered by insurance. When eligible, implants can be placed at the time of initial surgery or after appropriate healing time following radiation. Patients with large mucosal or external skin defects in combination to the bone may require two flaps or a fibula flap with two skin paddles for proper reconstruction (Kuo et al. 2010) (Fig. 1).

Anatomy

The popliteal artery bifurcates into the anterior tibial artery and the tibial/peroneal trunk. The tibial/peroneal trunk subsequently divides into the posterior tibial artery and the peroneal artery. The latter runs medially along the entire fibula remaining stable in caliber. The anterior tibial vessels lie in the anterior compartment and course down the leg medial to the tibia on the interosseous membrane. Distally, it is palpated on the dorsum of the foot between the 1st and 2nd toes as the dorsalis pedis.

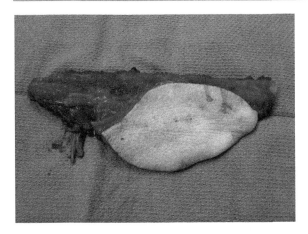

Fibula Free Flap, Fig. 1 The fibula has been harvested. Note the thick bone and the skin that is tethered to the bone by the septum, through which the vascular supply runs

The posterior tibial vessels lie in the posterior compartment deep in the leg and course down the leg between the posterior tibialis and soleus muscles. Distally, it is palpated posterior to the medial malleolus.

After bifurcating from the posterior tibial artery/vein, the peroneal vessels lie in close proximity to the fibula, coursing the entire distance of the bone along its medial aspect. The artery is accompanied by paired venae comitantes. Pedicle diameter generally allows for straightforward anastomosis. The paired venae comitantes are often 4.0 mm or larger. Rarely do the two veins come together into a single vessel. Thus, one should prepare two large veins in the neck. The peroneal artery is consistently 2.5–3.5 mm in diameter.

The peroneal artery provides the blood supply to the fibula via an endosteal and periosteal supply with the latter being crucial for the creation of wedge osteotomies that allow the bone to be contoured for mandibular reconstruction. The fibular bone may be harvested with a portion of proximal or distal skin with the underlying cuff of flexor hallucis longus and soleus muscles along the medial aspect of the leg.

The skin paddle is supplied by perforators from the peroneal vessels that enter the skin via the posterior crural septum as septocutaneous perforators or as musculocutaneous perforators that pierce the flexor hallucis longus and soleus muscles. The septum is identified just lateral to the flexor hallucis longus muscle on the posterior aspect of the fibula. One to three perforators are identified for skin harvest. They

can be identified preoperatively with formal angiogram or can usually be identified just prior to incision with a handheld Doppler.

Following anterior skin incision, the septocutaneous perforators usually are directly visualized lateral to the fibula in the fasciocutaneous posterior crural septum, but may supply the skin as musculocutaneous perforators that enter the septum more laterally to supply the skin, sometimes referred to as septomuscular perforators (Schusterman et al. 1992). Others report that these perforators are musculocutaneous in nature and may not enter the septum and can only be preserved by harvesting a cuff of flexor hallucis longus and soleus muscles. The soft tissue can be used for intraoral and/or external skin resurfacing which affects the selection of ipsilateral vs. contralateral fibula selection.

Preoperative Evaluation

Because of the high prevalence of peripheral vascular disease in head and neck cancer patients, preoperative examination of the legs for signs of vascular insufficiency is required. Besides palpating the patient's dorsalis pedis and tibialis posterior pulses, one can obtain bilateral arterial duplex blood flow studies using ultrasonography to assess collateral perfusion of the foot. Other methods include magnetic resonance angiography or CT angiogram to assess the adequacy of collateral circulation to the foot.

While variations of the lower leg anatomy are uncommon, they are important to identify if a fibular flap is planned. When a dominant peroneal artery exists, pedal circulation is more dependent on this vessel. Sacrifice of the peroneal artery in such cases renders the foot susceptible to ischemia when the fibula flap is harvested.

Contraindications

Older individuals may also have diffuse vascular disease of the fibula. The lower limb and foot may have adequate vascular supply, both input and output, on examination. However, sacrifice of the peroneal vessel with extensive dissection of the lower leg may lead to prolonged healing issues. Any sign of abnormal skin or vascular status in the lower limb should prompt a preoperative vascular analysis, or consideration of a different flap.

Abnormalities of the lower leg vascular anatomy may preclude safe harvest of the fibula; these include a dominant peroneal circulation with underdeveloped anterior tibial vessels or an enlarged peroneal artery which provides the dominant blood supply to the foot. Alternate flap selection is recommended when the peroneal artery is the dominant source of inflow, for patients with absent anterior tibial vessels, or for those with significantly impaired circulation to the leg.

Caution is advised in patients who have had extensive leg trauma or surgery. Patients with significant comorbidity, such as poorly controlled diabetes, severe venous stasis, or other circulation disorders, may not be ideal candidates for this flap.

Flap Harvest

The choice of which leg to use for reconstruction depends on the part of the bone and where the skin/mucosal defect is. In general, the ipsilateral fibula is chosen for mandibular defects that include the ascending ramus of the mandible and/or condyle (Wax et al. 2000). This allows for optimal placement of the pedicle so as to allow it to reach into the ipsilateral neck with no need to vein graft. In this setting, the skin is used for intraoral replacement. When the recipient vessels in the neck are contralateral to the mandibular defect, an ipsilateral flap should also be used. A contralateral fibula is selected for anterior and lateral mandibular defects to improve recipient vessel geometry. To orient the peroneal pedicle anteriorly, one should select an ipsilateral fibula, whereas orienting the peroneal pedicle posteriorly leads the surgeon to select a contralateral fibula (Table 2).

One must also consider the soft tissue defect with fibular selection as intraoral skin defects are more easily reconstructed with a contralateral fibula while external skin defects may be easier to reconstruct with an ipsilateral fibula. Recipient artery and vein location remains the primary determinant to ipsilateral or contralateral fibula selection. A mandibular reconstructive plate which may be prebent to a sterolithographic model or contoured to the mandible prior to resection is used for the reconstruction.

Rarely is it necessary to use a tourniquet for fibula harvest. Occasionally, one will encounter a patient that

Fibula Free Flap, Table 2 Determining which leg to harvest the fibula from depends on the side of the neck that you will use to perform the anastomosis and the location of the bony defect

Bony defect	Soft tissue defect	Side fibula is harvested from
TMJ, ascending ramus	Mucosa	Ipsilateral
TMJ, ascending ramus	Skin	Contralateral
Lateral mandible	Mucosa	Contralateral
Lateral mandible	Skin	Ipsilateral
Anterior mandible	Mucosa	Contralateral to side of neck where anastomosis is to be performed
Anterior mandible	Skin	Ipsilateral to side of neck where anastomosis is to be performed

has large venous varicosities that make dissection difficult. In these instances, a tourniquet may help. The other alternative is to use a different flap.

A Doppler may be used along the posterior-lateral aspect of the fibula at the junction of the middle and lower third of the fibula to identify cutaneous perforators. Prior to beginning the fibula harvest, the split thickness skin graft is harvested from over the expected soft tissue skin island defect, thereby eliminating a skin graft donor site that was previously harvested from the thigh (Kim et al. 2008). An anterior linear incision along the lateral aspect of the fibula including the skin/dermal paddle overlying the identified cutaneous perforators that run within the posterior crural septum is performed next. The skin paddle is harvested slightly larger than the anticipated defect.

With the anterior portion of the skin paddle outlined, you than reflect the peroneus muscles and extensor hallucis longus muscles anteriorly off the fibula being careful to remain close to the fibula to avoid inadvertent injury to the more medial anterior tibial artery which is subsequently identified and preserved. Osteotomies are made thru the fibula with a sagittal saw, while harvesting the maximal amount of fibula. Be sure to preserve 8 cm of proximal and distal fibula to avoid injuring the peroneal nerve and maintaining support of the ankle mortise, respectively. The interosseous membrane is divided which affords lateral retraction of the fibula. Incising the interosseous membrane brings one to the posterior compartment and exposes the chevron-shaped posterior tibialis muscle.

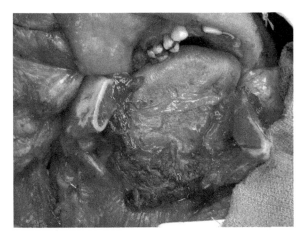

Fibula Free Flap, Fig. 2 An anterior mandible defect is present. The mandible has been resected from the angle to angle

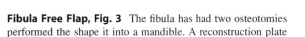

Fibula Free Flap, Fig. 3 The fibula has had two osteotomies performed the shape it into a mandible. A reconstruction plate has been used to stabilize it until it heals

Two Dingman bone clamps are placed on the osteotomized ends of the fibula for lateral retraction. The peroneal artery and vein are identified just deep to the chevron-shaped posterior tibialis muscle adjacent to the distal fibula osteotomy. Next, dissect the vascular pedicle, transecting the posterior tibialis from distal to proximal until the posterior tibial artery/vein bifurcation is encountered. Following completion of the head and neck ablation, preparation of recipient cervical vessels, and proper placement of a reconstruction plate, the vascular pedicle is ligated and the fibula is osteotomized on the back table to fit the mandibular defect (Fig. 2).

Osteotomies are performed on a back table making sure that precise fibula to mandible contact will occur to ensure postoperative healing and avoidance of bony nonunion. The fibula is inset and plated with 8-mm monocortical screws with the vascular pedicle lying lingual to the flap (Fig. 3). The soft tissue portion of the flap is used to close the oral cavity defect, and the microvascular anastomosis is completed using standard techniques. The leg is then closed, either with the previously harvested split thickness skin graft with topical Xeroform dressing, or closed primarily if no soft tissue was harvested with fibula.

Postoperative Care

Postoperatively, the flap is monitored utilizing clinical signs of viability with the aid of either an implantable arterial or venous Doppler monitor. Using an arterial or venous implantable Doppler decreases the frequency of return trips to the operating room for undetected intraoperative partial arterial and venous thromboses (Wax and Angelos 2011). By using the implantable Doppler intraoperatively, you can improve the accuracy of the arterial and venous anastomosis patency assessment. The use of the Doppler device allows one to detect problems with the anastomosis prior to the patient leaving the operating suite. It is possible to decrease the postoperative revision rate by 50% using these instruments. These reconstructions almost always involve a skin paddle that is easily accessed. The skin paddle is examined in addition to the Doppler. Any sign of vascular compromise, venous or arterial, prompts a return to the operating room for possible anastomotic revision. Many different anticoagulating pharmaceuticals have been used in an attempt to improve flap survival. There has not been much published to demonstrate there is any efficacy in using them. Giving prophylactic aspirin, heparin, or low molecular weight heparin postoperatively is not necessary unless there is recurrent arterial or venous thromboses intraoperatively that is independent of microvascular technique.

A below-the-knee walking boot or CAM boot is used postoperatively for 4–6 weeks until the donor site is completely healed. Patients are encouraged to be partial weight-bearing status on postoperative day 2 and full weight bearing with the use of a walker if necessary on postoperative day 5. The skin graft site

Fibula Free Flap,
Fig. 4 This panorex
demonstrates a well-healed
fibula prior to placements of
dental implants

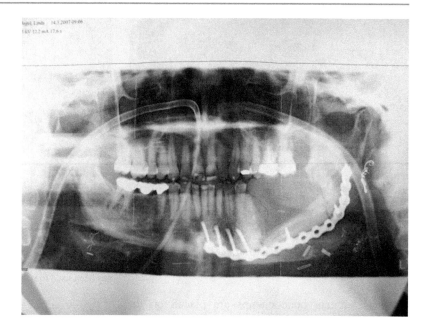

is taken down on postoperative day 5. Physical therapy is instituted and continued postoperatively to limit donor site morbidity. If no complications arise, oral diet is generally initiated 2–3 weeks postoperatively (Fig. 4).

Complications

Harvesting a fibula flap is generally well tolerated in this patient population with a low major complication rate and acceptable minor complication rate (Virgin et al. 2010). Flap loss is by far the most morbid complication that is encountered. The incidence of flap failure is not significantly higher with this flap than with other free flaps used in reconstruction of head and neck defects. The majority of complications are related to the donor site. Minor complications include complete or partial loss of skin graft and local infections. Major donor site complications include compartment syndrome which is generally avoided by using a split thickness skin graft for closure and suction drains to avoid hematoma formation. Foot ischemia rarely occurs, but mandates urgent assessment and management. Ankle instability is avoided by preserving the distal 6–8 cm of fibula for the ankle mortise. Gait changes may occur and are often related to harvesting large portions of soleus and gastrocnemius that is sometimes used for soft tissue filler in the neck to avoid additional flaps. Chronic lower extremity pain is rarely reported. Overall, harvest of the fibula is generally well tolerated. Even in patients that have both fibulas, harvested the expected lower limb function can be quite good (Ghaheri et al. 2005).

Head and neck complications are lower when only an osseous fibula flap is used. However, plate exposure or extrusion, infection, and nonunion can still occur with free tissue transfer. Patients may report postoperative pain or clicking with mastication or jaw opening which may be a sign of nonunion. Exposed or extruded hardware is generally removed after an appropriate, but unknown, period has elapsed to allow for bony union.

Future Directions

Preoperative computer design and sterolithographic modeling has been developed to allow precise placement of osteotomies and planning for bony reconstruction in select patients. This technology is helpful in both routine and difficult post-ablative reconstructions.

Preoperative planning is performed on a virtual three-dimensional CT model where the resection margins and mandibular and fibular osteotomies are chosen. This provides the ablative surgeon with cutting guides fit to the native mandible for osteotomies. A prebent reconstructive plate based on

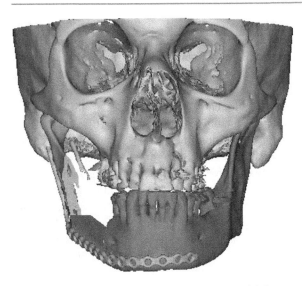

Fibula Free Flap, Fig. 5 This 3D stereolithic model demonstrates a computer-generated photo of the mandible with the tumor removed. The bony defect is demarcated and a proposed plate and fibula are demonstrated

a sterolithographic model from the virtual reconstruction is matched to a sterolithographic model based on the CT model. A planned virtual fibula is then inset which again allows planned osteotomies and provides the reconstructive surgeon with a cutting guide to place on the fibula (Fig. 5). This assists with fibular insetting and provides greater operative efficiency. Few outcomes data and cost analyses are available, but certain benefits to the surgeon and patient are readily evident and include decreased operative time, possibly more accurate occlusion, and improved facial projection. Exactly where this will fit in the reconstructive paradigm is not yet known.

Conclusions

The fibula free flap continues to be a workhorse flap for mandibular reconstruction following post-ablative resection, osteoradionecrosis, or severe facial trauma. It provides restoration of mandibular contour after appropriate osteotomies and plating are completed. The soft tissue skin island can be used for intraoral or external skin reconstruction with improvement in skin color often seen following irradiation or continued sun exposure. Patients often have an excellent functional outcome, although this is somewhat dependent on the extent of resection and whether the patient is a candidate for dental implants or dentures. The donor site morbidity is reasonable, with most patients returning to their preoperative activity level.

References

Bozec A, Poissonnet G, Chamorey E et al (2008) Free-flap head and neck reconstruction and quality of life: a 2-year prospective study. Laryngoscope 118:874–880

Ghaheri BA, Kim JH, Wax MK (2005) Second osteocutaneous fibular free flaps for head and neck defects. Laryngoscope 115(6):983–986

Head C, Alam D, Sercarz JA et al (2003) Microvascular flap reconstruction of the mandible: a comparison of bone grafts and bridging plates for restoration of mandibular continuity. Otolaryngol Head Neck Surg 129(1):48–54

Hidalgo D (1989) Fibula free flap: a new method of mandible reconstruction. Plast Reconstr Surg 84(1):71–79

Kim P, Fleck T, Heffelfinger R, Blackwell K (2008) Avoiding secondary skin graft donor site morbidity in the fibula free flap harvest. Arch Otolaryngol Head Neck Surg 134(12):1324–1327

Kuo YR, Shih HS, Chen CC, Boca R, Hsu YC, Su CY, Jeng SF, Wei FC (2010) Free fibula osteocutaneous flap with soleus muscle as a chimeric flap for reconstructing mandibular segmental defect after oral cancer ablation. Ann Plast Surg 64(6):738–742

Schusterman M, Reece G, Miller M, Harris S (1992) The osteocutaneous free fibula flap: is the skin paddle reliable? Plast Reconst Surg 90:787–793

Smith RB, Sniezek JC, Weed DT, Wax MK (2007) Utilization of free tissue transfer in head and neck surgery. Microvascular surgery subcommittee of American academy of otolaryngology – head and neck surgery. Otolaryngol Head Neck Surg 137:182–191

Virgin F, Iseli T, Iseli C, Sunde J, Carroll W, Magnuson J, Rosenthal E (2010) Functional outcomes of fibula and osteocutaneous forearm free flap reconstruction for segmental mandibular defects. Laryngoscope 120:663–667

Wax MK, Angelos P (2011) The use of the Doppler in monitoring free flaps in the head and neck. Laryngoscope (Submitted)

Wax MK, Winslow CP, Hansen J, MacKenzie D, Cohen J, Andersen P, Albert T (2000) A retrospective analysis of temporomandibular joint reconstruction with free fibula microvascular flap. Laryngoscope 110(6):977–981

Wei FC, Celik N, Yang W, Chen I, Chang Y, Chen H (2003) Complications after reconstruction by plate and soft-tissue free flap in composite mandibular defects and secondary salvage reconstruction with osteocutaneous flap. Plast Reconstr Surg 112:37

Field Cancerisation

▶ Field Cancerization

Field Cancerization

Steven J. Frampton[1,2] and Emma V. King[1,2]
[1]Poole Hospital NHS Foundation Trust, Poole, Dorset, UK
[2]Cancer Sciences Division, University of Southampton, Southampton, Hampshire, UK

Synonyms

Field cancerisation

Definition

Field cancerization is the development of an abnormal area of epithelium in which cells share a collection of early changes in the process of transformation towards malignancy.

Head and Neck Squamous Cell Carcinoma (HNSCC)

Head and neck squamous cell carcinoma is the sixth most common cancer in the world with a yearly incidence of 600,000 cases (Leemans et al. 2011). The average age of patients at diagnosis is ~65 years. The main aetiological risk factors were traditionally the smoking of tobacco and consumption of alcohol, with the chewing of betel quid an additional factor on the Indian subcontinent. Heavy smokers under the age of 46 suffer a 20-fold increased risk of oral or oropharyngeal cancer compared to nonsmokers, and heavy drinkers attract a fivefold increased risk. Interestingly, smoking and alcohol use act synergistically to produce a 50-fold risk if used together (Hunter et al. 2005). Microarray experiments in smokers have shown changes in the expression of recognized genes involved in adhesion, invasion, and antioxidant regulation. While most of these genes' expression normalizes 2 years after cessation, some only normalize after 30 years (Hunter et al. 2005). Human papilloma virus (HPV) transmitted through oral sex has been recognized as causative in recent years and is now producing a cohort of younger patients (Leemans et al. 2011). The average 5-year survival rate, pooled for all stages

of disease, is 40–50% for HNSCC and despite advances in management producing improved local tumor control, mortality figures have not improved significantly for over 2 decades (Leemans et al. 2011). Early stage cancers, accounting for a third of presentations, carry a better prognosis with the majority of treatments resulting in cure (Braakhuis et al. 2005). In addition, the HPV-related group appear to respond more favorably to treatment although the exact reasons for this are under investigation.

The external skin of the head and neck is a further site for carcinoma development. Nonmelanomatous skin cancers are the most common cancers in humans, and mostly arise from exposure to ultraviolet radiation in sunlight (Apalla et al. 2010). Basal cell carcinomas are normally relatively slow growing and invade locally with low metastatic potential. Conversely, squamous cell carcinomas grow more rapidly and metastasize with greater frequency. While basal cell carcinomas tend to arise without a visible precursor lesion, SCCs commonly arise from actinic keratoses.

The Multistep Process of Carcinogenesis

Carcinoma develops when cells of epithelial origin undergo successive genetic mutations resulting in a change in their appearance and behavior. This change is characterized by unregulated replication, altered cell-to-cell interactions, invasion through basement membranes, and stimulation of the surrounding stroma to provide a nutrient blood supply. The multistep hypothesis of carcinogenesis, originally arising from Knudson's "two hit hypothesis" describes how the cellular DNA accumulates an estimated 3–12 successive significant changes in order to generate this change in cell phenotype (Rhiner and Moreno 2009). The DNA mutations modify the expression of both *proto-oncogenes* and cell-cycle-regulating *tumor suppressor genes*, and depending on the particular cell functions affected, a variable number of mutations are required to produce the malignant phenotype. Exogenous carcinogens act as *initiators* to bring about a direct change in the DNA while *promoters* increase the frequency of cell turnover maximizing on the effect of the initiator and increasing the likelihood of further mutation. The multistep hypothesis has been validated in many organ systems and equally holds true in the head and neck (Chai and Brown 2009).

Residual Disease, Recurrent Disease and the "Second Primary"

Unfortunately, despite the best efforts of a surgeon, histological examination of an excised tumor does sometimes reveal tumor abutting the surgical margin. In such cases it must be assumed that tumor remains in the patient, and further treatment is indicated. The remaining area of primary tumor, which must be addressed, is termed *residual disease.*

Despite effective treatment of early mucosal SCCs with surgery or radiotherapy, further tumors still frequently arise in the aerodigestive tract following treatment. If the lesion arises within 2 cm of the location of the primary tumor and within 3 years of its diagnosis it has traditionally been termed *recurrent* disease, while lesions developing after 3 years or more than 2 cm from the primary site have been termed *"second primary"* tumors (Braakhuis et al. 2005). On occasion, a geographically separated mucosal tumor can be found at the same time, or within 6 months, of the diagnosis of a primary tumor. This is termed a *synchronous* tumor and differs from *metachronous* tumors, which are temporally separated by at least 6 months.

The annual incidence of second primary SCC tumors in the head and neck is approximately 3% for all sites, but has been documented as high as 8.5% per year following oropharyngeal primary tumors (Yamamoto et al. 2002). Combined with genuine locoregional recurrence and distant metastatic spread, they account for much of the mortality associated with head and neck SCC, and singularly for most of the mortality following successfully treated early stage primary disease.

The Original "Field Cancerization" Hypothesis

In 1953, 783 specimens of excised SCC from the lip, oral cavity, and pharynx were retrospectively examined (Slaughter et al. 1953). It was found that around the visibly abnormal tumor tissue lay areas that appeared normal to the naked eye but histologically displayed epithelial hyperplasia, hyperkeratinization, dyskaryosis, and capillary telangiectasia. In addition, in some specimens, there were further separate foci of carcinoma in situ or invasive SCC within the tissue surrounding the main specimen. The subsequent records of these patients were then reviewed and 88 (11.2%) were found to have developed at least one further SCC in the upper aerodigestive tract. This frequency was far higher than was statistically likely by chance alone. They concluded that there was "*a regional carcinogenic activity of some kind, in which a preconditioned epithelium has been activated over an area in which multiple cell groups undergo a process of irreversible change towards cancer.*" They went on to predict that "*oral epidermoid carcinoma arises from multifocal areas of precancerous change and not from one cell that suddenly becomes malignant.*" This was the first suggestion that SCCs arose from a premalignant "field" of cells.

Molecular Developments

It has proven difficult, on the basis of histology alone, to assess the risk of these visibly dysplastic fields proceeding to cancer. Although patches of oral erythroplakia have a significantly higher risk than leukoplakia (50% vs. 2–5% over 10 years), reliable prognostication for different severities of leukoplakia has been elusive (Hunter et al. 2005).

Various laboratory techniques have allowed us to explore the abnormalities in pre-neoplastic cells more fully. Fluorescence in situ hybridization (FISH) can be used to identify losses or translocations of DNA segments from chromosomes. DNA sequencing of known genes can allow comparison between tumor and non-tumor DNA. This enables identification of the site and nature of the mutations. DNA and micro RNA arrays are used to analyze the expression profiles of a number of genes simultaneously. The protein product of DNA and RNA can also be analyzed by various techniques (aka proteomics) allowing identification of changes in protein architecture and expression.

Studies have shown that lesions at successive points along the normal-dysplasia-neoplasia pathway show an increasing number of sites of loss of heterozygosity (LOH) (Califano et al. 1996). Common reasons for these mutations include chromosomal losses, which occur in many HNSCCs at 3p21, 9p21, 13q21, and 17p13 loci. Chromosomal length increases have been seen at 3q26 and 11q13 (Braakhuis et al. 2005). 17p13 mutations are thought to include TP53, the gene

Field Cancerization, Table 1 The current *established* HNSCC proto-oncogenes (PO) and tumor suppressor genes (TSG)

Gene	Location	Protein	Role	Normal protein function	Features in HNSCC
erbB-1	7p11	EGFR	PO	Transmembrane tyrosine receptor kinase	Overexpressed in 67% HNSCC
					Variable effect depending on mutation
MET	7q31	HGFR	PO	Receptor tyrosine kinase	Effect on cell growth, motility and angiogenesis
CCND1	11q13	CyclinD1	PO	Cyclin protein – complexes with cyclin-dependant kinases	Amplified in 20–80% HNSCC
					May push cell through G1/S
PIK3CA	3q26	P110α	PO	Cell signaling, phosphorylation	Mutations in 10–20% HNSCC
					Role in migration and invasion
p16^{INK4A}	9p21	p16	TSG	Inhibits cyclin-CDK complex	Lost in 52–82% HNSCC
					Associated with metastasis
TP53	17p13	p53	TSG	Cell-cycle control at G1/s	Mutated in 40–50% of HNSCC
				Apoptosis and DNA repair	Overexpression = poor prognosis
PTEN	10q23	PTEN	TSG	Inhibition of PI3K pathway	Mutations/deletions in 10% HNSCC
SMAD4	18q21	SMAD4	TSG	Gene transcription regulation	Mutated in 2/8 HNSCC cell lines
					Knockout in mice produces HNSCC

encoding P53, which is a key regulator of the cell cycle and apoptosis. The 9p21 locus is thought to include INK4a, the tumor suppressor gene encoding the key cell regulator protein p16. Mutations at this locus and 3p21 appear to be frequent *early* sites of mutation in the multistep process of carcinogenesis (Califano et al. 1996) (Table 1).

Using these molecular techniques it has become possible, to some extent, to stratify the risk of malignant transformation of some premalignant lesions. Oral leukoplakias demonstrating aneuploidy have been shown to be more likely to progress to malignancy, and to do so with aggressive features. P16 and combined p16/p53 status have been shown to have some prognostic value in laryngeal dysplasia, and p53 expression above the basal epithelial layer, or allelic imbalance at certain key genes (e.g., 3p14) is thought to have some predictive value for oral dysplasia (Hunter et al. 2005). In dysplastic oral lesions, loss of heterozygosity at 3p and/or 9p is associated with a 25% 3-year risk of malignant progression, but interestingly, excision of the clinically visible lesion does not reduce the risk (Lippman and Heymach 2007). Following excision of an oral tumor, 3p and 9p loss of heterozygosity in an area of adjacent leukoplakia carries a 26-fold increased risk of a second oral malignancy, while the histological identification of moderate or severe dysplasia only carries a 1.7-fold risk (Rosin et al. 2002). Clearly, these molecular markers offer better prospects for risk stratifying preneoplastic lesions. Our knowledge of the genes

encoded at many of these and other foci, and their role in carcinogenesis is yet to be elucidated but is the subject of ongoing research.

The histologically abnormal tissue immediately surrounding tumor has been shown to possess many of the same genetic abnormalities present in the primary tumor. The primary tumor has additional mutations, above and beyond those of the surrounding tissue, presumably accounting for its additional malignant behavior (Califano et al. 1996). It has subsequently been identified that a yet wider field exists, which histologically appears normal but contains genetic and molecular markers of progressing carcinogenesis. These genetically abnormal fields are often incompletely excised by surgical treatment of the primary tumor as they are large and invisible to the naked eye (Braakhuis et al. 2005). What is more, they are not seen on histological inspection of a surgical specimen since insufficient genetic mutations have accumulated to cause visible changes in cell architecture or position. As a result, a pre-neoplastic field, containing some mutations on the pathway toward carcinogenesis, remains in situ around the excised tumor, with potential to collect further genetic damage and progress toward invasive cancer. Efforts to improve the intraoperative visualization of abnormal mucosa have utilized autofluorescence and toluidine blue stain (Pai and Westra 2009), but the most promising work involves the development of confocal microscopy with exogenous fluorescent probes. These can potentially be targeted to any biomarker within the abnormal cells

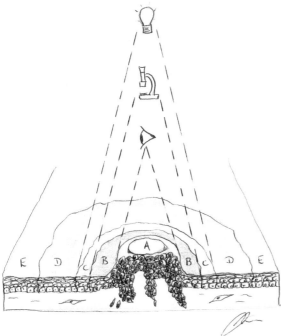

Field Cancerization, Fig. 1 This is a diagrammatic representation of the fields of cancerization. Only the central portion of a tumor (*A*) will be visible to the naked eye. Surrounding dysplastic tissue (*B*), often is not, and will only show atypical features on histological examination. The use of autofluorescence or confocal microscopy during surgery may increase the sensitivity to cellular atypia even beyond simple histological inspection (*C*). The surrounding tissue (*D*) has normal appearances but possesses molecular abnormalities that are only currently detectable using laboratory molecular techniques. As specific molecular probes are developed for confocal microscopy, (*C*) will approach (*D*). Finally, molecularly normal tissue (*E*) will be present, but this may be a sizeable distance (>7 cm) from the primary tumor

and enable their identification, and inclusion in the excised specimen, at the time of surgery (Fig. 1).

The "Second Field Tumor" Modification

With improved understanding of the molecular field of cancerization, it was proposed that there may be two distinct origins of the second tumors that can arise after treatment of a primary HNSCC (Braakhuis et al. 2005). Second tumors arising within the same genetically abnormal field as the primary tumor were distinguished from those that arose from outside of this field. While the latter were referred to as true *second primary* tumors they termed the first "*second field*" tumors.

Evidence for this arose from several studies. In one study the surgical excision specimens of oral/oropharyngeal tumors from 28 patients were analyzed. Samples 0.5 cm from the tumor edge and from the surgical margin were compared with the tumor itself. In ten cases there was evidence of a field of cancerization by LOH analysis. In four of these cases the field biopsy showed additional mutations, not present in the initial tumor, suggesting that the field was in places undergoing subsequent mutation independently of the primary tumor (Tabor et al. 2001). In a further study, 6 out of 10 second tumors and their associated margins were shown to share genetic similarity with the primary tumor (and its margins) suggesting that they arose from the same pre-neoplastic field of cancerization. Their patterns of genetic mutations were compared by sequencing their TP53 mutations and comparing their locations of LOH. The remaining 4 second tumors were significantly different in their genetic makeup to suggest that they were statistically unlikely to have arisen from a common precancerous field (Tabor et al. 2002).

Even though each field of genetically altered cells may be large, with diameters over 7 cm (Braakhuis et al. 2005), it has been shown that in any particular patient exposed to carcinogens there may be multiple separate fields of cancerization, interspersed by unaffected mucosa (Roesch-Ely et al. 2010). Each field is believed to have arisen from separate initial progenitor cells that have undergone different initial mutations, and subsequently accumulate differing profiles of DNA modification, shown by DNA sequencing and protein profiling (Roesch-Ely et al. 2010). A second tumor arising in a separate and genetically different field to that containing the primary tumor would be classified, therefore, as a true second primary tumor.

Some of the tumors previously regarded as recurrent tumors should not automatically be reclassified as second field tumors. Genuine local recurrences of the primary tumor do occur. These are thought to result from the invasion of small numbers of malignant cells beyond the boundaries of the surgical specimen despite histologically "clear" surgical resection margins. In 13 cases of presumed recurrent tumor (within 2 cm of the primary tumor, within 3 years of diagnosis), 8 of the primary tumor specimens displayed a pre-neoplastic field abnormality common to the second tumors (Tabor et al. 2004). This was evidenced by common mutations in the TP53 DNA sequence, a similar microsatellite shift, or a similar pattern of

LOH in specimens taken from the tumors and the surrounding excised tissue. In five of these cases, the genetic patterns (assessed by LOH) of the second tumor were sufficiently different from the first tumor for them to be identified as second field tumors. The analysis of the remaining three patients could not clearly differentiate between them being recurrent tumors or second field tumours. The five patients that experienced a second tumor *without* evidence of a field of cancerization were shown to have recurrent tumors. Analysis using the same techniques demonstrated a higher degree of similarity between the primary and second tumor than statistically could have occurred by chance (Tabor et al. 2004).

Development of a Field

In order for sufficient genetic mutations to be accumulated to produce a tumor, exposure to common carcinogens must occur over months or years. The rate of renewal of human oral epithelium is 14–24 days, suggesting that the cell of origin of these tumors is a stromal stem cell rather than a differentiated keratinocyte (Zhou and Jiang 2008). However, the alternative hypothesis of de-differentiation of mature keratinocytes by early mutations cannot, at present, be excluded. In health, each stem cell in the epithelium produces a daughter *clonal unit* or *patch*, ~200 cells (~2 mm) in diameter, containing transit-amplifying and differentiated cells. Mutations in the progenitor stem cell will be present in the whole colony. In order for the patch to spread to become a *field* further mutations must occur within the stem cell providing it with a competitive advantage over its neighbours through the process of *clonal selection* (Braakhuis et al. 2003). Subsequent DNA alterations in a subset of the resultant abnormal cells eventually produce histologically and then macroscopically visible abnormalities of the epithelium. Finally, when sufficient key mutations have accumulated, the full invasive phenotype is created (Fig. 2).

Epigenetic Factors and the "Epigenetic Field"

Epigenetic changes are chemical changes to the DNA of a cell without changes in the primary DNA sequence. One of the most well-known epigenetic mechanisms is DNA methylation. Methylation at specific points on a gene promoter sequence can modify the transcription of that gene, for example, reducing the expression or "silencing" a tumor suppressor gene (Chai and Brown 2009). This can facilitate further DNA damage while the regulatory gene is inactivated. Studies involving subjects with colorectal, prostate, and breast cancer have demonstrated a greater frequency of hypermethylation of specific genes in tumor cells. In addition they have demonstrated a field of hypermethylation in histologically normal tissue surrounding primary cancers (Niwa and Ushijima 2010).

In many organ systems gene-specific DNA hypermethylation has been seen and proposed to result from chronic inflammation (Niwa and Ushijima 2010). Examples include Barrett's esophagus following prolonged gastroesophageal reflux, the liver following viral hepatitis, and gastric mucosa following helicobacter pylori infection. Furthermore, a higher percentage of samples from ulcerative colitic mucosa were found to contain hypermethylated p16 if they were taken from areas that had progressed to dysplasia or frank carcinoma (Niwa and Ushijima 2010). Extent of hypermethylation therefore seems to correlate with the severity of cell dysfunction or injury. Evidence for a causative role for inflammation in hypermethylation has arisen from blockade of helicobacter-induced hypermethylation in gerbil gastric mucosa by the use of the immunosuppressive agent cyclosporin A. In humans, where smoking is a recognized risk factor for esophageal carcinoma, the duration of smoking history has been shown to correlate with hypermethylation levels of specific genes in esophageal mucosa (Oka et al. 2009). There is little documented work on hypermethylation in the rest of the head and neck but we might expect smoking, alcohol, and HPV infection to be associated with hypermethylation of specific genes. Interestingly, aging causes a background level of hypermethylation in a different subset of genes and this is markedly increased in those cells that develop into cancer, perhaps due to the increased number of cell cycles through which these cells have gone.

Currently, the role of hypermethylation in carcinogenesis has not been thoroughly investigated. It is unclear whether hypermethylation changes are a consequence of cellular inflammation from tumor

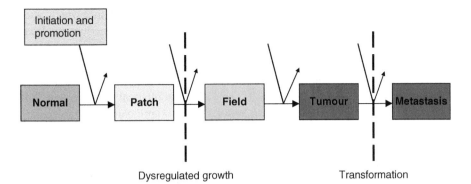

Field Cancerization, Fig. 2 The multistep theory of carcinogenesis and development of a field of cancerization. An initial mutation converts a normal stem cell into a progenitor cell producing a clonal patch of modified daughter cells (<200 cells wide). Subsequent mutations or epigenetic changes confer a competitive advantage, allowing the patch to spread laterally, no longer limited by regulating factors. Further changes produce further dysregulation of growth and cell adhesion, and an increased invasive tendency. Finally, the ability to metastasize is acquired. There is no fixed order to the progression of mutations; it is their accumulation and combined effect that confers the phenotype to the cell. However, 9p, 3p, and 17p mutations tend to occur earlier in the sequence while 13q, 18q, and 8p occur later

presence or whether they actively contribute to carcinogenesis. If proven to be causative, hypermethylation may provide a novel therapeutic target in cancer therapy.

Role of the Stroma

The stroma surrounding an epithelial tumor and precancerous change has been shown to accumulate similar genetic and epigenetic changes to the epithelium itself. It has been demonstrated that smokers with HNSCC exhibit stromal p53 mutations and loss of heterozygosity (Ge et al. 2010). Furthermore, it has been proposed that the stroma surrounding a field may not only change in response to the field or the carcinogen, but may actively feedback to exert influence on the epithelial field. Fibroblasts adjacent to the field are often activated and transdifferentiated into carcinoma-associated fibroblasts (CAFs). They have been shown to express growth factors associated with both tumor proliferation and the prevention of apoptosis and are capable of inducing epithelial tumors in xenografts (Ge et al. 2010). Transgenic mouse models in which a type of TGF-B receptor is knocked out in stromal fibroblasts produced epithelial tumors with 100% penetrance. It has been shown previously that the immune system has a role in tumor surveillance and its dysfunction or inhibition can increase the frequency of some carcinomas (Pai and Westra 2009).

It is likely that more complex interactions between modified epithelial tissue and its neighbouring tissues play a role in tumor survival.

Treatments for Field Cancerization

Current head and neck cancer treatment does not identify or intentionally treat the histologically normal, molecularly abnormal field. Routine molecular testing of excised tumors does not occur since we currently have insufficient evidence to support altered surveillance programs or treatment regimes on the basis of the findings of such tests. Surgical treatment currently aims to achieve clear tumor excision margins while the presence of any remaining dysplasia in the specimen is noted. Routine surveillance occurs for all HNSCC patients although routine mucosal inspection is limited to those areas visible in the clinic with a headlight and flexible nasendoscope.

Interestingly, there may be an inadvertent effect of radiotherapy on pre-neoplastic fields associated with primary tumors. In a retrospective study following patients for at least 10 years, 247 patients with oral cancer undergoing radiotherapy either with ($n = 38$) or without ($n = 209$) surgery were compared with 99 undergoing surgery alone (Rennemo et al. 2009). Radiotherapy was given to the primary site and levels I and II of the neck. For the first 5 years post treatment, there were significantly less second upper aerodigestive tract (UADT) mucosal tumors in the irradiated group (10.3% vs. 62.5%, $p < 0.001$). The average time to develop a second tumor was also significantly longer in the irradiated group (8.6 vs. 3.9 years). However, beyond 5 years the relative risk of a second tumor in the irradiated group returned to that of the nonirradiated group. Overall and cancer-specific survival was no different between the groups over the whole time period. It is presumed that the radiotherapy had some beneficial action against the pre-neoplastic field, but the cause for the accelerated deterioration beyond 5 years is unclear. It is possible that the delayed recurrences in the radiation group were due to the effect of continued smoking (which was not assessed), or possibly a result of radiation-induced second tumors.

EGFR inhibitors have shown efficacy alone or when used with chemoradiotherapy and are well tolerated. Cetuximab is currently licensed in the UK in combination with radiotherapy in patients with locally advanced HNSCC, a Karnofsky performance score of over 90%, and where platinum-based chemotherapy is contraindicated. Studies looking at lung carcinomas have identified EGFR tyrosine kinase domain mutations that predict sensitivity, and *ras* mutations that predict resistance, to EGFR inhibitors. Such molecular analysis in HNSCC could help to select patients who might experience greater benefit, and save ineffective administration to those with relative resistance to treatments (Lippman and Heymach 2007).

Cutaneous precancerous fields are regularly treated. Where there are multiple actinic keratoses (which can develop into SCC) in a close distribution, topical treatments are often tried including diclofenac gel, fluorouracil cream, or imiquimod. Alternatively, photodynamic therapy is sometimes used. In one trial aminolevulinic acid photodynamic therapy (ALA-PDT) was used to treat areas of the skin of the face and scalp (Apalla et al. 2010). Following two treatments separated by a week there was a significant reduction in the number of new lesions in that area compared to placebo for the subsequent 6 months. However, beyond 6 months the development of new lesions occurred at a similar incidence to the placebo group. This suggests that the treatment temporarily halts the development of new lesions but that further mutations do accumulate with time.

Further treatments for pre-neoplastic lesions and fields have been trialled but are not currently in clinical use. Oral n-acetyl cysteine, which acts as an antioxidant has been shown to reduce the frequency of DNA adducts and abnormal micronuclei in oral mucosa in healthy smokers (Hunter et al. 2005). Retinoids have been used to treat oral leukoplakia and produce clinical and histopathological improvement. However, the side effects are significant, the molecular abnormalities persist despite treatment, and most patients relapse on stopping treatment (Tanaka et al. 2011). COX-2 expression has been shown to be increased in HNSCC but while COX-2 inhibitors have prevented the progression from leukoplakia to carcinoma in animal models, they were no more clinically effective than placebo in humans when administered as a mouthwash (Hunter et al. 2005).

The morbidity and mortality associated with head and neck SCC and its treatment provides a pressing need for us to improve targeted treatment. Increasing knowledge of the key genes, the role and reversibility of epigenetic mechanisms, and the potential influence of the stroma will potentially open up novel therapeutic approaches. Once sufficient gene mapping has occurred in the areas that are frequently mutated in HNSCC, we may be able to use these genes for targeted treatment to currently invisible cells. Chemical or genetic therapies may be developed to specifically target some of the key mutations, while biomarkers with attached fluorescent probes would aid surgical visualization of the abnormal field. One of the major difficulties lies in identifying and locating an early field in "at-risk" patients before it has developed macroscopic abnormalities. Current studies are examining whether analysis of sputum or epithelial brushings could be analyzed in this patient group but this is currently in the very early stages of development.

References

Apalla Z, Sotiriou E, Chovarda E, Lefaki I, Devliotou-Panagiotidou D, Ioannides D (2010) Skin cancer: preventive photodynamic therapy in patients with face and scalp cancerization. A randomized placebo-controlled study. Br J Dermatol 162(1):171–175, epub 2009 Oct 26

Braakhuis BJ, Brakenhoff RH, Leemans CR (2005) Second field tumours: a new opportunity for cancer prevention? Oncologist 10(7):493–500

Braakhuis BJ, Tabor MP, Kummer A, Leemans CR, Brakenhoff RH (2003) A genetic explanation of Slaughter's concept of field cancerization: evidence and clinical implications. Cancer Res 63(8):1727–1730

Califano J, Van der Riet P, Westra W, Nawroz H, Clayman G, Piantadosi S, Corio R, Lee D, Greenberg B, Koch W, Sidransky D (1996) Genetic progression model for head and neck cancer: implications for field cancerization. Cancer Res 56(11):2488–2492

Chai H, Brown RE (2009) Field effect in cancer – an update. Ann Clin Lab Sci 39(4):331–337

Ge L, Meng W, Zhou H, Bhowmick N (2010) Could stroma contribute to field cancerization? Med Hypotheses 75(1):26–31, epub 2010 Feb 9

Hunter KD, Parkinson EK, Harrison PR (2005) Profiling early head and neck cancer. Nat Rev Cancer 5(2):127–135

Leemans CR, Braakhuis BJ, Brakenhoff RH (2011) The molecular biology of head and neck cancer. Nat Rev Cancer 11(1):9–22, epub 2010 Dec 16

Lippman SM, Heymach JV (2007) The convergent development of molecular-targeted drugs for cancer treatment and prevention. Clin Cancer Res 13(14):4035–4041

Niwa T, Ushijima T (2010) Induction of epigenetic alterations by chronic inflammation and its significance on carcinogenesis. Adv Genet 71:41–56

Oka D, Yamashita S, Tomioka T, Nakanishi Y, Kato H, Kaminishi M, Ushijima T (2009) The presence of aberrant DNA methylation in non-cancerous esophageal mucosae in association with smoking history: a target for risk diagnosis and prevention of esophageal cancers. Cancer 115(15): 3412–3426

Pai SI, Westra WH (2009) Molecular pathology of head and neck cancer: implications for diagnosis, prognosis and treatment. Annu Rev Pathol 4:49–70

Rennemo E, Zatterstrom U, Evensen J, Boysen M (2009) Reduced risk of head and neck second primary tumours after radiotherapy. Radiother Oncol 93(3):559–562, epub 2009 Sep 9

Rhiner C, Moreno E (2009) Super competition as a possible mechanism to pioneer precancerous cells. Carcinogenesis 30(5):723–728, epub 2009 Jan 6

Roesch-Ely M, Leipold A, Nees M, Holzinger D, Dietz A, Flechtenmacher C, Wolf T, Zapatka M, Bosch FX (2010) Proteomic analysis of field cancerization in pharynx and oesophagus: a prospective pilot study. J Pathol 221(4):462–470

Rosin MP, Lam WL, Poh C, Le ND, Li RJ, Zeng T, Priddy R, Zhang L (2002) 3p14 and 9p21 loss is a simple tool for predicting second oral malignancy at previously treated oral cancer sites. Cancer Res 62:6447–6450

Slaughter DP, Southwick HW, Smejkal W (1953) Field cancerization in oral stratified squamous epithelium; clinical implications of multicentric origin. Cancer 6(5):963–968

Tabor MP, Brakenhoff RH, Ruijter-Schippers HJ et al (2002) Multiple head and neck tumors frequently originate from a single pre-neoplastic lesion. Am J Pathol 161:1051–1060

Tabor MP, Brakenhoff RH, van Houten VM et al (2001) Persistence of genetically altered fields in head and neck cancer patients: biological and clinical implications. Clin Cancer Res 7(6):1523–1532

Tabor MP, Brakenhoff RH, Ruijter-Schippers HJ et al (2004) Genetically altered fields as origin of locally recurrent head and neck cancer: a retrospective study. Clin Cancer Res 10:3607–3613

Tanaka T, Tanaka M, Tanaka T (2011) Oral carcinogenesis and oral cancer chemoprevention: a review. Patholog Res Int:431246

Yamamoto E, Shibuya H, Yoshimura R, Miura M (2002) Site specific dependency of second primary cancer in early stage head and neck squamous cell carcinoma. Cancer 94(7):2007–2014

Zhou ZT, Jiang WW (2008) Cancer stem cell model in oral squamous cell carcinoma. Curr Stem Cell Res Ther 3(1):17–20

Fine Needle Aspiration Biopsy (FNAB)

▶ Fine Needle Aspiration for Head and Neck Tumors

Fine Needle Aspiration Cytology (FNAC)

Majid A. Khan and Todd A. Nichols
Division of NeuroRadiology, University of MS
Medical Center, Jackson, MS, USA

Definition

Fine needle aspiration cytology (FNAC) is a method used to take palpable or guided specimen for pathological diagnosis.

Cross-References

▶ Fine Needle Aspiration for Head and Neck Tumors
▶ Imaging Cystic Head and Neck Masses

Fine Needle Aspiration for Head and Neck Tumors

Feriyl Bhaijee and Anwer Siddiqi
Department of Pathology, University of Mississippi
Medical Center, Jackson, MS, USA

Synonyms

Aspiration; Aspiration biopsy; Aspiration cytology; Diagnostic aspiration; Fine needle aspiration biopsy (FNAB); Fine needle aspiration cytology (FNAC)

Definition

Fine needle aspiration (FNA) is defined as the removal of a sample of cells, using a fine needle, from a suspicious mass for diagnostic purposes (DeMay 2007a).

Purpose

FNA is widely recognized as the first step in diagnosis of malignant tumors of the head and neck, as well as ▶ Oropharyngeal Malignancies (DeMay 2007b). It is particularly useful in this region, as the ▶ Differential Diagnosis of Adult Neck Masses ranges from innocuous inflammation to aggressive malignancies. FNA may be used for both superficial and deep-seated lesions in the head and neck; the latter often requires radiologic guidance.

FNA is useful in the diagnosis of neoplasms, infections (e.g., fungal, protozoal), inflammation (e.g., granulomatous), or infiltrations (e.g., amyloidosis) (DeMay 2007a). For more information on specific entities found on FNA, see also: ▶ Benign Salivary Gland Neoplasms, ▶ Salivary Gland Malignancies, ▶ Minor Salivary Gland Neoplasms, ▶ Benign Sinonasal Neoplasms, ▶ Sinonasal Neoplasms, ▶ Cervical Esophageal Squamous Cell Carcinoma, ▶ Primary Neck Neoplasms, ▶ Follicular Thyroid Cancer, ▶ Papillary Thyroid Cancer, ▶ Medullary Thyroid Cancer, ▶ Benign Tumors of Larynx, ▶ Cervical Node Metastases from Squamous Cell Carcinomas, Patterns of, ▶ Unknown Primary Squamous Cell Carcinoma of Neck, ▶ Lymphomas Presenting in Head and Neck, ▶ Deep Neck Infections, ▶ Granulomatous Disorders.

Principle

Informed Consent

As with any surgical procedure, informed consent must be obtained from the patient or the patient's surrogate prior to FNA. Informed consent consists of explaining (1) the indication for FNA, (2) the risks and benefits of the procedure, and (3) alternative diagnostic procedures. Any questions or concerns should also be addressed. It is advisable to obtain *written* consent prior to commencing the FNA.

FNA Equipment

Superficial FNA requires the following equipment: a variety of fine needles, 25–22 gauge, of various lengths; a 10 cc syringe; a syringe pistol handle (optional), such as the 10 ml Cameco syringe pistol/gun™ (Belpro Medical) or Tao aspirator™ (Tao &Tao Technology); alcohol swabs; sterile gauze; topical anesthetic or skin refrigerant (optional), such as Gebauer's Ethyl Chloride® (Gebauer Company); plain glass slides; cellular fixatives, such as Fix-Rite 2™ (Thermo Scientific); protective gear (e.g., gloves, face shield); and resuscitative equipment. FNA of deep-seated lesions frequently requires radiologic guidance and needle guides, as well as specialist supervision (Fig. 1).

For most superficial FNAs, a 23 gauge, 1″ needle is sufficient to make about half a dozen cellular smears. A syringe pistol handle allows the operator to stabilize the lesion with one hand, and operate the syringe with the other – so while it is not essential, it often enhances operator comfort. Before the FNA, the needle is fitted on the syringe, and both are loaded in the syringe pistol handle.

Topical anesthesia (e.g., ethyl chloride) is preferred to local anesthetic agents (e.g., parenteral lidocaine), because the latter causes patient discomfort and local swelling, which may obscure the biopsy site. (See ▶ Anesthetic Techniques for Otolaryngologic Patient for more information).

When a pathologist is present for immediate FNA evaluation, additional equipment is necessary, e.g., 95% alcohol, staining solutions (e.g., Diff-Quik™), and a microscope. For subsequent cell block preparation, tissue culture transport media (e.g., Roswell Park Memorial Institute [RPMI] medium) or CytoLyt™ preservative solutin (Hologic, Inc.) may be used.

FNA Technique

Prior to FNA, the patient should be positioned in order to facilitate palpation of the suspicious mass (DeMay 2007a). The optimal approach to the mass, as well as its depth, consistency, and size should be carefully assessed. Any proximate pulsation should alert the operator to the risk of vascular injury (Fig. 2).

The procedure for sampling superficial lesions begins with cleaning the intended biopsy site with alcohol swabs. Next, the operator immobilizes the mass lesion with his non-dominant hand, ensuring a taut skin surface. Topical anesthesia, such as ethyl

Fine Needle Aspiration for Head and Neck Tumors, Fig. 1 FNA Equipment: syringe pistol handle/gun, 10 cc syringe, skin refrigerant (ethyl chloride), alcohol swabs, needles (25-22 gauge), sterile gauze, plain glass slides, cellular fixative

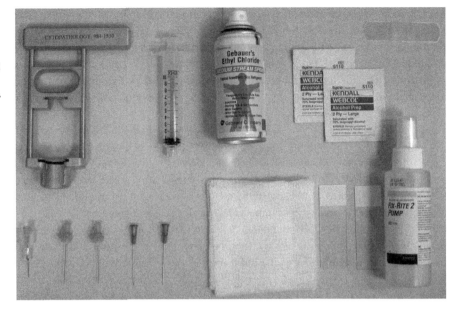

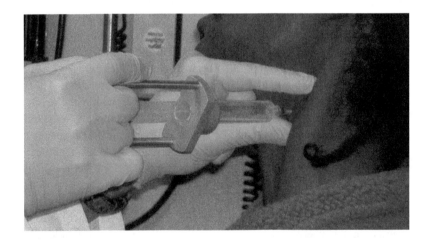

Fine Needle Aspiration for Head and Neck Tumors, Fig. 2 FNA of lateral neck mass using syringe pistol handle and 25 gauge needle

chloride, is then sprayed onto the biopsy site. The syringe, or the syringe pistol handle, is held in the operator's dominant hand, and the needle is inserted perpendicularly into the lesion. (A tangential approach is rarely used, but may be necessary when the mass is in close proximity to a vascular structure.) Once in the lesion, the plunger is withdrawn, or the syringe pistol handle is squeezed, thereby creating negative pressure in the barrel. Staying within the lesion, the needle is then advanced and withdrawn in a single axis, at three strokes per second for 5–10 s (DeMay 2007a). The movement of the needle is adjusted for the consistency of the mass: firm, sclerotic masses will require more force than soft, cystic lesions. The needle may be rotated during this step, in order to loosen the cores of tissue for aspiration. Biopsy material in the hub of the syringe suggests an adequate sample.

When the operator completes the back-and-forth rotating movements, the negative pressure on the syringe is released before the needle is withdrawn from the lesion. Failure to release the suction before withdrawing the needle will cause the aspirated material to enter the barrel of the syringe, where it may not be accessed for immediate pathologic evaluation. The biopsy site is covered with sterile gauze, and firm pressure is applied until satisfactory hemostasis is achieved. (This also prevents hematoma formation).

For deep-seated lesions, the FNA procedure is performed by an interventional radiologist under radiologic guidance (e.g., fluoroscopy, ultrasound, or computed tomography). Once obtained, the specimen is given to the pathologist, who offers an immediate assessment of adequacy.

Gross Findings

The immediate gross findings following FNA determine further actions (DeMay 2007a). If the material is inadequate, the FNA is repeated. If fluid is aspirated, the lesion is drained and any residual mass is reaspirated. If the aspirate is purulent, culture is indicated; if necrotic, the periphery of the lesion is reaspirated. If the aspirate is bloody, the FNA should be stopped, and reaspiration may be indicated.

Slide Preparation

Following FNA, the specimen obtained is handled carefully, with appropriate labeling, fixation, preparation, staining, and transport, as needed.

The frosted end of the plain glass slide should be labeled with the patient's identification and the date of the procedure. A tiny drop of the specimen in the syringe is then placed onto a glass slide, and a second slide is used to smear the aspirate across the first slide. The slides may then be (1) air-dried and stained for immediate evaluation by the pathologist, or (2) fixed with spray fixatives or 95% alcohol and transported to the laboratory. While spray fixatives are convenient, alcohol immersion results in better fixation. The smears should be fixed as soon as they are made.

Following smear preparation, the remainder of the aspirate in the needle may be rinsed in a cellular medium, such as RPMI. This medium is then transported to the laboratory, and used to prepare a cell block for further pathologic analysis.

Immediate staining is usually performed by the pathologist, using a Romanowski-type stain (such as Diff-Quik™). Diff-Quik™ staining takes about a minute, and the slides can be examined under the microscope without a coverslip. The pathologist assesses adequacy and, in certain cases, renders an immediate pathologic diagnosis.

Diagnostic Interpretation

The slides and cell media sent to the laboratory are processed according to institutional guidelines, and the processed slides are given to the pathologist for cytologic evaluation. Thereafter, immunocytochemical stains may be used to facilitate diagnosis. In some cases, cytogenetic or molecular studies are possible. The cellular aspirate in RPMI may be submitted for flow cytometry to further characterize lymphoid cell populations.

FNA of Thyroid Nodules

FNA is an integral part of the diagnostic work-up of thyroid nodules (see also ▶ Thyroid Nodules, Evaluation). The main purpose of thyroid nodule FNA is to identify malignancy and subsequent direct clinical management. While the technique of thyroid FNA follows the same general principles of FNA elsewhere in the head and neck, certain methods increase diagnostic yield (Galera-Davidson and Gonzalez-Campora 2008). The patient should be placed in a supine position, with a pillow under the shoulders, to facilitate extension of the neck. The operator stands on the side opposite to the thyroid lesion, and immobilizes the thyroid against the trachea with the non-dominant hand, while inserting the needle with the dominant hand (Fig. 3). Only 5–10 mL of suction is necessary, as excessive negative pressure will result in hematoma formation. The needle is advanced and withdrawn within the lesion in a single plane, until an aspirate appears in the hub of the needle. Moving the needle in different planes of the lesion will result in a painful, bloody aspirate, which is often non-diagnostic.

Fine-needling sampling without aspiration (cytopuncture) is often utilized for highly vascular organs, or very small lesions, in which FNA may yield a bloody specimen. Cytopuncture is based on the principle of capillarity. A fine needle is inserted in the lesion with the thumb and forefinger of the operator's dominant hand, and manually advanced and withdrawn for 5–10 s, as in conventional FNA. After withdrawing the needle, a syringe filled with air is attached to the base of the needle. The specimen is expelled onto plain glass slides, and the needle is rinsed in cellular medium.

The nature of the thyroid lesion will dictate the number of aspirations for each nodule (Galera-Davidson and Gonzalez-Campora 2008). Solitary nodules less than 3 cm in greatest diameter usually require one to four aspirations, while larger lesions may require up to eight aspirations to achieve diagnostic accuracy. In multinodular goiters, several lesions should be sampled.

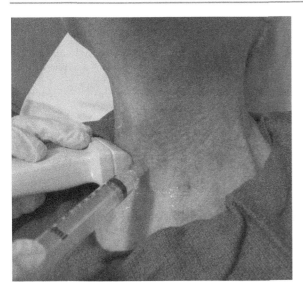

**Fine Needle Aspiration for Head and Neck Tumors,
Fig. 3** Ultrasound-guided FNA of thyroid mass using 10 cc
syringe and 25 gauge needle

Ultrasound-guided thyroid FNA is recommended
for nodules ≥1.0 cm in size, which demonstrate radiographic features of malignancy, e.g., calcifications or
solid areas (see Thyroid Ultrasound). Palpable lesions,
however, do not necessarily require ultrasound guidance, as an expert operator is likely to obtain an adequate specimen without ultrasound guidance. On-site
assessment of specimen adequacy is strongly
recommended for thyroid FNAs, as it decreases the
number of needle passes and assists less-experienced
operators in obtaining adequate specimens.

Indication

FNA has both diagnostic and therapeutic indications: it
facilitates diagnosis of suspicious masses and drainage
of cystic lesions.

Following careful consideration of the risks and
benefits, FNA should only be performed when the
outcome will affect patient management.

Contraindication

Contraindications to FNA include: patient refusal or
uncooperative patient, bleeding diatheses (including
anticoagulant therapy), inaccessible or ill-defined

masses, highly vascular lesions (e.g., Vascular Tumors
of the Head and Neck, Arteriovenous Malformations),
suspected hydatid cyst, and lack of necessary medical
resources (including resuscitative equipment). Also,
patients who cannot suppress a cough should not
undergo thyroid FNA.

Like most provider-performed tests, FNA is opera-
tor-dependent, and an inexperienced or unsure operator is a relative contraindication to FNA. Knowledge of
the embryology and anatomy of the neck and face is
essential. Specialist supervision is recommended until
competence and confidence are achieved.

Advantage/Disadvantage

Advantages of FNA
FNA is safe, accurate, fast, and cost-effective. When
performed correctly, FNA is highly sensitive and
highly specific. It has few risks, complications are
uncommon, and the diagnostic yield is often sufficient
to direct further clinical management. Despite the
cytologic nature of FNA specimens, histologic features
can also be evaluated, e.g., cellular architecture and
stromal composition.

FNA can be performed in almost any clinical setting
(e.g., office, bedside, etc.), and does not require expensive or complicated equipment. FNA biopsies can be
processed faster than any other surgical biopsy, including frozen sections. The entire FNA process – from
obtaining informed consent to rendering a pathologic
diagnosis – can be completed in less than an hour.

In addition to providing an early diagnosis, FNA
may also replace various radiologic investigations,
thus decreasing cost and facilitating therapeutic planning (DeMay 2007a).

Disadvantages of FNA
FNA-related complications are uncommon, and
include pain, anxiety, hematoma, hemorrhage, vasova-
gal reaction, nerve damage, infection, damage to vital
organs, and tumor necrosis (DeMay 2007a). These
risks increase with FNA of deep-seated lesions, especially those in close relation to vascular structures.
There is a hypothetical risk of tumor seeding along
the FNA tract, but this has not been reported in the
medical literature to date, and there is no direct evidence that FNA has an adverse effect on patient
survival.

Health care providers performing FNAs face the risk of needle stick injuries and subsequent infections, but appropriate safety measures and patient cooperation likely ameliorate this risk.

The main disadvantage of FNA is its limited diagnostic yield, as compared to surgical biopsy and histopathologic evaluation. As in any biopsy procedure, it is assumed that the target lesion is homogeneous, and that the biopsy sample is representative of the entire lesion (DeMay 2007a). However, the aspiration needle may not always enter the malignant focus, resulting in a false-negative diagnosis. Radiographic imaging reduces the likelihood of false negatives by characterizing the lesion before FNA is attempted, or by guiding the aspirating needle during the procedure. (See also: ▶ Imaging Cystic Head and Neck Masses). Moreover, operator inexperience may contribute to non-diagnostic aspirations. The many advantages of FNA, however, often outweigh this limitation, and its use should be tailored to the individual clinical context.

Cross-References

- ▶ Anesthetic Techniques for Otolaryngologic Patient
- ▶ Arteriovenous Malformations
- ▶ Benign Salivary Gland Neoplasms
- ▶ Benign Sinonasal Neoplasms
- ▶ Benign Tumors of Larynx
- ▶ Cervical Esophageal Squamous Cell Carcinoma
- ▶ Deep Neck Infections
- ▶ Differential Diagnosis of Adult Neck Masses
- ▶ Follicular Thyroid Cancer
- ▶ Granulomatous Disorders
- ▶ Imaging Cystic Head and Neck Masses
- ▶ Lymphomas Presenting in Head and Neck
- ▶ Medullary Thyroid Cancer
- ▶ Minor Salivary Gland Neoplasms
- ▶ Oropharyngeal Malignancies
- ▶ Papillary Thyroid Cancer
- ▶ Primary Neck Neoplasms
- ▶ Salivary Gland Malignancies
- ▶ Sarcoidosis
- ▶ Sinonasal Neoplasms
- ▶ Thyroid Nodules, Evaluation
- ▶ Unknown Primary Squamous Cell Carcinoma of Neck

References

DeMay RM (2007a) Introduction to FNA biopsy. In: DeMay RM (ed) Practical principles of cytopathology, revised edition. ASCP Press, Chicago, pp 131–136

DeMay RM (2007b) Head and neck. In: DeMay RM (ed) Practical principles of cytopathology. ASCP Press, Chicago, pp 179–185

Galera-Davidson H, Gonzalez-Campora R (2008) Thyroid. In: Bibbo M, Wilbur DC (eds) Comprehensive cytopathology, 3rd edn. Saunders Elsevier, Philadelphia, pp 633–670

First and Second Brachial Arch Syndrome

▶ Congenital Craniofacial Malformations and Their Surgical Treatment

First and Second Branchial Arch Syndrome

▶ Hemifacial Microsomia

First Arch Syndrome

▶ Hemifacial Microsomia

First Branchial Cleft Anomalies

M. Taylor Fordham and Paul R. Lambert
Otolaryngology-Head and Neck Surgery, College of Medicine, Medical University of South Carolina, Charleston, SC, USA

Synonyms

First branchial cleft cyst; First branchial cleft fistula; First branchial cleft sinus; Type I or Type II first branchial cleft anomaly

Definition

A first branchial cleft anomaly forms from the incomplete closure of the ventral portion of the first branchial cleft. These anomalies may present as cysts, sinuses, or fistulas, depending on the degree of cleft closure. A cyst is an encapsulated, epithelium-lined sac without any connections to the external environment. A sinus presents as a blind sac with a single connection to the external environment, typically the external auditory canal. A fistula is a patent tract that consists of two openings, typically the external auditory canal and the anterior triangle of the neck.

Epidemiology

Branchial cleft anomalies are the second most common cause of congenital neck masses, preceded in incidence only by thyroglossal duct cysts. Second branchial cleft anomalies are the most common of the branchial remnants, followed by first cleft anomalies. While some tertiary referral centers have reported that first branchial defects account for 18–25% of their branchial cleft practice (Choi et al. 1995; Bajaj et al. 2011), it is generally recognized that the first cleft anomalies account for less than 10% of all branchial cleft pathology (Olsen et al. 1980; Finn et al. 1987). Both the two largest case series to date noted an approximate 2:1 female predominance of these lesions (Olsen et al. 1980; Triglia et al. 1998) with an estimated annual incidence of 1 per million births (Arndal et al. 1995).

History

The natural history of first branchial cleft anomalies can be quite variable, largely as a result of frequent initial misdiagnosis. Nonetheless, these lesions typically come to the attention of the physician due to an obvious sinus tract or recurrent infections in the periauricular region (Solares et al. 2003). In a large literature review, the mean age at diagnosis was just under 19 years of age with the age range being from 20 days to 82 years (D'Souza et al. 2002). Other studies report lower mean ages at diagnosis, but it is worthwhile to note that older adults may present with these congenital lesions due to both prior misdiagnosis and/or mismanagement. A large case series showed that nearly half of the patients diagnosed with first branchial cleft anomalies had undergone at least one procedure including incision and drainage, incomplete

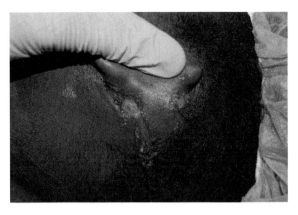

First Branchial Cleft Anomalies, Fig. 1 Left postauricular sinus associated with a first branchial cleft anomaly

excision, or injection of sclerosing agent. Prior procedures on these patients render future complete surgical resection more difficult. Given the challenges in diagnosis, most pediatric patients experience a delay of about 3.5–4 years from the time of presentation to the time of adequate treatment (Ford et al. 1992; Triglia et al. 1998).

Presenting symptoms have been classified into cervical, parotid, and auricular. Cervical symptoms include a draining tract in the neck, a neck mass, or a pit noted along the mandible. Parotid symptoms include a mass or cyst overlying the gland or the mastoid. Persistent otorrhea is the most common auricular symptom. Cervical symptoms are generally the most common (41%), followed by parotid (35%) and auricular (24%) symptoms (Triglia et al. 1998; Nicollas et al. 2000) (Fig. 1). One important distinction to note is that preauricular cysts or sinuses are distinct entities and are unrelated to first branchial cleft anomalies. These lesions arise from failure of fusion of the auricular hillocks of His and are more common than branchial cleft lesions, thus representing a separate developmental pathology (Finn et al. 1987; Hickey et al. 1994).

Clinical Features

First branchial cleft anomalies generally come to the attention of the otolaryngologist secondary to recurrent infections or recalcitrant drainage that has not responded to medical therapy or prior procedural interventions. Swelling in the periauricular or parotid

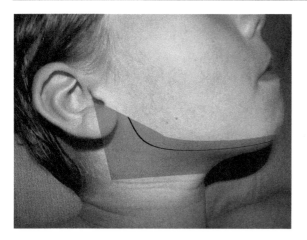

First Branchial Cleft Anomalies, Fig. 2 Note the triangular anatomic and embryologic boundaries within which most all first branchial cleft lesions arise

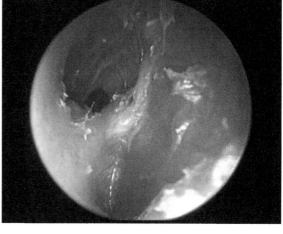

First Branchial Cleft Anomalies, Fig. 3 Note the membranous attachment from the external canal to the umbo highly suggestive of a first branchial cleft anomaly

region and drainage from the ear are common complaints, and yet these presenting signs are not specific to first cleft defects. For this reason, a thorough history and physical examination are critical to appropriately diagnose these lesions.

When examining these patients, certain findings can assist in securing the correct diagnosis. A sinus opening in the cervical neck in the triangular region bound by the external auditory canal, symphysis menti, and the hyoid bone is highly suggestive of a first cleft anomaly (Sichel et al. 1998) (Fig. 2). Depending on the nature of these lesions, there may also be a tract that communicates with the external auditory canal. This tract most commonly opens into the region of the bony-cartilaginous junction but may potentially open into the concha, postauricular skin, or rarely into the middle ear as reported once in the literature (Olsen et al. 1980). For these reasons, a draining ear in the presence of a normal tympanic membrane and middle ear space should raise suspicion for a possible first cleft lesion (D'Souza et al. 2002). Additionally on physical exam, one may discover a myringeal web or an epidermal extension from the floor of the external auditory canal to the umbo or portion of the tympanic membrane (Fig. 3). While this finding is not present in all first cleft pathology, some argue that it is pathognomonic for this diagnosis. These webs are hypothesized to be associated malformations not requiring removal during the surgical excision of the first cleft anomaly (Sichel et al. 1998).

Numerous attempts at formulating a classification system for first branchial cleft anomalies have been undertaken. In the early 1970s, Arnot proposed a system that classified these lesions into Types I and II. Type I lesions, as he described, presented in early-to-mid adult life and consisted of a cyst or sinus in the area of the parotid gland and lined exclusively by simple squamous epithelium. Arnot hypothesized that these lesions formed from cell rest buried during obliteration of the first cleft of the branchial apparatus. Type II lesions, on the other hand, presented in infancy or early childhood and consisted of a sinus or superficial cyst in the anterior neck with possible external openings just below the angle of the mandible and/or in the external auditory canal. These defects are histologically lined by keratinizing squamous epithelium consisting of hair follicles and sebaceous glands and originate secondary to failure of complete closure of the first branchial cleft (Arnot et al. 1971). Not long after Arnot's classification system, Work published his own system for defining these lesions. He described Type I lesions as ectodermal duplications of the membranous external auditory canal. He suggested that these pass deep to the lobule, superior to the facial nerve, and parallel to the external canal, ending in a cul-de-sac at the bony plate of the mesotympanum. Type II defects, as he suggested, are duplication anomalies of the external auditory canal and pinna. Unlike Type I, Type II defects

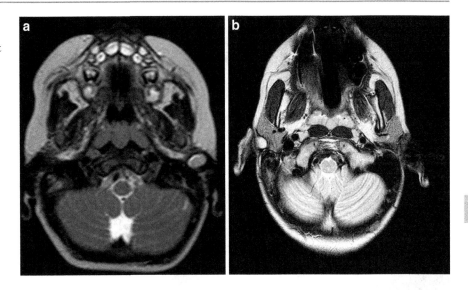

First Branchial Cleft Anomalies, Fig. 4 T2 MRI images of first branchial cleft lesions. (**a**) Note the cyst confined to the region of the left external auditory canal. (**b**) A right first branchial lesion intimately associated with the external canal and parotid gland

contain skin and cartilage (mesoderm). They pass over the angle of the mandible in variable relation to the facial nerve and terminate just inferior to the membranous external canal or form a sinus with it (Work et al. 1972). Yet another classification scheme was proposed by Olsen in 1980, and this system is arguably the simplest and most clinically useful. Olsen proposed dividing first branchial anomalies into cysts (tract with no external opening), sinuses (tract with one opening to external canal), and fistulas (tract with opening to external canal and cervical neck) (Olsen et al. 1980). Most recent literature on first branchial anomalies describes the lesions in this way.

Reports have yielded discrepancies as to which of the three lesions (cyst, sinus, and fistula) is the most common (Olsen et al. 1980; Triglia et al. 1998). While each type of lesion can run superficial to, deep to, or between the branches of the facial nerve, multiple studies have shown that over half of the first cleft tracts lie lateral to the nerve. The majority of isolated cysts are located lateral to the facial nerve, and there has been evidence to suggest that fistulas are more likely to pass deep to the facial nerve; however, it is important to remember that this relationship is variable and should never be taken for granted (Triglia et al. 1998; D'Souza et al. 2002; Del Pero et al. 2007). While these lesions are benign, there are rare reports of indwelling carcinoma, further supporting surgical management when appropriate for the patient (Roche et al. 2010).

Tests

Once the history and physical presentation of the patient have been reviewed, radiographic imaging can be very helpful in the workup and preoperative planning of a patient suspected of having a first branchial cleft anomaly. In fact, in one study, the history, physical examination, and imaging together led to the correct diagnosis in 92% of patients presenting with first cleft lesions (Schroeder et al. 2007). Computed tomography (CT) and ultrasonography (US) are the most commonly utilized radiographic modalities for the evaluation of these entities, with contrasted CT being arguably the most useful. MRI, while avoiding radiation exposure, may be helpful in assessing intraparotid lesions but adds little else to the information allowed by computed tomography alone (Fig. 4). Preoperative imaging is helpful not only in confirming the diagnosis, but also in possibly defining any fistulous or sinus tract in relation to its surrounding structures.

When using CT, the most common radiographic finding is a thin-rimmed unilocular or multilobular cystic lesion near or within the parotid gland with lack of significant post-contrast rim-enhancement (Fig. 5). Rim-enhancement around the cyst frequently indicates recent or ongoing infection. Fine cut CT images, furthermore, may delineate bony detail as well as a sinus tract to the external auditory canal, assisting the surgeon in his operative planning (Mukherji et al. 1993). It must be noted, however,

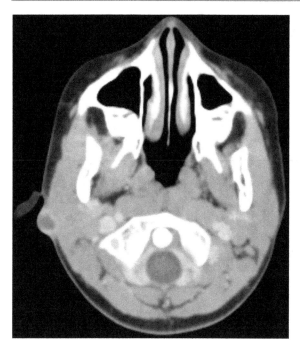

First Branchial Cleft Anomalies, Fig. 5 CT image showing a right first branchial cleft lesion

that in one study looking at all branchial anomalies, CT imaging correctly identified cysts in 95% of cases, sinuses in 81% of cases, and fistulas in only 50% of cases (Schroeder et al. 2007). Thus, imaging is utilized as a guide to the surgeon, recognizing its limitations in identifying the subtleties of these lesions, and is not intended to replace careful surgical dissection.

Ultrasonography has also been used to evaluate first cleft lesions although its use is less frequent. US findings would classically include smooth, well-defined, anechoic lesions; however, they may have variable appearances on US leading to confusion. Perhaps its greatest utility is in differentiating a cystic lesion from a lymph node which can be accomplished using color flow Doppler (Schroeder et al. 2007).

Other medical comorbidities should be considered in the evaluation of patients with a branchial cleft anomaly. These lesions, for example, may occur in conjunction with entities such as branchio-oto-renal syndrome, where patients have hearing loss and renal dysfunction in addition to branchial cleft cysts. The workup for these patients would naturally include an audiogram as well as blood work and/or a renal ultrasound to assess renal function. This syndrome should not be forgotten when evaluating patients with suspected branchial cleft lesions especially when the patient presents with bilateral brachial lesions.

Differential Diagnosis

The differential diagnosis for a first branchial cleft anomaly is broad and largely contingent on the presenting symptoms. The chief presenting symptoms can be divided into auricular, cervical, and parotid. Some patients will present with otorrhea (auricular), others with a draining cutaneous neck tract (cervical), and even others with a lesion overlying or involving the parotid gland (parotid). Thus, the differential diagnosis should be considered for each of these presenting symptoms and/or complaints, acknowledging that patients may present with a combination of these.

For a patient presenting with auricular symptoms, ▶ chronic otitis media with perforation, cholesteatoma, preauricular cyst or sinus, foreign body, and otitis externa must also be entertained. In the presence of a relatively normal ear exam, first branchial cleft anomalies should be considered high on the differential.

For patients presenting with cervical symptoms, scrofula, inflammatory lymphadenitis, skin or metastatic carcinoma, lymphoma, iatrogenic fistula, and trauma should also be considered.

Finally, in patients presenting with parotid symptoms, the differential becomes broader. Diagnoses to consider would include benign inflammatory lymphadenitis, recurrent sialadenitis with or without abscess, dermoid cysts, lymphangioma, lipoma, neurofibroma, hemangioma, metastatic carcinoma, primary parotid tumor, lymphoma, sarcoidosis, and tuberculosis (McRae et al. 1983).

Although the differential diagnosis is broad, a good history and physical exam in addition to proper imaging will correctly diagnose a first branchial anomaly in the vast majority of cases.

Etiology

The etiology of first branchial cleft anomalies requires knowledge of the ▶ embryology of the branchial apparatus. By the fourth week of fetal life, the branchial apparatus begins to form, consisting of six branchial arches separated externally by ectodermal clefts (or grooves) and internally by pharyngeal pouches. A number of head and neck structures develop from this apparatus, and errors in their development can explain numerous pathologies observed in the field of otolaryngology. As embryos develop, each branchial arch gives rise to muscular and cartilaginous components as well as to an artery and nerve. The first arch is composed of two processes, mandibular and maxillary, known collectively as Meckel's cartilage. While Meckel's cartilage gives rise to portions of the malleus and incus, the stylomandibular ligament, and a portion of the mandible, the first arch also yields the mandibular branch of the fifth cranial nerve, the muscles of mastication, the anterior belly of the digastric and the tensor tympani muscles. The second branchial arch gives rise to Reichert's cartilage which yields the malleus handle, long process of incus, stapes superstructure, styloid process, and lesser cornu and superior portion of the hyoid bone. The facial nerve and the muscles of facial expression are also associated with the second branchial arch. The first branchial cleft is the invagination between the first and second branchial arches. The dorsal portion of this groove deepens to form the external auditory canal and the lateral surface of the tympanic membrane while the middle portion forms the cavum conchae. The ventral portion of the cleft typically disappears. The first pouch also contributes to ear formation by developing into the middle ear cleft and Eustachian tube (Hyndman et al. 1929; Olsen et al. 1980).

First branchial anomalies are hypothesized to form due to the failure of complete closure of the ventral portion of the first branchial cleft. Thus, given the embryology, one would expect these lesions to be located somewhere between the structures of the first and second arch and likely in close proximity to the external auditory canal given its derivation from the dorsal portion of the first branchial cleft. Indeed, this is often what is discovered clinically when these lesions are diagnosed. As a general rule, branchial cleft anomalies lie inferior to the embryologic structures of their associated arch and superior to the derivatives of the subsequent arch (Schroeder et al. 2007). Thus, what has been mapped out clinically is a roughly triangular region in which these lesions are found. This region is demarcated by a line traveling from the external auditory canal along the lower edge of the mandible to the tip of the chin, inferiorly to the greater horn of the hyoid bone, and then back laterally and superiorly along the cervical neck to the external canal. In one of the largest case series to date, no lesion extended inferior to the horizontal plane passing through the hyoid bone, thus obeying the embryologic developmental patterns (Triglia et al. 1998).

What is of utmost importance to the surgeon treating these patients is the relationship of these lesions to the facial nerve. The embryologic development of the parotid gland and facial nerve help one to understand why first branchial cleft anomalies may be superficial to, deep to, or within the branches of this important structure (Solares et al. 2003). While the first branchial apparatus completes its differentiation by the sixth or seventh week of gestation, the parotid gland does not appear until the sixth week of development. During the seventh and eighth weeks, the gland migrates cranially and dorsally to achieve its final location. Similarly, the facial nerve and its associated muscles migrate upward around the sixth to eighth weeks. Furthermore, during the second month, the pinna migrates dorsolaterally, and the mandible progressively elongates. The later development of the parotid gland and facial nerve in relation to the first branchial cleft structures as well as the progressive elongation of the mandible as a first branchial arch structure all account for the variability one finds in the relationship of first branchial cleft anomalies to the facial nerve (Olsen et al. 1980; Mukherji et al. 1993).

Treatment

It is widely accepted that the only definitive treatment for first branchial cleft anomalies is complete surgical excision. Surgical management of these lesions can, nonetheless, be challenging given their proximity to the facial nerve as well as patients' frequent history of prior procedures and/or infections. Studies have suggested that multiple preoperative infections increase the risk of recurrence following surgical excision (Schroeder et al. 2007). Therefore, the ideal timing of surgery would be prior to the onset of infection or any attempt at incomplete removal. Unfortunately, this is often not the case. Many patients presenting to an otolaryngologist will not only have had prior infection(s), but also are likely to have had at

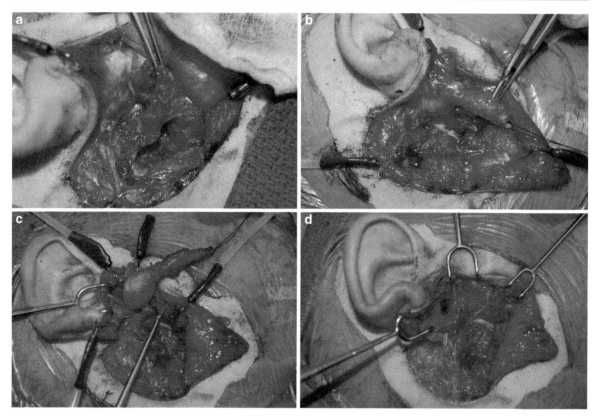

First Branchial Cleft Anomalies, Fig. 6 (**a–d**) Serial photographs taken during a first branchial cleft fistula excision. (**a**) Note the forceps grasping the partially dissected fistula as extensions run deep to an exposed branch of the facial nerve. (**b**) Further dissection of the tract clearly showing its medial course to the frontal branch of the facial nerve. (**c**) The fistula has been passed under the facial nerve (identified by nerve hook), and it continues posteriorly until it involves the external auditory canal. (**d**) Surgical field following complete excision of the fistulous tract. Note the exposed facial nerve branches as well as the necessary defect in the external auditory canal

least an incision and drainage performed (Triglia et al. 1998). Surgical excision is technically more difficult in the face of active infection; thus, it is considered judicious to postpone surgical excision of these lesions until any active or residual infection has cleared (Del Pero et al. 2006).

With few exceptions, wide exposure using a standard parotidectomy incision should be the approach for first cleft surgery. The two overarching goals of this operation are facial nerve preservation and complete surgical excision. Given the variability of the cyst, sinus, or fistula in its relationship to the facial nerve, exposure of the nerve is critical prior to attempting resection of these congenital anomalies (Fig. 6a–d). To obtain this exposure, a partial parotidectomy is likely to be performed (Work et al. 1972). This dissection rarely extends more than 1–2 cm beyond the pes anserinus of CN VII. A literature review of first branchial clefts revealed that the incidence of temporary facial nerve palsy was 21% in cases where the facial nerve was identified and 29% in cases where the nerve was not identified. Similarly, the incidence of permanent facial nerve paralysis in these cases was 1% when the nerve was identified and 12% when the nerve was not identified. These statistics were statistically significant and highlight the importance of nerve identification during this procedure (D'Souza et al. 2002). Most surgeons advocate the use of facial nerve monitoring although the literature does not necessarily address whether this helps preserve facial nerve function during surgery.

Following the exposure and identification of the facial nerve, dissection of the branchial anomaly is

F

undertaken. Lesions may be superficial, deep, or run between the facial nerve branches, and dissection along the sinus or fistulous tracts is important for complete excision. For those lesions with tracts approaching but of questionable involvement of the external auditory canal, it is recommended that a portion of the canal cartilage and skin surrounding the tract be removed in order to assure the lesion does not recur (Olsen et al. 1980; Triglia et al. 1998). If this is performed, some authors advocate packing the external canal for several weeks to allow appropriate healing and prevent canal stenosis (Work et al. 1972; Schroeder et al. 2007). With wide surgical exposure, facial nerve identification, and careful, thorough dissection, the recurrence rate of these lesions is exceedingly low.

Cross-References

▶ Chronic Otitis Media
▶ Congenital Cysts, Sinuses, and Fistulae
▶ Primary Malignancies of Head and Neck in Children (Non-hematologic)

References

Arndal H, Bonding P (1996) First branchial cleft anomaly. Clin Otolaryngol 21:203–207
Arnot RS (1971) Defects of the first branchial cleft. S Afr J Surg 9:93–98
Bajaj Y, Ifeacho S, Tweedie D, Jephson CG, Albert DM, Cochrane LA, Wyatt ME, Jonas N, Hartley BJ (2011) Branchial anomalies in children. Int J Pediatr Otorhinolaryngol 75(8):1020–1023
Choi SS, Zalzal GH (1995) Branchial anomalies: a review of 52 cases. Laryngoscope 105:909–913
Del Pero MM, Majumdar S, Bull PD (2007) Presentation of first branchial cleft anomalies: the Sheffield experience. J Laryngol Otol 121:455–459
D'Souza AR, Uppal HS, De R, Zeitoun H (2002) Updating concepts of first branchial cleft defects: a literature review. Int J Pediatr Otorhinolaryngol 62:103–109
Finn DG, Buchalter IH, Sarti E, Romo T, Chodosh P (1986) First branchial cleft cysts: clinical update. Laryngoscope 97:136–140
Ford GR, Balakrishnan A, Evans JNG, Bailey CM (1992) - Branchial cleft and pouch anomalies. J Laryngol Otol 106:137–143
Hickey SA, Scott GA, Traub P (1994) Defects of the first branchial cleft. J Larygol Otol 108:240–243
Hyndman OR, Light G (1929) The branchial apparatus. Arch Surg 19:410–452

McRae RG, Lee KJ, Goertzen E (1983) First branchial cleft anomalies and the facial nerve. Otololaryngol Head Neck Surg 91:197–202
Mukherji SK, Tart RP, Slattery WH, Stringer SP, Benson MT, Mancuso AA (1993) Evaluation of first branchial anomalies by CT and MR. J Comp Assist Tomogr 17:576–581
Nicollas R, Guelfucci B, Roman S, Triglia JM (2000) Congenital cysts and fistulas of the neck. Int J Pediatr Otorhinolaryngol 55:117–124
Olsen KD, Maragos NE, Weiland LH (1980) First branchial cleft anomalies. Laryngoscope 90:423–436
Roche JP, Younes MN, Funkhouser WK, Weissler MC (2010) Branchiogenic carcinoma of a first branchial cleft cyst. Otolaryngol Head Neck Surg 143:167–168
Schroeder JW, Mohyuddin N, Maddalozzo J (2007) Branchial anomalies in the pediatric population. Otolaryngol Head Neck Surg 137:289–295
Sichel JY, Halperin D, Dano I, Dangoor E (1998) Clinical update on type II first branchial cleft cysts. Laryngoscope 108:1524–1527
Solares CA, Chan J, Koltai PJ (2003) Anatomical variations of the facial nerve in first branchial cleft anomalies. Arch Otolaryngol Head Neck Surg 129:351–355
Triglia JM, Nicollas R, Ducroz V, Koltai PJ, Garabedian EN (1998) First branchial cleft anomalies. Arch Otolaryngol Head Neck Surg 124:291–295
Work WP (1972) Newer concepts of first branchial cleft defects. Laryngoscope 106:137–143

First Branchial Cleft Cyst

▶ First Branchial Cleft Anomalies

First Branchial Cleft Fistula

▶ First Branchial Cleft Anomalies

First Branchial Cleft Sinus

▶ First Branchial Cleft Anomalies

First Echelon Lymph Node

▶ Sentinel Lymph Node

Fisch Classification of Glomus Tumors

Brian C. Gartrell and Samuel P. Gubbels
Department of Surgery, Division of Otolaryngology,
University of Wisconsin Hospital and Clinics,
Madison, WI, USA

Definition

A classification system (A-D) describing glomus tumors based on anatomic location and size, with larger lettering representing more extensive tumors.

Cross-References

▶ Benign Neoplasia, Paragangliomas-Glomus Jugulare
▶ Paragangliomas
▶ Skull Base Neoplasms
▶ Surgical Approaches and Anatomy of the Lateral Skull Base
▶ Vascular Anomalies of Head and Neck

Fisch Infratemporal Fossa Approach

▶ Infratemporal Fossa Approach

Fisch Type A Approach

▶ Jugular Foramen, Approaches

Fisch Type B Approach

▶ Jugular Foramen, Approaches

Fisch Type C Approach

▶ Jugular Foramen, Approaches

Fissures of Santorini

Derek Robinson and Bradley W. Kesser
Department of Otolaryngology-Head and Neck
Surgery, University of Virginia Health System,
Charlottesville, VA, USA

Definition

Vertical fissures in the anterior portion of the external auditory canal cartilage in the region of the bony-cartilaginous junction.

Cross-References

▶ Pinna and External Auditory Canal, Anatomy

Flap Checks

▶ Free Flap Monitoring in Head and Neck Reconstruction

Flap Delay

▶ Delay of Flap

Flexible Esophagoscopy

▶ Transnasal and Rigid Esophagoscopy

Fluency Disorders

Carol Dinnes and Melissa Ghiringhelli
Massachusetts General Hospital, Revere and Chelsea
Healthcare Centers, Department of Speech-Language,
Swallowing Disorders and Reading Disabilities,
Revere/Chelsea, MA, USA

Synonyms

Dysfluency; Stammering; Stuttering

Definition

▶ Stuttering is a communication disorder that is characterized by interruption in the flow of speaking. Dysfluent speech can present as atypical rate, rhythm and/or sound, and word or phrase repetitions, with more serious symptoms including speech prolongations, blocking, or accessory behaviors (e.g., eye blinking, facial grimaces). In addition to physical tension and struggle in their speech muscles, people who stutter often experience embarrassment, anxiety, and fear about speaking. Perception of others' reaction to dysfluent speech may exacerbate stuttering or impact verbal interaction. People who stutter may limit verbal participation in certain activities, or try to hide their dysfluent speech using circumlocution, or pretend to forget what they wanted to say. In everyday conversations, most people produce brief dysfluencies from time to time, such as "um" or "uh." Stuttering is considered a problem when disruptions in the flow of speech are frequent enough to impede communication. The severity of stuttering can range from mild to severe; communication may be impacted in isolated events or pervade communication in all daily activities.

Epidemiology

More than 68 million people worldwide stutter, which is about 1% of the population. In the United States, that is over three million Americans who stutter. Stuttering affects four times as many males as females. Approximately 5% of all children go through a period of stuttering that lasts 6 months or more. Three-quarters of those will recover by late childhood, leaving about 1% with a long-term problem.

Clinical Features

Stuttering can manifest at sound, syllable, word, phrase, sentence, and/or conversational levels. There are many types of dysfluencies. People may present with one, several, or all stuttering patterns. Common features include: interjections such as "um" or "like"; repetitions of words or parts of words (li-li-like this); prolongations of speech sounds (lllllike this), or completely blocked speech (no sound). Some people who stutter appear very tense or "out of breath" when talking. Dysfluent speech can be accompanied by extraneous movements of lips, jaw, or tongue while attempting to speak.

▶ Stuttering may also present "covertly." That is, stuttering may not be visible or audible even to a trained listener as some people who stutter develop strategies to enable smooth communication. However, they report extreme awareness and anxiety in their effort to avoid ▶ dysfluency.

Tests

Fluency disorders are diagnosed using both informal observation and standardized testing with a speech-language pathologist. Standardized test measures, assess speech fluency in speaking and reading tasks as well as the patient's self perception as a verbal communicator. Test scores reflect an individual's performance in comparison to normative data for people at the same age.

Differential Diagnosis

Neurogenic stuttering is a type of fluency disorder which typically appears following an injury or disease to the central nervous system, i.e., the brain and spinal cord, including cortex, subcortex, cerebellar, and even the neural pathway regions. In the majority of cases, the injury or disease that caused the ▶ stuttering can be identified.

Neurogenic stuttering behaviors are similar to those associated with classic fluency disorder (repetitions, prolongations, blocks). However, most people appear unaware of or at least unconcerned with the disruptions in their speech. People speak without apparent effort or struggle, although speech sounds fragmented, halting, or is frequently interrupted. Neurogenic stuttering may occur in any position of a word or sentence, in any class of words and with equal frequency in any type of speaking situation. It can also occur in any vocal behavior such as singing or reciting well-learned passages. Classic strategies to alleviate stuttering are typically not effective for neurogenic stuttering.

Normal nonfluency Between the ages of 2 and 5 years many children experience a period of ▶ dysfluency, which most children will outgrow naturally versus classic stuttering which is likely to worsen. Normal nonfluency often accompanies rapid growth in speech and language development and is typically characterized by easy repetitions of whole words and phrases, and interjections of words or hesitations like "and" or "um."

Psychogenic dysfluency is a disorder of speech fluency that occurs when no medical factors or history of classic stuttering are present. Its appearance may be linked to emotional stress or trauma that the individual has recently experienced.

Cluttering is characterized by an abnormally rapid or irregular speaking rate which may result in excessive dysfluencies (interjections, incomplete phrases/words, revisions), imprecise articulation, frequent pauses, or atypical speech prosody. Cluttering is frequently linked to poor linguistic planning, whereas classic stuttering occurs at the motoric level.

Etiology

There are four factors most likely to contribute to the development of ▶ stuttering:

Genetics: Approximately 60% of those who stutter have a family member who also stutters.

Child development: Children with other speech and language problems or developmental delays are more likely to stutter.

Neurophysiology: Recent neurological research has shown that people who stutter process speech and language slightly differently than those who do not stutter.

Family dynamics: High expectations and fast-paced lifestyles can contribute to stuttering. Children and adults who stutter are no more likely to have psychological or emotional problems than children and adults who do not. There is no reason to believe that emotional trauma causes stuttering.

Treatment

Fluency treatment focuses on teaching specific strategies or behaviors to promote fluent verbal communication. People may learn to monitor and control speech rate, for example, saying words in a slightly slower, prolonged or "easy" manner. They may also learn to coordinate breathing and speaking to reduce and eliminate physical tension. Sessions often begin at the level of syllable or single words and progress to short phrases and sentences. People gradually learn to increase to natural speech rate and fluency in longer and more complex sentences and conversations. Another important treatment approach is increasing positive feelings and attitudes re: self and others, with respect to stuttering. Periodic "maintenance" or "check-in" sessions are often recommended following formal intervention to support continued speech fluency.

Cross-References

▶ Stuttering

References

http://asha.org/public/speech/disorders/stuttering.htm
http://www.nsastutter.org/stutteringInformation/generalInformation.html
http://www.stutteringhelp.org

Flush-Tip Insulated Probe

Angela E. Downes and A. Samy Youssef
Department of Neurosurgery, University of South
Florida, Tampa, FL, USA

Definition

Monopolar electrode composed of a malleable insulated wire on a probe handle with the insulation being continuous to the flush tip and thus minimizes the spread of current to adjacent structures besides the nerve.

Cross-References

▶ Intraoperative Neurophysiologic Monitoring of the Facial Nerve (VII)

Follicular Thyroid Cancer

▶ Well-Differentiated Thyroid Cancer

Follicular Unit Transplantation

Kofi Derek O. Boahene
Department of Otolaryngology-Head and Neck
Surgery, Johns Hopkins University School of
Medicine, Baltimore, MD, USA

Synonyms

Hair transplantation

Definition

Hair follicles naturally occur in a group of 1–4 hair shafts with associated nerves, muscle, sebaceous gland, and blood vessels. This distinct anatomic unit forms the basis of contemporary follicular unit hair transplantation. In follicular unit transplantation (FUT), donor hair is harvested using a long, thin donor strip that is subsequently dissected into individual follicular units with the aid of special microscopes. Under microscopic magnification, extra soft tissue around the harvested follicles is dissected off leaving an intact follicular unit. Alternatively, the donor hair can be extracted with a small, round, 1-mm punch-like instrument which avoids a long scar at the donor site. Follicular unit extraction (FUE) can also be performed with robotic assistance. After preparing the follicular units, the grafts are transplanted into the recipient site created with a 18–20 gauge needle ensuring a snug fit.

Food Intolerance

▶ Feeding Disorders

Food Selectivity

▶ Feeding Disorders

Foramen of Huschke

Derek Robinson and Bradley W. Kesser
Department of Otolaryngology-Head and Neck
Surgery, University of Virginia Health System,
Charlottesville, VA, USA

Definition

Naturally occurring opening in the anterior portion of the bony external auditory canal, resulting from incomplete ossification during development.

Cross-References

▶ Pinna and External Auditory Canal, Anatomy

Forehead Flap

▶ Interpolation Flaps

Foreign Bodies of Esophagus and Airway

Ari DeRowe
Pediatric Otolaryngology Unit, Dana-Dewek
Children's Hospital, Tel Aviv Sourasky Medical
Center, Tel Aviv University, Sackler School
of Medicine, Tel-Aviv, Israel

Airway

Foreign body aspiration in children can be a life-threatening accident. In children under 1 year old it is the most common cause of accidental death (Mofenson and Greensher 1985; Digoy 2008). Primary care physicians can help prevent such tragedies by educating parents regarding the hazards of small objects and nuts in the child's environment (Karatzanis et al. 2007). The child's anatomy; lack of teeth, specifically molar

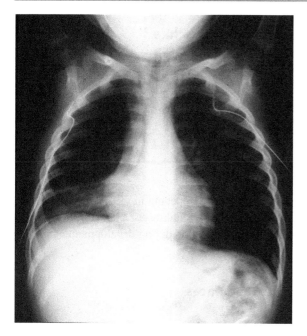

Foreign Bodies of Esophagus and Airway, Fig. 1 AP chest x-ray of plastic foreign body in right main bronchus of 7 year old

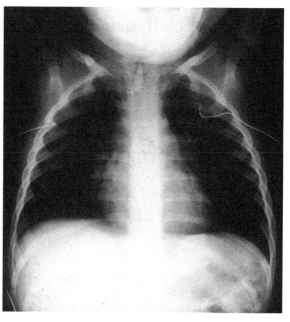

Foreign Bodies of Esophagus and Airway, Fig. 2 Same child shortly after presentation with respiratory distress. The foreign body has dislodged into the trachea

for chewing; the tendency to explore the surroundings orally; and yet undeveloped neuromuscular swallowing and breathing reflexes put the child at risk.

The evaluation of a child with suspected foreign body aspiration requires initial evaluation of urgency. If the child is in respiratory distress or has a suspected laryngotracheal foreign body, urgent intervention is required. Otherwise careful history and diagnostic workup are important. The type of foreign body should be ascertained. Great emphasis should be placed on history. When a choking event is followed by persistent respiratory symptoms, a foreign body aspiration is suspected and rigid bronchoscopy for diagnosis and management is indicated. Physical exam including auscultation is performed. One-sided decreased breath sounds are common in bronchial foreign bodies but the physical exam may be normal putting emphasis on the clinical history. Additional workup may include chest x-ray or fluoroscopy. Figures 1 and 2 show how unpredictable foreign body management can be. In Fig. 1, the foreign body appears to be in the right main bronchus. Following deteriorated breathing, another chest x-ray (Fig. 2) was performed, revealing a tracheal foreign body requiring emergent management. Figure 3 is an example of a laryngeal foreign

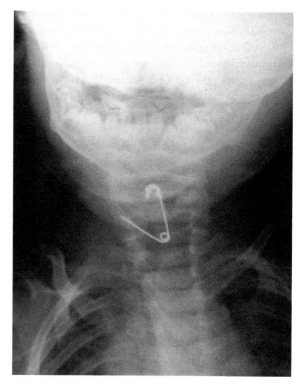

Foreign Bodies of Esophagus and Airway, Fig. 3 Laryngeal foreign body (safety pin) in a 6 month old

body in an 8 month old requiring emergent management. In the emergent situation, management is best carried out in the operating room with trained staff and appropriate equipment. Fasting status is not relevant.

Batteries, especially the small disk variety, are foreign bodies that are highly corrosive to the aerodigestive tract. Emergent removal is also indicated in these cases.

Rigid bronchoscopy remains the gold standard in the evaluation of tracheobronchial pathologies. In therapeutic interventions such as foreign body removal, the ability to manipulate the foreign body while simultaneously ventilating the patient through the rigid bronchoscope allows for safe and expedient removal. The introduction of rigid optics and video-endoscopic monitoring provided a quantum leap in diagnostic accuracy and safety of the procedure.

The decision to perform rigid bronchoscopy can be difficult. Risks of the procedure include damage to vocal cords, laryngeal edema, perforation of tracheobronchial tree, pneumothorax, tension pneumothorax, pneumomediastinum, hemorrhage into the airway causing respiratory failure, and damage to teeth. Also, anesthetic risks should be considered, especially in a small child with concurrent respiratory disease. On the other hand, the risk of a retained foreign body is considerable and can lead to respiratory failure, bronchiectasis, lung sequestration, and even death. Careful preoperative planning and setup for all possible scenarios can help avoid these complications allowing for a safe rigid bronchoscopy.

The classic history of a healthy child, a choking event followed by persistent respiratory symptoms is not always the case. Many times the choking incident is not witnessed and respiratory symptoms can mimic an URTI, asthma, or persistent pneumonia. In these cases a high level of suspicion is required to avoid delayed diagnosis and subsequent complications. This high index of suspicion is even more important in neurologically impaired children who are at increased risk for foreign body aspiration and delay of diagnosis (DeRowe et al. 2002). Aspirated vegetable material such as nuts is especially dangerous as the hydrophilic material expands and a severe reaction in the bronchus results in complete obstruction, granulation tissue formation, and great difficulty during bronchoscopy for extraction.

Chest x-rays may help with the diagnosis especially when history is inadequate. Hyperinflation on

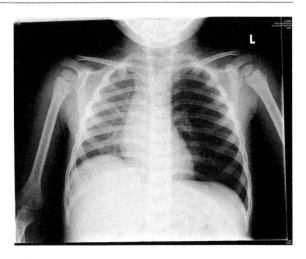

Foreign Bodies of Esophagus and Airway, Fig. 4 Chest x-ray showing hyperinflation of the left lung and mediastinal deviation to the right. Hallmarks of a radio-opaque foreign body in the left main bronchus

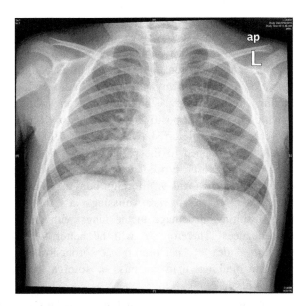

Foreign Bodies of Esophagus and Airway, Fig. 5 Same child as in Fig. 4 following removal of peanut from the left main bronchus

the effected side with mediastinal deviation to the healthy side is a classic finding as seen in Fig. 4. This effect is relieved after removal on follow-up x-ray in Fig. 5. However, in many cases the chest x-ray can initially appear normal. Auscultation may

Foreign Bodies of Esophagus and Airway, Fig. 6 Operating room setup for rigid bronchoscopy

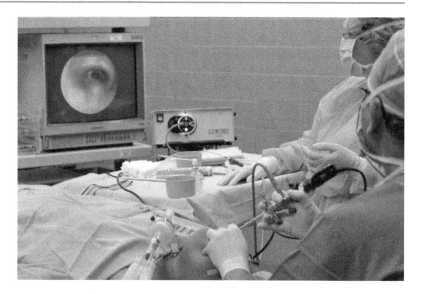

reveal decreased breath sounds or unilateral wheezing; however, normal breath sounds may also be misleading. This makes the diagnosis difficult. When the history of a choking episode is evident and there are persistent symptoms such as cough, fever, or dyspnea or any physical or radiographic findings, bronchoscopy is indicated. In an asymptomatic child with a positive choking history bronchoscopy can be deferred (Cohen et al. 2009). It should be explained to the parents that bronchoscopy is a diagnostic procedure with the possibility of therapeutic removal of a foreign body. Avoiding bronchoscopy may risk missing a foreign body resulting in damage to the lungs with grave consequences. Therefore, it will be better to err on the side of performing a bronchoscopy with no findings than to miss a foreign body (Cohen et al. 2009).

The diagnostic conundrum increases when there is no history of a choking episode. More subtle symptoms such as pneumonia unresponsive to antibiotics, wheezing unresponsive to treatment, or incidental physical or radiographic signs exist. Again a high index of suspicion is warranted. In such a situation flexible bronchoscopy under sedation may be the diagnostic procedure of choice. If a foreign body is found, the patient can proceed directly to rigid bronchoscopy for removal. Some centers suggest flexible

bronchoscopy is adequate for foreign body removal. However, the precarious nature of some foreign bodies and lack of control of the airway raise doubt regarding safety (Nicolai 2001). Communication between the pediatric otolaryngologist and pediatric pulmonologist is essential in these difficult cases.

The procedure is undertaken in the operating room preferably in a tertiary pediatric center with experienced staff, facilities, and equipment. The Otolaryngologist and Anesthesiologist share the airway and during all stages of the procedure communication is imperative (Zur and Litman 2009). Figure 6 is an example of the operative setup. Rigid bronchoscopy allows for simultaneous visualization, suctioning, manipulation of the foreign object, and ventilation. Documentation for academic and medicolegal considerations should be recorded via the video-endoscopic monitor. When dealing with a difficult airway always consider inability to secure the airway with the bronchoscope. A setup should include the possibility for emergency tracheotomy.

The bronchoscope is introduced while visualizing the vocal cords with the laryngoscope and observed on the video monitor. When the whole team can follow the procedure on the screen anxiety in the OR is reduced, increasing the safety of the procedure.

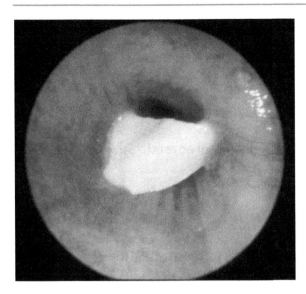

Foreign Bodies of Esophagus and Airway, Fig. 7 Peanut in left main bronchus as seen in rigid bronchoscopy

Retrieval of the foreign body is performed with optical forceps. The endoscopic view of Fig. 7 is the peanut that caused the left bronchial obstruction first seen in Fig. 4.

Esophagus

Many incidents of swallowed foreign bodies go unnoticed since there is not necessarily a choking incident. The peak incidence is 3 years of age. Many blunt and small items can pass through the digestive track without sequel. Impaction results in symptoms of dysphagia and drooling. In cases of large foreign body impaction respiratory symptoms may coexist due to tracheal compression (Reilly et al. 1996). Sharp foreign body and disk battery ingestion are emergencies because of risk of esophageal perforation. Coins are a common offender. Smaller coins such as dimes may pass the digestive system uneventfully and can be followed by serial x-rays. Children at risk include those who underwent previous esophageal surgery, e.g., tracheoesophageal fistula repair, and neurologically impaired children. In any case of suspicion a diagnosis should be made expediently. The risks of a retained esophageal foreign body include esophageal perforation, mediastinitis, sepsis, and stricture

formation. Rare complications include tracheoesophageal fistula and erosion into major vessels such as the aorta possibly leading to fatal hemorrhage. Chest x-ray AP+LAT are adequate for a radio-opaque foreign body; however, since many are plastic or food material plain x-rays may not be enough. A modified barium swallow may help in such cases. Computed Tomography may also help. However, even with negative studies and a reasonable suspicion, esophagoscopy should be performed as a diagnostic and therapeutic modality. There is ongoing debate regarding the optimal endoscopic management of esophageal foreign bodies. As endoscopic techniques improve there is a shift toward flexible esophagoscopy by pediatric gastroenterologists as modality of choice (Katsinelos et al. 2006). However, this is largely dependent on institution policies. Rigid esophagoscopy may have more of a risk to damage of teeth and trauma to the esophagus. In skilled hands these risks are negligible. Other techniques such as blind bougienage or balloon catheter extraction should be avoided especially in small children where the risk of airway compromise outweighs the advantages. Risks of the procedure must be discussed with the child's caregivers and weighed against the risks of a retained foreign body (Uyemura 2005).

Summary

Choking is life threatening in children. If the child survives the event, other complications, such as anoxic brain damage, sepsis, and respiratory failure, may occur. Great efforts should be made to avoid such incidents with severe regulations regarding small parts in the child's surroundings and feeding children with age appropriate foods. Balloons, latex gloves, and similar objects are especially deadly. Airway compromise, disk batteries and sharp objects require emergent management. Advances in endoscopic diagnostic and removal techniques have improved management and outcomes in these cases. Since not all episodes are witnessed a high level of suspicion is required when children present with suggestive symptoms. Parents should be educated regarding choking dangers.

References

Cohen S, Avital A, Godfrey S, Gross M, Kerem E, Springer C (2009) Suspected foreign body inhalation in children: what are the indications for bronchoscopy? J Pediatr 155:276–280

DeRowe A, Massick D, Beste DJ (2002) Clinical characteristics of aero-digestive foreign bodies in neurologically impaired children. Int J Pediatr Otorhinolaryngol 62(3):243–248

Digoy GP (2008) Diagnosis and management of upper aerodigestive tract foreign bodies. Otolaryngol Clin N Am 41:485–496

Karatzanis AD, Vardouniotis A, Moschandreas J et al (2007) The risk of foreign body aspiration in children can be reduced with proper education of the general population. Int J Pediatr Otorhinolaryngol 71:311–315

Katsinelos P, Kountouras J, Paroutoglou G, Zavos C, Mimidis K, Chatzimavroudis G (2006) Endoscopic techniques and management of foreign body ingestion and food bolus impaction in the upper gastrointestinal tract: a retrospective analysis of 139 cases. J Clin Gastroenterol 40:784–789

Mofenson HC, Greensher J (1985) Management of the choking child. Pediatr Clin North Am 32:183–192

Nicolai T (2001) Pediatric bronchoscopy. Pediatr Pulmonol 31:150–164

Reilly JS, Cook SP, Stool D, Rider G (1996) Prevention and management of aerodigestive foreign body injuries in childhood. Pediatr Clin North Am 43(6):1403–1411

Uyemura MC (2005) Foreign body ingestion in children. Am Fam Physician 72:287–291, 292

Zur KB, Litman RS (2009) Pediatric airway foreign body retrieval: surgical and anesthetic perspectives. Pediatric Anesthesia 19(suppl 1):109–117

Fossa of Rosenmuller

Ojas A. Shah and Ravindhra G. Elluru
Department of Otolaryngology, Cincinnati Children's Hospital and University of Cincinnati College of Medicine, Cincinnati, OH, USA

Definition

Pharyngeal recess which lies directly posterior and superior to the torus tubarius.

Cross-References

▶ Eustachian Tube, Anatomy and Physiology

Four-Flap Z-Plasty

▶ Z-plasty

Frameless Stereotactic Surgery

▶ Computer Assistance in Sinus Surgery

Frankfort Horizontal Plane

Derek Robinson and Bradley W. Kesser
Department of Otolaryngology-Head and Neck Surgery, University of Virginia Health System, Charlottesville, VA, USA

Definition

In profile view, a plane connecting the highest point of the opening of the external auditory canal with the lowest point on the lower margin of the orbit, used to orient a human skull or head so that the plane is horizontal.

Cross-References

▶ Pinna and External Auditory Canal, Anatomy

Free Flap

▶ Free Tissue Transfer in the Head and Neck, Complications

Free Flap Complications

▶ Donor Site Complications in Free Flap Surgery

Free Flap Monitoring in Head and Neck Reconstruction

Miriam O'Leary
Department of Otolaryngology, Tufts Medical Center, Boston, MA, USA

Synonyms

Doppler monitoring; Flap checks

Definition

Free flap monitoring is continuous or intermittent assessment of a free flap's blood supply in the early postoperative period.

Purpose

The purpose of free flap monitoring is early detection of venous congestion or arterial insufficiency, so that the patient may be brought back to the operating room as soon as possible to attempt flap salvage. In the operating room, the donor and recipient arteries and veins are closely examined for obstruction; the causes (thrombosis, kinking or twisting of the pedicle, extrinsic compression) are corrected as quickly as possible to restore normal arterial inflow and venous outflow for the flap.

Principle

The principle of free flap monitoring is to evaluate for changes in the arterial supply and venous drainage of the free flap in the early postoperative period. The most common cause of free flap failure is venous thrombosis, followed by arterial thrombosis. These events almost always occur within the first 72 h after surgery, so this is the critical period for frequent monitoring.

Indication

Free flap monitoring is indicated for every microvascular free tissue transfer.

Contraindication

There is no contraindication to free flap monitoring. However, certain methods of monitoring may not be appropriate or feasible in specific cases. The microsurgeon decides at the time of surgery which method(s) of monitoring to employ.

Advantage/Disadvantage

The advantage of free flap monitoring is early detection of free flap vascular compromise, which can facilitate flap salvage. New flap monitoring techniques allow "buried" flaps to be monitored, even though they cannot be visually inspected. Indirect methods of monitoring evaluate parameters such as flap oxygen saturation and metabolic byproducts.

The disadvantage of free flap monitoring is that some methods of monitoring may give false-negative and/or false-positive results. Some methods are unreliable and may not work or stop working even if the flap is viable. This could result in unnecessary return to the operating room for exploration. Doppler monitoring of the arterial signal may provide a false sense of security since the arterial pulse will persist for some time even in the presence of venous congestion. The team may not determine that the flap is failing until it is too late to attempt salvage.

Introduction

Microvascular free tissue transfer has revolutionized head and neck surgery, and is now widely utilized by head and neck surgeons throughout the world. The success of free flaps depends upon technically sound, functional anastomoses between donor and recipient arteries and veins, as well as adequate microcirculation within the tissues of the flap. Multiple studies have reported a 95% success rate of free flaps in head and neck reconstruction. However, flap failure can still occur in the early postoperative period due to occlusion of the vascular pedicle. Careful and intensive monitoring during this time allows rapid detection of compromised blood supply, and facilitates flap salvage rates of up to 50%. Protocols vary from surgeon to surgeon, but generally free flaps are monitored every 1–2 h for the first 48–72 h after surgery

(Wang et al. 2009). Over the past few decades, free flap monitoring has evolved from simple bedside clinical assessments to use of sophisticated instrumentation. Choice of free flap monitoring method depends on multiple factors, including the surgeon's experience and preference, type and location of flap, and availability of resources.

Clinical Parameters of Skin Paddle

For free flaps that contain a skin paddle, direct inspection of the skin is a mainstay of flap monitoring (Table 1). A skin paddle with adequate blood supply will be slightly pink in color. This may be difficult to assess if the natural skin color of the flap is pale compared to the surrounding tissues (e.g., oral cavity mucosa), or conversely if the patient has darkly pigmented skin. When testing for capillary refill, the skin will blanch and then the color will return in 1–2 s. The skin paddle will be warm to touch, although this can be a misleading parameter, especially for an intraoral skin paddle, which is surrounded by warm mucosal surfaces on all sides. Pricking the skin paddle with a needle will yield bright red blood from the dermis within 5 s. The parameters of color, warmth, tissue turgor, and response to pinprick can also be assessed by direct inspection in muscle-only flaps (Table 1).

Partial or complete obstruction of the venous anastomosis will become evident as venous congestion of the skin paddle. An early sign of venous congestion is abnormally fast capillary refill (less than 1 s). The skin color will become dusky and eventually turn blue-purple. The skin will appear and feel distended, swollen, and tense. Pricking the skin with a needle will produce immediate return of dark-colored blood from the dermis. Partial or complete obstruction of the arterial supply to the flap will manifest as ischemia. This is much less common than venous congestion. In the case of arterial occlusion, the skin paddle will be pale or mottled blue and cool to the touch. Capillary refill will be slow (more than 2 s) or absent. The tissue turgor will be decreased and the skin may have a "prune-like" appearance. Pinprick of the skin will not yield any blood, but may yield serum (Table 1).

A sudden arterial or venous obstruction such as a thrombosis will cause an abrupt and marked change

Free Flap Monitoring in Head and Neck Reconstruction, Table 1 Clinical parameters of skin paddle

Clinical parameter	Normal circulation	Venous occlusion	Arterial occlusion
Color	Pink	Blue/purple	Pale or mottled blue
Capillary refill time	1–2 s	<1 s	>2 s, or absent
Dermal bleeding	Bright red blood within 5 s	Immediate dark blood	No bleeding
Tissue turgor	Full	Tense/distended/ swollen	Hollow, "prunelike"
Temperature	Warm	Warm to cool	Cool

in these parameters from one flap check to the next. A gradual or partial obstruction will cause more subtle changes over time. For buried flaps with a skin paddle, a portion of the skin paddle can be exteriorized to allow visual inspection. Serial digital images or video footage can be taken to monitor skin paddle color over time, and can even be transmitted to the surgeon at home via the internet, although this permits evaluation of only one parameter of the flap. The disadvantage of using clinical parameters to monitor a free flap is that experience and good clinical judgment are necessary to properly interpret these findings. The experience of nursing staff and residents performing these flap checks may vary widely, and ultimately impact the ability to detect vascular compromise at an early, potentially salvageable, stage.

Doppler Monitoring

Serial evaluation of arterial and venous Doppler signals is another mainstay of free flap monitoring. Loss of the Doppler signal heralds occlusion of the venous or arterial pedicle. The simplest way to monitor Doppler signals is to mark sites on the patient's skin and/or on the flap itself, where the flap artery and vein(s) can be detected by a Doppler probe. A normal arterial Doppler signal is strong, staccato, and triphasic. A normal venous signal is fainter, more continuous, and may sound like rushing wind. It is optimal to monitor both the artery and vein separately; this may not always be possible due to the geometry of the vascular pedicle and the thickness of the overlying tissues. But it is imperative to understand that an arterial signal will persist for several hours in the face of complete venous obstruction, since the arterial system is high pressure and the venous system is low pressure (Funk et al. 2010).

Doppler signals can also be monitored continuously with the use of an implantable device. This consists of a 20 MHz ultrasonic probe mounted on a silicone cuff which the surgeon wraps around the venous pedicle. The probe is connected to a thin wire which is brought out through the wound and plugged into a monitor at the patient's bedside. The venous Doppler signal is continuously audible to anyone at the patient's bedside, and therefore simple to follow. Between postoperative day 5 and 10, the probe can be separated from the cuff and removed from the wound by gently pulling on the wire. Sudden loss of the Doppler signal can indicate venous occlusion, but changes in patient position may alter the position of the probe and lead to loss of signal. Proper placement of the cuff and securing of the wire are crucial to the success of this monitoring modality. Notable false-positive and false-negative rates have been reported using implantable Doppler probes (Farwell and Luu 2009). This system is used most commonly for buried flaps, such as in pharyngoesophageal reconstruction, but is applicable to any free flap.

Color Duplex Sonography

Color duplex ultrasonography is another method for monitoring free flap vascularity. This noninvasive modality records blood flow velocity and direction, and can be examined both within the flap and in the recipient vessels. The combined color flow and spectral images provide a precise and quantitative analysis of blood inflow and outflow for the flap. However, this monitoring modality necessitates ultrasonography expertise, as well as knowledge of the flap vessel geometry for that patient. Practically speaking, the microvascular surgeon and a radiologist both have to be present during the ultrasound to yield useful information from this study. Therefore, it is not feasible to use this monitoring modality more than once a day (Smit et al. 2010).

Laser Doppler Flowmetry

Laser Doppler flowmetry is a continuous noninvasive monitoring modality. In this system, a coherent laser light is delivered through a fiber-optic cable to illuminate flap tissue. The same probe collects the light that is reflected back, and a frequency shift is detected by the system. The power-spectral density of shifted light varies with the velocity of moving cells in the tissue. Therefore, the probe can follow trends in the velocity of flap blood flow in order to identify an anastomotic occlusion. The probe can detect blood flow to a depth of 8 mm in the flap tissue. With this monitoring modality, trends in blood flow velocity are more important than absolute measurements, especially in cases of venous congestion. The probe must secure firmly to the flap tissue, and motion of the probe or tissue can interfere with readings. Laser Doppler flowmetry has been combined with tissue spectrometry and temperature sensors to improve the monitoring accuracy (Smit et al. 2010).

Near-Infrared Spectroscopy

Near-infrared spectroscopy (NIS) is another noninvasive continuous method for evaluating flap vascularity. NIS functions similar to a pulse oximeter in following free flap vascularity. It uses optical spectrometry to measure the hemoglobin content and oxygenation of tissues. A probe is attached to the flap which delivers specific wavelengths of near-infrared light to the flap tissue. Hemoglobin in the tissue selectively absorbs the light and therefore reduces the light intensity; this altered optic signal from the flap tissue is analyzed to determine the hemoglobin concentration in the tissues. The near-infrared light can penetrate tissue up to a depth of 2 cm. The monitor displays the result as an oxygen saturation, which is a familiar and easy parameter for all levels of health care providers to follow (Wang et al. 2009). Studies have demonstrated that NIS can detect vascular compromise before it is clinically evident. The measurements are apparently not affected by movements of the probe, although obviously the probe needs to be attached to the flap in a secure manner, which must also be easy to remove when it is no longer needed; this may be challenging in flaps which are difficult to access. Also, the probe only covers a small area of the flap, which may not be representative of the whole (Farwell and Luu 2009). These NIS systems are fivefold more expensive than the implantable Doppler system, and twice as expensive as the laser Doppler flowmeter.

Microdialysis

Microdialysis is an invasive monitoring modality which is not in widespread clinical use. For this system, a double-lumen microdialysis catheter the size of an 18-gauge needle is placed into the flap tissues. This catheter is connected to a small pump which instills physiologic fluid through the catheter and across a dialysis membrane, where it equilibrates with interstitial fluid of the flap tissues. Samples of the perfusate are analyzed for levels of glucose, lactate, pyruvate, and glycerol metabolites, which indicate the metabolic status of the flap. If the glucose level decreases and the lactate to pyruvate ratio increases, it indicates that anaerobic metabolism is occurring, which signifies arterial compromise. Increasing glycerol levels indicate cell membrane damage, which can occur in either venous congestion or arterial insufficiency. Like NIS, microdialysis can identify vascular compromise before clinical signs develop. However, it takes practice to learn how to use the system, and each fluid analysis takes 30 min (Smit et al. 2010). It is also much more expensive than other monitoring system currently in use.

Conclusion

There are multiple different ways of monitoring arterial supply and venous drainage of a free flap in the early postoperative period. The most basic method, and still most widely used, is clinical inspection of the flap with attention to specific clinical parameters. But several other modalities are available which can detect vascular compromise before it is clinically apparent, and therefore optimize the surgeon's ability to salvage a compromised flap. Use of more than one monitoring modality can provide complementary data about the flap's vascularity. Most head and neck microvascular surgeons in this country utilize clinical inspection plus Doppler monitoring (Spiegel and Polat 2007). Sophisticated instruments have been developed

to analyze many other indicators of a flap's viability. However, more information must be balanced against cost-effectiveness, as the newer technologies are many times more expensive than clinical inspection or use of a handheld Doppler. Ultimately, no matter what method is used to monitor a free flap in the early postoperative period, the microsurgeon's experience and clinical judgment will determine which flaps return to the operating room for exploration and potential salvage.

Cross-References

► Angiosome
► Fasciocutaneous Flaps
► Fibula Free Flap
► Free Tissue Transfer in Head and Neck
► Free Tissue Transfer in the Head and Neck, Complications
► Musculocutaneous Flap
► Osseocutaneous Flaps
► Perforator Flaps
► Subscapular System Flaps

References

Farwell DG, Luu Q (2009) Advances in free flap monitoring: have we gone too far? Curr Opin Otolaryngol 17:267–269

Funk GF, Blackwell KE, Heffelfinger RN (2010) Complications of free tissue transfer in head & neck reconstruction. In: Urken ML (ed) Multidisciplinary head & neck reconstruction a defect-oriented approach. Lippincott Williams & Wilkins, Philadelphia, pp 45–80

Smit JM, Zeebregts CJ et al (2010) Advancements in free flap monitoring in the last decade: a critical review. Plast Reconstr Surg 125:177–185

Spiegel JH, Polat JK (2007) Microvascular flap reconstruction by otolaryngologists: prevalence, postoperative care, and monitoring techniques. Laryngoscope 117:485–490

Wang SJ, Teknos TN, Chepeha DB (2009) Complicatinos of free-tissue transfer. In: Eisele DW, Smith RV (eds) Complications in head and neck surgery, 2nd edn. Mosby, Philadelphia, pp 795–811

Free Flaps

► Classification of Flaps

Free Tissue Transfer in Head and Neck

Mark K. Wax[1], Daniel S. Schneider[2] and
Lindau Robert H. III [3,4]
[1]Department of Otolaryngology-Head and Neck
Surgery, Oregon Health and Science University,
Portland, OR, USA
[2]Microvascular/Facial Plastic Surgery, Oregon
Health & Science University, Portland, USA
[3]Univeristy of Nebraska Medical Center, Omaha,
NE, USA
[4]Nebreska Methodist Estabrook Cancer Center,
Omaha, NE, USA

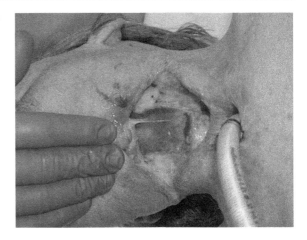

Free Tissue Transfer in Head and Neck, Fig. 1 This patient has had a laryngectomy with bilateral neck dissections. He was reconstructed primarily, but his wounds did not heal. Given time he could be reconstructed

Introduction

Reconstruction of ablative defects of the head and neck has undergone an evolutionary shift and growth over the last decades. Prior to the introduction of antibiotics, surgical treatment of head and neck mucosal cancer, while successful in small volume disease, was fraught with multiple complications due to the high rate of infection. With the advent of good antibiotic prophylaxis and improved anesthesia techniques, the ability to resect tumors in the head and neck area with acceptable morbidity and mortality was markedly improved. Many of the ablative procedures that are performed today can trace their routes to anatomical dissection and ablations that were performed many decades ago. While there have been many innovations in the technique of surgical ablation, the anatomic foundation that underlies the tissue blocks to be removed has not changed. Unfortunately, removal of composite tissue of the head and neck for oncologic reasons is complicated by the reconstructive process. The structures that are often times resected are involved in many of the important functions of the upper aerodigestive tract. Communication is an essential aspect of quality of life. Proper communication involves not only the production of sound but it is modulation to form understandable language. In order to produce acceptable and understandable sounds many structures of the upper aerodigestive tract are involved. These start at the larynx with the production of sound and then it is modulation by the structures of the oral cavity and

tongue. The abilities to chew, swallow, and eat are all intricately related to the structures starting in the lips and proceeding down into the cervical esophagus. Any reconstructive modality of these structures must consider these multiple functions. The composite tissues involved in these functions; mucosa with its supple motion, the underlying soft tissue, the soft tissue supportive structures whether they are cartilage or bone, and the muscular three-dimensional movements that are required for these functions all have important ramifications when considering reconstruction.

Using minimal reconstructive techniques with local tissue, most patients will still heal although the functional and cosmetic sequelae can be quite considerable. The Andy Gump deformity and the chronic fistula patient are all familiar to older surgeons who have lived through the era prior to the introduction of improved reconstructive techniques (Fig. 1) (Briant 1977). The priority of reconstructive surgeons is now to functionally rehabilitate the patient. To do this, it has been found that the best method of reconstruction involves replacement of the composite soft tissue defects with composite soft tissue. The use of a pedicled flap with the pectoralis major muscle revolutionized reconstruction in that it brought vascularized tissue from an untreated area that was remarkably healthy and allowed for healing and closure of many of the chronic wounds seen in our head

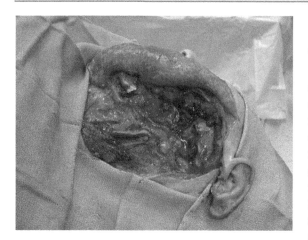

Free Tissue Transfer in Head and Neck, Fig. 2 This defect includes the mandible, maxilla, lateral temporal bone, and skull base. The volume and complexity of the defect requires multiple high volume composite tissues

and neck oncologic practice (Liu et al. 2001). This flap became the work horse for reconstruction. It allowed patients to leave the hospital at much earlier times and remarkably decreased the morbidity of the procedure in the postoperative period. However, the lack of ability to conform this tissue to a three-dimensional structure, a lack of bone, and limitations on its arc of rotation meant that it was still limited in the functional rehabilitation and somewhat in its reconstructive use. There remained a number of problem area in head and neck reconstruction that were poorly addressed by regional pedicled flaps. Pharyngo-esophageal reconstruction, ▶ mandibular reconstruction, and ▶ skull base reconstruction were all compromised, although improved, with the use of the pectoralis major flap (Fig. 2). Improvements in intra- and postoperative care along with the expansion of radiation and chemotherapy techniques saw the complexity of reconstructive needs multiply dramatically. Free tissue transfer allowed for replacement of the composite tissue defect with a vascularized source of composite tissue. Bone and large volume soft tissue defects could be replaced with bone and soft tissue from distal parts of the body. A multitude of donor sites allowed one to tailor the replacement tissue with similar structured tissue and volumes (Rosenthal et al. 2007). Thus, as the continued use of free tissue transfer progressed, the functional and aesthetic outcomes were improved.

Historical Perspectives

The history of microvascular surgery extends back to 1759 when Howell employed a pin and circumferential suture technique (Watts 1907). Up until the early 1900s, several different materials were used as a permanent intravascular stent. Vascular structures were then tied over the top of these stents. The continued exposure to foreign bodies, along with the decreasing cross-sectional diameter, did not allow for much success or for long-term patency. Alex Currell, in 1902, successfully transplanted a segment of small bowel into the neck of a dog, using the jugular and carotid artery as recipient vessels (Carrel 1902). The subsequent introduction of the operating room microscope set the stage for expanded application for small vessel work. In 1957 Sitenberg et al. was credited with the first successful clinical application of a free tissue transfer (Seidenberg et al. 1959). While the patient died on postoperative day seven, the autopsy confirmed a patent anastamosis. Continued work over the next decades involved incorporation of microsurgical techniques with an operating room microscope and better suture placement in the laboratory. Reports of 100% patency rates in dogs and rabbits became quite common.

Refinements in the use of end-to-end and end-to-side anastamosis in the late to mid-60s allowed for consistent patency and survival of transferred tissues with dissimilar vessel diameters. Refinements in instrumentation introduced by Buncky and Ackland set the state for a consistent free tissue experience in the human setting (Acland 1977). In the 1970s, many authors explored and described the vascular anatomy in sites ranging from the radial forearm to the iliac crest, composite bone and soft tissue and muscle flap, based on a single vascular pedicle. In 1977 Panje and colleagues are credited with the first groin transfer flap for oral pharyngeal reconstruction following cancer ablation (Panje et al. 1977). Subsequent to that, the introduction of free tissue transfer was popularized in the Otolaryngology literature (Urken 1991; Hayden 1991). With the advent of increasing technical expertise available in Otolaryngology, free tissue transfer became a reliable and highly successful alternative to pedicle flap reconstruction.

Today, the majority of Otolaryngology – Head and Neck Surgery programs have a number of microvascular trained head and neck oncologic, ablative, and reconstructive surgeons on faculty who perform the majority of the reconstructions.

Characteristics of Free Tissue Used in the Head and Neck

Tissues available for composite free tissue transfer can be harvested from almost any anatomic site. A characteristic of the human anatomy is that significant anatomic structures are often supplied proximally by a named arterial vessel that is accompanied by venous outflow from that area. Thus most anatomic sites can trace their dominant blood supply to a single named vascular pedicle. Another fortunate characteristic is that many soft tissue structures have anastomotic plexus with local tissues supplied by different vascular plexus. Thus sacrifice of the main vascular pedicle does not adversely affect the local surrounding tissues. This concept of overlapping vascular supply is often referred to as the angiosome concept. In this model, the primary area of supply is considered the first ► angiosome, while the overlapping area is considered the second angiosome. The adjacent tissues that are independent of the neighboring vascular supply are considered the third angiosome (Taylor et al. 2011).

One must remember that the tissue that is being used for reconstruction comes from a distant site. While in that site it had a certain function. Harvesting this tissue for transfer can leave a functional deficit based on the tissues removed or the dissection process itself. For example, harvesting the radial forearm fasciocutaneous flap involves removal of skin, subcutaneous tissue, and fascia, along with the radial artery from the forearm. Similarly harvesting the ► fibula osteocutaneous free flap involves extensive dissection of all compartments of the lower leg. It also involves sacrifice of one of the vascular supplies to the leg and the placement of a split thickness skin graft in a compromised bed. Thus there are a number of factors that determine the anatomic donor sites that one can or wishes to use for reconstruction.

Donor Site Considerations

The first and foremost consideration in deciding which donor site to use is can that particular donor site tolerate the sacrifice of a vascular and anatomic unit. The ► fibular flap is an excellent replacement for bony and soft tissue components in the jaw or maxilla; however, harvesting from that site requires removal of the peroneal artery which is one of the three vessels supplying the lower leg and foot. Unfortunately, a significant number of patients in the head and neck oncologic practice also have peripheral vascular disease due to underlying comorbidities. In these patients, vascular supply to the distal extremity may be compromised from the normal. Sacrifice of the peroneal artery may significantly affect the wound healing characteristics of the lower leg. Loss of the foot or toes has been rarely reported.

Another consideration in deciding which tissue site to use in free flap reconstruction is what the ablative defect encompasses. Composite tissue defects are best reconstructed with composite free tissue flaps. Thus, resection of the bone and soft tissue is best replaced with bone and soft tissue. Removal of soft, three-dimensional structures such as the tongue or soft palate, require replacement with a supple three-dimensional structure. Large volume defects, such as skull base, maxillectomy, or orbital exenterations require large volume replacement with tissues that can be supplely manipulated to obliterate the defect. Each of these particular defects brings with it reconstructive needs that must be addressed by the tissue that is to be harvested from a distant site. Oftentimes it is possible to match the donor site tissue characteristics and volume to the tissues that were removed from the ablative sites (Smith et al. 2007). In many patients, exact matches are not possible. An excellent example of this is the antero lateral thigh flap. This is the primary reconstructive modality in many Asian institutions. The typical Asian patient has a very thin, pliable, anterolateral soft tissue and skin component, making it moldable and high volume. It can be used to reconstruct many soft tissue defects in the head and neck regions. In many North American Caucasians the adipose component is higher, and thus the tissue characteristics are not similar (Fig. 3). A radial forearm flap is often better suited for reconstruction of these three-dimensional defects. A drawback to the radial forearm flap is the volume of tissue that can be transplanted is limited (Fig. 4).

Finally, when deciding on a donor site, one must consider what the functional and healing morbidity will be to the patient. As an example, the radial forearm

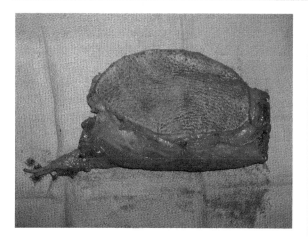

Free Tissue Transfer in Head and Neck, Fig. 3 The Antero Lateral Thigh flap can yield a high volume tissue replacement that is limited in its ability to be folded in three dimensions

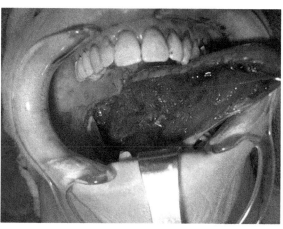

Free Tissue Transfer in Head and Neck, Fig. 5 This intraoperative photo demonstrates a hemi glossectomy defect

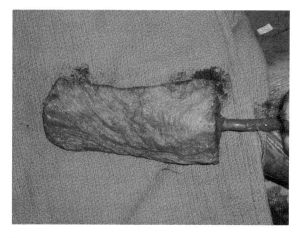

Free Tissue Transfer in Head and Neck, Fig. 4 The radial forearm fasciocutaneous flap is a low volume flap with excellent three-dimensional mobility

free flap involves extensive dissection of muscle and soft tissue the forearm. Using modern reconstructive techniques, a skin graft can be harvested with minimal morbidity and be placed on a wound bed that is receptive. In the majority of patients, healing can take place with a little long-term functional morbidly. However, long-term functional morbidity is not the same as short-term functional morbidity. Most of these patients will have marked decreased mobility and function of the arm. Coupled with extensive procedures in the head and neck area and the requirement to care for

tracheotomy tubes and feeding tubs, significant morbidity can be encountered. Thus, the determination of the appropriate donor site must take into account all of the above considerations.

Fasciocutaneous Free Flaps

Fasciocutaneous free flaps are a group of free flaps that consist of variable amounts of skin, subcutaneous tissue, and fascia. They are named fasciocutaneous because the vascular supply is through a named artery that runs in the fascia. The perforators that supply the skin come through the subcutaneous tissue and then through the subdermal plexus supply the overlying skin. These flaps can be thin and pliable, such as the radial forearm or they can be thick and essentially two dimensional such as rectus skin perforator flaps or anterolateral thigh flaps. The skin is an excellent replacement for mucosa and the variable amounts of subcutaneous tissue lets one choose among the various options depending on the volume and the three-dimensional requirements for reconstruction (Figs. 5, 6). The tissue characteristics are delineated in the table for the various fasciocutaneous flaps. (Table 1) It should be mentioned that a number of fasciocutaneous flaps may be transferred with other composite tissues such as the ▶ fibula osteocutaneous, the radial osteocutaneous, or the ▶ scapula.

One characteristic of the various fasciocutaneous free flaps is that their anatomy and vascular

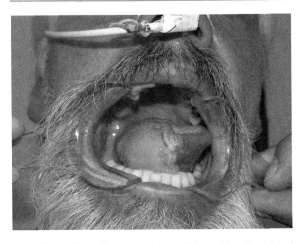

Free Tissue Transfer in Head and Neck, Fig. 6 A hemi glossectomy defect has been repaired with radial forearm free flap. The supple forearm skin is an excellent replacement for a hemi tongue

Free Tissue Transfer in Head and Neck, Table 1 Similarities and differences among the different fasciocutaneous flaps used in reconstruction of head and neck defects

Fasciocutaneous flap	Advantages	Disadvantages
Radial forearm	Thin, pliable tissue paddle	Donor site visible
	Large caliber, long vascular pedicle	Requires skin graft
	Consistent anatomy	Potential for vascular compromise of hand
	Technically straightforward	
	Two-team approach possible	
Ulnar flap	Thin, pliable tissue paddle	Potential for ulnar nerve injury
	Relatively hairless	Smaller, shorter vascular pedicle than radial forearm flap
	Two-team approach possible	Two venous anastomoses
		Donor site visible
		Requires skin graft
Anterolateral thigh	Large skin paddle available	Inconsistent vascular anatomy
	Versatile in volume	Technically challenging
	Primary closure usually possible	Poor color match
	Low donor site morbidity	Lateral thigh numbness
	Two-team approach possible	
Lateral arm	Thin, pliable tissue paddle	Small caliber, short vascular pedicle
	Donor site easily hidden	Potential for radial nerve injury
	Primary closure usually possible	Poor color match
		Two-team approach difficult
Scapular flap	Large skin paddle available	Repositioning patient in operating room
	Soft, pliable tissue paddle	Bulky, thick skin
	Large caliber, long vascular pedicle	Low potential for transfer as sensate flap
	Good color match	Two-team approach difficult
	Versatile three-dimensional positioning in donor site	
	Low donor site morbidity	
	Versatile in volume	

size are relatively consistent. The most popular fasciocutaneous flaps that are currently used are the radial forearm (Table 2), the anterolateral thigh (Table 3), and the ▶ scapula (Table 4). The tissue characteristics are all different so it is possible to tailor the reconstructive tissue to the ablative defect with some precision.

In some instances, such as the scapula or radial osteocutaneous, the fasciocutaneous flaps can be transferred by themselves. In others, such as the latissimus dorsi or the fibula free flap, the tissues require composite fascia and skin as well as the underlying bone or muscle to preserve the perforators.

Myocutaneous Free Flaps

Another common type of free tissue that is utilized in head and neck reconstruction are myogenous or myocutaneous free flaps. These flaps have a vascularized muscle with a named artery. The vessel traverses into the muscle for a variable distance and then divides in a variable fashion. While this intramuscular branching can be variable the vascular supply to the muscle and the skin overlying it is consistent. Thus the muscle can be utilized on a consistent basis. The vascular supply to the muscle then exits the muscle and sends perforators to the skin overlying the muscle. This allows the skin and muscle to be transferred as a

Free Tissue Transfer in Head and Neck, Table 2 The radial forearm free fasciocutaneous flap

Artery	Artery diameter	Vein(s)	Pedicle length	Nerve
Radial artery	2.5–3 mm	Paired venae comitantes (may converge into one) and/or cephalic vein	Up to 20 cm	Lateral antebrachial cutaneous nerve

Free Tissue Transfer in Head and Neck, Table 3 The anterolateral thigh free fasciocutaneous flap

Artery	Artery diameter	Vein(s)	Pedicle length	Nerve
Descending branch of lateral femoral circumflex artery	1.5–3.5 mm	Paired venae comitantes	Up to 7 cm	Lateral femoral cutaneous nerve

unit, as a myocutaneous free flap. Alternatively the muscle can be covered with a split thickness skin graft (Figs. 7, 8). The Rectus Abdominus and Latissimus Dorsi myocutaneous flaps are the most commonly utilized muscle flaps in head and neck reconstruction. Other flaps such as the Gracilis, Serratus Anterior, and Vastus Lateralis have also been used occasionally in the head and neck.

Both the myocutaneous or muscle only free flaps are ideal for a number of purposes in head and neck reconstruction. The muscle provides a high volume replacement for some large volume oncologic ablations. The ability of the muscle to fold into three-dimensional structures, and fit into nooks and crannies, allows it to seal many areas where the inelasticity of other flaps causes problems. This is a particular need in reconstruction of skull base defects (Chiu et al. 2008). The multitude of potential spaces and "nooks and crannies" that need to be filled to obliterate the dead space and isolate the intracranial contents are great. A large volume flap that can fit into many spaces is required. The rich vascularity of the myocutaneous flap also allows replacement in patients who have seen multiple previous treatment paradigms, including radiation, surgery, and previous chemotherapy. The muscle heals rapidly and adheres to the previously treated surfaces quite well. While

the choice between one muscle flap or another may depend on surgeon preference there are disadvantages and advantages to each that should be considered (Table 5).

Bony Free Flaps

Disturbing the continuity of the mandible or maxilla is associated with a significant functional, rehabilitative, and cosmetic deformity. These structures play a critical role in the self perception that we have and what we present to the world. Any deformity no matter how slight is immediately perceived by an observer and more importantly by the patient. All the functional aspects of the upper aerodigestive tract are dependent on a functional and anatomically intact mandible and maxilla. Disturbing this bony continuity can have devastating functional outcomes. This issue has been addressed since the first oncologic or traumatic ablation presented to the reconstructive surgeon. Mandibular and maxillary reconstruction was a difficult problem for reconstructive surgeons until the advent of vascularized bone was introduced into the reconstructive field. The use of free bone grafts has worked well for uncontaminated or small mandibular defects. It is well documented as being efficacious in the oral-maxillofacial surgery literature for their reconstructive procedures. Unfortunately, head and neck oncology often involves a large bony as well as tissue resection. The opening of the neck tissues with resection of the bony structures of the mandible or maxilla exposed the underlying surgical bed to the infected or contaminated surface of the aerodigestive tract. This led to a high incidence of extrusion or infection when nonvascularized bone grafts were utilized. Further compounding the issue is the frequent use of preoperative or postoperative radiation in these patients. This added considerably to the morbidity.

▶ Mandibular reconstruction was introduced by Ostrup and Frederickson in 1974 in a canine model (Ostrup and Fredrickson 1974) and then by McKee et al. who used a revascularized rib. The ▶ fibula and radial forearm osteocutaneous flaps are now the most commonly utilized bony-soft tissue flaps for reconstruction of mandibular defects in the head and neck. Iliac crest was extremely popular in the past, but has been less utilized because of donor site

Free Tissue Transfer in Head and Neck, Table 4 The scapula free fasciocutaneous flap

Artery	Artery diameter	Vein(s)	Pedicle length	Nerve
Circumflex scapular artery (may be followed to subscapular artery)	4 mm (6 mm if followed to subscapular artery)	Paired venae comitantes	7–10 cm (11–14 cm if followed to subscapular vessels)	(dorsal cutaneous rami of T1 and T2 experimental)

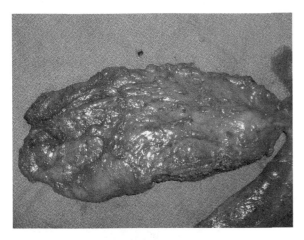

Free Tissue Transfer in Head and Neck, Fig. 7 This Latissimus Dorsi muscle is going to used as a replacement for a scalp defect. Only the muscle has been elevated

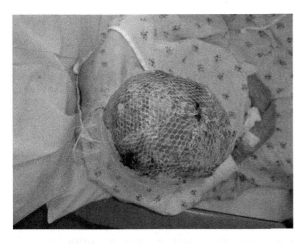

Free Tissue Transfer in Head and Neck, Fig. 8 The scalp has been reconstructed with the Latissimus Dorsi muscle. A split thickness skin graft has been used to provide external coverage

Free Tissue Transfer in Head and Neck, Table 5 Differences and similarities between the common myocutaneous flaps used in head and neck reconstruction

Myocutaneous flap	Advantages	Disadvantages
Latissimus dorsi	Large caliber, long vascular pedicle	Repositioning patient in operating room
	Large surface area available	Two-team approach difficult
	Versatile in volume	Unpredictable final volume after atrophy
	Transferred as free or pedicled flap	Frequently requires revision
	Low donor site morbidity	Poor color match
	Primary closure usually possible	
	Technically straightforward	
Rectus abdominus	Large caliber, long vascular pedicle	Potential for ventral hernia
	Large surface area available	Requires abdominal wall reconstruction
	Versatile in volume	Unpredictable final volume after atrophy
	Consistent anatomy	May require revision
	Primary closure usually possible	Poor color match

morbidity, unreliability of the skin paddle, and better composite tissue options. A scapular free tissue transfer allows for a limited length of bone of good stock, but because of technical difficulties and inability to perform as a two-team procedure, has also fallen out of favor in most microvascular reconstructive surgeons' hands (Table 6).

Radial forearm osteocutaneous flap allows for supple skin to be transferred with the bone. A small piece of bone up to 10 cm can be utilized (Fig. 9) and is thin but with sufficient plating will routinely heal well (Fig. 10). The radial forearm osteocutaneous flap fell into disfavor a decade or so ago because of the high incidence of radial forearm bone fractures. With revisions in surgical technique and routine plating, this no longer happens and the flap has been shown to be reliable for many head and neck reconstructions (Waits et al. 2007) (Table 7).

Free Tissue Transfer in Head and Neck, Table 6 Similarities and differences between the osteocutaneous free flaps that are commonly used in head and neck reconstruction

Osteocutaneous flap	Advantages	Disadvantages
Fibular	Up to 25 cm of bone available	Usually requires skin graft
	Large caliber, long vascular pedicle	Potential for vascular compromise of lower extremity
	Ideal bone height	Skin paddle fixed to bone
	Multiple osteotomies possible	Moderate donor site morbidity
	May be used for total mandibular reconstruction	May be difficult to fit with dental prostheses (dentures)
	Accepts endosseous dental implants	
	Two-team approach possible	
Radial forearm	Thin, pliable tissue paddle	Limited bone length and height
	Large caliber, long vascular pedicle	Donor site visible
	Consistent anatomy	Requires skin graft
	Versatile positioning in recipient site	Potential for vascular compromise of hand
	Supports dental prostheses (dentures)	Risk of radius fracture
	Two-team approach possible	Plating of radius recommended
Scapular	Large skin paddle available	Repositioning patient in operating room
	Skin paddle may be oriented independent of bone axis	Limited bone height
	Versatile in volume	Bulky, thick skin
	Multiple osteotomies possible	Potential for long-term shoulder dysfunction
	Primary closure usually possible	Low potential for transfer as sensate flap
	Minimal atrophy	Two-team approach difficult
	Good color match	
Iliac crest	Large skin paddle available	Bulky skin paddle
	Contour similar to mandible	Short pedicle
	Donor site easily hidden	Not pliable in three dimensions

(continued)

Free Tissue Transfer in Head and Neck, Table 6 (continued)

Osteocutaneous flap	Advantages	Disadvantages
	Primary closure usually possible	Donor site morbidity – pain, hernia
	Supports endosseous dental implants	Requires abdominal wall reconstruction
	Two-team approach	Technically challenging
		Small caliber, short vascular pedicle
		Poor color match

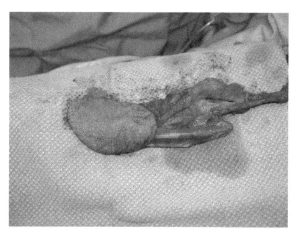

Free Tissue Transfer in Head and Neck, Fig. 9 A radial osteocutaneous free flap has been harvested. Notice the bone is attached to a mobile thin supple cutaneous portion

The ▶ fibula supplies the best and most diverse options for reconstruction of large bony defects (Table 8). Up to 25 cm of bone with a large skin paddle can be harvested (Fig. 11). The donor leg does not require any reconstruction or prophylactic plating. The cutaneous defect is best reconstructed with a split thickness skin graft that can be harvested from the donor site prior to harvesting the flap. Functional morbidity can be quite high with many patients requiring extensive rehabilitation and physiotherapy before they regain their preoperative functional status. Peripheral vascular disease is frequently encountered in this patient population. While some feel that having one vessel left to supply the leg is adequate, with the plethora of other flaps available it is best to look elsewhere for bone if there is any doubt about the vascularity of the leg and foot (Fig. 12) (Miller et al. 2011).

The bone of the fibula is hardy and can withstand the multiple osteotomies that may be required to shape it to fit the contour of the resected mandible or maxilla. The skin paddle is not as flexible as that of the radial forearm but it can be used to reconstruct the soft tissue defect adequately.

Use of bone allows for tissue implants and rehabilitation with denture implants (Fig. 13). This has been well documented and described in the literature and is quite efficacious. Unfortunately the cost is prohibitive in this patient population and this must also be considered.

Selective Issues in Free Tissue Transfer

Many of the specialized functions of the upper aerodigestive tract rely on normal sensation of the mucosal and deeper structures. The ability to talk, swallow, chew, and phonate all depend on adequate sensory feedback being available and interpreted in an efficacious manner. Any resection or oncologic ablation will have an effect on this function since the ablation will remove the sensing tissue. During neck dissection or tumor ablation, many sensory nerves that primarily innervate structures of the head and neck area can be resected or removed. Adding to this are the effects of ancillary treatments such as radiation or chemotherapy which can have a denervation effect on the linings or deep structures of the head and neck. One only has to recall the feeling of dental anesthesia to realize the morbidity that lack of sensation in the lip, tongue, or other structures can induce. The ability to reinnervate or provide sensation to areas of the head and neck from which it has been removed is a rehabilitative potential that is being explored. It has been noted that spontaneous reinnervation will occur from the nerves either deep in the bed of the resection margin or as in growth from the periphery.

In thin flaps, such as the radial forearm flap, recovery and the pattern of recovery can be quite variable. Almost half of patients will recover some

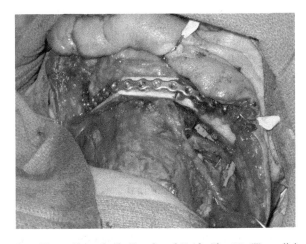

Free Tissue Transfer in Head and Neck, Fig. 10 The radial forearm osteocutaneous flap has been used to reconstruct a mandibular defect. The bone of the forearm has been osteotomized to conform to the mandibular contour

Free Tissue Transfer in Head and Neck, Table 7 The radial forearm osteocutaneous free flap

Artery	Artery diameter	Vein(s)	Pedicle length	Nerve	Bone
Radial artery	2–2.5 mm	Paired venae comitantes (may converge into one) and/or cephalic vein	Up to 20 cm	Lateral antebrachial cutaneous nerve	Radius (up to 12 cm length)

Free Tissue Transfer in Head and Neck, Table 8 The fibula osteocutaneous free flap

Artery	Artery diameter	Vein(s)	Pedicle length	Nerve	Bone
Peroneal artery	1.5–4 mm	Paired peroneal veins (may converge into one)	Up to 8 cm	Lateral sural cutaneous nerve	Fibula (up to 25 cm length)

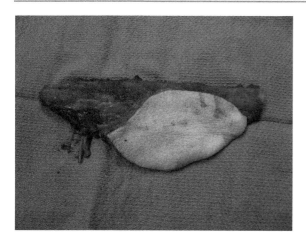

Free Tissue Transfer in Head and Neck, Fig. 11 The fibula osteocutaneous free flap provides the most bone with a large skin paddle for composite tissue reconstruction

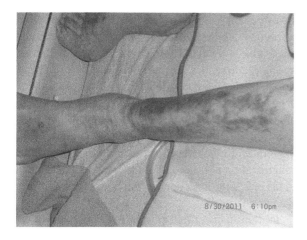

Free Tissue Transfer in Head and Neck, Fig. 12 This leg demonstrates many of the signs of vascular insufficiency and should not be considered as a donor site for bone

sort of sensation in a thin flap. Thicker flaps will not recover as well.

Many of the fasciocutaneous free flaps that are used for reconstruction in the head and neck, such as the radial forearm, ulnar, and even scapula can be harvested with a sensory nerve that supplies the skin of the donated area. Anastamosis to the supplying sensory nerve of the head and neck is usually something that can be performed and is well within the armamentarium of most reconstructive surgeons. Urken et al. looked at 17 patients who underwent sensate radial forearm flaps for glossectomy defects (Urken 2004). Objective testing demonstrated that return of sensation was excellent. One of the issues that arose during the evaluation of these patients was that the recovery of sensation in the transferred tissue seemed to be greater than one would expect from the neural representation in forearm tissue. It may be that the forearm did indeed become more like mucosa in the head and neck from a sensory input perspective.

While there have been many studies that show that reinnervation of the radial forearm flaps provides good two point discrimination, such as light touch and temperature, very little has been done to describe the effect of reinnervation on functional or quality of life outcomes. It is well within the armamentarium of the reconstructive surgeon to reinnervate these flaps. As to whether this provides better function or not is unknown. It has been well established that degree of resection of the tongue volume is one of the greatest determinants of oral rehabilitative potential; whether reinnervated flaps will affect this is undergoing study.

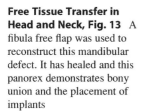

Free Tissue Transfer in Head and Neck, Fig. 13 A fibula free flap was used to reconstruct this mandibular defect. It has healed and this panorex demonstrates bony union and the placement of implants

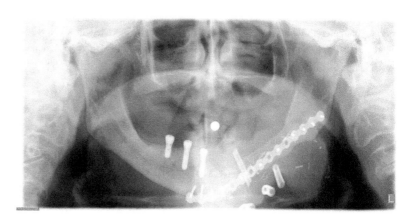

References

Acland RD (1977) Instrumentation for microsurgery. Orthop Clin North Am 8:281–294

Briant TD (1977) The treatment of cancer of the head and neck. J Otolaryngol 6(5):349–352

Carrel A (1902) The operative technique of vascular anastomosis and transplantation of organs. Lyon Med 98:859–864

Chiu ES, Kraus D, Bui DT, Mehrara BJ, Disa JJ, Bilsky M, Shah JP, Cordeiro PG (2008) Anterior and middle cranial fossa skull base reconstruction using microvascular free tissue techniques: surgical complications and functional outcomes. Ann Plast Surg 60(5):514–520

Hayden RE (1991) Microvascular free flaps for soft-tissue defects. Otolaryngol Clin North Am 24(6):1343–1366

Liu R, Gullane P, Brown D, Irish J (2001) Pectoralis major myocutaneous pedicled flap in head and neck reconstruction: retrospective review of indications and results in 244 consecutive cases at the Toronto General Hospital. J Otolaryngol 30(1):34–40

Miller ME, Moriarty JM, Blackwell KE, Finn JP, Yiee JH, Nabili V (2011) Preoperative magnetic resonance angiography detection of septocutaneous perforators in fibula free flap transfer. Arch Facial Plast Surg 13(1):36–40

Ostrup LT, Fredrickson JM (1974) Distant transfer of a free, living bone graft by microvascular anastomoses. An experimental study. Plast Reconstr Surg 54(3):274–285

Panje WR, Krause CJ, Bardach J, Baker SR (1977) Reconstruction of intraoral defects with the free groin flap. Arch Otolaryngol 103(2):78–83

Rosenthal E, Couch M, Farwell DG, Wax MK (2007) Current concepts in microvascular reconstruction. Otolaryngol Head Neck Surg 136(4):519–524

Seidenberg B, Rosenak SS, Hurwitt ES, Som ML (1959) Immediate reconstruction of the cervical esophagus by a revascularized isolated jejunal segment. Ann Surg 149(2):162–171

Smith RB, Sniezek JC, Weed DT, Wax MK (2007) Microvascular surgery subcommittee of American academy of otolaryngology–head and neck surgery. Utilization of free tissue transfer in head and neck surgery. Otolaryngol Head Neck Surg 137(2):182–191

Taylor GI, Corlett RJ, Dhar SC, Ashton MW (2011) The anatomical (angiosome) and clinical territories of cutaneous perforating arteries: development of the concept and designing safe flaps. Plast Reconstr Surg 127(4):1447–1459

Urken ML (1991) Composite free flaps in oromandibular reconstruction. Review of the literature. Arch Otolaryngol Head Neck Surg 117(7):724–732

Urken ML (2004) Targeted sensory restoration to the upper aerodigestive tract with physiologic implications. Head Neck 26(3):287–293

Waits CA, Toby EB, Girod DA, Tsue TT (2007) Osteocutaneous radial forearm free flap: long-term radiographic evaluation of donor site morbidity after prophylactic plating of radius. J Reconstr Microsurg 23(7):367–372

Watts SH (1907) The suture of blood vessels. Implantation and transplantation of vessels and organs. An historical and experimental study. Ann Surg 46(3):373–404

Free Tissue Transfer in the Head and Neck, Complications

Gina D. Jefferson
Department of Otolaryngology and Communicative Sciences, University of Mississippi Medical Center, Jackson, MS, USA

Synonyms

Free flap; Microvascular free flap

Since the 1970s, the use of free tissue transfer to reconstruct complex head and neck defects became popular with the realization that regional flaps do pose specific limitations. The success rate of microvascular free tissue transfers to the head and neck region is reportedly greater than 95% in larger series (Bui et al. 2007; Suh et al. 2004; Bianchi et al. 2009). Despite the reported success rates, it is important to remain vigilant in the postoperative monitoring of free flaps in order to recognize vascular compromise early to achieve salvage. Any flap loss negatively impacts both the patient and the surgeon.

Reconstruction of the head and neck region utilizing free tissue transfer most commonly suffers from venous thrombosis rather than arterial thrombosis at a ratio of 3:1 due to low-flow and low-pressure (Bui et al. 2007; Bianchi et al. 2009). Free flaps with a visible and accessible skin paddle are regularly inspected for color, refill, and turgor by both nursing and the surgeons. An external suture is also usually placed into the skin that overlies the anastomosed vessels for nursing to regularly check the Doppler signal. The surgeon also performs needle pin prick of the accessible skin paddle. If the reconstruction has no accessible skin paddle, i.e., when placing a free flap patch in reconstruction of a neopharynx, the surgeon may choose to place an implantable Doppler device or a flow coupler device. This allows monitoring of the blood flow across the microvascular anastomosis. A flap demonstrating venous congestion is notable for edema, ecchymosis, petechiae and brisk dark red blood ooze upon pin prick. Arterial insufficiency, on the other hand, is exhibited by cold pallor of the skin paddle and poor turgor. There is an absent Doppler signal and little to no bleeding is elicited from the tissue upon pin prick. The skin paddle appears pale or mottled.

Microvascular free tissue transfer complications of the head and neck region related to the vasculature typically occur within the first 5 days of reconstruction (Bui et al. 2007; Suh et al. 2004). Consistent with the most common cause of vascular compromise resulting from venous obstruction, patients become more mobile during postoperative days 3–5 when increased head movements may cause kinking or repositioning of the anastomosed vessels beneath the mandible. The salvage rate for venous thrombosis is also higher than that for arterial thrombosis (Bui et al. 2007; Bianchi et al. 2009). The ability to detect venous compromise and rapidly return to the operating room for salvage is likely greater due to more obvious signs of venous compromise than if arterial insufficiency is present. In addition, the pathophysiology behind venous congestion differs from that of arterial insufficiency. Arterial insufficiency more rapidly results in the *no-reflow phenomenon* of the microcirculation. Ischemia results in the release of oxygen free radicals which is directly toxic to the endothelial layer of the microvasculature. This incites the release of proinflammatory mediators and ultimately results in thrombosis of the microcirculation despite patency of the anastomosed vessels.

There should remain a low threshold for surgical reexploration when vascular thrombosis is suspected. Explore the neck to examine the vascular pedicle for kinks, external compression, hematoma, and vasospasm. Perform a *second* venous anastomosis if possible to create additional flap drainage. If an early thrombus is appreciated, heparinize and perform a thrombectomy using vessel dilators or Fogarty catheters. When an organized thrombus is present, heparinize the patient and perform thrombectomy. In the event of an established, late thrombosis thrombolytics infused throughout the flap vasculature are useful to remove clot within the microvasculature. The involved segment of vessel with thrombus may necessitate excision and reanastomosis in the setting of late thrombosis. Revision of an anastomosis may also require a vein graft. Thrombectomy with or without thrombolysis result in flap salvage approximately 60–70% of the time (Bui et al. 2007; Suh et al. 2004). If the flap is not salvageable and the patient remains medically stable a second free flap is considered. When the patient is unstable, there is a lack of recipient vessels and an exposed vital structure

exists, a local pedicle flap is used. Delayed reconstruction is an option for the medically unstable patient with no local pedicle flap options, who has no recipient vessels and there are no exposed vital structures (Bui et al. 2007; Wei and Mardini 2009). Of note, an antithrombotic agent, or a combination of agents, is frequently administered by microvascular surgeons prophylactically. However, there is no established recommended regimen. We use 7 days of low dose aspirin and low molecular weight heparin subcutaneously.

Although vascular compromise causing total or partial necrosis of the flap is arguably the most devastating complication, wound dehiscence is the most common. Recipient site local skin necrosis and infection ultimately leading to wound dehiscence is frequently encountered in the salvage surgical setting due to previous radiotherapy. Radiation exposure induces local tissue hypoxia thereby compromising the local wound healing process. Conservative management with local wet to dry packing encourages granulation tissue formation and healing of the wound. When major wound dehiscence and local necrosis results, a new free tissue transfer or regional flap becomes necessary.

Likewise, an orocutaneous or pharyngocutaneous fistula, or simply an infection in the vicinity of the vascular supply of the flap, predisposes the flap to thrombosis. Systemic and local inflammatory mediators activate the complement cascade and ultimately the arachidonic acid pathway leading to platelet activation and potential thrombus organization. Early reexploration of the wound permits assessment of the wound and vessel situation. Creation of a controlled fistula as well as placement of a dermal graft or regional flap for protection of the carotid sheath are considered at the time of operative evaluation of the wound.

Complications at the donor site may also occur. The radial forearm flap should not result in vascular compromise of the hand as the surgeon is mandated to *preoperatively* assess adequate ulnar circulation to the thumb and index finger via an Allen's test. If this test is equivocal in the clinic then the patient should undergo Doppler assessment of the deep palmar arch integrity with Allen's test. Prior to ligation of the radial artery intraoperatively, the Allen's test is performed once more by clamping the radial artery distally after elevating the skin paddle then releasing the tourniquet and assessing the capillary refill within the thenar eminence, thumb, and index finger distribution. Less than 100% skin graft adherence to the recipient site can lead to exposure of the flexor tendons and is managed conservatively with local wound care. When an osteocutaneous radial forearm flap is utilized there is a risk for radius fracture. This is avoided by scalloping the bone during the harvest and by plating the remaining segments of radius for stability. Complications related to the fibula free flap include ischemia of the lower extremity, knee or ankle instability, foot or great toe weakness. Ischemia to the leg is prevented by preoperative assessment of adequate 3-vessel run-off, i.e., peroneal, anterior tibial, and posterior tibial arterial supply, into the distal lower extremity. Assessment by physical exam and color flow Doppler, CT angiogram or MR angiogram is sufficient. The surgeon should leave 6 cm of fibula both proximally and distally to ensure stability of the knee and ankle joint which also protects the common peroneal nerve from injury proximally. When harvesting a rectus abdominis myocutaneous flap, the surgeon must restore the integrity of the rectus sheath. The anterior rectus sheath is harvested to some degree when including the skin as a component of the flap. Direct closure of the remaining anterior rectus sheath with nonabsorbable suture, or placement of mesh is necessary when reapproximation of the sheath remnants is not feasible in order to prevent abdominal herniation.

The success rate of microvascular free tissue transfer to reconstruct major head and neck defects is largely successful. Vascular complications are avoided by paying strict attention to detail, by meticulously handling vessels, and by carefully planning the vessel arrangement in the neck wound. Flap salvage is usually possible to some degree when vascular compromise is recognized early and the patient is promptly returned to the operating room. Finally, a microvascular surgeon always should have a back-up plan.

References

Bianchi B, Coopelli C, Ferrari S, Ferri A (2009) Free flaps: outcomes and complications in head and neck reconstructions. J Cranio-Maxillofac Surg 37:438–442

Bui DT, Cordeiro PG, Hu QY et al (2007) Free flap reexploration: indications, treatment, and outcomes in 1193 free flaps. Plast Reconstr Surg 119:2092–2100

Patel RS, McCluskey SA, Goldstein DP et al (2010) Clinicopathologic andn therapeutic risk factors for perioperative complications and prolonged hospital stay in free flap reconstruction of the head and neck. Head Neck 32:1345–1353

Pattani KM, Byrne P, Boahene K, Richmon J (2010) What makes a good flap go bad?: a critical analysis of the literature of intraoperative factors related to free flap failure. Laryngoscope 120:717–723

Perisanidis C, Herberger B, Papadogeorgakis N et al (2011) Complications after free flap surgery: do we need a standardized classification of surgical complications? Br J Oral Maxillofac Surg 50:113–118

Suh JD, Sercarz JA, Abemayor E et al (2004) Analysis of outcome and complications in 400 cases of microvascular head and neck reconstruction. Arch Otolaryngol Head Neck Surg 130:962–966

Wei F, Mardini S (2009) Flaps and reconstructive surgery. Elsevier, Philadelphia

Frey's Syndrome

John Drew Prosser[1] and Jimmy James Brown[2]
[1]Department of Otolaryngology, Georgia Health Sciences University, Augusta, GA, USA
[2]Department of Otolaryngology-Head and Neck Surgery, Georgia Health Sciences University, Augusta, GA, USA

Synonyms

Auriculotemporal syndrome; Baillarger's syndrome; Dupuy's syndrome; Frey-Baillarger syndrome; Gustatory hyperhidrosis; Gustatory sweating

Definition

Frey's syndrome involves the experience of facial flushing and sweating during mastication or activities that increase salivary flow (hence the name gustatory sweating). These symptoms are most commonly noted following parotidectomy, but may follow other surgical procedures, traumatic injuries or inflammatory processes of the parotid gland, submandibular gland, upper thoracic or cervical sympathetic trunk (Calzada and Hanna 2010). Symptoms may range in severity from patient to patient, from the barely perceptible to persistently bothersome.

Etiology

Although widely referred to by the common name of Frey's syndrome, the first case was originally reported by Baillarger in 1853 (Sok and Rosen 2008). In 1897 the first case of bilateral Frey's syndrome was reported by Weber and it was not until 1923 that the neurologist Lucie Frey described the classical symptoms of facial sweating and flushing with meals in a 25-year-old soldier who suffered a gunshot wound to the parotid region (Sok and Rosen 2008). The neurologist to whom the syndrome is commonly attributed might have not been the first to describe the syndrome; however she should be given credit for correctly identifying the autonomic innervation of both the parotid gland and overlying facial skin which lead to the implication of the auriculotemporal nerve in its pathogenesis (Sok and Rosen 2008).

The underlying cause of the symptomatology is purported to be due to aberrant regeneration of severed postganglionic parasympathetic secretomotor neurons of the parotid salivary gland innervating or reconnecting with severed postganglionic sympathetic fibers of sweat glands in the facial skin overlying the parotid bed. Since both nerve fibers utilize the neurotransmitter acetylcholine, this stimulates facial sweating and flushing during mastication. Most commonly this syndrome is found following parotid surgery, but has also been reported several weeks or months after varied injuries to the parotid gland including blunt and penetrating trauma, infectious and inflammatory diseases, as well as condylar fractures (Sok and Rosen 2008).

Clinical Presentation

This condition usually presents several weeks to months following surgery of the parotid gland, but can present many years later. The patient complains of unilateral (on the same side of surgical dissection) facial sweating and flushing and occasional warmth which is brought on by mastication. This is occasionally associated with generalized discomfort over the same area. Often this is noticed after sweat marks appear on the ipsilateral collar during a meal. The signs and symptoms are present overlying the parotid bed and upper part of the neck, where skin flaps are elevated for surgical excision. Symptoms can also involve the post-auricular area and external auditory canal, which can be confused with cerebrospinal fluid if concomitant mastoid surgery was performed.

On physical examination one can notice flushing and sweating, particularly if the patient is given

a sialagogue. There is occasional warmth but the area is without discrete tenderness to palpation. Minor's starch/iodine test will be positive and can be used to both confirm the diagnosis and map the involved area if targeted treatment (i.e., Botox injection) is being considered. Even though presentation may be rapid or delayed, once gustatory sweating and flushing are present this signifies aberrant cross reinnervation has occurred, and therefore symptoms will remain persistent if no treatment is provided.

Diagnosis

The diagnosis of Frey's syndrome can be made by patients' history, however, should treatment be considered, objective tests including mapping of the area, should be pursued. The initial objective test is the Minor's starch iodine test. To perform this test the ipsilateral side of the face and neck are first cleaned thoroughly with an alcohol solution and allowed to dry. Next the suspected involved area is painted with a 2% iodine solution, traditionally a mixture of 2 g of iodine in 10 mL of almond or castor oil and 90 mL of alcohol. Alternatively povidone-iodine with alcohol (Betadine) swabs can be used. This solution is allowed to completely dry. Following this starch powder (typically potato or rice starch) is then applied evenly to the painted area. A sialagogue (typically a lemon wedge or lemon candy) is given and chewed for several minutes to stimulate salivary flow. Dark blue or purple spots will form along the area of gustatory sweating, and is a result of a reaction of the sweat dissolving the starch with iodine. Interestingly if this test is used to evaluate every patient following parotidectomy, up to 95% will show signs of positive reaction, indicative of subclinical disease in patients which are asymptomatic (Calzada and Hanna 2010). If treatment is being considered, the area can then be marked with a surgical pen and photographed with surgical ruler for reference.

Differential Diagnosis

The differential diagnosis includes primary hyperhidrosis, which typically would present with more generalized sweating, and not associated with surgical or other injury to the parotid region. Hyperhidrosis most commonly involves the back or arms but can involve focal body regions such as the face. Gustatory sweating can often be confused for a food allergy or adverse reaction which can lead to unnecessary food restrictions or diet modifications. Further salivary fistulas or infections could give erythema and drainage over the parotid area, particularly from the post-auricular incision site, but the patient would also likely have associated fever, warmth, tenderness, and a malodor to the drainage not characteristic of sweat.

Prophylaxis

Many surgical techniques have been proposed to reduce the incidence of Frey's syndrome following parotidectomy. These methods mainly rely on placing a barrier (either biologic or artificial) between the regenerating free nerve endings and the aberrant targeted sweat glands. The main techniques include transposition of sternocleidomastoid (SCM) muscle flaps, superficial musculoaponeurotic system (SMAS) flap interposition, temporoparietal flap transposition, acellular dermal barrier, partial superficial parotidectomy, and maintenance of a thick skin flap. There is much controversy regarding these techniques and the proposed benefits. The most often studied has been the SCM muscle flap technique. A recent meta-analysis performed of studies on the use of the SCM flap concluded that there is of date inconclusive evidence to recommend the use of the SCM flap to prevent the incidence of Frey's syndrome following parotidectomy (Sanabria et al. 2011). A meta-analysis of varied surgical techniques to reduce the incidence of post-parotidectomy Frey's syndrome favored utilization of an operative technique but did not assess individual techniques (Curry et al. 2009). Most authors agree that maintenance of a thick skin flap and performing a limited superficial parotidectomy seem to be the most consistent operative techniques to minimize the risk of developing symptomatic disease (de Bree et al. 2007).

Therapy

Once the diagnosis is confirmed and the patient is symptomatic, management consists of initial application of topical anticholinergic products, such as scopolamine and glycopyrrolate, and nonscented

Frey's Syndrome, Table 1 Hyperhidrosis disease severity scale

Question: How would you rate the severity of your hyperhidrosis?	Score
My sweating is never noticeable and never interferes with my daily activities	1
My sweating is tolerable but sometimes interferes with my daily activities	2
My sweating is barely tolerable and frequently interferes with my daily activities	3
My sweating is intolerable and always interferes with my daily activities	4

deodorants. For most mild cases this medical therapy will result in symptomatic improvement to the point where no further intervention is warranted. In refractory cases it is recommended that the patient be evaluated with a qualitative hyperhidrosis severity questionnaire (Sok and Rosen 2008). Although many validated questionnaires exist, the most current and simplest is the Hyperhidrosis Disease Severity Scale (HDSS), Table 1. This is a single-question, 4-point scale for assessing the severity of hyperhidrosis. Patients rate their tolerability of hyperhidrosis symptoms based on the extent to which it interferes with their daily activities. A score greater than 2 has been used as a criteria for consideration of Botox injections. The goal being reduction of symptom scores below 2 (Sok and Rosen 2008).

Once conservative therapy has failed, botulinum toxin (Botox) injections as previously mentioned are delivered into the superficial dermis to chemodenervate purported aberrant nerve connections. The diffusion radius is approximately 5 mm and intradermal injections should be spaced to allow overlap of these diffusion zones across the involved skin. The techniques starts with performing a Minor's starch iodine test as described above. The affected skin area is marked with a surgical pen and divided into 5 mm boxes in the form of a grid over the involved area. Lyophilized botulinum toxin type A (Botox, 100 units per vial) is then reconstituted with 1 mL of sterile, preservative-free saline to a final concentration of 10 U/0.1 mL. This solution is then drawn into a 1 ml tuberculin syringe with a 30 gauge needle (utilized for patient comfort). Intradermal injections are performed within five to ten units of Botox injected in the center of each 5-mm^2 grid. The injection must be performed slowly to confirm a visible wheal, which is indicative of a proper plane of injection. Injection into this plane not only improves efficacy but also decreases the likelihood of unwanted facial weakness. Gentle pressure is then applied for evening of toxin distribution and hemostasis. Following the injections, the markings may be removed and the patient observed briefly for any complications. If weakness of the facial muscles is noted from a deep injection or too large of a quantity, the patient is informed that the weakness should be temporary and will resolve after a few weeks (Sok and Rosen 2008).

If both medical and injection therapies fail, surgical interventions should be considered. Previously tympanic neurectomy has been performed to interrupt the presynaptic neurons responsible for the cross reinnervation. Although successful in a majority of cases, this procedure has been widely abandoned due to its invasive nature and low efficacy. In advanced cases today, surgical management revolves around re-elevation of a skin flaps and interposition of vascularized tissue, free tissue graft, or acellular dermis between the parotid bed and skin flap. However the risk of complications including injury from re-elevation of the flap from a previously dissected facial nerve should be considered (Johnson 2008). Given these factors as well as their ease and repeatability, Botox injections have become the standard first line treatment in cases refractory to medical management.

Prognosis

Once aberrant cross reinnervation has occurred it is permanent, however with treatment a majority of patients achieve symptomatic relief. Botox injections have been reported to have 80–100% efficacy among patients treated for the first time (de Bree et al. 2007). Recurrence of symptoms is common but repeated treatments can be performed with ease and minimal morbidity without increasing complications.

Epidemiology

The incidence of Frey's syndrome following parotidectomy varies across reports. This is likely due to the inconsistency with which the diagnosis is sought postoperatively. When unsolicited, approximately 10% of patients will admit to gustatory sweating, however if specifically asked the number rises to approximately 30–40%. If a Minor's starch iodine test is performed on all patients following parotidectomy, up to 95% will show signs of a positive test (de Bree et al. 2007).

Another hindrance to determining the true incidence of Frey's syndrome following parotidectomy is the varied time of presentation. Regeneration of the postganglionic parasympathetic nerve fibers to the skin is not instantaneous and this latent period is reported to take from 2 weeks to >8 years. Approximately 50% will present within 12 months, which rises to 83% within 24 months (de Bree et al. 2007). Further it has been observed that the facial skin area involved with gustatory sweating tends to gradually enlarge during follow-up. This progressive nature lends support to the varied lengths of time required by regenerating nerve fibers to reach sweat glands which are of varied distance from the proximal nerve endings.

Cross-References

▶ Benign Salivary Gland Neoplasms
▶ Botulinum Toxin
▶ Parotidectomy
▶ Salivary Gland Physiology

References

Calzada GG, Hanna EY (2010) Benign neoplasms of the salivary glands. In: Flint PW et al (eds) Cummings otolaryngology head and neck surgery, 5th edn. Mosby Elsevier, Philadelphia, pp 1162–1177

Curry JM, King N, Reiter D, Fisher K, Heffelfinger RN, Pribitkin EA (2009) Meta-analysis of surgical techniques for preventing parotidectomy sequelae. Arch Facial Plast Surg 11(5):327–331

de Bree R, van der Waal I, Leemans CR (2007) Management of Frey syndrome. Head Neck 29(8):773–778

Johnson JT (2008) Parotidectomy. In: Myers EN (ed) Operative otolaryngology: head and neck surgery, 2nd edn. Saunders Elsevier, Philadelphia, pp 511–524

Sanabria A, Kowalski LP, Bradley PJ, Hartl DM, Bradford CR, de Bree R, Rinaldo A, Ferlito A (2011) Sternocleidomastoid muscle flap in preventing Frey's syndrome after parotidectomy: a systematic review. Head Neck 34(4): 589–598

Sok JC, Rosen CA (2008) Treatment of gustatory sweating (Frey's syndrome) with botulinum toxin A. In: Myers EN (ed) Operative otolaryngology: head and neck surgery, 2nd edn. Saunders Elsevier, Philadelphia, pp 495–498

Frey-Baillarger Syndrome

▶ Frey's Syndrome

Frontoethmoidectomy

▶ Paranasal Sinuses in Contemporary Surgery, External Approaches to

Functional Endonasal Sinus Surgery

▶ Endoscopic Sinus Surgery in Children

Functional Endoscopic Sinus Surgery (FESS)

▶ Endoscopic Sinus Surgery in Children
▶ Primary Sinus Surgery

Functional Neck Dissection

▶ Neck Dissection Anatomy

G

Galea Aponeurotica

▶ Epicranial Aponeurosis

Gamma Globulin

▶ Otolaryngologic Allergy/Immunology

Gamma Probe-Guided Lymphadenectomy

▶ Sentinel Lymph Node Biopsy for Head and Neck Cancer

Gastroesophageal Reflux

▶ Reflux Disease and LPR

Gastroesophageal Reflux in Children

Samra S. Blanchard[1] and Anjali Malkani[2]
[1]Division of Pediatric Gastroenterology, University of Maryland, School of Medicine, Baltimore, MD, USA
[2]Department of Pediatric Gastroenterology and Nutrition, University of Maryland, School of Medicine, Baltimore, MD, USA

Definition

Gastroesophageal reflux (GER) is defined as the involuntary retrograde passage of gastric contents into the esophagus with or without regurgitation or vomiting. It is a frequently experienced physiological condition occurring several times a day mostly postprandially and causing no symptoms. Gastroesophageal disease (GERD) occurs when reflux of the gastric contents causes symptoms that affect the quality of life or pathological complications.

Regurgitation is defined as effortless passage of gastric contents into the mouth. Other terms such as "spitting up" and "spilling" are also used for regurgitation. When regurgitation occurs in healthy, thriving, happy infants, it is always physiological.

Epidemiology

The prevalence of GERD in infants and children is in the range of 1–10%. The prevalence of GER is age dependent. About 70–85% of infants have regurgitation within 2 months of life, and GER resolves without intervention in about 95% of infants by 1 year of age. Children with chronic respiratory and neurological diseases have a higher incidence of GERD.

Pathophysiology

Two major elements that compose the anti-reflux barrier are the lower esophageal sphincter (LES) and the crural diaphragm. The LES is a thickened ring of tonically contracted smooth muscle in the distal esophagus that generates a high-pressure zone at the gastroesophageal junction and serves as a mechanical barrier between the stomach and the esophagus. The right crura of diaphragm encircle the LES and provide

S.E. Kountakis (ed.), *Encyclopedia of Otolaryngology, Head and Neck Surgery*, DOI 10.1007/978-3-642-23499-6,
© Springer-Verlag Berlin Heidelberg 2013

additional support. Both structures generate a high-pressure zone in the distal esophagus. Failure of one or both mechanisms predisposes GER.

Transient lower esophageal sphincter relaxation (TLESR) is the predominant mechanism of GERD in all ages. TLESR is defined as an abrupt decrease in LES pressure to the level of intragastric pressure, unrelated to swallowing and of relatively longer duration than the relaxation triggered by a swallow. TLESR is a neural reflex, mediated through the brainstem, and the vagus nerve is the efferent pathway. Gastric distention and pharyngeal stimulation have been demonstrated to elicit relaxation. In addition to TLESRs, mechanical support of the hiatal crura, delayed esophageal clearance, and noxious characteristics of the refluxate contribute to GERD. Hiatal hernia is not as common in children as compared to adults but has been reported in cases of severe reflux, cystic fibrosis, and in children with neurological impairment.

Delayed gastric emptying has been associated with GERD in infants and children. Gastric emptying depends on the volume, osmolality, and caloric density of the meal consumed. The receptive relaxation of the fundus in response to a meal also impacts the occurrence of TLESRs. Recently, gastric emptying was shown to be delayed in patients with cow's milk protein allergy in comparison with control subjects and infants with GER. It should be kept in mind that secondary GERD occurs with cow's milk protein allergy and contributes to pathophysiology of GERD.

The refluxate (gas, liquid, or mixed contents) provokes esophageal distention or acidification, and this may trigger delayed esophageal clearance.

The pathogenicity of the refluxate is determined by its constituents: acid, pepsin, and bile salts. Acid in combination with pepsin has been found to be the most noxious to esophageal mucosa. Esophageal mucosal injury in GERD occurs when mucosal defensive factors are overwhelmed by the refluxate.

There is a higher incidence of GER in infants, which is physiological. It is due to shorter esophagus, wider angle of His, frequent feedings, and more time in the supine position.

Clinical Presentations

Regurgitation and vomiting are the most common symptoms of infant reflux. The typical presentation of uncomplicated infant GER is effortless, painless regurgitation in a healthy infant with normal growth – the so-called happy spitter. It is usually effortless and non-bilious with no or minimum irritability. A thorough history and physical examination with attention to warning signals suggesting other diagnosis is generally sufficient to establish a clinical diagnosis of uncomplicated infant GER. Detailed feeding history including amount and frequency of formula or breast feeding, position during feeding, burping, and behavior during feeding should be obtained. Choking, gagging, coughing with feedings, or significant irritability can be warning signs for GERD or other diagnosis. If there is a forceful vomiting of gastric contents, laboratory and radiographic investigation (upper gastrointestinal series) is warranted to exclude other causes of vomiting.

Unexplained crying and distressed behavior are nonspecific symptoms and associated with a variety of pathological and non-pathological conditions in infants. Healthy young infants fuss or cry an average of 2–2.5 h daily. Consideration should be given to individual variation of crying in infants and parental perception of the crying. Irritability coupled with arching in infants is thought to be a nonverbal equivalent of heartburn and chest pain in older children. Other causes of irritability including cow's milk protein allergy, neurologic disorders, constipation, and infection should be ruled out. The presentation of cow's milk protein allergy overlaps with GERD, and both conditions may coexist in 42–58% of infants.

Failure to thrive or poor weight gain can be the result of recurrent regurgitation and is a warning sign for GERD that alters clinical approach and management. A detailed feeding history should be obtained including the amount of intake, frequency of feedings, and description of infant sucking and swallowing behavior. Poor weight gain despite an adequate intake of calories should prompt evaluation for causes of regurgitation and weight loss other than GERD.

Heartburn is a symptom of GERD with or without esophagitis. Although older children can verbalize pain, the exact description may not be reliable until at least 8 years of age or later. In adolescents heartburn and regurgitation are reliable indicators of GERD. The guidelines recommend lifestyle changes initially, followed by 2–4-week empiric trial of acid suppression. If symptoms persist, then endoscopic evaluation is warranted to determine the presence of esophagitis and exclude other diagnosis such as eosinophilic esophagitis or infections.

Dysphagia can be the presentation of GERD; however, anatomic abnormalities, neurologic disorder, inflammatory conditions of mouth and esophagus, and psychological conditions should be ruled out. Imaging studies and endoscopic evaluation with histology can help to define the etiology.

Odynophagia or pain caused by swallowing can occur in GERD and eosinophilic esophagitis but also can be seen in oropharyngeal inflammation.

Food refusal has often been a considered a symptom of GER, but there is no evidence that supports a causal relationship.

Extraesophageal Symptoms of GER

Dental erosions can be associated with acid reflux, especially on occlusive surfaces of posterior teeth. Dental erosion, also known as perimylolysis, is the irreversible loss of dental hard tissue by a chemical process in the absence of bacteria. This differentiates it from caries. It is characterized as a hard "dished out" area with a smooth, glistening base. Ingestion of acidic beverages and poor hygiene are the external contributory factors, but this usually affects anterior surfaces.

Sandifer's syndrome is spasmodic torsional dystonia with arching of the back and opisthotonic posturing. It is an uncommon but specific presentation of GERD. Other neurological disorders including seizures, infantile spasm, and dystonia should be ruled out. The true pathophysiologic mechanisms of this condition remain unclear, but it is speculated to be secondary to vagally mediated reflex due to esophageal acid exposure. It responds well to anti-reflux treatment.

Apnea and *apparent life-threatening events (ALTEs)* are frequently considered extraesophageal manifestations of GERD in infants, but causality is rarely established. Apnea of prematurity (AOP) is a developmental sleep disorder which is yet to be completely understood. Feeding is an important trigger for AOP. While hypoxemia during feeding is most likely related to an immature coordination between sucking/swallowing and breathing, it is potentially due to an immature laryngeal chemoreflex. Hypoxemia after feeding may be caused by diaphragmatic fatigue, and GER only rarely plays a role. Although a clear temporal relation based on history suggests GER, the current evidence supports that GER is not related to apnea or to ALTEs. It is also reported that anti-reflux medications do not reduce the frequency of apnea in premature infants.

Otolaryngologic presentations include stridor, chronic cough, hoarseness and lump in the throat, recurrent sinusitis, pharyngitis, and serous otitis media. Postglottic edema, vocal cord edema, arytenoid edema, and tracheal cobblestoning during laryngoscopy and bronchoscopy have been associated with GERD. There is no proven mechanism by which GER can cause these symptoms, although direct injury by the refluxate, neural reflexes mediated by intraesophageal acid, and stimulation of laryngeal chemoreceptors have been speculated. Pepsin has been identified in the middle-ear fluid of children with effusion.

Asthma and GER commonly coexist, and children with asthma were reported to have a high prevalence of GER. Sixty to eighty percent of children with asthma have abnormal pH or pH/impedance studies. Esophageal acidification in healthy individuals has minimal effect on pulmonary function; however, in patients with asthma, it can cause airway hyperresponsiveness and airway obstruction. Nocturnal wheezing appears related to GERD. Proposed mechanisms for GER inducing asthma are direct aspiration, vagally mediated laryngeal and bronchial spasm, and neurally mediated inflammation through the release of tachykinins.

Conversely, asthma can induce GER. Chronic hyperinflation can flatten the diaphragms, alter crural function, reduce resting LES pressure, and change the angle of His.

In patients where symptoms of asthma and GERD coexist, we can consider a 3-month trial of aggressive acid suppression. In patients with persistent asthma and no GERD, 24-h pH probe and impedance study can be helpful in determining the presence of GERD for possible treatment with acid suppression.

Recurrent pneumonia and interstitial lung disease may be complications of GER due to the failure of airway defense mechanisms to protect the lungs against aspirated stomach contents. The most common cause of recurrent pneumonia in children is primary aspiration compared to GERD in 6% in reported series. Other causes of pneumonia in children (direct aspiration due to dysfunctional swallow, immune deficiencies, congenital heart disease, anatomic abnormalities, and asthma) are more common than GERD and should be ruled out first. No test can determine whether GER is causing recurrent pneumonia. Lipid-laden alveolar macrophages have been used as indicator of aspiration, but the sensitivity and specificity are low. Elevated pepsin content of alveolar lavage fluid is reported from patients with GER; however, evidence is inconclusive for routine use. A trial of nasogastric feeding may be used to exclude aspiration during swallowing as a cause of pneumonia. A trial of nasojejunal feeding may help in determining whether surgical therapy is likely to be beneficial. In patients with severely impaired lung function, surgery can help to prevent further pulmonary damage despite lack of definite proof that GER is causative.

Complicated GERD

Barrett's esophagus, esophageal strictures, and adenocarcinoma are the most important complications of chronic GERD.

Esophageal strictures are typically located in the distal third of the esophagus and should be distinguished from other causes of strictures. Chronic exposure to acid and pepsin, hiatal hernia, and esophageal dysmotility predispose to strictures. Reflux strictures are treated with a series of dilations in conjunction with aggressive medical therapy. Surgical therapy is reserved for recalcitrant strictures.

Barrett's esophagus (BE) is the condition in which normal esophageal squamous epithelium is replaced by a metaplastic columnar epithelium with goblet cells that predisposes cancer development. It occurs in children with less frequency than in adults. Cystic fibrosis, severe neurological impairment, and repaired esophageal atresia are associated with BE in children. Symptoms are a poor guide to the severity of acid reflux and esophagitis. Aggressive acid suppression is recommended. Dysplasia surveillance is managed according to adult guidelines to help identify patients who may progress to develop dysplasia and adenocarcinoma.

Adenocarcinoma is extremely rare in childhood but reported in a child in the setting of BE.

Diagnosis

The diagnosis of uncomplicated GER is usually established with a detailed history and physical exam. In infants, there is no symptom which is diagnostic for GERD or predicts response to treatment. Because of these inconsistencies, parent-reported infant GERD questionnaires based on symptoms have been developed. The questionnaire has been shown to be reliable for documentation and monitoring of reported symptoms, but the correlation between the results of reflux investigation is poor. Atypical presentations, complicated GER, or failure to respond to empiric management are indications for further diagnostic evaluations. These include radiography, endoscopy with esophageal biopsy, esophageal pH monitoring, and combined pH and esophageal impedance measurements.

Fluoroscopic evaluation of the upper gastrointestinal tract has low sensitivity and specificity for diagnosing GERD, but it may be useful in identifying other anatomic abnormalities such as strictures, hiatal hernia, intestinal malrotation, or pyloric stenosis. Modified barium swallow studies can be helpful in diagnosing aspiration during swallowing in patients with airway symptoms.

Nuclear scintigraphy is generally utilized in infants to quantify gastric emptying and obtain information regarding reflux-related aspiration. The study in infants is performed using liquid labeled with technetium 99 m. In children and adults, the standard protocol involves a low-fat, egg-white meal with imaging at 0, 1, 2, and 4 h after meal ingestion. Gastric emptying may be delayed in some children who have GERD.

Esophageal pH monitoring is widely accepted as a safe method of detecting acid reflux. GERD episode during pH monitoring is defined as a sudden decrease in intraesophageal pH to below 4.0. Based on the cutoff value of pH 4, several parameters can be defined to quantify the amount of GERD: number of episodes/24 h of drop in pH below 4, number of episodes of certain duration (i.e., above 5 min), and percentage of time during a 24-h period that esophageal pH is below 4. These parameters are also correlated to awakeness or state of sleep, meal time, and body position. The percentage of time in a 24-h study that the esophageal pH is less than 4, also called the "reflux index" (RI), is considered the most valid measure of reflux because it reflects the cumulative exposure of the esophagus to acid. Commonly, an RI greater than 11% is considered abnormal in infants, while RI greater than 7% is abnormal in older children. The greatest utility of pH monitoring is to correlate the specific symptom in relation to intraesophageal pH reading at the time of the "event" (apnea, stridor, or Sandifer's syndrome) and to assess efficacy of antisecretory therapy.

Esophageal impedance monitoring is a sensitive tool for evaluating overall GERD and particularly in detecting nonacid reflux episodes. Multichannel intraluminal impedance (MII) detects reflux episodes based on changes in electrical resistance to the flow of an electrical current between two electrodes on the probe when a liquid or gas bolus moves between them. When combined with esophageal pH monitoring, the MII test allows detection of both acid and nonacid episodes of GER.

Endoscopic evaluation with histology is the most accurate method of detecting esophageal injury by reflux and diagnosing Barrett's esophagus. Macroscopic lesions associated with GERD include erosions, exudate, ulcers, strictures, and hiatal hernia. Histologic findings of reflux esophagitis include basal cell hyperplasia, increase papillary length, basal layer spongiosis (edema), and erosion and ulcerations in severe cases. None of the histologic findings listed are specific for reflux esophagitis. There is also a poor correlation between the severity of symptoms and presence and absence of esophagitis. There is insufficient evidence to support the use of histology to diagnose or exclude GERD.

Treatment

For noncomplicated reflux, no intervention is required for most infants. Effective parental **reassurance** and educating parents regarding regurgitation and lifestyle changes are usually sufficient to manage infant reflux. This includes adjusting feeding regimens, positioning after feeds, and avoiding environmental smoke exposure. Review of 14 randomized controlled trials and practice guidelines summarized that **thickening feeds** does not seem to reduce measurable reflux, but it decreases the frequency of overt regurgitation and vomiting. It also increased the infant's weight gain per day. Agents such as rice cereal (more popular in North America), corn or potato starch, carob-bean gum (also called locust-bean gum – more popular in Europe), carob-seed flour, and sodium carboxymethylcellulose are often used. Thickening a 20-kcal/oz formula with one tablespoon of rice cereal increases the caloric density to 34 kcal/oz which can cause excessive weight gain in infants and may induce constipation.

A subset of infants with cow's milk protein allergy have regurgitation and vomiting, mimicking GER.

Forty percent of patients with GER were shown to have cow's milk protein allergy. In these infants, symptoms decrease significantly within 2 weeks time after elimination of cow's milk protein from the diet. In breast-fed infants, milk and milk products should be eliminated from maternal diet. In formula-fed infants, hydrolyzed or amino-acid-based formulas should be considered for 2–4-week trial. Studies have shown that prone positioning resulted in decreased frequency of reflux, but due to the risk of sudden infant death syndrome (SIDS), the American Academy of Pediatrics recommends that all infants younger than 12 months of age generally be placed in supine position for sleep even they have GERD.

In older children, mild symptoms of reflux without complications are often well managed by lifestyle changes such as weight loss, if appropriate, and by avoidance of fatty foods, caffeinated beverages, and chocolate and not eating before bedtime.

Pharmacotherapeutic agents used in GERD encompass antisecretory agents, antacids, surface barrier agents, and prokinetics (Table 1). Antisecretory agents include histamine-2 receptor antagonists (H2RAs) and proton pump inhibitors (PPIs).

Histamine-2 receptor antagonists decrease acid secretion by inhibiting histamine-2 receptors on gastric parietal cells. H2RAs (cimetidine, ranitidine, famotidine, and nizatidine) are effective in healing reflux esophagitis in infants and children. The fairly rapid development of tachyphylaxis in all H2RAs is a drawback for chronic use, and tolerance can be seen as early as 14 days of repeated administration. All H2RAs require dose adjustment in renal impairment. All can cause irritability and abnormal liver function tests. Gynecomastia and drug interactions have been reported with cimetidine.

Proton pump inhibitors (PPI) inhibit acid secretion by blocking Na+-K+-ATPase of the "proton pump" that performs the final step in the acid secretory process of the parietal cell. They thereby inhibit both basal and stimulated secretion of gastric acid, independent of the parietal cell stimulation. The superior efficacy of healing by PPIs is largely due to their ability to maintain intragastric pH at or above 4 for longer periods of time and to inhibit meal-induced acid secretion for which H2RAs do not have any effect. All PPIs are usually well tolerated; common adverse effects reported for all proton pump inhibitors include headache, diarrhea, rash, nausea, and constipation.

Gastroesophageal Reflux in Children, Table 1 Drugs used in treatment of GERD

Medication	Pediatric dose	Comments
H₂ receptor antagonists		
Cimetidine	20–40 mg/kg/day divided 2–4 times a day (Adult dose: 800–1,200 mg/dose 2–3 times daily)	Rash, bradycardia, dizziness, nausea, vomiting, hypotension, gynecomastia, reduces hepatic metabolism of theophylline and other medications, neutropenia, thrombocytopenia, agranulocytosis, doses should be decreased with renal insufficiency
Ranitidine	2–10 mg/kg/day divided 2–3 times a day (Adult dose:300 mg twice daily)	Headache, dizziness, fatigue, irritability, rash, constipation, diarrhea, thrombocytopenia, elevated transaminases, doses should be decreased with renal insufficiency[a]
Famotidine	1 mg/kg/day divided 2 times a day (Adult dose: 20 mg twice daily)	Headache, dizziness, constipation, diarrhea, nausea, doses should be decreased with renal insufficiency[a]
Nizatidine	10 mg/kg/day divided 2 times a day (Adult dose: 150 mg twice daily)	Headache, dizziness, constipation, diarrhea, nausea, anemia, urticaria, doses should be decreased with renal insufficiency
Proton pump inhibitors		
All should be given 20–30 min before meals		
Not approved for infants		
Omeprazole	1.0–3.3 mg/kg/day <20 kg: 10 mg/day >20 kg: 20 mg/day	Headache, diarrhea, abdominal pain, nausea, rash, constipation, vitamin B12 deficiency
Lansoprazole	0.8–4 mg/kg/day <30 kg: 15 mg/day >30 kg: 30 mg/day Approved for >1 year of age	Headache, diarrhea, abdominal pain, nausea, elevated transaminase, proteinuria, angina, hypotension
Pantoprazole	No pediatric dose available (Adult dose: 40 mg once daily) IV dose same as oral dose (adults)	Headache, diarrhea, abdominal pain, nausea
Rabeprazole	No pediatric dose available (Adult dose: 20 mg once daily) (Adult dose: 20 mg once daily) Adult dose: 40 mg/day Adult dose: 40 mg/day Adult dose: 40 mg/day Adult dose: 40 mg/day Adult dose: 40 mg/day Approved for use in those >1 year old	Headache, diarrhea, abdominal pain, nausea
Omeprazole with sodium bicarbonate	Recognizing that this formulation has not received FDA approval for use in children despite an approved dosage for omeprazole in children and considering that omeprazole has been used safely in children as an extemporaneous formulation with sodium bicarbonate, the following dosage is recommended: 5 to <10 kg: 5 mg once daily 10 to ≤20 kg: 10 mg once daily >20: 20 mg once daily Alternate dosing: 1 mg/kg/day once or twice daily	Avoid using in patients on sodium-restricted diets due to high content of sodium bicarbonate Headache, diarrhea, abdominal pain, nausea
Esomeprazole	1–11 years 10–20 mg daily 12–17 years 20–40 mg daily Adult dose:20–40 mg/day	Headache, diarrhea, constipation, abdominal pain, somnolence

(continued)

Gastroesophageal Reflux in Children, Table 1 (continued)

Medication	Pediatric dose	Comments
Barrier agents		
Sucralfate	40–80 mg/kg/day divided 4 times/day	Vertigo, constipation, aluminum toxicity, decreases the absorption of concurrently administered drugs
Alginate	0.2–0.5 ml/kg/dose 3–8 times/day	Tablets need to be chewed before swallowing Need to separate from other medications by 2 h
Prokinetic drugs		
Metoclopramide	0.1 mg/kg/dose 4 times/day	Drowsiness, restlessness, dystonia, tardive dyskinesia, gynecomastia, galactorrhea
Cisapride	0.8 mg/kg/day divided into four doses daily	Rare cases of serious cardiac arrhythmia (FDA recommends ECG before administration)
	(Adult dose: 10–20 mg/dose four times daily)	Beware of drug interactions (macrolide antibiotics, imidazoles, protease inhibitors)
		Very restricted use in the USA
		Do not use in patients with liver, cardiac, or electrolyte abnormalities (FDA recommends checking K^+, Ca^{++}, Mg^{++}, and creatine before administration)
Domperidone	No pediatric dose available	Hyperprolactinemia, dry mouth, rash, headache, diarrhea, nervousness
Bethanechol	0.1–0.3 mg/kg/dose 4 times/day	Hypotension, bronchospasm, salivation, cramps, blurred vision, bradycardia
Baclofen	<2 years 10–40 mg/day Divided 2–3 times daily 2–7 years 20–60 mg/day Divided 2–3 times daily >7 years 30–120 mg/day Divided 2–3 times daily	Somnolence, confusion, depression, hypotension, weakness, diaphoresis, hematuria

PPIs currently approved for use in children in North America are omeprazole, lansoprazole, and esomeprazole for above 1 year of age and pantoprazole above 5 years of age. At this time in Europe, only omeprazole and esomeprazole are approved. No PPIs have been approved for use in infants younger than 1 year of age. Although not approved, PPIs are commonly used for the treatment of infants with GERD. Multiple studies have shown that a trial of PPI in infants with reflux-like symptoms produced similar improvement in irritability while taking placebo or PPI, despite documented reduction of esophageal acidification in the PPI group. This concluded that PPI therapy is not beneficial for the treatment of infants with symptoms that were purported but not proven to be due to GERD.

PPIs are highly efficacious and safe for the treatment of GERD-related symptoms and signs, including the most severe degrees of reflux esophagitis in older children and adolescents. Several open label treatment studies have found even higher rates of healing of erosive esophagitis in children compared with studies in adults. A failure to respond to PPI should raise consideration of insufficient dosing, improper administration, or incorrect diagnosis. Experience indicates that the most common error in PPI prescribing in children is underdosing. Another common error in prescribing PPIs in children is splitting the total daily dose into twice-daily dosing. The optimal administration mode for PPIs is once per day, just before the first meal of the day, since that is when acid pumps or proton pumps are generated and can then be efficiently blocked.

Antacids work by neutralizing gastric acid and decreasing the exposure of gastric acid to esophagus during episode of reflux. Most available products contain the combination of magnesium and aluminum hydroxide or calcium carbonate. The use of aluminum-containing antacids in infants can lead to elevated aluminum levels and cause osteopenia, microcytic anemia, and neurotoxicity as complications.

Surface barrier agents contain either alginate or sucralfate. **Sodium alginate (Gaviscon)** forms a surface gel that creates physical barrier against refluxate and protects the mucosa. It appears to be relatively safe, as only a limited number of side effects have been reported. Occasional formation of large bezoar-like masses of agglutinated intragastric material has been reported in infants with the use of Gaviscon. **Sucralfate** is a compound of sucrose, sulfate, and aluminum, which forms a gel in an acidic environment. North American and European Pediatric Gastroenterology Society (NASPGHAN/ESPGHAN) GER guidelines committee concluded that there is no adequate data of efficacy or safety of sucralfate in the treatment of infant GERD, especially with the risk of aluminum toxicity. In older children, its main use is in erosive and ulcerative esophagitis.

Prokinetic agents improve regurgitation via their effects on lower esophageal sphincter pressure, esophageal peristalsis, and acid clearance or promoting gastric emptying. The current NASPGHAN and ESPGHAN practice guidelines concluded that there is insufficient evidence to justify the routine use of prokinetic agents. **Bethanechol** seems to increase muscarinic cholinergic drive, resulting in increased LES tone and esophageal peristaltic amplitude and velocity. Because it is a cholinergic agonist, it increases salivary and bronchial secretions and may contribute to bronchospasm. **Domperidone** is a peripheral dopamine-D2 receptor antagonist that facilitates gastric emptying and esophageal motility. NASPGHAN working group concluded that the effectiveness of domperidone is unproven. **Cisapride** is a benzamide derivative and is a non-dopamine-receptor-blocking, non-cholinergic prokinetic drug with 5HT4-antagonistic properties. It stimulates motility in lower esophagus, stomach, and small intestine by increasing acetylcholine release in the myenteric plexus. Despite the vast majority of the clinical trials, the efficacy of cisapride demonstrated that at least one of the end points changes favorably as a result of the intervention. Due to reports of fatal cardiac arrhythmias or sudden death, from July 2000 in the USA and Europe, cisapride has been restricted to a limited access program supervised by a physician.

Metoclopramide has cholinomimetic and mixed serotonergic effects. Adverse effects of irritability, drowsiness, and extrapyramidal reactions can be seen up to 34% of children taking metoclopramide. **Erythromycin**, a macrolide antibiotic, also has prokinetic effects by its ability to act on motilin receptors and initiate phase 3 activity of the migrating motor complexes. Erythromycin does not have effects on esophageal or LES motility, but may improve gastric emptying in selective cases in infants and children. There is also a concern of development of infantile hypertrophic pyloric stenosis with use of erythromycin in newborn period, especially first 14 days of life. **Baclofen** is a gamma-aminobutyric acid B (GABA B) receptor agonist; it inhibits the occurrence of transient lower esophageal sphincter relaxations. Baclofen has been shown to decrease the frequency of emesis and improve reflux episodes in neurologically impaired children. Potential side effects include drowsiness and lowered seizure threshold.

Endoscopic Treatment

Endoluminal gastroplication (EG) is emerging as a minimally invasive procedure for the treatment of gastroesophageal reflux disease in children. Endoscopic gastroplication using the EndoCinch endoscopic suturing device was developed by Swain and colleagues. The basis of this procedure is to construct plications in the gastric mucosa/submucosa below the lower esophageal sphincter with the intent to improve its function by augmenting the anti-reflux barrier. It is shown to reduce transient lower esophageal sphincter relaxations and slightly increase lower esophageal sphincter pressure. The largest pediatric series reported by one center followed up 16 children after endoluminal gastroplication. Four had recurrent symptoms requiring a repeat procedure within 2–24 months. Three years after procedure, nine patients were doing well with no medications.

Other endoscopic GERD treatments have not been studied in children.

Surgical Treatment

Despite the availability and proven efficacy of PPIs for severe GERD, anti-reflux surgery remains widely used in children. In the United States, fundoplication is among the most commonly performed operations by pediatric surgeons. The widely performed wrap is Nissen fundoplication which involves passage of gastric fundus behind the esophagus to encircle the distal esophagus. Laparoscopic Nissen fundoplication has largely replaced open Nissen fundoplication due to its decreased morbidity, shorter hospital stays, and fewer postoperative complications, but a somewhat higher reoperation rate is reported in laparoscopic

Nissen fundoplication. A partial, 270° wrap (Toupet) is used in patients with severe esophageal motor dysfunction.

Fundoplication prevents GER by increasing LES pressure, increasing the length of the intra-abdominal esophagus, accentuating the angle of His, and reducing hiatal hernia if present. However, fundoplication has no impact on poor esophageal clearance or delayed gastric emptying and may cause dysphagia, bloating, and retching in these settings. In general, outcomes of fundoplication have been more carefully evaluated in adults than children. Most of the literature on anti-reflux surgery in children with GERD consists of retrospective case series in which documentation of diagnosis and details of previous treatments are deficient, making it difficult to assess the outcome of surgery. The symptom improvement has been described between 60% and 90% of children, but also failure rate varies between 2% and 50% depending on reported series. Complications after surgery are due to alterations in fundic capacity and compliance that may persist from months to years. These include retching and gagging, gas-bloat syndrome, early satiety, and dumping syndrome.

The problems with anti-reflux surgery occur especially in children with neurologic impairment (NI), repaired esophageal atresia, or chronic lung disease and to a lesser degree in otherwise normal children. The children with NI have more than twice the complication rate, three times the morbidity, and four times the reoperation rate compared to otherwise healthy children.

Anti-reflux surgery may be of benefit in children with confirmed GERD who have failed optimal medical therapy or are dependent on medical therapy over a long period of time or who have life-threatening complications of GERD. Children with respiratory complications including asthma or recurrent aspiration are generally considered most likely to benefit from surgery when medical therapy fails, but additional studies are required to confirm this.

References

Chang AB, Lasserson TJ, Kiljander TO et al (2006) Systematic review and meta-analysis of randomized controlled trials of gastro-oesophageal reflux interventions for chronic cough associated with gastro-oesophageal reflux. BMJ 332:11–17

Gibbons TE, Gold BD (2003) The use of proton pump inhibitors in children: a comprehensive review. Paediatr Drugs 5:25–40

Gold BD (2005) Asthma and gastroesophageal disease in children: exploring the relationship. J Pediatr 146:S13–S20

Gold BD (2010) Gastroesophageal reflux disease. In: Bishop WP (ed) Pediatric practice gastroenterology, 1st edn. McGrawHill, New York, pp 160–189

Hassall E (2005) Outcomes of fundoplication: causes of concern, newer options. Arch Dis Child 90:1047–1052

Khan S, Orenstein SR (2006) Gastroesophageal reflux disease in infants and children. In: Granderath FA, Kamolz T, Pointner R (eds) Gastroesophageal reflux disease. Principles of disease, diagnosis and treatment, 1st edn. Springer, Wien/New York, pp 45–64

Orenstein SR, Hassall E (2007) Infants and proton pump inhibitors: tribulations, no trials. J Pediatr Gastroenterol Nutr 45:395–398

Sherman PM, Hassall E, Fagundes-Neto U et al (2009) A global, evidence-based consensus on the definition of gastroesophageal reflux disease in the pediatric population. Am J Gastroenterol 104:1278–1295

Thakkar K, Boatright RO, Gilger M et al (2010) Gastroesophageal reflux and asthma in children: a systematic review. Pediatrics 125:e925–e930

Thomson M, Antoa B, Hall S et al (2008) Medium term outcome of endoluminal gastroplication with the EndoCinch device in children. J Pediatr Gastroenterol Nutr 46:172–177

Vandenplas Y, Rudolph CD, Di Lorenzo C, Hassall E, Liptak G, Mazur L, Sondheimer J, Staiano A, Thomson M, Veereman-Wauters G, Wenzl TG (2009) Pediatric gastroesophageal reflux clinical practice guidelines: joint recommendations of the North American society for pediatric gastroenterology, hepatology, and nutrition (NASPGHAN) and the European society for pediatric gastroenterology, hepatology, and nutrition. J Pediatr Gastroenterol Nutr 49(4):498–547

Gene Therapy

Gerald T. Kangelaris and Lawrence R. Lustig
Department of Otolaryngology-Head and Neck Surgery, University of California, San Francisco, San Francisco, CA, USA

Definition

The insertion, alteration, or removal of genes within an individual's cells and biological tissues to treat disease.

Cross-References

▶ Sensorineural Hearing Loss

Genes

▶ Genetics of Hearing Loss

Genetic Deafness

▶ Genetic Sensorineural Hearing Loss

Genetic Hearing Loss

▶ Genetic Sensorineural Hearing Loss

Genetic Heterogeneity

Matthew Ng[1] and Drew M. Horlbeck[2]
[1]Department of Surgery, Division of Otolaryngology, University of Nevada School of Medicine, Las Vegas, NV, USA
[2]Department of Surgery, Division of Pediatric Otolaryngology, Nemours Children's Clinic, Jacksonville, FL, USA

Definition

Different mutated genes causing the same phenotype.

Cross-References

▶ Sensorineural Hearing Loss-Congenital-Genetics

Genetic Mixed Hearing Loss

▶ Congenital Mixed Hearing Loss

Genetic Sensorineural Hearing Loss

Aurash S. Alemi and Lawrence R. Lustig
Department of Otolaryngology-Head and Neck Surgery, University of California, San Fransisco, San Fransisco, CA, USA

Synonyms

Congenital deafness; Genetic deafness; Genetic hearing loss; Inherited hearing loss; Nonsyndromic hearing loss; Syndromic hearing loss

Definition

Hearing loss is the most common disorder of the sensory system, affecting between 1 and 3 in 1,000 children at birth (http://www.nidcd.nih.gov/health/statistics/Pages/quick.aspx). Severe hearing loss, which occurs prior to acquisition of spoken language (termed *prelingual* hearing loss), can have profound effects on oral communication. The treatment of severe and profound hearing loss thus remains an important therapeutic challenge. A thorough understanding and appreciation for the genetic mechanisms of hearing loss is paramount to the work-up and management of patients as it informs both diagnostic and therapeutic approaches.

Classification

Hearing loss (HL) is broadly classified as sensorineural (SNHL), which is caused by dysfunction of the inner ear, and conductive (CHL), which is caused by the impedance of sound waves from the external and middle ear to the cochlea. Sensorineural hearing losses can in turn be subdivided into acquired (i.e., environmental) and inherited (i.e., genetic) forms (Fig. 1). This entry will focus upon genetic causes of SNHL.

In addition to location of the anatomic defect and the clinical presentation, age of onset and severity of symptoms are two other commonly used classification schemes. *Prelingual* refers to the onset of hearing loss prior to the acquisition of speech, whereas *postlingual* represents hearing loss that develops after the acquisition of speech. As noted earlier, this has profound

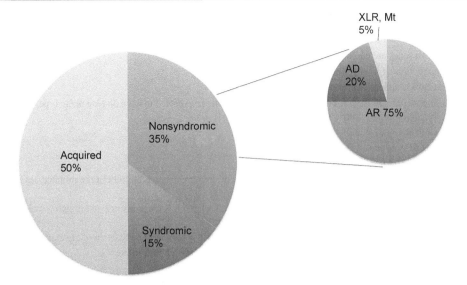

Genetic Sensorineural Hearing Loss, Fig. 1 Causes of acquired and inherited hearing loss. Acquired and inherited causes of hearing loss each comprise 50% of all cases. There are several causes of acquired HL including infection (e.g., CMV, Toxoplasmosis, Rubella, Herpes, Syphilis), trauma, noise exposure, and ototoxicity (e.g., aminoglycosides, loop diuretics, cisplatin). Of causes of inherited hearing loss, the two subcategories are syndromic (accounting for 30% of inherited hearing loss) and nonsyndromic (accounting for about 70% of inherited hearing loss). Of causes of nonsyndromic hearing loss (inset), autosomal recessive (AR) forms are the most common, accounting for 75–80% of cases. Autosomal dominant (AD) inheritance comprises approximately 20%. X-linked (XLR), Y-linked and mitochondrial (Mt) inherited genes together comprise approximately 5% of cases of nonsyndromic hearing loss (Morton and Giersch 2010)

implications on the development of oral communication. Severity of hearing loss is also defined by the degree of hearing impairment as mild (20–40 dB), moderate (41–55 dB), moderately severe (56–70 dB), severe (71–90 dB), and profound (>90 dB).

Etiology

Genetics of Hearing Loss

As referenced in Table 1, there are several mechanisms by which hearing loss can be inherited. Autosomal recessive, where a mutation in both alleles is required to cause disease phenotype, is the most common form. Autosomal dominant, by contrast, only requires that one allele be mutated to lead to the disease phenotype. X-linked inheritance generally behaves as a recessive trait, however, since males only have one X-chromosome, it manifests at a disproportionally higher rate in men than women. Mitochondrial disorders are inherited via mutations of the mitochondrial DNA and are hence only passed from mother to child. (See Table 2 for more in depth discussion of modes of inheritance.)

Clinical Presentation: Syndromic Versus Nonsyndromic Hearing Loss

The classification of hearing loss into several subcategories has important clinical applications. *Syndromic* hearing losses are those that are associated with additional organ system involvement. In contrast, in *nonsyndromic* forms of hearing loss, no other clinical features are associated with the hearing deficit. This distinction is important since it can have severe ramifications on the future health of the individual. Indeed, discovery of hearing impairment in children should prompt a thorough investigation for manifestations of a syndromic disorder.

Nonsyndromic Hearing Loss

Nonsyndromic hearing loss accounts for approximately 70% of all hereditary cases of hearing loss (Minárik et al. 2012) and to date over 70 loci have been identified in the pathogenesis of nonsyndromic hearing loss (HHL website). Autosomal recessive

Genetic Sensorineural Hearing Loss, Table 1 Inheritance modes

Inheritance mode	General features
Autosomal recessive	Both sexes are equally affected
	Only homozygotes express disease phenotype
	Child is generally born to two asymptomatic carriers
	If both parents are carriers, roughly 25% of children are expected to have disease phenotype, 50% are expected to be asymptomatic carriers and 25% are unaffected
Autosomal dominant	Both sexes are equally affected
	Heterozygotes express disease phenotype
	One parent generally has disease phenotype
	If one parent has the disease, roughly 50% of children are expected to inherit the mutated allele and hence the disease phenotype
X-linked	Males are affected more frequently because females have 2 X chromosomes, although females may exhibit variable degrees of disease because of Lyonization
	Affected man will pass allele to all daughters, who will be asymptomatic carriers. He cannot pass disease to sons
	Affected woman will pass allele to 50% of her daughters and 50% of her sons will have the disease phenotype
Mitochondrial	Non-Mendelian inheritance pattern
	Because genes are in mitochondria, which are inherited from the egg, disease can only be transmitted from mother to child
	All offspring of affected female are expected to inherit disease phenotype, although severity may differ

Genetic Sensorineural Hearing Loss, Table 2 Selected causes of autosomal recessive nonsyndromic hearing loss (Source: Hereditary Hearing Loss website)

Locus	Chromosomal location	Gene
DFNB1	13q12	GJB2
DFNB2	11q13.5	MYO7A
DFNB3	17p11.2	MYO15A
DFNB4	7q31	SLC26A4
DFNB6	3p14-p21	TMIE
DFNB7/11	9q13-q21	TMC1
DFNB8/10	21q22	TMPRSS3
DFNB9	2p22-p23	OTOF
DFNB12	10q21-q22	CDH23
DFNB16	15q21-q22	STRC
DFNB18	11p14-15.1	USH1C
DFNB21	11q	TECTA
DFNB22	16p12.2	OTOA
DFNB23	10p11.2-q21	PCDH15
DFNB28	22q13	TRIOBP
DFNB29	21q22	CLDN14
DFNB30	10p11.1	MYO3A
DFNB31	9q32-q34	WHRN
DFNB36	1p36.3	ESPN
DFNB37	6q13	MYO6
DFNB72	19p13.3	GIPC3
DNFB91	6p25	SERPINB6

patterns of inheritance of nonsyndromic hearing loss are the most common, accounting for 75–80% of cases. Autosomal recessive deafness tends to be prelingual, stable and severe, whereas autosomal dominant hearing loss tends to have a postlingual onset, be progressive and less severe (Morton and Giersch 2010). Thus, because autosomal recessive modes of inheritance comprise the largest portion of cases of nonsyndromic hearing loss, approximately 75–80% of cases are prelingual and severe.

Nonsyndromic hearing loss is given a specialized nomenclature. The prefix DFN (shortened for *deafness*) is given to each gene locus, and is then followed by either A or B, which represent autosomal dominant and autosomal recessive inheritance, respectively. Finally, the order in which the genes were discovered is reflected numerically with an integer number following DFN. For example, DFNB1, the nonsyndromic human form of deafness caused by the Connexin 26 mutation, represents an autosomal recessive mutation, which was the first autosomal recessive locus to be identified. While the gene candidates of many loci have been identified, not all have, and the precise cause of many cases of nonsyndromic deafness remain unknown (Hereditary Hearing Loss website).

Autosomal Recessive Nonsyndromic Hearing Loss

To date, 71 loci have been identified as causing autosomal recessive nonsyndromic hearing loss, of which 41 genes have been cloned (Hereditary Hearing Loss website). The protein products of these genes include ion channels, membrane proteins, transcription factors, and various cytoskeletal elements. Because of the large number of mutations causing autosomal recessive nonsyndromic hearing loss, only the most common DFNB1 will be discussed below.

Connexin 26

Autosomal recessive mutations in Connexin 26, causing DFNB1, accounts for 30–40% of all cases of deafness in most populations (Zelante et al. 1997; Denoyelle et al. 1999; Dodson et al. 2011). There are as many as 21 genes belonging to the connexin family, 5 of which are involved in deafness (Connexins-deafness, homepage, http://davinci.crg.es/deafness). Connexins are a homogeneous family of transmembrane proteins which are expressed in a variety of tissues and play a role in intercellular signaling by forming channels called gap junctions, which are especially prevalent in the auditory epithelium and cardiac myocytes. The mutant gene in DFNB1 is *GJB2*, which has been mapped to chromosome 13. As the genotype is highly variable by population, phenotype can also vary in severity from moderate to profound deafness depending on mutation type (Gürtler 2012).

Autosomal Dominant Nonsyndromic Hearing Loss

Fifty-four loci have been identified which cause autosomal dominant nonsyndromic hearing loss, from which 25 genes have been cloned (Hereditary Hearing Loss website). As a general rule, most autosomal dominant forms of nonsyndromic hearing loss are postlingual, whereas most cases of autosomal recessive nonsyndromic hearing loss are prelingual (Hildebrand et al. 2010) (Table 3).

X-Linked and Mitochondrial Nonsyndromic Hearing Loss

Together, X-linked and mitochondrial inheritance patterns account for less than 5% of causes of nonsyndromic hearing loss (Table 4). Five loci and three genes have been mapped for the X-linked form and seven loci and several gene point-mutations have been identified for the mitochondrial form (HLL

Genetic Sensorineural Hearing Loss, Table 3 Selected causes of autosomal dominant nonsyndromic hearing loss (Source: Hereditary Hearing Loss website)

Locus	Chromosomal location	Gene
DFNA1	5q31	*DIAPH1*
DFNA2A	1p34	*KCNQ4*
DFNA2B	1p35.1	*GJB3*
DFNA3A	13q11-q12	*GJB2*
DFNA3B	13q12	*GJB6*
DFNA4	19q13	*MYH14*
DFNA5	7p15	*DFNA5*
DFNA6	4p16.3	*WFS1*
DFNA9	14q12-q13	*COCH*
DFNA10	6q22-q23	*EYA4*
DFNA11	11q12.3-q21	*MYO7A*
DFNA12	11q22-24	*TECTA*
DFNA13	6p21	*COL11A2*
DFN51	9q21	*TJP2*

Genetic Sensorineural Hearing Loss, Table 4 Causes of X-linked recessive nonsyndromic hearing loss (Source: Hereditary Hearing Loss website)

Locus	Chromosomal location	Gene
DFNX1	Xq22	*PRPS1*
DFNX2	Xq21.1	*POU3F4*
DFNX3	Xp21.2	Unknown
DFNX4	Xp22	*SMPX*
DFNX5	Xq23-q27.3	Unknown

website). Mitochondrial nonsyndromic deafness is of particular clinical relevance because the A1555G mutation in 12S rRNA is believed to predispose to aminoglycoside-induced deafness in addition to nonsyndromic hearing loss (Prezant et al. 1993; Estivill et al. 1998).

Syndromic Hearing Loss

In contrast to the more commonly seen nonsyndromic forms of hearing loss, syndromic hearing loss accounts for about 30% of inheritable hearing loss. The term *syndromic* hearing loss refers to hearing loss that presents with a constellation of other systemic findings. The severity of hearing loss varies across different syndromes, ranging from minor cases of hearing impairment to profound deafness. Like nonsyndromic deafness, syndromic forms can also be inherited in autosomal recessive, autosomal dominant, X-linked, and mitochondrial patterns (Table 5). A discussion of some of the more common syndromes follows.

Autosomal Recessive Syndromic Hearing Loss

Pendred Syndrome
Pendred syndrome is the most common form of syndromic deafness, and accounts for almost 10% of all cases of hereditary hearing loss (Everett et al. 1997; Dror et al. 2011). Pendred syndrome is most commonly caused by a mutation in *SLC26A4* – a gene encoding pendrin – an anion transporter present in the kidney, thyroid, and inner ear (Genetics Home Reference 2012; Everett et al. 1997; Dror et al. 2011). As such, patients present with varying severity of sensorineural hearing loss, bilateral enlargement of the vestibular aqueducts and endolymphatic sacs as well as thyroid goiter, which may develop later in life. Of note, mutations in *SCL26A4* have also been isolated as a cause of nonsyndromic hearing loss in DFNB4 (Dror et al. 2011).

Usher Syndrome
Usher syndromes are a very common cause of autosomal recessive syndromic hearing loss and are the most common disorders affecting hearing and vision, accounting for approximately 50% of all deafness-blindness cases (NIDCD website; Bonnet and El-Amraoui 2012). Three subtypes of Usher syndrome have been identified, termed USH1, USH2, and USH3, that have varying degrees of early onset, hearing and vestibular dysfunction and retinitis pigmentosa, a progressive degeneration of the retina (Table 6) (Bonnet and El-Amraoui 2012). USH1 is characterized by profound bilateral deafness accompanied by severe vestibular dysfunction which present at birth. Retinitis pigmentosa generally manifests as decreased night vision and becomes apparent before age 10. In contrast to USH1, USH2, and USH3 are characterized by normal to near normal vestibular function. USH2 has moderate to severe hearing loss at birth with *normal* vestibular function and retinitis pigmentosa that manifests later in childhood closer to the teenage years.

Genetic Sensorineural Hearing Loss, Table 5 Selected causes of syndromic hearing loss (Source: Hereditary Hearing Loss website)

Syndrome	Chromosomal locus	Gene
Autosomal dominant		
Branchio-oto-renal		
BOR1	8q13.3	*EYA1*
BOR2	19q13.3	*SIX5*
	1q31	Unknown
BOS3	14q21.3-q24.3	*SIX1*
Neurofibromatosis		
NF2	22q12	*NF2*
Stickler		
STL1	12q13.11q13.2	*COL2A1*
STL2	1p21	*COL11A1*
STL3	6p21.3	*COL11A2*
	6q13	*COL9A1*
	1p34.2	*COL9A2*
Treacher Collins		
TCOF1	5q32-33.1	*TCOF1*
Autosomal recessive		
Alport		
	2q36-37	*COL4A3*
		COL4A4
Jervell and Lange-Nielsen		
JLNS1	11p15.5	*KCNQ1*
JLNS2	21q22.1-22.2	*KCNE1*
Pendred		
PDS	7q21-34	*SLC26A4*
PDS	5q35.1	*FOXI1*
X-linked recessive		
Alport		
	Xq22	*COL4A5*

USH3 children are born with normal hearing at birth, with progressive impairment throughout childhood and teenage years. Like the hearing deficits, severity of vision impairment also varies with problems generally arising by the teenage years (Bonnet et al. 2011). Of note, like Pendred syndrome, gene mutations causing Usher syndrome are also responsible for nonsyndromic hearing loss.

Jervell and Lange-Nielsen Syndrome
Jervell and Lange-Nielsen syndrome (JLNS) classically involves sensorineural hearing loss and elongated QTc on electrocardiogram (EKG) testing (>500 ms). The prolongation of QTc predisposes to syncope from ventricular tachyarrhythmias, most notably *torsades*

Genetic Sensorineural Hearing Loss, Table 6 Types of Usher syndrome (Source: Hereditary Hearing Loss website)

Type	Subtype	Gene	Disease phenotype
1.	USH1B	MYO7a	Profound congenital hearing loss
	USH1C	USH1C	Absent vestibular responses
	USH1D	CDH23	Retinitis pigmentosa within first decade of life
	USH1E	Unknown	
	USH1F	PCDH15	
	USH1G	SANS	
	USH1H	Unknown	
2.	USH2A	USH2A	Moderate to severe congenital hearing loss
	USH2B	Unknown	Normal vestibular responses
	USH2C	VLGR1b	Retinitis pigmentosa within first two decades of life
	USH2D	WHRN	
3.	USH3	USH3	Progressive hearing loss
		PDZD7	Variable vestibular responses
			Variable onset of retinitis pigmentosa

Genetic Sensorineural Hearing Loss, Table 7 Subtypes of Waardenburg Syndrome. Pigmentation abnormalities and sensorineural hearing loss are associated with all subtypes. Only distinguishing features are listed above

Subtype	Gene[a]	Clinical manifestations
Type I	PAX3	Presence of dystopia canthorum[b]
Type II	MITF SNAI2	Lack of dystopia canthorum[b]
Type III (Klein-Waardenburg Syndrome)	PAX3	Type I + upper limb hypoplasia or contracture
Type IV (Waardenburg-Shah Syndrome)	EDNRB EDN3 SOX10	Type II + Hirschsprung disease (congenital colonic aganglionosis)

[a]Genes cited from OMIM. For additional reading, see Hereditary Hearing Loss homepage
[b]Dystopia canthorum is a displacement of the inner canthi and lacrimal puncta

de pointes. JLNS should be distinguished from the closely related and more common Romano-Ward syndrome, which lacks sensorineural hearing loss. The genetic cause of JLNS has been localized to two genes, KCNQ1 and KCNE1, which encode subunits of potassium channels expressed in cardiac and auditory tissue (OMIM #220400). Because of JLNS, newborns and children diagnosed with a sensorineural hearing loss should be screened with an EKG.

Autosomal Dominant Syndromic Hearing Loss

Branchio-Oto-Renal Syndrome
As the name implies, branchio-oto-renal (BOR) syndrome is characterized by the constellation of branchial arch, otologic, and renal defects. Unlike other hearing loss syndromes discussed thus far, otologic involvement in BOR may affect the external, middle or inner ear, and as a result hearing loss can be sensorineural, conductive, or mixed. Major otologic manifestations generally include preauricular pits and external ear abnormalities as well as a lower incidence of microtia, ossicular malformation, and cochlear hypoplasia (Chang et al. 2004). Branchial anomalies manifest as fistulae, pits, or sinuses, while renal

abnormalities are extremely variable and can range from renal hypoplasia to complete agenesis. Mutations have been isolated to three different genes – EYA1 as well as two additional genes SIX1 and SIX5 (OMIM), which act to regulate organogenesis.

Waardenburg Syndrome
Waardenburg syndrome is a rare autosomal dominant syndrome characterized by sensorineural hearing loss, and pigmentation abnormalities of the eyes, skin and hair, including the classic "white forelock" and iris pigmentary disturbances (Table 7) (Zhang et al. 2012). There are four clinically described subtypes of Waardenburg syndrome with slight variations in clinical features and different responsible genes (see Table 3).

X-Linked Recessive Syndromic Hearing Loss

Alport Syndrome
Alport syndrome is caused by a hereditary defect in the synthesis of type IV collagen, resulting in sensorineural hearing loss, nephritis, and ocular defects. While predominantly X-linked recessive, it can also occur by autosomal transmission (Artuso et al. 2012). Type IV collagen is a principal component of the basement membrane, and thus its mutation causes defective glomerular basement membrane formation, which

leads to gross or microscopic hematuria and eventually end-stage renal disease. Ocular manifestations include anterior lenticonus, perimacular flecks, and corneal lesions. Several genes have been identified, *COL4A5*, which encodes the α_5 chain of type IV collagen, is inherited via X-linked recessive transmission. Mutations in *COL4A3* and *COL4A4*, which encode α_3 and α_4 chains, respectively, are also implicated in the pathogenesis of Alport syndrome, but are transmitted by autosomal recessive inheritance.

Diagnostics

Initial Evaluation
The evaluation of child with significant hearing loss should ideally take place by a multidisciplinary team involving geneticists, audiologists, and otolaryngologists as well as other specialists depending on the systemic findings. A complete clinical history including details about the pregnancy and postpartum periods can help identify environmental causes such as intrauterine infections, which are known to cause hearing loss. A well-documented family history including evidence of consanguinity is also important for the evaluation of possible inheritable forms of hearing loss. A well-performed physical exam is also necessary to evaluate for cases of syndromic hearing loss, which, as previously discussed, can affect a wide range of organ systems. For reasons explained above, thorough evaluation of the head and neck, endocrine, renal, and cardiac systems are necessary. Because of the common association of otologic and ophthalmologic manifestations, a thorough eye examination should also be performed on children with hearing loss.

Newborn Hearing Screening
Newborn hearing screening programs have played an instrumental role in the diagnosis of infants born with hearing impairment. Technological advances have also facilitated this increase in prominence of the hearing test, as they have made it possible to make audiologic diagnosis at an earlier age. In fact, the development of technologies such as evoked otoacoustic emissions and auditory brainstem response testing has substantially reduced the number of infants falsely identified as having hearing impairment (i.e., false positives), and likewise increased the number of infants correctly identified as having hearing impairment (i.e., true positives) (Norton et al. 2000). Additionally, because not all forms of inheritable hearing impairment manifest immediately at birth, routine screening and follow-up throughout childhood are necessary to ensure timely diagnosis. Screening typically takes the form of an otoacoustic emissions test in the nursery with a follow-up scheduled for several weeks if the child fails the test. Confirmation with auditory brainstem evoked testing ensues if the loss persists.

Genetic Testing
As previously discussed, genetic causes are implicated in about 50% of cases of hearing loss in children, providing a rationale for genetic testing in infants born with congenital hearing loss.

As more culprit genes are discovered, the battery of genetic tests that could potentially be ordered by clinicians continues to grow. However, it is important that genetic screening be done in a reproducible and efficient manner. If syndromic hearing loss is suspected based on the constellation of symptoms, gene-specific mutation screening should be done to confirm the etiology. In cases where nonsyndromic hearing loss is suspected, environmental causes (i.e., intrauterine infection with CMV or rubella) should first be ruled out with the proper serologic testing. In the absence of serologic evidence of intrauterine infection, genetic testing for *GJB2* is advisable (ACMG statement: Genetic evaluation of congenital hearing loss expert panel, from ACMG website). Because of the high prevalence of DFNB1, the autosomal recessive mutation in the connexin26 gene *GJB2*, it is prudent to screen for this mutation first. Additionally, the choice and order of genetic tests will depend on the pedigree constructed by the medical geneticist, as the inheritance pattern of hearing impairment can inform the diagnostic approach to a certain extent. Computed tomography scans can also be used to visualize the temporal bones. In cases where vestibular aqueducts appear dilated, genetic screening for Pendred syndrome is warranted, given that it is another common cause of inherited deafness. Most importantly, it must be conveyed to patients that a negative genetic test does *not* rule out a genetic cause for the hearing loss. Lastly, an EKG is recommended due to the remote possibility of Jervell and Lange-Nielsen syndrome.

The Molecular Approach: Utility of the Mouse Model

The vast numbers of transgenic mice that have been created and studied has contributed greatly to the understanding of auditory function. Mouse models of deafness have emerged in part because genetic linkage analyses are difficult to execute in small families and histologic observation of the human cochlea is only possible in postmortem studies. Thus, many investigators are turning to the mouse model to answer molecular and genetic questions related to hearing loss.

In depth histologic, immunohistochemical, and electron microscopic examinations of cochleae have allowed for a more concrete understanding of the functions of the inner ear and the repercussions of single or multiple gene mutations. Additionally, molecular studies have allowed for proper identification of the genes involved, which has helped pave the way for therapeutic approaches.

As technology and genomics continue to evolve, so too will the capacity to deliver targeted therapies for genetic causes of hearing loss.

Differential Diagnosis

Hearing loss is an objective finding that can be confirmed with formal audiologic techniques such as pure tone audiometry as well as electrophysiological modes such as measured acoustic brainstem responses (ABR). Once confirmed, the differential diagnosis includes all genetic and environmental causes of hearing loss. Conductive hearing loss must be differentiated from sensorineural and mixed forms. Disruption of the external or middle ear canal can lead to a conductive hearing loss. In addition to genetic forms of sensorineural hearing loss other congenital forms can be caused by prenatal infectious etiologies, structural malformations, or ototoxic trauma.

Prophylaxis

Because of the variable genetic mechanisms of sensorineural hearing loss, the best prevention can be achieved by appropriate screening of potential parents. As discussed, autosomal recessive forms of hearing loss are generally from parents who are asymptomatic, thus a thorough genetic screening of couples with a history of hereditary hearing impairment is warranted.

Therapy

General Considerations

The general approach to treatment should closely follow the suspected diagnosis. In cases where multiorgan syndromic involvement is apparent, treatment and proper follow-up of associated comorbidities is paramount. In cases of nonsyndromic hearing loss, this is less of a concern.

An important issue that must be considered is the approach to genetic counseling. Because many deaf infants are born to non-deaf parents, it is extremely important to ensure information is delivered by the most qualified health care professional. In these circumstances, it is advisable to consult a medical geneticist who can accurately relay recurrence risk to the parents.

Specific Treatments

Currently, the two main treatment possibilities for patients with significant hearing loss are hearing aids and cochlear implants.

Hearing aids amplify ambient sounds to the cochlea and are helpful in patients with mild to severe sensorineural hearing losses. The three general types of hearing aids include behind the ear (BTE), in the ear (ITE), and completely within the canal (CIC) aids. The location depends on the severity of the hearing loss as well as the functionality of the patient. For example, hearing aids completely in the canal are less desirable for young children because of the risk of damage to the ear.

For patients with severe to profound hearing loss, cochlear implantation is an excellent option (Kral and O'Donoghue 2010). It is an internally implantable electronic device that directly stimulates the auditory nerve afferent fibers, bypassing the damaged organ of Corti. Implants do not completely restore "normal" hearing, but they can provide significant benefit for speech understanding. Studies have clearly demonstrated that appropriately placed cochlear implants in children born with deafness can provide near-normal to normal speech and language development, and younger implantation leads to steeper growth rates of vocabulary (Svirsky et al. 2004; Hayes et al. 2009).

Timing of initiation of rehabilitation is also critical. Hearing amplification should be instituted as soon as possible. The Joint Committee on Infant Hearing recommended in 2007 the initiation of rehabilitation no later than 6 months of age to minimize the impact on language development (JCIH 2007). Studies have also documented that earlier cochlear implantation (under 18 months) results in markedly improved performance compared to children implanted later in life (Kral and O'Donoghue 2010).

Prognosis

Genetic sensorineural hearing loss comprises approximately 50% of congenital cases of hearing loss, and is a problem with social, economic, and medical repercussions. As has been discussed, there are several causes of genetic hearing loss and proper identification is necessary to prevent untoward health complications. Prognosis is highly dependent upon etiology and severity of hearing loss, but as discussed above, early intervention has shown promise for improvement (Kral and O'Donoghue 2010). A well-coordinated approach by a comprehensive medical staff is crucial to the delivery of adequate medical care to patients with hearing loss from genetic causes.

Cross-References

▶ Bone-Anchored Hearing Aids in Conductive and Mixed Hearing Loss
▶ Cochlea, Anatomy
▶ Cochlear Implantation, Revision – Adult
▶ Cochlear Implants in Patients with Multiple Disabilities
▶ Cochlear Nerve, Anatomy
▶ Congenital Conductive Hearing Loss
▶ Embryology of Ear (General)
▶ Genetic Sensorineural Hearing Loss
▶ Genetics in Otolaryngology
▶ Genetics of Hearing Loss
▶ Genetics of Presbycusis
▶ Hearing Aid
▶ Hearing Assessment in Infancy and Childhood
▶ Hearing Exam
▶ Hearing (Sensorineural Hearing Loss – Pediatric)
▶ Hearing Testing, Auditory Brainstem Response (ABR)
▶ Implantable Hearing Devices
▶ Middle Ear Anatomy
▶ Physiology of Cochlea
▶ Presbycusis
▶ Sensorineural Hearing Loss
▶ Sensorineural Hearing Loss-Congenital-Genetics
▶ Surgical Devices (Cochlear Implantation, Pediatric)
▶ Surgical Devices (Cochlear Implantation, Revision – Pediatric)
▶ Vestibular and Central Nervous System, Anatomy

References

Artuso R, Fallerini C, Dosa L, Scionti F, Clementi M, Garosi G, Massella L, Epistolato MC, Mancini R, Mari F, Longo I, Ariani F, Renieri A, Bruttini M (2012) Advances in Alport syndrome diagnosis using next-generation sequencing. Eur J Hum Genet 20(1):50–57
Bonnet C, El-Amraoui A (2012) Usher syndrome (sensorineural deafness and retinitis pigmentosa): pathogenesis, molecular diagnosis and therapeutic approaches. Curr Opin Neurol 25(1):42–49
Bonnet C, Grati M, Marlin S, Levilliers J, Hardelin JP, Parodi M, Niasme-Grare M, Zelenika D, Délépine M, Feldmann D, Jonard L, El-Amraoui A, Weil D, Delobel B, Vincent C, Dollfus H, Eliot MM, David A, Calais C, Vigneron J, Montaut-Verient B, Bonneau D, Dubin J, Thauvin C, Duvillard A, Francannet C, Mom T, Lacombe D, Duriez F, Drouin-Garraud V, Thuillier-Obstoy MF, Sigaudy S, Frances AM, Collignon P, Challe G, Couderc R, Lathrop M, Sahel JA, Weissenbach J, Petit C, Denoyelle F (2011) Complete exon sequencing of all known Usher syndrome genes greatly improves molecular diagnosis. Orphanet J Rare Dis 6:21
Chang EH, Menezes M, Meyer NC, Cucci RC, Vervoort VS, Schwartz CE, Smith RJH (2004) Branchio-Oto-renal syndrome: the mutation spectrum in EYA1 and its phenotypic consequences. Hum Mutat 23:582–589
Connexins and Deafness homepage. http://davinci.crg.es/deafness/. Cited 15 Feb 2012
Denoyelle F, Marlin S, Weil D, Moatti L, Chauvin P, Garabedian EN, Petit C (1999) Clinical features of the prevalent form of childhood deafness, DFNB1, due to a connexin-26 gene defect: implications for genetic counseling. Lancet 353:1298–1303
Dodson KM, Blanton SH, Welch KO, Norris VW, Nuzzo RL, Wegelin JA, Marin RS, Nance WE, Pandya A, Arnos KS (2011) Vestibular dysfunction in DFNB1 deafness. Am J Med Genet A 155:993–1000
Dror AA, Brownstein Z, Avraham KB (2011) Integration of human and mouse genetics reveals pendrin function in hearing and deafness. Cell Physiol Biochem 28(3): 535–544
Estivill X, Govea N, Barceló E, Badenas C, Romero E, Moral L, Scozzri R, D'Urbano L, Zeviani M, Torroni A (1998) Familial progressive sensorineural deafness is mainly due to the mtDNA A1555G mutation and is enhanced by treatment of aminoglycosides. Am J Hum Genet 62(1):27–35
Everett LA, Glaser B, Beck JC, Idol JR, Buchs A, Heyman M, Adawi F, Hazani E, Nassir E, Baxevanis AD, Sheffield VC,

Green ED (1997) Pendred syndrome is caused by mutations in a putative sulphate transporter gene (PDS). Nat Genet 17(4):411–422

Genetics Home Reference, NIH. http://ghr.nlm.nih.gov/condition/pendred-syndrome. Cited 16 Feb 2012

Gürtler N (2012) Hereditary hearing impairment. In: Lalwani AK (ed) Current diagnosis & treatment in otolaryngology – head & neck surgery, 3rd edn. McGraw-Hill, New York, pp 713–720

Hayes H, Geers AE, Treiman R, Moog JS (2009) Receptive vocabulary development in deaf children with cochlear implants: achievement in an intensive auditory-oral educational setting. Ear Hear 30:128–135

Hereditary Hearing Loss Website. http://hereditaryhearingloss.org/main.aspx?c=.HHH&n=86162. Cited 15 Feb 2012

Hildebrand MS, Husein M, Smith RJH (2010) Genetic sensorineural hearing loss. In: Niparko J (ed) Cummings otolaryngology head & neck surgery, vol 3, 5th edn. Mosby Elsevier, Philadelphia, pp 2086–2099

JCIH (2007) http://pediatrics.aappublications.org/content/120/4/898.full?ijkey=oj9BAleq21OlA&keytype=ref&siteid=aapjournals. Accessed February 15, 2012

Kral A, O'Donoghue GM (2010) Profound deafness in childhood. N Engl J Med 363:1438–1450

Minárik G, Tretinárová D, Szemes T, Kádasi L (2012) Prevalence of DFNB1 mutations in Slovak patients with non-syndromic hearing loss. Int J Pediatr Otorhinolaryngol 76:400–403

Morton CC, Giersch AB (2010) Genetics of hearing loss. In: Fuchs P (ed) The Oxford handbook of auditory science: the ear, 1st edn. Oxford University Press, Oxford, pp 377–407

National Institute on Deafness and Other Communication Disorders. http://www.nidcd.nih.gov/health/statistics/Pages/quick.aspx. Cited 15 Feb 2012

Norton SJ, Gorga MP, Widen JE, Folsom RC, Sininger Y, Cone-Wesson B, Vohr BR, Fletcher KA (2000) Identification of neonatal hearing impairment: summary and recommendations. Ear Hear 21:529–535

Prezant TR, Agapian JV, Bohlman MC, Bu X, Oztas S, Qiu WQ, Arnos KS, Cortopassi GA, Jaber L, Rotter JI et al (1993) Mitochondrial ribosomal RNA mutation associated with both antibiotic-induced and non-syndromic deafness. Nat Genet 4(3):289–294

Svirsky MA, Teoh SW, Neuburger H (2004) Development of language and speech perception in congenitally, profoundly deaf children as a function of age at cochlear implantation. Audiol Neurootol 9:224–233

Zelante L, Gasparini P, Estivill X, Melchionda S, D'Agruma L, Govea N, Mila M, Monica MD, Lutfi J, Shohat M, Mansfield E, Delgrosso K, Rappaport E, Surrey S, Fortina P (1997) Connexin26 mutations associated with the most common form of non-syndromic neurosensory autosomal recessive deafness (DFNB1) in Mediterraneans. Hum Mol Genet 6:1605–1609

Zhang H, Chen H, Luo H, An H, Sun L, Mei L, He C, Jiang L, Jiang W, Xia K, Li JD, Feng Y (2012) Functional analysis of Waardenburg syndrome-associated PAX3 and SOX10 mutations: report of a dominant-negative SOX10 mutation in Waardenburg syndrome type II. Hum Genet 131:491–503

Genetics in Otolaryngology

Selena E. Heman-Ackah[1], Sabrina M. Heman-Ackah[2] and Anil K. Lalwani[1]
[1]Department of Otolaryngology-Head and Neck Surgery, New York University, New York, NY, USA
[2]School of Medicine, University of North Carolina, Chapel Hill, NC, USA

Synonyms

Inheritance; Otolaryngic genetics; Otolaryngologic genetics

Definition

1. *Allele*: one of two or more versions of a gene.
2. *Autosomal dominant*: a pattern of inheritance by which one copy (allele) of an autosomal gene is required for expression of a trait.
3. *Autosomal recessive*: a pattern of inheritance by which two copies (alleles) of an autosomal gene are required for expression of a trait.
4. *Chromosome*: an organized package of DNA and associated proteins found in the nucleus of the cell.
5. *Deoxyribonucleic acid* (*DNA*): a double-stranded helix comprised of two paired nucleotides with a phosphate-deoxyribose backbone joined by ester bonds.
6. *Epigenetics*: inheritable changes in gene expression caused by mechanisms other than DNA mutations.
7. *Expressivity*: the variation in phenotype among individuals carrying a particular genotype.
8. *Gene*: a molecular unit of inheritance consisting of a sequence of DNA that occupies a specific location on a chromosome coding for a specific protein.
9. *Genetics*: a discipline which studies the science of genes, heredity, and variation.
10. *Genotype*: the genetic makeup of an organism or individual with reference to a single trait, set of traits, or entire complex of traits.
11. *Mitochondrial inheritance*: inheritance of a trait encoded in the mitochondrial genome.

12. *Penetrance*: the variation in whether individuals carrying a particular gene mutation also express an associated trait or phenotype.

13. *Phenotype*: the observable constitution of an organism or individual resulting from the interaction of the genotype and the environment.

14. *Ribonucleic acid*: a single-stranded molecule comprised of a nucleotide with a phosphate-ribose backbone.

15. *Sex-linked inheritance*: inheritance of a trait encoded on the X or Y chromosome.

16. *Mendelian genetics*: patterns of inheritance initially described by Charles Mendel including autosomal dominant, autosomal recessive, and sex-linked inheritance.

Basic Characteristics

Introduction

The concept of genetics as a means for inheritance of traits and disease was first introduced by Gregor Mendel in his work *Experiments in Plant Hybridization* in 1865 presented on February 8 and March 8 before the *Naturforschender Verein* (Natural Science Association) in Brunn. In this publication, described patterns of inheritance are based upon transmission of specific physical characteristics in the pea plant offspring including variegation in color and seed form. In 1869, Friedrich Miescher discovered a weak acid in the nuclei of white blood cells which later was found to represent deoxyribonucleic acid (DNA). In the late 1800s, Walther Flemming, Eduard Strasburger, and Edouard van Beneden described the chromosome distribution during cellular division. Around the same time, Hugo de Vries as well as Correns and Tschermak rediscovered the previously ignored works of Mendel and postulated that the inheritance of specific traits in organisms was transmitted in particles named (pan)genes at that time. In 1903, Sutton hypothesized that chromosomes, described by Flemming, Strasburger, and van Beneden, form the hereditary units in a Mendelian fashion, and in 1905, William Bateson was the first to coin the term genetics with regard to this method of inheritance. Since these discoveries, human genetics has expounded exponentially in terms of the current body of knowledge and understanding.

Human genetics forms the basis of existence and the backbone of basic human development function. With the deciphering of the human genome, the understanding of gene fundamentality, critical genetic pathways, and deleterious genetic disorders continues to grow. The complex interaction between environmental factors and genetics in the manifestation and evolution of genetic disorders is the current focus of investigation. Within otolaryngology – head and neck surgery, a number of genetic disorders have been elucidated and are commonly encountered in the practice. A keen understanding of genetics, therefore, is essential for the practicing otolaryngologist. As the body of knowledge regarding the interaction of genetics in disease as well as the propensity for its use in disease prevention and treatment expands, genetics will become even more fundamental to the practice of otolaryngology.

DNA

The basic means for transmission of inheritance is transferred via the genetic code. The genetic code provides the basic information from which proteins and transcription factors are transmitted which are essential to cellular function and life. The basic genetic material and code are transmitted via DNA. DNA is a double-stranded helical molecule comprised of two paired nucleotides with a phosphate-deoxyribose backbone joined by ester bonds. Four nucleotides are included within DNA which binds with a specific pattern: adenine (A) pairs with thymine (T), and cytosine (C) pairs with guanine (G). Each DNA molecule is comprised of a sense or coding strand ($5'$ to $3'$) that is paired with a complementary antisense or template strand ($3'$ to $5'$). Each triplet of nucleotides corresponds to a specific amino acid. This unit is known as a codon. Genes represent a sequence of codons which are transcribed into corresponding ribonucleic acid (RNA), proteins, and polypeptides. Within the cell, DNA is housed within two specific locations, the nucleus and the mitochondria.

The vast majority of DNA is housed within the nucleus and is referred to as autosomal DNA. The structure of autosomal DNA is linear, and it becomes packaged into chromosomes during certain stages of the cell cycle. Housed within the 0.06 μm in diameter nucleus of the cell is approximately 2 m of DNA comprised of 3×10^9 base pairs. However, less than 5% of the entire genome codes for genes which are transcribed, accounting for a total of approximately 19,000 genes translating into proteins. Approximately half of all autosomal DNA is inherited from each parent, respectively.

A minor proportion of DNA is housed within the mitochondria known as mitochondrial DNA. Mitochondrial DNA is a single circular double-stranded helix molecule comprised of 16,569 base pairs. Each mitochondrion contains multiple copies – from 100 to 10,000 – of this circular DNA which consists of 37 genes coding for 2 rRNA, 22 tRNA, and 13 polypeptides (Taanman 1999). Mitochondrial DNA is essential in its contribution to enzyme complexes critical for oxidative phosphorylation. Unlike autosomal DNA, mitochondrial DNA is inherited solely of maternal origin.

Chromosomes

Autosomal DNA is organized into chromosomes following DNA replication and preceding cellular division. Within chromosomes, the DNA molecules are tightly coiled and surrounded by support proteins known as histones. Together, the DNA molecules and support proteins form dense DNA-protein complexes known as chromatin. The typical structure of a chromosome consists of two chromatids fused at the centromere. The centromere divides the chromosome into two sections – a shorter portion known as the short arm (p) and a longer portion known as the long arm (q). The location of the centromere also provides each chromosome with its characteristic shape and is utilized in the location and description of specific genes. The telomere is a repetitive sequence of DNA at the end of the chromosome which protects the end chromosome from deterioration or fusion with neighboring chromosomes. The human genome contains 23 paired chromosomes of maternal and paternal origin for a total of 46 chromosomes: female (46,XX) and male (46,XY).

RNA

RNA is an essential molecule in the translation of information coded within the genome into vital proteins. RNA is made up of a single sugar-phosphate backbone with a nucleotide base comprised of the following nucleotide base pairs: adenine (A), guanine (G), cytosine (C), and uracil (U). During the transcription process, adenine pairs with guanine, and uracil pairs with cytosine. There are multiple types of RNA which are critical to cellular function.

RNA functions to aid in the transcription of the DNA code and the translation of the genetic code into protein and polypeptide products. During transcription, messenger RNA (mRNA) pairs with DNA utilizing the sense strand as a template configuring the RNA in a $3'$ to $5'$ orientation which is identical to the antisense strand of DNA with the exception of the thymine to uracil substitutions. Transcription occurs within the nucleus of the cell following which the mRNA exits the nucleus. Along with transfer RNA (tRNA), the code is translated into protein with the assistance of a ribosome (a complex of protein and ribosomal RNA). Translation describes the process by which the information encoded within the tRNA is converted to corresponding amino acids. Specific tRNA nucleotide triplets are covalently bound to individual amino acid. Each nucleotide triplet represents a codon, of which there are 64, corresponding to a specific amino acid or a stop signal. The peptide produced by the tRNA ultimately forms proteins and polypeptides which are critical to virtually every cellular function.

In addition to mRNA, rRNA, and tRNA, there are various forms of RNA that are essential to cellular function. MicroRNAs (miRNAs) are posttranscriptional regulators that function in translation repression and gene silencing. Small interfering RNAs (siRNAs) are a group of RNAs including inhibitory RNA, silencing RNA, and short interfering RNA. siRNAs have multiple functions including interfering with specific gene expression, antiviral mechanisms, and shaping chromatin structure of the genome. Small nuclear RNAs (snRNAs) participate in RNA splicing, regulation of transcription factors, and maintenance of the telomeres. Finally, signal recognition particle RNA (SRP RNA) is essential to translation translocation, membrane integration, and posttranslational transport.

Proteins

Proteins are essential to tissue structure, cellular function, and enzymatic activity. The entire human genome is housed within every cell; however, only proteins are produced within the cell pursuant to its specific function. To accomplish this, only specific genes within the cell are expressed according to the specific cellular needs. The transcription and translation process is therefore a highly regulated and specific process governed by tissue and cellular types.

Patterns of Inheritance

Various patterns of inheritance have been described to date. Alleles refer to a specific copy of a gene. Two copies of each allele are inherited by each individual, one from each parent. Homozygous describes an individual with two of the same alleles of the gene. Heterozygous describes an individual with two different copies of an allele. Mendelian genetics refers to the patterns of inheritance first described by Charles Mendel including autosomal recessive inheritance, autosomal dominant inheritance, and X-linked inheritance.

With *autosomal recessive* inheritance, two copies of the mutated alleles are required for the transmission of the specific phenotype (i.e., a specific trait or disease process). Therefore, in order for an individual to inherit an autosomal recessive disease, they must inherit two copies of the disease allele. Regarding autosomal recessive disorders, individuals with only one copy of the disease genotype are considered disease carriers. The following parental genotypes may produce offspring with the autosomal recessive genotype: two heterozygous parents, one heterozygous parent, and one homozygous abnormal parent or two homozygous abnormal parents. For offspring of two heterozygous individuals, there is a 50% chance of inheriting the disease genotype, a 25% chance of inheriting the disease carrier state, and a 25% chance of having the normal genotype. There is no sexual predilection with regard to autosomal recessive disease inheritance. Examples of autosomal recessive disorders encountered in otolaryngology – head and neck surgery include cystic fibrosis, Kartagener syndrome, Werner syndrome, Gardner syndrome, Usher syndrome, Refsum disease, Jervell and Lange-Nielsen syndrome, Pendred syndrome, and most forms of nonsyndromic hearing loss. Tables 1, 2, 3, and 4 highlight some of the genetic disorders encountered in otolaryngology by subspecialty with the most commonly associated genes, function, and characteristic clinical phenotype. Genetic disorders with lethal phenotypes more commonly are inherited via an autosomal recessive mode of inheritance owing to the normal phenotypical presentation of the carrier individuals at childbearing age. Autosomal recessive disorders with lethal phenotypes, such as Tay-Sachs disease and Bowen-Conradi syndrome, most often occur in patient with no prior family history of disease. The lethal phenotypes tend to occur more frequently among consanguineous families in which the parents are genetically related. The founder effect describes the expression of a mutation initially occurring in one or few founding members of a group which has been propagated by the tendency for marriages to occur within the same group. This is believed to be the source of the tendency for many autosomal recessive disorders to have racial and ethnic predilections (i.e., sickle-cell anemia, β-thalassemia, and Gaucher disease).

With the *autosomal dominant* form of inheritance, only one allele with the mutated gene is required for the transmission of the specific phenotype (i.e., a specific trait or disease process). Therefore, the offspring of one homozygous normal parent and one heterozygous parent with one have a 50% chance of inheriting the disease allele. Additionally, the offspring of two heterozygous parents with the disease phenotype have a 75% chance of inheriting the disease and only a 25% chance of being normal. There is no carrier state in autosomal dominant inheritance. Alternatively, in extremely rare cases, if one parent possesses two diseased alleles (homozygous dominant) and the other parent possess two normal alleles, the offspring have a 100% chance of inheriting the disorder. There is no sexual predilection in the pattern of inheritance with autosomal dominant disorders. Therefore, inheritance of one disease allele confers the phenotype of disease unless there is "incomplete penetrance." *Penetrance* describes the variation in whether individuals carrying a particular gene mutation also express an associated trait or phenotype. With complete penetrance, every individual with the disease allele expresses the disease phenotype; with incomplete penetrance, a certain proportion of individuals with the disease allele do not express the disease phenotype. Because of the nature of transmission, autosomal dominant disorders are rarely associated with fatal mutations. This is because the presentation of fatal mutations with autosomal dominant inheritance would preclude its transmission. Examples of autosomal dominant disorders in otolaryngology – head and neck surgery include DiGeorge syndrome, Osler-Weber-Rendu syndrome, Gorlin syndrome, branchiootorenal syndrome, Stickler syndrome, neurofibromatosis type I, neurofibromatosis type II, Treacher-Collins syndrome, Gardner syndrome, and Pallister-Hall syndrome.

Genes expressed on the X or Y chromosomes are responsible for *sex-linked inheritance*. The vast majority of sex-linked genetic disorders are carried on the X chromosome. Females inherit two X chromosomes,

Genetics in Otolaryngology, Table 1 Genetic disorders in otology and neurotology

Disease name	Most common gene responsible	Gene function	Mode of inheritance	Clinical phenotype
Genetic disorders in otology and neurotology				
Alport syndrome	COL4A5	Type IV collagen	XR	Sensorineural hearing loss, renal anomalies, ocular anomalies
Branchiootorenal syndrome	EYA1	EYA1 protein (transcription factor/ coactivator)	AD	Mixed hearing loss, pinna deformities, preauricular pits, fistulas and tags, Mondini malformation
Jervell and Lange-Nielsen syndrome	KCNE1, KCNQ1	Potassium channel	AR	Sensorineural hearing loss, cardiac dysfunction (prolong QT interval)
Keipert syndrome	q22.2–q28	Unknown	XR	Sensorineural hearing loss, facial dysmorphisms, broad thumbs and halluces, brachydactyly
Neurofibromatosis type II	NF2	Merlin (tumor suppressor)	AD	Bilateral vestibular schwannomas, meningiomas, gliomas, schwannomas, juvenile cataracts
Nonsyndromic hearing loss	GJB2	Gap junction protein (connexin 26)	AR	Sensorineural hearing loss
Norrie syndrome	NDP	Norrin protein (tissue development)	XR	Sensorineural hearing loss, blindness, cataracts
Pendred syndrome	SLC26A4	Transporter protein (pendrin)	AR	Sensorineural hearing loss, EVA, Mondini malformation, euthyroid goiter
Refsum disease	PHYH	Peroxisomal enzyme (phytanoyl-CoA hydroxylase)	AR	Sensorineural hearing loss, peripheral polyneuropathy, cerebellar ataxia, retinitis pigmentosa, ichthyosis
Stickler syndrome	COL2A1	Type II collagen, alpha 1 unit	AD	Sensorineural hearing loss, Marfanoid habitus, ocular abnormalities, arthritis abnormalities, Pierre Robin sequence
Treacher-Collins syndrome	TCOF1	Treacle protein (prenatal bone and soft tissue development)	AD	Sensorineural, mixed or conductive hearing loss, aural atresia, auricular deformities, EVA, Mondini malformation, zygomatic and mandibular hypoplasia, downward slanting palpebral fissures, lower lid coloboma, palatal defects
Usher syndrome	USH2A	Basement membrane protein (usherin)	AR	Sensorineural hearing loss, vestibular dysfunction, retinitis pigmentosa
Von Hippel Lindau syndrome	VHL	Tumor suppressor	AD	Endolymphatic sac tumors, pheochromocytoma, hemangioblastomas, cysts in the kidney, pancreas, and male genital tract, clear cell renal cell carcinoma, retinal angiomas
Waardenburg syndrome	PAX3	Gene regulation and neural crest cell signaling	AD	Sensorineural hearing loss, pigmentary anomalies (i.e., heterochromatic iritis, skin depigmentation, white forelock), craniofacial anomalies (i.e., canthorum, synophrys, broad nasal dorsum)
Wildervanck syndrome	Unknown	Unknown	XD	Sensorineural or mixed hearing loss, abducens palsy, cervical fusion

AD autosomal dominant inheritance, *AR* autosomal recessive inheritance, *XD* X-linked dominant inheritance, *XR* X-linked recessive inheritance, *EVA* enlarged vestibular aqueduct

one from each parent, respectively. Therefore, a female may inherit a mutated allele on the X chromosome from either parent. Males, however, only inherit one copy of the X chromosome which is maternally derived. Therefore, among males, all X-linked genetic disorders must be maternally inherited. X-linked disorders are further subdivided into *X-linked dominant* disorders which are exceedingly rare and *X-linked recessive* disorders which are the most common. X-linked dominant disorders require only one diseased allele for the disease phenotype. All females born to a male with an X-linked dominant disorder will inherit the disease mutation as the father has only the single affected X chromosome.

Genetics in Otolaryngology, Table 2 Genetic disorders in otolaryngology – head and neck surgery

Disease name	Most common gene responsible	Gene function	Mode of inheritance	Clinical phenotype
Genetic disorders in head and neck cancer				
Cowden syndrome	*PTEN*	Tumor suppressor gene	AD	Thyroid cancer; thyroid adenomas; multiple trichilemmomas; gingival fibromatosis; hamartomas of the breast, thyroid, and gastrointestinal tract; breast cancer
Gardner syndrome	*APC*	Peroxisomal enzyme (phytanoyl-CoA hydroxylase)	AR	Thyroid cancer, multiple epidermal cysts, facial bone osteomas, cutaneous fibromas, lipomas, leiomyomas of the gastrointestinal tract, adenomatous polyps of the colon
Gorlin syndrome	*PTCH1*	Tumor suppressor	XD	Multiple basal cell carcinomas, odontogenic keratocysts, bifid ribs, scoliosis, frontal bossing, mental retardation
Multiple endocrine neoplasia IIA (MEN IIA)	*RET*	Proto-oncogene	AD	Medullary thyroid carcinoma, pheochromocytoma, parathyroid adenoma/hyperplasia
Multiple endocrine neoplasia IIB (MENIIB)	*RET*	Proto-oncogene	AD	Medullary thyroid carcinoma, pheochromocytoma, Marfanoid habitus, multiple mucosa neuromas, hyperplastic corneal nerves
Neurofibromatosis type I	*NF1*	Neurofibromin (tumor suppressor)	AD	Café-au-lait spots, cutaneous neurofibromas, scoliosis, optic gliomas, axillary and groin freckles, malignant peripheral nerve sheath tumors, increased risk of malignancy (i.e., brain tumors or leukemias), Lisch nodules, hypertension, macrocephaly, attention deficit hyperactivity disorder, pheochromocytoma
Tylosis	*TOC*	Cytoglobin protein	AD	Esophageal cancer and hyperkeratosis of the palms and soles
Werner syndrome	*WRN*	Werner protein (DNA maintenance and repair)	AR	Thyroid cancer, accelerated aging, short stature, propensity for multiple malignancies

AD autosomal dominant inheritance, *AR* autosomal recessive inheritance, *XD* X-linked dominant inheritance

Genetics in Otolaryngology, Table 3 Genetic disorders in rhinology

Disease name	Most common gene responsible	Gene function	Mode of inheritance	Clinical phenotype
Genetic disorders in rhinology				
Osler-Weber-Rendu syndrome	*ENG*	Defective contractile elements in vessels	AD	Arteriovenous malformations of the nose, lung, liver, gastrointestinal tract, and brain
Cystic fibrosis	*CFTR*	Transmembrane chloride channel	AR	Chronic sinusitis, respiratory dysfunction, pancreatic insufficiency, and infertility
Kartagener syndrome	*KTU*	Peroxisomal enzyme (phytanoyl-CoA hydroxylase)	AR	Ciliary dyskinesia, impaired mucociliary clearance, otitis media, sinusitis, situs inversus, bronchiectasis, chronic cough, male infertility

AD autosomal dominant inheritance, *AR* autosomal recessive inheritance

Because the father only passes the Y chromosome to the male offspring, paternal possession of X-linked dominant disorders has no influence on the genotype or phenotype of male offspring. Half of all offspring born to a female with an X-linked dominant disorder will inherit the disease genotype and phenotype. In certain X-linked dominant disorders (i.e., focal dermal hypoplasia), expression of the genetic mutation within

Genetics in Otolaryngology, Table 4 Genetic disorders in laryngology

Disease name	Most common gene responsible	Gene function	Mode of inheritance	Clinical phenotype
Genetic disorders in laryngology				
Opitz-Frias syndrome	*MID1*	TRIM motif (microtubule anchoring)	XR	Laryngeal cleft, hypertelorism, cleft lip, cleft palate, hypospadias
	22q11.2	Transcription factor	AD	
Pallister-Hall syndrome	*GLI3*	Zinc finger protein	AD	Laryngeal cleft, hypothalamic hamartoblastoma, hypopituitarism, imperforate anus, postaxial polydactyly, bifid epiglottis
Congenital (hereditary) angioedema	*C1NH*	C1 esterase inhibitor	AD	Angioedema

AD autosomal dominant inheritance, *XD* X-linked dominant inheritance

males is highly or uniformly fatal. X-linked hypophosphatemia, CHILD syndrome, Lujan-Fryns syndrome, Aicardi syndrome, and incontinentia pigmenti are all examples of X-linked dominant disorders. With X-linked recessive disorders, one functional form of the gene precludes the phenotypical presentation of disease. As with autosomal recessive disorders, a carrier state may occur with X-linked recessive disorders. Females possessing only one copy of the disease allele are carriers and typically do not have the disease phenotype. Females may inherit this diseased X-linked allele from either or both parent. For a female to express the disease phenotype, both copies of the allele must have the disease genotype which is extremely uncommon. However, because the X chromosome in male offspring is maternally derived, males may only inherit X-linked recessive disorders from their mother. Also because males lack a second X chromosome, the disease allele represents the only functional X chromosome allele, leading to the phenotypical expression of disease. There are various X-linked recessive diseases encountered in otolaryngology including X-linked stapes gusher syndrome, X-linked Alport syndrome, idiopathic hypoparathyroidism, X-linked agammaglobulinemia of Bruton, Lesch-Nyhan syndrome, severe combined immunodeficiency disease, Wiskott-Aldrich syndrome, Norrie disease, X-linked ichthyosis, Keipert syndrome (nasodigitoacoustic syndrome), and Fragile X syndrome.

In addition to the classical Mendelian forms of genetic inheritance, additional modes of genetic inheritance have been identified. These include mitochondrial inheritance, digenic inheritance, chromosomal anomalies, genetic imprinting, epigenetic influences, and complex genetics. In addition to mutations to the autosomal genome, mutations may occur within the mitochondrial genome. The mitochondrial DNA is solely maternally inherited; therefore, diseases derived from mitochondrial genomic deletions are maternally inherited as well. Additionally, mutations within the mitochondrial genome may be acquired. Mitochondrially inherited disorders are less frequently encountered in otolaryngology than autosomal inherited disorders and range in severity from asymptomatic to fatal. Because the mitochondrial genome is essential to cellular energy production, tissues with high energy demand are preferentially affected including the nervous system, muscle, heart, and endocrine systems (Wallace 2010). Within otolaryngology practice, mitochondrially inherited genetic disorders that may be encountered include aminoglycoside induce ototoxicity, mitochondrially inherited nonsyndromic hearing loss, NARP (neuropathy, ataxia, and retinitis pigmentosa), Leber hereditary neuropathy, and MELAS (mitochondrial encephalomyopathy, lactic acidosis, and stroke-like episodes). Oxidative injury has been described as a major potential source of acquired mitochondrial genomic mutations. Decreased endogenous antioxidants (i.e., glutathione), decreased reducing enzymes (i.e., superoxide dismutase), and increased free radical species have been identified as potentially contributing to the development of mutations within the mitochondrial genome (de Grey 2005; Seidman et al. 2004). Acquired mitochondrial mutations have been implicated in phenotypical changes with aging in many organ systems including the inner ear, skin, and retina. In addition, carcinogenic mutations within the mitochondrial genome have been identified which may be germline related or de novo. Most commonly within the head and neck, thyroid tumors and adenocarcinoma have been associated with mitochondrial mutations (Brandon et al. 2005; Mancini-DiNardo et al. 2006).

Coinheritance of mutations at two distinct genetic loci producing the phenotype of disease is known as digenic or diallelic inheritance. Certain forms of Usher type I may be transmitted via digenic inheritance patterns including mutations in the *CDH23* and *PCDH15* genes (Zheng et al. 2005). Waardenburg syndrome type II with ocular albinism in certain cases has been associated with digenic inheritance (Chiang et al. 2009). Additionally, digenic inheritance of mutation in gap junction proteins genes *GJB2* and *GJB6* has been demonstrated in certain forms of nonsyndromic hearing loss (Liu et al. 2009).

Genetic imprinting is an additional non-Mendelian pattern of inheritance by which certain genes are expressed in a parent-of-origin-specific manner. Alleles inherited by a specific parent are silenced via mechanisms including methylation of cytosine within DNA and histone acetylation which produces monoallelic gene expression without alteration of the genetic sequence. This may occur on either the maternally derived or paternally derived allele. The markers for genetic imprinting are established through the germline and are maintained throughout all somatic cells. Utilizing noncoding RNA and differentially methylated regions as imprinting control regions, imprinted genes are typically grouped within clusters to allow for sharing of these regulatory units (Mancini-DiNardo et al. 2006). The most common examples of genetic imprinting in otolaryngology are Beckwith-Wiedemann syndrome, Angelman syndrome, Prader-Willi syndrome, and Silver-Russell syndrome. Beckwith-Wiedemann syndrome is characterized by gigantism, macroglossia, anterior abdominal wall defects (most commonly congenital exomphalos), neonatal hypoglycemia, organomegaly, and the development of multiple tumors during childhood, most commonly Wilms tumors. Beckwith-Wiedemann syndrome may be transmitted via silencing of the paternally derived *BWS* gene, silencing of the maternally derived *IF2* gene, or paternal silencing of the *CDKN1C* gene. Angelman syndrome and Prader-Willi syndrome

are related genetic disorders. Both disorders are associated with genetic imprinting involving the normal *UBE3A* gene located on chromosome 15q11–13 (Horsthemke and Wagstaff 2008). However, Angelman syndrome is associated with paternal imprinting where only the mutated maternally derived *UBE3A* gene is expressed. With Prader-Willi syndrome, the maternally derived *UBE3A* gene is imprinted and only the mutated paternally derived *UBE3A* gene is expressed. Angelman syndrome is characterized by developmental delay, sleep disturbance, seizures, movement and balance disorders, microcephaly, and an unusually happy demeanor. Prader-Willi syndrome is characterized by hypotonia, short stature, hyperphagia, obesity, behavioral issues, hypogonadism, and mental retardation. Silver-Russell syndrome is a disorder of aberrant genetic imprinting. Hypomethylation of the imprinting control region 1 (ICR1) in 11p15.5 has been demonstrated to affect the expression of *IGF2* and *H19* in association with Silver-Russell syndrome (Nativio et al. 2011; Grønskov et al. 2011). Silver-Russell syndrome is characterized by intrauterine growth restriction, dwarfism, hypoglycemia, failure to thrive, blue sclera, hemihypertrophy, craniofacial dysostoses, clinodactyly, hypotonia, precocious puberty, and cardiac defects.

Recently, the study of epigenetics has revealed the etiology of a variety of hereditary disorders. Epigenetics refers to inheritable changes in phenotype or gene expression caused by mechanisms other than changes in the underlying DNA sequence. Various epigenetic phenomena have been identified including gene silencing, bookmarking, X chromosome inactivation, paramutation, position effect, and reprogramming. Gene silencing refers to the inactivation of certain genes by mechanisms other than genetic modifications including DNA methylation, histone acetylation, transposon silencing, transgene silencing, transcriptional gene silencing, and RNA-directed DNA methylation. Bookmarking is an epigenetic mechanism by which cellular memory is passed to subsequent cellular generations through mitosis. Patterns of gene expression in the cell are transmitted through cellular memory by bookmarking though mitosis via noncompaction of gene promoters which are marked for expression during mitosis. Bookmarking may occur via gene silencing by DNA methylation, transcriptional regulation by histone modifications, regulation of gene expression by noncoding small RNA molecules, and retention of regulatory machinery on target gene loci for activation and repression (Sarge and Park-Sarge 2009; Zaidi et al. 2011). X chromosome inactivation describes the process by which one of the two inherited copies of the X chromosome in females is inactivated or silenced by packaging it into heterochromatin which prevents active transcription. With X chromosome inactivation either the maternal or paternally derived copy can become inactivated. DNA methylation and histone acetylation are often involved (Ng et al. 2007). Interactions between two different alleles of a single locus which induce inheritable changes of one allele induced by the other allele are referred to as paramutation. Position effect describes the effect of change in chromosome location on the expression of a gene. Reprogramming describes the process by which epigenetic markers are erased and remodeled.

The pattern of inheritance by which multiple genes in combination lead to the phenotype of disorders or disease is known as complex genetics or polygenic inheritance. In polygenic inheritance, multiple factors including lifestyle and environment influence the phenotype of disease. This makes it difficult to quantify the probability by which inheritance may be conferred. Within otolaryngology, the most commonly cited disorders with polygenic inheritance are cleft lip and cleft palate which are thought to be secondary to complex involvement of both major and minor genetic influences with variable interactions from environmental factors (Stanier and Moore 2004).

Chromosomal anomalies may occur sporadically, or they may be transmitted from generation to generation, leading to various disorders. Sporadically occurring chromosomal anomalies are more likely to be genetically lethal than inherited anomalies. Chromosomal anomalies take many forms including aneuploidy, chromosomal losses, microdeletions, or rearrangements. Aneuploidy (an abnormal number of chromosomes) is the most common form of chromosomal anomaly typically occurring sporadically. Trisomy (inheritance of one extra copy of a chromosome) is the most common form of aneuploidy. Trisomies, however, are often incompatible with life. Trisomies 9, 13, 16, 18, 21, and X are the exceptions. Table 5 provides an overview of the clinical presentation of the trisomies which are compatible with life as well as

Genetics in Otolaryngology, Table 5 Clinical characteristics of aneuploidy

Aneuploidy	Clinical phenotype
Trisomy 9	Micrognathia, low-set ears, upslanting palpebral fissures, high-arched palate, webbed neck, microcephaly, cranial dysostosis, cleft palate, short sternum, rocker bottom feet, cardiac anomalies, mental retardation, and renal anomalies
Trisomy 13 (Patau syndrome)	Craniosynostosis; upslanting palpebral fissures; broad nose; cleft lip; cleft palate; anteverted nares; micrognathia; small, dysplastic, and low-set ears; severe mental retardation; intrauterine growth restriction; cardiac anomalies; and postaxial polydactyly
Trisomy 16	Intrauterine growth retardation, delayed development, cardiac defects, facial dysmorphisms, hypotonia, and cognitive delay
Trisomy 18	Intrauterine growth restriction, clenched hands, rocker bottom feet, low-set or malformed ears, facial clefts, esophageal atresia, renal anomalies, cardiac defects, scalp anomalies, and central nervous system deformities, life span less than 1 year
Trisomy 21 (Down syndrome)	Impairment in cognitive ability, microgenia, macroglossia, epicanthic folds, upslanting palpebral fissures, short limbs, single transverse palmar crease, high-arched palate, short stature, hypotonia, Eustachian tube dysfunction, otologic anomalies and cardiac anomalies, and increased risk of developing certain malignancies
Trisomy X	Hypertelorism, broad nasal dorsum, and recurrent infection, with otherwise physically and cognitive development

other forms of aneuploidy. Other forms of sex-linked aneuploidy may occur most commonly including XYY, XXY, and XXYY; rarely, XXYY, XXXY, and XXXXY have been described (Tartaglia et al. 2011). Like aneuploidy, chromosomal losses are typically not well tolerated, resulting in death in utero. Turner syndrome (45,X) is the most commonly encountered exception in which one copy of sex chromosome is lost. However, even in the case of Turner syndrome, the vast majority of fetuses succumb prior to term birth. Characteristic findings in Turner syndrome include short stature, webbed neck, broad chest, low frontal hairline, low-set ears, gonadal dysfunction, amenorrhea, infertility, cardiac anomalies, renal anomalies, hypothyroidism, hearing loss, visual disturbance, diabetes, and cognitive deficits. Chromosomal anomalies may also take the form of rearrangement including deletions, duplications, translocations, or inversions. Mental retardation, growth restriction, and multiple congenital malformations are most commonly associated with deletions and duplications. Translocations and inversions most commonly produce a normal phenotype. Microdeletion refers to the duplication or deletion of small chromosomal segments containing a limited number of linked, but functionally unrelated genes which typically occur sporadically; however, inheritance of microdeletions may occur if the microdeletion results in a balanced chromosomal rearrangement. There are various microdeletion syndromes that are encountered within otolaryngology practice. Of particular interest is microdeletion within the short arm of chromosome 22, the 22q11.2 deletion, which is associated with a constellation of symptoms. Deletions within this region of chromosome 22 have been linked to numerous syndromes including DiGeorge syndrome, velocardiofacial syndrome, CHARGE, and Shprintzen syndrome as well as certain forms of craniocerebellocardiac syndrome, Bernard-Soulier syndrome, Opitz-Frias syndrome, and Cayler cardiofacial syndrome (Ben-Shachar et al. 2008; Jyonouchi et al. 2009; Hay 2007; Nakagawa et al. 2001; McDonald-McGinn et al. 1995). The variability in breakpoints and degree of involvement of the microdeletion are responsible for the presence of various syndromes in association with microdeletions.

Cross-References

▶ Benign Neoplasia-Schwannoma-Neurofibromatosis Type 1
▶ Benign Neoplasia-Schwannoma-Neurofibromatosis Type 2
▶ Congenital Laryngeal and Tracheal Anomalies
▶ Congenital Aural Atresia
▶ Congenital Conductive Hearing Loss
▶ Congenital Craniofacial Malformations and Their Surgical Treatment
▶ Congenital Cysts, Sinuses, and Fistulae
▶ Congenital Mixed Hearing Loss
▶ Facial Paralysis in Children
▶ Genetics of Hearing Loss
▶ Head and Neck Squamous Cell Carcinoma, Risk Factors

References

Ben-Shachar S, Ou Z, Shaw CA et al (2008) 22q11.2 distal deletion: a recurrent genomic disorder distinct from DiGeorge syndrome and velocardiofacial syndrome. Am J Hum Genet 82(1):214–221

Brandon M, Baldi P, Wallace DC (2006) Mitochondrial mutations in cancer. Oncogene 25(34):4647–4662

Chiang PW, Spector E, McGregor TL (2009) Evidence suggesting digenic inheritance of Waardenburg syndrome type II with ocular albinism. Am J Med Genet 149A (12):2739–2744

de Grey AD (2005) Reactive oxygen species production in the mitochondrial matrix: implication for the mechanism of mitochondrial mutation accumulation. Rejuvenation Res 8(1):13–17

Grønskov K, Poole RL, Hahnemann JM et al (2011) Deletions and rearrangements of the H19/IGF2 enhancer region in patients with Silver-Russell syndrome and growth retardation. J Med Genet 48(5):308–311

Hay BN (2007) Deletion 22q11: spectrum of associated disorders. Semin Pediatr Neurol 14(3):136–139

Horsthemke B, Wagstaff J (2008) Mechanisms of imprinting of the Prader-Willi/Angelman region. Am J Med Genet A 146A (16):2041–2052

Jyonouchi S, McDonald-McGinn DM, Bale S et al (2009) CHARGE (coloboma, heart defect, atresia choanae, retarded growth and development, genital hypoplasia, ear anomalies/deafness) syndrome and chromosome 22q11.2 deletion syndrome: a comparison of immunologic and nonimmunologic phenotypic features. Pediatrics 123(5): e871–e877

Liu XZ, Yuan Y, Yan D et al (2009) Digenic inheritance on nonsyndromic deafness caused by mutations at the gap junction proteins Cx26 and Cx31. Hum Genet 125(1):53–62

Mancini-DiNardo D, Steele SJ, Levorse JM et al (2006) Elongation of the Kcnq1ot1 transcript is required for genomic imprinting of neighboring genes. Genes Dev 20(10):1268–1282

McDonald-McGinn DM, Driscoll DA, Bason L et al (1995) Autosomal dominant "Opitz" GBBB syndrome due to a 22q11.2 deletion. Am J Med Genet 59(1):103–113

Nakagawa M, Okuno M, Okamoto N et al (2001) Bernard-Soulier syndrome associated with 22q11.2 microdeletion. Am J Med Genet 99(4):286–288

Nativio R, Sparago A, Ito Y et al (2011) Disruption of genomic neighbourhood at the imprinted IGF2-H19 locus in Beckwith-Wiedemann syndrome and Silver-Russell syndrome. Hum Mol Genet 20(7):1363–1374

Ng K, Pullirsch D, Leeb M et al (2007) Xist and the order of silencing. EMBO Rep 8(1):34–39

Sarge KD, Park-Sarge OK (2009) Mitotic bookmarking of formerly active genes: keeping epigenetic memories for fading. Cell Cycle 8(6):818–823

Seidman MD, Ahmad N, Joshi D, Seidman J, Thawani S, Quirk WS (2004) Age-related hearing loss and its association with reactive oxygen species and mitochondrial DNA damage. Acta Otolaryngol Suppl 552:16–24

Stanier P, Moore GE (2004) Genetics of cleft lip and palate: syndromic genes contribute to the incidence of nonsyndromic clefts. Hum Mol Genet 13:R73–R81

Taanman JW (1999) The mitochondrial genome: structure, transcription, translation and replication. Biochim Biophys Acta 1410(2):103–123

Tartaglia N, Natalie A, Howell S et al (2011) 48,XXYY, 48, XXXY and 49,XXXXY syndromes: not just variants of klinefelter syndrome. Acta Paediatr 100(6):851–860

Wallace DC (2005) Mitochondria and cancer: Warburg address. Cold Spring Harb Symp Quant Biol 70:363–374

Wallace DC (2010) Mitochondrial DNA mutations in disease and aging. Environ Mol Mutagen 51(5):440–450

Zaidi SK, Young DW, Montecino M et al (2011) Bookmarking the genome: maintenance of epigenetic information. J Biol Chem 286(21):18355–18361

Zheng QY, Yan D, Ouyang XM et al (2005) Digenic inheritance of deafness caused by mutations in genes encoding cadherin 23 and protocadherin 15 in mice and humans. Hum Mol Genet 14(1):103–111

Genetics of Adult Sensorineural Hearing Loss

Gerald T. Kangelaris and Lawrence R. Lustig
Department of Otolaryngology-Head and Neck Surgery, University of California, San Francisco, San Francisco, CA, USA

Introduction

Hearing loss is one of the most common clinical conditions affecting adults. An estimated 45% of individuals over age 60 have clinically relevant hearing loss in at least one ear. Rates significantly increase with advanced age, such that approximately 70% of individuals over age 70 suffer from hearing loss. Patients suffering from untreated hearing loss suffer from social isolation, loss of autonomy, depression, and loss of self-esteem. The magnitude of the problem is expected to increase with time; in the USA, the number of people over 65 years of age is expected to grow from 13% of the population in 2010 to 20% in 2040, representing 80 million people. The primary treatment modality for adult sensorineural hearing loss is auditory amplification; however, fewer than 25% of those who would benefit from hearing aids use them. Cost is the primary cited reason for nonuse, with 64% of nonusers stating that they can simply not afford hearing aids. Furthermore, their benefit in auditory rehabilitation is limited. Despite the ability of hearing aids to amplify sound, users often note that improvements in speech recognition are poor, particularly in noisy environments. Taken together, hearing loss represents a widespread disease process with an increasing prevalence that is not adequately treated on the population level. The development of new therapeutic strategies is needed.

Presbycusis, or age-related hearing loss (ARHL), is the most frequent cause of adult sensorineural hearing loss. ARHL is typically characterized by a progressive, bilateral, and symmetrical hearing loss varying in severity and predominantly affecting the high frequencies. The hearing loss may be central or peripheral in origin and patients most commonly note difficulty in speech discrimination, hearing in noise, and sound detection and localization. Clinical and histological studies of patients with ARHL fail to show uniform pathology, suggesting the disease represents a multifactorial process reflecting the contributions of accumulated damage to the auditory system. Commonly suggested causative factors include noise exposure, environmental and medical ototoxic agents, trauma, vascular insults, metabolic changes, hormones, dietary factors, and host immune factors, all interacting variably with the context of an individual's personal genetic susceptibility (Liu and Yan 2007).

Given the scope of the problem and the overall poor treatment options available to patients, research has recently begun to focus on exploring the underlying genetic causes and predispositions giving rise to ARHL. This entry explores the prominent factors contributing to ARHL, with a specific focus on the discovered genetic mechanisms underpinning ARHL, and discuss potential future gene and molecular-based therapies.

Pathophysiology of ARHL

Pathologic Findings

Dr. Harold Schuknecht offered the first classification schema of presbycusis through histopathologic investigations of temporal bones. Comparing histopathologic findings in the human inner ear to pre-mortem hearing tests, he categorized presbycusis into the following four groups: sensory, metabolic, neural, and cochlear conductive. The latter represents basilar membrane stiffness and is generally regarded as a hypothetical subtype. Noting that many patients have a mixture of the four pathologic subtypes and that approximately 25% of cases show no specific pathologic findings, Schuknecht would later add two additional categories: mixed and indeterminate (Liu and Yan 2007).

Sensory presbycusis is characterized by a high-frequency sensory hearing loss with normal low-frequency hearing thresholds. Histological findings demonstrate hair cell loss within the basal end of the cochlea. Audiometry reveals a steeply sloping high-frequency loss, often with a notch or dip in the 4 kHz region. These findings have led researchers to hypothesize a link between sensory presbycusis and noise-induced hearing loss. While there is agreement that noise exposure contributes to progressive hearing loss, its association with and contributions to age-related hearing loss is poorly understood. Due to the complex interactions of environmental influences and genetic factors, results of studies examining hearing losses in noise-exposed and aging ears are contradictory and variable.

In contrast, metabolic, or strial, presbycusis is characterized by an increase in audiometric thresholds across all frequencies. This flat audiometric pattern is the most typical finding in cohort studies of elderly people. Histologic examination reveals degeneration of the stria vascularis and lateral cochlear wall. This degeneration is believed to lead to an alteration of endolymph resulting in elevated pure tone thresholds across the auditory spectrum. There is a loss of expression of key ion transport enzymes such as the sodium-potassium ATPase and the sodium-potassium-chloride cotransporter, as well as a decrease in the -80–100 mV endocochlear potential within the scala media. While aging and environmental factors – predominantly noise exposure – appear to be key factors in the development of sensory presbycusis, strial presbycusis is felt to result primarily from aging independent of exogenous influences.

Neural presbycusis refers to degeneration of the spiral nerve ganglion. The defining patient symptom is reduced word recognition and comprehension. The clinical presentation is that of auditory dyssynchrony, where outer hair cell function is preserved as shown by otoacoustic emissions, but the auditory brainstem responses are reduced or absent. It remains difficult to distinguish auditory nerve dysfunction caused by a decreased endocochlear

potential from that caused by degeneration of spiral nerve ganglion neurons.

Contribution of Genetic Factors

Age-related hearing loss is commonly believed to be a complex interplay between an individual's genetic predisposition and environmental exposures. While every individual with presbycusis will experience a continual decline in hearing sensitivity with aging, there are large variations in age of onset, severity of hearing loss, and progression of disease. There are a number of exogenous factors including noise exposure, ototoxic medications, trauma, and diet that influence the phenotype of ARHL. It is not well understood whether environmental exposures produce an accelerating effect of aging in the ear or whether they act on specific physiologic pathways (Van Eyken et al. 2007).

The contribution of genetic factors to ARHL has been demonstrated. Epidemiologic studies show that presbycusis clusters in families and that genetic factors account for approximately half of the variance of ARHL (Fransen et al. 2003). A Swedish study on 250 monozygotic and 207 dizygotic twin males (age 36–80) evaluated hearing loss via a questionnaire and audiometric data (Karlsson et al. 1997). Twin similarity between monozygotic twins decreased with age, while that of the dizygotic twins increased suggesting that environmental effects become more important with age. Hearing thresholds above 3 kHz showed a heritability value of 0.47 for the age group above 64 years, indicating that genetic factors account for approximately half of the population variance for high-frequency hearing loss in this demographic. A study using the Framingham cohort compared audiometric data from genetically related individuals (e.g., sibling pairs, parent-child pairs) with those from genetically unrelated individuals (spouse pairs) (Gates et al. 1999). The data showed a clear familial aggregation for ARHL and that genetic factors account for 35–55% of the variance of ARHL, depending on the frequencies analyzed. In this study, the genetic effects were more pronounced in females compared to males and for the strial presbycusis phenotype compared to the sensory phenotype. Finally, a Danish twin study investigated the heritability of self-reported hearing loss in mono- and dizygotic twins aged 75 and older and identified a heritability index of approximately 40% (Christensen et al. 2001).

Nongenetic Causes of ARHL

Noise Exposure

Noise exposure is a commonly recognized and well-studied environmental factor contributing to presbycusis. Various intensities of noise stimulation result in the audiologic phenomena of adaptation, temporary threshold shifts, and incomplete recovery, the latter or which results in permanent damage and hearing loss. Acoustic trauma leads to cochlear damage via both mechanical and metabolic damage. Mechanical damage results from noise exposures of short duration and high intensity, while metabolic cochlear damage is seen with decreased noise levels over a longer period of time. Exposures to acoustic intensities greater than 130 dB can disrupt portions of the cochlea, leading to hair cell loss through mechanical disruption of the stereocilia and direct damage to supporting and sensory cells. This mechanical damage has little individual variability. In contrast, there is large individual variability among individuals exposed to long-term noise levels between 90 and 130 dB. These conditions lead to metabolic cochlear damage, which is initially characterized by outer hair cell loss, then followed by inner hair cell degeneration if exposure continues. The auditory system is capable of sound conditioning, which is the process of decreased susceptibility to noise-induced hearing loss by previous exposure to nontraumatic noise.

It is difficult to distinguish either audiometrically or histologically between noise-induced and genetically influenced age-related hearing loss. Although models exist to predict the amount of hearing loss based on cumulative lifetime noise exposure, susceptibility to noise exposure in the development of hearing loss displays tremendous individual variability. It has been hypothesized that the susceptibility of an individual to noise-mediated hearing loss occurs due to individual differences in vulnerability at the level of the hair cell or via protective mechanisms of the middle and inner ear.

Animal studies suggest that noise exposure has an additive or interactive effect on age-related hearing loss. One study, for example, demonstrated that noise exposure early in life may predispose to ARHL (Erway et al. 1996). A study utilizing a mouse model found an increased vulnerability to age-related cochlear changes among mice exposed to noise at a young age (Kujawa and Liberman 2006). Additional support for this finding came from another study investigating the BALB/C and C57Bl/6 J mouse models, which show pronounced age-related hearing loss (Ohlemiller et al. 2000). This study found that these mice were more vulnerable to noise exposure compared to control mice, suggesting that genes associated with ARHL confer hearing loss vulnerability to noise exposure.

Ototoxic Medications

A variety of medications are potentially toxic to the inner ear. Elderly subjects are particularly affected by these medications due to both the increased exposure of harmful drugs and higher circulating blood levels because of altered renal and hepatic functioning. Commonly cited examples of ototoxic medications include aminoglycoside antibiotics, the chemotherapeutic agent cisplatin, loop diuretics, and salicylates.

Aminoglycoside antibiotics work by inhibiting bacterial ribosomal protein synthesis and remain a popular choice of therapy due to its continued effectiveness against infections by Gram-negative bacteria. Certain drugs within this medication class are preferentially vestibulotoxic (streptomycin, gentamicin, and tobramycin), while others are predominately ototoxic (neomycin, kanamycin, amikacin, and sisomicin). Despite these tendencies, all are capable of injuring either the vestibular or auditory organs with sufficiently high doses. The ototoxicity manifests as an apoptotic loss of outer hair cells with preferential loss at the basal turn of the cochlea. Consequently, the expressed phenotype is that of a nonreversible hearing loss predominantly affecting the high frequencies.

Aminoglycoside antibiotics appear to potentiate the ototoxic effects of noise and vice versa. While aminoglycoside-induced ototoxicity is generally considered to be dose-dependent, some individuals display an abnormal sensitivity to their toxic effects. Seventeen to thirty-three percent of patients with aminoglycoside-induced hearing loss display a mutation in the mitochondrial 12 S ribosomal RNA gene (Prezant et al. 1993). Carriers of this mutation not exposed to aminoglycoside antibiotics are also more likely to experience a high-frequency progressive hearing loss.

Platinum-based chemotherapeutic medications, including cisplatin, similarly lead to outer hair cell death, predominantly at the basal turn of the cochlea. Approximately 7% of patients will have a clinically relevant high-frequency, bilateral, and permanent hearing loss, although hearing threshold changes have been reported in up to 100% of patients undergoing ultra-frequency audiometric testing. The underlying mechanism of aminoglycoside- and cisplatin-induced ototoxicity is hypothesized to be via the formation of free radicals leading to permanent sensory cell and neuronal damage. Accordingly, antioxidant treatment has been shown to help preserve hearing in aminoglycoside- and cisplatin-treated subjects.

Salicylates and loop diuretics most commonly result in reversible threshold shifts that improve following medication cessation. Interestingly, long-term salicylate use may actually improve hearing. The mechanism of this process is unclear, however there is evidence that salicylates may have a protective effect on aminoglycoside-induced hearing loss through an antioxidant effect.

Alcohol and Smoking

Heavy alcohol use has been associated with an increased risk of ARHL, while light alcohol use may actually be protective against hearing loss. The effects of smoking on the auditory system are less clear. Cigarette smoke leads to hypercoagulability, vasoconstriction, and hemodynamic effects. These effects, in combination with carbon monoxide-induced hypoxia, have been hypothesized to lead to decreased oxygen supply in the inner ear resulting in cochlear damage, mitochondrial mutations, and ultimately hearing loss. The results of numerous studies, however, have failed to show consistent results.

Chemical Exposures

Industrial chemicals such as toluene, trichloroethylene, styrene, and xylene have been shown to contribute to ARHL. Exposure to these chemicals displays a nonlinear effect in combination with noise exposure, meaning that the risk of developing hearing loss increases with age but also with a lifetime exposure to solvents (Van Eyken et al. 2007). Dockworkers exposed to noise and organic solvents – predominantly xylene isomers – showed an increased risk of hearing loss compared to those exposed to noise alone. The risk increased for every year of age, for additional noise exposure, and for lifetime exposure to the organic solvents. Similarly, a higher prevalence of high-frequency hearing loss in styrene-exposed and styrene and noise-exposed workers was seen compared to noise-exposed and non-exposed workers.

Additionally, elevated hearing thresholds have been demonstrated in workers exposed to even small doses of toluene.

Medical Factors

Several medical conditions have been hypothesized to contribute to age-related hearing loss. An association between diabetes mellitus and high-frequency sensorineural hearing loss exits among age-matched controls. Commonly postulated mechanisms include microangiopathic lesions of the inner ear leading to cochlear damage and primary neuropathy of the acoustic neuronal pathways. Diabetic patients up to 60 years of age have higher rates of high-frequency hearing loss compared to healthy age-matched controls, but the difference in hearing loss between the groups diminishes after age 60. Mitochondrial DNA mutations leading to a combination of late-onset diabetes and sensorineural hearing loss have been described. Approximately 1–2% of all diabetic cases in Europe and Japan exhibit these mutations.

A number of studies have evaluated the influence of cardiovascular disease on age-related hearing loss. The Framingham cohort found an association between low-frequency hearing loss and cardiovascular events (stroke, coronary artery disease, or intermittent claudication) (Gates et al. 1993). This low-frequency hearing loss is thought to be associated with microvascular disease-induced damage to the stria vascularis. Hypertension and systolic blood pressure are also associated with increased hearing thresholds. An inverse relationship of high-density lipoprotein levels and hearing thresholds has been demonstrated, particularly in women. A gender-specific association between cardiovascular disease and hearing loss has also been shown; specifically, the risk of age-related hearing loss is twice as likely in women with a self-reported history of myocardial infarction compared to those without. Mouse studies have also demonstrated the association of cardiovascular disease on AHRL. The effects of cardiovascular disease on inner ear function may stem from cochlear hypoxia ultimately causing mitochondrial oxidative stress and cochlear damage (Van Eyken et al. 2007).

Genetic Causes of ARHL

Sound perception is a complex interplay of physical, neural, and molecular pathways. Alterations in any of these pathways can lead to hearing loss. While a variety of nongenetic causes of ARHL and their impacts on these pathways have been described, little is known about the genetic underpinnings of this disease in humans as investigations into the genetic basis of ARHL have only begun in earnest in the last decade. It is expected, however, that numerous genetic influences will affect the phenotypic presentation of ARHL.

Genetically complex traits are determined by a combination of three factors: a genetic background that comprises a large number of genetic factors each with small effects, several major genes each with moderate to large effects, and environmental effects. Phenotypic variation of complex traits is influenced by incomplete penetrance and variable expressivity. Incomplete penetrance is defined as the lack of phenotypic expression of a particular allele in an individual who carries that allele. In contrast, variable expressivity occurs when most or all of the individuals who carry a certain allele express its phenotype, but expression occurs to a greater or lesser degree in each individual.

Two major approaches exist to identify susceptibility genes for complex disorders like ARHL. Linkage analysis is a familial-based investigation in which co-segregation of the disease and an allele of a genetic marker at a certain locus is examined. These studies are preferred in identifying rare genetic variants with large effects. In contrast, association studies examine the co-occurrence of a disease and an allele of a genetic marker. These studies can be performed in unrelated and familial-based samples, but the majority of studies utilize unrelated samples in a case-control study design. This method is ideal in identifying common genetic variants with small effects.

Linkage Analysis

Linkage analysis identifies regions of the genome that contain susceptibility genes by relating inheritance patterns of a disease found in families with those of genetic markers. If marker alleles are co-inherited with the disease more than can be expected by chance, the alleles are liked to the disease under investigation. A large collection of families is a prerequisite for linkage studies. This prerequisite is problematic for late-onset diseases like ARHL because the elder generations are often deceased. The statistical outcome of linkage analysis is the LOD score, which is the

logarithm of the odds of linkage versus no linkage. A LOD score above +3 is significant evidence for linkage, and a score below −2 is significant evidence against linkage.

To date, several linkage studies for ARHL have been published, only one of which has reached genome-wide significance. The first linkage study utilized the Framingham cohort (DeStefano et al. 2003). Audiometric data was collected from parents during a first phase (1973–1975) and compared to their children (1995–1999). After correcting for age and gender, the authors analyzed the average pure-tone hearing thresholds for the middle and low frequencies. Linkage for ARHL was found at six different loci on four chromosomes, with the 11q13 locus demonstrating the highest LOD score of 2.1.

The 3q22 region was identified as another possible linked allele (Garringer et al. 2006). The study investigated a sample of male dizygotic twins with self-reported hearing loss. The linkage generated a LOD score of 2.5 and corresponds to a region of the chromosome 3q where the *DFNA18* locus resides, which has been reported to cause a form of progressive hereditary hearing loss.

Finally, a cross-sectional family-based genetic study by Huyghe et al. examined audiometric data from 200 sibships (Huyghe et al. 2008). The study found a linkage peak on 8q24.13–q24.22 for a trait correlated to audiogram shape. The signal based on simulations reached genome-wide significance, as did the maximal LOD score of 4.2 for chromosome 8 ($p = 0.017$). The identified region on chromosome 8 represents the first statistically significant locus associated with an ARHL phenotype.

Association Studies

Association studies analyze genetic variations in unrelated individuals and investigate variations that are more frequent in affected individuals compared to unaffected individuals. The ideal association study is the genome-wide association study (GWAS), in which hundreds of thousands of single nucleotide polymorphisms (SNPs) across the genome are compared in unrelated individuals. Unfortunately, GWAS are expensive and therefore association studies are typically limited to pre-selected sets of candidate genes. However, costs are continually coming down for these studies, making increasingly larger numbers of genetic traits candidates for this powerful genetic approach.

Huyghe et al. conducted a genome-wide association and linkage analysis as previously described (Huyghe et al. 2008). While the linkage analysis was notable for a linkage peak on 8q24.13–q24.22 for a trait correlated to audiogram shape, the GWAS did not detect any association signals that reached genome-wide significance.

An association study by Friedman et al. investigated 846 cases and 846 controls selected from 3,434 individuals across eight centers in six European countries (Friedman et al. 2009). Analyzing over 500,000 SNPs, the 23 most interesting SNPs among 138 samples were genotyped. This resulted in the identification of a highly significant and replicated SNP located within *GRM7*, a gene that encodes for a metabotropic glutamate receptor type 7. This receptor is expressed in human and mouse hair cells and in spiral ganglion, and is believed to modulate hair cell excitability and synaptic efficacy.

A GWAS by Van Laer et al. used audiometric data from 352 individuals aged 50–75 years in the genetically isolated Finnish Saami population (Van Laer et al.). They applied principle component (PC) analysis to the multivariate audiometric phenotype as a data reduction technique; the first three PCs captured 80% of the hearing threshold variation with preservation of biologically important audiometric features. The top-ranked SNP, rs457717, was localized in an intron of the IQ motif-containing GTPase activating-like protein (IQGAP2). IQGAP2 is a member of the Ras superfamily of GTPases and helps regulate a wide variety of cellular signaling pathways. It is expressed inside the cochlea and has been implicated in cadherin-mediated cell adhesion. Additionally, the seventh-ranked SNP, rs161927, was positioned immediately downstream of the metabotropic glutamate receptor 7 gene (*GRM7*). This finding appears to support the findings of Friedman et al. (2009) that *GRM7* variants may cause an increased susceptibility to glutamate excitotoxicity, which may lead to ARHL.

Reactive Oxygen Species

Oxidative stress from free radicals and other reactive metabolites of aerobic metabolism plays a causative role in the overall aging process and the diseases associated with aging. The cochlea comprises metabolically active tissues that naturally generate reactive oxygen species (ROS) during reduction of O_2 to H_2O including hydrogen peroxide, hydroxyl radicals, and superoxide anions. ROS can cause DNA, cellular, and tissue damage if not neutralized by antioxidant scavenger systems. The cochlea has two active classes of antioxidant enzymes: enzymes involved in glutathione (GSH) metabolism (glutathione *S*-transferase, GST; glutathione peroxidase, GPX1; and glutathione reductase, GSR) and enzymes involved in the breakdown of superoxide anions and hydrogen peroxide (e.g., catalase, CAT; superoxide dismutase, SOD). Genetic variation leading to impaired ROS antioxidant enzymatic functioning has been postulated to result in cellular injury (Uchida et al.).

A number of human and animal studies support the claim that inner ear oxidative stress results in both cellular injury and hearing loss. The superoxide anion is the most common ROS and causes auditory sensory damage, resulting in auditory neuron and hair cell apoptosis. Under normal circumstances, the copper/zinc superoxide dismutase (SOD1) is highly expressed within the cochlea. However, studies of mouse knockout models of SOD1 have demonstrated cochlear hair cell degeneration and loss of spiral ganglion cells and nerve fibers, resulting in findings consistent with ARHL (McFadden et al. 2001). Similarly, knockout models of GPX1 show that deletion in this antioxidant gene can lead to both age-related and noise-induced hearing loss. Glutathione *S*-transferases (GST) consist of several gene classes including *GSTM* and *GSTT*, and function in antioxidant pathways and ROS detoxification. *GSTM1* and *GSTT1* genes show genetic variability in humans, with up to 50% of Caucasian individuals displaying the null genotype for the *GSTM1* gene. These null genotypes cannot conjugate metabolites specific for these enzymes, making them more susceptible to oxidative stress. High-frequency otoacoustic emissions in *GSTM1* individuals have been shown to have lower amplitudes compared to individuals possessing the gene, suggesting that affected individuals may be more prone to ARHL (Rabinowitz et al. 2002). Finally, polymorphisms of *NAT2*6A* show an increased risk of ARHL, with homozygotic and heterozygotic individuals conferring a 15- and 3-fold risk compared to wild type (Unal et al. 2005). *NAT2*6A* belongs to the enzymatic family of N-acetyltransferase (NAT), which is involved in the metabolism and detoxification of cytotoxic and carcinogenic compounds as well as reactive oxygen species.

Mitochondrial Mutations

Mitochondria are intracellular organelles that play a number of cellular roles including oxidative phosphorylation for cellular energy production, the mediation of apoptosis, and control of cellular oxidative stress. Given their high metabolic requirements, cochlear tissues contain an abundance of mitochondria. Mitochondria and mitochondrial DNA (mtDNA) are particularly vulnerable to damage from reactive oxidative species. A number of mouse models for aging have shown that an accumulation of mtDNA mutations may contribute to ARHL. In humans with ARHL, a significant increase in mitochondrial mutations in auditory tissue has been demonstrated in comparison to controls. Specific deletions within mtDNA, known as common aging deletions, have been demonstrated to accumulate with age in human and rodent tissues, including the cochlea. The most frequently acquired mitochondrial common aging deletion in humans is mtDNA^{4977}, which deletes 4,977 base pairs (bp) between two 13-bp repeats starting at nucleotides 8470 and 13447. Investigations of human temporal bones reveal that the common aging deletion is frequently found in patients with ARHL while nearly absent in age-matched control patients without a history of ARHL. Similarly, the equivalent common aging deletion in rodents, mtDNA^{4834}, has also been linked to ARHL (Uchida et al.).

An accumulation of mitochondrial mutations leads to metabolically deficient cellular functioning and ultimately results in cellular death. This phenomenon is particularly problematic in postmitotic tissue, such as the inner ear, where cellular regeneration is not possible, leading to permanent sensory cellular loss. Mitochondrial metabolites, such as alpha-lipoic acid and acetyl L-carnitine, upregulate mitochondrial function and improve energy-producing capabilities within the cell. These metabolites reduce age-associated deterioration in auditory sensitivity and improve cochlear function presumably via their abilities to protect and repair age-induced cochlear mtDNA damage.

Candidate-Gene Investigations

A number of targeted candidate-gene investigations have been performed to identify genetic associations with ARHL. The *KCNQ4* gene is one gene that has been identified as playing a role in ARHL. This gene encodes for a voltage-gated potassium channel and is expressed in both inner and outer hair cells of the cochlea and the vestibular organs. It is theorized to play a role in the release of potassium from the hair cells and the recycling of potassium in the inner ear. An autosomal-dominant pattern of non-syndromic hearing loss, DFNA2, results from a mutation in the *KCNQ4* gene. Patients afflicted with DFNA2 display phenotypic similarities to ARHL, and therefore Van Eyken et al. examined *KCNQ4* as a candidate gene for ARHL. They were able to demonstrate several SNPs in a region spanning 13 kb in the middle of this gene to be significantly associated with ARHL in two independent Caucasian populations (Van Eyken et al. 2006).

Associations to ARHL have also been found with the gene *GRHL2*, which is responsible for the autosomal dominant hearing loss DFNA28. This gene encodes a transcription factor widely expressed in a variety of epithelial tissues including tissue within the inner ear lining the cochlear duct, where it is most prominent during embryonic development and less so during early postnatal stages. Significant associations in *GRHL2* variants and ARHL susceptibility have been observed and replicated in two independent populations (Van Laer et al. 2008).

The role of uncoupling proteins (UCPs) in hearing loss has also been investigated. These represent a family of mitochondrial proton transporters and are thought to be regulators of thermal control and energy metabolism. A population-based aging study found polymorphisms in UCP2 to be significantly associated with hearing impairment (Sugiura et al.).

Therapies

The identification of molecular and genetic causes of hearing loss allows for new therapeutic possibilities beyond the currently available approaches of amplification and cochlear implantation. Gene therapy is one possible future strategy. Initial attempts at adenovector introduction of the transcription factor *Math1* into the cochlea to incite regeneration of hair cells have been successful and resulted in the recovery of hearing abilities in mature deaf mice (Izumikawa et al. 2005).

A number of different possibilities exist for administration of gene therapy including infusion with osmotic mini-pumps, direct microinjection into the cochlea, and application of a vector-transgene infused medium, such as Gelfoam, directly onto the round window. These approaches can also be used to administer therapeutic or otoprotective pharmacologic substances into the inner ear such as antioxidants and growth factors.

Stem cells represent another exciting possibility for biologic treatment of ARHL. After its grafting into rat cochlea, neural stem cells have been shown to survive and adopt the correct hair cell morphologies and positions. Stem cells and embryonic neurons introduced to the inner ear can survive, migrate, differentiate and grow into the neuroauditory system of adult mammals. Embryonic stem cells have also been shown to differentiate into hair cells and potentially also into other inner ear cell types (Van Eyken et al. 2007). These findings give hope that new treatments for ARHL may arise in the future.

References

Christensen K, Frederiksen H et al (2001) Genetic and environmental influences on self-reported reduced hearing in the old and oldest old. J Am Geriatr Soc 49(11):1512–1517

DeStefano AL, Gates GA et al (2003) Genomewide linkage analysis to presbycusis in the Framingham Heart Study. Arch Otolaryngol Head Neck Surg 129(3):285–289

Erway LC, Shiau YW et al (1996) Genetics of age-related hearing loss in mice. III. Susceptibility of inbred and F1 hybrid strains to noise-induced hearing loss. Hear Res 93(1–2):181–187

Fransen E, Lemkens N et al (2003) Age-related hearing impairment (ARHI): environmental risk factors and genetic prospects. Exp Gerontol 38(4):353–359

Friedman RA, Van Laer L et al (2009) GRM7 variants confer susceptibility to age-related hearing impairment. Hum Mol Genet 18(4):785–796

Garringer HJ, Pankratz ND et al (2006) Hearing impairment susceptibility in elderly men and the DFNA18 locus. Arch Otolaryngol Head Neck Surg 132(5):506–510

Gates GA, Cobb JL et al (1993) The relation of hearing in the elderly to the presence of cardiovascular disease and cardiovascular risk factors. Arch Otolaryngol Head Neck Surg 119(2):156–161

Gates GA, Couropmitree NN et al (1999) Genetic associations in age-related hearing thresholds. Arch Otolaryngol Head Neck Surg 125(6):654–659

Huyghe JR, Van Laer L et al (2008) Genome-wide SNP-based linkage scan identifies a locus on 8q24 for an age-related hearing impairment trait. Am J Hum Genet 83(3):401–407

Izumikawa M, Minoda R et al (2005) Auditory hair cell replacement and hearing improvement by Atoh1 gene therapy in deaf mammals. Nat Med 11(3):271–276

Karlsson KK, Harris JR et al (1997) Description and primary results from an audiometric study of male twins. Ear Hear 18(2):114–120

Kujawa SG, Liberman MC (2006) Acceleration of age-related hearing loss by early noise exposure: evidence of a misspent youth. J Neurosci 26(7):2115–2123

Liu XZ, Yan D (2007) Ageing and hearing loss. J Pathol 211(2):188–197

McFadden SL, Ohlemiller KK et al (2001) The influence of superoxide dismutase and glutathione peroxidase deficiencies on noise-induced hearing loss in mice. Noise Health 3(11):49–64

Ohlemiller KK, Wright JS et al (2000) Vulnerability to noise-induced hearing loss in 'middle-aged' and young adult mice: a dose-response approach in CBA, C57BL, and BALB inbred strains. Hear Res 149(1–2):239–247

Prezant TR, Agapian JV et al (1993) Mitochondrial ribosomal RNA mutation associated with both antibiotic-induced and non-syndromic deafness. Nat Genet 4(3):289–294

Rabinowitz PM, Pierce Wise J Sr et al (2002) Antioxidant status and hearing function in noise-exposed workers. Hear Res 173(1–2):164–171

Sugiura S, Uchida Y et al The association between gene polymorphisms in uncoupling proteins and hearing impairment in Japanese elderly. Acta Otolaryngol 130(4):487–492

Uchida Y, Sugiura S et al Molecular genetic epidemiology of age-related hearing impairment. Auris Nasus Larynx 38(6):657–665

Unal M, Tamer L et al (2005) N-acetyltransferase 2 gene polymorphism and presbycusis. Laryngoscope 115(12):2238–2241

Van Eyken E, Van Laer L et al (2006) KCNQ4: a gene for age-related hearing impairment? Hum Mutat 27(10):1007–1016

Van Eyken E, Van Camp G et al (2007) The complexity of age-related hearing impairment: contributing environmental and genetic factors. Audiol Neurootol 12(6):345–358

Van Laer L, Huyghe JR et al A genome-wide association study for age-related hearing impairment in the Saami. Eur J Hum Genet 18(6):685–693

Van Laer L, Van Eyken E et al (2008) The grainyhead like 2 gene (GRHL2), alias TFCP2L3, is associated with age-related hearing impairment. Hum Mol Genet 17(2):159–169

Genetics of Hearing Loss

Angela Peng and Kelley Dodson
Department of Otolaryngology-Head and Neck Surgery, Virginia Commonwealth University, Richmond, VA, USA

Synonyms

Autosomal dominant deafness; Autosomal recessive deafness; Genes; Inheritance; Nonsyndromic deafness; Syndromic deafness

Basic Characteristics

Introduction

Hearing loss is the most frequent sensory impairment, with roughly 1/1,000 being profoundly impaired at birth. For every child born with profound deafness, there are 1–2 born with lesser but clinically significant bilateral or unilateral losses (Nance 2003). A genetic etiology is the cause in at least 50% of congenitally affected individuals (Marazita et al. 1993). Syndromic deafness, or deafness associated with additional clinical abnormalities, accounts for about 30% of genetic cases, while genes for nonsyndromic hearing loss explain for the remaining 70% (Toriello et al. 2004). Inheritance is autosomal dominant in 15–20%, autosomal recessive in about 80%, X-linked in 1–5%, and mitochondrial in 1–10%, depending upon the population (Marazita et al. 1993). Despite the mode of inheritance, the gene expressivity may vary within families such that the same gene may not manifest the same degree of hearing loss (Tomaski and Grundfast 1999). Environmental or infectious etiologies are implicated in the remaining 30–40% of children with "nongenetic" hearing loss. Of these etiologies, prenatally acquired cytomegalovirus (CMV) is most often implicated.

When categorizing the type of hearing loss, it is important to distinguish the onset (congenital, later onset in childhood, or in adulthood), inheritance pattern, laterality, progressive features, vestibular involvement, audiologic phenotype, and association with any other clinical abnormalities (Tomaski and Grundfast 1999). Apart from identifying and treating the hearing deficit, it is of great importance to establish the etiology whenever possible.

Research in the field of hearing impairment and deafness has undergone exciting new developments within the past 10 years. Great strides have been made in deciphering the molecular basis of deafness, yet many aspects of this heterogeneous disorder remain to be clarified. Although more than 150 nonsyndromic loci have already been identified, new genes continue to be described (Van Camp and Smith 2011) (*Hereditary Hearing Loss Homepage*, www.hereditaryhearingloss.org). It is estimated that 1% of the human genome, or over 300 genes, will be involved in auditory perception.

Syndromic Hearing Loss

Hearing loss is associated with more than 400 inherited syndromes (Hone and Smith 2001). This is part of the classification that may include the involvement of craniofacial, skeletal, ocular, neurological, renal, or cardiovascular systems (Mhatre and Lalwani 1996).

Table 1 summarizes some common forms of syndromic hearing loss, including the mode of inheritance, type of hearing loss, and gene involved in prominent syndromes.

The following reviews the syndromes in detail (Toriello et al. 2004).

Alport's Syndrome

Type of deafness: Bilateral SNHL which is progressive and variable in degree (males more affected)

Age of onset: Late childhood to young adulthood (progressive)

Clinical symptoms: Progression to end-stage glomerulonephritis (early microscopic hematuria and renal insufficiency), lenticonus and perimacular flecks, hypertension

Radiologic finding: External auditory canal, ossicular and middle ear anomalies

Heredity: Heterogeneity based upon genetic mutation and mode of inheritance. All involve defect of type IV collagen causing abnormalities in basilar membrane, part of spiral ligament, and stria vascularis (loss of basement integrity). Locus(Gene): Xq22 (*COL4A5*)/6 (X-linked), 2q36-q37(*COL4A3/4*) (autosomal dominant and recessive)

Apert's Syndrome

Type of deafness: CHL

Age of onset: At birth (1 in 160,000)

Clinical symptoms: Craniosynostosis, syndactyly of hands and feet, variable mental retardation, short anterior cranial fossa, depressed nasal bridge, downslanting palpebral fissues with proptosis and hypertelorism, high arched palate, cervical fusion

Radiologic finding: Craniosynostosis, ventriculomegaly, hydrocephalus, cervical fusion

Heredity: Autosomal dominant; Locus(Gene): 10q26(FGFR2) – fibroblast growth factor receptor 2

Branchio-oto-renal Syndrome

Type of deafness: Hearing loss in 75% of cases, CHL in 30%, SNHL in 20%, mixed in 50%, may be progressive

Genetics of Hearing Loss, Table 1 Syndromic hearing loss

Mode of inheritance	Name	Type of hearing loss	Gene
AR	Jervell & Lange-Nielsen	SNHL	KCNQ1, KCNE1
	Norrie[a]	SNHL	NDP
	Pendred	SNHL	SLC26A4, FOXI1, KCNJ10
	Pierre Robin[a]	CHL/Mixed	SOX9
	Usher	SNHL	MYO7A, CDH23, PCDH15, SANS, VLGR1, SHRN, USH1C, USH2A, WHRN, USH3A, PDZD7
AD	Alports[a]	SNHL	COL4A5, COL4A3/4
	Aperts	CHL	FGFR2
	Branchio-oto-renal	CHL/SNHL/mixed	EYA1, SIX1, SIX5
	Treacher Collins	CHL	TCOF1
	Stickler	CHL/mixed	COL2A1, COL11A2, COL11A1, COL9A1, COL9A2
	Waardenburg[a]	SNHL	PAX3, MITF, SNAI2, PAX3, EDNRB, EDN3, SOX10
X-linked	Alport[a]	SNHL	COL4A6, COL4A3/4
	Norrie[a]	SNHL	NDP
	Pierre Robin[a]	CHL/Mixed	SOX9

[a]Mode of inheritance may be variable
SNHL sensorineural hearing loss, *CHL* conductive hearing loss

Age of onset: Early childhood to young adulthood

Clinical symptoms: Hearing loss, preauricular pits or sinuses, branchial cleft cysts or fistulas, pinna malformations, inner ear deformities, renal anomalies, elevated creatinine or proteinuria
Radiologic finding: Various anomalies have been reported including malformed ossicles, malformed cochlea, and enlarged vestibular aqueduct
Heredity: Autosomal dominant; Locus(Gene): BOR1 (*EYA1*), BOS3(*SIX1*), BOR2(*SIX5*)

Jervell and Lange-Nielsen Syndrome
Type of deafness: Profound bilateral SNHL
Age of onset: At birth

Clinical symptoms: Recurrent syncope, torsade de pointe arrhythmia, sudden death from cardiac conduction delay, electrocardiogram shows prolonged QT interval, high mortality rate

Important clinical finding: EKG showing prolonged QT interval

Heredity: Autosomal Recessive; Locus(Gene): JLNS1(*KCNQ1*), JLNS2(*KCNE1*); potassium channel on apical cell layer of stria vascularis; dominant forms of Long QT syndromes cause cardiac abnormalities without deafness

Norrie Syndrome (Oculoacousticocerebral Dysplasia)
Type of deafness: Progressive SNHL, asymmetric (males more affected) in 35–40%

Age of onset: Early childhood to adolescence

Clinical symptoms: Very early onset of progressive blindness during infancy due to retinal detachment, secondary cataracts, leukocoria, 50% with progressive mental disorders, including psychosis

Heredity: X-linked, autosomal recessive; Locus (Gene): NDP(*NDP*) – "Norrie disease (pseudoglioma)" gene; norrin protein is involved in specialization of the retina and blood supply to inner ear and retina

Pendred's Syndrome
Type of deafness: bilateral SNHL, often later onset and progressive, may fluctuate
Age of onset: At birth (1–7.5 per 100,000 births)

Clinical symptoms: thyroid goiter (may be euthyroid), vestibular hypofunction

Radiologic finding: Enlarged vestibular aqueduct, Mondini dysplasia

Heredity: Autosomal recessive; Locus(Gene): PDS(*SLC26A4*), PDS(*FOXI1*) – "Pendrin"; pendrin protein affects the transport of iodine and chloride ions

Pierre Robin Syndrome
Type of deafness: Primarily CHL although may be mixed
Age of onset: At birth (1 in 8500–1 in 30,000)

Clinical symptoms: cleft lip and palate, micrognathia, glossoptosis, malformed ears, subglottic stenosis, mobius syndrome, may be associated with other syndromes, most commonly associated with Stickler's syndrome

Radiologic finding: middle ear malformations

Heredity: X-linked, autosomal recessive, or sporadic; Locus(Gene): Most common mutation in 17q24.3-q25.1(SOX9), multiple genes may also be involved (11q23-q24(PVRL1), 2q31(GAD67))

Stickler's Syndrome (Hereditary Progressive Arthroophthalmopathy)

Type of deafness: High frequency SNHL, progressive bilateral

Age of onset: Early childhood

Clinical symptoms: Pierre Robin sequence (cleft palate, micrognathia), flat nasal bridge, myopia, retinal detachment, cataracts, arthropathy, marfanoid habitus, scoliosis

Heredity: Autosomal dominant with variable expression; collagen type II and XI affected

Locus(Gene): STL1(*COL2A1*): most common; STL3(*COL11A2*), STL2(*COL11A1*), STL3(*COL9A1*)

Treacher Collins Syndrome (Mandibulofacial Dysostosis)

Type of deafness: Variable, usually conductive and bilateral (present in 55%)

Age of onset: At birth

Clinical symptoms: Downsloped palpebral fissures with hypoplastic zygomas, large downturned mouth, mandibulofacial dysostosis, cleft lip/palate, normal intelligence, malformed auricles, microtia/atresia, coloboma of lower eyelids, dental malformation

Radiologic findings: Ossicular malformations, aural atresia, absent/obliterated middle ears, inner ear may be normal

Heredity: Autosomal dominant with variable expression. Treacle – intracellular protein defects, affecting crest cell migration and pharyngeal arch development. Locus(Gene): TCOF1(*TCOF1*)

Usher Syndrome

Type of deafness: Variable onset depending on type

Age of onset: At birth (4.4/100,000)

Clinical symptoms: progressive degeneration of retina leading to blindness ("retinitis pigmentosa") where loss of night vision is first, followed by loss of visual fields, then finally blindness

Type I (most common): congenital deafness (profound), vestibular dysfunction, early onset of retinitis pigmentosa

Type II: congenital deafness (moderate, sloping), normal vestibular function, early adult onset of retinitis pigmentosa

Type III: progressive hearing loss (born with good or mild hearing loss), variable vestibular function present and variable onset of retinitis pigmentosa

Radiologic finding: none

Heredity: Autosomal recessive; Locus(Gene): *Type I:* USH1B-G(*MYO7A, CDH23, PCDH15, SANS*), *Type II:* USH2A-D(*VLGR1, WHRN*), *Type III*: USH3 (*USH3A, PDZD7*)

Waardenburg's Syndrome (Type I-IV)

Type of deafness: Variable, may be unilateral or bilateral. Type II most commonly associated with hearing loss

Age of onset: Early childhood to young adulthood

Clinical symptoms: Pigmentation changes (from neural crest cell defects) including heterochromia iridis, white eyelashes, pinched nose, flattened nasal root

Type I: dystopia canthorum (widely spaced medial canthi), white forelock, 58–75% have HL

Type II: absence of dystopia canthorum, 80–90% have HL

Type III "Klein-Waardenburg Syndrome": Type I + limb abnormalities

Type IV "Shah-Waardenburg Syndrome": Type II + Hirschsprung disease; autosomal recessive

Radiologic finding: Usually normal, may have abnormalities of the semicircular canals especially in Type 2

Heredity: Autosomal dominant although type IV is autosomal recessive

Locus(Gene): *Type I*: WS1(*PAX3*); *Type II*: WS2A (*MITF*), WS2D(*SNAI2*); *Type III*: WS3(*PAX3*); *Type IV*: WS4(*EDNRB, EDN3, SOX10*)

Otosclerosis

Although otosclerosis is not necessarily a syndrome, it is an inherited disorder that causes hearing loss. It is autosomal dominant although the penetrance and degree of expressivity vary. To date, several loci have been described in families with otosclerosis; however, no genes have yet been identified. Patients usually present with mild to severe conductive hearing loss, although they may have a sensorineural component. Typical clinical presentation occurs in the third decade and most people will manifest the hearing loss by age 50. Caucasians are most commonly affected. Physiologically, the endochondral bone formation and sclerosis of the temporal bone at the oval and round window cause dampening of the transmission of sound to the inner ear. Surgical management with stapedectomy or stapedotomy is highly successful at reversing the hearing loss. It is important in young males with "otosclerosis" to rule out with CT imaging the X-linked condition DFN3, or stapes gusher syndrome. This entity is caused by widening of the internal auditory canal and associated pressure transmission to the oval window, creating an "inner ear" conductive hearing loss. Stapedectomy in these cases would result in a dead ear (Tomaski and Grundfast 1999).

Nonsyndromic Hearing Loss

Nonsyndromic hearing loss accounts for 70% of genetic deafness. Thus far, at least 86 autosomal recessive, 62 autosomal dominant, and 5 X-linked loci have been reported (www.hereditary-hearingloss.org). Some loci may hold multiple genes responsible for deafness, yet some genes may share multiple loci assignments (Schrijver 2004). Unlike syndromic deafness, nonsyndromic hearing loss is not associated with any clinical findings apart from the hearing impairment. The hearing loss is primarily sensorineural; prelingual in autosomal recessive inheritance patterns and more often postlingual in autosomal dominant patterns (Schrijver 2004). In patients with profound hearing loss (> 90 dB), a nonsyndromic genetic diagnosis was more common than in those with lesser forms of hearing loss (Morzaria et al. 2004).

Classification of the deafness loci is based on mode of inheritance, and the HUGO Gene Nomenclature committee has established this categorization: DFNA (dominant), DFNB (recessive), DFNX (X-linked), DFNY (Y-linked), and DFNM (modifier). Additional symbols such as mitochondrial (MRTNR, MTTS) may specify the form of hearing loss (Dror and Avraham 2010). Each locus has an associated number which identifies the sequential order of its discovery (Van Camp and Smith 2011) (www.hereditaryhearingloss. org). Please refer to Table 2 for a listing of some of the known and named nonsyndromic deafness genes, as discussion of each entity is beyond the scope of this entry.

Genetics of Hearing Loss, Table 2 Nonsyndromic hearing loss[a]

Mode of inheritance	Gene
AR	GJB2, MYO7A, MYO15A, SLC26A4, TMIE, TMC1, TMPRSS3, OTOF, CDH23, GIPC3, STRC, USH1C, TECTA, OTOA, PCDH15, RDX, GRXCR1, TRIOBP, CLDN14, MYO3A, WHRN, GPSM2, ESRRB, ESPN, MYO6, HGF, ILDR1, MARVELD2, COL11A2, PJVK, SLC26A5, LRTOMT/COMT2, LHFPL5, GIPC3, BSND, MSRB3, LOXHD1, TPRN, PTPRQ, SERPINB6, GIPC3
AD	DIAPH1, GJB2, KCNQ4, GJB3, GJB6, MYH14, CEACAM16, DFNA5, WFS1, COCH, EYA4, MYO7A, TECTA, COL11A2, POUF3, MYH9, ACTG1, MYO6, SLC17A8, GRHL2, TMC1, DSPP, CCDC50, MYO1A, TJP2, SMAC/DIABLO
X-linked	PRPS1, POU3F4, SMPX

[a]Listed in the order of discovery (Van Camp and Smith 2011)

Connexin-26 and −30 (DFNB1)

Mutations of the DFNB1 locus on the long arm of chromosome 13, containing the *GJB2* (connexin 26) and *GJB6* (connexin 30) genes, are the most common genetic cause of profound prelingual hearing loss in this country. Despite the large number of genes (>100 at present) known to cause hearing impairment, the discovery that deafness resulting from mutations at this locus is so common in most populations was an important breakthrough. Many mutations have been discovered, ranging from the common 35delG mutation in Caucasian populations to novel mutations found only in single families. Connexin 26 and 30 are structurally related subunits of a gap junction protein, which can aggregate to form homomeric and heteromeric connexons, facilitating the passage of ions and small molecules between cells. Although most connexin deafness is congenital and profound, there is audiometric variability, even within some families with the same mutation. Truncating mutations, which result in a shortened defective protein, are associated with greater degrees of hearing loss than nontruncating mutations, which result from amino acid substitutions with no change in protein size (Snoeckx et al. 2005). More recent data suggests that temporal bone anomalies may be more common than previously recognized. The DFNB1 locus also contains an adjacent gene, GJB6, in which a 309 kb deletion, common in certain ethnic groups, can cause digenic deafness in association with a heterozygous connexin 26 mutation.

Mitochondrial Deafness

Mitochondrial genes, as well as their mutations, are solely the result of maternal inheritance. It is believed that mitochondrial hearing loss is due to alteration of ATP metabolism thus disturbing the ion gradient required by cochlear hair cells (Schrijver 2004). Mitochondrial mutations associated with hearing loss may also be syndromic or nonsyndromic. Most mitochondrial deafness is sensorineural in nature.

Some of the more commonly acquired syndromic mitochondrial diseases associated with hearing loss involve neuromuscular syndromes such as Kearns-Sayre Syndrome (deletions in multiple genes), Myoclonic epilepsy and ragged red fibers (mutation in *MTTK* gene), Mitochondrial encephalophathy, lactic acidosis and stroke like episodes (mutation in *MTTL1*), and Maternally inherited diabetes and deafness (mutations and deletions in multiple genes including *MTTL1, MTTK, MTTE*). However, most mitochondrial deafness is nonsyndromic in nature. Of note, are several mutations in the mitochondrial 12 S rRNA subunit, encoded by the MTRNR1 gene, including the well-known A1555G mutation, the C1494T mutation, and the 961 mutations. These mutations induce or cause worsening of hearing loss due to a dose independent susceptibility to aminoglycoside ototoxicity, which results in severe to profound deafness, even after a single exposure to an aminoglycoside antibiotic. Other mutations in the mitochondrial serine t-RNA MTTS1 gene, including the A7445G mutation, have also been associated with hearing loss although the penetrance varies, depending on other genetic and environmental modifiers (Schrijver 2004).

Genetics Evaluation and Counseling

Upon the diagnosis of hearing loss, a thorough evaluation is of utmost importance to establish an etiologic diagnosis. A thorough history (including prenatal, perinatal, and family history), physical examination, and audiologic work-up should be performed for each patient. Existing evidence suggests that in addition to a Human Genetics consultation, CT scanning of the temporal bone and molecular testing for *GJB2* mutations are generally indicated, if the specific etiology is not apparent by the initial history and physical examination (Preciado et al. 2004). Additional tests, such as an EKG, or other laboratory tests or molecular studies should be ordered on a case by case basis. Consultation with other specialists such as an ophthalmologist may also be warranted.

The medical geneticist and genetic counselor assist with the evaluation, diagnosis, and family counseling. Although limited options for genetic therapy are currently available, it is important to establish a genetic etiology when present, and educate the family, particularly with regard to future pregnancies (Robin et al. 2005). It is also important to consider the ethical dilemmas that the parents and children may face after learning about the diagnosis. Current technology allows for the screening of single genes, or in combination on newer "gene chips." In order to be cost effective, directed testing is important based upon sound clinical acumen.

Conclusion

At least half of all congenital and early onset hearing loss is genetic in nature. The field of genetic hearing loss has made great strides within the past decade, as we presently recognize over 150 loci associated with nonsyndromic hearing loss and hundreds of syndromes which include hearing loss as one component. As we continue to refine and apply this genetic knowledge, we hope to develop promising therapeutic and preventative applications.

Cross-References

▶ Otosclerosis

References

Dror AA, Avraham KB (2010) Hearing impairment: a panoply of genes and functions. Neuron 68:293–308

Hone SW, Smith RJ (2001) Genetics of hearing impairment. Semin Neonatol 6:531–541

Marazita ML, Ploughman LM, Rawlings B et al (1993) Genetic epidemiological studies of early-onset deafness in the U.S. school-age population. Am J Med Genet 46:486–491

Mhatre AN, Lalwani AK (1996) Molecular genetics of deafness. Otolaryngol Clin North Am 29:421–435

Morzaria S, Westerberg BD, Kozak FK (2004) Systematic review of the etiology of bilateral sensorineural hearing loss in children. Int J Pediatr Otorhinolaryngol 68:1193–1198

Nance WE (2003) The genetics of deafness. Ment Retard Dev Disabil Res Rev 9:109–119

Preciado DA, Lim LH, Cohen AP et al (2004) A diagnostic paradigm for childhood idiopathic sensorineural hearing loss. Otolaryngol Head Neck Surg 131:804–809

Robin NH, Prucka SK, Woolley AL et al (2005) The use of genetic testing in the evaluation of hearing impairment in a child. Curr Opin Pediatr 17:709–712

Schrijver I (2004) Hereditary non-syndromic sensorineural hearing loss: transforming silence to sound. J Mol Diagn 6: 275–284

Snoeckx RL, Huygen PL, Feldmann D et al (2005) GJB2 mutations and degree of hearing loss: a multicenter study. Am J Hum Genet 77:945–957

Tomaski SM, Grundfast KM (1999) A stepwise approach to the diagnosis and treatment of hereditary hearing loss. Pediatr Clin North Am 46:35–48

Toriello HV, Reardon W, Gorlin R (2004) Hereditary hearing loss and its syndromes. Oxford University Press, Oxford

Van Camp G and Smith RJH (2011) Hereditary hearing loss homepage. www.hereditaryhearingloss.org

Genetics of Presbycusis

Amy Lawrason, Jessica Weiss and Kourosh Parham
Division of Otolaryngology, Department of Head and Neck Surgery, University of Connecticut Health Center, Farmington, CT, USA

Definition

Presbycusis: A general term used to describe hearing loss from a lifetime of insults to the auditory system (Gates and Mills 2005).

Introduction

Age-related hearing loss, or presbycusis, has adverse effects on the physical, cognitive, behavioral, and social functions of the geriatric population. Presbycusis is likely the product of a lifetime of insults to the auditory system. The key insults include aging and noise damage, genetic susceptibility, otologic disorders, and exposures to ototoxic agents. The identification of genetic factors has been difficult because of the inability to separate the genetic influences on presbycusis from the environmental variables.

Few estimates exist of the proportion of age-related hearing loss that arises from genetic or familial causes.

The literature estimates a heritability range between 25% and 75% with a significant proportion being influenced by gender (McMahon et al. 2008). The following review discusses the roles of heritability, genetic factors, and mitochondrial pathways in the development of presbycusis.

Pathophysiology

Age-related hearing loss is characterized by a decrease in hearing sensitivity and speech understanding in noise as well as slowed central auditory processing. Typically, hearing loss begins in the higher frequencies and progresses to include middle frequencies which are important in the comprehension of voiceless consonants. It is partially for this reason that patients with presbycusis complain that they can hear, but have difficulty understanding what is being said. Please refer to the Springer Link entry on Presbycusis for additional information on the pathophysiology.

Heritability of Presbycusis

The specific genes involved in age-related hearing loss are still relatively unknown, specifically in humans. Similarities between the auditory systems of mice and humans have allowed researchers to use mice as a model for the better understanding of presbycusis.

Murine Studies

A genetic component for presbycusis has been shown with inbred and hybrid strains of mice. Erway and colleagues used auditory-evoked brainstem responses to assess hearing loss in five strains of inbred mice and ten combinations of hybrids (Erway et al. 1993). Their results supported a genetic model for presbycusis and they identified recessive alleles at three different loci contributing to presbycusis. Subsequent work in C57BL/6 J mice identified the Ahl1 gene (age-related hearing loss gene 1). Ahl1 was mapped to chromosome 10 with a mutation in this gene being associated with elevated hearing thresholds at high frequencies in middle- and older-aged mice (Johnson et al. 1997). Cadherin 23 is the gene associated with this locus and has been localized to stereocilia (Noben-Trauth et al. 2003). Based on this finding, it is hypothesized that cadherin 23 plays a critical role in signal transduction

Genetics of Presbycusis, Table 1 *Correlations of age-adjusted pure-tone average (PTA) hearing thresholds in ears with sensory presbycusis phenotype or normal hearing.* The sensory presbycusis phenotype showed a familial aggregation of hearing threshold levels, with spouse-spouse, parent-child, and sibling-sibling PTA hearing threshold correlations shown in the table (Data from Gates et al. 1999)

Correlation coefficient						
	Mid-frequency PTA		High-frequency PTA		Low-frequency PTA	
Family group	Better ear	Worse ear	Better ear	Worse ear	Better ear	Worse ear
Spouse-Spouse	0.08	0.02	0.09	0.03	0.09	0.08
Parent-Child	0.26	0.26	0.20	0.21	0.22	0.22
Sibling-Sibling	0.39	0.37	0.17	0.20	0.35	0.39
Heritability	0.55	0.53	0.35	0.38	0.50	0.53

Genetics of Presbycusis, Table 2 *Correlations of age-adjusted pure-tone average (PTA) hearing thresholds in ears with clinical strial presbycusis phenotype or normal hearing.* The strial presbycusis phenotype demonstrated a strong familial association in the sister-sister and mother-daughter pairs. Displayed in the table are the spouse-spouse, parent-child, and sibling-sibling PTA hearing threshold correlations (Data from Gates et al. 1999)

Correlation coefficient						
	Mid-frequency PTA		High-frequency PTA		Low-frequency PTA	
Family group	Better ear	Worse ear	Better ear	Worse ear	Better ear	Worse ear
Spouse-Spouse	−0.87	−0.63	−0.76	−0.83	−0.85	−0.75
Parent-Child	0.25	0.25	0.01	0.06	0.21	0.25
Sibling-Sibling	0.32	0.38	0.25	0.27	0.35	0.36
Heritability	0.26	0.42	0.25	0.28	0.28	0.35

in the inner ear. It is currently unknown whether a mutation in Ahl1 is responsible for hearing loss in humans as well.

Human Studies

Individuals with presbycusis often report a family history of hearing loss among parents, siblings, and close relatives. Given this information, it has been presumed that presbycusis has a genetic component that influences the age of onset and severity of the loss. Documenting the role of genetics in the development of presbycusis has been difficult, and it is suggested that examination of large-population-based cohorts is a useful method for detecting the role of inheritance in presbycusis (Gates et al. 1999).

In the Framingham cohort, heritability of presbycusis phenotypes was estimated to be 0.35–0.55 (Gates et al 1999). In that study, hearing levels in genetically unrelated and genetically related individuals were measured and compared. The audiometric pure-tone thresholds at 250–8,000 Hz were obtained, and the pure tone average hearing thresholds were calculated for all frequencies in 2,311 subjects. In general, women had a lower pure-tone average threshold than men. Sensory and strial presbycusis phenotypes were analyzed (Tables 1 and 2, respectively). The sensory presbycusis phenotype showed a familial aggregation of hearing threshold levels, which were greatest for mother-daughter pairs, sister pairs, and brother pairs. The correlations for the father-child pairs were not significant, which was suggestive of extrinsic factors playing a larger role in the father's hearing loss patterns. The strial presbycusis phenotype demonstrated a strong familial association in the sister-sister and mother-daughter pairs. Overall, the heritability estimates suggest that 35–55% of the variance of the sensory presbycusis phenotype and 25–42% of the strial presbycusis phenotype are attributable to genes. The results of this study demonstrated that in a large group of biologically related people, hearing sensitivity is more similar than in a group in the same general environment, but unrelated.

In a study conducted in Sydney, Australia, the association between the magnitude of hearing loss

Genetics of Presbycusis, Table 3 *Prevalence and odds of hearing loss in subjects with and without a family history of hearing loss.* After adjusting for known risk factors, a positive family history was shown to be statistically significantly associated with hearing loss. The findings support a strong association between family history and presbycusis, with the association seemingly stronger the more severe the hearing loss (Data from McMahon et al. 2008)

	Age-standardized percentage with hearing loss (%)	Multivariate-adjusted odds ratio (95% confidence interval)	Significance (P)
Any hearing loss			<0.0001
No family history	27.9	1.0 (referent)	
Any family history	34.1	1.68 (1.38–2.05)	
Mild hearing loss			0.0006
No family history	20.0	1.0 (referent)	
Any family history	21.4	1.46 (1.18–1.82)	
Moderate-to-severe hearing loss			0.0001
No family history	7.8	1.0 (referent)	
Any family history	12.7	2.40 (1.76–3.28)	

and self-report family history after adjusting for age, sex, industrial exposure, smoking, and diabetes was obtained. Pure-tone audiometry was performed and a forced choice questionnaire to assess family history of hearing loss was distributed to an aged population of 50 years or older (McMahon et al. 2008). The prevalence of hearing loss among this population was 33%, with 68.2% classified as mild and 31.8% classified as moderate-to-severe. Of the 2,669 subjects, 46.7% gave a family history of hearing loss. Participants reporting a family history of hearing loss were significantly slightly younger than those who reported no family history. Participants with increased severity of hearing loss were also more likely to report a family history of hearing loss among parents or siblings. After adjusting for known risk factors (age, sex, history of noise exposure, diabetes, smoking) a positive family history was shown to be statistically significantly associated with hearing loss. This association was true regardless of whether the loss was reported in the mother, father, or siblings. The findings from this study support a strong association between family history and presbycusis, with the association seemingly stronger the more severe the hearing loss (Table 3). In addition, a strong association between a positive maternal family history and moderate-to-severe hearing loss in women as well as between a positive paternal family history and moderate-to-severe hearing loss in men was observed.

In 2001, a study of Danish twins focusing on the relative importance of genetic and environmental factors in self-reported reduced hearing among an older population was published (Christensen et al. 2001). Both monozygotic and dizygotic twins were included. Monozygotic twins have identical genotypes and dizygotic twins share half their genes. In 1995, twins aged 75 or greater were identified from the Danish Twin Registry. Interviews were conducted among 2,401 individuals. In 1997 and 1999, follow-up interviews took place and at the end of the study a total of 3,928 twins of age 70 or greater had been interviewed. The questions that were posed included "Do you have reduced hearing?" (yes/no) and "Do you have a hearing aid?" (yes/no). The similarity in hearing outcomes was measured using proband-wise concordance rates, odds ratios, and correlations for reduced hearing. The proband-wise concordance rate reflected the probability of disease for one twin given that the partner is affected. The odds ratio can be interpreted as the increased risk of reduced hearing for one twin given the presence versus the absence of reduced hearing in the partner twin. Data analysis showed the statistics to be higher in the monozygotic twin pairs than in the dizygotic twin pairs, indicating a heritable effect. The heritability was estimated to be 40%.

Genetic Factors

To aid in the identification of genetic factors important in human presbycusis, there are two major approaches for gene identification: linkage studies and association studies. Linkage studies are a family-based approach which investigate the co-segregation of the disease and an allele of a genetic marker at a specific locus. An association study investigates the co-occurrence of a disease and an allele of a genetic marker (Van Eyken et al. 2007). Both study types analyze genetic markers, or variants within the genome. Microsatellite markers and single nucleotide polymorphisms (SNPs) are the frequently used variants. SNPs are genetic variants that occur frequently in the human genome and are thought to be responsible for the variation seen between individuals. Some are also considered causative for complex disorders. Linkage studies require a large collection of families, which can be difficult when researching a late-onset disease such as presbycusis, as many of the parents of the subjects are deceased. In association studies, the disease is described as a dichotomous trait, where a specific SNP allele confers susceptibility to the disease and occurs more often in affected individuals. Currently association studies are performed on candidate genes, which are genes selected based on the biological and physiological properties and the biochemical pathways in which they act.

Using the Framingham Heart Study population, DeStefano and colleagues evaluated the genetic linkage between measures from audiometric examinations and markers from a genome-wide scan (Destefano et al. 2003). Subjects were excluded if they had chronic ear infections, sudden deafness, Meniere's disease, or any known non-presbycusic conditions. Pure-tone averages were used as a quantitative measure of hearing, and a genome-wide scan was conducted to identify genes that affect age-related hearing loss. The scan identified multiple chromosomal locations with evidence of linkage to presbycusis, with some of these locations corresponding with genes implicated in congenital deafness. Genetic linkage was measured by the logarithm of odds (LOD) score. LOD scores greater than 3.6 have been shown to be significant and scores from 2.2 to 3.6 suggest evidence of linkage. The analysis revealed three distinct regions on chromosome 11 (2, 79, 143 cM), as well as a region on chromosomes 10 (171 cM), 14 (126 cM), and 18 (116 cM) that showed evidence of linkage. Several of the locations that were identified contain genes that are known to cause congenital forms of deafness. This suggests that congenital and age-related hearing loss may share common genes. The LOD scores in this study were suggestive, but did not reach significance.

A linkage analysis for presbycusis was also performed using members of the National Academy of Sciences–National Research Council (NAS–NRC) twin panel (Garringer et al. 2006). The subjects completed an eight-question survey (Q8) and provided a blood sample for DNA analysis in a study of genes related to healthy aging. Concordance for hearing loss among the twins was considered if both answered yes to the question: "Do you have hearing loss?" LOD scores were computed. Among this study population an LOD score of 2.5 for hearing loss was observed at chromosome 3 for the 50 affected sibling pairs. This suggests an increased allele sharing at this marker region, which is mapped to the DFNA18 locus. Finally, using the same analytical method as the Danish Twin study, hearing loss based on the Q8 survey responses demonstrated a heritability of 61%.

Mitochondrial Contribution

Mitochondria are essential organelles within which intracellular energy production takes place. They produce energy through oxidative phosphorylation and store energy in the form of adenosine triphosphate. Unlike other organelles, mitochondria contain their own DNA which is maternally inherited and is distinct from nuclear DNA. Mitochondrial DNA (mDNA) contains no introns; thus, expression of the entire genome is vital for normal mitochondrial function. Each cell contains thousands of copies of mDNA, which encodes 13 proteins essential for oxidative phosphorylation as well as 22 transfer RNAs and two ribosomal RNAs.

Mutations in mDNA accumulate over time due to replication errors and oxidative damage. The proximity of mDNA to the oxidative phosphorylation process (which yields reactive oxygen species) makes it especially susceptible to oxidative damage. Given the large number of copies of mDNA in each cell, a certain number of mutations may be tolerated without compromising function; however, when the number of mutated copies exceeds a threshold level, the phenotype expressed by the cell shifts from that of normal function to one of aging through cell dysfunction and death. The tissues that are most susceptible to dysfunction due to mDNA mutation are those with the highest energy demand. The cochlea is highly metabolically active and thus vulnerable to the effects of mDNA damage. The mutation most commonly associated with aging is a 4,977 base pair deletion known as the Common Deletion (CD). This deletion involves an area of the mitochondrial genome that encodes for cytochrome c oxidase, an essential protein in oxidative phosphorylation. The CD can be found in high levels in diseases such as Kearns-Sayre Syndrome, Chronic Progressive External Ophthalmoplegia, and Pearson Syndrome. Several studies have been performed quantifying the CD in relation to presbycusis (see Markaryan et al. 2009, for references).

In 1997, Bai and colleagues used PCR technique to evaluate for the presence of the CD in mDNA from temporal bones. They determined that the deletion was found in a higher frequency in temporal bones from individuals known to have been affected by presbycusis compared to those unaffected. Markaryan et al. (2009) also completed a PCR study aimed at quantifying the CD in age-matched temporal bones of those with and without presbycusis. They found that with increasing age, the quantity of the CD increased and that at 8,000 Hz the amount of the CD directly and significantly correlated with the severity of hearing loss.

The CD is not the only recognized mutation in mDNA. Mutations can be acquired in the form of deletions, point mutations, and duplications. In 2008, in an attempt to elicit additional mutations possibly contributing to the development of presbycusis, Markaryan and colleagues evaluated the mitochondrial genome of two temporal bones affected by presbycusis and two of those not affected. In addition to the CD, three novel deletions were identified, each of which involved an area of the genome that encodes for cytochrome c oxidase. A correlation between these novel deletions and presbycusis was not found, but the authors theorized that these deletions may contribute to pushing a cell's mitochondrial genome above threshold such that mitochondrial dysfunction is ensued and tissue aging is expressed.

In summary, mitochondrial function is essential for highly metabolic tissues such as the cochlea. Mutations in the mitochondrial genome accumulate with age and once they reach a threshold level, oxidative phosphorylation and tissue function are compromised. The current literature supports the hypothesis that mDNA mutations likely play a role in the development of some types of presbycusis.

Future Directions

Gene therapeutic studies hold promise. Izumikawa et al. showed that the introduction of the developmental gene Math1 resulted in the recovery of hearing abilities of mature deaf mice (Izumikawa et al. 2005). Similar approaches in the aged organism may successfully address genes targeted in presbycusis, be they inherited or acquired mutations.

Conclusion

The contribution of genetics to age-related hearing loss has been difficult to quantify because of the inability to separate genetic factors from environmental factors. Murine research, large-population-based cohort studies, and gene studies using linkage and association analysis have led to estimations of heritability and have identified several genetic foci which are thought to contribute. Additionally, research has demonstrated a potential role of mDNA mutations in the development of presbycusis. With the identification of specific genetic factors, gene therapy is a potentially promising treatment for presbycusis. In addition, patients with a family history of presbycusis can take preventive measures from a young age to help avoid or delay the development of age-related hearing loss.

References

Christensen K, Frederiksen H, Hoffman HJ (2001) Genetic and environmental influences on self-reported reduced hearing in the old and oldest old. J Am Geriatr Soc 49:1512–1517

Destefano AL, Gates GA, Heard-Costa N et al (2003) Genomewide linkage analysis to presbycusis in the Framingham Heart Study. Arch Otolaryngol Head Neck Surg 129:285–289

Erway LC, Willot JF, Archer JR, Harrison DE (1993) Genetics of age-related hearing loss in mice: I. Inbred and F1 hybrid strains. Hear Res 65:125–132

Garringer HJ, Pankratz ND, Nichols WC et al (2006) Hearing impairment susceptibility in elderly men and the DFNA18 locus. Arch Otolaryngol Head Neck Surg 132:506–510

Gates GA, Couropmitree NN, Myers RH (1999) Genetic associations in age-related hearing thresholds. Arch Otolaryngol Head Neck Surg 125:654–659

Izumikawa M, Minoda R, Kawamoto K et al (2005) Auditory hair cell replacement and hearing improvement by Atoh1 gene therapy in deaf mammals. Nat Med 11:271–276

Johnson KR, Erway LC, Cook SA, Willot JF, Zheng QY (1997) A major gene affecting age-related hearing loss in C57BL/6 J mice. Hear Res 114:83–92

Markaryan A, Nelson E, Hinojosa R (2009) Quantification of the mitochondrial DNA common deletion in presbycusis. Laryngoscope 119:1184–1189

McMahon CM, KiXey A, Rochtchina E et al (2008) The contribution of family history to hearing loss in an older population. Ear Hear 29:578–584

Noben-Trauth K, Zheng QY, Johnson KR (2003) Association of cadherin 23 with polygenic inheritance and genetic modification of sensorineural hearing loss. Nat Genet 35:21–23

Van Eyken E, Van Camp G, Van Laer L (2007) The complexity of age-related hearing impairment: contributing environmental and genetic factors. Audiol Neurotol 12:345–358

Glomus Jugulare

▶ Tumors of Jugular Foramen

Glomus Tumor

Brian C. Gartrell and Samuel P. Gubbels
Department of Surgery, Division of Otolaryngology, University of Wisconsin Hospital and Clinics, Madison, WI, USA

Synonyms

Paraganglioma

Definition

Neoplastic lesions derived from cells of neural crest origin that represent the most common benign tumors of the middle ear (glomus tympanicum) and the jugular foramen (glomus jugulare).

Cross-References

▶ Benign Neoplasia, Paragangliomas-Glomus Jugulare
▶ Benign Neoplasia, Paragangliomas-Glomus Tympanicum

▶ Benign Neoplasia, Paragangliomas-Glomus Vagale
▶ Imaging for Parapharyngeal Space Tumors, Poststyloid Parapharyngeal Space Paraganglioma
▶ Magnetic Resonance Imaging, Paraganglioma of the Skull Base
▶ Paragangliomas
▶ Primary Neck Neoplasms
▶ Skull Base Neoplasms
▶ Surgical Approaches and Anatomy of the Lateral Skull Base
▶ Vascular Anomalies of Head and Neck

Glomus Tumor (Glomus Jugulare, Glomus Tympanicum, Glomus Vagale)

▶ Osteoradionecrosis of Skull Base (Benign Neoplasia-Paragangliomas)

Glottic Web

▶ Adult Glottic Stenosis

Glue Ear

▶ Chronic Otitis Media
▶ Otitis Media with Effusion

Goldenhar Syndrome

▶ Congenital Craniofacial Malformations and Their Surgical Treatment
▶ Hemifacial Microsomia

Goldenhar-Gorlin Syndrome

▶ Hemifacial Microsomia

Gradenigo's Syndrome

▶ Petrous Apicectomy

Granulomatous Diseases of Head and Neck in Adults

Alexis Jackman Hope[1], Caitlin P. McMullen[1] and Kenneth Bagwell[2]
[1]Department of Otorhinolaryngology, Albert Einstein College of Medicine/Montefiore Medical Center, Bronx, NY, USA
[2]Albert Einstein College of Medicine, Bronx, NY, USA

Synonyms

Allergic granulomatosis with angitis; Granulomatosis with polyangiitis

Definition

Granulomatous diseases are a diverse group of pathologies that share a common finding of granulomatous inflammation. The pathologic hallmark is a granuloma, which is a focal area of macrophages that can fuse to form multinucleated giant cells. This tight collection of cells is often described as appearing microscopically similar to epithelial cells and therefore, the term epithelioid is often used to describe these macrophages. The inflammatory background of these epithelioid macrophages varies depending upon the specific etiology of the disease and can include cells such as lymphocytes, neutrophils, eosinophils, and fibroblasts.

A wide variety of diseases are known to cause granulomatous inflammation in the head and neck, and they are often broadly categorized into infectious and noninfectious etiologies. Infectious etiologies include various bacterial and mycotic organisms, such as syphilis and histoplasmosis. The noninfectious etiologies include a wider variety such as idiopathic, immunologic, and foreign body-type reactions. This chapter will discuss the presentation, diagnosis, and management of commonly encountered granulomatous diseases of the head and neck.

Noninfectious Etiologies

Sarcoidosis

Sarcoidosis is a granulomatous disease of unknown etiology that affects multiple organ systems. While the exact immunopathogenesis of sarcoidosis remains elusive, the accumulation of inflammatory cells and granuloma formation are thought to be the result of an exaggerated Th-1 cell-mediated immune response to an unidentified antigen. The incidence of sarcoidosis is variable globally. There is a relatively high prevalence in Nordic countries, such as Sweden. However, sarcoidosis occurs in approximately 20 of 100,000 people in the United States. This rate is significantly higher in African-Americans with this population commonly developing more severe disease. The highest-risk population in the USA appears to be African-American women ages 30–39, which has an annual incidence of 107 per 100,000 (Rybicki et al. 1997). Particular polymorphisms within the cytokine TNF-alpha and ACE genes have been linked with higher risk and increased severity of disease (Medica et al. 2007).

Symptomatically, many diseases may mimic sarcoidosis. Therefore, a complete history and physical are critical in the evaluation of suspected patients. The respiratory system is most commonly involved, but multiple organ systems may be affected. Constitutional symptoms may include fatigue, weight loss, low-grade fever, and night sweats. Other symptoms are organ specific, such as dyspnea and dry cough in patients with respiratory involvement. Erythema nodosum and lupus pernio are common cutaneous lesions, and joint symptoms such as joint pain are common musculoskeletal complaints (Rybicki et al. 1997).

Sarcoidosis of the head and neck can afflict essentially any structure in the region. Structures most often involved are the cervical lymphatics, skin, and salivary glands (Fig. 1). Ocular, laryngeal, and otologic sarcoidosis has been described, in addition to disease of the nose and paranasal sinuses. Approximately one-third of patients develop ocular disease. Chronic uveitis is the most common manifestation, but all anatomic aspects of the eye may be affected, including the eyelids, ocular nerve, and lacrimal glands.

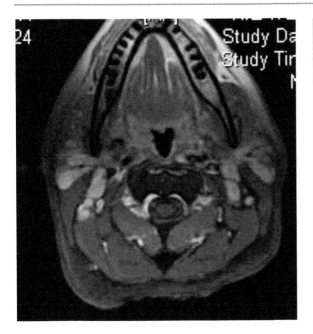

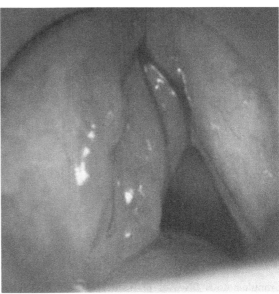

Granulomatous Diseases of Head and Neck in Adults, Fig. 1 Axial post contrast fat-suppressed T1 MR of the neck in a patient with sarcoidosis involving the cervical lymphatics and parotid glands

Granulomatous Diseases of Head and Neck in Adults, Fig. 2 Endoscopic view of laryngeal sarcoidosis

Patients may have dryness, nodules, photophobia, erythema of the eye, pain, and vision changes. Treatment of ocular sarcoidosis with topical or systemic corticosteroids is critical to prevent complications such as cataracts and glaucoma (Jones and Mochizuki 2010).

Laryngeal sarcoidosis is rare, but evaluation of the larynx is critical as this manifestation may progress to airway obstruction. A high degree of suspicion is necessary for early diagnosis. Symptoms include stridor, hoarseness, dyspnea, sleep apnea, and coughing. Most commonly, sarcoidosis affects the supraglottic larynx. Laryngoscopy may demonstrate changes such as mucosal edema, nodularity, and cobblestoning (Fig. 2). Vocal fold paralysis can occur and is typically due to compression of the left recurrent laryngeal nerve by lymphadenopathy. Nonetheless, atypical presentations such as direct vocal fold involvement and bilateral vocal fold paralysis have also been reported (Mayerof and Pitman 2010).

Involvement of the pinna, external auditory canal, middle ear, and neurootologic structures has been described. Symptoms may include cutaneous lesions of the helix, hearing loss, tinnitus, aural fullness,

dizziness, and otalgia. The presentation and course of sarcoidosis-related hearing loss are extremely variable (Shah et al. 1997).

Paranasal sinus sarcoidosis is rare. However, rhinologic sarcoidosis is almost always symptomatic. Patients may present with headache, facial pain, anosmia, obstruction, epistaxis, crusting, and chronic infection. Endoscopic exam of the nasal cavity may demonstrate erythema, edema, nodular mucosa, crusting, polyps, friability, hypertrophied mucosa, synechiae, and septal perforations. The most common sites of involvement are the septum and inferior turbinates. The submucosal nodules typically observed in the initial stage of the disease represent the macroscopic manifestation of the granuloma (Fig. 3). As the disease progresses, submucosal glands are progressively replaced by granuloma and fibrosis, resulting in the decreased production of secretions and nasal crusting.

The diagnosis of rhinogenic sarcoidosis can be difficult as the signs and symptoms are nonspecific. deShazo et al. proposed a set of diagnostic criteria to aid in its diagnosis. Accordingly, the patient should demonstrate (1) radiologic evidence of sinusitis, (2) sinus tissue demonstrating noncaseating granuloma with negative staining for fungus and acid-fast bacilli, (3) negative serology for similarly presenting diseases such as syphilis and Wegener's, and (4) no

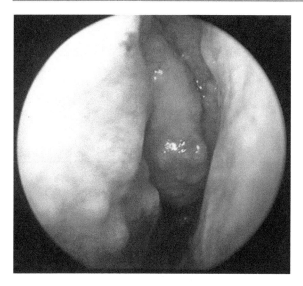

Granulomatous Diseases of Head and Neck in Adults,
Fig. 3 Endoscopic view of nasal sarcoidosis

evidence of other granulomatous disease processes of the nose and paranasal sinuses. Although widespread acceptance of these criteria has not been adopted, the fulfillment of these criteria may guide the physician's evaluation of patients with suspected sinonasal sarcoidosis.

Radiological findings of paranasal sarcoidosis are variable and nonspecific. Computed tomography (CT) and magnetic resonance imaging (MRI) may demonstrate partial or complete opacification of the sinuses, sinonasal masses, mucosal nodularities, thickening of the turbinates, and destruction of nasal cartilage and bone (Knight et al. 2006). If systemic disease is suspected, adjunctive imaging of other organ systems may be useful in diagnosis. Classically, imaging of the chest demonstrates bilateral hilar adenopathy and parenchymal infiltrates.

Laboratory studies can contribute to the evaluation of patients with suspected sarcoidosis, help exclude other diseases that have similar clinical presentations, and manage those with known disease. A full panel of studies, including antineutrophil cytoplasmic antibodies (ANCA), erythrocyte sedimentation rate (ESR), antinuclear antibodies (ANA), rapid plasma regain (RPR), and angiotensin I-converting enzyme (ACE), should be performed. Tuberculosis should be ruled out with purified protein derivative (PPD) and cultures. ANA levels are elevated in approximately 30% of patients, and serum ACE level is elevated in 60–80%. Although the rates of false positives of these tests limit their diagnostic utility, ACE levels can be helpful in monitoring disease activity and response to therapy (Shah et al. 1997).

Histopathologic analysis is a key component in making the diagnosis of sarcoidosis. Tissue specimens characteristically demonstrate multiple noncaseating granulomas, hyaline fibrosis, multinucleated giant cells, and leukocyte infiltration (Fig. 4). The granulomas are composed of mature mononuclear cells in organized collections. They may be found surrounded by plasma cells as well as various other inflammatory cells.

Multiple treatment modalities exist in the management of sarcoidosis of the head and neck. In the case of laryngeal involvement, treatment may involve systemic corticosteroids or other immunomodulating medications such as methotrexate, azathioprine, and etanercept and/or local therapies such as steroid injections and laser ablation. Mild, limited rhinologic disease may respond to topical corticosteroids and saline irrigation, but more often paranasal sinus disease requires systemic therapy. The role of endoscopic sinus surgery in the management of paranasal sinus disease is limited as the short-term results of improved quality of life and decreased steroid requirements have not been shown to persist over time.

The prognosis of sarcoidosis is generally good. Most patients have a benign course, and in up to 70%, the disease resolves spontaneously. Mortality from this disease has been shown to be less than 3%. Complications of pulmonary and cardiac involvement are the most common causes of sarcoidosis-related mortality (Shah et al. 1997).

Granulomatosis with Polyangiitis (Wegener's Granulomatosis)

Granulomatosis with polyangiitis (GPA), formerly known as Wegener's granulomatosis, is a rare autoimmune disease characterized by antineutrophil cytoplasmic antibody (ANCA)-associated necrotizing vasculitis of small- and medium-sized vessels and granulomatous inflammation. The exact etiology of GPA remains unknown. However, recent studies have demonstrated that tissue injury in GPA results from the interaction of a specific IgG-class ANCA directed at the enzyme proteinase 3 (PR3). Subsequent activation of the inflammatory cascade by these antibodies against monocytes and neutrophils has been

Granulomatous Diseases of Head and Neck in Adults, Fig. 4 Low and high powered views of histological section of sarcoidosis involving the inferior turbinate

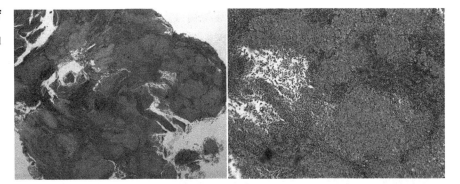

shown to be directly related to the development of focal necrotizing perivascular lesions with marked accumulation of lymphocytes and macrophages typical of granulomas.

Several studies have suggested a rising incidence of GPA. A recent large population-based study in Sweden reported a mean increase in incidence from 3.3 per million in 1975–1984 to 7.7 in 1985–1990 and 11.9 in 1991–2001(Knight et al. 2006). Although advances in laboratory testing have likely contributed to the rising incidence, other factors such as increased physician awareness and recognition of more limited forms of disease may also be playing a role.

Typically, patients with GPA present with vague symptoms such as fever, malaise, and weight loss before organ-specific symptoms become apparent. The most commonly affected organs are the upper and lower respiratory tracts and the kidneys. Renal disease manifests as glomerulonephritis. Pulmonary disease may present with cough, dyspnea, wheezing, hemoptysis, and pleuritic chest pain. Any organ system can be involved, and the disease may be limited to one site for many months or years before disseminating.

Otorhinolaryngologic findings are common in GPA and, in a case series of 199 patients with GPA, the initial site of presentation was within the head and neck in 63% of patients. Sinonasal findings include nasal cavity crusting, purulent and bloody rhinorrhea, septal perforation, and saddle nose deformities (Fig. 5). Orbital masses are another common head and neck manifestations of GPA. They occur in 15–40% of patients, and symptoms include proptosis, facial swelling, double vision, and loss of vision (Srouji et al. 2007). Otologic manifestations of GPA, such as otitis media, are common and are often the result of granuloma formation in the middle ear, Eustachian tube, and nasopharynx. In a recent study of hearing loss in GPA,

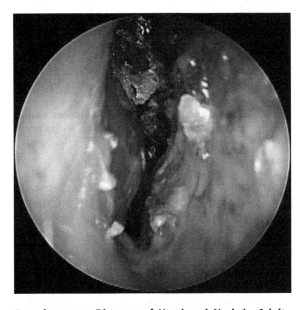

Granulomatous Diseases of Head and Neck in Adults, Fig. 5 Endoscopic view of nasal granulomatosis with polyangitis (Wegener's granulomatosis)

56% of patients were found to have hearing impairment, which included varying degrees of conductive, sensorineural, and mixed hearing loss (Bakthavachalam et al. 2004). Laryngeal and tracheal diseases, such as subglottic and tracheal stenosis, are less common but can be fatal. Initially, airway lesions are characterized by a friable and/or ulcerated mucosa that is eventually replaced by fibrotic scar tissue during resolution of active disease (Fig. 6).

In 1990, the American College of Rheumatology proposed a classification system for Wegener's granulomatosis. This system includes oral ulcers or nasal discharge, radiographic findings of infiltrates or cavitary lesions on chest radiographs, abnormal urinary sediment with red blood cell casts or more than

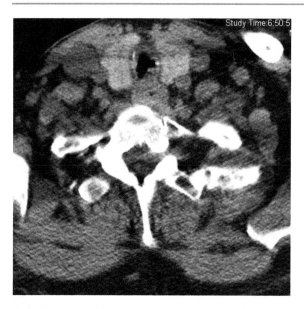

Granulomatous Diseases of Head and Neck in Adults,
Fig. 6 Axial CT scan of a patient with granulomatosis with
polyangitis (Wegener's granulomatosis) involving the trachea

five red blood cells per high power field, and granulomatous inflammation on biopsy (Leavitt et al. 1990).
Although the classification system is helpful in understanding GPA, no specific diagnostic criteria has been
developed. Therefore, the diagnosis is made using
clinical suspicion together with radiographic, laboratory, and pathologic findings.

In the evaluation of a patient with suspected GPA, it
is important to distinguish this disease entity from
similar diseases in the differential diagnosis. These
include sarcoidosis, Churg-Strauss syndrome, syphilis,
extranodal NK/T cell lymphoma (formerly known as
lethal midline granuloma), and cocaine-induced midline destructive lesions. Additionally, it is important to
recognize nonotolaryngologic manifestations that may
cause irreversible organ damage or be life threatening.
In many patients, a multidisciplinary approach is
warranted.

Laboratory testing is critical in the evaluation of
patients with suspected GPA. In particular, serologic
testing for c-ANCA plays an important role in the
diagnosis of GPA, and a combination of sensitive or
specific tests are used to detect its presence. Initially,
an indirect immunofluorescence assay, a particularly
sensitive test, is performed to demonstrate the
cytoplasmic staining pattern (c-ANCA) typical of
GPA. This is followed by a more specific test, the

enzyme-linked immunosorbent assay (ELISA), to
further identify c-ANCA. In GPA, the target antigens
of the autoantibodies are proteinase 3 (PR3) and
myeloperoxidase (MPO). Both of these antigens are
present in the azurophilic granules of neutrophils and
the peroxidase-positive lysosomes of monocytes. Of
the two antigens, PR3 is more closely associated with
the diagnosis of GPA and is present in 80–90% of
ANCA-positive patients with GPA.

ANCA sensitivity and specificity are difficult to
measure as testing is not standardized. Additionally,
the sensitivity of ANCA-PR3 varies in GPA with the
activity and extent of disease. A wide range of both
sensitivity and specificity of ANCA testing has been
reported. In a large meta-analysis of the clinical utility
of ANCA testing in the diagnosis of GPA, the sensitivity
ranged from 34% to 92% and specificity ranged from
88% to 100%, with a pooled sensitivity of 66% (95%
CI) and specificity of 98% (97–99%) (Rao et al. 1995).
In more limited forms and inactive disease, the sensitivity of ANCA testing is decreased. False-positive
ANCA testing may occur in the presence of other systemic autoimmune diseases, drug-induced vasculitis,
inflammatory bowel disease, and bacterial endocarditis
as well as other infections. ANCA testing may also be
positive in Churg-Strauss syndrome and cocaine-
induced vasculitis. However, in CSS, ANCA testing is
more likely to be directed at myeloperoxidase, whereas
in cocaine-induced vasculitis, it is directed at human
neutrophil elastase.

Additional laboratory testing in the workup of GPA
includes a complete blood count, basic metabolic tests,
and urine analysis, which are helpful to identify hematologic, renal, and metabolic abnormalities. Hematologic abnormalities in GPA include a normochromic,
normocytic anemia, leukocytosis, thrombocytosis, and
elevated erythrocyte sedimentation rate. The presence
of markedly elevated peripheral blood eosinophils,
particularly in the setting of nasal polyposis, is suggestive of CSS. Laboratory signs of renal involvement in
GPA include elevated concentrations of plasma creatinine, proteinuria, and urine sediment with red and
white blood cells and casts.

Radiographic findings may also aid in the diagnosis
of GPA. Radiographic findings in patients with head and
neck involvement are often nonspecific. In the paranasal
sinuses, CT findings include mucosal thickening,
mucocele, orbital mass and bony destruction, and sclerosis. In patients presenting with limited upper

respiratory tract disease who do not have any constitutional symptoms, imaging of the chest is recommended since up to a third of patients may have asymptomatic lower respiratory disease. Pulmonary findings on imaging are highly variable and include nodules, which may be cavitary, diffuse lung and pleural opacities, atelectasis, and hilar adenopathy (Cordier et al. 1990).

Histopathologic evidence of GPA is often difficult to obtain in patients with disease limited to the upper respiratory tract. In a study of 30 specimens from 17 patients with well-documented disease, active vasculitis was seen in 41% of patients and extravascular necrosis was present in 12% of patients; samples larger than 5 mm were more likely to contain diagnostic material (Del Buono and Flint 1991). Unlike sarcoidosis, where numerous noncaseating granulomas are seen on histopathology, necrotizing granulomas are only occasionally present in GPA. In patients with systemic disease, histopathologic confirmation of GPA may need to be obtained from other sites of involvement such as the skin, lungs, or kidney. Histopathology is also important in differentiating GPA from extranodal NK/T cell lymphoma, which requires biopsies to characterize tumor morphology and to perform immunohistochemical stains and genetic studies for Epstein-Barr virus.

GPA is managed with immunosuppressive therapy, which is administered as an initial induction phase followed by maintenance therapy for a variable period of time. The goal of the initial therapy, which typically consists of cyclophosphamide and glucocorticoids, is complete remission with the absence of disease activity. In patients who have a contraindication to or refuse to take cyclophosphamide, rituximab has been shown to be as effective as cyclophosphamide in short-term studies (Stone et al. 2010). Although more commonly used in maintenance therapy, methotrexate may be an initial therapeutic option in patients with mild, limited disease without kidney involvement. For maintenance therapy, the use of the least toxic drug is desirable. This may include methotrexate, azathioprine, and/or glucocorticoids.

Churg-Strauss Syndrome (Allergic Granulomatosis and Angiitis)

Churg-Strauss syndrome (CSS), also known as allergic granulomatosis and angiitis, is a vasculitis of the small and medium vessels. This syndrome was first described in 1951 by Churg and Strauss as an angiitis featuring asthma, eosinophilia, and granulomas. The mean age of onset is variable, and no sex predominance has been clearly demonstrated. Studies in the United Kingdom have demonstrated the prevalence of this disease to be 2.7–3.4 per million, depending on the criteria used in diagnosis (Watts et al. 2000).

The natural progression of CSS proceeds in three stages. The initial prodromal phase presents with asthma, allergic rhinitis, polyposis, and recurrent rhinosinusitis. The second phase involves peripheral blood eosinophilia and eosinophilic tissue infiltrates. Systemic vasculitis occurs later in the third stage of CSS. The predominant organ systems affected include the lungs, paranasal sinuses, and skin. However, multiple organ systems can be involved. The major morbidity and mortality associated with allergic granulomatosis and angiitis arises largely from cardiovascular, gastrointestinal, and kidney disease.

History and physical exam are critical in the evaluation of patients with suspected CSS. Systemic symptoms include weight loss, fever, and fatigue, but they may also be organ specific. Pulmonary symptoms of dyspnea and cough may clinically mimic asthma. These symptoms are often quite severe and hemoptysis may also be present. Neuropathies, specifically mononeuritis multiplex, are the second most common finding. Skin findings include nodules, palpable purpura, eczema, and urticaria. Patients may also complain of migratory joint pain and joint swelling.

Despite the rarity of this disease, the majority of patients with confirmed CSS have otorhinolaryngologic manifestations. As a result, otolaryngologists should be aware of the clinical presentation and management of these patients. Unilateral or bilateral sensorineural hearing loss, conductive hearing loss, aural discharge, vertigo, tinnitus, otitis media, temporal bone involvement, and facial nerve paralysis have all been described. CSS of the nose and paranasal sinuses usually involves recurrent or chronic rhinosinusitis, allergic rhinitis, and nasal polyposis (Fig. 7). Three-quarters of patients with otolaryngologic manifestations of CSS will have polyposis, which can be severe. Further physical examination may also reveal nasal crusting.

Diagnosis of CSS can be made by clinical criteria alone, as histopathology is not necessarily pathognomonic. Lanham et al. proposed a set of criteria for its diagnosis. According to their criteria, asthma history, peripheral blood eosinophilia greater

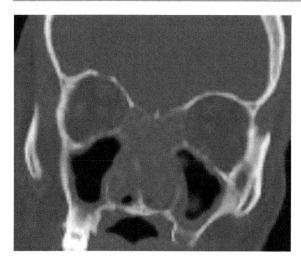

Granulomatous Diseases of Head and Neck in Adults,
Fig. 7 Coronal CT scan of patient with allergic granulomatosis
and angiitis (Churg-Strauss syndrome)

than 1,500 cells/mm^3, and systemic vasculitis affecting
at least two organ systems define the syndrome. In
1990, the American College of Rheumatology
established the following clinical criteria for the diagnosis of CSS, of which the patient should exhibit at
least four of the following: asthma history, eosinophilia greater than 10% on blood count differential,
mononeuropathy or polyneuropathy, nonfixed pulmonary infiltrates on x-ray, paranasal sinus abnormalities,
and biopsy-proven extravascular eosinophilia. These
criteria yielded a sensitivity of 85% and a specificity of
99.7% (Masi et al. 1990).

Laboratory and imaging studies are useful adjuncts
in the diagnosis of CSS. Eosinophilia will be demonstrated in the differential of a complete blood count.
Erythrocyte sedimentation rate and C-reactive protein
levels are elevated in the majority of patients.
Antineutrophil cytoplasmic antibodies (ANCA) have
been reported to occur in 40–60% of patients with
CSS. Although antibodies to both PR3 and MPO
have been detected, there is a predilection for MPO-
ANCA; this reportedly occurs in up to 70% of patients
(Sinico et al. 2005). Hepatitis serology, antinuclear
antibody, anti-double-stranded DNA antibody testing
to rule out other diseases with similar presentation
should be obtained. Chest x-ray is a useful adjunctive
study as pulmonary infiltrate is an ACR criterion for
diagnosis. Computer tomography (CT) imaging of the
nose and paranasal sinuses may demonstrate
nonspecific findings consistent with sinusitis and

nasal polyposis. If angiography is performed for symptomatic vasculitis, characteristic stenosis may be
visualized.

Biopsy of affected mucosa reveals eosinophilic and
inflammatory cell infiltrates. Histopathologic examination of nasal polyps will demonstrate eosinophilic
infiltrate and areas of necrosis. Unlike sarcoidosis,
histopathology is not pathognomonic and the diagnosis
can be made by clinical criteria alone (Masi et al.
1990).

Corticosteroids are the mainstay in the treatment of
CSS. Immunosuppressant therapy with cyclophosphamide is also used to manage patients with CSS. In
patients with polyposis and refractory rhinosinusitis,
endoscopic sinus surgery can relieve symptoms, but
recurrence of sinonasal polyps is not uncommon.
Relapse may occur early in the course of treatment or
many years later. Cardiac involvement and complications of vasculitis are the most common causes of
death in CSS.

Cholesterol Granuloma

Cholesterol granulomas are expansile cystic lesions
containing   intramucosal   cholesterol   crystals
surrounded by giant and chronic inflammatory cells
within a fibrous capsule. These rare lesions have been
found originating in the paranasal sinuses and the
petrous apex of the temporal bone. The etiology of
these lesions was once thought to be caused by
impaired sinus ventilation; however, recent studies
suggest that aggressive pneumatization of the petrous
apex during adolescence leads to coaptation of bone
marrow and mucosa, causing hemorrhage into the apical air cells (Jackler and Cho 2003). Symptoms of
cholesterol granuloma will depend on its location.
Compression of local structures such as adjacent cranial nerves will result in specific manifestations.
Workup should include CT and MRI studies, which
will reveal a non-contrast-enhancing, soft tissue density, expansile lesion with or without surrounding bony
erosion. High T1 and T2 signals are characteristic of
cholesterol granuloma; however, areas of low signal
may be observed when hemosiderin deposition is
present (Fig. 8). Histopathology is necessary for diagnosis, and tissue biopsy will reveal cholesterol clefts
surrounded by fibrous granulation tissue with foreign
body giant cells and hemosiderin-laden macrophages.
Treatment depends on symptomatology and location.
In relatively asymptomatic patients, regular follow-up

Granulomatous Diseases of Head and Neck in Adults, Fig. 8 (a) Nasal endoscopy of patient who presented with a right nasal mass who was diagnosed with cholesterol granuloma. (b) T1 and T2 MR of the same patient, with the lesion involvement the right sphenoid sinus and ipsilateral petrous apex

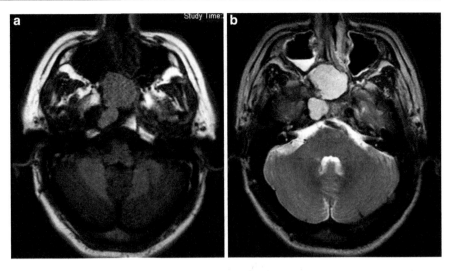

and serial imaging are appropriate; however, surgical treatment may become necessary.

Infectious Etiologies

Bacterial

Syphilis

Syphilis, caused by the spirochete *Treponema pallidum*, is clinically divided into three stages, all of which, although rare, can affect nearly all structures in the head and neck. Infection can be either congenital, from passage of spirochetes across the placenta, or acquired. The chancre of acquired primary syphilis has been reported in various locations throughout the upper respiratory tract, such as in the nasal cavity, middle ear, tonsil, and larynx. Sinonasal symptoms of secondary syphilis include rhinitis with thick discharge and irritation of the anterior nares, while the gummatous lesions of tertiary syphilis often involve and erode the nasal septum, resulting in saddle nose deformity. Congenital syphilis is often remembered for the rash it causes; however, nasal discharge can occur 1–2 weeks prior to the appearance of the rash. The nasal discharge contains infectious spirochetes in high concentrations. Diagnosis of syphilis relies on serologic tests, and parenteral penicillin G is the treatment of choice.

Mycobacterial

Mycobacterial infections of the head and neck can be categorized into tubercular and nontubercular. The most common site of involvement is the cervical lymph nodes, but disease has been reported to occur in almost all structures in the head and neck such as the salivary glands, oral cavity, and paranasal sinuses. Patients may report a history of tuberculosis and treatment, past positive PPD, or exposure to infected individuals. Constitutional symptoms are present only in a minority of patients; therefore, localizing symptoms should direct appropriate diagnostic testing such as tissue biopsy and culture. For example, the most common symptom of nasal tuberculosis is nasal obstruction, and other symptoms include nasal crusting, epistaxis, and rhinorrhea. Chest radiography may or may not reveal active disease or evidence of prior disease. Findings on nasal endoscopy can include granulomatous tissue proliferation, ulceration, and reddish nodularity. Tissue biopsy, necessary for diagnosis, will reveal the typical picture of caseating granulomas with or without evidence of AFB on staining or culture; the use of PCR for detection is becoming more commonplace in aiding the diagnosis. Nevertheless, positive response to 6–12-months of multidrug antituberculous chemotherapy may eventually be the only indication of final diagnosis.

Nontubercular disease caused by other *Mycobacterial* species has been reported. Some species described include *Mycobacterium avium-intracellulare, chelonae, marinum,* and *kansasii.* Manifestations depend upon the area of involvement and are often similar to tuberculous infections. Depending on the species, certain aspects of the history may be helpful; for example, *Mycobacterium marinum* is associated with close exposure to fish or contaminated water.

Biopsy is usually required for diagnosis, and the choice of antimycobacterial agents for treatment will vary with species' sensitivities.

Mycobacterium leprae has various manifestations depending upon the host immune response. In the case of lepromatous leprosy, symptoms of infection include nasal obstruction and discharge, epistaxis, nasal deformity, and anosmia. This infection is clinically divided into three stages. In the early stage, the nasal mucosa may appear dry, pale, and yellowish with scattered granulomas. During the intermediate stage, the mucosa becomes thickened and produces mucoid purulent or bloody secretions teeming with AFB. In the late stage, the mucosa becomes dry and encrusted and destruction of the septal cartilage and inferior turbinates will be apparent. Treatment with antimycobacterial agents is appropriate once the diagnosis is made.

Rhinoscleroma

Rhinoscleroma is a chronic destructive granulomatous disease cause by *Klebsiella rhinoscleromatis* that affects the upper aerodigestive tract. The nose and nasal cavity are most commonly involved, but infections of the nasopharynx, larynx, and trachea have also been reported (Tami 2005). It is endemic in Egypt, Southeast Asia, Mexico, Central and South America, and Eastern Europe. This infection usually begins at an early age and progresses through three stages: atrophic, granulomatous, and fibrotic/sclerotic. The most common symptom is nasal obstruction. Other reported symptoms include epistaxis, rhinorrhea, and chronic rhinitis. On nasal endoscopy, a mixed picture of nodular and atrophic mucosa with destruction of the nasal architecture may be observed. Diagnosis involves tissue biopsy and culture. In the early stages of the disease, tissue biopsy will reveal Mikulicz's cells and Russell's bodies. A prolonged course of antibiotics is necessary until there is no longer tissue evidence of infection.

Fungal

Histoplasmosis

Histoplasmosis capsulatum is a dimorphic fungus endemic to the Ohio and Mississippi River Valleys that usually causes asymptomatic infection of the lungs; however, infections have been known to disseminate, with the majority of these occurring in immunocompromised hosts. Hematogenously disseminated infections can spread throughout the head and neck. Presenting symptoms are largely dependent upon the location of the infection. In the oral cavity and along the respiratory tract, findings can range from indurated ulcers to proliferative lesions. In the nose and paranasal sinuses, symptoms include nasal obstruction, pain, and cutaneous sores with destruction of the nares. On intranasal examination, ulcerative lesions with crusting may be observed and can involve any portion of the nasal cavity; severe infections result in destruction of the nasal architecture. Diagnosis can be made with incisional biopsy and fungal staining, which will show the *H. capsulatum* yeast forms along with noncaseating granulomas. Once diagnosed, appropriate therapy with itraconazole can be initiated; amphotericin is reserved for more severe destructive disease.

Cryptococcus

Cryptococcus neoformans is an encapsulated, opportunistic fungal organism that can infect the paranasal sinuses in HIV-positive patients. Nevertheless, cryptococcal infections has been reported throughout the upper respiratory tract as well as in the salivary glands. *C. neoformans* sinusitis typically presents in late-stage HIV infection when patients have impaired immunity, but symptomatology may be similar to the immunocompetent host. However, these patients are at higher risk for multiple sinus involvement and extension beyond the paranasal sinuses. Methods of diagnosis include culture, biopsy, and PCR for detection of the cyptococcal antigen.

Coccidioidomycosis

Coccidioidomycosis is a disease caused by the dimorphic fungus *Coccidioides immitis* that has been most commonly associated with the southwestern United States, often specifically cited in the San Joaquin Valley of California. Certain demographic groups are at higher risk for developing this disease, including the very young and elderly and the immunocompromised. While the majority of infected individuals are asymptomatic, many present with flu-like illness. Disseminated coccidioidomycosis is a known complication, and cutaneous involvement such as granulomatous plaques is often present. Other presentations in the head and neck include neck mass and laryngeal and sinonasal granulomas. Diagnosis relies on tissue biopsy, which will reveal *C. immitis* endospores surrounded by a granulomatous reaction. Serologic studies will be positive in 75% of patients with IgM antibodies present in the first 1–3 weeks and IgG antibodies thereafter until the disease abates (Arnold et al. 2004). The majority of cases resolve without treatment; however, itraconazole and fluconazole can be used for prolonged disease; amphotericin is typically reserved for severe disease.

Aspergillus

Aspergillus, a fungal genus, is the most common cause of fungal sinusitis, and the species *Aspergillus flavus* is associated with a particular type of fungal sinusitis known as granulomatous invasive fungal sinusitis (GIFS). The classification schema of fungal sinusitis has undergone many changes throughout its documented history; chronic invasive forms are further subdivided into granulomatous and nongranulomatous based upon histopathology, yet the clinical presentations of the two types tend to be similar. Unlike in other forms of invasive fungal sinusitis due to other fungal species, these patients are typically immunocompetent. Reports of this disease are primarily from Sudan; however, there are case reports from other countries in diverse geographical areas such as India, Pakistan, and the United States. Histological findings include invasive fungal hyphae, noncaseating granulomas, and a fibrinous inflammatory infiltrate.

Granulomatous invasive fungal sinusitis tends to remain indolent until surrounding anatomic structures are involved. Presenting signs and symptoms can include proptosis, palatal erosions, chronic headache, seizures, altered mental status, and focal neurologic findings; more fatal complications have been reported, including mycotic aneurysm, internal carotid artery rupture, and cavernous sinus thrombosis. Endoscopic findings may include severe mucosal edema, polyps, and a mass lesion, which may be ulcerated. Radiologic findings may reveal mucosal thickening, focal sinus hyperattenuation, thick mucin plugs, and bony erosion (Stringer and Ryan 2000). Treatment centers on use of antifungal agents in combination with surgical debridement.

Cross-References

References

Arnold MG, Arnold JC, Bloom DC, Brewster DF, Thiringer JK (2004) Head and neck manifestations of disseminated coccidioidomycosis. Laryngoscope 114:747–752

Bakthavachalam S, Driver MA, Cox C, Spiegel JH, Grundfast KM, Merkel PA (2004) Hearing loss in Wegener's granulomatosis. Otol Neurotol 24:833–837

Cordier JF, Valeyre D, Guillevin L, Loire R, Brechot JM (1990) Pulmonary Wegener's granulomatosis, a clinical and imaging study of 77 cases. Chest 97:906–912

Del Buono EA, Flint A (1991) Diagnostic usefulness of nasal biopsy in Wegener's granulomatosis. Hum Pathol 22:107–110

Jackler RK, Cho M (2003) A new theory to explain the genesis of petrous apex cholesterol granuloma. Otol Neurotol 24:96–106

Jones N, Mochizuki M (2010) Sarcoidosis: epidemiology and clinical features. Ocul Immunol Inflamm 18:72–79

Knight A, Ekbom A, Brandt L, Askling J (2006) Increasing incidence of Wegener's granulomatosis in Sweden 1975–2001. J Rheumatol 33:2060–2063

Leavitt RY, Fauci AS, Bloch DA, Michel BA, Hunder GG, Arend WP, Calabrese LH, Fries JF, Lie JT, Lightfoot RW,

Masi AT, McShane DJ, Mills JA, Stevens MB, Wllace SL, Zvaifler NJ (1990) The American College of Rheumatology 1990 criteria for the classification of Wegener's granulomatosis. Arthritis Rheum 33:1101–1107

Masi AT, Hunder GG, Lie JT, Michel BA, Bloch DA, Arend WP, Calabrese LH, Edworthy SM, Fauci AS, Leavitt RY et al (1990) The American College of Rheumatology 1990 criteria for the classification of Churg-Strauss syndrome (allergic granulomatosis and angiitis). Arthritis Rheum 133:1094–1100

Mayerof RM, Pitman MJ (2010) Atypical and disparate presentations of laryngeal sarcoidosis. Ann Otol Rhinol Laryngol 119:667–671

Medica I, Kastrin A, Maver A, Peterlin B (2007) Role of genetic polymorphisms in ACE and TNF-alpha gene in sarcoidosis: a meta-analysis. J Hum Genet 52:836–847

Rao JK, Weinberger M, Oddone EZ, Allen NB, Landsman P, Feussner JR (1995) Role of antineutrophil cytoplasmic antibody (c-ANCA) testing in diagnosis of Wegener's granulomatosis. A literature review and meta-analysis. Ann Intern Med 123:925–932

Rybicki BA, Major M, Popovich J Jr, Maliarik MJ, Iannuzzi MC (1997) Racial differences in sarcoidosis incidence: a 5-year study in a health maintenance organization. Am J Epidemiol 145:234–241

Shah UK, White JA, Gooey JE, Hybels RC (1997) Otolaryngologic manifestations of sarcoidosis: presentation and diagnosis. Laryngoscope 107:67–75

Sinico RA, Di Toma L, Maggiore U, Bottero P, Radice A, Tosoni C, Grassseli C, Pavone L, Gregorini G, Monti S, Frassi M, Vecchio F, Corace C, Venegoni E, Buzio C (2005) Prevalence and clinical significance of antineutrophil cytoplasmic antibodies in Churg-Strauss syndrome. Arthritis Rheum 52:2926–2935

Srouji IA, Andrews P, Edwards C, Lund VJ (2007) Patterns of presentations and diagnosis in patients with Wegener's granulomatosis: ENT aspects. J Laryngol Otol 121:653–658

Stone JH, Merkel PA, Spiera R, Seo P, Langford CA, Hoffman GS, Kallenberg CGM, St Clair W, Turkiewicz A, Tchao NK, Webber L, Ding L, Sejismundo LP, Mieras K, Weitzenkamp D, Ikle D, Seyfert-Margolis V, Mueller M, Brunetta P, Allen NB, Fervenza FC, Geetha D, Keogh KA, Kissen EY, Monach PA, Peikert T, Stegeman C, Ytterberg SR, Specks U (2010) Rituximab versus cyclophosphamide for ANCA associated vasculitis. N Engl J Med 363:221–232

Stringer SP, Ryan MW (2000) Chronic invasive fungal rhinosinusitis. Otolaryngol Clin N Am 33:375–387

Tami TA (2005) Granulomatous diseases and chronic rhinosinusitis. Otolaryngol Clin N Am 38:1267–1278

Watts RA, Lane SE, Bentham G, Scott DG (2000) Epidemiology of systemic vasculitis: a ten-year study in the United Kingdom. Arthritis Rheum 43:414–419

Granulomatous Disorders

▶ Granulomatous Infections of Head and Neck in Childhood

Granulomatous Infections of Head and Neck in Childhood

Ravi C. Nayar[1] and Usha Kini[2]
[1]Department of Otolaryngology-Head and Neck Surgery, St John's Medical College Hospital, Bangalore, Karnataka, India
[2]Department of Pathology, St John's Medical College, Bangalore, Karnataka, India

Synonyms

Benign lymphoproliferative disorder; Granulomatous disorders

Definition

Granulomatous disease is caused by a tissue response, in the form of a granuloma, characterized by macrophages, epithelioid cells, and lymphocytes, in which the etiological agent is often identifiable.

Introduction

Granulomatous disease is not a term specific to a particular disease. It is instead a term describing a granulomatous response, which is a form of chronic inflammation. It is a response to a variety of stimuli, infective, noninfective, or neoplastic while, some include lymphoproliferative disorders such as Kikuchi disease, Kimura disease, etc. A further confounding factor is that both granulomatous reaction and lymphoproliferative disorders may coexist in the same patient. The coexistence of a granulomatous response with a carcinoma is also described.

These diseases present primarily as nodules, mass, or an ulcerative lesion, with symptoms secondary to the lesion, such as pressure symptoms, etc., or associated with systemic symptoms.

The classical histopathological picture of a granuloma (Fig. 1) is characterized by focal aggregates of activated macrophages having an epithelioid (epithelial-like) appearance surrounded by lymphocytes with or without necrosis. Giant cells are usually present. The etiological agent is often identifiable in the section,

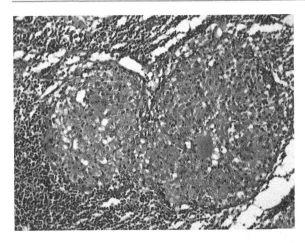

Granulomatous Infections of Head and Neck in Childhood, Fig. 1 Low power view showing a classical granuloma composed of epithelioid cells and occasional multinucleate giant cell and surrounded by lymphocytes (Hematoxylin and Eosin x 200)

though special stains may be necessary. A classical picture of a lymphoproliferative condition is characterized by sheets of atypical lymphoid cells distorting the normal lymph nodal architecture.

The pediatric otolaryngologist is primarily concerned in ruling out malignancy, and unless the index of suspicion for a specific disease is high, the histopathology often comes as a surprise. The frequency of occurrence of a particular condition may vary in different geographical areas. Nevertheless, close cooperation between the clinician and pathologist is the key to an expeditious diagnosis, and an iterative loop involving these two specialties may often result in realizing the need to review the diagnosis, especially if treatment response is poor.

Establishing a definitive diagnosis and ruling out malignancy is but the first step, as the treatment is specific and needs to be individualized to the condition identified (Barnes 2008; Mahadevia and Brandwein-Gensler 2008; Newman and Hayes-Jordan 2006; O'hare 1999).

Classification

Granulomatous lesions classified based on histopathology, etiology, and site of origin are as follows:
Infective
- Bacterial
  - Actinomycosis
  - Nocardiosis
  - Brucellosis

- Cat scratch disease
- Rhinoscleroma
- Syphilis
- Tularemia
- Mycobacterial – Tuberculosis, leprosy
- Fungal
  - Fungal granuloma
- Parasitic
  - Toxoplasmosis, leishmaniasis
- Indeterminate
  - Rhinosporidiosis

Inflammatory diseases
- Crohn's Disease
- Giant cell granuloma,
- Sarcoidosis

Vasculitic diseases
- Kawasaki's disease,
- Wegener's Granulomatosis

Miscellaneous conditions
- Eosinophilic ulcer,
- Foreign body granuloma
- Gouty granuloma,
- Malakoplakia,
- Malignancy-associated granuloma

Lymphoproliferative Disease
- Angioimmunoblastic lymphadenopathy with dysproteinemia
- Anticonvulsant-associated lymphadenopathy
- Castleman's disease
- Inflammatory pseudotumor
- Kikuchi-Fujimoto Disease
- Kimura Disease
- Langerhans cell Histiocytosis
- Pseudolymphoma
- Rosai-Dorfman Disease
- Midline Destructive Process – due to T cell lymphoma
- Lymphoproliferation secondary to immunodeficiency states such as AIDS, posttransplant, etc.
- Hodgkin's lymphoma
- Nodes draining a primary squamous cell carcinoma (In the interests of brevity, the following diseases have been singled out for description in this entry.)

Bacterial Infections:
1. Actinomycosis and Nocardia
2. Cat scratch disease
3. Syphilis
4. Mycobacterial

Inflammatory disease
5. Fungal granuloma
6. Giant cell granuloma
7. Sarcoidosis
Vasculitic Disease
8. Kawasaki's Disease
9. Wegener's Granulomatosis
Lymphoproliferative Disease
10. Castleman's Disease
11. Langerhans cell Histiocytosis
12. Rosai-Dorfman Disease

Actinomycosis

Bacteriology
Though a bacteria, the name "Actinomycosis" is derived from Greek for "Ray Fungus." It was first described by Israel in 1878 who noted sulfur granules in a case of "Lumpy jaw," hence the name of the organism "*Actinomyces israelii*." This Gram-positive anaerobic bacteria and other bacteria of the same genus are commensals of the oral cavity, which act as opportunistic pathogens.

Clinical Presentation
The commonest region involved is the cervicofacial, though the abdominal and thoracic regions may also be affected. A mandibular lump and lymphadenopathy is the most frequent presentation. However, it can present anywhere in the head and neck to include nasal cavity, temporal bone, oral cavity, larynx, cheek, and parotid gland. The clinical presentation is often mistaken for a squamous cell carcinoma.

Pathology
Cervical lymphadenopathy is common. This usually suppurates and causes multiple sinuses in the skin overlying the area with production of "sulfur granules." They are readily identified by their pattern of growth in colonies made up of dense masses of hematoxylin-stained tangled filaments that radiate outward and tend to be eosinophilic at the periphery, highlighted by silver stains giving it a cotton-wool appearance (Fig. 2a–d).

Diagnosis
The organisms should be demonstrated on FNAC from the lesion or proved invasive at histology.

Treatment
The treatment is usually both medical and surgical. The organism is sensitive to penicillin and others of the same group. However, intravenous antibiotics have to be given over a protracted period (2 or 3 weeks) and oral antibiotics for a further period of 3–6 months to affect a cure. Surgical treatment is often individualized, but incision and drainage of the neck lesion is often necessary.

Nocardiosis

Bacteriology
This is a condition similar to actinomycosis in clinical presentation, though less common and less invasive. It was described by Nocard in 1888, hence the causative organism was first named *Nocardia brasiliensis*, though others of the same genus were identified subsequently.

Clinical Presentation
This condition is more common in immunologically compromised patients, and in the healthy pediatric age group patients. It mimics actinomycosis and its clinical manifestations vary depending on the portal of entry either after a skin prick or affecting the mucous glands of the nasal, oral, or oropharyngeal region.

Pathology
The biopsy of the lesion is characterized by microabscesses and ill-defined granulomas characterized by aggregates of epithelioid cells and lymphocytes. The Gram's stain shows slender slightly beaded, branching filamentous bacilli that are Gram-positive and resembles actinomyces, but it does not form the "sulphur granules" characteristic of actinomyces. Culture of these lesions is difficult though these organisms are aerobic.

The patient, in addition, may have involvement of the lung wherein the diagnosis probably requires an open lung biopsy or the brain resulting in abscesses with capsules less developed than pyogenic abscesses.

Treatment
Treatment is with antibiotics, such as sulfonamides, trimethoprim, and long-term medication is called for.

Granulomatous Infections of Head and Neck in Childhood, Fig. 2 Colony of actinomycetes surrounded by fibroblastic stroma in (**a**) (Hematoxylin and Eosin x 200). (**b–d**) showing the colony stained positive with Periodic acid-Schiff stain (**b**) and Gomori's Methenamine Silver (**c**) and negative with Ziehl-Neelsen stain (**d**)

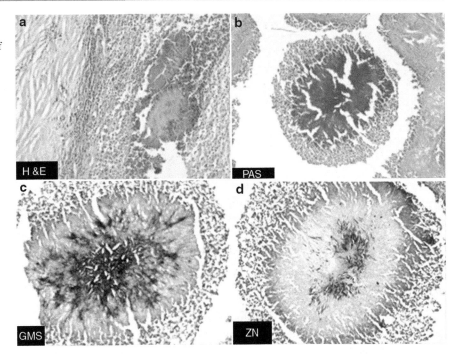

Cat Scratch Disease (CSD)

Bacteriology
A disease of immunocompetent individuals, CSD is caused by a Gram-negative bacillus (Rickettsial-like), originally called *Rochalimaea henselae* now renamed *Bartonella henselae*, an obligate intracellular organism. This is picked up by the cats paw from soil and is introduced through a breach in the skin caused by the cats scratch. Its incidence is about 9.3 per 100,000 in the USA.

It was described by Debre in 1950, but the bacteria was identified by Wear in 1988. Initially it was named Afipia felis (after the Armed Forces Institute of Pathology), but was renamed subsequently.

Clinical Presentation
The disease is directly related to contact with cats and hence the eponymous name associated with it. However, rose thorns, dogs, monkeys, fish bones, etc., have also been implicated. At the site of inoculation, an erythematous lesion develops within 3–10 days of the scratch, and progresses to vesicular and papule formation. It resolves within a week. A further month or two later, a painful regional lymphadenopathy develops, and that may be the stage at which the patient presents,

unless as is the case in up to 25%, systemic illness, such as fever, headache, myalgia, encephalitis, hepatitis, etc., develops. The disease is usually self-limiting and for lasts 6–8 weeks.

Pathology
Histopathology (Fig. 3) shows changes in the nodes, which vary with the evolution of the disease. The early stage lesions show follicular hyperplasia with significant histiocytes, while intermediate stage lesions have granulomatous changes. In the late stages, these lesions show abscesses of various sizes characterized by central, stellate necrosis with neutrophils surrounded by palisading histiocytes. The proliferating histiocytes in the sinusoids is quite characteristic.

Diagnosis
The causative bacterium can be identified with the Warthin-Starry silver stain, particularly in stage III lesions, which exhibit necrosis. The diagnosis can be confirmed by serology, immunofluorescence, and PCR.

Treatment
Treatment is supportive and symptomatic, except in cases with systemic illness, where antibiotics, such as Ciprofloxacin, Gentamicin, etc, may be indicated.

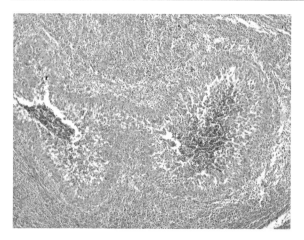

Granulomatous Infections of Head and Neck in Childhood, Fig. 3 Granulomata in Cat scratch disease showing central necrosis with neutrophils and surrounded by palisading epithelioid cells (Hematoxylin and Eosin x 200)

Incision and drainage may lead to fistula formation, hence aspiration of purulent material may be a preferred method.

Parinaud's syndrome (oculoglandular syndrome): This syndrome is an atypical presentation of CSD, and consists of conjunctivitis associated with lymphadenopathy of the parotid, submandibular, and preauricular group of nodes.

Note that in patients with acquired immunodeficiency syndrome, subcutaneous nodules with similar histology caused by the same organism (Bartonella) have been described. These are termed as bacillary angiomatosis, but are neither granulomatous or lymphoproliferative disorders.

Syphilis

Bacteriology

This sexually transmitted disease, called the "Great Pox" in the fifteenth century, is caused by *Treponema pallidum* (the term derived from Greek, means "Pale turning thread"). It may be a mutated form of *Treponema pertenue*, which is endemic to Africa, causing the disease yaws, which is spread through nonveneral contact. The disease bejel is caused by *T. endemicum* is endemic to the Middle East and Pinta caused by *T carateum* is endemic to Mexico and South America. The incidence of syphilis dropped in the 1940s consequent to the widespread use of antibiotic.

Clinical Presentation

Clinical stages, namely, primary, secondary, and tertiary and congenital forms are described.

The primary stage develops as an ulcer at the site of inoculation, within 1 week to 3 months as a "chancre." Cutaneous chancres are typically painless and hard raised lesions. Mucosal chancres are gray erosions, or nonspecific deep ulcers with a reddish base and irregular raised border. They heal within 3–6 weeks, without scarring, or leaving a thin "cigarette paper" scar and hence not often detected.

The secondary stage results from systemic dissemination. It manifests 6–8 weeks later presenting as fever and generalized rash. These rashes coalesce to form annular mucosal lesions, or hyperplastic lesions such as condyloma lata.

If untreated, these patients lapse into a latent stage characterized by cervical lymphadenopathy with a predilection for periarticular areas such as epitrochlear and inguinal.

Tertiary syphilis, which may develop after many years, is characterized by neurological illness, cardiac lesions, or gummatous lesions. These gummatous lesions may mimic Wegener's granulomatosis in the sinonasal area.

Congenital Syphilis

Though the incidence is diminishing in the West, this is still a worldwide problem world wide. There are two types of presentations: *early* which presents with condyloma, mucocutaneous lesions, and extensive erythematous rash and the *late* form presenting with interstitial keratitis, neurosyphilis, gummas, and bony lesions.

The characteristic features of congenital syphilis have been described as a medical student's nightmare, consisting of lesions causing a saddle nose deformity, anterior tibial saber shin deformity. Hutchinson's notched incisors, mulberry molars, frontal bossing of Parrot, shortened maxilla, concave midface, sternoclavicular thickening (Higoumenakis sign), mandibular prognathia, rhagades (circumferential wrinkles of peroral skin), Hutchinson's triad – notched incisors, ocular interstitial keratitis, and VIII nerve deafness. Note that the natural history is altered in HIV patients with each stage being more prolonged.

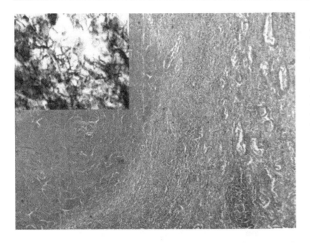

Granulomatous Infections of Head and Neck in Childhood, Fig. 4 Gumma in syphilis showing granuloma with large area of necrosis (Hematoxylin and Eosin x 100), which with Warthin-Starry stain show numerous spirochetes (*inset*)

Pathology

Three stages are noted at pathology. In the first stage, dense infiltrates of plasma cells and lymphocytes is prominently noted, while in the second stage, plasma cells and lymphocytes with giant cells are observed with non-caseous granulomas. Gummatous lesions are noted in the tertiary stage.

Regional lymph node enlargement is seen in the primary and tertiary disease stages, whereas generalized lymphadenopathy is a common finding in secondary syphilis. It is characterized by diffuse plasma cell infiltration, fibrosis, capsular and pericapsular inflammation with associated phlebitis. Occasionally, granulomas are noted. A Warthin-Starry or Levaditi stains highlight the spirochete *T. pallidum*. A Southern blotting and PCR are helpful on lymph node aspirates and lymph node biopsies. In secondary syphilis, the changes classically are of follicular hyperplasia. In tertiary lesions, classical gummata are noted having central necrosis and show numerous spirochetes when stained with silver stain (Fig. 4).

Diagnosis

T. pallidum is seen on dark field microscopy and with immunofluorescence of smear from primary and secondary lesions.

Serological Tests

VDRL and RPR tests – sensitive but high false positive rates.

Specific antitreponemal antibodies tests: FTA-ABS, MHA-TP, TPI tests are more specific. They remain positive indefinitely.

Treatment

Penicillin remains the drug of choice. Benzathine penicillin is given intramuscularly in most stages. The Jarisch-Herxheimer reaction is an acute febrile illness developing within 24 hours of giving treatment with penicillin for syphilis.

Mycobacterial Infection

Historical

Tuberculosis was called White Plague or Consumption until its causative organism was identified. Robert Koch proved the validity of his "Kochs postulates" on the bacteria *Mycobacterium tuberculosis* in 1882. Though treatment of this condition has been successful in many individual cases, in the domain of public health, there is concern at the increasing incidence in urban poor, immigrants, and those with AIDS being affected by this disease, and the development of drug resistant strains. Extrapulmonary tuberculosis and non-tuberculous mycobacteria is now increasingly identified in culture isolates.

Bacteriology

M. tuberculosis is a strict aerobic bacillus and once stained is resistant to decolorization by acid alcohol, and hence is called acid-fast bacillus. *M. bovis* and *M. africanum* also cause similar disease. *M. tuberculosis* is transmitted by inhalation of aerosol droplets, ingestion, and skin trauma.

Clinical Presentation

The classical picture is of a subclinical pulmonary infection in the upper lobes (Simons Focus), as oxygen tension is highest in that region of the lung. This infection and enlargement of the draining hilar lymph nodes is called the Ghon's Complex. The primary infection often heals followed by radiologically detectable calcification as a calcified granuloma (Ranke complex), but it remains a risk for reactivation lifelong.

Presentations in the head and neck include primary sinonasal TB, mucocutaneous TB – lupus vulgaris, laryngeal tuberculosis, lymphadenopathy, and lesions in any region of the head and neck.

Granulomatous Infections of Head and Neck in Childhood, Fig. 5 Granulomatous lymphadenitis due to mycobacterial infection showing early granuloma in (**a**), with progression to form central necrosis in (**b**); fine needle aspirate showing the classical granuloma composed of epithelioid cells having slipper-shaped nuclei. (**d**) shows both intracellularly and extracellularly located multiple acid-fast bacilli with Ziehl Neelsen stain (x 1000)

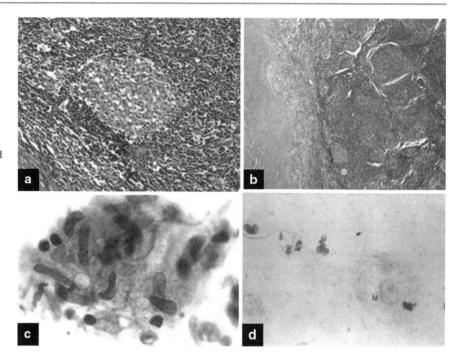

Pathology

The lymph nodes show multiple discrete small to large epithelioid granulomas characterized by central necrosis forming large caseous masses surrounded by Langhans giant cells and lymphocytes (Fig. 5a–d). The acid-fast bacilli in these lesions can be demonstrated by special stains, such as Ziehl Neelsen stain, cultures, or PCR to establish the diagnosis.

Diagnosis

Mantoux test is an intradermal test based on cell-mediated immunity. Testing is carried out with, 0.1 ml containing 0.04 microgram tuberculin units of a purified protein derivative of *M. tuberculosis* (1/1,000 strength). The Test is read for induration and is positive if it is equal to or more than 10 mm in diameter, after 72 hours.

Treatment

In order to increase compliance, the WHO has recommended special clinics to supervise treatment regimens directly, called DOTS (Directly observed therapy short course). The primary treatment regimen for a newly diagnosed case of tuberculosis consists of Rifampicin 600 mg for 6 months once daily, Isoniazid 300 mg, with Pyridoxine 10 mg once daily for 6 months, supplemented by pyrazinamide 1.5 g daily for 2 months. Ethambutol 50 mg daily is added if the risk of drug resistance is high. Multidrug resistance (MDR) and extensive drug resistance (XDR) is currently a worldwide therapeutic problem.

Surgery is for tuberculous lymphadenitis and it consists of a modified neck dissection addressing the lymph node groups in the neck.

MOTT (Mycobacteria other than *M. tuberculosis*)

These comprise *M. Kansasii, M. marinum*, in Group I, *M. scrofulaceum, M. Szulgai*, in Group II, *M. avium, M. intracellulare*, and *M. xenopi* in Group III, and *M. fortiutum* and *M. chelonei* in Group IV as per the Runyon classification.

The diseases with MOTT is increasingly common, not in the least due to improved methods of identification. It can present in any of the four clinical forms.
1. Cervical lymphadenitis
2. Ulcerative granuloma
3. Pneumonias in patients with underlying pulmonary disease such as emphysema
4. Pneumonias and generalized infections in patients with AIDS.

Pathology

Caseating granulomatous disease of cervical lymph node without pulmonary involvement is likely to be caused by atypical mycobacteria (MOTT) organisms. Florid suppuration overshadowing granulomatous response with numerous acid-fast bacilli is quiet characteristic. A simple acid-fast staining in these cases will clinch the diagnosis.

In immunosuppressed patients, a florid spindle cell proliferation simulating a neoplastic process could also be noted.

Treatment

MOTT is less sensitive to standard anti-TB drugs. Macrolides, such as clarithromycin, are effective. Cervical lymphadenitis due to MOTT is better treated by surgical resection.

Fungal Granuloma

Fungi are eukaryotic organisms with rigid cell walls – existing as yeast or molds, mainly causing infections opportunistically in debilitated hosts. Many fungi cause disease in the head and neck, though not all lead to a granulomatous infection.

Mycoses (infections due to fungus) are of four types

1. Superficial – Pityriasis versicolor and dermatophytosis. Causes mainly skin infections.
2. Subcutaneous – Sporotrichosis, Mycetoma (Rhinosporidiosis used to be classified in this category). These cause diseases mainly in lower extremities but can present in head and neck.
3. Systemic – These fungi are called dimorphic because they can exist as yeast at body temperature and as molds in room temperature This enables them to form spores, and the mode of transmission is by inhalation. Ex. Histoplasmosis, Blastomycosis, Coccidiomycosis and Para coccidiomycosis.
4. Opportunistic – Aspergillosis, Cryptococcosis, Zygomycosis.

Host immunity, both specific and nonspecific and other factors such as blood sugar level and pH can affect the growth of fungi.

Fungal infections can involve lymph nodes and present as chronic suppurative lesions of all the conditions listed above. The most common fungal infections associated with a granulomatous response are mucormycosis, cryptococcosis, and histoplasmosis.

When suspected, Giemsa stains, Gomori Methenamine Silver (GMS) stains, or Periodic acid-Schiff (PAS) stains help in demonstrating the fungal organisms and when they are too few, they can only be detected by either culture using Sabouraud's medium impregnated with antibiotics or immunological testing with estimating levels of antibodies and molecular testing.

Zygomycosis

Bacteriology

This disease can occur as either rhinocerebral, pulmonary, gastrointestinal, cutaneous, or disseminated forms. Nosocomial factors and increased incidence in transplant centers are being noted.

Clinical Presentation

Clinically, the predominant manifestation is as an invasive rhinocerebral infection. If the patient is granulocytopenic, the disease is acute and fulminant; in diabetics, the disease is chronic though invasive. AIDS patients rarely develop zygomycosis as their neutrophil cell function is intact.

Pathology

Histopathology reveals evidence of characteristic broad hyphae with no septation. The stromal reaction varies if the disease is invasive or chronic granulomatous in nature (Fig. 6). The presence of vascular invasion and thrombotic infarction is pathognomonic.

Treatment

The goals of treatment are debridement, systemic antifungal therapy, correction of underlying hyperglycemia or neutropenia. Amphotericin B is the drug of choice, but Azoles such as the triazoles – fluconazole, voriconazole, and itraconazole also have a role.

Cryptococcosis

Bacteriology

This is an infection caused by *Cryptococcus neoformans*, and *C. gatti*. These are round to oval cysts, 3–10 μ with thick mucinophilic capsule involving skin and mucosa of nasopharyngeal area. The cysts are best demonstrated in aspirates and tissue biopsies

Granulomatous Infections of Head and Neck in Childhood,
Fig. 6 (**a**) Granuloma in zygomycosis showing central necrosis with characteristic hyphae (Hematoxylin and Eosin x 400), which can also be distinctly noted in a fine needle aspirate (**b**, PAP stain)

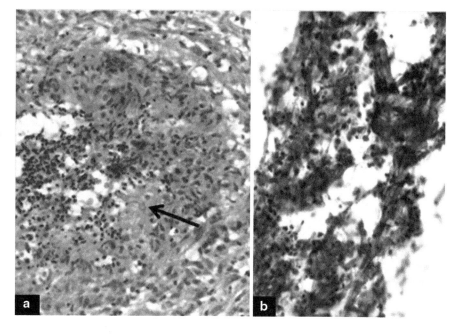

Granulomatous Infections of Head and Neck in Childhood,
Fig. 7 Granulomata in cryptococcal lymphadenitis showing numerous cryptococci in pale staining macrophages (**a** and **b**) (Hematoxylin and Eosin x 200). Note capsular staining in (**c**) (Grimelius silver stain) and (**d**) (Periodic acid-Schiff stain)

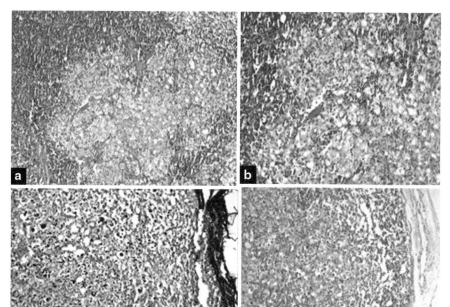

by Gomori methenamine silver stain and accentuated by Periodic acid-Schiff stain (Fig. 7). Collapsed cysts may appear boat-like.

Clinical Presentation

The clinical presentation is as skin lesion, pulmonary nodule, or meningitis. It becomes disseminated and potentially fatal in immunosuppressed individuals but remains self-limiting in immunocompetent individuals.

Treatment

Intravenous Amphotericin B, combined with oralflucytosine, may be effective. When the disease coexists with AIDS, oral fluconazole can be used in addition.

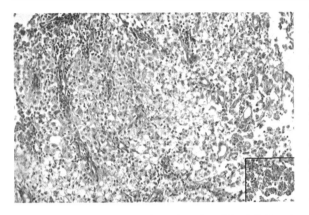

Granulomatous Infections of Head and Neck in Childhood, Fig. 8 Granulomata in histoplasmosis showing aggregates of macrophages with intracytoplasmic budding yeast forms (*inset*) (Hematoxylin and Eosin x 400)

Histoplasmosis

Bacteriology

It is an infection caused by *Histoplasma capsulatum*. The disease is spread via an avian vector (the European Starling).

Clinical Presentation

Most individuals exposed to the infection develop subclinical pneumonia, but exposure to large doses of inhaled fungi leads to acute fulminant pneumonia. In immunosuppressed and immunocompetent individuals, infection of the gingiva, tongue, palate, and larynx may occur. The lesion shows oval intracellular cysts measuring 2–5 μ and are found in histiocytes.

Pathology

The lesion is most often subclinical and remains as pulmonary infection in individuals with normal immunity but becomes disseminated in immunosuppressed individuals. Strangely, both immunocompetent and immunosuppressed individuals, irrespective of age, may develop infection of the gingiva, tongue, palate, and larynx.

The mucosal biopsies characteristically show intrahistiocytic location of the cysts, the "halo" effect around each organism (artifact of tissue processing), and its nuclei (Fig. 8). The oropharyngeal infections may serve as the sentinel of disseminated infection. They are best diagnosed in aspirates and touch preparations of tissue biopsies. Positive staining of cysts

with Periodic acid-Schiff stain and negative staining with Gomori Methenamine Silver (GMS) stain is classical. When they are too few, they can only be detected by either culture using Sabouraud's medium impregnated with antibiotics or immunological testing with estimating levels of antibodies and molecular testing.

Treatment

Itraconazole is the drug of choice, and fluconazole is the second-line agent. Posaconazole is also effective in refractory cases.

Miscellaneous

Rhinosporidiosis

Bacteriology

Rhinosporidiosis is a granulomatous disease caused by *Rhinosporidium seeberi* affecting the mucous membrane of nasopharynx, oropharynx, conjunctiva, rectum, and external genitalia.

This organism was previously considered to be a fungus, and rhinosporidiosis is classified as a fungal disease under ICD-10. But, it is now considered to be a parasite, classified under Mesomycetozoea.

Clinical Presentation

The disease affects humans and animals such as cattle, horses, and goat. Though found predominantly in India and Sri Lanka, migration and ease of travel has resulted in cases being described in many geographical areas including Europe and the USA.

The disease characteristically presents with large, friable polypoidal growths in the nasal cavity. Though the floor of the nose and inferior turbinate are the commonest sites, the lesions may appear elsewhere too. Traumatic inoculation from one site to others is common. Laryngeal rhinosporidiosis too has been described and may be due to inoculation from the nose during endotracheal intubation. After inoculation, the organisms replicate locally resulting in the hyperplasia of host tissue and localized immune response.

Pathology

On histopathological examination, the lesion shows hyperplastic epithelium with numerous globular cysts of varying shape, representing sporangia in different stages of development and transelimination. The

Granulomatous Infections of Head and Neck in Childhood,
Fig. 9 Hyperplastic squamous epithelium (**a**) showing sporangia containing spores (**b**) in a case of rhinosporidiosis (Hematoxylin and Eosin x 400)

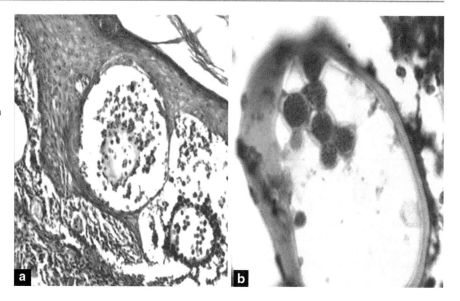

sporangia are sharply defined globular thick-walled cysts measuring up to 0.5 mm in diameter, which contain numerous rounded endospores, 6–7 μ in diameter (Fig. 9). Immature and collapsed sporangia are also present. It is not necessary to perform special staining because of the characteristic microscopy of the lesion.

Treatment
The lesion can be surgically excised with cautery of the base. The procedure is often associated with severe bleeding the use of Dapsone has been suggested empirically to prevent systemic spread, which though rare does occur.

Toxoplasmosis

Bacteriology
One of the most common parasitic infections affecting the young is caused by the protozoan *Toxoplasma gondii*.

Clinical Presentation
In immunocompetent patients, the most common presentation is of a firm moderately enlarged posterior cervical lymphadenopathy.

Pathology
Microscopically, the nodal architecture is well preserved. There are characteristic clusters of small histiocytic cells with abundant cytoplasm and eccentric oval nuclei, forming microgranulomas.

Treatment
Cytology and serology can avoid a surgical procedure for this self-limiting process. However, in severe forms of infection in immunocompromised patients, specific antibiotics are prescribed. (Pyrimethamine and sulfadiazine, for 4–5 weeks; dosage to be increased in HIV positive patients).

Nonspecific Inflammatory Diseases

Giant Cell Granuloma
Historical
Described by H Jaffe in 1953, this is a benign granulomatous lesion of the facial and calvarial bones.

Clinical Presentation
It presents as an expanding mass lesion with evidence of bone destruction. Though not malignant, it can be progressive with local extension and tissue destruction. It is most likely a form of reparative granuloma where there is injury to the periodontal membrane especially after tooth removal and a mass of fibroblastic granulation tissue develops.

Pathology
The lesion is characterized by cystic lesion in the bone, which shows large aggregates of multinucleate giant

cells and spindle cells in a cellular vascular stroma and new bone formation rimmed by osteoblasts. The giant cells have patchy distribution and are associated with large areas of hemorrhage.

Clinical Presentation

Clinically, it presents as either arising from the periphery of the bone (Peripheral type), presenting as a gingival lesion in the maxilla as a pedunculated or sessile mass. Or less commonly, it presents as an endosteal lesion, usually in the mandible anterior to the first molar (Central type).

Treatment

It is by excision and/or curettage of the lining epithelium. The surgical challenge lies in the reconstruction of the defect, as these lesions affect the bones of the facial skeleton. The advent of microvascular surgery has improved the cosmetic results of reconstruction.

Sarcoidosis

First described by C Boeck in 1899, this disease is more common in African Americans and affects females more than males.

Clinical Presentation

In the Sinonasal system, it presents in the following stages:

Stage I: With nonspecific reversible, mucosal edema and turbinate hypertrophy.

Stage II: With crusting friable mucosa, synechae, and vestibular granuloma.

Stage III: With irreversible changes, ulceration, synechae, nasal stenosis, and saddle nose deformity.

The disease leads to salivary gland enlargement and dysfunction of secretory glands resulting in the Sicca syndrome, called Heerfordts syndrome or uveoparotid fever. Laryngeal involvement starts in the supraglottic region. In the central nervous system, neurosarcoidosis most commonly affects the VII cranial nerve.

Pathology

An inverse relationship with susceptibility to *M. tuberculosis* has been described. A link with HLA Class haplotype BB, and a familial association is also noted. It is a multisystemic chronic, non-caseating granulomatous disease of unknown etiology. Though most common in the lungs, it can

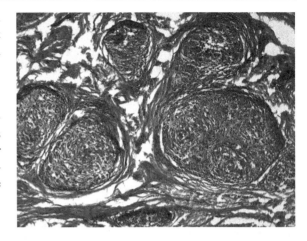

Granulomatous Infections of Head and Neck in Childhood, Fig. 10 Sarcoid granulomas shown here are non-necrotizing, distinctly discrete and numerous (Hematoxylin and Eosin x 100)

involve both the upper and lower respiratory systems, skin, and reticuloendothelial system.

The hallmark of sarcoidosis is the presence of a non-caseating granuloma with epithelioid cells and Langhans giant cells (Fig. 10). These giant cells are smaller and have fewer nuclei than that seen in tuberculosis. Intracytoplasmic inclusion bodies such as Schauman bodies, Hamazaki Wesenberg inclusion bodies, and Asteroid bodies are seen in some. However, none of them are specific for sarcoidosis. Hence, the diagnosis of sarcoidosis is always one of the exclusion. When all the possibilities for granulomatous inflammation are excluded and the clinical picture is characteristic, there is a justification in labeling a case as sarcoidosis.

The etiology and pathogenesis of sarcoidosis remains elusive and whether it is a pattern of reaction or a distinct disease entity itself is not clear. It has been shown that certain types of genetic polymorphisms are associated with increased risk of disease and is thought to represent a dysfunction of circulating T cells with over activity of B cells – an altered immune response to antigens. It is currently believed that cell-mediated immunity is enhanced at the sites of lesions. The other features include cutaneous anergy, decreased T cell function, and increased humoral immunity with increased B cell hypersensitivity, and polyclonal hypergammaglobulinemia. EBV virus relations are suspected. Elevated ACE levels is a feature of this condition. Kveim Siltzbach test using intradermal inoculation of sarcoid extract was previously used but is not recommended nowadays.

Treatment

Systemic steroids, such as prednisolone, at 30–40 mg per day are prescribed for stage II and III, extrathoracic disease, and symptomatic patients in any stage. Other regimes using cytotoxic agents, such as methotrexate, azathioprine, cyclophosphamide, etc., are also described.

Vasculitic Disease

Kawasaki Disease/Syndrome

An acute febrile illness of childhood affecting the vascular, integumentary, and reticuloendothelial system (Synonym: Mucocutaneous lympadenopathy syndrome) First described by B Kawasaki from Japan in 1967, where epidemics have occurred, the disease has a worldwide distribution.

Clinical Presentation

The disease presents with a fever, and truncal rash, which occurs within a week of the commencement of the illness. Ocular symptoms, such as conjunctival injection, which is nonexudative, and oral symptoms, such as mulberry tongue, annular chelitis, tonsillar hypertrophy, xerostomia, and mouth ulcers, are also described.

Cervical lymphadenopathy occurs in more than 80% of patients, causing neck stiffness and pain. Though large, does not suppurate. The lymph nodes appear matted on CT scans.

The hands and feet become erythematous, then desquamation occurs. Cardiovascular involvement, particularly cardiac arrhythmias, prolonged QT intervals, and coronary artery aneurysms may occur This occurs in over 25% of untreated children, and accounts for most of the mortality described for this condition. The blood tests reveal anemia and raised ESR levels.

Pathology

The disease is characterized by reactive proliferative changes in the media, panarteritis, fibrin thrombi in small vessels and aneurysm dilatations of medium-sized arteries. Perivasculitis and marked fibrosis following infarcts is noted in the healed stage. These pathologic changes are thought to be immune mediated. Coronory arteritis may lead to fatal complications.

Treatment

The condition is largely self-limiting. Intravenous immunoglobulin and aspirin for its anti-inflammatory properties are used. The use of steroids is contraindicated.

Wegener's Granulomatosis (WG)

This disease is a necrotizing granulomatous vasculitis of an unknown etiology, involving the upper aerodigestive tract, lower respiratory tract, and kidneys. It is infrequent in young patients less than 10 years of age, commoner in adults around 40 years. A predilection for the Caucasian race is marked. It may be limited to one site or multifocal. Each patient has an unpredictable course. WG has many clinical manifestations and may masquerade as a variety of other conditions. Without treatment, it is progressive and fatal.

History

Klinger 1931 described two postmortem cases. He thought it was an atypical polyarteritis nodosum. Wegener, in 1936, described the triad of granulomatous vasculitis of the upper and lower respiratory tract, systemic vasculitis, and focal necrotizing glomerulonephritis.

Clinical Presentation

Nonspecific constitutional symptoms, such as weight loss, easy fatiguability, fever, headache, weakness, and poor wound healing, may be the only presenting symptoms. Granulomas in head and neck may be seen in the eye and orbit, musculoskeletal, integumentary, and nervous system. Rhinitis, epistaxis, rhinorrhea, anosmia, and nasal obstruction are common symptoms. They present with polypoidal masses, crusting, and friable mucosa. Cartilage destruction may be noted followed by saddle nose deformity and septal perforations. Ear problems are very common such as SOM, external otitis and VII nerve dysfunction. The lesion can involve the cochlear apparatus but generally spares the vestibular apparatus.

Radiography shows nodules, infltrates, cavitation, and hilar adenopathy. These patients have cough, dyspnea, chest pain, and hemoptysis. Signs of renal involvement, such as hematuria, renal failure, and histopathological findings of aggressive glomerular-nephritis are characteristic. In the musculoskeletal type, ankle edema and knee effusions may be seen. In the nervous system, mononeuritis monoplex, with weakening of isolated cranial nerves is common.

Pathology

This lesion is characterized by necrotizing granulomatous inflammation involving the upper and lower respiratory tract such as the nose and lungs. Necrotizing vasculitis affecting small- to medium-sized vessels, especially the lungs and the upper airways, is observed as is renal disease manifesting as focal necrotizing glomerulonephritis. Limited WG is considered when patients do not manifest the full triad.

Granulomatous vasculitis is seen as vasculitis of small- and medium-sized arteries and veins and is characterized by palisading epithelioid histiocytes, multinucleated giant cells, and an inflammatory infiltrate.

Necrotizing vasculitis: It is a microvasculitis involving small vessels, which display either granuloma or necrosis. Renal biopsy shows focal segmental necrotizing glomerulonephritis with crescent formation.

Elevated ESR, circulating immune complexes, anemia, thrombocytosis, hypergammaglobulinemia, positive cANCA, with specificity for proeinase-3 in granulocytes and PR3, are characteristic for WG and is 90% sensitive.

Treatment

Steroids and cylcophosphamide, trimethoprim (sulfamethoxazole), plasmapheresis of circulating immune complexes in renal system dysfunction is indicated as a temperorary measure.

Lymphoproliferative Disease

Castleman's Disease

It was first reported by Castleman in 1954, who described 13 patients with intrathoracic lymphadenopathy. Two types, localized and multicentric were described by Keller in 1972.

Clinical Presentation

This is an uncommon disease usually seen in young adults. It mainly causes lymph node enlargement in the intrathoracic region and less often in the extrathoracic region, mainly head and neck.

Pathology

The lymph nodal involvement represents a distinct form of hyperplasia rather than a neoplasm. The hyaline vascular/angiofollicular type shows large follicles with marked vascular proliferation and hyalinization of their germinal centers. In the lymphoid subtype, there is marked expansion of the mantle zone with inconspicuous germinal centers. The plasma cell type is characterized by diffuse plasma cell proliferation in the interfollicular tissue, accompanied by Russell bodies. Lack of a nodal sinus within the main lesion is quite characteristic.

Treatment

Localized Castleman's disease occurs in younger patients and has a good prognosis. This condition can be cured by surgical excision, though the lesion tends to bleed heavily and preoperative embolization has been described as being useful. An increased serum interleukin has been described as being responsible for the symptomatology, and has been treated with a specific monoclonal antibody. It is associated at times with an acquired immunodeficiency syndrome.

The multicentric Castleman's disease, found in older individuals, tends to progress, causes systemic symptoms, and is associated with paraneoplastic conditions such as amyloidosis, myaesthenia, pemphigus, refractory anemia, and peripheral neuropathy. Monoclonal antibodies, rituximab and steroids, and have been used for the treatment of this condition. The prognosis of this variety is poor with a reported median survival of about 2 years.

This disease entity is considered by many as a lymphoproliferative disorder rather than a reactive/inflammatory condition. Associated neoplasms, such as angiomatous hamartoma and vascular neoplasm, may develop and hence a close follow-up is warranted.

Kikuchi and Fujimoto's Disease

Two Japanese pathologists- Kikuchi and Fujimoto and colleagues in 1972 first described this entity which occurred in patients of any age, or ethnic background with involvement of any anatomic site, including nodal and extranodal locations. The female: male ratio is approximately 3 to 4:1 and the mean age is 25 to 29 years.

The typical presentation is unilateral cervical lymphadenopathy with fever, myalgias and skin rashes. The histology shows partially maintained lymph node architecture with patchy but mainly paracortical involvement. Areas of fibrinoid necrosis with abundant extracellular apoptotic bodies is noted

**Granulomatous Infections
of Head and Neck in
Childhood,**
Fig. 11 Langerhans cell
histiocytosis: (**a**) shows
ulcerative lesions on the neck
with the biopsy in (**b**) showing
sheets of Langerhans cells
having vesicular nucleus with
nuclear groves in the long axis
highlighted in (**c**) (fine needle
aspirate). Electron microscopy
(**d**) confirms the diagnosis by
demonstrating Birbeck
granules in the cytoplasm

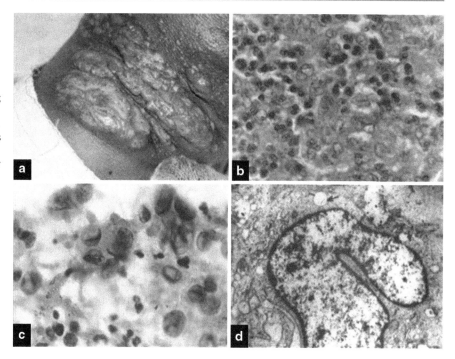

while the parafollicular area shows a mixture of benign histiocytes, so called crescentic or C shaped forms, immunoblasts and plasmacytoid monocytes surrounding the necrotic areas. The neutrophils are prominently absent and the plasma cells are few or absent. The uninvolved areas show paracortical hyperplasia. The histiocytes characteristically express CD 68, lysozyme and myeloperoxidase – a feature unique to histiocytes in Kikutchi- Fujimoto's disease.

Langerhans Cell Histiocytosis

The term Langerhans Cell Histiocytosis is a specific clinicopathologic entity characterized by the proliferation of Langerhans cells. These cells are components of the dendritic cell system, which functions as antigen-processing cells in the immune system.

Clinical Presentation

A variety of clinical types are described such as:

Unifocal (initially called Eosinophilic granuloma) – which is a slowly progressive disease, occurring in bone without extraskeletal involvment. It may be monostotic or polyostotic due to an expanding proliferation of Langerhans cells.

Multifocal unisystem (initially called Hand-Schuller-Christian disease) – which is seen mostly in children, presenting with fever, bone lesions, and skin eruptions in the scalp, and ear canals. There is involvement of the pituitary stalk, leading to diabetes insipidus. The bone lesions lead to exopthalmos.

Multifocal multisystem (initially called Letterer-Siwe Disease) – which is a rapidly progressive disease in which Langerhans cells proliferate in many tissues. It is seen mostly in children under the age of 2, and the prognosis is poor even with chemotherapy.

Pathology

At histology, the pathognomonic cells of Langerhans are unique with irregular elongated nuclei with characteristic grooves and arranged in sheets. Their cytoplasm is abundant and acidophilic. The sinuses are distended by these Langerhans cells admixed with a variable number of eosinophils; foci of necrosis is common with eosinophils forming eosinophilic microabscesses, always confined to sinuses (Fig. 11). The lesion may be confused with a tuberculous granuloma or deep fungal infections. The presence of Birbeck granules under electron microscopy is diagnostic.

Classically, the Langerhans cells are positive for CD1a, S-100, CD 68 vimentin, and negative for CD45 RA and EMA.

Treatment

The unifocal variety may be surgically excised, and the prognosis is excellent.

The multifocal, single system variety is treated with steroids either systemic or as a cream for the skin lesions.

The multifocal, multisystem variety is treated with vinca alkaloids, antimetabolites, and alkylating agents either singly or in combination, but it has a poor prognosis.

Rosai-Dorfman Disease (Sinus histiocytosis with Massive Lymphadenopathy)

A rare, idiopathic, benign disorder of the reticuloendothelial system characterized by painless reactive histiocyte proliferation of unknown etiology. It usually affects children and young adults, but people of any age may also be affected. The etiology of this condition remains unknown. Infection by a virus such as EBV and HHV6 are suspected by some.

Clinical Presentation

Most patients have a gigantic lymph nodal disease, in addition 40% show an extranodal disease. The nasal cavity, facial soft tissues, eyelids may be involved. In the head and neck, a cervical mass, or symptoms such as sinusitis, epistaxis, facial pain, or saddle nose deformity may be present. Subglottic lesions are common.

Pathology

The lymph nodes show sinusoidal distension with distinctive type of histiocytes, with very large, round nuclei, distinct central nucleoli, and voluminous lightly eosinophilic pale cytoplasm. Numerous plasma cells with emperipolesis, due to cytophagocytosis, is characteristic. Although, the cervical lymph nodes are by far the most common and most prominent site of involvement, other peripheral or central lymph node groups may be affected with or without cervical disease.

Immunohistochemically, Rosai-Dorfman histiocytes express positvity for S100 and CD68 markers. Extranodal disease shows dark staining areas of lymphocytes, and pale foci of histiocytes.

Treatment

Excision of the lesion and steroids form the mainstay. Radiation therapy, once popular, is now not part of the

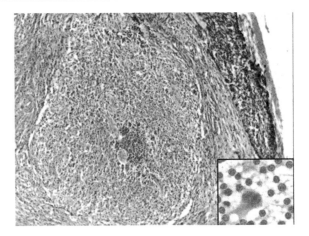

Granulomatous Infections of Head and Neck in Childhood, Fig. 12 Hodgkin's lymphoma showing classical Reed Sternberg cells (*inset*) amidst granulomatous background (Hematoxylin and Eosin x 100)

protocol. This lesion is relatively unaffected by therapy although chemotherapy has proved effective in some cases. Prognosis is excellent except in about 10% of patients who worsen secondary to immune system involvement.

Malignant Lymphomas

In cases of granulomatous lymphadenitis, one has to be aware that some malignant conditions are rarely associated with granulomatous inflammation (Fig. 12) and in a very extensive manner that may mask the malignant component. One among them are lymphomas. Lymphomas associated with marked granulomatous reaction are well documented in the literature including association with primary presentation or in relapse.

Tuberculosis is the most common cause of caseating granulomas in the East. However, patients with suboptimal response to antituberculous treatment and those with non-caseating granulomas should be evaluated carefully to exclude all the possible associated tumors.

Immunohistochemistry is of great help in highlighting the malignant cell of interest and confirming the diagnoses. Tissue culture and molecular studies for mycobacteria are helpful to confirm or exclude the diagnosis of tuberculosis, particularly with a nonclassic morphological appearance.

References

Barnes L (2008) Miscellanous disorders of the head and neck. In: Barnes L (ed) Surgical pathology of the head and Neck, vol 3, 2nd edn. Informa Health Care, New York, pp 1717–1734, Chapter 26

Mahadevia P, Brandwein-Gensler M (2008) Infectious diseases of the head and neck. In: Barnes L (ed) Surgical pathology of the head and Neck, vol 3, 2nd edn. Informa Health Care, New York, pp 1609–1715, Chapter 25

Newman K, Hayes-Jordan A (2006) Lymph node disorders. In: Grosfeld J, Neill JO, Coran AG, Fonkasrud EW (eds) Pediatric surgery, 6th edn. Mosby Elsevier, Philadelphia, pp 844–849, Chapter 54

O'hare TJ (1999) Granulomatous and lymphoproliferative diseases of the head and neck. In: Thawley SE, Panje WR, Batsakis JG (eds) Comprehensive management of head and neck tumours, vol 2, 2nd edn. W B Saunders, Philadelphia, pp 1931–1981, Chapter 84

Gray

Sébastien Schmerber[1,2,3], Arnaud Attye[1,2,4], Ihab Atallah[5], Cédric Mendoza[1,2,4] and Alexandre Karkas[1,2,6]

[1]Department of Otolaryngology-Head and Neck Surgery, Otology/Neurotology Unit, University Hospital of Grenoble, Grenoble, France

[2]Service ORL. Hôpital A. Michallon, Grenoble, France

[3]Otology, Neurotology and Auditory Implants Department, University Hospital of Grenoble CHU A. Michallon, Grenoble, France

[4]Department of Neuroradiology, University Hospital of Grenoble, Grenoble, France

[5]Department of Otolaryngology-Head and Neck Surgery, University Hospital of Grenoble, Grenoble, France

[6]Clinique Universitaire Oto–Rhino–Laryngologie, Centre Hospitalier Universitaire A. Michallon, Grenoble, France

Definition

(Abbreviation: Gy): A unit of absorbed radiation equal to the dose of 1 J of energy absorbed per kilogram of matter (human tissue), or 100 rad.

Grisel's Syndrome

Chris Sanders Taylor
Department of Neurological Surgery, University of Cincinnati, Cincinnati, OH, USA

Definition

A nontraumatic atlantoaxial subluxation thought to be infectious in etiology.

Cross-References

▶ Craniocervical Junction, Abnormalities

Gustatory Hyperhidrosis

▶ Frey's Syndrome

Gustatory Sweating

▶ Frey's Syndrome

H

Habitual Snoring

▶ Snoring Without Apnea, Evaluation

Hair Cells

Gerald T. Kangelaris and Lawrence R. Lustig
Department of Otolaryngology-Head and Neck
Surgery, University of California, San Francisco, San
Francisco, CA, USA

Definition

Sensory receptors of the auditory and vestibular systems. Auditory hair cells are located within the organ of Corti and come in two anatomically and functionally distinct types: outer and inner hair cells.

Cross-References

▶ Sensorineural Hearing Loss

Hair Follicle Unit

▶ Apopilosebaceous Unit

Hair Transplantation

▶ Follicular Unit Transplantation

Hairy Polyps

▶ Heterotopias, Teratoma, and Choristoma

Haller's Cell, Infraorbital Ethmoid Cell

▶ Radiologic Evaluation/Diagnostic Imaging of Paranasal Sinuses and Chronic Rhinosinusitis

Handicapped

▶ Cochlear Implants in Patients with Multiple Disabilities

S.E. Kountakis (ed.), *Encyclopedia of Otolaryngology, Head and Neck Surgery*, DOI 10.1007/978-3-642-23499-6,
© Springer-Verlag Berlin Heidelberg 2013

Hard Failure

Selena E. Heman-Ackah[1] and J. Thomas Roland Jr.[2]
[1]Department of Otolaryngology-Head and Neck Surgery, New York University, New York, NY, USA
[2]Department of Otolaryngology, New York University School of Medicine, New York, NY, USA

Definition

Device malfunction leading to loss of function which can be confirmed by integrity testing or a loss of link with the external apparatus.

Cross-References

▶ Cochlear Implantation, Revision – Adult
▶ Surgical Devices (Cochlear Implantation, Revision – Pediatric)

Harelip

▶ Cleft Lip

Hay Fever

▶ Allergic Rhinitis

Head and Neck Cancer Pain Management

Timothy J. Beacham
Department of Anesthesiology, University of Mississippi, Jackson, MS, USA

Definition

Pain is a very prevalent symptom in cancer patients, especially in those with advanced disease. Seventy-five to ninety percent of them will deal with pain on a daily basis, and this is a major detriment to their quality of life and their ability to function normally. We can classify pain in many ways. One example is describing it in terms of its chronicity. There are acute, intermittent, and chronic types of pain. Chronic pain is the most common type of pain in cancer patients, and this is often caused by direct tumor involvement of the neighboring tissues. Cancer patients also experience procedural pain, which tends to be more acute in nature, and is related to surgery or procedures such as lumbar puncture. Toxicity related to the anticancer treatment modalities, especially chemotherapy, can also induce painful neuropathies in some patients.

Head and neck pain may arise due to tissue damage from multiple sources such as mucosal injury, invasion of the tumor into somatic tissue (skin, muscle, bone) with inflammation or ischemia, and nerve infiltration or compression. Treatment for head and neck cancer involves single or multimodal therapy employing surgery, chemotherapy (CT), and/or radiation (RT), all of which can damage somatic tissues and nerves. These multiple sources of somatic tissue and neural damage from the tumor and cancer treatment result in pain being experienced by all head and neck cancer patients.

One type of pain is nociceptive, which is direct activation of the pain receptors called nociceptors. These send input along unmyelinated C fibers directly to the CNS, which is perceived as pain. There is also neuropathic pain, which is caused by abnormal function of the somatic sensory neurons, and this can be caused by nerve compression or invasion of the nerve by the tumor. This causes release of action potential despite the fact that the nociceptors at the nerve endings are not being activated. There is also a subcellular level derangement of function that can occur with treatment modalities such as chemotherapy that would cause these nerves to be firing and sending pain signals to the brain without direct activation of the nociceptors. The third type of pain is idiopathic, which cannot be explained by any identifiable pathology. This may be because of an organic process that the treating physician simply cannot identify. The other possibility is that it is more of a functional issue and the pain symptoms are being produced by some psychological process. A functional source of pain is relatively rare, especially in cancer patients.

In many circumstances, severe pain that is associated with the initial presentation of head and neck cancer is suggestive of more advanced disease. The prevalence of pain among patients with advanced disease is 80–100%; almost all patients with head and neck cancer will experience some pain during the course of their disease. In advanced head and neck cancer, pain is frequently multidimensional.

One of the most feared consequences of cancer is the possibility of severe and uncontrolled pain in patients with advanced cancer. In patients with head and neck cancer, pain is reported in up to 85% of cases at diagnosis. Pain due to soft tissue and bone destruction and nerve injury may involve inflammatory and/or neuropathic mechanisms. Further, it is estimated that 45–80% of all cancer patients have inadequate pain management. Barriers to adequate pain management include patients' reluctance to report pain, current pain management practices by health-care providers, and providers' negative ideas about and regulatory barriers to the use of opioids. In addition, limited understanding of the frequency and role of neuropathic pain mechanisms and the lack of use of management approaches for neuropathic pain may compromise symptom management in cancer patients.

As for management, the World Health Organization published its recommendations for cancer pain management with something called the analgesic adder. Multiple studies over the last two decades have sought to validate this model, some have criticized it, but mostly it has stood the test of time and proved to be an adequate treatment model for the vast majority of cancer patients. It is certainly not perfect, but it does form an effective conceptual framework to work with creating an individualized plan that can address their pain concerns. The first step of the ladder is non-opioid analgesics including Tylenol, aspirin, and some of the NSAIDs such as ibuprofen and naproxen. These often work for a short time in the early stages, but quickly become inadequate as cancer progresses. The next step would be to move to a weak opioid. These include codeine, low doses of oxycodone, propoxyphene, Darvocet, and hydrocodone. These are often prepared as combination products with the NSAIDs. For example, Lortab, Norco, and Tylenol No.3 are all a very common combination drugs with a weak opioid and an NSAID as an adjuvant. The next rung on the ladder is a strong opioid, which is for severe pain, not controlled by the previous step. Morphine, higher doses of oxycodone, hydromorphone, methadone, and fentanyl are all much stronger in terms

of their ability to relieve pain and their activation of the opioid receptors. Even at this step, it is worth considering continuing a non-opioid adjuvant such as ibuprofen or Tylenol as these can often open your therapeutic window by decreasing the amount of opioid that you are requiring for the same level of pain relief and decreasing the likelihood that your patients can be experiencing side effects related to that high opioid dose.

The WHO recommends usage of analgesic medication "by mouth," "by the clock," and "by the ladder." Drug administration by mouth is often the most convenient form for patients and does not require any high level of nursing care like intermittent muscular injections or IV medication would. "By the clock" refers to a round-the-clock schedule with rescue doses for acute breakthrough pain to ensure the patient is never left uncovered. Finally, "by the ladder" refers to the gradual stepwise progression through the therapeutic ladder to avoid unnecessary side effects related to high opioid doses. As a practical matter, it's important to know that dosage of non-opioid medication is limited by therapeutic ceiling. In other words, you cannot expect much higher Tylenol doses to provide more and more pain relief. There is simply a maximum effect that Tylenol can have in terms of pain relief. There is also the toxicity issue where usually between 4 and 6 g of Tylenol in 1 day could induce hepatotoxicity. Using high doses of other NSAIDs is associated with gastric ulcer problems and bleeding issues. The dosage of opioid/NSAID combo products can therefore be increased until you believe that maximum dose of non-opioid component has been reached. At that point, in order to give your patient more opioid medication, you may have to switch to different formulation of the combination drug or switch to a stronger opioid.

The opioids themselves are limited only by side effects. So with increasing doses of opioid medication, you expect an increasing level of pain relief in a fairly linear pattern. Opioid dosages are limited by their side effects. So at very high doses, you could expect respiratory depression, sedation, and altered mental status. You must often use adjuvants to account for the nonlethal opioid side effects at lower doses. Constipation is the most common. Prescribing the patients stool softeners and laxatives will help them avoid this. Nausea and vomiting is typically a transitory symptom related to activation of central chemoreceptors in the nausea center of the brain, as well as by GI dysmotility. It tends to resolve as tolerance to the opioid develops, but in the short term can be treated with anti-emetics and pro-motility agents. Sedation is very prominent with initiation or escalation of opioids, and one should follow a stepwise approach in dealing with this problem. Stopping of other CNS depressants, especially alcohol or sleeping pills, is an important step. You may also consider adding a stimulant. There are popular ADHD medicines that may give the patient just that little bump up that they need to get through the acute period of increased sedation related to the increasing opioid medication. The same stepwise approach can be used to deal with confusion as a side effect. First, eliminate other medicines that might be exacerbating the problem, then try to decrease your opioid dose if possible. If confusion persists, you need to rule out other causes of confusion such as sepsis. If all these are ruled out and the patient continues to have delirium related to the high doses of opioids, you can try a neuroleptic such as Haldol at low doses. Rotating your opioids on a fairly regular schedule may help you avoid tolerance to individual medicines and side effects related to metabolic accumulation which at higher levels can become toxic to patients.

You should expect that you are going to be escalating the dose of opioids over time because the patients will develop tolerance to the effects of these medicines and their disease may progress to cause more pain. Often people get scared to escalate an opioid dose because they feel like it may be a sign of the patient becoming addicted to the medicine. Addiction is extremely rare in cancer patients. However, it can be identified through the continued craving of the opioids for the psychologic effects rather than the relief of pain; off-prescription use of the drugs; obtaining from multiple sources such as other physicians, friends, and parents; and use of these medicines despite harm to self or others. Dependence, on the other hand, is extremely common and simply refers to the physical development of withdrawal symptoms after rapid dose reduction. It has nothing to do with addiction; it is simply the biologic process. It is also important to be aware of pseudo addiction, which may be seen in a patient where some sort of increasing psychological stress that leads them to seek out and perseverate about where their pain medication is coming from as they fear it will be cut off from them, even though they truly need it. This can be eliminated by the physician working to establish an effective therapeutic relationship with the patient, in order to give them the confidence

that you, as the physician, care about relieving their pain and will not abandon them to suffer alone. This may break the cycle of constantly worrying about where the pain medicine will come from.

Cancer pain causes increased morbidity, reduced performance status, increased anxiety and depression, and diminished quality of life (QOL). Head and neck and oral pain management may be particularly challenging due to the rich innervation of the orofacial region and because oral intake, swallowing, speech, and other motor functions of the head and neck and oropharynx are constant pain triggers. In addition, the oral mucosa is susceptible to the effects of systemic chemotherapy and regional radiotherapy, resulting in painful mucositis. The oral microbial flora may cause secondary infection with attendant pain and morbidity. Pain may be the first symptom in 20–50% of all cancer patients due to the malignancy, and oral pain may arise from head and neck cancer in up to 85% from metastatic disease in the head and neck or due to oral involvement in systemic cancers (e.g., leukemia). In a recent study, investigators identified pain in 56% of patients with head and neck cancer at diagnosis and found mixed nociceptive and neuropathic pain in 93% of those with pain. In large surveys of pain characteristics in cancer including head and neck cancer, patients suffered pain associated with the tumor (87–92.5%) or cancer therapy (17–20.8%) or both. In head and neck cancer, 78% of patients report pain in the head, face, or mouth and 54% in the cervical region or shoulder. In head and neck cancer, pain is the major reason (up to 85%) for seeking care, but at diagnosis pain is usually of low intensity (mean 10-cm visual analogue scale [VAS] = 3). Pain due to oral mucositis is the most frequently reported patient-related complaint impacting quality of life during cancer therapy and often results in severe pain for which opioid analgesics are prescribed sometimes with additional impaired quality of life. Successful pain management requires knowledge of, and attention to, multiple pain mechanisms that may culminate in the patient's pain. In head and neck cancer patients, neuropathic pain has not been well characterized in terms of sensory report (location, intensity, quality, and pattern) or sensory quantification (allodynia and hyperalgesia). In addition to neuroplasticity as a mechanism for neuropathic pain, other mechanisms may play a role in producing neuropathic pain associated with mucositis that may be conditioned by inflammatory mediators (e.g., tumor necrosis factor alpha [TNF-α]), which play a central role in the activation of cytokines and are elevated in mucositis TNF-α is known to be involved in mediation of neuropathic pain and hyperalgesia. Other chemical mediators implicated in neuropathic pain include reactive oxygen/nitrogen species, bradykinin, substance P, and other cytokines that are upregulated in mucositis. Investigators also have demonstrated changes in dorsal horn processing of nociceptive stimuli that result in neuropathic pain. These mechanisms may result in neuropathic pain associated with tissue damage that occurs from head and neck cancer or its treatment.

Conclusion

In conclusion, pain is an extremely common symptom in patients with head and neck cancer, and it is far too often undertreated. Attention should be paid to the patient's particular emotional and cultural circumstances which may limit their reporting of pain. The analgesic ladder provides an effective framework for the establishment of a treatment plan that can be individualized your patient's needs through your empathic, therapeutic relationship with them. As your patient's personal and disease-related circumstances change, alterations in the pain relief plan should be made. Careful attention to the relief of opioid-related side effects and reassuring your patient that you are dedicated to relieving their cancer-related pain will help the patient avoid behaviors which may be construed as addiction and possibly limit the physician's ability to appropriately escalate the opioid dosage.

Head and Neck Cancer Staging

Sarah Elizabeth Bailey
Department of Otolaryngology and Communicative Sciences, University of Mississippi Medical Center, Jackson, MS, USA

Introduction

The extent of cancer at the time of diagnosis is a key factor used to define treatment and to gauge the probability of a successful outcome after treatment. Cancer staging systems allow for an objective assessment of the anatomical extent of disease, which gives a meaningful and functional description. By codifying the extent of cancer, data recording is standardized and this imparts precision on both the clinical description and the histopathological classification of malignant neoplasms. Through achieving this, staging systems serve multiple functions, which include predicting prognosis, assisting with treatment planning, assessing treatment results, allowing comparisons to be made of clinical data, facilitating information exchange between treatment centers, and contributing to the ongoing investigation of cancer (Edge et al. 2010).

Accurate staging of a cancer is based on all available clinical information including physical and endoscopic examination, radiographic imaging, intraoperative findings, and histopathological findings. There are three staging systems used in the United States, with the TNM (tumor, node, and metastasis) staging system being the most widely used among clinicians (Edge et al. 2010).

The TNM Staging System

The TNM staging system was developed in France between 1943 and 1952. It has since undergone multiple revisions, such that the most recent seventh edition, published in 2010, is currently in use. It is based on published evidence, with international consensus being utilized in areas of controversy. The TNM staging system is applicable to all sites and helps prognosticate by documenting the disease burden at the primary site, in the neck (metastatic lymphadenopathy), and at distant sites (distant metastases). It is comprised of three categories: T – the characteristics of the primary site tumor including size, location, or both; N – the degree of regional lymph node involvement; and M – the presence or absence of distant metastases. The addition of numbers to each category is indicative of the extent of malignant disease (Edge et al. 2010).

Furthermore, the specific TNM status of each patient may be tabulated to a numerical status of Stage I, II, III, or IV with specific subdivisions for each stage denoted with an A, B, or C status. In general, early stage disease is denoted as Stage I with advanced stage disease denoted Stage IV. The grouping is adopted in order to ensure that each group is essentially homogeneous with respect to survival, and that the survival rates of these groups for each cancer site are unique (Edge et al. 2010).

Cancers were first divided into groups according to stages based on the fact that localized disease had higher survival rates than more extensive or disseminated disease. Traditionally, these groups were referred to as early cases and late cases, implying progression with time. Although the anatomical extent of disease, as categorized by TNM, is a very powerful prognostic indicator in cancer, it is recognized that many factors have a significant impact on predicting outcomes. So in actuality, the stage of disease at the time of diagnosis may be related to multiple other factors such as tumor type, unique tumor characteristics, concurrent comorbidities, and the tumor-host relationship, rather than simply the growth rate and extension of the malignancy. To that end, some prognostic factors have already been incorporated into stage grouping, such as grade in soft tissue sarcoma and age in thyroid cancer. One such potential prognostic marker that may have a significant impact is the human papillomavirus status in oropharyngeal malignancies. Therefore, with advances in cancer knowledge and in other prognostic markers, the TNM classification and stage groupings will continue to be updated periodically in order to remain clinically relevant (Edge et al. 2010).

General Rules of the TNM System

The first general rule of the TNM system dictates that all cases should be confirmed microscopically. The second general rule describes two classifications for each anatomic site. These two classifications include a *clinical* classification or a pretreatment clinical classification, designated TNM or cTNM, and a *pathological* or postsurgical histopathological classification, designated pTNM. In general, cTNM is the basis for the choice of treatment and pTNM is the basis for prognostic assessment and may determine adjuvant treatment. The clinical classification is based on evidence collected from physical examination, imaging, endoscopy, biopsy, or surgical exploration, while the pathological classification is based on the pretreatment

evidence supplemented or modified by the additional evidence acquired from surgery and pathological examination. The pathological assessment of the primary tumor (pT) involves resection of the primary tumor or biopsy adequate to evaluate the highest pT category. The pathological assessment of the regional lymph nodes (pN) involves removal of nodes adequate to confirm the absence of regional lymph node metastasis (pN0) and sufficient to evaluate the highest pN category. The pathological assessment of distant metastasis (pM) involves microscopic examination (Edge et al. 2010).

The third general rule states that once the TNM classification and stage grouping are established for a malignant lesion, they cannot be changed. This is because the clinical stage is essential to select and evaluate efficacy of therapy, while the pathological stage provides the most accurate data to approximate prognosis and calculate outcomes (Edge et al. 2010). Next, the fourth general rule states that if there is uncertainty regarding the correct T, N, or M category for a particular case, then the less advanced category should be chosen, which will then be reflected in the stage grouping.

The fifth general rule outlines the staging in the instance of multiple simultaneous tumors in one organ and states that the tumor with the highest category should be classified and the multiplicity or the number of tumors should be designated in parentheses, e.g., T2(m) or T2(3) (Edge et al. 2010). Finally, the sixth general rule states that definitions of TNM categories and stage grouping may be telescoped or expanded for clinical or research purposes providing the basic definitions recommended are not changed. For example, any T, N, or M can be divided into subgroups (Edge et al. 2010).

TNM Classifications

For all sites of the head and neck, the TNM clinical and pathological classification systems share the same general definitions for the primary tumor (T), regional lymph node metastasis (N), and distant metastases (M). Subdivisions of some main categories are described for sites requiring greater specificity (e.g., T1a, 1b or N2a, 2b or M1a, 1b) (Edge et al. 2010) (Table 1).

Head and Neck Cancer Staging, Table 1 General definitions of clinical and pathological classifications for primary tumors, regional lymph nodes, and distant metastases of all head and neck sites (Edge et al. 2010)

Primary tumor

Clinical classification (T or cT)		Pathological classification (pT)	
TX	Primary tumor cannot be assessed	pTX	Primary tumor cannot be assessed histologically
T0	No evidence of primary tumor	pT0	No histological evidence of primary tumor
Tis	Carcinoma in situ	pTis	Carcinoma in situ
T1 ↓ T2 ↓ T3 ↓ T4	Increasing size and/or local extent of the primary tumor	pT1 ↓ pT2 ↓ pT3 ↓ pT4	Increasing size and/or local extent of primary tumor histologically

Regional lymph nodes[a]

Clinical classification (N or cN)		Pathological classification (pN)[b]	
NX	Regional lymph nodes cannot be assessed	pNX	Regional lymph nodes cannot be assessed histologically
N0	No regional lymph node metastasis	pN0	No regional lymph node metastasis histologically
N1 ↓ N2 ↓ N3	Increasing involvement of regional lymph nodes	pN1 ↓ pN2 ↓ pN3	Increasing involvement of regional lymph nodes histologically

Distant metastasis[c]

Clinical classification (M or cM)		Pathological classification (pM)	
M0	No distant metastasis	pM1[d]	Distant metastasis microscopically confirmed
M1	Distant metastasis		

[a]Midline nodes are considered ipsilateral except in the thyroid
[b]Histological examination of selective neck dissection specimen ordinarily includes ≥6 lymph nodes, while radical or modified neck dissection specimen ordinarily includes ≥10 lymph nodes. If the nodes are negative, but the specimen is inadequate, the classification is pN0
[c]The MX category is considered inappropriate because clinical assessment of metastasis can be based on physical examination alone; thus, by using MX, exclusion from staging may occur
[d]pM0 is not a valid category

Further guidelines for pathological classification of regional lymph nodes outline that direct extension of the primary tumor into lymph nodes is classified as lymph node metastasis. Additionally, tumor deposits (satellites), i.e., macro- or microscopic nests or nodules, in the lymph drainage area of a primary carcinoma without histological evidence of residual lymph node in the nodule, may represent discontinuous spread, venous invasion (V1/2), or a totally replaced lymph node. If a nodule is considered by the pathology to be a totally replaced lymph node, it is documented as a positive lymph node, and each such nodule is counted separately as a lymph node in the final pN determination (Edge et al. 2010).

Furthermore, metastasis in any lymph node other than regionally is classified as a distant metastasis. In addition, when size is a criterion for pN classification, measurement is made of the metastasis, not of the entire lymph node. Also, for cases with micrometastasis only, i.e., no metastasis larger than 0.2 cm, can be identified by the addition of "(mi)," e.g., pN1(mi) or pN2(mi). Finally, the number of resected and positive nodes should be documented (Edge et al. 2010).

Head and Neck Cancer Staging, Table 2 Designations when sentinel lymph node assessment is attempted (Edge et al. 2010)

Sentinel lymph nodes (sn)	
pNX (sn)	Sentinel lymph node could not be assessed
pN0 (sn)	No sentinel lymph node metastasis
pN1 (sn)	Sentinel lymph node metastasis

Head and Neck Cancer Staging, Table 3 Histopathological grading is the same for all head and neck sites except for thyroid and mucosal malignant melanoma (Edge et al. 2010)

Histopathological grading (G)	
GX	Grade of differentiation cannot be assessed
G1	Well differentiated
G2	Moderately differentiated
G3	Poorly differentiated
G4	Undifferentiated

Head and Neck Cancer Staging, Table 4 Additional descriptors in the TNM system (Edge et al. 2010)

Additional descriptors	
m	Indicates the presence of multiple primary tumors at a single site
y	Identifies cases in which classification is performed during or following initial multimodality therapy and categorizes the extent of disease actually present at the time of that examination and not prior to multimodality therapy
r	Identifies recurrent tumors classified after a disease-free interval
a	Indicates that classification is first determined at autopsy

Head and Neck Cancer Staging, Table 5 Optional descriptors for the TNM system (Edge et al. 2010)

Lymphatic invasion (L)	
LX	Lymphatic invasion cannot be assessed
L0	No lymphatic invasion
L1	Lymphatic invasion
Venous invasion (V)	
VX	Venous invasion cannot be assessed
V0	No venous invasion
V1	Microscopic venous invasion
V2	Macroscopic venous invasion[a]
Perineural invasion (Pn)	
PnX	Perineural invasion cannot be assessed
Pn0	No perineural invasion
Pn1	Perineural invasion is present

[a]Note: Macroscopic involvement of the wall of veins (without tumor inside the veins) is classified as V2

Head and Neck Cancer Staging, Table 6 Classification of residual tumor in the TNM system (Edge et al. 2010)

Residual tumor (R)	
RX	Presence of residual tumor cannot be assessed
R0	No residual tumor
R1	Microscopic residual tumor
R2	Macroscopic residual tumor

Sentinel Lymph Node

The sentinel lymph node(s) is the first lymph node to receive lymphatic drainage from a primary tumor. If it contains metastatic disease, this indicates that other lymph nodes may contain tumor and vice versa (Edge et al. 2010) (Table 2).

Isolated Tumor Cells

Isolated tumor cells (ITC) are single tumor cells or small clusters of cells not more than 0.2 mm in greatest dimension that are usually detected by routine H and E stains or immunohistochemistry. ITC typically lack evidence of metastatic activity and penetration of vascular or lymphatic walls; therefore, cases with ITC in lymph nodes or at distant sites should be classified as N0 or M0, respectively (Edge et al. 2010).

Histopathological Grading

In most sites, further information regarding the primary tumor may be recorded by histopathological grading. Grades 3 and 4 can be combined in some circumstances as G3-4, indicating poorly differentiated or undifferentiated cancers. The bone and soft tissue sarcoma classifications also use "high grade" and "low grade" (Edge et al. 2010) (Table 3).

Head and Neck Cancer Staging, Table 7 Staging of primary tumors of the oral cavity (Edge et al. 2010)

Primary tumor (T)	
TX	Primary tumor cannot be assessed
T0	No evidence of primary tumor
Tis	Carcinoma in situ
T1	Tumor ≤2 cm in greatest dimension
T2	Tumor >2 cm but ≤4 cm in greatest dimension
T3	Tumor ≥4 cm in greatest dimension
T4a	*Moderately advanced local disease* Lip: tumor invades through cortical bone (not superficial erosion alone of bone/tooth socket by gingival primary), inferior alveolar nerve, floor of mouth, or skin of face (i.e., chin or nose) Oral cavity: tumor invades adjacent structures only (cortical bone of mandible or maxilla, deep (extrinsic) muscle of tongue [genioglossus, hyoglossus, palatoglossus, and styloglossus], maxillary sinus, or skin of face)
T4b	*Very advanced local disease* Tumor invades masticator space, pterygoid plates, or skull base and/or encases internal carotid artery

Head and Neck Cancer Staging, Table 8 Staging of regional lymph nodes of all head and neck sites except thyroid, nasopharynx, cutaneous melanoma, cutaneous carcinoma of the eyelid, and Merkel cell carcinoma (Edge et al. 2010)

Regional lymph nodes (N)	
NX	Regional lymph nodes cannot be assessed
N0	No regional lymph node metastasis
N1	Metastasis in a single ipsilateral lymph node, ≤3 cm in greatest dimension
N2	Metastasis in a single ipsilateral lymph node >3 cm but ≤6 cm in greatest dimension; or multiple ipsilateral lymph nodes, none ≥6 cm in greatest dimension; or bilateral or contralateral lymph nodes, none ≥6 cm in greatest dimension
N2a	Metastasis in a single ipsilateral lymph node >3 cm but ≤6 cm in greatest dimension
N2b	Metastasis in multiple ipsilateral lymph nodes, none >6 cm in greatest dimension
N2c	Metastasis in bilateral or contralateral lymph nodes, none >6 cm in greatest dimension
N3	Metastasis in a lymph node >6 cm in greatest dimension

Head and Neck Cancer Staging, Table 9 Staging of distant metastases in all head and neck sites except cutaneous melanoma, bone sarcoma, and Merkel cell carcinoma (Edge et al. 2010)

Distant metastasis (M)	
M0	No distant metastasis
M1	Distant metastasis

Head and Neck Cancer Staging, Table 10 Anatomic stage and prognostic groups of all head and neck sites except nasopharynx, cutaneous carcinoma of the eyelid, sarcomas, and thyroid (Edge et al. 2010)

Anatomic stage/prognostic groups			
Stage 0	Tis	N0	M0
Stage I	T1	N0	M0
Stage II	T2	N0	M0
Stage III	T3	N0	M0
	T1	N1	M0
	T2	N1	M0
	T3	N1	M0
Stage IVA	T4a	N0	M0
	T4a	N1	M0
	T1	N2	M0
	T2	N2	M0
	T3	N2	M0
	T4a	N2	M0
Stage IVB	T4b	Any N	M0
	Any T	N3	M0
Stage IVC	Any T	Any N	M1

Additional Descriptors

For identification of special cases in the TNM or pTNM classification, the r, a, m, and y symbols are used to indicate cases needing different analysis and do not affect the stage grouping (Table 4).

Optional Descriptors

See Table 5.

Residual Tumor Classification

The absence or presence of residual tumor after treatment is described by the symbol R, which supplements

Head and Neck Cancer Staging, Table 11 Staging of oropharyngeal primary tumors (Edge et al. 2010)

Primary tumor (T)	
TX	Primary tumor cannot be assessed
T0	No evidence of primary tumor
Tis	Carcinoma in situ
T1	Tumor ≤2 cm in greatest dimension
T2	Tumor >2 cm but ≤4 cm in greatest dimension
T3	Tumor ≥4 cm in greatest dimension or extension to lingual surface of epiglottis
T4a	*Moderately advanced local disease* Tumor invades the larynx, extrinsic muscle of tongue, medial pterygoid, hard palate, or mandible[a]
T4b	*Very advanced local disease* Tumor invades lateral pterygoid muscle, pterygoid plates, lateral nasopharynx, or skull base or encases carotid artery

[a]Mucosal extension to lingual surface of epiglottis from primary tumors of base of tongue and vallecula does not constitute invasion of larynx

Head and Neck Cancer Staging, Table 12 Staging of hypopharyngeal primary tumor (Edge et al. 2010)

Primary tumor (T)	
TX	Primary tumor cannot be assessed
T0	No evidence of primary tumor
Tis	Carcinoma in situ
T1	Tumor limited to one subsite of hypopharynx and/or ≤2 cm in greatest dimension
T2	Tumor invades more than one subsite of the hypopharynx or an adjacent site, or measures >2 cm but ≤4 cm in greatest dimension without fixation of the hemilarynx
T3	Tumor ≥4 cm in greatest dimension or with fixation of hemilarynx or extension to esophagus
T4a	*Moderately advanced local disease* Tumor invades thyroid/cricoid cartilage, hyoid bone, thyroid gland, or central compartment soft tissue[a]
T4b	*Very advanced local disease* Tumor invades prevertebral fascia, encases carotid artery, or involves mediastinal structures

[a]Central compartment soft tissue includes prelaryngeal strap muscles and subcutaneous fat

TNM and pTNM and indicates tumor status following treatment. It reflects the effects of therapy, influences further therapeutic procedures and is a strong prognostic predictor (Edge et al. 2010) (Table 6).

Classification of Anatomic Sites

Tumors of the head and neck encompass a variety of cancers, arising from a variety of sites. Head and neck cancers are organized according to the major anatomic sites of origin, which may be further subdivided into anatomic subsites. The major sites include the oral cavity, the pharynx (oropharynx, hypopharynx, nasopharynx), the larynx (supraglottis, glottis, and subglottis), the nasal cavity and ethmoid sinus, the maxillary sinus, the salivary glands, and the thyroid gland, as well as the cervical esophagus, mucosal malignant melanoma, and those tumors arising in the soft tissues and bone, and skin of the head and neck (Edge et al. 2010).

Oral Cavity
The anterior border of the oral cavity is the junction of the skin with the vermilion border of the lips and the posterior border is the junction of the hard and soft palates superiorly, the anterior tonsillar pillars laterally, and the circumvallate papillae inferiorly. The major subsites of the oral cavity are the lip, gingiva, anterior two third tongue, floor of mouth, buccal mucosa, upper and lower alveolar ridges, hard palate, and retromolar trigone, which consists of the mucosa overlying the anterior aspect of the ascending ramus of the mandible (Tables 7–10).

Oropharynx
The oropharynx begins at the junction of the hard and soft palates superiorly and the circumvallate papillae inferiorly and extends from the level of the soft palate superiorly, which separates it from the nasopharynx and to the level of the hyoid bone inferiorly, where the hypopharynx begins. The subsites of the oropharynx are the tonsil, the anterior and posterior tonsillar pillars, the glossotonsillar sulci, base of tongue, soft palate and uvula, and the lateral and posterior pharyngeal walls (Table 11).

Hypopharynx
The superior boundary of the hypopharynx is the hyoid bone, where it is contiguous with the oropharynx and it extends inferiorly to the cricopharyngeus muscle, where it meets the cervical esophagus. The major subsites are the pyriform sinuses, the postcricoid

Head and Neck Cancer Staging, Table 13 Staging of laryngeal primary tumors (Edge et al. 2010)

Primary tumor (T)	
TX	Primary tumor cannot be assessed
T0	No evidence of primary tumor
Tis	Carcinoma in situ
Supraglottis	
T1	Tumor limited to one subsite of supraglottis with normal vocal cord mobility
T2	Tumor invades mucosa of more than one adjacent subsite of supraglottis or glottis or region outside of supraglottis (mucosa of base of tongue, vallecula, medial wall of pyriform sinus) without fixation of larynx
T3	Tumor limited to larynx with vocal cord fixation and/or invades any of the following: postcricoid area, preepiglottic space, paraglottic space, and/or inner cortex of thyroid cartilage
T4a	*Moderately advanced local disease* Tumor invades through the thyroid cartilage and/or invades tissues beyond the larynx (trachea, soft tissue of neck including deep extrinsic muscles of the tongue, strap muscles, thyroid, or esophagus)
T4b	*Very advanced local disease* Tumor invades prevertebral space, encases carotid artery, or invades mediastinal structures
Glottis	
T1	Tumor limited to vocal cord(s) (may involve anterior or posterior commissure) with normal mobility
	T1a — Tumor limited to one vocal cord
	T1b — Tumor involves both vocal cords
T2	Tumor extends to supraglottis and/or subglottis, and/or with impaired vocal cord mobility
T3	Tumor limited to the larynx with vocal cord fixation and/or invasion of paraglottic space, and/or inner cortex of the thyroid cartilage
T4a	*Moderately advanced local disease* Tumor invades through the outer cortex of the thyroid cartilage and/or invades tissues beyond the larynx (trachea, soft tissues of neck including deep extrinsic muscle of tongue, strap muscles, thyroid, or esophagus)
T4b	*Very advanced local disease* Tumor invades prevertebral space, encases carotid artery, or invades mediastinal structures
Subglottis	
T1	Tumor limited to the subglottis
T2	Tumor extends to vocal cord(s) with normal or impaired mobility
T3	Tumor limited to larynx with vocal cord fixation
T4a	*Moderately advanced local disease* Tumor invades cricoid or thyroid cartilage and/or invades tissues beyond the larynx (trachea, soft tissues of neck including deep extrinsic muscles of tongue, strap muscles, thyroid, or esophagus)
T4b	*Very advanced local disease* Tumor invades prevertebral space, encases carotid artery, or invades mediastinal structures

region, and the lateral and posterior pharyngeal walls (Table 12).

Larynx

The larynx is bordered by the oropharynx superiorly, the trachea inferiorly, and the hypopharynx laterally and posteriorly. The larynx is subdivided vertically by the vocal cords into the supraglottic, glottic, and subglottic subsites. The supraglottic larynx includes the epiglottis, which has both lingual and laryngeal surfaces, the false vocal cords, the arytenoid cartilages, and the aryepiglottic folds. The glottic larynx includes the true vocal cords, the anterior and posterior commissures, and the region 1 cm below the plane of the true vocal cords. The vocal cords are lined with stratified squamous epithelium, which contrasts with the pseudostratified ciliated respiratory mucosa lining the remainder of the larynx. The subglottic larynx starts 1 cm below the vocal folds and continues to the inferior aspect of the cricoid cartilage.

The TNM classification system for the larynx applies to epithelial malignancies only and

Head and Neck Cancer Staging, Table 14 Staging of primary tumors in the nasopharynx (Edge et al. 2010)

Primary tumor (T)	
TX	Primary tumor cannot be assessed
T0	No evidence of primary tumor
Tis	Carcinoma in situ
T1	Tumor confined to nasopharynx, or tumor extends to oropharynx and/or nasal cavity without parapharyngeal extension[a]
T2	Tumor with parapharyngeal extension[a]
T3	Tumor involves bony structures of skull base and/or paranasal sinuses
T4	Tumor with intracranial extension and/or involvement of cranial nerves, hypopharynx, orbit, or with extension to the infratemporal fossa/masticator space

[a]Parapharyngeal extension denotes posterolateral infiltration of tumor

Head and Neck Cancer Staging, Table 16 Anatomic stage and prognostic groups of the nasopharynx (Edge et al. 2010)

Anatomic stage/prognostic groups			
Stage 0	Tis	N0	M0
Stage I	T1	N0	M0
Stage II	T1	N1	M0
	T2	N0	M0
	T2	N1	M0
Stage III	T1	N2	M0
	T2	N2	M0
	T3	N0	M0
	T3	N1	M0
	T3	N2	M0
Stage IVA	T4	N0	M0
	T4	N1	M0
	T4	N2	M0
Stage IVB	Any T	N3	M0
Stage IVC	Any T	Any N	M1

Head and Neck Cancer Staging, Table 15 Staging of regional lymph nodes of the nasopharynx (Edge et al. 2010)

Regional lymph nodes (N)		
NX	Regional lymph nodes cannot be assessed	
N0	No regional lymph node metastasis	
N1	Unilateral metastasis in cervical lymph node(s), ≤6 cm in greatest dimension, above the supraclavicular fossa, and/or unilateral or bilateral, retropharyngeal lymph nodes ≤6 cm in greatest dimension	
N2	Bilateral metastasis in cervical lymph node(s), ≤6 cm in greatest dimension, above the supraclavicular fossa	
N3	Metastasis in a lymph node >6 cm in greatest dimension and/or to supraclavicular fossa	
	N3a	>6 cm in greatest dimension
	N3b	Extension to the supraclavicular fossa

nonepithelial tumors such as those of lymphoid tissue, soft tissue, cartilage, or bone are not included (Edge et al. 2010) (Table 13).

Nasopharynx

The nasopharynx is bounded anteriorly by the choanae at the back of the nose and at the level of the soft palate inferiorly, the nasopharynx meets the superior oropharynx. The nasopharynx includes the vault, the lateral and posterior walls, and the superior surface of the soft palate.

Nasopharyngeal carcinoma differs from other head and neck carcinomas in a variety of ways including epidemiology, histology, natural history, and response to treatment. Therefore, the TNM staging system varies from the majority of other head and neck carcinomas (Edge et al. 2010) (Tables 14–16).

Nasal Cavity and Paranasal Sinuses

The paranasal sinuses consist of the maxillary, frontal, ethmoid, and sphenoid sinuses. This region includes the lining of the nasal cavity (medial maxillary walls) as well as the nasal septum (Table 17).

Salivary Glands

The major salivary glands include the parotid, submandibular, and sublingual glands. These types of cancers include mucoepidermoid carcinoma, adenocarcinoma, adenoid cystic carcinoma, acinic cell carcinoma, carcinoma ex-pleomorphic adenoma, polymorphous low grade carcinoma, salivary duct carcinoma, primary squamous cell carcinoma, and primary small cell carcinoma. Minor salivary gland tumors are classified according to the anatomic site of origin such as the oral cavity or larynx (Edge et al. 2010) (Table 18).

Thyroid Gland

The four major histopathological types of thyroid cancer include papillary carcinoma, follicular

Head and Neck Cancer Staging, Table 17 Staging of nasal cavity and paranasal sinus primary tumors (Edge et al. 2010)

Primary tumor (T)	
TX	Primary tumor cannot be assessed
T0	No evidence of primary tumor
Tis	Carcinoma in situ
Maxillary sinus	
T1	Tumor limited to maxillary sinus mucosa without erosion or destruction of bone
T2	Tumor causing bone erosion or destruction including extension into hard palate and/or middle nasal meatus, except extension to posterior wall of maxillary sinus and pterygoid plates
T3	Tumor invades any of the following: bone of posterior wall of maxillary sinus, subcutaneous tissues, floor or medial wall of orbit, pterygoid fossa, ethmoid sinuses
T4a	*Moderately advanced local disease* Tumor invades anterior orbital contents, skin of cheek, pterygoid plates, infratemporal fossa, cribriform plate, sphenoid or frontal sinuses
T4b	*Very advanced local disease* Tumor invades any of the following: orbital apex, dura, brain, middle cranial fossa, cranial nerves other than maxillary division of trigeminal nerve (V_2), nasopharynx, or clivus
Nasal cavity and ethmoid sinus	
T1	Tumor limited to any one subsite, with or without bony invasion
T2	Tumor invading two subsites in a single region or extending to involve an adjacent region within the nasoethmoidal complex, with or without bony invasion
T3	Tumor extends to invade the medial wall or floor of the orbit, maxillary sinus, palate, or cribriform plate
T4a	*Moderately advanced local disease* Tumor invades any of the following: anterior orbital contents, skin of nose or cheek, minimal extension to anterior cranial fossa, pterygoid plates, sphenoid or frontal sinuses
T4b	*Very advanced local disease* Tumor invades any of the following: orbital apex, dura, brain, middle cranial fossa, cranial nerves other than V_2, nasopharynx, or clivus

Head and Neck Cancer Staging, Table 18 Staging of primary tumors of the major salivary glands (Edge et al. 2010)

Primary tumor (T)	
TX	Primary tumor cannot be assessed
T0	No evidence of primary tumor
Tis	Carcinoma in situ
T1	Tumor ≤2 cm in greatest dimension without extraparenchymal extension
T2	Tumor >2 cm but ≤4 cm in greatest dimension without extraparenchymal extension
T3	Tumor ≥4 cm in greatest dimension and/or extraparenchymal extension
T4a	*Moderately advanced local disease* Tumor invades the skin, mandible, ear canal, and/or facial nerve
T4b	*Very advanced local disease* Tumor invades the skull base and/or pterygoid plates, and/or encases carotid artery

Head and Neck Cancer Staging, Table 19 Staging of well-differentiated primary tumors of the thyroid gland (Edge et al. 2010)

Primary tumor (T)		
TX	Primary tumor cannot be assessed	
T0	No evidence of primary tumor	
Tis	Carcinoma in situ	
T1	Tumor ≤2 cm in greatest dimension and limited to thyroid	
	T1a	Tumor ≤1 cm
	T1b	Tumor >1 cm but ≤2 cm
T2	Tumor >2 cm but ≤4 cm in greatest dimension and limited to thyroid	
T3	Tumor ≥4 cm in greatest dimension, and is limited to the thyroid or any tumor with minimal extrathyroid extension (extension to sternothyroid muscle or perithyroid soft tissues)	
T4a	*Moderately advanced local disease* Tumor of any size extends beyond the thyroid capsule to invade subcutaneous soft tissues, larynx, trachea, esophagus, or recurrent laryngeal nerve	
T4b	*Very advanced local disease* Tumor invades prevertebral fascia or encases carotid artery or mediastinal vessels	

carcinoma, medullary carcinoma, and anaplastic (undifferentiated) carcinoma. The TNM staging system of cancers incorporates the age at diagnosis into stage designation for well-differentiated thyroid cancer. Additionally, all anaplastic carcinomas are considered T4 tumors and Stage IV (Edge et al. 2010) (Tables 19–24).

Head and Neck Cancer Staging, Table 20 Staging of anaplastic carcinomas of the thyroid gland (Edge et al. 2010)

Primary tumor (T)	
T4a	Intrathyroidal anaplastic carcinoma (surgically resectable)
T4b	Extrathyroidal anaplastic carcinoma (surgically unresectable)

Head and Neck Cancer Staging, Table 21 Staging of regional lymph nodes of the thyroid gland (Edge et al. 2010)

Regional lymph nodes (N) – include central compartment, lateral cervical, and upper mediastinal lymph nodes		
NX	Regional lymph nodes cannot be assessed	
N0	No regional lymph node metastasis	
N1	Regional lymph node metastasis is present	
	N1a	Metastasis to level VI (pretracheal, paratracheal, and prelaryngeal/Delphian lymph nodes)
	N1b	Metastasis to unilateral, bilateral, or contralateral cervical or superior mediastinal lymph nodes

Head and Neck Cancer Staging, Table 22 Anatomic stage and prognostic groups of well-differentiated thyroid cancer (Edge et al. 2010)

Anatomic stage/prognostic groups			
Papillary or follicular: <45 years old			
Stage I	Any T	Any N	M0
Stage II	Any T	Any N	M1
Papillary or follicular: >45 years old			
Stage I	T1a	N0	M0
	T1b	N0	M0
Stage II	T2	N0	M0
Stage III	T3	N0	M0
	T1	N1a	M0
	T2	N1a	M0
	T3	N1a	M0
Stage IVA	T1	N1b	M0
	T2	N1b	M0
	T3	N1b	M0
	T4a	N0	M0
	T4a	N1	M0
Stage IVB	T4b	Any N	M0
Stage IVC	Any T	Any N	M1

Cervical Esophagus

The cervical esophagus is the portion of the esophagus that extends to the thoracic inlet with 0the cricopharyngeus muscle representing the transition between the hypopharynx and the cervical esophagus. The majority of cervical esophageal malignancies are comprised of squamous cell carcinoma, while adenocarcinoma occurs most commonly in the distal esophagus (Tables 25–27).

Head and Neck Cancer Staging, Table 23 Anatomic stage and prognostic groups of medullary carcinoma of the thyroid gland (Edge et al. 2010)

Anatomic stage/prognostic groups			
Stage I	T1a	N0	M0
	T1b	N0	M0
Stage II	T2	N0	M0
	T3	N0	M0
Stage III	T1	N1a	M0
	T2	N1a	M0
	T3	N1a	M0
Stage IVA	T1	N1b	M0
	T2	N1b	M0
	T3	N1b	M0
	T4a	Any N	M0
Stage IVB	T4b	Any N	M0
Stage IVC	Any T	Any N	M1

Head and Neck Cancer Staging, Table 24 Anatomic stage and prognostic groups of anaplastic carcinoma of the thyroid gland (Edge et al. 2010)

Anatomic stage/prognostic groups			
Anaplastic carcinoma			
Stage IVA	T4a	Any N	M0
Stage IVB	T4b	Any N	M0
Stage IVC	Any T	Any N	M1

Head and Neck Cancer Staging, Table 25 Staging of primary tumors of esophageal squamous cell carcinoma (Edge et al. 2010)

Primary tumor (T)		
TX	Primary tumor cannot be assessed	
T0	No evidence of primary tumor	
Tis	High grade dysplasia[a]	
T1	Tumor invades lamina propria, muscularis mucosae, or submucosa	
	T1a	Tumor invades lamina propria or muscularis mucosae
	T1b	Tumor invades submucosa
T2	Tumor invades muscularis propria	
T3	Tumor invades adventitia	
T4	Tumor invades adjacent structures	
	T4a	Resectable tumor invading pleura, pericardium, or diaphragm
	T4b	Unresectable tumor invading other adjacent structures, such as the aorta, vertebral body, and trachea

[a]High grade dysplasia (HGD) includes all noninvasive neoplastic epithelia that were formerly called carcinoma in situ, which is no longer used for columnar mucosa

Cutaneous Cancers

The TNM classification system applies to carcinomas of the skin (squamous and basal cell carcinomas), malignant melanoma of the skin, and to Merkel cell carcinoma. The anatomical sites include the lip (excluding the vermillion border), eyelid, external ear, the scalp and neck, and all other areas of the face (Edge et al. 2010).

Cutaneous malignant melanoma classifications apply to all skin sites including eye. Histologic factors incorporated into the TNM staging are well known prognostic factors and include the thickness of the primary tumor in cutaneous melanoma, the presence or absence of mucosal ulceration, and the mitotic rate.

Additionally, serum LDH is an important, independent prognostic factor in patients with disseminated melanoma and is thus incorporated into the M staging (Edge et al. 2010) (Tables 28–39).

Mucosal Melanoma

Mucosal melanomas are recognized as a distinct subtype from cutaneous melanoma and are associated with a worse prognosis; therefore, no stage I or stage II is recognized. Additionally, tumor of any size limited to the epithelium is T3 disease (Edge et al. 2010) (Tables 40–42).

Bone and Soft Tissue

Head and neck sarcomas are classified according to their site of origin: soft tissues such as cartilage and peripheral nerve tissue or bone. Soft tissue sarcomas include angiosarcoma, hemangiopericytoma, malignant fibrous histiocytoma, synovial sarcoma, chrondrosarcoma, rhabdomyosarcoma, malignant schwannoma, liposarcoma, leiomyosarcoma, fibrosarcoma, alveolar soft part sarcoma, and Kaposi sarcoma. Bone sarcomas include osteosarcoma and Ewing sarcoma. Sarcomas are staged based on a two-tiered grading system, either high or low grade (Edge et al. 2010) (Tables 43–49).

Head and Neck Cancer Staging, Table 26 Staging of regional lymph nodes in esophageal squamous cell carcinoma (Edge et al. 2010)

Regional lymph nodes (N)	
NX	Regional lymph node(s) cannot be assessed
N0	No regional lymph node metastasis
N1	Metastasis in 1–2 regional lymph nodes
N2	Metastasis in 3–6 regional lymph nodes
N3	Metastasis ≥7 regional lymph nodes

Head and Neck Cancer Staging, Table 27 Anatomic stage and prognostic groups for esophageal squamous cell carcinoma (Edge et al. 2010)

Anatomic stage/prognostic groups					
Stage 0	Tis (HGD)	N0	M0	G 1, X	Any tumor location
Stage IA	T1	N0	M0	G 1, X	Any tumor location
Stage IB	T1	N0	M0	G 2,3	Any tumor location
	T2-3	N0	M0	G 1, X	Lower tumor location, X
Stage IIA	T2-3	N0	M0	G 1, X	Upper, middle tumor location
	T2-3	N0	M0	G 2-3	Lower tumor location, X
Stage IIB	T2-3	N0	M0	G 2-3	Upper, middle tumor location
	T1-2	N1	M0	Any G	Any tumor location
Stage IIIA	T1-2	N2	M0	Any G	Any tumor location
	T3	N1	M0	Any G	Any tumor location
	T4a	N0	M0	Any G	Any tumor location
Stage IIIB	T3	N2	M0	Any G	Any tumor location
Stage IIIC	T4a	N1-2	M0	Any G	Any tumor location
	T4b	Any N	M0	Any G	Any tumor location
	Any	N3	M0	Any G	Any tumor location
Stage IV	Any	Any N	M1	Any G	Any tumor location

Head and Neck Cancer Staging, Table 28 Staging of primary tumor cutaneous carcinomas with the exception of the eyelid (Edge et al. 2010)

Primary tumor (T)	
TX	Primary tumor cannot be assessed
T0	No evidence of primary tumor
Tis	Carcinoma in situ
T1	Carcinoma <2 cm in greatest dimension, with <2 high-risk features[a]
T2	Carcinoma >2 cm in greatest dimension, or tumor of any size with at least 2 high-risk features[a]
T3	Tumor invasion of the maxilla, mandible, orbit, or temporal bone
T4	Tumor invasion of the skeleton (appendicular or axial) or with perineural involvement of the skull base

[a]High-risk features for the primary tumor (T) staging:
Depth/invasion: >2 mm thickness, Clark level ≥IV, perineural invasion
Anatomic location: primary site ear, primary site non-hair-bearing lip
Differentiation: poorly differentiated or undifferentiated

Head and Neck Cancer Staging, Table 29 Staging of primary tumor cutaneous carcinomas of the eyelid (Edge et al. 2010)

Primary tumor (T)	
TX	Primary tumor cannot be assessed
T0	No evidence of primary tumor
Tis	Carcinoma in situ
T1	Tumor ≤5 mm in greatest dimension not invading the tarsal plate or eyelid margin
T2a	Tumor >5 mm but ≤10 mm in greatest dimension or any tumor invading the tarsal plate or eyelid margin
T2b	Tumor >10 mm but ≤20 mm in greatest dimension or involves full thickness eyelid
T3a	Tumor >20 mm in greatest dimension or any tumor invading adjacent ocular or orbital structures or any tumor with perineural invasion
T3b	Tumor whose complete resection requires enucleation, exenteration, or bone resection
T4	Tumor is not respectable due to extensive invasion of ocular, orbital, craniofacial structures, or brain

Conclusion

The TNM system has standardized the description and reporting of cancers throughout the world. It is primarily an anatomic system that helps prognosticate by

Head and Neck Cancer Staging, Table 30 Staging of regional lymph nodes in cutaneous carcinomas of the eyelid (Edge et al. 2010)

Regional lymph nodes (N)	
NX	Regional lymph nodes cannot be assessed
N0	No regional lymph node metastases
N1	Regional lymph node metastases present

Head and Neck Cancer Staging, Table 31 Anatomic stage and prognostic groups of cutaneous carcinomas of the eyelid (Edge et al. 2010)

Anatomic stage/prognostic groups			
Stage 0	Tis	N0	M0
Stage IA	T1	N0	M0
Stage IB	T2a	N0	M0
Stage IC	T2b	N0	M0
Stage II	T3a	N0	M0
Stage IIIA	T3b	N0	M0
Stage IIIB	Any T	N1	M0
Stage IIIC	T4	Any N	M0
Stage IV	Any T	Any N	M1

Head and Neck Cancer Staging, Table 32 Staging of cutaneous melanoma primary tumors (Edge et al. 2010)

Primary tumor (T)		
TX	Primary tumor cannot be assessed	
Tis	Melanoma in situ	
T1	≤1.0 mm thickness	
	T1a	Without ulceration and mitosis <1/mm^2
	T1b	With ulceration or mitoses ≥1/mm^2
T2	1.01–2.0 mm thickness	
	T2a	Without ulceration
	T2b	With ulceration
T3	2.01–4.0 mm thickness	
	T3a	Without ulceration
	T4b	With ulceration
T4	>4.0 mm thickness	
	T4a	Without ulceration
	T4b	With ulceration

Head and Neck Cancer Staging, Table 33 Staging of regional lymph nodes of cutaneous melanoma (Edge et al. 2010)

Regional lymph nodes (N)		
NX	Regional lymph nodes cannot be assessed	
N0	No regional lymph node metastasis	
N1	One lymph node	
	N1a	Micrometastasis[a]
	N1b	Macrometastasis[b]
N2	Two or three lymph nodes	
	N2a	Micrometastasis
	N2b	Macrometastasis
	N2c	In transit metastases/satellites without metastatic nodes
N3	≥4 metastatic nodes, or matted nodes, or in transit metastases/satellite(s) with metastatic node(s)	

[a]Micrometastases are diagnosed after sentinel lymph node biopsy and completion lymphadenectomy if performed
[b]Macrometastases are defined as clinically detectable lymph node metastases confirmed by therapeutic lymphadenectomy or when any lymph node metastasis exhibits extracapsular extension

Head and Neck Cancer Staging, Table 34 Staging of distant metastases in cutaneous melanoma (Edge et al. 2010)

Distant metastasis (M)		
M0	No distant metastases	
M1a	Distant skin, subcutaneous, or nodal metastases	Normal LDH
M1b	Lung metastases	Normal LDH
M1c	All other visceral metastases	Normal LDH
	Any distant metastasis	Elevated LDH

Head and Neck Cancer Staging, Table 35 Anatomic stage and prognostic groups for cutaneous melanoma (Edge et al. 2010)

Clinical staging			
Stage 0	Tis	N0	M0
Stage IA	T1a	N0	M0
Stage IB	T1b	N0	M0
	T2a	N0	M0
Stage IIA	T2b	N0	M0
	T3a	N0	M0
Stage IIB	T3b	N0	M0
	T4a	N0	M0
Stage IIC	T4b	N0	M0
Stage III	Any T	N1, N2, or N3	M0
Stage IV	Any T	Any N	M1

Head and Neck Cancer Staging, Table 36 Staging of primary tumors in Merkel cell carcinoma (Edge et al. 2010)

Primary tumor (T)	
TX	Primary tumor cannot be assessed
T0	No evidence of primary tumor
Tis	Carcinoma in situ
T1	≤2 cm in greatest dimension
T2	>2 cm but ≤5 cm in greatest dimension
T3	>5 cm in greatest dimension
T4	Tumor invades bone, muscle, fascia, or cartilage

Head and Neck Cancer Staging, Table 37 Staging of regional lymph nodes in Merkel cell carcinoma (Edge et al. 2010)

Regional lymph nodes (N)		
NX	Regional lymph nodes cannot be assessed	
N0	No regional lymph node metastasis	
N1	Metastasis in regional lymph node(s)	
	N1a	Micrometastasis[a]
	N1b	Macrometastasis[b]
N2	In transit metastasis[c]	

[a]Micrometastases are diagnosed after sentinel or elective lymphadenectomy
[b]Macrometastases are defined as clinically detectable nodal metastases confirmed by therapeutic lymphadenectomy or needle biopsy
[c]In transit metastasis: a tumor distinct from the primary lesion and located either (1) between the primary lesion and the draining regional lymph nodes or (2) distal to the primary lesion

Head and Neck Cancer Staging, Table 38 Staging of distant metastases in Merkel cell carcinoma (Edge et al. 2010)

Distant metastasis (M)		
M0	No distant metastasis	
M1	Metastasis beyond regional lymph nodes	
	M1a	Metastasis to skin, subcutaneous tissues, or distant lymph nodes
	M1b	Metastasis to lung
	M1c	Metastasis to all other visceral sites

Head and Neck Cancer Staging, Table 39 Anatomic stage and prognostic groups of Merkel cell carcinoma (Edge et al. 2010)

Anatomic stage/prognostic groups			
Stage 0	Tis	N0	M0
Stage IA	T1	pN0	M0
Stage IB	T1	cN0	M0
Stage IIA	T2	pN0	M0
	T3	pN0	M0
Stage IIB	T2	cN0	M0
	T3	cN0	M0
Stage IIC	T4	N0	M0
Stage IIIA	Any T	N1a	M0
Stage IIIB	Any T	N1b	M0
	Any T	N2	M0
Stage IV	Any T	Any N	M1

Head and Neck Cancer Staging, Table 40 Staging of primary tumors in mucosal melanoma (Edge et al. 2010)

Primary tumor (T)	
TX	Primary tumor cannot be assessed
T3	Mucosal disease
T4a	Tumor involving deep soft tissue, cartilage, bone, or overlying skin
T4b	Tumor involving brain, dura, skull base, lower cranial nerves (IX, X, XI, XII), masticator space, carotid artery, prevertebral space, mediastinal structures

Head and Neck Cancer Staging, Table 41 Staging of regional lymph nodes in mucosal melanoma (Edge et al. 2010)

Regional lymph nodes (N)	
NX	Regional lymph nodes cannot be assessed
N0	No regional lymph node metastases
N1	Regional lymph node metastases present

documenting the burden of disease at the primary site, the neck, and distant metastases. As beneficial as this system is, it is still limited in that it does not encompass all factors known to have significant bearing on tumor behavior and thus prognosis. It is expected that the TNM system will continue to be periodically updated with advances in prognostic efficiency through the use of markers of poor prognosis other than anatomic stage.

Head and Neck Cancer Staging, Table 42 Anatomic stage and prognostic groups in mucosal melanoma (Edge et al. 2010)

Anatomic stage/prognostic groups			
Stage III	T3	N0	M0
Stage IVA	T4a	N0	M0
	T3	N1	M0
	T4a	N1	M0
Stage IVB	T4b	Any N	M0
Stage IVC	Any T	Any N	M1

Head and Neck Cancer Staging, Table 43 Staging of primary soft tissue sarcomas except Kaposi sarcoma and angiosarcoma (Edge et al. 2010)

Primary tumor (T)		
TX	Primary tumor cannot be assessed	
T0	No evidence of primary tumor	
T1	Tumor ≤5 cm in greatest dimension	
	T1a	Superficial
	T1b	Deep
T2	Tumor >5 cm in greatest dimension	
	T2a	Superficial
	T2b	Deep

Head and Neck Cancer Staging, Table 44 Staging of regional lymph nodes in soft tissue and bone sarcomas (Edge et al. 2010)

Regional lymph nodes (N)	
NX	Regional lymph nodes cannot be assessed
N0	No regional lymph node metastases
N1	Regional lymph node metastases present

Head and Neck Cancer Staging, Table 45 Translation from three- and four-grade systems to two-grade (high and low grade) system for histopathological grade of soft tissue and bone sarcomas (Edge et al. 2010)

Histopathological grade (G)		
TNM two-grade system	Three-grade systems	Four-grade systems
Low grade	Grade 1	Grade 1
		Grade 2
High grade	Grade 2	Grade 3
	Grade 3	Grade 4

Head and Neck Cancer Staging, Table 46 Anatomic stage and prognostic groups for soft tissue sarcomas (Edge et al. 2010)

Anatomic stage/prognostic groups				
Stage IA	T1a	N0	M0	Low grade
	T1b	N0	M0	Low grade
Stage IB	T2a	N0	M0	Low grade
	T2b	N0	M0	Low grade
Stage IIA	T1a	N0	M0	High grade
	T1b	N0	M0	High grade
Stage IIB	T2a	N0	M0	High grade
Stage III	T2b	N0	M0	High grade
	Any T	N1	M0	Any grade
Stage IV	Any T	Any N	M1	Any grade

Head and Neck Cancer Staging, Table 47 Staging of primary tumors in bone sarcomas (Edge et al. 2010)

Primary tumor (T)	
TX	Primary tumor cannot be assessed
T0	No evidence of primary tumor
T1	Tumor ≤8 cm in greatest dimension
T2	Tumor >8 cm in greatest dimension
T3	Discontinuous tumors in the primary bone site

Head and Neck Cancer Staging, Table 48 Staging of distant metastases in bone sarcomas (Edge et al. 2010)

Distant metastases (M)		
M0	No distant metastases	
M1	Distant metastases present	
	M1a	Lung
	M1b	Other distant sites

Head and Neck Cancer Staging, Table 49 Anatomic stage and prognostic groups of bone sarcomas (Edge et al. 2010)

Anatomic stage/prognostic groups				
Stage IA	T1	N0	M0	Low grade
Stage IB	T2	N0	M0	Low grade
Stage IIA	T1	N0	M0	High grade
Stage IIB	T2	N0	M0	High grade
Stage III	T3	N0	M0	Any grade
Stage IVA	Any T	N0	M1a	Any grade
Stage IVB	Any T	N1	Any M	Any grade
	Any T	Any N	M1b	Any grade

Cross-References

► Cervical Esophageal Squamous Cell Carcinoma
► Hypopharyngeal Squamous Cell Carcinoma
► Malignant Laryngeal Neoplasms
► Malignant Neoplasms of the Oral Cavity
► Medullary Thyroid Cancer
► Merkel Cell Cancer of Head and Neck
► Minor Salivary Gland Neoplasms
► Nasopharyngeal Carcinoma
► Neoplasia, Malignant Neoplasia-Metastatic Disease
► Nonmelanoma Skin Cancers of Head and Neck
► Oropharyngeal Malignancies
► Salivary Gland Malignancies
► Sinonasal Malignancies
► Well-Differentiated Thyroid Cancer

References

Edge SE, Byrd DR, Compton CC et al (2010) AJCC (American Joint Committee on Cancer) cancer staging manual, 7th edn. Springer, New York

Head and Neck Cancer Surveillance

Bruce Ashford
Department of Head & Neck Surgery, Liverpool Hospital, Liverpool, Sydney, NSW, Australia

The advantages of improved treatment outcomes for cancer and generally increasing longevity are mirrored by the challenges of surveillance for cancer survivors. This is particularly true for head and neck cancer survivors. What are the key issues in surveillance of head and neck cancer and what are the current best approaches for early detection of recurrence of cancer for our patients? (Fig. 1).

The spectrum of cancers of the head and neck is broad. With this breadth is inherited a variety of oncologic behavior. The scope of surveillance of basal cell carcinoma (BCC) is patently different from that of larynx squamous cell carcinoma (SCC) or even papillary thyroid carcinoma (PTC). As a consequence, the scope of expectations of the patient and practitioner

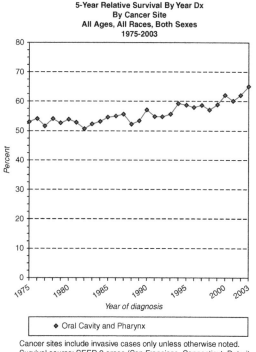

Cancer sites include invasive cases only unless otherwise noted.
Survival source: SEER 9 areas (San Francisco, Connecticut, Detroit, Hawaii, Iowa, New Mexico, Seattle, Utah, and Atlanta).
The 5-year survival estimates are calculated using monthly intervals.

Head and Neck Cancer Surveillance, Fig. 1 SEER survival data thyroid, oral cavity/pharynx and larynx

within each disease group is different, and the modalities of most facilities likewise will be different.

In addition to the generic behavior of broad groups of malignancies is the individual expression within each patient. Initial stage, pathological grade, and response to treatment all influence the likely pattern of recurrence and automatically expect from the treating physician a level of circumspection regarding surveillance.

Cancers with clear and persisting etiological causes can both persist and recur following standard therapy. The possibility of second primary tumor needs always to be considered in addition to any recurrence.

In a time when patients are more exposed to information, the patient themselves can play a powerful role in cancer surveillance. A very powerful ally in the fight against cancer is the motivated patient. Both in terms of compliance with surveillance schedule and with respect to sinister symptoms and lesions, the patient plays a key role in early detection of recurrence. So too, other caregivers, including family doctors and nurse practitioners,

will, as health budgets contract, need to assume greater roles in ongoing care and review of patients. This can only safely be built on a commitment to education on the part of the head and neck cancer specialist, and a willingness on the part of governments to fund such education.

Historical Context

Management of head and neck cancer, indeed all cancer, has undergone major changes in the last two decades. The multidisciplinary model of care has many advantages, including the sharing of burden of surveillance. A group approach to surveillance of head and neck cancers can utilize most efficiently the skills of each member of the team to enhance detection methods. Along with the internal audit process inherent in this model, the discussion of difficult cases and recalcitrant disease can be more broadly canvassed and more uniformly approached (Fig. 2) (SEER Program 1973–2008).

Patients with a new diagnosis of head and neck cancer need to have their surveillance tailored to the pathology. For patients with SCC of the upper aerodigestive tract, a 3-monthly review schedule in the first year following treatment is recommended. Thereafter, a widening of interval in between surveillance visits is reasonable.

The duration of surveillance is not clear. In an ideal setting, all cancer patients would be followed at least annually for life. The burden of disease and the limitations of resources demand that the most intense surveillance occurs in the years immediately following diagnosis and treatment. Most recurrent disease occurs in the first 3 years. However, the specter of new primary malignancy in patients who survive initial treatment for head and neck cancer increases over time.

Strategies for Surveillance Need to Encompass Local, Regional, and Distant Disease

Local Surveillance
Local recurrence of head and neck cancer is the least occult. We are always interested and most attentive to the site of primary disease. Both mucosal and skin changes in areas of previous treatment, whether

Head and Neck Cancer Surveillance, Fig. 2 Seer oral cancer survival by stage

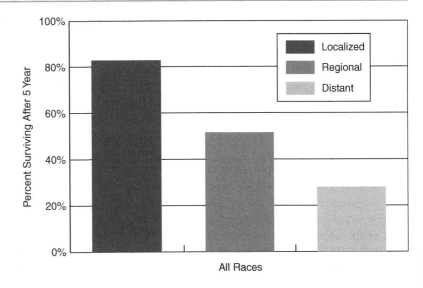

surgical or radiation, can be deceptive. Contour changes, altered pigmentation, and ulceration need to be found and submitted to both examination and, as appropriate, investigation. Fine needle and punch biopsy may be used to exclude recurrent malignancy.

Of special interest is the not uncommon phenomenon of the ▶ unknown primary SCC. Emergence of the hitherto unknown primary can be expected at a rate of between 5% and 10% per annum. For those patients in this group, who are most likely to have emergence in difficult areas to assess and access (e.g., pharynx/hypopharynx), meticulous attention and adherence to a surveillance regimen is paramount. This may involve physical examination, fiberoptic examination, and potentially examination under anesthesia. Prior radiation to the most likely areas of primary SCC can further complicate surveillance and interpretation.

Also of special interest is the immunosuppressed patient. As transplant and chronic immunosuppressive disease survival become more common, we need to consider this group differently. All those who care for this group have been amazed by the rapidity of onset of both recurrent and new malignancy. This will influence not only treatment paradigms, but also approaches to surveillance. A more regular review schedule needs to be adopted and followed and ideally other caregivers need to be sensitive to the need for a group approach to surveillance.

Regional Surveillance

Regional failure following definitive treatment of head and neck cancer is a key indicator of effectiveness of

primary therapy. With the advent of organ preservation in the management of head and neck cancer, nonoperative measures and intensity-modulated radiotherapy have revolutionized dose and extent of treatment of lymph node basins. Our understanding of patterns of nodal spread of head and neck cancer has been based on early work by Shah and lately by O'Brien (Shah et al. 1993; O'Brien et al. 2001). Mucosal and cutaneous carcinoma, and subsites within these broad categories, have predictable patterns of nodal involvement, and surveillance can be tailored with prosecution of specific areas.

Clinical examination has always been the cornerstone of surveillance of regional control. Recently, the advent of clinician-operated portable ultrasound has expanded the sensitivity of such examination, and has been employed both in screening, and to increase the efficacy of needle biopsy of suspicious nodes. When the normal tissue qualities are lost following either surgery or chemo/radiotherapy, the ultrasound acts as a force-multiplier in enhancing surveillance.

Distant Surveillance

Distant failure carries a more dismal prospect than either local or regional failure following head and neck cancer treatment. Whether it be true distant emergence of metastatic disease uncontrolled by primary therapy, or it be a second primary, the identification of such disease is most commonly a turning point from curative to palliative intent.

Surveillance of distant sites in the management of the survivor of head and neck cancer is heavily dependent upon resources. The identification of distant disease at the time of clinical deterioration due to such disease is not ideal. The best chance of survival is when distant failure is seen well before clinical manifestation. In these instances, early, isolated disease is still able to be managed with cure being the aim. So the capability of each unit, and the relative wealth of each community will dictate the modalities at the disposal of the multidisciplinary group.

Again, thorough clinical examination and a history of change in constitutional symptoms will be key to early diagnosis. But clearly, the use of investigation is a major part of surveillance of distant sites. The use of plain chest radiography, computed tomography, and PET will all be used to a varying degree at different times and within different geographic settings.

Lifestyle Surveillance

The understanding of the effects of known carcinogens in effecting the immune system of cancer sufferers has changed our approach in advising patients of future risk following cancer therapy. The key modifiable carcinogens in head and neck cancer are tobacco and alcohol use. Smoking rates vary from country to country, but rates are highest in Asia with the encroachment of western influence and newfound affluence. Smoking rates are declining in the West, but not in the Middle East. There is no question that an active smoking cessation program must be part of effective surveillance and prevention strategies.

Specific Modalities

Serological Markers

Of all the malignancies affecting the head and neck, it is the thyroid diseases (differentiated thyroid cancer (DTC) and medullary thyroid cancer (MTC)) that have the most useful serological markers for surveillance. The routine use of both thyroglobulin and calcitonin in these diseases has changed the regimen and sensitivity of surveillance. No such serological markers are in established use in mucosal, cutaneous, or salivary gland malignancies.

Ultrasound

Ultrasound has now become a widely employed adjunct to physical examination in the office setting. Once the domain of radiologists alone, both surgeons

and physicians have discovered the relative ease of use and great facility of ultrasound.

Ultrasound is very useful for nodal surveillance in the neck. Given the predilection of many head and neck malignancies for lymphatic dissemination, the survey of nodal basins is of great value when combined with clinical examination.

The combination of US with fine needle aspiration biopsy can further add value to cancer surveillance. Yield and anatomical accuracy are increased when FNA is combined with US. In addition, biochemical analysis of aspirations can help in surveillance of particular malignancies, e.g., MTC and DTC's. Calcitonin and thyroglobulin analysis of cell blocks, respectively, can confirm the diagnosis of recurrence in such cases and help plan operative strategies.

Fiberoptic Transnasal Pharyngolaryngoscopy

Direct fiberoptic surveillance of the upper aerodigestive tract has become entrenched within the armamentarium of the head and neck oncologist. This has been borne of traditional indirect inspection of the pharynx and larynx via a reflected image. Portable, less expensive devices exist to provide the practitioner the facility to survey the nasal cavity, post nasal space, pharynx, hypopharynx, and larynx including the subglottis. More sophisticated capability can be afforded using transnasal esophagoscopy. This allows clinic-based panendoscopy and biopsy with multiport scopes and itself is also borne of the shift toward outpatient care models that combine well with the multidisciplinary model of head and neck cancer care.

Particular groups in whom direct fibreoptic surveillance is of use include larynx cancer and the unknown primary. Survey of the larynx is not only less involved on the awake patient, but allows functional assessment that is not possible in the obtunded state. In addition, the dynamic assessment of the tongue base and pharyngeal wall in the likely sites of the emergence in the unknown primary will prompt, as in the larynx, surveillance of the appropriate sites for biopsy, whether at the same time with a sophisticated multiport scope, or in the operating room.

Positron Emission Tomography (PET)

The current popularity of PET in the staging of head and neck cancer has lead to its introduction as a tool in surveillance imaging, particularly in the early post treatment phase. Fluorodeoxyglucose (FDG)-PET is the most commonly used modality and is often combined with either CT or MRI to enhance the anatomical guidance afforded.

As early as 2000, Lowe et al. showed the facility of PET in the post therapy surveillance of advanced head and neck cancers (Lowe et al. 2000). In keeping with many studies since, they prospectively demonstrated the high sensitivity of PET in detecting recurrent disease, and its superiority in this setting to other techniques.

A comprehensive review of the use of PET in monitoring response to therapy (Schoder et al. 2009) highlights some of the key factors to consider in the use of PET following nonoperative therapy in particular. The timing of PET in assessing response to therapy is important. The later the PET/CT is undertaken (commonly at 3 months), the less likelihood of false positive results due to normal post treatment inflammatory/granulomatous reactions.

It is worth restating their view that the true value of FDG PET in the post treatment setting is the high negative predictive value (NPV). NPV's in the order of 100% are of great reassurance to both clinician and patient.

Future Developments

Novel Markers

It is now standard care for serum surveillance of a growing number of malignancies. These include colonic adenocarcinoma (CEA), pancreatic (CA19.9), and prostate cancer (PSA). A number of serum proteins are currently either under investigation or in use in SCC surveillance. These include squamous cell carcinoma antigen (SCCA) and anti-SFXN3-auto Ab. Feng et al. (2010) have explored the use of SCCA, Cyfra 21–1, EGFR, and Cyclin D1 in both diagnosis and response to treatment in oral SCC. Murase et al. (2008) published findings on the use of serum markers to survey oral cancer. They assert that serum anti-SFXN3-autoAb is worthy of clinical evaluation as a novel tumor maker for the early detection of oral squamous cell carcinoma. The surveillance, particularly of SCC of deep or regional disease where inspection of mucosal disease, or even standard imaging modalities are deficient, would be greatly enhanced if an available and sensitive serum marker were available.

Summary

The surveillance of head and neck cancer in the future will be built on clinical examination and its adjuncts. Of all the sophistication and technological advances in diagnosis and therapy, the cancer survivor needs most a committed and skilled clinician who understands the appropriate use of investigations within ever-shrinking financial constraints. Overuse of investigations is wasteful. Strict levels of evidence should dictate the adjuncts to clinical examination outside of trials. Too often, the responsibility of clinicians is subjugated by the allure of technology which in truth is not as good as the clinician. As such, it behooves the head and neck cancer specialist to be active in both data collection and original research, so that inroads can continue to be made against the most debilitating and disfiguring of cancers.

Cross-References

▶ Unknown Primary

References

Feng X, Li J, Han Z, Xing R (2010) Serum SCCA, Cyfra 21–1, EGFR and Cyclin D1 levels in patients with oral squamous cell carcinoma. Int J Biol Marker 25(2):93–98

Lowe VJ, Boyd JH, Dunphy FR, Kim H, Dunleavy T, Collins BT, Martin D, Stack BC Jr, Hollenbeak C, Fletcher JW (2000) Surveillance for recurrent head and neck cancer using positron emission tomography. J Clin Oncol 18(3):651–658

Murase R, Abe Y, Takeuchi T, Nabeta M, Imai Y, Kamel Y, Kagawa-Miki L, Ueda N, Sumida T, Hamakawa H, Kito K (2008) Serum autoantibody to sideroflexin 3 as a novel tumor marker for oral squamous cell carcinoma. Proteomics Clin Appl 2(4):517–527

O'Brien CJ, McNeil EB, McMahon JD, Pathak I, Lauer CS (2001) Incidence of cervical node involvement in metastatic cutaneous malignancy involving the parotid gland. Head Neck 23:744–748

Schoder H, Fury M, Lee N, Kraus D (2009) PET monitoring of therapy response in head and neck squamous cell carcinoma. J Nucl Med 50(1):74S–88S

Shah JP, Medina JE, Shaha AR, Schantz SP, Marti J (1993) Cervical lymph node metastasis. Curr Prob Surg 30

Surveillance, Epidemiology, and End Results (SEER) Program. Research Data (1973–2008), National Cancer Institute, DCCPS, Surveillance Research Program, Cancer Statistics Branch

Head and Neck Manifestations of AIDS

Andrew H. Murr
Department of Otolaryngology-Head and Neck
Surgery, University of California, San Francisco
School of Medicine, San Francisco, CA, USA

Synonyms

AIDS; HIV; HTLV-III; LAV

Definition

HIV, AIDS, CDC, WHO, CD4

HIV: Human immunodeficiency virus. This is the causative infectious agent which causes AIDS. HIV has several strains and is a retrovirus in the subfamily of lentiviruses.

AIDS: Acquired immunodeficiency syndrome. This disease is caused by the HIV virus which diminishes T-cell immunity and causes opportunistic infections and malignancies.

CDC: Center for Disease Control in Atlanta, Georgia. This institution is responsible for tracking cases of HIV infection. They also create criteria for diagnosis of the condition.

WHO: World Health Organization. An international disease control and monitoring body that has created a staging system for AIDS.

CD4: A type of T-cell that mirrors the severity of HIV infection.

CMV: Cytomegalovirus.

HPV: Human papilloma virus.

HSV: Herpes simplex virus.

MALT: Mucosa-associated lymphoid tissue.

HAART: Highly active antiretroviral therapy. Consists of protease inhibitors and reverse transcriptase inhibitors.

Geniculate ganglion: A ganglion located in the temporal bone which is part of the facial nerve which can harbor neurotropic viruses.

T-cell count: White-blood thymus-processed cells which have immunity dysfunction due to HIV infection.

Seropositivity: Conversion to positive from negative on the HIV blood test.

Pneumocystis carinii: Now known as *Pneumocystis jeroveci*, this is a fungal pneumonia that was extremely uncommon prior to the era of HIV. Prior to antiretroviral treatment, it was often a cause of death in the end stages of AIDS.

Aphthous ulcers: Discrete oral ulcers in the oral cavity or on the lips. Often there is an erythematous border and a white center. Thought to be caused by CMV or EBV.

EBV: Epstein Barr Virus is a virus associated with various diseased including oral ulceration and nasopharyngeal carcinoma. It can be associated with pathology in the HIV population.

Aspergillus: Ubiquitous fungus that can cause infection in immunocompromised hosts.

Cryptococcus: A type of fungus that can cause pneumonia, meningitis, or other types of infections in patient infected with HIV and who is immunocompromised in late-stage AIDS.

Blastomycosis: A type of fungus that can afflict people who are immunocompromised.

Leishmaniasis: A type of parasitic infection that is spread by the sand fly.

Kaposi's sarcoma: A rare cutaneous malignancy that was a hallmark of AIDS. KS in the HIV setting could affect the upper aerodigestive tract. It is thought to be caused by HIV and human herpes virus-8.

Otosyphilis: *Treponema pallidum* infection of the inner ear.

Malignant otitis externa: Bacterial or fungal infection of the ear canal that progresses to skull base bone infection (osteomyelitis).

ABR: Auditory brainstem response. An electrical hearing test elicited by presentation of specific auditory frequency sound that promotes a reproducible and measurable brain wave.

NHL: Non-Hodgkin's lymphoma. A type of lymphoma associated with HIV infection.

Thrush: Candida infection or overgrowth of the oral cavity or upper aerodigestive tract.

NRTI: Nucleoside reverse transcriptase inhibitors. This class of drugs is part of highly active antiretroviral therapy (HAART) and is very effective in preventing the progression of HIV infection.

Protease inhibitor: This class of drugs is part of highly active antiretroviral therapy (HAART) and is very effective in preventing the progression of HIV infection.

MAC: *Mycobacterium avium* complex. A type of nontuberculous mycobacterial infection that can afflict immunocompromised patients.

Facial lipoatrophy: A characteristic fat redistribution thought to be due to a side effect of HAART therapy. Results in cheek and temporal facial hollowing in the head and neck.

Lymphoepithelial cyst: A specific type of parotid cyst associated with Sjogren's disease and also commonly with HIV infection.

Etiology

HIV infection is due to the dissemination of the human immunodeficiency virus of which there are several subtypes. The virus itself is classified as a retrovirus and is in the subfamily of lentiviruses. The organism most likely existed as a primate virus, and it is possible that it was transferred to the human population in epidemic rather than sporadic form from a location in sub-Saharan Africa in the 1970s. The current epidemic outside the African continent was highly epidemiologically linked to a single patient, patient zero, who was a steward working for Air Canada and who was both highly sexually promiscuous and also had the ability to travel extensively. Many early cases of HIV in North America could be linked to this single patient (Shilts, And the Band Played On). As early as 1982, the only reported cases of what was to be called AIDS in the United States were limited to patients in California, New Jersey, and New York. At this time, the viral etiology of the disease, although suspected, had not been definitively identified (Gottlieb et al. 1981; Masur et al. 1981). As such, the disease had many different monikers including gay bowel disease, gay men's disease, and other erroneous and misleading names. Nevertheless, senior astute physicians in epicenter locations for the disease, like San Francisco, California, could recall in the depths of their memories cases of young otherwise healthy men who developed rare and puzzling opportunistic infections like *Pneumocystis carinii* pneumonia and pulmonary aspergillosis and who subsequently succumbed rapidly to the ravages of the infection. The second population affected by the epidemic in North America was the intravenous drug use segment of society in metropolitan areas. It was later understood that sharing infected needles among this group of addicted people who used

heroin and cocaine intravenously was as risky as unprotected anal sex as a behavioral vector for viral transmission. Women initially falsely appeared to be spared from the disease in North America. However, in Africa, the disease spread through the female population through heterosexual contact as rapidly as it did through the gay male population in the USA. Prior to the virus being definitively identified, there was controversy as to whether AIDS could be transferred in a maternal-fetal fashion. This was further confounded by the fact that the virus was a latent and neurotropic virus that could exist in a patient for years, undetected, and without causing symptoms, much like the varicella zoster virus can cause shingles many decades after it caused chicken pox (Ho et al. 1985). In Newark, New Jersey, Dr. James Oleske courageously postulated that a constellation of symptoms that he identified in the infant children of drug-addicted African American women actually represented the effects of the maternal-fetal transmission of what was to be known as AIDS (Oleske et al. 1983). The last early identified population pool of AIDS patients was in hemophilia patients who underwent transfusions on a frequent basis. Often, the development of immunodeficiency could be linked to blood that was tainted with hepatitis B or C virus. Patients requiring transfusion during routine surgery were also found to be at risk for developing the immunodeficiency constellation which then called the safety of the nation's blood supply into question (Shilts 1987). Finally, in 1983, two groups identified the virus behind the disease: a French group identified the LAV (lymphadenopathy-associated virus) and a group at the NIH in the USA identified the HTLV-III (human T-lymphotropic virus-III) (Barre-Sinoussi et al. 1983; Gallo et al. 1983). This is now known as HIV or human immunodeficiency virus. Other major landmarks in the effort to control spread of the disease include the development of a test to identify the virus in patients or in blood, the emphasis on education of the public so that it is commonly understood that unprotected sex can lead to transmission of the virus, and the development of a treatment in the form of HAART therapy. HAART stands for highly active antiretroviral therapy. This therapeutic cocktail of several medications substantially delays the progression from HIV infection to the syndrome known as AIDS where opportunistic infections and cancers can develop as a result of the immune dysregulation caused by the chronic viral infection.

HAART therapy has substantially reduced the incidence of the head and neck manifestations of HIV and AIDS in clinical practice (Stephenson 1997).

Epidemiology

HIV and AIDS affect a wide cross section of the population including men, women, and children of all ages and backgrounds. It is estimated by the CDC that the incidence of HIV in the United States is 56,300 new infections for 2006. The incidence is probably stable over the past 10 years. The prevalence of HIV is estimated to be 1,106,400 people. Blacks/African Americans account for 46% of all people with HIV in the USA while whites account for 35% and Hispanic/Latino persons account for 18%. The rate of infection for black males and black females also outstrip the rates for white persons or Hispanic persons. The diagnosis rate for black males is 115.7/100,000 and for black females is 55.7/100,000. The diagnosis rate for white males is 19.7/100,000 and for Hispanic males is about 40/100,000. Three quarters of the HIV population is male and one quarter is female. The age group with the highest rate of new HIV infection is age 30–39 with a rate of 42.6/100,000. Although the lowest rate of new cases is in the age group greater than age 50, with a rate of 6.5/100,000, the number of people living with HIV/AIDS in this age category account for 24% of all cases. Transmission of the virus is most commonly through men who have sex with men. This transmission accounts for 48% of all cases or 532,000 people. Twenty-eight percent of people are infected through high-risk heterosexual sex, and 72% of women with HIV were infected through high-risk heterosexual sex. Injection drug use accounted for 19% of patients living with HIV. High-risk heterosexual contact accounted for 31% of new cases in 2006, and injection drug use accounted for 12% of new cases. Men who have sex with men accounted for 53% of new HIV infection in 2006 (Moore 2011).

Basic Characteristics

All areas of the head and neck can be afflicted with disease processes that are caused by HIV infection. The clinical problems can be divided in general into inflammatory or infectious disorders and malignancy.

A third category of problems can be related to treatment of the disease itself. A marker for anticipating opportunistic infections is the CD4 T-cell count. When the CD4 count is above the range of approximately 250 cells/μl or so, patients often have fairly normal immunity compared with the general population. When the CD4 count falls below this range, the risk of developing unusual infections becomes higher.

Acute Infection

The acute acquisition of HIV infection often follows on the heels of some form of exposure. This exposure can come in the form of unprotected sex, exposure to infected material such as blood or other bodily fluid, direct injection of infected material from illicit substance use, or exposure through transfusion (although this is extremely rare due to blood bank screening) (Workowski et al. 2010). The initial manifestations are indistinguishable from a common cold. Upper respiratory symptoms such as a runny nose and nasal congestion, body aches, cough, and fatigue are common. Lymphadenopathy in the neck or elsewhere in the body may be present. Often, the symptoms subside in a week or two, and the patient returns to normal appearing health. On history, the risk circumstances may be recalled after the fact by the patient. The virus at this stage can then go into a latent phase. In fact, there is a variable latency of several weeks to several months or longer where even the blood test to detect the HIV virus will be negative. It is possible that the virus is able to elude immune surveillance and blood test detection by existing in a latent fashion in the central nervous system. A model for this is the manner in which varicella virus can remain in the geniculate ganglion and avoid the immune system's protective mechanisms which were developed by the initial exposure to the acute infection by the virus. In fact, with acute HIV infection, it can be possible for the initial clinical hallmark of conversion from seronegativity to a seropositive status to be acute facial nerve paralysis. This typically can occur several weeks or months after the initial exposure. It can be postulated that, like varicella, the HIV virus remains dormant in the geniculate ganglion as well (Murr and Benecke 1991).

Chronic Infection

Like many other chronic viral infections, HIV can coexist with the host in a quiescent phase. At this stage, the blood test would be positive for viral exposure, and the patient would be able to communicate the disease to another individual, but actual AIDS would not yet exist. The immune condition is generally mirrored by the T-cell count at this stage. As long as the T-cell count, specifically the CD4:CD8 ratio, remains in balance, typically the patient will not have any more susceptibility to infection than a normal adult from a head and neck standpoint. However, as the T-cell count drops and the CD4 count decreases, the risk of developing HIV- or AIDS-related infections and AIDS-related malignancies increases. The diagnostic criteria for AIDS from a condition of seropositivity are assessed from one of several staging systems. The two most commonly used staging systems in the USA include the CDC staging system and the WHO clinical staging and disease classification system (CDC 1993). The CDC staging system utilizes assessment of the CD4 count and the presence of HIV-related conditions to assess the diagnostic presence of AIDS. In this system, the CD4 count is <200 cells/µl (or a CD4 percentage less than 14%). AIDS-related conditions include symptomatic conditions (category B) or indicator conditions (category C). There are many examples in each category, but examples of category B conditions include oropharyngeal candidiasis, hairy leukoplakia, idiopathic thrombocytopenia purpura, and herpes zoster involving two or more episodes or more than one dermatome. Examples of C category AIDS-indicator conditions include recurrent pneumonia; candidiasis of the bronchi, trachea, or lungs; esophageal candidiasis; chronic herpetic ulcers; Kaposi's sarcoma; mycobacteria tuberculosis or atypical mycobacterial infections; lymphoma; or chronic wasting syndrome among other problems. The WHO classification defines an asymptomatic primary phase and then stages the disease into four clinical stages and does not rely on a CD4 count but rather divides various associated medical conditions into categories that if present will define advancing stages of the syndrome (WHO 2006). These stages are then used to determine the appropriateness of beginning antiretroviral therapy. From a head and neck point of view, stage 1 involves generalized lymphadenopathy. Stage 2 can be manifested by recurrent upper respiratory infections such as tonsillitis, sinusitis, otitis media, herpes zoster, angular cheilitis, or recurrent oral ulcers. Stage 3 can be manifested by persistent oral candidiasis, oral hairy leukoplakia, acute necrotizing ulcerative stomatitis,

gingivitis, periodontitis, or chronic thrombocytopenia (<50,000 cells/µl). Stage 4 is defined by chronic herpes simplex infections; esophageal candidiasis, Kaposi's sarcoma; CMV infection; mycobacterial infection; candidiasis of the trachea, bronchi, or lungs; disseminated mycosis; or lymphoma among other diseases (CDC and WHO).

Head and Neck Manifestations

Infection: Unusual secondary infections are a hallmark of the HIV effect on the immune system. In the early era of AIDS, *Pneumocystis carinii* pneumonia was highly suggestive of the presence of the disease. Susceptibility to sinusitis and generalized lymphadenopathy were very common reasons for referral to the otolaryngologist – head and neck surgeon. Today, the classification system and staging systems for HIV/AIDS utilize the presence of certain types of infections to determine progression of the immune system damage and also the need for antiretroviral therapy.

Oral Cavity: The oral cavity is a common site for HIV-related infection. Oral candidiasis or thrush can affect any site in the upper aerodigestive tract including the lips, oral cavity, oropharynx, hypopharynx, larynx, trachea, bronchi, and esophagus. *Candida albicans* is a common organism which can cause erythema and discomfort of the mucous membrane. Pseudomembranous patches may be present, and biopsy may reveal the organism itself on silver staining or reveal pseudoepitheliomatous hyperplasia which must be distinguished from frank dysplasia. Treatment can began with clotrimazole oral troches and can progress to systemic antifungals such as fluconazole if needed. Intravenous antifungal therapy is sometimes required. Aphthous stomatitis or aphthous ulcers are a common finding in HIV-infected patients. The cause of aphthous ulcers is unknown, but it may be related to CMV or EBV secondary infection. While aphthous ulcers are not typically dangerous, they can be very annoying to patients because of pain which may limit oral dietary intake. Treatment usually involves local care including topically applied mouthwashes or over-the-counter gel products that form a temporary shell over the ulcer to diminish pain and promote earlier healing. Thalidomide has been reported as a treatment for severe and recurrent aphthous ulcers in the HIV population (Shetty 2007). Herpes simplex viral infection is another commonly encountered opportunistic infection and can affect the oral cavity in HIV patients. HSV can produce painful vesicular lesions of the oral cavity mucous membrane or around the lips or mouth. Diagnosis can be made on clinical grounds or by utilizing viral cultures or direct fluorescent antibody testing. Although HSV certainly afflicts non-HIV-infected patients, the extent of involvement can be more severe in the HIV population than in the general population. Treatment utilizes antiviral drugs such as acyclovir, valacyclovir, and famciclovir. Hairy leukoplakia can involve the oral cavity or tongue and may be related to EBV infection. White to gray patches are the hallmark of this condition, and while the condition may be disturbing to the patient, it usually does not cause much discomfort. Hairy leukoplakia is a category B indicator in the CDC documentation system and a stage 3 indicator in the WHO system, so astute observation of the presence of this condition may have impact on decisions to begin antiretroviral treatment (Marcusen and Sooy 1985).

Sinuses: In the early era of the AIDS epidemic, sinusitis was a common reason for referral to the otolaryngologist. Despite years of clinical investigation including culture studies and pathology review of surgical specimens, no discrete unusual cause of sinusitis was elucidated where the CD4 T-cell count was above the 250 cells/μl range. Of course, the incidence of sinusitis and allergy in the general population is extremely high, and it is not certain that sinusitis is definitely different in the HIV-infected patient when compared to the normal population when the T-cell count is high. The bacteriology included Staphylococcus, Streptococcus, Moraxella, and Haemophilus species as is seen in the general population. Treatment was similar to the treatment of sinusitis in the general population, and surgical indications were similar as well. Nevertheless, as the CD4 T-cell count drops below approximately the 200 cells/μl level, strange opportunistic infections can occur in the sinuses including *Aspergillus*, *Pseudoallescheria boydii*, and *Cryptococcus*. Interestingly, as opposed to the rapidly advancing rhinocerebral mucormycosis associated with uncontrolled diabetes or with severely immunosuppressed bone marrow transplant patients, the HIV population often manifested a type of indolent invasive fungal sinusitis. Indolent invasive fungal sinusitis may eventually cause orbital or intracranial complications, but it does so in a very slowly progressive fashion. Still, a high suspicion for diagnosis can be based

on endoscopic examination with the hallmark being avascular and insensate areas of dead ethmoid bone or septum in a patient with skin changes or orbital or brain invasion on CT and MRI imaging studies. While debridement and intravenous and topical antifungal therapy can temporarily slow the progression of this infection, it is the recovery of the immune function that is the key to treating this problem successfully. Fortunately, the use of antiretroviral therapy has dramatically decreased the incidence of this type of devastating infection (Shah et al. 2005).

Ear: Otitis media may be present in the HIV-infected individual but like sinusitis, the presentation and bacteriology is similar to that seen in the general population. Skull base osteomyelitis known as malignant otitis externa can rarely be seen in HIV-infected patients with low T-cell counts and is associated with *Pseudomonas aeruginosa* or *Aspergillus fumigatus*. Symptoms include deep-seated and boring ear pain, otorrhea, and cranial nerve neuropathies. An elevated erythrocyte sedimentation rate and imaging studies showing soft tissue in the ear canal and findings consistent with skull base erosion are frequently present. Systemic culture-directed antimicrobial therapy is usually the treatment of choice. Recovery of immune function typically restores the patient's ability to halt the progression of the osteomyelitic infection and portends an improved outcome (Grandis et al. 2004). Early HIV infection is often accompanied by generalized lymphadenopathy, and the adenoid pad which has a role in Eustachian tube dysfunction is nothing more than mucosally associated lymphoid or MALT tissue. Lymphoid hypertrophy of the adenoid pad can impinge upon the Eustachian tube and secondarily cause otitis media. Indications for myringotomy tube placement perhaps with a greater emphasis on concomitant adenoidectomy can be very helpful in treating this problem. As the immune damage from the virus progresses as indicated by a low T-cell count, unusual opportunistic infections can affect the middle ear including pneumocystis or mycobacterial infections of the middle ear. These types of unusual infections are manifested by a polyp in the ear canal or by a large perforation of the tympanic membrane with drainage or polyp in the middle ear. A CT scan may reveal a destructive process. Mastoidectomy may be considered, but attention should be paid to biopsy and pathological examination as a method of securing the diagnosis. The incidence of sensorineural hearing loss is not necessarily elevated in the HIV population; however, antiretroviral therapy may be accompanied by ototoxicity, so audiometric evaluation is important when indicated. HAART therapy may be associated with auditory brainstem response (ABR) conduction delays with either low amplitude wave forms or waveform abnormalities as shown in a study of children receiving either three-drug or four-drug HAART regimens. Likewise, some vestibular abnormalities may be present in patients with HIV and receiving HAART therapy. Whether this pathology is due to HIV infection, treatment of HIV, or coincident HIV-related pathologies is currently not known. However, some temporal bone pathology observations have recorded microscopic derangements of the hair cells and other ultrastructural changes (Palacios et al. 2008). Another related cause of sensorineural hearing loss in the HIV population is otosyphilis. Otosyphilis is not specifically a risk related to HIV infection except that patients who engage in risky sex behavior are more at risk to contract both types of infection, so it is prudent to have an elevated suspicion in patients with HIV who also manifest a sensorineural hearing loss and/or tinnitus and/or vestibular symptoms. Diagnosis is suggested by a positive fluorescent treponemal antibody absorption (FTA-ABS) test. Cerebrospinal fluid examination may be nonspecific and in fact is frequently noncontributory in otosyphilis but may help differentiate between otosyphilis and neurosyphilis. Treatment of otosyphilis is often patterned after neurosyphilis treatment regimens and centers around the use of prolonged intravenous penicillin therapy and steroid therapy. The CDC often has the most up-to-date treatment recommendations with regard to otosyphilis as specific treatment is often controversial because patients are subject to relapses due to incomplete therapy (Yimtae et al. 2007). Finally, facial nerve paralysis either unilateral or bilateral may be a sequelae of HIV seroconversion or HIV infection (Murr and Benecke 1991). While sporadic cases have been reported in the USA, this appears to be a more common phenomenon in Africa. Whether this is due to herpes virus infection or due to the neurotropic characteristic of some strains of HIV is not known.

Neck: Lymphadenopathy is one of the most common presenting symptoms of HIV infection. It is often present as one of the manifestations of acute HIV infection or present immediately after seroconversion.

Lymph nodes may be enlarged in any area of the head and neck including all of Waldeyer's ring (tonsils, adenoids, base of tongue), nodes of Rouviere, and levels 1 through 6 of the neck. In the early days of the AIDS epidemic, the lymphoid hypertrophy of the neck was an easily accessible physical examination finding and so was furiously subjected to medical diagnostic attempts. Research on lymph tissue in HIV patients to identify the virus or to find some pathognomonic characteristic was pursued. Nevertheless, the lymph tissue did not seem to harbor a particular characteristic on pathological examination that pointed specifically to HIV infection. Rather, the pathological findings were similar to that found in any viral lymphadenitis and were therefore nonspecific. Furthermore, there was no distinguishing finding between Waldeyer's ring lymph tissue and lymph tissue taken from the neck itself. The general lack of productiveness of node sampling of the lymph tissue reservoir of the head and neck should be balanced by the increased incidence of lymphoma, squamous cell carcinoma, and opportunistic infections that can plague HIV-infected or AIDS patients, especially those with low T-cell counts (Shapiro et al. 1992). Opportunistic infections of the neck include *Mycobacterium tuberculosis* or scrofula, and atypical mycobacterial infections such as *Mycobacterium avium* complex (MAC). TB is often treated with prolonged antibiotic therapy, and the diagnosis can be made with PPD placement and fine needle aspiration examination and culture. MAC infection is diagnosed using the same techniques; however, surgery is sometimes used adjunctively to control the infection in the neck (Lee et al. 1992). Fungal neck infections can be caused by Cryptococcus, Histoplasmosis, and Coccidioidomycosis. The incidence of these severe infections has decreased dramatically with the advent of antiretroviral therapy.

Salivary Glands: Salivary glands and especially the parotid gland can be affected in HIV and AIDS. The common presenting symptom is that of a unilateral or frequently bilateral parotid mass in the tail of the parotid gland. Imaging reveals characteristics consistent with a fluid-filled cyst. Fine needle aspiration diagnosis will usually affirm the presence of straw-colored fluid which is pathologically consistent with a benign lymphoepithelial cyst. This type of cyst is similar to that seen in Sjogren's disease but does not appear to have a propensity for malignant transformation to lymphoma in general. Observation alone is an acceptable strategy for the management of lymphoepithelial cysts secondary to HIV infection. Treatment for these cysts can be undertaken if they are causing discomfort or physical deformity. Sclerotherapy has been described with a number of different agents. Doxycycline is a sclerosing agent that can be injected into the cyst via an 18-gauge intravenous catheter after withdrawing the straw-colored fluid that is present. The doxycycline injection has been shown to temporarily sclerose the cyst which decreases its size, and decompression afforded by the fluid removal improves the physical deformity caused by the presence of the cyst. Surgical excision can be contemplated, but lateral parotidectomy has risk to the facial nerve and also poses its own physical deformity potential from loss of tissue volume. Also, the cysts may recur even after parotidectomy. Lymphoepithelial cysts are so associated with HIV infection that if an otherwise asymptomatic patient presents with a lymphoepithelial cyst, the next clinical diagnostic test should be HIV testing (Lustig et al. 1998).

Facial Lipoatrophy: Facial lipoatrophy is not technically associated with HIV infection; rather it is associated with the treatment of HIV infection. The condition of lipoatrophy was first widely reported contemporaneously with the development of protease inhibitors which were available around 1997. The development of HAART therapy with its combination of protease inhibitors and nucleoside reverse transcriptase inhibitors (NRTIs) seemingly has some ability to effect this change in fat distribution. In addition, treatment sequelae can include hyperlipidemia and even the development of type II diabetes mellitus. The hallmark of the disorder is atrophy of the fat of the face, limbs, and buttocks, and accumulation of fat in the breasts, neck, and abdomen. In the face, the fat atrophy produces a characteristic "sallow" appearance with hollowing of the cheeks and relative prominence of the orbicularis oris muscle. Also, periorbital and temporal wasting can occur. These physical changes are often distressing to the patient because of the alteration of normal appearance and also because the appearance itself is characteristic of people undergoing treatment for HIV. It is estimated that about half of the patients who are on protease inhibitors will develop lipoatrophy, and the condition appears to affect males in greater proportion than females. Treatment can include antidiabetes drugs or switching the

combination of antiretroviral drugs. Unfortunately, however, discontinuation of antiretroviral medications does not reverse the changes in fat distribution that were produced by the treatment. Surgical correction using implants or fillers seem to offer the best cosmetic correction results (Funk et al. 2007).

Larynx: The larynx can become involved with any of the above mentioned processes. The patient may present with an altered voice or pain and difficulty with swallowing. Otalgia may be present as a referred pain due to the innervation of the larynx by the ninth and tenth cranial nerve which also can connect through Arnold's nerve to the external auditory canal. The most common HIV-related infection of the larynx is likely candidiasis or thrush. CMV ulceration can be very painful and may interfere with swallowing and therefore nutrition. Biopsy may reveal cytoplasm inclusions characteristic of CMV infection. Treatment may include intravenous ganciclovir or cidofovir if symptoms are unrelenting or airway compromise is of concern or if an invasive form of CMV is present. Herpes simplex virus types I and II will often respond to antivirals like acyclovir, but biopsy and culture of the lesion is often necessary to establish the diagnosis. Of course, bacterial infections such as *Haemophilus influenza* related epiglottis or streptococcal infection may sporadically occur, especially in nonimmunized individuals, but this type of infection is probably not more frequent than in the general population especially if the T-cell count is intact. Mycobacterial infections including MAC and tuberculosis can be related to HIV and AIDS and in the larynx present as hoarseness and granulation tissue on physical examination which may progress to obstructive airway symptoms. Frequently, patients will also manifest known pulmonary involvement with mycobacterial infection and laryngeal involvement will represent a site of extrapulmonary spread. Diagnosis will be suspected by a positive PPD skin test (greater than 5-mm reaction). Biopsy may show caseating granulomas with acid-fast organisms. MAC infections usually have biopsies showing many more organisms than what is commonly seen in tuberculosis infections. Cultures are important to help direct antibiotic therapy which is the primary treatment of both types of mycobacterial infections. Fungal infections of the larynx such as Aspergillus, Cryptococcus, Histoplasmosis, Coccidioidomycosis, and Blastomycosis have been reported in the past but are now extremely rare in the USA due to antiretroviral therapy. Treatment would consist of intravenous anti-fungal antibiotics. In any case, these types of infections would not typically be encountered unless the T-cell count was below 100 cells/μl. Finally, parasitic laryngeal leishmaniasis has been rarely reported in patients who have traveled to endemic areas like South America, Africa, or Asia. Hoarseness and swallowing complaints will prompt a laryngeal examination which is likely to show a mass that may be indistinguishable from malignancy on physical appearance. Routine hematoxylin-eosin staining should reveal the parasite, or staining with Giemsa stain. Cultures sometimes also reveal the organism. Antimonial therapy or possibly amphotericin B would be expected to treat the disease (Gurney et al. 2009).

Malignancy: Malignancies of the head and neck are known to be present in increased incidence in patients with HIV infection. These types of cancers are generally thought to be immunity-related cancers rather than cancers related to prolonged exposure to carcinogens, such as alcohol or cigarette smoke.

Kaposi's Sarcoma (KS) is the most common HIV-related malignancy of the head and neck. KS was a rare skin cancer seen in men of Mediterranean decent prior to the AIDS epidemic. In 1986, KS was noted to be so commonly associated with AIDS that it became an AIDS-defining diagnosis. KS can involve organ systems in addition to the head and neck but, in the head and neck, may involve any site of the upper aerodigestive tract or the skin. The lesions appear to be purple and raised and may become necrotic and bleed. They may also create obstruction depending on their exact site which may lead to airway symptoms, swallowing symptoms, or both. The diagnosis of KS is so highly suggested by its physical appearance that biopsy is not always necessary; however, biopsy would be expected to show spindle cells with abundant vascular channels and inflammatory infiltrates. Immunohistochemical staining may be positive for factor VIII antigen. The presence of KS has been linked to the synergy between HIV and human herpes virus-8. Treatment of KS is undertaken if the lesions are symptomatic. Not all KS requires treatment as it may be self-limited. Low-dose radiation of about 2,000 Gy has been used to control symptomatic upper aerodigestive tract KS. Systemic chemotherapy has also demonstrated response including the use of etoposide, liposomal doxorubicin, paclitaxel, and bleomycin. Intralesional injection of vinblastine has also been reported to produce improvement. Surgical excision or debulking may also be indicated.

Squamous Cell Carcinoma of the upper aerodigestive tract is also associated with HIV infection. Often, patients do not have the usual risk factors for the disease. Human papilloma virus (HPV), especially types 6 and 11 which are associated with recurrent respiratory papillomatosis, may be associated with the increased propensity for HIV patients to develop squamous cell carcinomas of the head and neck. These cancers are often seen in late-stage AIDS and have a poor survival even with standard treatment. There may be an association between HIV, HPV, and anogenital carcinoma. Treatment of these cancers involves application of surgery, chemotherapy, and radiation therapy like it does in patients without HIV infection. It is not certain that antiretroviral therapy has improved the overall prognosis of patients who develop squamous cell carcinomas, but it is possible that antiretroviral therapy delays the expression of squamous cell carcinoma.

Lymphoma, especially non-Hodgkin's lymphoma (NHL), is seen with increased incidence in the upper aerodigestive tract of patients with HIV. It seems to appear in end-stage AIDS and is a category C AIDS-indicator in the CDC system and a clinical stage 4 indicator in the WHO system. Central nervous system lymphoma is an especially troublesome clinical problem in the management of patients with AIDS. Lymphoma can afflict any area of the head and neck including the sinuses or nasal cavity, the larynx, the oral cavity or oropharynx, and the neck. Fine needle aspiration biopsy may be diagnostic or open biopsy may be required depending upon the needs of the pathologist. The NHL subtype is higher in the AIDS population than it is in the general population. Forty percent of NHLs in AIDS are the Burkitt's type which is associated with a chromosome 8–14 translocation. Thirty percent are categorized as immunoblastic lymphoma, and 30% are categorized as large-cell lymphoma. It is likely that these malignancies are related to Epstein-Barr virus infection in the setting of HIV infection. It is also possible that human herpes virus-8 plays a role in the development of NHL. Chemotherapy protocols are usually selected for treating these malignancies, but the prognosis for AIDS patients with NHL is poor (Gurney et al. 2009).

Cross-References

▶ Acute and Chronic Rhinosinusitis
▶ Acute Otitis Media
▶ Antibiotics and Medical Management of ABRS
▶ Benign Salivary Gland Neoplasms
▶ Facial Nerve Paralysis Due to Viral Etiology
▶ Facial Paralysis
▶ Fine Needle Aspiration for Head and Neck Tumors
▶ Granulomatous Disorders
▶ Head and Neck Cancer Staging
▶ Head and Neck Squamous Cell Carcinoma, Risk Factors
▶ Idiopathic Facial Nerve Paralysis
▶ Imaging Cystic Head and Neck Masses
▶ Invasive Fungal Sinusitis
▶ Laryngeal Papillomatosis
▶ Lymphomas Presenting in Head and Neck
▶ Malignant Laryngeal Neoplasms
▶ Malignant Neoplasms of the Oral Cavity
▶ Molecular Markers in Head and Neck SCCA
▶ Oral Mucosal Lesions
▶ Oropharyngeal Malignancies
▶ Positive Vector
▶ Primary Neck Neoplasms
▶ Salivary Gland Disorders, Sialorrhea
▶ Stomatitis

References

(1992) 1993 revised classification system for HIV infection and expanded surveillance case definition for AIDS among adolescents and adults. MMWR Recomm Rep 41(RR-17):1–19. PubMed PMID: 1361652

Barré-Sinoussi F, Chermann JC, Rey F, Nugeyre MT, Chamaret S, Gruest J, Dauguet C, Axler-Blin C, Vézinet-Brun F, Rouzioux C, Rozenbaum W, Montagnier L (1983) Isolation of a T-lymphotropic retrovirus from a patient at risk for acquired immune deficiency syndrome (AIDS). Science 220(4599):868–871

Funk E, Brissett AE, Friedman CD, Bressler FJ (2007) HIV-associated facial lipoatrophy: establishment of a validated grading scale. Laryngoscope 117(8):1349–1353

Gallo RC, Sarin PS, Gelmann EP, Robert-Guroff M, Richardson E, Kalyanaraman VS, Mann D, Sidhu GD, Stahl RE, Zolla-Pazner S, Leibowitch J, Popovic M (1983) Isolation of human T-cell leukemia virus in acquired immune deficiency syndrome (AIDS). Science 220(4599):865–867. PubMed PMID: 6601823

Grandis JR, Branstetter BF, Yu VL (2004) The changing face of malignant (necrotising) external otitis: clinical, radiological, and anatomic correlations. Lancet Infect Dis 4:34–39

Gottlieb MS, Schroff R, Schanker HM, Weisman JD, Fan PT, Wolf RA, Saxon A (1981) Pneumocystis carinii pneumonia and mucosal candidiasis in previously healthy homosexual men: evidence of a new acquired cellular immunodeficiency. N Engl J Med 305(24):1425–1431

Gurney TA, Lee KC, Murr AH (2009) Laryngeal manifestations of acquired immunodeficiency syndrome. In: Fried MP, Ferlito A (eds) The larynx, vol 1. Plural Publishing, San Diego, pp 853–857

Ho DD, Rota TR, Schooley RT, Kaplan JC, Allan JD, Groopman JE, Resnick L, Felsenstein D, Andrews CA, Hirsch MS (1985) Isolation of HTLV-III from cerebrospinal fluid and neural tissues of patients with neurologic syndromes related to the acquired immunodeficiency syndrome. N Engl J Med 313(24):1493–1497

Lee KC, Tami TA, Lalwani AK, Schecter G (1992) Contemporary management of cervical tuberculosis. Laryngoscope 102(1):60–64

Lustig LR, Lee KC, Murr A, Deschler D, Kingdom T (1998) Doxycycline sclerosis of benign lymphoepithelial cysts in patients infected with HIV. Laryngoscope 108(8 Pt 1):1199–1205

Marcusen DC, Sooy CD (1985) Otolaryngologic and head and neck manifestations of acquired immunodeficiency syndrome (AIDS). Laryngoscope 95(4):401–405

Masur H, Michelis MA, Greene JB, Onorato I, Stouwe RA, Holzman RS, Wormser G, Brettman L, Lange M, Murray HW, Cunningham-Rundles S (1981) An outbreak of community-acquired Pneumocystis carinii pneumonia: initial manifestation of cellular immune dysfunction. N Engl J Med 305(24):1431–1438

Moore RD (2011) Epidemiology of HIV infection in the United States: implications for linkage to care. Clin Infect Dis 52(Suppl 2):S208–S213

Murr AH, Benecke JE Jr (1991) Association of facial paralysis with HIV positivity. Am J Otol 12(6):450–451, Review. PubMed PMID: 1805637

Oleske J, Minnefor A, Cooper R Jr, Thomas K, dela Cruz A, Ahdieh H, Guerrero I, Joshi VV, Desposito F (1983) Immune deficiency syndrome in children. JAMA 249(17):2345–2349, PubMed PMID: 6834633

Palacios GC, Montalvo MS, Fraire MI, Leon E, Alvarez MT, Solorzano F (2008) Audiologic and vestibular findings in a sample of human immunodeficiency virus type-1-infected Mexican children under highly active antiretroviral therapy. Int J Pediatr Otorhinolaryngol 72(11):1671–1681. Epub 2008 Sep 23. PubMed PMID: 18814921

Popovic M, Sarin PS, Robert-Gurroff M, Kalyanaraman VS, Mann D, Minowada J, Gallo RC (1983) Isolation and transmission of human retrovirus (human t-cell leukemia virus). Science 219(4586):856–859. PubMed PMID: 6600519

Shah AR, Hairston JA, Tami TA (2005) Sinusitis in HIV: microbiology and therapy. Curr Allergy Asthma Rep 5(6):495–499, Review. PubMed PMID: 16216176

Shapiro AL, Shechtman FG, Guida RA, Kimmelman CP (1992) Head and neck lymphoma in patients with the acquired immune deficiency syndrome. Otolaryngol Head Neck Surg 106(3):258–260. PubMed PMID: 1589218

Shetty K (2007) Current role of thalidomide in HIV-positive patients with recurrent aphthous ulcerations. Gen Dent 55(6):537–542, PubMed PMID: 18050580

Shilts R (1987) And the band played on. St. Martin's Press, New York

Stephenson J (1997) The art of "HAART": researchers probe the potential and limits of aggressive HIV treatments. JAMA 277(8):614–616

WHO (2006) WHO case definitions of HIV for surveillance and revised clinical staging and immunological classification of HIV-related disease in adults and children. http://www.who.int/hiv/pub/vct/hivstaging/en/index.html. Accessed 29 Mar 2011

Workowski KA, Berman S; Centers for Disease Control and Prevention (CDC) (2010) Sexually transmitted diseases treatment guidelines, 2010. MMWR Recomm Rep 59(RR-12):1–110. (2011) Erratum in: MMWR Recomm Rep 60(1):18. Dosage error in article text. PubMed PMID: 21160459

Yimtae K, Srirompotong S, Lertsukprasert K (2007) Otosyphilis: a review of 85 cases. Otolaryngol Head Neck Surg 136(1):67–71. PubMed PMID: 17210336

Head and Neck Sarcoma

Bruce Ashford
Department of Head & Neck Surgery, Liverpool Hospital, Liverpool, Sydney, NSW, Australia

Definition

Sarcomas of the head and neck comprise a heterogeneous compilation of tumors, all derived from the mesenchyme. Sarcomas account for 1% of all malignancies. There are more than 30 separate sarcomas. Eighty percent of sarcomas arise from soft tissues (muscle, endothelial cells, cartilage, and nerve) (de Bree et al. 2010).

Only 15% of sarcomas arise in the head and neck. Most sarcomas occur in adults, but of those arising in children, rhabdomyosarcoma (RMS) is by far the most common. In adults, malignant fibrous histiocytoma (MFH) is the most common.

Classification

Soft Tissue Sarcomas
Malignant fibrous histiocytoma
Angiosarcoma
Fibrosarcoma
Rhabdomyosarcoma
Angiosarcoma
Leiomyosarcoma
Alveolar soft part sarcoma
Kaposi sarcoma
Malignant schwannoma/Malignant peripheral nerve sheath tumor (MPNST)

Hard Tissue Sacomas
Chondrosarcoma
Bone sarcoma
Osteosarcoma
Ewing sarcoma

Etiology

Genetic Syndromes
Li-Fraumeni syndrome is an autosomal dominant disorder resulting in a germline mutation of the tumor suppressor gene *p53*. Affected individuals may develop breast cancer, leukemia, adrenocortical carcinoma, and a variety of soft tissue sarcomas.

Inherited retinoblastoma, due to *Rb1*, confers susceptibility to both bone and soft tissue sarcomas.

Neurofibromatosis type I results in greater rates of sarcoma, particularly rhabdomyosarcoma in childhood and malignant peripheral nerve sheath tumors in adulthood.

Radiation **induced** – sarcoma is one of the malignancies associated with a lag following external beam radiotherapy (EBRT). Limited survival and inadequate follow-up data from longer-term survivors have impacted on a clear appreciation of the incidence of radiation-induced sarcoma. MFH, angiosarcoma and osteosarcoma have been implicated in postradiation malignancy observational studies. Average latency between treatment and emergence of radiation implicated sarcoma is 11–14 years. Perhaps 0.1% of patients treated with standard wide-field EBRT will develop a sarcoma in field. The applicability of this estimate in the era of IMRT and altered fractionation is questionable.

Clinical Presentation

The presentation of sarcoma is dependent upon the site. In the head and neck, sarcomas arising within or close to the skin will present earlier than those arising

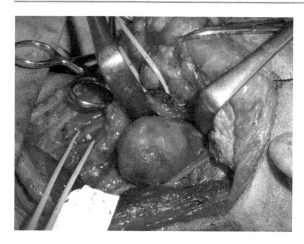

Head and Neck Sarcoma, Fig. 1 MPNST parapharynx

in bone or deep soft tissues. The usual painless lump presentation spoken of in limb sarcoma still applies. Given the complexity of anatomical arrangement within the head and neck, often the growing sarcoma presents late after an effect on function, for example, occlusion or swallowing.

Worthy of mention in clinical presentation is the degree to which the cutaneous sarcoma may give a gross underestimation of the extent based on appearance only. Their proclivity for dermal spread and involvement of nerves and the lymphovascular space dictates a far more sinister course than initial appearance suggests (Sturgis et al. 2003).

With deeper sarcomas of soft tissue, a painless mass in the neck is the usual presentation. With growth, impingement on the airway has an effect on both speech and swallowing (Fig. 1). Often the internal effect is more gross than any external component. Bone sarcomas of the head and neck may involve the jaws or skull base. Destruction of the mandibular or maxillary structure can present as a painless swelling or malocclusion. Skull base involvement may present with a cranial nerve palsy, otalgia, or ocular effects.

Clinical examination (including where indicated fiberoptic examination of the upper aerodigestive tract) should raise suspicion of sarcoma if the usual diagnosis seems unlikely. Most important is to entertain the potential diagnosis when the appearance is out of the ordinary. This is easier with the deep soft tissue sarcomas, but clinical examination for some cutaneous sarcomas (esp MFH) will be less suggestive, the diagnosis often only with histopathology.

Angiosarcoma has a more characteristic appearance, whereas MFH can look surprisingly benign.

Diagnostics

Ideally, diagnostic modalities will augment the clinical findings. Diagnosis is eventually reliant on tissue diagnosis, but often radiologic prosecution of a lesion is employed to include sarcoma within the differential.

Cutaneous sarcomas, including MFH and angiosarcoma will be diagnosed on biopsy of a less sinister appearing lesion or within an area of suspected recurrence. Histopathology will reveal poorly defined or anaplastic spindle cells, mitoses, and poorly defined margins. Initial review of the histology may allow the inclusion of non-sarcomatous lesions within the differential, for example, lymphoma, carcinoma, and melanoma. The degree of cytological malignancy, combined with the clinical picture, should help to rule out benign conditions.

	Myogenin	CD31	CD34	HHV8	SMA	Desmin	Vimectin	Hcaldesman	S100	CK
Most useful										
Rhabdomyosarcoma	+									
Angiosarcoma		+								+
Kaposi Sarcoma		+	+	+						
Somewhat useful										
Leiomyosarcoma					+	+	+	+		
MPNST									+	+
Not useful										
Fibrosarcoma										
MFH										
Osteosarcoma										

Immunohistochemistry (IHC) will sharpen the focus on sarcoma and differentiate between poorly differentiated non-sarcomas from tumors of mesenchymal origin. As many of the sarcomas have subtypes (e.g., epithelioid, glandular, endothelioid), some IHC markers will have variability within sarcoma types.

Imaging is employed to determine the extent and anatomical relations of the tumor. This is particularly true of computed tomography (CT). In addition, CT is of added benefit in assessment of bone involvement (Fig. 2). Magnetic resonance imaging (MRI) is of added benefit in assessing soft tissue tumors, or

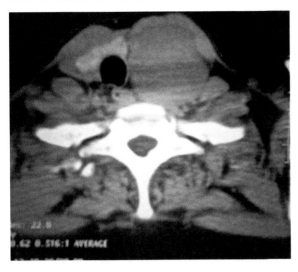

Head and Neck Sarcoma, Fig. 2 Fibrosarcoma of carotid sheath, non-contrasted CT

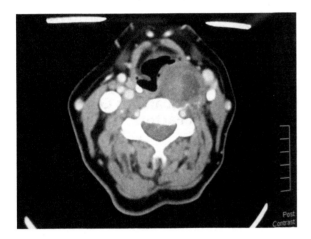

Head and Neck Sarcoma, Fig. 3 MPNST of parapharynx, contrast CT

assessing involvement of muscle, nerve, or skin. Of less value is using MRI for accurate assessment of grade. Often the combined use of CT and MRI with the use of contrast is used to exclude other diagnoses and to include sarcoma in the differential (Fig. 3). Positron emission tomography (PET) is of value in the staging of malignancy to determine distant disease.

Differential Diagnosis

Differential diagnoses are best considered with regard to the site of origin.

Cutaneous sarcoma – including MFH, angiosarcoma, leiomyosarcoma, Kaposi sarcoma

Benign – Infective ulcer (pyogenic granuloma), dermatofibroma

Malignant – Pigmented basal cell carcinoma (BCC), squamous cell carcinoma (SCC), melanoma

Deep soft tissue sarcoma

Benign – benign salivary gland tumors (pleomorphic/ monomorphic adenoma), lipoma, vascular malformations, benign schwannoma, benign lymph-adenopathy (reactive/infective, e.g., mycobacterial)

Malignant – metastatic carcinoma, melanoma, adenocarcinoma

Bone sarcoma

Benign – fibrous dysplasia, aneurysmal bone cyst, radicular cyst, ameloblastoma

Malignant – primary bone SCC

Staging Systems

American Joint Committee Cancer

NB – Histological Grade as a component of Staging

- Primary tumor
  - Tx – Primary tumor cannot be assessed
  - T0 – No evidence of primary tumor
  - T1 – Tumor less than 5 cm in greatest dimension (T1a, superficial; T1b, deep)
  - T2 – Tumor greater than 5 cm in greatest dimension (T2a, superficial; T2b, deep)
- Regional lymph nodes
  - Nx – Lymph nodes cannot be assessed
  - N0 – No lymph nodes metastases
  - N1 – Lymph nodes metastases present
- Distant metastases
  - Mx – Distant metastases cannot be assessed
  - M0 – No distant metastases
  - M1 – Distant metastases present
- Histopathologic grade
  - Gx – Grade cannot be assessed
  - G1 – Well differentiated
  - G2 – Moderately differentiated
  - G3 – Poorly differentiated
  - G4 – Undifferentiated
- Combined
  - IA (G1-2, T1a-b, N0, M0) – Low-grade, small, and superficial or deep tumor
  - IB (G1-2, T2a, N0, M0) – Low-grade, large, and superficial tumor

- IIA (G1-2, T2b, N0, M0) – Low-grade, large, and deep tumor
- IIB (G3-4, T1a-b, N0, M0) – High-grade, small, and superficial or deep tumor
- IIC (G3-4, T2a, N0, M0) – High-grade, large, and superficial tumor
- III (G3-4, T2b, N0, M0) – High-grade, large, and deep tumor
- IV (any G, any T, N1, M0) – Any metastasis

Memorial Sloan-Kettering staging system for soft tissue sarcomas

- Size (cm): Less than 5 cm is favorable; greater than 5 cm is unfavorable.
- Depth of invasion: Superficial is favorable; deep is unfavorable.
- Grade: Low is favorable; high is unfavorable.

Stage grouping based on Memorial Sloan-Kettering staging system for soft tissue sarcomas

- Stage 0–3 Favorable signs
- Stage I – 2 Favorable signs
- Stage II – 1 Unfavorable sign or 1 favorable sign and 2 unfavorable signs
- Stage III – 3 Unfavorable signs
- Stage IV – Distant metastases

Therapy

Therapy for sarcoma needs to be discussed in the context of a group of interested and experienced clinicians (Grimer et al. 2010). Most large population centers will have access to a specialized sarcoma group which is best resourced to properly assess and manage the patient with sarcoma. This is best achieved with a multidisciplinary framework and often with regional, national, or international collaboration. In the case of head and neck sarcoma, a combined approach between the head and neck multidisciplinary team and the sarcoma group is the ideal model.

Management of head and neck sarcoma is primarily surgical (Hoffman et al. 2004). Generously clear margins are the aim, but this is hampered by anatomical constraints. Adjuvant radiation is occasionally employed in an effort to augment margin status. Chemotherapy may be indicated, as in limb sarcoma, as neoadjuvant therapy in borderline resectable cases. Chemotherapy is most commonly employed in the setting of attempted control of metastatic disease. Its role in adjuvant therapy aimed at cure is not established, except in rhabdomyosarcoma and Ewings sarcoma. Doxorubicin-based chemotherapy following surgery for localized sarcoma in adults may confirm a 6–10% benefit on recurrence and 4% benefit on survival over 10 years (Sarcoma Meta-analysis Collaboration 2000).

References

de Bree R, van der Waal I, de Bree R, Leemans CR (2010) Management of adult soft tissue sarcomas of the head and neck. Oral Oncol 46(11):786–790

Grimer R, Judson I, Peake D, Seddon B (2010) Guidelines for the management of soft tissue sarcomas. Sarcoma

Hoffman HT, Robinson RA, Spiess JL, Buatti J (2004) Update in management of head and neck sarcoma. Curr Opin Oncol 16:333–341

Sarcoma Meta-analysis Collaboration (SMAC) (2000) Adjuvant chemotherapy for localised resectable soft tissue sarcoma in adults. Cochrane Database Syst Rev 4:CD001419

Sturgis EM, Potter BO (2003) Sarcomas of the head and neck region. Curr Opin Oncol 15:239–252

Head and Neck Squamous Cell Carcinoma, Risk Factors

Sarah Elizabeth Bailey
Department of Otolaryngology and Communicative Sciences, University of Mississippi Medical Center, Jackson, MS, USA

Definition

Betel nut: The product of the Areca catechu tree, is also known as areca nut, and is chewed habitually and acts as a mild stimulant.

Betel quid: The combination of betel leaf, areca nut, and slaked lime with or without other ingredients or flavorants.

Introduction

In 1993, a statistical model suggested that between six and ten independent genetic alterations were needed to accumulate prior to the development of head and neck squamous cell carcinoma (HNSCC)

(Chang and Ha 2010). It is generally accepted that this series of genetic changes must occur for frank malignancy to arise and account for the 20- to 25-year latency period seen in the majority of HNSCC. During this time, cumulative exposure to carcinogens is the principal cause of the specific genetic changes acquired during progression toward malignancy. The interaction between lifetime carcinogen exposure and genetic predisposition results in markedly different risks of developing HNSCC among individuals.

While the vast majority of head and neck cancers in the United States are squamous cell carcinomas of the upper aerodigestive tract, multiple factors have been shown to contribute to the development of this type of cancer (Sturgis et al. 2004). It is well known that the primary risk factors for HNSCC are the environmental toxins tobacco and alcohol, with tobacco exposure being a much higher risk factor. Each is a risk factor independent of the other, but they combine synergistically and in a dose–response fashion to further increase the risk of HNSCC (Hashibe 2010). Other known risk factors to the development of HNSCC include viral infections, occupational exposures, diet, genetics, and ultraviolet (UV) light exposure, among other risk factors. Other factors such as laryngopharyngeal reflux (LPR) remain controversial (Chang and Ha 2010).

Tobacco Exposure

It has been shown that processed tobacco contains more than 30 known carcinogens, whereas tobacco smoke contains high concentrations of reactive oxygen species and over 50 known carcinogens and procarcinogens (Chang and Ha 2010). The major carcinogens in cigarette smoke include polycyclic aromatic hydrocarbons (PAHs) and tobacco-specific nitrosamines (TSNA). Key events in malignant transformation of tobacco-associated tumors involve mutations in the p53 tumor suppressor gene, which is directly damaged by tobacco smoke constituents or metabolites, resulting in loss of normal cell growth mechanisms (Baez 2008).

Tobacco use includes smoking tobacco products such as cigarettes, cigars, and pipes, chewing smokeless tobacco products, and using snuff tobacco. Local smoking tobacco products such as bidi and chutta, both of which are hand-rolled Indian cigarettes, are also important risk factors for HNSCC. Chewing betel nut (areca nut) and betel quid with or without tobacco is widespread in certain regions of Asia and India and is an independent risk factor for the development of HNSCC with the effects being synergistic with tobacco and alcohol. Other types of tobacco use include water pipes in North Africa, the Mediterranean region, and parts of Asia; kreteks (clove-flavored cigarettes) in Indonesia; and suipa, chillum, or hookli (clay pipes) in Southeast Asia (Hashibe 2010).

Smoking is well known to increase the risk of developing HNSCC. There is a dose–response relationship for tobacco smoking, which is indicated by the fact that the relative risk for the development of HNSCC increases with the frequency, duration, and pack years of smoking in current tobacco users. Furthermore, the relative risk gradually declines after smoking cessation with no excess risk at 20 years. Other high risk factors for the development of HNSCC include age at onset of smoking less than 18 years of age and a duration of smoking more than 35 years (Hashibe 2010).

In comparison to nonsmokers, smoking has been shown to confer a 1.9-fold risk to males and a threefold risk to females for development of HNSCC. Individuals who smoke (2 packs daily) and drink alcohol (4 units of alcohol daily) are 35 times more likely to develop HNSCC than nonusers (Chang and Ha 2010). Other studies indicate between a 5- and 25-times greater risk for developing HNSCC in heavy smokers compared to nonsmokers (Baez 2008). Smokers that have been treated for cancer and who continue to smoke have been found to have a two- to six-times greater risk of developing a second primary tumor than those patients who stop smoking. Furthermore, epidemiologic studies have suggested that smokeless tobacco users (both chewing tobacco and snuff) have a fourfold increase in the risk of oral cavity carcinoma compared to nonusers (Chang and Ha 2010). This carcinogenic effect is attributed to the nitrosamines in the smokeless tobacco products of betel quid with tobacco, snuff, and chewing tobacco (Baez 2008).

Involuntary smoking, also known as environmental tobacco smoke exposure or passive smoking, is a proven risk factor for lung cancer, and studies indicate a relation between secondhand smoke and HNSCC. The literature has demonstrated that long-term involuntary smoke exposure is a risk factor for HNSCC, particularly of the pharynx and larynx, independent of tobacco smoking or alcohol drinking. Patients with HNSCC have been shown to have a significantly higher long-term exposure to involuntary tobacco smoke in both the workplace and home than controls without cancer. The larynx and pharynx experience higher rates of direct contact with involuntary smoking than the oral cavity, and thus, study results are consistent with the expectations supported by anatomic differences (Yuan-Chin et al. 2008).

Marijuana Exposure

Marijuana contains carcinogens similar to tobacco smoke, such as aromatic hydrocarbons, but in higher concentrations (Sturgis et al. 2004). It has generally been considered a risk factor for head and neck cancer; however, evidence regarding the association of smoking marijuana and the development of HNSCC is somewhat conflicting. It has been shown that marijuana is often smoked with tobacco or used along with alcohol, resulting in confounding and making confirmation or exclusion of this relationship more difficult. One study demonstrated a tobacco-adjusted risk of 2.6 for HNSCC associated with marijuana use, with evidence of a dose–response relationship (Sturgis et al. 2004). In contrast, a more recent meta-analysis demonstrated an increased risk of HNSCC in patients who have smoked marijuana for over 20 years and never used alcohol while adjusting for tobacco use, although the potential for confounding by tobacco use still exists (Berthiller et al. 2009). Therefore, studies have failed to show a strong association between marijuana smoking and an increased risk for HNSCC independent of tobacco smoking.

Alcohol Exposure

Although it is often difficult to separate the effects of smoking and alcohol, research has consistently shown that alcohol consumption independently increases the risk of squamous cell carcinoma in the upper aerodigestive tract. In addition, the risk of developing HNSCC is dose dependent. As an example, one study reported that alcohol alone confers a 1.7-fold risk of developing HNSCC to males drinking 1–2 beverages per day compared with nondrinkers, with a rise to more than threefold for heavy drinkers (Chang and Ha 2010).

Alcohol is proposed to cause HNSCC through a variety of mechanisms including the creation of DNA-damaging free radicals, immune suppression, the formation of a solvent effect on tobacco, and nutritional deficiencies (Baez 2008). Studies have also tried to correlate the type of alcoholic beverage with specific cancer risks, but the causative factor remains ethanol (Sturgis et al. 2004).

Increasing evidence indicates that the major carcinogenic effect of alcohol is acetaldehyde, which forms toxic-free radicals and is known to induce chromosomal aberrations and has also been linked to cancer development in animal models (Baez 2008).

Viral Infections

Human papillomaviruses (HPVs) are DNA viruses that specifically target the basal cells of epithelial mucosa with a family composed of more than 100 genotypes. It is well known that viral-type HPV 6, 11, 16, and 18 infect mucosal epithelial cells of the oral cavity, oropharynx, anogenital tract, and uterine cervix. Knowledge gained from cervical cancer has demonstrated that persistent infection with high-risk HPVs is required for cancer development. Several high-risk HPV types have been identified in HNSCCs, although there is a predominance of HPV type 16 (Chang and Ha 2010).

It has been demonstrated that oral HPV infection increases the risk for oropharyngeal cancer. Both molecular and epidemiologic evidence points to a causal role for HPV, primarily type 16, in a subgroup of head and neck cancers, namely, invasive tumors of the oropharynx and oral cavity. HPV-associated head and neck cancers have a different risk profile from non-HPV-associated head and neck cancers, including a high lifetime number of vaginal-sex partners, a high lifetime number of oral-sex partners, and seropositivity for HPV 16. Furthermore, patients are typically younger, are nonusers of tobacco and alcohol, and have a better prognosis, perhaps because of better radiation responsiveness and the absence of field cancerization (Chang and Ha 2010). Additionally, a strong association has been demonstrated between marijuana and HPV-16-positive HNSCC even after adjusting for sexual history, tobacco, and alcohol, although residual confounding may be reflected in this finding (Berthiller et al. 2009).

The strongest association between a virus and head and neck cancer has been demonstrated between Epstein-Barr virus (EBV) and nasopharyngeal carcinoma (NPC). EBV is a herpes DNA virus that infects the majority of the population worldwide during childhood or adolescence. After infection, immunity is developed, but EBV is present for lifetime. In acute and convalescent phases of infection, IgM and IgG antibodies to EBV antigens are raised. The EBV antigens include the nuclear core early antigen (Ea) and the viral capsid antigen (VCA). In the majority of the population, IgG VCA and IgG Ea are raised. However, in NPC, IgA VCA and IgA Ea are raised, making these antibodies useful as markers for NPC (Chang and Ha 2010).

Additionally, EBV antigens are found on NPC cells and not on normal nasopharyngeal cells. EBV expresses both lytic and nuclear antigens, with lytic antigens including latent membrane proteins 1, 2, and 3 (LMP-1, -2, -3) and nuclear antigens including Epstein-Barr nuclear antigens 1–6 (EBNA-1 to -6). In NPC, the EBNA-1 is always expressed, while LMP-1 is consistently expressed; neither of these latent proteins are expressed in normal nasopharyngeal cells. Furthermore, Epstein-Barr-encoded ribonucleic acids (EBERs) are expressed in the cytoplasm of NPC cells and not in normal nasopharyngeal cells (Chang and Ha 2010).

While the majority of population worldwide have been infected with EBV, most do not develop NPC. It is postulated that EBV is not the initiating event in NPC, but rather its role results from a latent infection of the genetically susceptible and environmentally transformed nasopharyngeal epithelial cells. NPC is a relatively rare malignancy in most populations, but is a much more common cancer in the Chinese population, supporting a genetic link or shared dietary habits (Chang and Ha 2010).

Patients infected with the human immunodeficiency virus (HIV) present with a variety of malignancies, and there has been a link made between HIV and HNSCC, although this has not been consistently demonstrated. Therefore, HIV remains most notably associated with non-Hodgkin's lymphoma and Kaposi's sarcoma of the head and neck. Moreover, herpes simplex virus (HSV) is less strongly correlated with the development of oral carcinomas than EBV or HPV, but these findings have never been confirmed (Chang and Ha 2010).

Occupational Exposures

Occupations or occupational hazards have been linked to head and neck cancer including asbestos, pesticides, polycyclic aromatic hydrocarbons, textile workers, wood workers, manufacturers of mustard gas, plastic, and rubber products, naphthalene refiners, ethanol, sulfuric acid mist, leather and paint workers, automobile mechanics, diesel exhaust, organic solvents, certain mineral oils, asphalt, stone dust, mineral wool, formaldehyde, construction workers (cement dust), farmers, metal workers (metal dust), the dry-cleaning agent perchloroethylene, and bartenders due to second-hand smoke. Although occupational exposures play a minor role overall, they are considered major risk factors for malignancies in the sinonasal region. The most important exposures occur in metalworking and refining, woodworking (wood dust), and leather or textile industries. Additionally, asbestos has been implicated as a risk factor for laryngeal cancer, although this association is weak (Chang and Ha 2010).

Diet

Dietary factors have been shown to contribute to the development of HNSCC. Studies have shown that the risk of nasopharyngeal carcinoma is increased with diets high in preservatives such as salted fish, eggs, and preserved meats, all of which contain high levels of nitrosamines (Chang and Ha 2010). An increased risk of HNSCC has also been associated with more frequent intake of red meat and animal fat (Chang and Ha 2010). Moreover, low folate levels may be a risk for HNSCC as shown in some studies, but not others (Sturgis et al. 2004).

Other studies have demonstrated an inverse association between beta-carotene and vitamin A intake, both of which are considered protective aspects of diets high in fruits and vegetables, and the risk of head and neck cancers. Among other possible protective factors are vitamins C and E, milk, vegetables, fruit, high-fiber diets, and increased zinc intake (Sturgis et al. 2004).

Diets are complex and highly variable, and it is difficult to translate foods into nutritional constituents. As a result, it is a challenge to precisely define the potential beneficial and detrimental compounds. Other factors confounding dietary assessment are the effects of smoking and alcohol. Smoking has been correlated with reduced dietary intake and serum carotenoid levels, while alcohol has been associated with low folate levels (Sturgis et al. 2004).

Genetics

Given that only a fraction of patients exposed to tobacco and alcohol develop HNSCC that some HNSCC occurs at unusually young ages and that some patients have no obvious exposure to known carcinogens, genetic susceptibility is implicated as a contributing factor to carcinogenesis (Baez 2008). Genetic susceptibility indicates that potentially inherited phenotypic differences in carcinogen-metabolizing systems, DNA repair systems, and cell cycle control or apoptosis all influence the risk for tobacco- and alcohol-induced cancers (Baez 2008).

Several observations are compatible with this hypothesis, although they do not exclude exposure to common environmental factors and may be a result of shared environmental factors (Chang and Ha 2010). One such observation is in first-degree relatives and siblings of patients with HNSCC, who have been shown to be more likely to develop HNSCC than controls (Chang and Ha 2010). Another such observation is in nasopharyngeal carcinoma, where it has been reported that the risk of NPC is up to eight times higher in a first-degree relative or up to 20 times higher compared to the general population (Chang and Ha 2010). Furthermore, certain HLA alleles have been consistently demonstrated to be more prevalent in NPC patients compared to the general population, while protective effects have been shown to be conferred by other alleles.

Ethanol is metabolized to acetaldehyde by alcohol dehydrogenase (ADH), which is then metabolized to acetate by aldehyde dehydrogenase (ALDH). Various alleles coding for the enzymes ADH and ALDH result in increased or decreased activity levels of the enzymes. Certain ADH alleles are thought to be protective because they are found in nonalcoholics or have significantly increased activity compared to other alleles, while other alleles are thought to increase the risk of HNSCC. Moreover, ALDH alleles which code for low enzyme activity result in increased accumulation of acetaldehyde and an increased risk of cancer;

other ALDH alleles code for an inactive ALDH, which results in high levels of acetaldehyde after drinking, which manifests as flushing, nausea, and tachycardia resulting in a tendency to limit alcohol intake (Baez 2008).

Not only is there a direct physical trauma resulting to the upper aerodigestive tract from smoking tobacco and drinking alcohol, but there may also be failure of deactivation of carcinogens or activation of procarcinogens as a result of genetic polymorphisms of intrinsic enzymatic systems that detoxify carcinogens (Chang and Ha 2010). One such system is the cytochrome P-450 enzyme system, which is responsible for oxidative metabolism of chemicals and consists of multiple subfamilies and approximately 60 separate P-450 genes. While these enzymes are found primarily in the liver, they are also found in the upper aerodigestive tract. One particular enzyme that has been studied is CYP1A1, which has been shown to have a mild risk association between one of its polymorphisms and the development of HNSCC. Other P-450 enzymes have been studied, and no conclusive data has been generated supporting or refuting an association with the development of HNSCC (Chang and Ha 2010).

Another such enzyme, glutathione S-transferase (GST), is a family of enzymes responsible for the detoxification of harmful chemicals such as polycyclic hydrocarbons of tobacco smoke. There are five separate loci that produce different GST subtypes, all of which are responsible for the detoxification of many different compounds. There are several polymorphisms within each subtype, which may account for certain patients being more at risk for HNSCC in the presence of tobacco smoke. Several studies have indicated that GSTM1 and GSTT1 have subtle effects contributing to an increased risk of HNSCC (Chang and Ha 2010; Baez 2008).

In addition, N-acetyl transferases, which metabolize aryl- and heterocyclic amines present in tobacco smoke, have polymorphisms causing variable levels of activity of the enzymes and thus have variable ability to detoxify carcinogens. It has been shown that the slow phenotype may result in an increased risk of oral squamous cell carcinoma (Baez 2008).

Altered DNA repair capacity has also been suspected to increase the risk of HNSCC. The nucleotide excision repair pathway, which is responsible for removing oxidative DNA damage, has been shown inconsistently to have certain polymorphisms associated with a risk of HNSCC (Baez 2008). While it is suspected that detoxification systems do contribute to the development of HNSCC, studies have also shown that these detoxification systems are functionally redundant such that only simultaneous deficiency in several enzyme systems increases the risk of HNSCC (Chang and Ha 2010).

Genetic susceptibility of individuals may be measured by mutagen sensitivity. Biomarkers are currently being developed that identify molecular changes associated with the development of HNSCC. These markers would therefore provide a means of measuring genetic susceptibility to cancer and potentially provide prognostic information. Through the use of biomarkers and genetic profiling, at-risk individuals could be identified, which could potentially impact early detection as well as primary and secondary prevention strategies (Sturgis et al. 2004).

Radiation

Previous ionizing radiation, whether for malignant or for benign disease, has not been linked to the development of HNSCC. There is, however, a strong association between gamma irradiation and head and neck sarcomas, salivary gland malignancies, thyroid cancers, and paranasal sinus cancers. Furthermore, the literature indicates that therapeutic radiation of head and neck malignancies does not increase the risk of second primary squamous cell carcinomas of the head and neck, but it does increase the rate of head and neck sarcomas. Environmental, medical diagnostic, and therapeutic radiation exposure to the head and neck are also associated with salivary gland malignancies and have a significant dose–response relationship with the risk increasing with increasing dose (Sturgis et al. 2004).

Other Risk Factors

Other factors that may contribute to the development of HNSCC in selected patients include poor oral hygiene and periodontal disease, which has been linked with carcinoma of the oral cavity, as well as immunosuppression, particularly lip cancer in the renal transplant recipient. Dental prostheses or poorly fitting dentures may also be an independent risk factor for the development of oral carcinoma. Likewise, mechanical irritation, thermal injury, and chemical exposure in pipe smoking may be etiologic factors contributing to the development of lower lip squamous cell carcinoma (Chang and Ha 2010).

There is controversy regarding the role of laryngopharyngeal reflux (LPR) and laryngeal cancer. Some studies have shown that LPR is associated with an elevated risk of laryngeal cancer after adjusting for age, gender, ethnicity, smoking, and alcohol. However, other literature supports that the relationship between LPR and laryngeal cancer is still unknown. Given these controversial findings thus far, it is still unknown whether or not LPR is an associated factor, a cocarcinogen, or an independent risk factor for laryngeal cancer (Chang and Ha 2010). In addition, *Helicobacter pylori* has been associated as a risk factor for laryngeal cancer, although these findings are lacking (Sturgis et al. 2004).

With regard to cutaneous squamous cell carcinoma, cumulative sun exposure, specifically to UV B radiation, is the most important environmental cause. In addition, age greater than 60 years is also a risk factor, while phenotypic characteristics such as fair skin, light-colored eyes, red hair, and Northern European origin also increase the risk of cutaneous squamous cell carcinoma. Furthermore, UV light exposure is associated with the development of lower lip squamous cell carcinoma (Chang and Ha 2010).

Conclusions

While there are many risk factors leading to the development of HNSCC, tobacco and alcohol exposure are known to account for the majority of cases. Further investigations into other factors known to modify the risk of HNSCC are needed for purposes of prevention efforts, early detection, and patient education in high-risk populations.

Cross-References

▶ Field Cancerization
▶ Tobacco and Head and Neck Cancer

References

Baez A (2008) Genetic and environmental factors in head and neck cancer genesis. J Environ Sci Health 26:174–200

Berthiller J, Yuan-Chin AL, Boffetta P et al (2009) Marijuana smoking and the risk of head and neck cancer: pooled analysis in the INHANCE consortium. Cancer Epidemiol Biomarkers Prev 18:1544–1551

Chang S, Ha P (2010) Biology of head and neck cancer. In: Flint PW, Haughey BH, Lund VJ, Niparko JK, Richardson MA, Robbins KT, Thomas JR (eds) Cummings otolaryngology head and neck surgery, 5th edn. Mosby/Elsevier, Pennsylvania, pp 1015–1029

Hashibe M (2010) Risk factors: tobacco and alcohol. In: Olshan EF (ed) Epidemiology, pathogenesis, and prevention of head and neck cancer, 1st edn. Springer, New York, pp 65–86

Sturgis EM, Wei Q, Spitz MR (2004) Descriptive epidemiology and risk factors for head and neck cancer. Semin Oncol 31:726–733

Yuan-Chin AL, Boffetta P, Sturgis EM et al (2008) Involuntary smoking and head and neck cancer risk: pooled analysis in the international head and neck cancer epidemiology consortium. Cancer Epidemiol Biomarkers Prev 17:1974–1981

Head Shadow Effect

Thomas J. Balkany[1] and Daniel M. Zeitler[1,2]
[1]Department of Otolaryngology-Head and Neck Surgery, University of Miami Miller School of Medicine, University of Miami Ear Institute, Miami, FL, USA
[2]Denver Ear Associates, Denver, CO, USA

Definition

When speech and competing noise are spatially separated, signal-to-noise ratio (SNR) at each ear is disparate due to the differential filtering of sound by the head. The listener can attend to the ear with the more favorable SNR in order to maximize speech recognition performance and sound localization. The head shadow effect does not rely on central auditory processing, and produces the most robust effect of binaural listening with improvements on the order of 4–7 dB.

Cross-References

▶ Adult Bilateral Cochlear Implantation

Headache and Facial Pain in Otolaryngology

Michael D. Lupa[1] and John M. DelGaudio[2]
[1]Department of Otolaryngology, Emory University, Atlanta, GA, USA
[2]Department of Otolaryngology-Head and Neck Surgery, Emory University School of Medicine, Atlanta, GA, USA

Synonyms

Migraine-associated vertigo; Migrainous vertigo; Vestibular migraine

Introduction

Headache is a near universal human experience. It is estimated that one person in three will develop a severe headache at some point during their life. The lifetime prevalence of all types of headaches is estimated to be 90% for males and 95% for women (Boes et al. 2008).

In addition to the considerable frequency of headache, the morbidity associated with headache can be significant. In a survey of 20,000 households in the USA, it was found that 18.2% of females and 6.5% of males were affected by migraine. More than 90% of those reporting migraines reported an impaired ability to function during attacks, and 53% reported severe disability requiring bed rest. About 30% had missed one day of work in the previous 3 months due to migraine (Lipton et al. 2001). This morbidity is a global phenomenon, with the World Health Organization listing migraine as one of the top 20 causes of disability (Leonardi et al. 2005).

Given its high prevalence, it is not surprising that migraine headaches and their variants have increasingly been implicated in many complaints seen in otolaryngology practices. One recent study highlighted this by looking at patients referred to a rhinology practice for "sinus" induced facial pain with negative computed tomography scans and normal nasal endoscopic exams. Basically, this group had no clear objective sign that their pain had an actual sinus etiology. In this group, the authors found that 58% of the patients improved with medical therapy for a variety of different types of headache after referral to a neurologist (Paulson and Graham 2004). In another study looking at patients presenting to a rhinology practice with facial pain or pressure, localized sinus headache, and physician- or self-diagnosed "sinus headache" with negative CT and nasal endoscopy exam, 92% had significant reduction in pain with empiric migraine-directed therapy (Kari and DelGaudio 2008).

The misdiagnosis of migraine as "sinus headache" can in part be due to the frequent occurrence of cranial autonomic symptoms in migraine patients. These symptoms include nasal congestion, rhinorrhea, lacrimation, conjunctival erythema, and eyelid edema and are frequently unilateral, although they can be bilateral. Barbanti et al. reported that 45.8% of patients suffering from migraine headaches reported cranial autonomic symptoms (Barbanti et al. 2002). The presence of these symptoms commonly leads to a misdiagnosis of "sinus headache." Schreiber et al. reported that of 80% of 2,991 patients with a self- or physician diagnosis of "sinus headache" were found to meet the IHS criteria for migraine headache (Schreiber et al. 2004).

In addition to being increasingly recognized as a cause "sinus headache," migraine and its variants have also been implicated as a common cause of vertigo in adults and children. This vertigo often appears without a concurrent headache (Lempert and Neuhauser 2005). It is estimated that this variant, termed vestibular migraine (also referred to as migraine-associated vertigo, migrainous vertigo), affects between 6% and 9% of patients seen in dizziness units. In one study of 100 patients with vestibular migraine or likely vestibular migraine as a cause of vertigo, migraine prophylactic medical therapy or conservative treatment was given consisting of physical therapy, lifestyle modification (migraine diet), and medication changes. The patients then retrospectively reported their symptoms. The medication group had significantly reduced duration, intensity, and frequency of episodic vertigo attacks once treatment was instituted (Baier et al. 2009). The conservative therapy group only had a reduction in the intensity of their vertigo symptoms. Though these results are promising, further study is required.

Headache Classification

Headache is a broad term encompassing most of the pain syndromes of the head and neck, and as such,

Headache and Facial Pain in Otolaryngology, Table 1 Classification of headaches from the International Headache Society

The primary headaches	The secondary headaches
Migraine	Headache attributed to head or neck trauma
Tension-type headache	Headache attributed to cranial or cervical vascular disorder
Cluster headache and other trigeminal-autonomic cephalgias	Headache attributed to a substance or its withdrawal
Other primary headache disorders	Headache attributed to infection
	Headache attributed to disturbance of hemostasis
	Headache attributed to disorder of cranium, neck, eyes, ears, nose, sinuses, teeth, mouth, or other facial or cranial structures
	Headache attributed to psychiatric disorder
	Cranial neuralgias and central causes of facial pain
	Other headache, cranial neuralgia, central or primary facial pain

From Headache Classification Committee of the International Headache Society (2004)

causes are diverse and for many instances, incompletely understood. All headache types however, share the commonality of involving the regions of the body innervated by the third cranial nerve and the upper cervical nerves (Oshinsky 2008).

The various types of headaches have been characterized by the International Headache Society into two broad groups, primary and secondary. Within these two main groups, the 14 main headache types are divided (see Table 1). Secondary headaches have a definable underlying pathologic cause. Causes include metabolic, infectious, inflammatory, traumatic, neoplastic, immunologic, endocrine, and vascular entities (Cady and Schreiber 2004). Though a headache can herald these serious conditions, it is important to remember that a significant secondary pathologic condition is rarely the cause of a headache, occurring approximately 1 in 250,000 cases (Cady and Schreiber 2004).

When no clearly identifiable cause can be found, then a headache is characterized as a primary headache syndrome. Headaches included in this group include migraine, probable migraine, tension-type headache, and cluster headache. These are far more common than

Headache and Facial Pain in Otolaryngology, Table 2 Findings suggesting secondary cause of headache

New onset of headache
Preceding trauma
Positional headache (initiated by standing, lying down, bending)
Systemic signs (fever, chills, weight loss)
Rapid onset of headache ("thunderclap headache")
Older age at onset
Focal neurologic symptoms (not consistent with typical migraine aura)
Headache due to transient increases in intracranial pressure (coughing, sneezing, Valsalva maneuver)

From Braun et al. (2010)

Headache and Facial Pain in Otolaryngology, Table 3 Migraine types and variants (International Headache Society Classification Committee)

Migraine without aura	Basilar-type migraine
Probable migraine without aura	Probable migraine with aura
Migraine with aura	Childhood periodic syndromes that are commonly precursors of migraine
Typical aura without headache	Cyclical vomiting
Familial hemiplegic migraine	Abdominal migraine
Sporadic hemiplegic migraine	Benign paroxysmal vertigo of childhood
Retinal migraine	Complications of migraine
Chronic migraine	Status migrainosus
Persistent aura without infarction	Migrainous infarction
Migraine – triggered seizures	

From Headache Classification Committee of the International Headache Society (2004)

secondary pathologies and will be the primary focus of this entry.

To differentiate between primary and secondary headache disorders, a thorough history, physical and neurologic examinations are required, with attention to potential "red flags" for a possible secondary headache disorder, which are listed in Table 2. Included with the usual physical exams must be examination of the eye, temporomandibular joint, cerebrovasculature (temporal arteries, carotid arteries for bruits), cervical paraspinal and trapezius muscles, and the sinuses. Abnormalities on exam should warrant consideration of whether a secondary headache disorder is present. If a secondary cause is suspected, a more thorough evaluation is required which may involve imaging (CT or MRI), blood work (complete blood count, complete metabolic count, erythrocyte sedimentation rate), angiography, or cerebrospinal fluid evaluation including opening pressure evaluation (Braun et al. 2010).

Migraine

As mentioned previously, migraine carries with it a significant burden of morbidity and is remarkably common. Patients will typically have their first headache by age 40. Up to 90% will also have a positive family history of migraine (Boes et al. 2008). No clear Mendelian genetic pathway has been isolated to date aside from the exceedingly rare autosomal dominant familial hemiplegic migraine (Schreiber 2006). Once migraine occurs, it tends to recur throughout a patient's life with variable frequency.

There are currently no reliable biological markers for migraine, so the disease is classified by its clinical features. These clinical features can be quite varied, and as such, migraine headaches and their variants have been grouped by the International Headache Society (IHS) into a number of different categories (see Table 3).

The 2004 IHS classification is extremely broad, and a description of all its subtypes is beyond the scope of this entry. One thing to note about the scheme is that it fails to address many of the migraine-related symptoms seen in otolaryngology practice. For instance, vertigo seen in migraine-associated vertigo is only described in the setting of basilar migraine and benign positional vertigo of childhood (Neuhauser and Lempert 2005). To rectify this, Lempert and Neuhauser proposed diagnostic criteria for migrainous vertigo in 2005 which are listed in Table 4. The IHS classification also fails to address the "sinus" symptoms seen in the likely migraine variant encompassing most sinus headaches (Cady and Schreiber 2004).

Migraine has been traditionally divided into those headaches with aura and those without aura. Both migraines without aura and with aura can be present in the same patient. Aura is the transient focal neurologic symptom that precedes headache in many patients with migraine. The most common symptom that patients with aura experience is termed scintillating scotoma or teichopsia. This is often described as a shimmering arc of white or colored light in the left or

Headache and Facial Pain in Otolaryngology, Table 4 Diagnostic criteria for migrainous vertigo or probable migrainous vertigo

Definite migrainous vertigo	Probable migrainous vertigo
Episodic vestibular symptoms of at least moderate severity	Episodic vestibular symptoms of at least moderate severity
Current or previous history of migraine according to 2004 criteria of the IHS	One of the following:
One of the following migrainous symptoms during ≥ 2 attacks of vertigo[a]: migrainous headache, photophobia, phonophobia, visual, or other auras	1. Current or previous history of migraine according to 2004 criteria of the HIS
	2. Migrainous symptoms during vestibular symptoms
	3. Migraine precipitants of vertigo in >50% of attacks
	4. Response to migraine medications in >50% of attacks
Other causes ruled out by appropriate investigations	Other causes ruled out by appropriate investigations

From Lempert and Neuhauser (2005)
[a]Vestibular symptoms are rotational or another illusory self or object motion. Vertigo maybe spontaneous or positional

right visual field homonymously. It will typically enlarge and may have a zigzag pattern. Commonly, it is followed by a spreading area of vision loss referred to as the negative scotoma (Boes et al. 2008). The next most common aura that patients may develop is the sensory aura which typically presents as a paresthesia. Less common auras include language auras (aphasia) and motor auras (transitory weakness).

The most common type of migraine headache is migraine without aura. According to the IHS, for a particular headache to achieve migraine status without aura, attacks must be recurrent (at least five previous attacks), last between 4 h and 72 h if untreated, and not be secondary to an underlying pathologic process (Cady and Schreiber 2004). In addition, the headache must meet at least two of the following four criteria: moderate to severe in intensity, unilateral, throbbing, and aggravated by activity. Finally, it must be associated with one of the following: nausea, vomiting, photophobia, or phonophobia.

Migraine with aura (also referred to as classic migraine) occurs in 15–20% of migraine sufferers (Boes et al. 2008). To meet the criteria for diagnosis, a patient must have had at least two headaches with aura, as defined above. The aura symptoms usually develop within 5–10 min and last less than 60 min.

A headache meeting criteria for migraine without aura typically will follow a patient's aura symptoms.

Basilar migraine is defined by the dramatic constellation of brainstem symptoms during its aura. It must be differentiated from vertebrobasilar insufficiency. To meet the criteria, a patient must have an aura encompassing two of the following symptoms according to the IHS: dysarthria, vertigo, tinnitus, hypoacusis, diplopia, visual symptoms, decreased level of consciousness, ataxia, or bilateral paresthesias. These aura symptoms are followed by a severe headache that is typically occipital in location. The headache may be associated with prolonged vomiting. Given the dramatic symptoms associated with this variant, an MRI and possible EEG are essential parts of the evaluation (Boes et al. 2008).

The IHS includes benign paroxysmal vertigo of childhood in its classification scheme. To meet the criteria, patients must be children that have at least five attacks of severe vertigo occurring without warning, lasting from minutes to hours. Vomiting and nystagmus are often associated with the vertigo symptoms, as are headaches. The evidence that the symptoms are migraine related is based on an epidemiological link with migraine in a series of these patients. Most of these series are small, and whether this is truly a migraine variant is still a matter of some debate (Krams et al. 2011).

Pathophysiology of Migraine
The understanding of the pathological changes causing migraine is still evolving. There is thought to be a genetic component, as mentioned above, but the exact nature is yet to be elucidated. The initial theory that headache is mediated by changes in vascular flow has been shown to be incomplete. Currently, most authors believe that the headache of migraine results from the activation of meningeal and other intracerebral blood vessel nociceptors in combination with a change in peripheral and central pain modulation (Silberstein 2008). This change in function is termed sensitization.

Headache and its associated neurovascular changes are all served by the trigeminal nerve. The trigeminal nerve has been found to secrete substance P, calcitonin gene-related peptide (CGRP), and neurokinin A at its branches on the intracranial vasculature. These peptides are thought to mediate neurogenic inflammation which is characterized by vasodilation, increased leakage of plasma proteins from dural vessels, increased platelet aggregation, as well as sensitization of surrounding nerve fibers (Boes et al. 2008). The role of CGRP has been shown by the efficacy of a CGRP antagonist in the treatment of migraine (Magis and Schoenen 2011). In addition, triptan medications, which are effective at treating migraine symptoms and discussed below, have been shown to inhibit the release of neuroinflammatory proteins at the peripheral branches of the trigeminal nerve (Schreiber 2006).

Once sensitization has occurred peripherally, it is thought to progresses toward the more central circuits of the trigeminal system including the trigeminal nucleus caudalis. A clinical marker of central pain sensitization is the presence of cutaneous allodynia (pain from a stimulus that is normally not painful). Evidence for this comes from the observation that triptan medications for migraine are vastly more effective if taken prior to the onset of cutaneous allodynia in patients, implying that central sensitization has yet to occur (Burstein et al. 2004).

Although research has focused on the intracranial portions of the trigeminal nerve, there is no reason to believe that the other branches of trigeminal nerve are immune to the pathological processes of migraine (Schreiber 2006). This may account for some of the symptoms seen in "sinus headache" which is now largely thought to be a migraine variant. Also, some authors have postulated that the pathologic changes seen in migraine are common to all primary headache disorders such as tension headaches and cluster headaches (Lipton et al. 2000). The model is based on the idea that the symptoms experienced during a given headache are determined by where the pathologic process terminates as it evolves through the peripheral and central portions of the trigeminal system. This cessation in headache evolution is thought to be from normal homeostatic mechanism present in the CNS countering the pathologic process leading to migraine headache. For instance, a headache that is terminated by normal homeostatic mechanisms in the peripheral sensitization phase would be experienced as either a probable migraine or a tension headache rather than an IHS-recognized migraine. This theory is termed the convergence hypothesis (Schreiber 2006).

Recent discoveries have also spread more light on the cause of aura, the defining symptom of classic migraine. As mentioned above, it is felt to be more of a neuronal process than a vascular one. Older research showed a spreading decrease in cerebral blood flow by xenon studies in patients with migraine beginning in the occipital lobe. This spread crossed vascular territories, decreasing the likelihood that it had solely a vascular cause. Newer studies with PET scans have also confirmed the presence of this phenomenon. This cortical spreading depression is widely thought to be the cause of visual aura. It has been linked to the headache of migraine by causing the activation of trigeminovascular afferents (Boes et al. 2008).

Treatment of Migraine

There is no cure for migraine, and treatment involves both lifestyle modification and medication. Lifestyle modification involves the avoidance of triggers. Triggers can be extremely varied and include things such as excessive stress, irregular sleep, and consumption of certain foods. Foods containing nitrites, red wine, and monosodium glutamate have all been linked to migraine. Medications such as caffeine, theophylline, and nifedipine have also been suspected of precipitating headaches.

Medical therapy is divided into prophylactic treatment and symptomatic treatment to relieve the pain, nausea, and other symptoms of an attack. Prophylactic therapy is needed when the frequency, duration, or simple dread of an attack interferes with a patient's lifestyle. Other indications for prophylaxis include control of prolonged neurologic symptoms and lack of response to symptomatic treatment (Boes et al. 2008).

Symptomatic treatment as stated above should be begun as early in the development of the migraine symptoms as possible. Some patients will get relief with simple nonspecific analgesics such as aspirin and acetaminophen. Other nonspecific treatments that are of value in the treatment of migraine include opioids and chlorpromazine (Silberstein 2008) and corticosteroids. Specific migraine medications include members of the triptan class and drugs of the ergotamine class. Triptans have strong agonist activity at 5-HT1B/D receptors in the CNS (Magis and Schoenen 2011). The 5-HT1B receptor mediates vascular constriction, whereas activation of the 5-HT1D receptor leads to inhibition of the release of sensory neuropeptides. Evidence indicates that activation of the 5-HT1D receptor leads to decreased excitability of the trigeminal nucleus caudalis which receives input from the trigeminal nerve.

The triptan family is diverse, and they come in a variety of different drug delivery methods including orally, subcutaneously, and intranasally. All are effective, and there is little guidance of which drug to use in a given clinical situation. Side effects of the oral triptans include tingling, flushing, and a feeling of heaviness in the head, neck, or chest. Side effects from injection of sumatriptan include local reaction, burning, and tingling sensation (local or generalized). These medications are contraindicated in patients with coronary insufficiency and also in patients with untreated hypertension and peripheral vascular disease (Silberstein 2008).

Ergot drugs are less specific for the 5HT receptor and have largely been replaced by the triptan drugs, though they still have a role in therapy. They are both vasoconstrictors and vasodilators depending on the dose. Ergotamine tartrate is available in an oral form as well as a rectal suppository. Dihydroergotamine, another member of this family, is very effective and is delivered by an intranasal or parenteral route. These drugs are contraindicated in women who are pregnant and, like the triptans, in patients with coronary artery disease and peripheral vascular disease (Boes et al. 2008).

Preventative medications include beta-adrenergic blockers, tricyclic antidepressants, and calcium channel blockers. In addition, anticonvulsants such as sodium valproate and gabapentin have both shown efficacy in migraine prophylaxis (Silberstein 2008). Other preventative measures tried include oral riboflavin and oral magnesium supplementation. The evidence for these measures is less robust than in some of the other preventative therapies listed. Of note, most studies looking at treatment for migrainous vertigo have utilized some combination or member of the preventative medications listed above in their treatment regimen (Baier et al. 2009).

Future therapies include CGRP antagonists termed the geptans which have the advantage of no vasoconstrictor properties, making them safer for a wider number of patients. Their efficacy has already been proven in a number of randomized controlled studies (RCTs), though their speed of action is slightly less than the triptans. Other future therapeutic options include a new 5HT1F agonist called lasmiditan which again lacks the vasoconstrictive effects of the triptans and nonpharmacologic therapies such as biofeedback (Magis and Schoenen 2011).

Tension-Type Headache

Tension-type headaches are the most common of the primary headache disorders (Braun et al. 2010). The lifetime prevalence of tension-type headache is between 30% and 70% (Ashina 2008). Numerous terms have been used for this headache in the past including tension headache, muscle contraction headache, psychomyogenic headache, stress headache, and ordinary headache. The IHS standardized the term tension-type headache and classified them into three types based on frequency: infrequent episodic, frequent episodic, and chronic tension-type headaches (Ashina 2008). The chronic form is the most debilitating and is present if a given headache is present for greater than 15 days in a given month.

The tension-type headache is bilateral, of a pressure-like quality, and of mild to moderate intensity. It is never associated with typical migrainous characteristics, such as aggravation by routine physical activity, severe nausea, vomiting, and severe photophobia or phonophobia. Mild nausea, phonophobia, and photophobia may however be associated with the chronic form of the disease. The headache may last anywhere from 30 min to 7 days.

The pathogenesis of tension-type headaches remains unclear. Research looking at peripheral myogenic causes from overuse, or prolonged positioning, has been unrevealing (Ashina 2008). Newer research has looked into the presence of central pain sensitization similar to the changes seen in migraine. Initial research has been encouraging.

Treatment is similar to migraine in that it is divided into acute therapy and preventative therapies. Common acute treatments include NSAIDs and acetaminophen. Interestingly, an RCT looking at the value of sumatriptan in patients meeting criteria for migraine, probable migraine, and tension-type headaches found that this drug was efficacious for all three types, again pointing to a common pathway in the three types of headaches (Lipton et al. 2000).

Preventative treatments are indicated for the disabling chronic variant. Evidence from randomized control trials supports the use of amitriptyline and the SSRI mirtazapine in this role (Ashina 2008).

Cluster Headache

Cluster headache also referred to as Horton's headache and histaminic cephalgia is the most painful of the recurrent headache disorders (Boes et al. 2008). They are rare when compared to migraine and tension-type headache and are four times more common in men than women (Braun et al. 2010). The headache belongs to a group of disorders referred to as trigeminal-autonomic cephalgias which include paroxysmal hemicranias and SUNCT (short-lasting unilateral, neuralgiform headache with conjunctival injection and tearing).

The headache is characterized by rapidly evolving, extremely painful attacks centered near the eye and temporal regions. The pain is accompanied by ipsilateral signs of autonomic nervous system activation which include conjunctival injection, lacrimation, nasal congestion, rhinorrhea, eyelid edema, sweating of the head or face, miosis, and ptosis. The other hallmark of the cluster headache is periodicity. This clustering period typically lasts between 2 and 12 weeks (Boes et al. 2008; Rozen 2009), though the timing of the cluster can vary. Also specific to this disorder is that the patients with cluster headache tend to be restless and agitated, as compared to migraine patients that prefer to stay still during their headaches. Per the IHS criteria, a patient must have suffered at least five attacks to be diagnosed with the disease. The pathophysiology of cluster headache is still being elucidated, and as with the other primary headache disorders, trigeminovascular connections are thought to play a central role.

Given the severity of cluster headaches, rapid relief of symptoms is required. The most commonly used treatments are oxygen, subcutaneous sumatriptan, and subcutaneous or intramuscular dihydroergotamine. Oxygen is thought to function through its vasoconstrictive effects. Other less frequently used therapies include octreotide and dripping 4% viscous lidocaine in the nostril ipsilateral to the pain (Rozen 2009).

Once the diagnosis is established, preventative therapy is imperative. Corticosteroids are excellent choice while establishing a diagnosis or if past history suggests that the patient's cluster will be of short duration. For longer-term prophylaxis, calcium channel blockers such as verapamil, lithium carbonate, melatonin, and topiramate can be employed (Rozen 2009).

Trigeminal Neuralgia

Trigeminal neuralgia, also referred to as *tic douloureux* is one of the most severe pains known. It has a slightly higher prevalence in women 1.5:1 and is generally seen between the fifth and seventh decade of life. The pain is described as shock like, shooting, or lancinating, and the duration is typically only seconds. The pain is felt in one or more divisions of the trigeminal nerve, most commonly the second and third divisions. The first division can be involved but only rarely (Braun et al. 2010). Though the tongue is innervated by the third branch of the trigeminal nerve, it is not typically involved by the process. Physical exam between attacks is normal with no sensory deficits in the range of the affected nerve. Once the disease has developed, it typically has an intermittent course with exacerbations and remittances. Spontaneous remission may occur.

The exact cause is unknown, but some have speculated that vascular loops around the Gasserian ganglion are the etiologic agent (Boes et al. 2008). Given this uncertainty, numerous medical and surgical therapies have been employed. Of the medical therapies, carbamazepine has been found to be the most efficacious, with up to 90% of patients responding (Prasad and Galetta 2009). Other medical therapies employed include phenytoin, baclofen, clonazepam, gabapentin, and valproate.

Nonmedical therapies involve ablation or blockade of the offending branch of the trigeminal nerve or the Gasserian ganglion itself. Simplest of these treatments is blockade of the affected nerve with alcohol. Longer-lasting treatment can be achieved with radiofrequency ablation of the peripheral nerve roots. Other treatments include middle fossa or posterior fossa section of the trigeminal sensory root and microvascular decompression of the Gasserian ganglion (Prasad and Galetta 2009).

Medication-Overuse Headache

Medication-overuse headache also referred to as "rebound headache and medication-induced headache" refers to the daily or near-daily headaches that are attributed to excessive use of acute headache medication. The disorder typically develops in patients who utilized medications greater than 10 days in a given month. All commonly used headache medications including triptans, ergots, and opioids may cause this disorder. The IHS criteria for the disorder involve having headaches on greater than 15 days on a given month coupled with overuse of an acute headache medication. The exact definition of what constitutes "overuse" per the IHS varies depending on the medication (Silberstein et al. 2005).

The difficult concept with this type of headache is that in order to treat it, and diagnose it, one must withdraw the patient from the very medications they are dependent on. In fact, one of the IHS criteria is that the headache resolves or reverts to its previous pattern within 2 months of discontinuation of the offending agent.

The treatment of these patients is difficult. The medication needs to be tapered and eventually discontinued. Steroids have shown some benefits during the transitional and acute withdrawal phase. If control cannot be achieved during the withdrawal, then prophylactic therapy needs to be initiated. At times during the withdrawal phase, patients may even need to be hospitalized for symptomatic control (Braun et al. 2010).

Summary

Headaches are an extremely common and extremely diverse group of disorders. The pathophysiology of primary headache disorders continues to be elucidated. Recent evidence has pointed to an increased role of migraine and migraine variants in many of the commonly seen complaints in otolaryngology practices. Effective treatments are available for these disorders and, when appropriately applied, can greatly improve the quality of life of an affected patient.

Cross-References

▶ Vertebrobasilar Insufficiency

References

Ashina M (2008) Tension-type headache. In: Scharpia A, Scharpia A (eds) Schapira: neurology and clinical neuroscience, vol 1, 1st edn. Mosby, St. Louis

Baier B, Winkenwerder E et al (2009) "Vestibular migraine": effects of prophylactic therapy with various drugs. A retrospective study. J Neurol 256(3):436–442

Barbanti P, Fabbrini G et al (2002) Unilateral cranial autonomic symptoms in migraine. Cephalalgia 22(4):256–259

Boes CJ, Capobianco DJ, Cutrer FJ, Cutrer FJ, Dodick DW, Garza I, Swanson JW (2008) Headache and other craniofacial pain. In: Bradley WJ (ed) Neurology in clinical practice, vol 2, 5th edn. Butterworth-Heinemann, Munich, pp 2,011–2,062

Braun ES, Schwedt JA, Swarm TJ, Hocking RA (2010) Pain management in the head and neck patient. In: Flint: cummings otolaryngology: head & neck surgery, vol 1, 5th edn. Mosby, St. Louis, pp 239–249

Burstein R, Collins B et al (2004) Defeating migraine pain with triptans: a race against the development of cutaneous allodynia. Ann Neurol 55(1):19–26

Cady RK, Schreiber CP (2004) Sinus headache: a clinical conundrum. Otolaryngol Clin North Am 37(2): 267–288

Headache Classification Committee of the International Headache Society (2004) The international classification of headache disorders: 2nd edition. Cephalalgia 24 Suppl 1:9–160

Kari E, DelGaudio JM (2008) Treatment of sinus headache as migraine: the diagnostic utility of triptans. Laryngoscope 118(12):2235–2239

Krams B, Echenne B et al (2011) Benign paroxysmal vertigo of childhood: long-term outcome. Cephalalgia 31(4): 439–443

Lempert T, Neuhauser H (2005) Migrainous vertigo. Neurol Clin 23(3):715–730, vi

Leonardi M, Steiner TJ et al (2005) The global burden of migraine: measuring disability in headache disorders with WHO's classification of functioning, disability and health (ICF). J Headache Pain 6(6):429–440

Lipton RB, Stewart WF et al (2000) Wolfe Award. Sumatriptan for the range of headaches in migraine sufferers: results of the spectrum study. Headache 40(10):783–791

Lipton RB, Stewart WF et al (2001) Prevalence and burden of migraine in the United States: data from the American Migraine Study II. Headache 41(7):646–657

Magis D, Schoenen J (2011) Treatment of migraine: update on new therapies. Curr Opin Neurol 24(3):203–210

Neuhauser HK, Lempert T (2005) Diagnostic criteria for migrainous vertigo. Acta Otolaryngol 125(11): 1247–1248

Oshinsky ML (2008) Headache pathogenesis. In: Silberstein SD (ed) Schapira: neurology and clinical neuroscience, 1st edn. Mosby, St Louis

Paulson EP, Graham SM (2004) Neurologic diagnosis and treatment in patients with computed tomography and nasal endoscopy negative facial pain. Laryngoscope 114(11): 1992–1996

Prasad S, Galetta S (2009) Trigeminal neuralgia: historical notes and current concepts. Neurologist 15(2):87–94

Rozen TD (2009) Trigeminal autonomic cephalalgias. Neurol Clin 27(2):537–556

Schreiber CP (2006) The pathophysiology of migraine. Dis Mon 52(10):385–401

Schreiber CP, Hutchinson S et al (2004) Prevalence of migraine in patients with a history of self-reported or physician-diagnosed "sinus" headache. Arch Intern Med 164(16):1769–1772

Silberstein SD (2008) Migraine. In: Scharpia A (ed) Schapira: neurology and clinical neuroscience, 1st edn. Mosby, St. Louis

Silberstein SD, Olesen J et al (2005) The international classification of headache disorders, 2nd Edition (ICHD-II)–revision of criteria for 8.2 Medication-overuse headache. Cephalalgia 25(6):460–465

Headache in Children

Howard S. Jacobs[1] and Jack Gladstein[2]
[1]Department of Pediatrics, University of Maryland School of Medical, Baltimore, MD, USA
[2]Department of Pediatrics and Neurology, University of Maryland School of Medical, Baltimore, MD, USA

Children with a primary headache disorder are often erroneously referred to otolaryngologists for evaluation/therapy of suspected ▶ sinusitis as the cause of their discomfort. A primary headache is defined as a headache intrinsic to the nervous system, that is, Migraine, Tension-Type Headache (TTH) or New Daily Persistent Headache (NDPH), as opposed to a secondary headache, which can be attributed to an extrinsic cause, such as sinusitis (Hershey et al. 2009). In a study by Senbil et al., 40% of patients diagnosed with migraine and 60% of patients with TTH had been previously misdiagnosed as a sinus headache (Senbil et al. 2008). Complicating the task of differentiating a primary headache from one caused by sinusitis is the fact that both sinus pain and primary headache pain are perceived through the trigeminal nerve; the upper branch, the ophthalmic branch, innervating the dura and the middle, maxillary branch, innervating the sinuses. The inferior, mandibular branch innervates the oral structures, which can also be associated with headache and neck pain.

Migraine Headaches

Migraine headaches are moderate to severe *episodic* headaches associated with *autonomic symptoms* (Table 1). For the purpose of this discussion we shall consider Migraine without Aura, Migraine with Aura, and Chronic (or Transformed) Migraine.

In 2004 the International Classification of Headache Disorders, 2nd edition (ICHD-II) was developed to allow clinicians and researchers to have established criteria for headache (Headache Classification Subcommittee of the International Headache Society 2004). The ICHD-II criterion for Migraine without Aura follows:

Description
Recurrent headache disorder manifesting in attacks lasting 4–72 h. Typical characteristics of the headache are unilateral location, pulsating quality, moderate or severe intensity, aggravation by routine physical activity and association with nausea and/or photophobia and phonophobia

Diagnostic Criteria
1. At least five attacks fulfilling criteria B-D
2. Headache attacks lasting 4–72 h (untreated or unsuccessfully treated)
3. Headache has at least two of the following characteristics
   (a) Unilateral location
   (b) Pulsating quality
   (c) Moderate or severe pain intensity
   (d) Aggravation by or causing avoidance of routine physical activity (e.g., walking or climbing stairs)
4. During headache at least one of the following
   (a) Nausea and/or vomiting
   (b) Photophobia and phonophobia
5. Not attributed to another disorder

Migraine with Aura is the same as the above but the headache is preceded by an aura. Auras are usually, but not always visual, usually described as the scintillating scotoma (Scotoma Fig. 1). But they may also be auditory, olfactory or gustatory.

Unfortunately ICHD-II criteria apply very well to the adult population, but not so well with children. Pediatric and adolescent migraineurs often present with bilateral pain, which may or may not be throbbing in nature and may be of shorter duration (Virtanen et al. 2007). From a clinical perspective when the headaches are *intermittent, moderate to severe* and associated with *autonomic symptoms* such as nausea, photophobia and/or phonophobia, they are migraine headaches, even if of shorter duration or not throbbing in nature. Often the child or her/his parent will describe the necessity of lying down in a darkened room when suffering from the headache. Usually, a family history of recurrent headache, which on detailed questioning is consistent with migraine, will be present. Further, pediatric patients seldom present with migraine with aura. A preceding aura makes the diagnostic process straightforward and easily distinguishes it from a secondary headache.

Chronic Migraine also called Transformed Migraine is characterized as a more frequent, even daily, lower

Headache in Children, Table 1 Comparison of Headache Types

	headache	Pattern	Autonomic Sx	Nasal discharge	Fever	Cough
Migraine	+++−++++	Intermittent	Present	+/− watery, self limited	None	None
TTH	+−++	Intermittent	None	Not present	None	None
NDPH	+−++++	Variable	Usually	+/− watery, self limited	None	None
Sinusitis	+/−	Persistent	None	Acute purulent *or* >10–14 days	+/−	Present

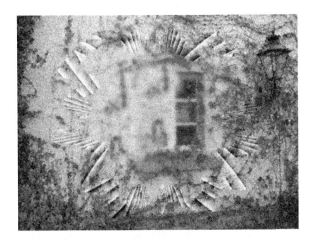

Headache in Children, Fig. 1 Scotoma (from Delia Machert at Migraineaura.com)

level headache, punctuated by spikes of severe headache pain. This type of migraine usually has developed over a period of time. However this time frame is much shorter in pediatric patients than it is in adults, as short as 6 months (Gladstein and Holden 1996).

Of note, as part of the autonomic symptom complex, a patient may experience nasal congestion or nasal discharge during an acute migraine headache, but migraine specific symptoms will also be present (Cady and Schreiber 2004; Senbil et al. 2008; Hershey et al. 2009).

Tension-Type Headaches (TTH)

TTH are also intermittent headaches but are less severe than migraines and are not associated with autonomic symptoms. The important key in differentiating this from sinus headache is (1) the intermittent nature of the headache and (2) the absence of symptoms referable to the upper respiratory tract. It should be noted

that TTH can, like migraine, evolve into a chronic form i.e., Chronic Tension Type Headache

New Daily Persistent Headache (NDPH)

New Daily Persistent Headache (NDPH) is a troubling disorder characterized by abrupt onset of daily headache with no history of head injury and without any preceding headache complaint. Often the patient can tell the care provider the exact day of onset (Winner et al. 2008). Again the absence of respiratory symptoms is of note (Table 1).

Sinusitis

The AAP published diagnostic criteria for pediatric sinusitis in 2001 (Subcommittee on Management of Sinusitis and Committee on Quality Improvement 2001),

> The diagnosis of acute bacterial sinusitis is based on clinical criteria in children who present with upper respiratory symptoms that are either persistent or severe

The persistent symptoms of significance were *nasal or post-nasal discharge, daytime cough* or *both* lasting at least ten to fourteen days, and the severe symptoms included a fever *of at least 39 °C with purulent nasal discharge for at least 3 days in an ill appearing child*. It should be noted that headache is not included here. The paper notes that unilateral frontal or periorbital head pain may be present, but is not a necessary part of the diagnosis.

In the adult literature, headache is a minor diagnostic criterion for sinusitis (Mucha and Baroody 2003). Further, headache alone is not sufficient to make a diagnosis of sinusitis and has been shown to have no relationship to the appearance of the sinuses on

Computerized Tomography (Shields et al. 2003; Cady and Schreiber 2004).

Unlike the primary headaches, the headache of sinus origin should be associated cough and acute purulent discharge or persistent nasal discharge of greater than 10–14 days (Table 1). Whereas the symptoms of primary headache are expected to be intermittent, the symptoms of sinus inflammation should be persistent.

The following table may be helpful:

Imaging

Can imaging help the practitioner? CT scans of the sinuses bear little relationship to the complaint of headache and multiple studies have shown that plain films and CT scans are usually not necessary for the diagnosis of sinusitis and often can confuse the picture (Newton 1996; Cady and Schreiber 2004).

What if the physician is confident that the headache is not secondary to a sinusitis; does imaging help further the diagnostic process? In the presence of a history consistent with primary headache for greater than 6 months duration and a normal neurologic exam the answer would be that it does not (Lewis et al. 2002). If, however, the history or exam raises concerns that this might not be a primary headache, then the study of choice would be an MRI. While a CT scan is very helpful in the emergency setting, an MRI allows views of the posterior fossa that cannot be obtained with CT. This is of great importance as pediatric tumors are often found in the posterior fossa.

Treatment

Once the diagnosis of migraine has been established, it is reasonable for the otolaryngologist to initiate treatment for the child if the headaches are still intermittent (less than one to two per week). Though it may be necessary to treat associated nausea with antiemetics and some migraines can be successfully treated with acetaminophen or NSAIDS, the mainstays of intermittent therapy are the triptans. Although almotriptan (Axert – Janssen Pharmaceuticals) is the only triptan currently FDA approved in the pediatric age range, and then only those 12 and above, the triptans have been used with acceptable tolerability and success in pediatric migraine (Hamalainen et al. 1997; Lewis et al. 2004;

Vollono et al. 2011). Triptans are 5HT1B/D agonists and as such are thought to mimic serotonin which gets temporarily depleted during an acute migraine attack. These drugs stop sterile inflammation and work best at the earliest onset of the headache. Using the "let's give it an hour and see what happens" approach will likely guarantee poor response to triptan therapy.

There are a number of triptans available for our use. In the preschool child, rizatriptan (Maxalt MLT – Merck) and zolmitriptan (Zomig ZMT – AstraZenica) offer the advantage of a meltaway tablet.

In school age and older patients, Sumatriptan, which is available in tablet, nasal spray, and air injectable or SQ injectable forms is often used. It should be noted however that the nasal spray, should not be sniffed into the oropharynx as the taste is quite bad. If the nasal spray is to be used, the patient should be instructed to use the spray with the head bent forward and not sniff the medicine back. Obviously, the drawback with a SQ form is the patient anxiety and discomfort. Unfortunately, though the air injectable form (Sumavel DosePro – Zogenix) is needle-less, it is not without local discomfort. The oral sumatriptan, in most cases, is the easiest to use, with three dosage strengths; 25 mg for the school age child, 50 mg for the young teen and 100 mg for the older teen or particularly large patient.

In addition to the use of prescription drugs, the otolaryngologist can recommend behavioral strategies that might decrease frequency and severity of attacks. Migraineurs can be often overscheduled, not get enough sleep, miss meals and suffer from stresses that may not be impacting their peers. Addressing the lifestyle issues is a key element of migraine care, as is referral of patients for relaxation therapy, self-hypnosis, biofeedback or behavioral modification programs.

Pediatric migraineurs with more frequent headaches should be referred to a pediatric headache specialist who will be able work with the patient and her/his family over a more extended period of time than may be practical for a busy otolaryngologist.

Cross-References

▶ Sinusitis

References

Cady RK, Schreiber CP (2004) Sinus headache: a clinical conundrum. Otolaryngol Clin North Am 37:267–288

Gladstein J, Holden EW (1996) Chronic daily headache in children and adolescents: a 2-year prospective study. Headache 36(6):349–351

Hamalainen M, Hoppu K, Santavuori P (1997) Sumatriptan for migraine attacks in children: a randomized, placebo-controlled study. Do children with migraine respond to oral sumatriptan differently from adults? Neurology 48(4):1100–1103

Headache Classification Subcommittee of the International Headache Society (2004) The international classification of headache disorders. Cephalalgia Int J Headache 24(suppl 1):1–160

Hershey A, Powers S, Winner P, Kabbouche M (2009) Pediatric headaches in clinical practice. Wiley-Blackwell, Hoboken

Lewis D, Ashwal S, Dahl G et al (2002) Practice parameter: evaluation of children and adolescents with recurrent headaches: report of the Quality Standards Subcommittee of the American Academy of Neurology and the Practice Committee of the Child Neurology Society. Neurology 59(4):490–498

Lewis D, Ashwal S, Hershey A et al (2004) Practice parameter: pharmacological treatment of migraine headache in children and adolescents. Neurology 63(12):2215–2224

Mucha SM, Baroody FM (2003) Sinusitis update. Curr Opin Allergy Clin Immunol 3:33–38

Newton DA (1996) Sinusitis in children and adolescents. Prim Care Clin Office Pract 23(4):701–717

Senbil N, Yavuz Gurer YK, Uner C, Barut Y (2008) Sinusitis in children and adolescents with chronic or recurrent headache: a case-control study. J Headache Pain 9:33–36

Shields G, Seikaly H, LeBoeuf M et al (2003) Correlation between facial pain or headache and computerized tomography in rhinosinusitis in Canadian and U.S. subjects. Laryngoscope 113:943–945

Subcommittee on Management of Sinusitis and Committee on Quality Improvement (2001) Clinical practice guidelines: management of sinusitis. Pediatrics 108:798–808

Virtanen R, Aromaa M, Rautava P et al (2007) Changing headache from preschool age to puberty. A controlled study. Cephalalgia Int J Headache 27(4):294–303

Vollono C, Vigevano F, Tarantino S, Valeriani M (2011) Triptans other than sumatriptan in child and adolescent migraine: literature review. Expert Rev Neurother 11(3):395–401

Winner P, Lewis D, Rothner D (2008) Headache in children and adolescents, 2nd edn. BC Decker, Hamilton

Hearing (Sensorineural Hearing Loss – Infection)

▶ Congenital Cytomegalovirus and Sensorineural Hearing Loss

Hearing (Sensorineural Hearing Loss – Pediatric)

▶ Congenital Cytomegalovirus and Sensorineural Hearing Loss

Hearing Aid

Karam Badran, Hossein Mahboubi and Hamid Djalilian
Department of Otolaryngology-Head and Neck, University of California, Irvine Medical Center, Orange, CA, USA

Definitions

1. ▶ *Sensorineural Hearing Loss*: Hearing loss due to cochlear hair cell or auditory nerve dysfunction in the inner ear or in the neural structure from ear to brain.
2. ▶ *Conductive Hearing Loss*: Sound conduction to the inner ear is diminished or nonoccurring due to a dysfunction in the external and/or the middle ear.
3. ▶ *Mixed Hearing Loss*: The presence of both sensorineural and conductive hearing loss.
4. ▶ *Single-Sided Deafness*: The presence of severe to profound hearing loss in one ear.
5. *Monaural/Binaural Hearing Aid*: One hearing aid (monaural). Two hearing aids (binaural).
6. *Analog Hearing Aid*: A type of hearing aid that utilizes analog audio processing to provides amplification by representing the voltage of sound signals as a continuous set of values. This amplification system creates an electrical signal that is analogous to the input acoustic signal in frequency, intensity, and temporal patterns.
7. *Digitally Programmable Analog Hearing Aid*: Contains an analog sound path that is modified by digital control circuits rather than an integrated circuit. The digital control circuits are programmed by an external device and do not require the hearing aid to possess any fitter controls allowing for large numbers of controls. The digital controller also contains more than one memory setting so that the user can access different programs than adjust

amplification levels according to the environmental setting surrounding the user.

8. *Digital Hearing Aid*: Contains an analog-to-digital converter, which changes sound to a series of numbers. These numbers are then manipulated before being converted back to an analog signal. By processing numbers, more complex and fine processing of sound to specific frequencies can be accomplished through the integrated circuit. This circuit is also smaller and therefore uses less power than the analog processing method.

Introduction

The treatment for hearing loss has several approaches depending on the location of the lesion and the degree of deficit across frequencies based on audiologic evaluation. Lesions in the external and middle ear result in ▶ conductive hearing loss, which is treated with medical or surgical treatment. Hearing loss due to inner ear or eighth cranial nerve lesions result in a sensorineural deficit treated through amplifying the signal. The decision to provide patients with amplification is based on the degree of hearing loss and the individual's self-perceived communication difficulty. For some individuals, a mild hearing loss has a severe impact on their ability to function, and for others, a moderate-to-severe hearing loss has little impact on their perceived day-to-day function. For pediatric patients, the American Academy of Audiology Pediatric Amplification Guidelines indicates that amplification with hearing instruments should be considered for a child who demonstrates a hearing loss, including sensorineural, conductive, or mixed hearing losses of any degree (Palmer 2009). The amplification of sound through the conversion of speech is made possible due to the hearing aid's ability to convert a speech signal into an electrical impulse directed and amplified toward the inner ear.

Individuals have suffered with hearing loss since the evolution of man. The earliest recorded forms of hearing aids as a method of sound amplification came in the form of large, horn-shaped, unpowered, ear trumpets used to direct sound into the ear of a hearing-impaired person in the late seventeenth century. Beginning in the eighteenth century, bone-conducting aids, unlike the former air conducting hearing aids, were noted in literature that described sound passing through a solid wooden object that the listener placed against their teeth. Bone conduction allowed sound to transmit to the inner ear via the vibration of the teeth and skull. By the 1920s, hearing aids began using an external power source to operate a microphone. The microphone converted the sound to an electrical signal that was transmitted to a carbon body, used to amplify the current to be released via speaker into the external ear canal. Vacuum tube hearing aids replaced the carbon body in the 1950s increasing the efficiency of amplification, yet units were still large. The development of the transistor paved the way for one piece, present-day analog hearing aids that can be placed behind the ear or deep within the external auditory canal. These analog hearing aids refer to the mechanism where the electrical voltage is similar to the sound pressure level entering the microphone.

The fundamental structure of a hearing aid is composed of a microphone, amplifier, and receiver. The microphone receives the acoustic signal (Fig. 1) and converts it to an electric or binary signal, depending on analog or digital technology, respectively. This signal is then passed through the amplifier that intensifies the signal and then converts it back into an acoustic signal through the receiver and is funneled to the eardrum.

Transmission of the signal, style, monaural versus binaural amplification, circuitry, signal processing and output, and program options dictate the type of hearing aid that is used by the individual. The sound signal can be delivered through bone conduction, for individuals suffering from middle and outer ear disease, or by air conduction when the deficit concerns only the inner ear. Bone conduction hearing aids, where surgical/medical treatment is not warranted or is declined by the individual, can come in the form of an external bone vibrator or as an implantable device, as seen in the bone-anchored hearing aid (BAHA). Transcranial contralateral routing through bone can also be of use in transmitting sound from the contralateral nonfunctioning ear to the functioning ear. Air conducting devices, utilized by the majority of patients, rely on air conduction in the outer and middle ear. Several air conduction models are present and selection of a specific style is based on the size and shape of the ear canal, power requirements, and features needed to compensate and address hearing loss, and the aesthetic needs of the patient. Styles include behind-the-ear, in-the-ear, in-the-canal, and completely-in-the-canal. Regardless the method of

Hearing Aid, Fig. 1 Digital versus analog hearing aids. Analog hearing aids follow the *top* path, while digital hearing aids take the *lower* path

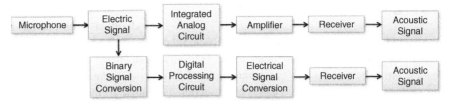

conduction, a choice between monaural and binaural compensation must be made. Monaural external hearing aid is best utilized when hearing losses are minimal, or unilateral hearing deficits are significant. Binaural amplification however, should be utilized in individuals with hearing loss in both ears. Binaural hearing aids elicit a significant advantage to noise suppression and enhancement in the signal-to-noise ratio (Kim and Barrs 2006).

Implantable devices are becoming more widely utilized to overcome compliance issues dealing with conventional external hearing aids. The conventional aid has had complaints of stigma, acoustic feedback, occlusion effect, difficult manipulation controls, and being easily lost or damaged. Regardless of the type of hearing aid, implantable or not, all aids require a fitting and verification process (Counter 2008).

Initially, an audiologic examination and a discussion of the individual's communication needs are undertaken. The optimal method of delivering a sound signal (air/bone conduction, programmability of the aid, monaural/binaural, bandwidth) is selected while still upholding the patient's preference in style and level of compliance. After the final decision is made on the type of hearing aid, an ear impression is made. The quality of the impression that captures the external auditory meatus and outer ear dictates the physical fit and comfort of the hearing aid. Once received, verification of hearing aid output that is in accordance to design parameters is assessed through electroacoustic function analysis done in a test chamber. The verification of output parameters leads to further customization as the hearing aid is programmed to the patient's audiometric needs and expectations. Decisions to be made while programming include memory options, feedback reduction, and gain responses. It is after programming that the physical fit of the device is assessed. If later the hearing aid does not meet the acoustic expectations of the user, the digital sound processing technology of modern hearing aids allows for programming to fit a wide

degree of hearing loss. The fitting process is uniform for most patients; however, certain circumstances surround the fitting of infants and the elderly (Stach and Ramachandran 2010).

Pediatric Hearing Aid Fitting

The fitting of an aid for a child or infant is challenging for several reasons. The smaller external ear anatomy and canal results in higher sound pressures, while the resonance qualities of the child are different from the adult making some frequencies appear louder than others (Stach and Ramachandran 2010). This has given rise to pediatric guidelines that are different from those of adults. With growth, anatomy and sound characteristics/environments change and must be regularly accounted for in hearing aid adjustment, selection, and fitting.

Aside from physical variances from adults, the child's hearing deficit is not as well characterized, which makes prescribing gain difficult. Provided the difficulties, it is crucial to ensure rehabilitation early in life as neural connections in the brain that allow speech to be understood are formed based on the signals they receive from the cochlea (Moodie 2004). In order to maximize expressive language ability, it is best if both cochleas are sending signals to the auditory cortex; for this reason, binaural hearing aids are essential unless there is a contraindicating concern or severe unilateral hearing loss.

The style of choice is a behind-the-ear hearing aid to allow for growing ears and a less costly replacement of only the ear mold rather than the entire aid. In addition to the economic practicality, BTE aids allow for assistive listening devices such as FM or other wireless systems to be utilized. This allows for wireless transmission from an external microphone to the receiver found in the ear, aiding in the ability to discriminate a sound signal from noise, found especially useful in the classroom. Difficulties in fitting continue as individuals become older (Palmer 2009).

Hearing Aid Fitting in the Elderly

As patients age, changes in neuronal activity and the central nervous system sometimes affect auditory senses. These neural changes compound earlier hearing deficits. If auditory nervous system function is extremely affected, these elderly patients do not appear to benefit as much from hearing aids as those adults with similar hearing deficits. These findings point to complementary components and assistive listening devices, in addition to hearing aids, for improved signal-to-noise ratio in the fitting guidelines for the elderly. Components include directional microphones, noise-reduction processing, and remote microphones. A diminished neural system can also cause cognitive deterioration resulting in the inability to correctly position the aid. In addition, manifestations of old age may result in difficulty while manipulating the hearing aid due to arthritis and a myriad of other complications (Kricos 2006).

Digital Hearing Aid Technology

Technological advances have greatly improved the usability of conventional air conducting aids. The most notable change in hearing aids has been the transition from the analog aid to the most recently developed digital signal processing technology. Analog aids produce electrical voltage from the microphone that is similar to the sound pressure that is received. Amplification in this method is not always ideal for individuals with decreased dynamic range resulting in the need for greater or lesser amplification and feedback.

Digital aids are programmable and provide preset programs to allow automatic changes in the output of the hearing aid depending on the acoustic situation. This is made possible through the converter that is placed within the microphone that modifies the original analog signal into one that is based on a series of numbers. This digital signal is then filtered for distortion and processed at specific frequency bands by means of a preset algorithm. The amplified binary information is then converted and filtered into sound energy prior to entering the external auditory canal. Through the filtration processes, the digital hearing aid is able to reduce the acoustic distortion. The ability to include a preset programmable algorithm, which controls the amplification of specific frequency channels,

compensates for a decreased dynamic range in those individuals with hearing loss. The decreased range is due to an increase in the threshold of audibility while the upper limit of discomfort stays the same.

Current digital hearing aids also attempt to remove noise from the speech signal by recognizing noise as a constant frequency and speech as a fluctuating one. In removing noise, speech is brought out of the background increasing the signal-to-noise ratio. Other breakthroughs have been made to boost the signal-to-noise ratio through advances in microphone modes. These advances have led to hearing aids with dual microphones rather than the single omnidirectional microphone. The dual microphones act to focus one microphone at a point anterior to the individual with greater sensitivity and the other microphone, pointing posteriorly, is used to acoustically delay and cancel the background noise. This allows a specific direction to preferentially become amplified while the other direction is preferentially suppressed producing an improved signal-to-noise ratio. With further automation providing high-fidelity amplification, hearing aid technology has made tremendous strides since the day of the ear trumpet.

Hearing Aid Styles

Behind-the-Ear Hearing Aids

Current Behind-the-Ear (BTE) hearing aids have evolved from the classic hearing aid models. They consist of a case that is situated behind the auricle and includes all three components of the hearing aid: microphone, amplifier, and receiver. A hollow tube, which passes over the pinna and connects to a custom-fitted ear mold inside ear canal, transmits the amplified sound. The tube and mold materials and shape can change the intensity and frequency gain. This enables providers to design customized hearing aids. Subcategories of BTEs include open-canal fittings and receiver-in-the-canal (RIC). The first one uses a thinner tube and a standard mold that does not occlude the canal completely. This model is suited for high-frequency hearing loss since it allows low-frequency sounds to pass the open ear canal. In RICs, the receiver is separate from microphone and it is connected to the main behind the ear case with a thin wire. This allows lower acoustic feedback and a smaller BTE case.

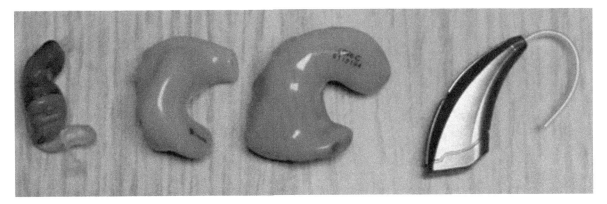

Hearing Aid, Fig. 2 Different styles of hearing aids. From *left*: completely-in-the-canal (CIC), in-the-canal (ITC), in-the-ear (ITE), and behind-the-ear (BTE)

BTEs are relatively larger than other styles (Fig. 2) and accommodate larger batteries that allow longer wearing time. User buttons to control volume or program options are located on the backside. Approximately 31% of hearing aid users wear BTE styles (Natalizia et al. 2010).

In-the-Ear (ITE)

ITE hearing aids contain the same components as BTEs, but they sit entirely in the concha and external auditory canal. They are custom-made based on the patient's anatomy. The customization makes these instruments inappropriate for young children and infants due to frequent changes in ear size and geometry. ITEs are relatively smaller than BTEs (Fig. 2) but are still able to utilize large batteries and are equipped with a directional microphone. The acoustic feedback is higher than BTEs but still reasonable. ITEs are the most popular hearing aids with about 38% of patients using them (Natalizia et al. 2010).

In-the-Canal (ITC)

While its name implies that this system lies in the canal, this hearing aid is actually a smaller version of the in-the-ear hearing aid that fills a smaller part of the concha not extending beyond the tragus. This style of hearing aid proves to be difficult to insert and remove from the ear canal (Fig. 2); however, its basic appeal is cosmetic and improves the communication abilities of those patients with marginal hearing loss. The placement of the aid gives the user the advantage of pinna acoustic effects and increases gain in the high

frequencies due to the location of the microphone being at the entrance of the ear canal (Bailey et al. 2006).

Completely-in-the-Canal (CIC)

The development and marketing of this type of aid was in response to the public's continual demand for a hearing aid that could not be detected when placed in the canal. Unlike the ITC hearing aids, the completely-in-the-canal (CIC) aid fits entirely within the ear canal, with no part protruding into the concha (Fig. 2). However, this comes with discomfort, as well as problems with inserting and removing the hearing aid. In order to obtain maximum benefits from CIC aids, certain fitting criteria must be met, including the distance of the lateral end of the hearing aid from the meatal opening, and the distance of the medial end of the hearing aid from the tympanic membrane. Its deep insertion takes full advantage of pinna and concha effects, boosting real gain in the high frequencies, and reduces occlusion effects (Bailey et al. 2006). This also eliminates feedback from telephone use as experienced by the more protruding ITE and ITC hearing aids; however, it also precludes the use of a directional microphone.

As body styles continue to decrease in size, so do their batteries. This comes with problems in replacing the battery and aid as greater dexterity becomes more important. Lyric (InSound Medical Inc., Newark, CA) is a continuous wear hearing aid developed to solve battery insertion and insertion/removal issues with CIC hearing aids. The Lyric aid remains 24 h a day

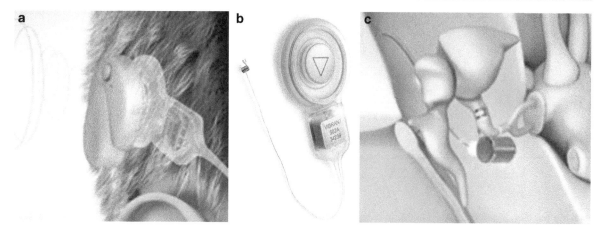

Hearing Aid, Fig. 3 The external processor (**a**) of the Vibrant Soundbridge contains the microphone. The subcutaneously placed implant with electronic lead to the Floating Mass Transducer (**b**). The Floating Mass Transducer is seen attached to the incus (**c**)

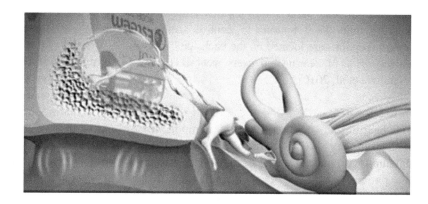

Hearing Aid, Fig. 4 The Envoy Esteem is completely implantable. The processor is subcutaneously inserted and the piezoelectric transducer is seen receiving and delivering mechanical stimuli

inserted into the bony part of the external auditory meatus for up to 4 months at a time. The fitting process is also designed without the need for ear canal impressions.

Partial and Complete Middle Ear Implant

Middle ear implants are aids for individuals with pure sensorineural and some mixed hearing loss. The implants are available in two categories: partially or totally implantable using either piezoelectric or electromagnetic systems. One of the strongest reasons for a middle ear implant over conventional amplification methods, used for sensorineural hearing loss, appears to be improved cosmetics (Chasin et al. 2002). In the partially implantable aid, the processor and microphone are held to the scalp and transmit a signal to the output transducer that converts an electrical signal into a vibration to the ossicular chain. These partial implants, where parts are found outside the middle ear, are driven by electromagnetic and electromechanical principles to signal the output transducer. Totally implantable devices have the system's microphone and transducer placed beneath the skin. Electromagnetic devices, working best at lower frequencies, are low mass and do not have a significant impact on the vibration of the middle ear as they are not rigidly attached (Spindel 2002). Piezoelectric crystal principles are optimal for high-frequency signals because when coupled to transducer and ossicle, the rigidity of the device will dampen the vibration of the middle ear (Spindel 2002).

The first FDA-approved partially implantable electromagnetic device is the ▸ Vibrant Soundbridge® device (MED-EL GmbH, Innsbruck, Austria), available since 2000. The Vibrant device (VSB)

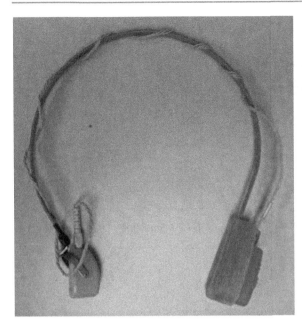

Hearing Aid, Fig. 5 Conventional Contralateral Routing of Signal (CROS)-bone conduction hearing aid

mechanically causes the ossicles to vibrate in the middle ear by directly driving the incus. The amplitude of vibrations can be adjusted for optimal hearing compensation. This semi-implantable device (Fig. 3) has an external microphone, Audio Processor (AP), and an internal Vibrating Ossicular Replacement Prosthesis (VSOP). The electromagnetic prosthesis is composed of a Floating Mass Transducer™ that is attached to the incus and its magnet aligns with the vibration of the stapes. The typical user must change the battery of the processor once a week.

An example of a totally implantable piezoelectric device is the Envoy Esteem (Envoy Medical, St. Paul, MN). This technology takes advantage of the acoustic features of the external ear as the eardrum is used as the microphone device. A piezoelectric transducer is placed on the body of the incus (Fig. 4) that sends an electric current to the processor when mechanically stimulated by ossicular chain vibrations. The electrical signal is processed, amplified, and sent back to the transducer. The transducer converts the electrical stimulus to a mechanical stimulus to vibrate the stapes by a piezoelectric driver. In order to implant the processor, a portion of the incus must be surgically removed. The completely implantable device does not have any external features and has a battery life of 3–5 years that

can be replaced during an outpatient procedure. (Haynes et al. 2009).

Bone Conduction Hearing Aids

It has been known for a long time that the cochlea is capable of hearing through bone conduction. Bone conduction hearing occurs when vibrations of sound are transmitted to the cochlea via vibrations of the skull. Bone conduction hearing occurs via: (1) sound radiated into the external auditory canal, (2) inertia of middle ear ossicles, (3) cochlear fluid inertia, (4) cochlear wall compression, and (5) transmission of pressure via the cerebrospinal fluid. The cochlear fluid inertia appears to be the most important factor (Stenfelt and Goode 2005). Hearing aids can stimulate the cochlea using bone conduction. Bone conduction hearing aids are generally indicated in cases where air conduction hearing aids cannot be used. These conditions include patients who suffer from chronic otitis externa or otitis media, or congenital atresia of the ear canal. Bone conduction hearing aids include a microphone, sound processor and bone oscillator. The hearing device has to be held tightly against the skull for efficient conduction of vibrations to the skull (Fig. 5). The bone conduction hearing device can be held to the skull with a headband or other means such as glasses, etc.

SoundBite Hearing System
In an effort to maintain cosmetic appeal and avoid the need for surgical procedures for a bone conduction device, the SoundBite Hearing System (Sonitus Medical, San Mateo, CA) has been developed. A behind-the-ear (BTE) microphone unit and removable in-the-mouth (ITM) hearing device are wirelessly connected to provide treatment for single-sided deafness or conductive hearing loss. The microphone is placed within the ear canal of the impaired ear and connected to a BTE digital signal processor that wirelessly transmits the signal to the ITM device. The ITM device is safely mounted (Fig. 6) to the molars of the maxilla (Murray et al. 2011) and delivers mechanical vibrations to both cochleas through the teeth once the wireless stimulus is received. This allows for simultaneous activation of both cochleas in a unilateral conductive defect and quickly transmits the sound signal to the contralateral cochlea in the case of unilateral hearing loss.

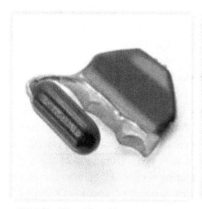

ITM (In-The-Mouth)
Hearing Device

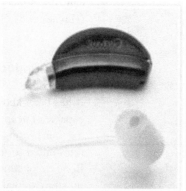

BTE (Behind-The-Ear)
Microphone Unit

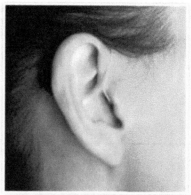

BTE Microphone Unit when worn

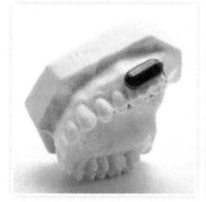

ITM Hearing Device
on Tooth Model (side view)

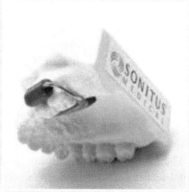

ITM Hearing Device
on Tooth Model (back view)

Hearing Aid, Fig. 6 SoundBite Hearing System

Bone-Anchored Hearing Aid (BAHA)

The BAHA device has two components: (1) a titanium abutment that is attached to the skull during a surgical procedure and (2) the external processor (Fig. 7). The processor contains the microphone, digital signal processing, and the bone oscillator. The oscillator's vibrations are transmitted to the skull via the surgically implanted screw. The BAHA device overcomes some of the cosmetic and functional problems of a traditional bone conduction hearing aid. First, the mechanical vibrations that are transmitted to the skull are more efficiently transmitted through an abutment which is attached via a titanium screw in the skull. This eliminates some of the loss of signal and distortion that occurs from transmitting vibrations through the skin. Second, without a headband, the device has the advantage of

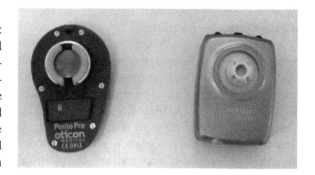

Hearing Aid, Fig. 7 External processor of the bone-anchored hearing aid (BAHA)

being less cosmetically visible. The ▶ BAHA device can be used for unilateral deafness. A BAHA on one side of the head transmits vibrations to both cochleas with minimal attenuation; therefore, bilateral BAHA

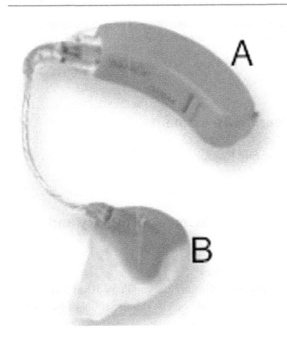

Hearing Aid, Fig. 8 The TransEar contains two components: (**A**) the processor and (**B**) the vibratory transfer unit

can not only provide bilateral output, but more beneficial input from two microphones (Dun et al. 2011).

Unilateral Deafness Devices

Single-sided sensorineural hearing loss is often treated with amplification to the side of the hearing defect. When this deficit becomes extremely significant or the individual is completely deaf in one ear, transmission of sound to the contralateral cochlea is the standard of care. A conventional Contralateral Routing of Signal (CROS) aid employs a microphone in or behind the ear of deficit. The microphone then transfers the signal via wire or FM transmission to a BTE or ITE processor to the more functional ear. The CROS arrangement leaves much to be desired in terms of cosmetics, comfort, head shadow, and satisfaction (Hol et al. 2005). Bone conducting devices such as the BAHA contralateral routing system and SoundBite device, explained above, transmit sound vibration to the skull for delivery to the better functioning cochlea. The development of this treatment for bi-and unilateral hearing loss also overcomes some aesthetic and functional features. Another nonsurgical bone conducting device is the TransEar (Ear Technology Corp., Johnson City, TN).

This hearing aid employs mechanical vibrations to the bony skull for contralateral routing of sound from within the ear canal of the deficient ear. The noninvasive design requires the creation of auditory canal impressions for the case that will house an oscillatory device. This device will make contact with the bony portion of the ear canal; the initial site of vibratory conduction. The TransEar processor is a BTE unit that also contains the microphone (Fig. 8).

Radio-Frequency Transmission/FM Transmission

As a type of assistive listening device, this technology can be either coupled to a hearing aid or used alone in order to aid a person's ability to hear and discriminate speech and environmental sounds. FM systems transmit auditory signals using radio waves. The device consists of an external microphone and transmitter, which is placed near the speaker. The microphone will obtain audio signal and send it to a receiver worn by the listener or those listeners wearing hearing aids with the receiver integrated into the aid. The delivery of the signal by the transmitter is done through frequency modulated (FM) signal to the receiver. The FM transmitter system may also be coupled directly to the output of a television, radio, or tape recorder, rather than external microphone (Bailey et al. 2006). Where FM transmission is used in combination with a hearing aid, the FM system provides the greatest signal-to-noise reduction enhancement relative to other auditory assistive devices (Stach and Ramachandran 2010). The large reduction in noise is due to the proximity of the speaker's mouth and the microphone, found inches away, and is sent directly to a listener's ear, thereby eliminating the impact of noise and distance, making it the ideal solution for the patient with difficulty hearing in noise. The FM transmitter device is best used for students in noisy classrooms or for the elderly in a restaurant, lecture, or church where external noises and distance from the speaker can cause distortion or interference with the speech signal.

Cross-References

▶ Acquired Mixed Hearing Loss
▶ Adult Bilateral Cochlear Implantation

▶ Bone Conduction
▶ Bone-Anchored Hearing Aid in Pediatrics
▶ Bone-Anchored Hearing Aid in Single-Sided Deafness
▶ Bone-Anchored Hearing Aids in Conductive and Mixed Hearing Loss
▶ Cochlear Implant
▶ Implantable Hearing Devices
▶ Sensorineural Hearing Loss
▶ Surgical Devices (Cochlear Implantation, Pediatric)
▶ Vibrant Soundbridge (VSB)

References

Bailey BJ, Johnson JT, Newlands SD (2006) Hearing aids and assistive listening devices. In: Head & neck surgery-otolaryngology, 4th edn. Lippincott Williams & Wilkins, Philadelphia, pp 2279–2293
Chasin M, Westerkull P, Kroll K (2002) Bone anchored and middle ear implant hearing aids. Trends Amplif 6:31–84
Counter P (2008) Implantable hearing aids. Proc Inst Mech Eng H 222:837–852
Dun CA, Faber HT, de Wolf MJ, Cremers CW, Hol MK (2011) An overview of different systems: the bone-anchored hearing aid. Adv Otorhinolaryngol 71:22–31
Haynes DS, Young JA, Wanna GB, Glasscock ME III (2009) Middle ear implantable hearing devices: an overview. Trends Amplif 13:206–214
Hol MK, Bosman AJ, Snik AF, Mylanus EA, Cremers CW (2005) Bone-anchored hearing aids in unilateral inner ear deafness: an evaluation of audiometric and patient outcome measurements. Otol Neurotol 26(5):999–1006
Kim HH, Barrs DM (2006) Hearing aids: a review of what's new. Otolaryngol Head Neck Surg 134:1043–1050
Kricos PB (2006) Audiologic management of older adults with hearing loss and compromised cognitive/psychoacoustic auditory processing capabilities. Trends Amplif 10:1–28
Moodie KS (2004) Individualized hearing instrument fitting for infants. In: Seewald RC (ed) A sound foundation through early amplification. Phonak AG, Switzerland, pp 213–217
Murray M, Miller R, Hujoel P, Popelka GR (2011) Long-term safety and benefit of a new intraoral device for single-sided deafness. Otol Neurotol 32:1262–1269
Natalizia A, Casale M, Guglielmelli E, Rinaldi V, Bressi F, Salvinelli F (2010) An overview of hearing impairment in older adults: perspectives for rehabilitation with hearing aids. Eur Rev Med Pharmacol Sci 14:223–229
Palmer CV (2009) A contemporary review of hearing aids. Laryngoscope 119(11):2195–2204
Spindel JH (2002) Middle ear implantable hearing devices. Am J Audiol 11:104–113
Stach BA, Ramachandran V (2010) Hearing aids: strategies of amplification. In: Flint PW (ed) Cummings otolaryngology: head & neck surgery, 5th edn. Mosby, Philadelphia, pp 2265–2275
Stenfelt S, Goode RL (2005) Bone-conducted sound: physiological and clinical aspects. Otol Neurotol 26:1245–1261
Waltzman SB, Roland JT (2006) Cochlear implants. Thieme Medical Publishers, New York

Hearing Assessment

▶ Hearing Exam

Hearing Assessment in Infancy and Childhood

LaGuinn Sherlock
Department of Otorhinolaryngology-Head and Neck Surgery, University of Maryland, School of Medicine, Baltimore, MD, USA

Definitions

1. Acoustic reflex: Contraction of the stapedial muscle in response to high-intensity acoustic stimuli.
2. Auditory brainstem response (ABR): Neural activity generated in the cochlea, auditory nerve, and brainstem in response to acoustic stimulation.
3. Auditory dys-synchrony: A condition in which auditory stimuli are not processed by the brain, characterized by abnormal ABR, absent acoustic reflexes, and normal otoacoustic emissions.
4. Behavioral observation audiometry (BOA): Non-reinforced procedure of evaluating behavioral responses to sound in infants and low-functioning children.
5. Closed-set word list: A word recognition test where the number of possible responses is restricted.
6. Conditioned play audiometry (CPA): A reinforced procedure for measuring behavioral responses to sound using objects to play with (e.g., dropping blocks in a bucket, putting pegs in a pegboard).
7. Cross-check principle: The results of a single component of the evaluation are cross-checked by one or more independent measures.
8. Early hearing detection and intervention (EHDI): An interdisciplinary and integrated system,

endorsed by the Joint Commission on Infant Hearing (JCIH), to ensure early detection of and subsequent intervention for hearing loss.

9. Malingering: Pretending to have hearing loss or exaggerating a true hearing loss.
10. Open-set word list: A word recognition test where the possible response is not restricted.
11. Otoacoustic emissions (OAEs): Sound produced by the motility of the cochlear outer hair cells.
12. Pure tone average (PTA): Average of thresholds obtained at 500, 1,000, and 2,000 Hz.
13. Speech awareness threshold (SAT): The lowest intensity of speech to which a behavioral response occurs.
14. Speech recognition threshold (SRT): The lowest intensity level where spondaic words are recognized 50% of the time.
15. Spondees: Two-syllable words with equal stress on each syllable (e.g., baseball, hotdog, outside).
16. Tympanometry: A measure of tympanic membrane and middle ear system compliance and pressure using an acoustic probe tone and pressure changes in a sealed ear canal.
17. Visual reinforcement audiometry (VRA): A method of measuring behavioral responses to sound based on the principles of operant conditioning, using a visual reinforcer.

Introduction

Hearing plays a critical role in the development of speech and language, as well as social and educational development. Early identification of hearing loss and subsequent intervention can significantly reduce the effects of hearing loss on overall development (Joint Committee on Infant Hearing (JCIH) 2007). Although mild and unilateral hearing losses generally do not affect speech and language development, they can significantly affect social and educational development (Anderson and Matkin 1991). Prior to universal newborn hearing screening, these losses were often not identified until the child was school-aged, and then only if the child was experiencing difficulty in school. The incidence of hearing loss is estimated at 3 in every 1,000 live births (NCHAM). Infants can be screened for hearing loss using electrophysiological tests. Behavioral assessment of hearing sensitivity can be conducted with children who are developmentally

6 months to 5 years old, using either behavioral observation audiometry (BOA), visual reinforcement audiometry (VRA), or conditioned play audiometry (CPA). Around the time the child is 5 years old, conventional audiometry can be conducted. Behavioral assessment is considered the "gold" standard because it is the only direct measure of hearing. While electrophysiological measures, such as tympanometry, acoustic reflexes, otoacoustic emissions (OAEs), and auditory brainstem response (ABR) testing, facilitate evaluation of structural function (e.g., tympanic membrane compliance, cochlear outer hair cell function), they are not direct measures of hearing sensitivity. Considering the limits of pediatric attention for behavioral assessment and the value of objective assessment of structural integrity and system function, using a test battery approach, combining behavioral and electrophysiological procedures, provides an essential cross-check of test results to determine the child's hearing status and subsequent need for intervention. Furthermore, assessment of functional auditory status (i.e., how the child responds to sound) facilitates appropriate intervention, especially in cases of minimal and unilateral hearing loss.

Objectives of Hearing (Audiologic) Assessment

The key objectives of audiological assessments in infants and children are to: (1) determine if hearing loss is present and to establish the type, degree, and configuration of hearing loss in each ear; (2) evaluate the functional use of hearing by the child and the potential impact of hearing loss on speech and language development, communication, and education; (3) identify risk factors for progressive or delayed-onset hearing loss that would indicate the need for ongoing audiological monitoring; (4) assess candidacy for sensory devices (e.g., hearing aids, assistive listening devices, or cochlear implants); (5) refer for medical evaluation and early intervention services as indicated; (6) counsel the parents about the hearing status in a culturally sensitive and empathetic manner, as well as to convey the outcome of the assessment to other healthcare providers (e.g., pediatrician, early intervention programs); and (7) determine the need for other assessments, such as speech/language, cognitive, or behavioral based on the case history and audiological assessment outcome (American Speech-Language-Hearing Association (ASHA) 2004).

Early Hearing Detection and Intervention (EHDI)

As of 2005, every state in the United States has an early hearing detection and intervention (EHDI) program. Early programs were referred to as universal newborn hearing screening (UNHS) programs, but the terminology has been modified to better reflect the purpose of these programs, which is to provide early intervention to reduce developmental delays (i.e., speech, language, social, and educational) secondary to unidentified or late-identified hearing loss.

Universal newborn hearing screening was initiated in the 1990s. Prior to implementation of UNHS, only infants identified as having a risk factor for hearing loss were screened, typically with an auditory brainstem response (ABR) test. Selectively screening only those children with a risk factor resulted in missing about 50% of children with hearing loss (Joint Committee on Infant Hearing (JCIH) 2007). The Joint Commission on Infant Hearing recommends that each child should have a hearing screening by the time they are 1 month old. If the infant does not pass the screening, a comprehensive audiological evaluation should be completed by the time the infant is 3 months old, and when hearing loss is identified, intervention should be initiated no later than 6 months of age. Intervention should not be delayed, however, for lack of behavioral evaluation of hearing; ear-specific electrophysiological data is sufficient to initiate intervention. Infants can be fitted with hearing aids as young as 1 month of age due to the availability of hearing aid fitting algorithms for infants. Although initial screening rates exceed 90% of all newborns (NCHAM), a significant number of infants who do not pass the screening test are lost to follow-up. Pediatric otolaryngologists can play a valuable role in facilitating audiological follow-up by reinforcing audiological recommendations.

Infant hearing screens are conducted with electrophysiological tests that measure otoacoustic emissions (OAE) and/or the auditory brainstem response (ABR). A simple probe assembly with a removable probe tip is used for OAE screening. The main advantages of OAE screening are the low cost and simple acquisition (i.e., no infant preparation is involved). OAEs, however, are sensitive to internal and external noise, and the presence of vernix or other debris in the ear canals can result in a false-positive screening result. Furthermore, OAEs are a measure of the integrity of the cochlear outer hair cells and therefore, represent a preneural response. Infants in the NICU are at higher risk for

auditory dys-synchrony, a disorder of auditory neural synchrony that affects speech and language development and education, because of concomitant risk factors such as premature birth, low birth weight, hyperbilirubinemia, exposure to ototoxic medications, and hypoxia. OAE screening will miss this condition and therefore, screening with ABR is recommended for this population (Joint Committee on Infant Hearing (JCIH) 2007). ABR screening requires more time to prepare the infant for testing, but as long as the infant is sleeping, the screening itself is completed rapidly. The costs associated with ABR screening are higher (supplies include electrodes and prep materials), thus some hospitals use OAE screening in the well-baby nursery and ABR screening the NICU. Other hospitals use a two-stage screening method, whereby infants who refer on OAE screening are rescreened using ABR.

Screening outcomes can be affected by outer and middle ear dysfunction, resulting in referral for follow-up, even in the presence of normal cochlear and neural function. Children who refer on one or both ears, or who have significant risk factors for progressive hearing loss, should be evaluated behaviorally as they get older, until normal hearing has been confirmed in both ears. Infants who refer on the initial screening should be rescreened within 1 month. Both ears should be rescreened even if only one ear is referred at the time of the initial screening (Joint Committee on Infant Hearing (JCIH) 2007). In cases where the infant is not screened at birth (e.g., home birth, hospital discharge, or transfer before screening conducted), the child should be screened no later than one month of age. Children who are at risk for delayed-onset or progressive hearing loss should have at least one audiological evaluation no later than 24–30 months of age. Some children with mild hearing loss will pass the newborn hearing screening; therefore, the presence of one or more risk indicators (listed below) should prompt referral for an audiological evaluation.

The risk indicators (Joint Committee on Infant Hearing (JCIH) 2007) associated with permanent congenital, delayed-onset, or progressive hearing loss are as follows:

1. Caregiver concern* regarding hearing, speech, language, or developmental delay.
2. Family history* of permanent childhood hearing loss.
3. NICU care of more than 5 days or any of the following regardless of length of stay: ECMO*,

assisted ventilation, exposure to ototoxic medications (gentamycin and tobramycin) or loop diuretics (furosemide/Lasix), and hyperbilirubinemia that requires exchange transfusion.

4. In utero infections, such as CMV, herpes, rubella, syphilis, and toxoplasmosis.
5. Craniofacial anomalies, including those that involve the pinna, ear canal, ear tags, ear pits, and temporal bone anomalies.
6. Physical findings, such as white forelock, that are associated with a syndrome known to include a sensorineural or permanent conductive hearing loss.
7. Syndromes associated with hearing loss or progressive or late-onset hearing loss*, such as neurofibromatosis, osteopetrosis, and Usher syndrome; other frequently identified syndromes include Waardenburg, Alport, Pendred, and Jervell and Lange-Nielsen.
8. Neurodegenerative disorders*, such as Hunter syndrome, or sensory motor neuropathies, such as Friedreich ataxia and Charcot-Marie-Tooth syndrome.
9. Culture-positive postnatal infections associated with sensorineural hearing loss*, including confirmed bacterial and viral (especially herpes viruses and varicella) meningitis.
10. Head trauma, especially basal skull/temporal bone fracture* that requires hospitalization.
11. Chemotherapy*.

*Risk indicators of greater concern for delayed-onset hearing loss.

Comprehensive Audiological Assessment

The goal of the audiological assessment is to determine the presence or absence of hearing loss, the degree and configuration of hearing loss, and the integrity of the auditory system. This goal is achieved using a test battery approach such that each test result is cross-checked with a separate and independent test. The use of multiple procedures is essential with infants and young children to develop an accurate picture of the child's hearing ability. A comprehensive audiological assessment is a process and should not be viewed as a single event.

Indications for a comprehensive audiological evaluation include referral on initial and secondary newborn hearing screens, the presence of a risk factor for progressive or delayed-onset hearing loss, and certain

behaviors that are indicative of hearing loss. These behaviors vary as a function of age. In infants, not startling to sudden and/or loud sounds, lack of change in sucking rate when sounds in the environment change, and not turning to look at new or sudden sounds may be signs that the infant has hearing loss. Toddlers who do not respond or respond inappropriately to verbal instructions, talk too softly or too loudly, or misarticulate speech may have hearing loss. Signs of hearing loss in school-aged children include frequently asking for repetition, turning up the television volume, having difficulty following directions in the classroom, lack of attention during class discussions, and isolation from other students. In addition, any time there is parental concern for hearing loss and/or delays in speech and language development, the child should receive a comprehensive audiological assessment.

Case History

The case history guides the strategy for the audiological assessment and for making subsequent recommendations and referrals. It is the first cross-check of the audiological test outcome (Diefendorf 2009). Information collected during the case history includes outcome of the newborn hearing screening; birth; otological and medical histories; evaluation of risk factors for congenital, progressive, and/or delayed-onset hearing loss, family history of hearing loss, and parental report of the child's responses to sound. Parents can provide meaningful information about the child's general listening behavior (e.g., startling to loud sounds, preferring a loud volume on the television, hearing the telephone ring, etc.). Information provided during the case history helps to determine the cognitive age of child (and whether or not it is different than chronological age), which is important for selecting the most appropriate test protocol. Information about general otological history also can influence the test protocol in terms of prioritizing test procedures. For example, when testing a child with suspected or confirmed ear infections, emphasis may be placed on measuring thresholds at fewer frequencies in order to enable testing by both air- and bone-conduction to determine the degree of the air-bone gap.

With older children, it is helpful to know if educators have expressed concern about the child's hearing. In some cases of mild or moderate hearing loss, the child may be compensating well for the hearing loss in the home environment but not in the classroom environment. Consequently, the parents may not have concerns for hearing loss but the child's educators may notice that the child does not respond well or consistently, especially when the educator is talking from a distance or when there is excessive competing noise in the classroom.

Behavioral Assessment

Behavioral assessment of hearing can be accomplished with children as young as 4 months old (Madell 1998). Responses to sound are reflexive at very early ages and can be conditioned in children up to 4–5 years old. Starting at about the age of 5 years old, depending on maturity and developmental level, children can be evaluated via conventional audiometry. Selection of the proper procedure with respect to the child's cognitive and physical development is important to achieve the most accurate test results and hence, facilitate appropriate management of the child.

Test results from behavioral testing can be affected by the state of the child during the assessment and the experience of the audiologist. Children who are overactive, hungry, or tired will be more difficult to test and response reliability may be adversely affected. The audiologist must have a thorough understanding of the principles of operant conditioning, including the correct use of distraction and reinforcement, the timing of stimulus presentation and response, and knowledge of the effects of developmental age on outcome. Behavioral assessment is often best conducted with two clinicians, one to control the audiometer and observe responses and one to monitor and/or condition the child and provide confirmation of observed responses; however, the assessment can be accomplished with a single experienced clinician.

Behavioral responses to sound in the test environment are influenced by a number of factors. The developmental age of the child affects the type of response that can be observed or conditioned whereas the child's chronological age affects whether or not the child has the neuromuscular coordination to make certain movements (e.g., eye shift, head-turn, handling small objects for play audiometry). Hearing level influences behavioral conditioning; the child with a severe/profound hearing loss may be considerably more difficult to condition due to their relative lack of experience with sound and difficulty achieving sufficient volume from the equipment to elicit

reflexive responses to sound. Previous experience with audiological evaluations can influence how readily the child responds during the test session. Placement of the test chair, test assistant, visual reinforcers and lighting in the test environment also can affect test outcome. If the test chair is not properly located for sound field testing, thresholds may be underestimated or overestimated. If the test assistant does not maintain the child's attention at midline and/ or is too distracting, response reliability will be affected. If the visual reinforcer is not placed sufficiently away from midline, head-turn response may not be readily detectable and therefore, may result in elevated thresholds. Poor lighting will affect observation of responses to sound.

Testing is frequently conducted in a sound-treated audiometric test suite. Behavioral testing of young children is often initiated in the sound field test condition because it is easier to condition the child. Although the test results will not indicate hearing sensitivity for each ear, they will provide an indication as to whether or not hearing is sufficient to develop speech and language. The younger the child, or more developmentally delayed, the more rapidly response fatigue sets in. Therefore, testing each individual ear can take place following sound field testing, or on a different day when necessary.

The test session is usually initiated with measurement of a speech awareness threshold (SAT) or speech recognition threshold (SRT), depending on the age and developmental level of the child because children generally respond more readily to speech than non-speech stimuli. The SAT is measured using live voice presentation of sounds such as "ba, ba, ba" or "shh." The presentation level is increased until a response occurs. The SAT should be in agreement with the best audiometric threshold by 5–10 dB. The SRT is measured using spondaic words. The child can respond either by pointing to corresponding pictures or by repeating the words. The SRT is the level at which the child correctly identifies or repeats the word 50% of the time. The SRT should be in agreement with pure tones at 500, 1,000, and 2,000 Hz by 6–8 dB. In cases of a sharply sloping upward or downward hearing loss, the best agreement between SRT and pure tones is usually with a two-frequency average (e.g., 500 and 1,000 Hz or 1,000 and 2,000 Hz).

Thresholds for non-speech stimuli are measured with pure tones, which may be frequency-modulated

Hearing Assessment in Infancy and Childhood, Fig. 1 Sample audiogram depicting behavioral thresholds to warbled puretone stimuli presented in the sound field test condition

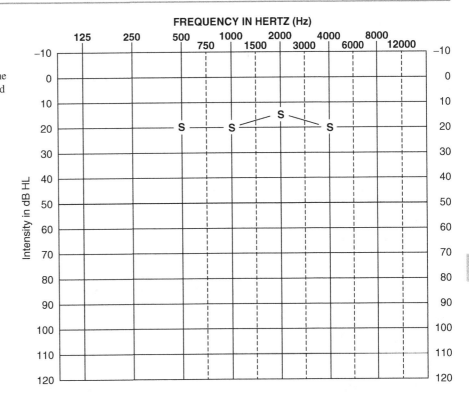

(a.k.a. warbled) to avoid standing waves in the sound field test condition. Standing waves occur when direct sound from the source (e.g., the loudspeaker) interacts with reflections of sound, causing cancellation of the original sound. Thresholds also may be measured using narrowband noise stimuli; this stimulus may elicit a response more readily than pure tone signals. Responses to narrowband noise typically occur at lower presentation levels (5–10 dB) than responses to pure tone signals, due to the broadband nature of the stimulus. Test results obtained in the sound field are conventionally denoted with an "S" on the audiogram (see Fig. 1). The goal of using non-speech stimuli is to measure thresholds across a range of frequencies to determine the configuration of hearing sensitivity across the frequency region most important for speech (500–4,000 Hz). At a minimum, thresholds are measured at 500 and 2,000 Hz.

In very young children, behavioral methods lack the precision to establish valid hearing thresholds. Consequently, responses may be described as minimum response levels (MRLs) (Roeser and Clark 2004). MRLs are generally lower for speech than for non-speech stimuli.

Behavioral Observation Audiometry (4–6 Months Old) Behavioral observation audiometry (BOA) is a non-reinforced subjective procedure and therefore, is subject to misinterpretation due to poor test-retest reliability and high intersubject and intrasubject variability (Northern and Downs 2002). Testing is almost exclusively conducted in the sound field test condition so specific-ear information cannot be obtained. The responses are usually suprathreshold, making it more difficult to definitively rule out hearing loss. For these reasons, the use of electrophysiological measures in conjunction with BOA is essential.

BOA is conducted by placing the infant in the test suite (a.k.a. sound field) at a calibrated location. The infant may be held by the parent, or more ideally remains in their infant carrier; this enables more accurate observation of behavioral changes that signal a response to sound. Changes in certain behaviors can be observed coincident with the presentation of sound (speech or nonspeech stimuli). In very young infants, the behavior that is most likely to coincide with threshold or near-threshold responses is changes in sucking rate (Madell 1998). Response fatigue occurs quickly to repeated presentation of signals (Northern and Downs 2002).

Visual Reinforcement Audiometry (6 Months to 2.5 Years Old) The infant is held in the parent's lap, oriented toward the clinician providing distraction from the reinforcement tower. There must be a sufficient angle between the child and the visual reinforcer (45°–90°) to ensure a head-turn response. Figure 2 is an illustration of the typical test room setup. Testing is often initiated in the sound field test condition, and may progress to earphones (insert or circumaural) to test each ear individually. The use of insert earphones is generally preferable to headphones in young children. The weight and/or placement of headphones over the ears can cause the canals to collapse, which can result in the measurement of a conductive hearing loss and adversely affect management of the child (Northern and Downs 2002). Inserts have a higher interaural attenuation than headphones, which reduces the incidence of crossover and need for masking. This is especially helpful in cases of asymmetrical or unilateral hearing loss.

As with younger children, the test session often begins with a speech detection or speech awareness threshold. At this age, many children are able to point to their body parts so the speech signal may be "Show me your nose," or "Touch your head." Testing progresses to the presentation of non-speech stimuli (e.g., warbled pure tones, narrowband noise). Testing is initiated at low presentation levels and increased until a spontaneous head-turn is observed. The head-turn response is reinforced by activating the visual reinforcer in the test suite. Higher starting levels can result in a greater false-positive response rate; therefore, it is important that the starting level is selected based on case history information and observation of the child. It is critical that false responses are not reinforced. In between responses, the child is oriented to the midline by a test assistant, or by the audiologist controlling the audiometer.

The order of frequency presentation is influenced by the state of the child, the presumed etiology of hearing loss, and the presence or absence of elevated hearing levels at each frequency. The frequency range that is most critical for speech and language development is 500–4,000 Hz so the most important frequencies to start with are 500 and 2,000 Hz; 1,000 Hz can often be interpolated, except when the slope between 500 and 2,000 Hz is very sharp. Once thresholds have been obtained from each ear in this frequency range, testing may continue with

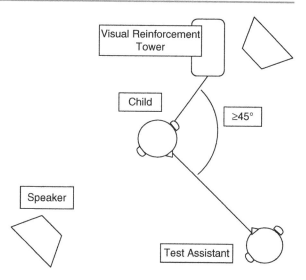

Hearing Assessment in Infancy and Childhood, Fig. 2 Typical room set-up for VRA testing. The visual reinforcement tower must be at an angle ≥45° from midline to ensure an identifiable head-turn

evaluation of 250 and 8,000 Hz, depending on the state of the child and whether or not bone-conduction testing is necessary.

Play Audiometry (3–5 Years Old) By the age of 3 years old, children can be conditioned to respond to sound with play activities. Younger children may be more comfortable sitting on the parent's lap, while older and/or more independent children can be seated in a chair. Testing should be initiated with insert earphones or headphones, but if the child is highly resistant to placement of phones or cannot be conditioned to respond appropriately with phones in place, testing can be switched to the sound field test condition. In this case, the child is placed at a location corresponding to the calibrated spot in the sound field.

The child is instructed on the action expected (e.g., dropping a block in a bucket, putting a peg in a pegboard, putting a ring on a stick) and trained to perform the action whenever the sound is heard (pure tone or narrowband noise). The timing of the signal presentation must be varied so that the child is not responding to a pattern of presentation rather than a sound. If the child becomes bored, a change in activity can facilitate ongoing response behavior. The order of signal presentation is similar to that described under VRA.

Conventional Audiometry (>4 years old) Some children who are at least 5 years old developmentally can be evaluated via conventional audiometry, depending on the maturity level of the child. By this age, testing can often be initiated with earphones. First, an SRT is measured by instructing the child to repeat words (e.g., "Say baseball, hotdog, oatmeal"). Pure tone thresholds are measured by instructing the child to raise his hand or push a button each time he hears the tone. Attention can potentially be maintained for longer periods of time by activating the visual reinforcement when the child presses the button.

Speech Testing There is no widely accepted method for evaluating word recognition ability with children; however, speech testing is an important component of the test battery because it helps to determine how well the child uses hearing for communicative function. Word recognition scores can be obtained using picture-pointing tests (closed-set test) with younger children and children with poor articulation. Older children can repeat words (open-set test). Consideration must be given to the receptive vocabulary level of the child. Word recognition scores may be depressed due to vocabulary deficits rather than deficits in speech perception. Consideration also must be given to the effects of an open-set versus closed-set test. Word recognition scores will typically be slightly better (~10%) with a closed-set test. Table 1 is a summary of commonly used pediatric speech tests.

Electrophysiological Assessment

Tympanometry Tympanometry is an objective test of middle ear system function which measures energy transmission through the middle ear system. Tympanometry is highly useful for distinguishing between intact and non-intact tympanic membranes, the presence of middle ear effusion, disarticulated ossicular chain or other middle ear pathology, and Eustachian tube dysfunction.

Tympanometric measures are conducted with a measurement probe containing a speaker to generate a probe tone, a microphone to monitor the level of the probe tone, and an air pump to generate changes in air pressure in the ear canal. The traditional probe tone frequency is 226 Hz, as specified in the ANSI S3.39 (1987) standard. However, this probe tone should not be used for infants younger than approximately 6 months old because the canal walls of infants are soft and susceptible to movement. The low-frequency probe tone can cause movement of the ear canal walls that makes the tympanometric test result appear normal. Consequently, a higher-frequency probe tone, 1,000 Hz, is recommended for infants.

The probe assembly is placed in the ear canal to create a hermetic seal. The air pressure is changed in the ear canal from positive (+200 daPa) to negative (−400 daPa) and as the pressure changes, the compliance of the middle ear system changes. This change in compliance is measured by changes in reflected energy. Tympanometry yields measures of equivalent ear canal volume, compliance, tympanometric peak pressure, and tympanometric width. Clinically, tympanograms are described quantitatively in terms of compliance (normal, high, or low), pressure peak (normal or negative), and volume (normal, small, or large). Compliance is interpreted in conjunction with ear canal volume. No measurable compliance with a very small ear canal volume is suggestive of a probe against the ear canal wall or impacted cerumen. No measurable compliance with normal ear canal volume indicates middle ear pathology, while no measurable compliance with a large ear canal volume is indicative of a tympanic membrane perforation or patent pressure equalization tubes. Normal compliance with significant negative pressure is indicative of Eustachian tube dysfunction. Tympanometric test results may also be described qualitatively using Jerger's classification system, which is based on compliance and peak pressure. Tympanograms by type are illustrated in Fig. 3. Type A tympanograms are characterized by normal compliance and a pressure peak near 0 daPa. Tympanograms with low compliance are classified as Type A$_S$ (shallow), while tympanograms with high compliance are classified as Type A$_D$ (deep). Flat tympanograms are classified as Type B. Type C tympanograms are characterized by normal compliance and negative pressure.

Most children will sit quietly for tympanometry. Some children, however, do not respond well to the placement of the probe in the ear canal. When this occurs, distraction techniques are implemented (e.g., a test assistant plays peek-a-boo, the child is given a toy to play with) (Northern and Downs 2002). In cases of highly resistant children, the parent is instructed to hug the child to their chest and wrap their arms around the child in such a way that the child cannot use her hands to prevent placement of

Hearing Assessment in Infancy and Childhood, Table 1 Speech tests commonly used for pediatric assessment of word recognition ability

Acronym	Test name	Author	Format and response mode	Age/application
ANT	Audio numbers test	Erber 1980	Closed-set picture pointing	Severe/profound hearing loss
NU-6	Northwestern University Auditory Test No. 6		Open-set word repetition	Children ≥ 12 years old
NU-CHIPS	Northwestern University children's perception of speech	Elliott and Katz 1980	Open-set word repetition	Children >2.5 years old
PBK	Phonetically balanced Kindergarten word lists	Haskins 1949	Open-set word repetition	4.5–12 years old
PSI	Pediatric speech intelligibility test	Jerger et al. 1980	Closed-set picture pointing	Children ≥ 3 years old
WIPI	Word intelligibility by picture identification	Ross and Lerman 1970	Closed-set picture pointing	Children ≥ 3 years old

the probe. The child's head is gently pressed against the parent to avoid excessive movement. The test procedure takes only a few seconds and can be completed in all but the most recalcitrant children.

Acoustic Reflexes The acoustic reflex is the contraction of the stapedial muscle in response to high-level acoustic stimuli. Acoustic reflexes are indirectly measured by presenting pure tone stimuli at high intensities (i.e., ≥ 70 dB HL) and measuring changes in reflected energy in the ear canal. The acoustic reflex arc involves the bilateral contraction of the stapedial muscle with ipsilateral stimulus presentation. Measurement of the reflex can be made ipsilaterally (uncrossed) in the ear being stimulated, and contralaterally (crossed) in the ear not being stimulated. Conventionally, the ear being stimulated is the reference ear (e.g., right contralateral reflexes are measured with the measurement probe in the left ear and the stimulus in the right ear). Conductive pathologies will result in elevated or absent reflexes due to the significant reduction in sound used to activate the reflex arc. Acoustic reflexes are usually present with sensorineural hearing loss, until hearing loss exceeds 65–70 dB HL, and then reflexes are typically absent or not measurable because the relative intensity of the sound (re: threshold) is insufficient to elicit a reflex, and/or because of the limits of equipment output. Pathology of the seventh cranial nerve affects contraction of the stapedial muscle and will, therefore, affect measurement of the reflex in the probe ear.

Table 2 summarizes the typical configuration of reflexes as a function of pathology.

There is little evidence to support the measurement of acoustic reflexes in infants younger than 4 months, and hence this test is not part of the test battery until children reach the age of about 6 months of age.

Otoacoustic Emissions Otoacoustic emissions (OAEs) are sounds produced by the motility of the outer hair cells in the cochlea. The sound travels through the middle ear system into the outer ear, where it can be measured by a microphone. OAEs are preneural and therefore, facilitate differentiation between cochlear hearing loss and neural dysfunction (Prieve and Fitzgerald 2009). OAEs are affected by middle ear pathology, and so must be interpreted in conjunction with tympanometry. OAEs are not a direct measure of hearing sensitivity but can be used with other objective tests of auditory function to grossly estimate hearing.

OAEs are measured with a probe assembly containing speakers for sound presentation and a microphone for measuring the emissions. Signal averaging methods are used because OAEs are low-level signals that can be easily obscured by noise internal and external to the probe. Internal noise (e.g., sucking, vocalizations, breathing) is lowest in children who are sleeping or sitting very quietly. OAE measurement can be very difficult and time-consuming with children who are noisy breathers and/or very active. External noise can be minimized by ensuring an adequate probe fit and testing in a quiet environment.

Hearing Assessment in Infancy and Childhood, Fig. 3 Jerger classification of tympanometry results. Type A tympanograms are characterized by normal compliance (i.e., peak admittance) and normal peak pressure, Type A$_D$ by high compliance with normal peak pressure, Type A$_S$ by low compliance with normal peak pressure, Type B by no compliance and Type C by normal compliance with negative pressure

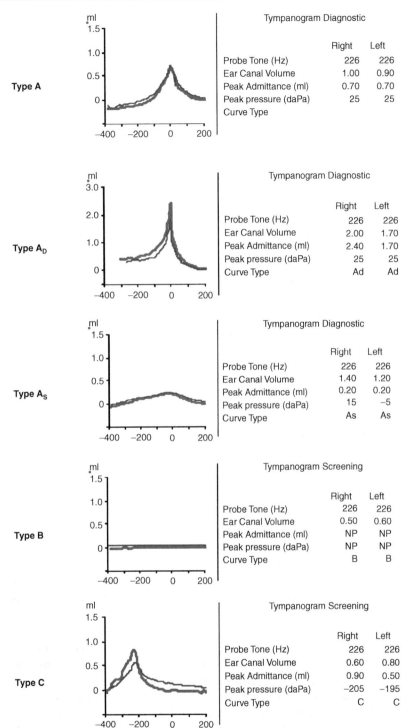

For clinical purposes, OAEs are evoked with external acoustic sources. Transient-evoked OAEs (TEOAEs) are usually evoked by a click signal, which activates the cochlea simultaneously from the base to the apex. TEOAEs are typically measured with an 80 dB pSPL (78–82 dB SPL) click. The click is not frequency-specific but analysis of the response occurs in specific frequency domains, providing information

Hearing Assessment in Infancy and Childhood, Table 2 Typical configuration of acoustic reflexes for ipsilateral and contralateral stimulation as a function of underlying pathology

	Ipsilateral	Contralateral	Pathology
Right	Present	Present	Hearing is within normal limits OR sensorineural hearing loss of slight, mild, or moderate degree
Left	Present	Present	
Right	Present	Elevated/absent	Conductive pathology in the left ear
Left	Elevated/absent	Elevated/absent	
Right	Elevated/absent	Elevated/absent	Conductive pathology in the right ear
Left	Present	Elevated/absent	
Right	Present	Absent	Possible left cranial nerve pathology
Left	Absent	Present	
Right	Absent	Absent	Bilateral conductive pathology OR bilateral sensorineural hearing loss of ≥ 70 dB HL
Left	Absent	Absent	

in the frequency region 500–5,000 Hz. For general clinical measurement, TEOAEs need to be at least 6 dB above the noise floor and have a reproducibility rate above 70% to be considered present (American Speech-Language-Hearing Association (ASHA) 2004). TEOAEs are illustrated in Fig. 4. TEOAEs are measurable in ears with hearing levels as high as 35 dB HL, but are generally absent when hearing loss exceeds 35 dB HL. Distortion product otoacoustic emissions (DPOAEs) are evoked by the simultaneous presentation of two closely spaced pure tones, referred to as primary frequencies that are conventionally referred to as f1 and f2. The interaction of the two primary frequencies on the basilar membrane results in cochlear output at other discrete frequencies (i.e., distortion products) that are mathematically related to the primary frequencies. The largest DP occurs at 2f1–f2 and is, therefore, the DP measured for clinical purposes. DPOAEs are analyzed in terms of the signal-to-noise ratio primarily, and in terms of the absolute amplitude secondarily (see Fig. 5). DPOAEs are measurable in ears with hearing levels as high as 40–45 dB HL, but are absent when hearing loss exceeds 45 dB HL. Both TEOAE and DPOAE amplitudes are significantly higher in infants than adults (Hall 2000) with amplitude decreasing significantly between the neonatal period and early childhood.

OAEs are susceptible to ototoxicity and hypoxia and hence, may provide evidence of cochlear damage in frequency regions (e.g., >4 kHz) not measured by other electrophysiological tests. They are particularly valuable for monitoring the effects of ototoxic treatment. Figure 6 illustrates DPOAEs measured pre-, peri- and posttreatment with cisplatin. The patient,

a 13-month-old child, was sleeping during the pretreatment assessment and so behavioral testing was not completed. DPOAEs were present and robust across the test frequency range in both ears. Three weeks after treatment was initiated, high-frequency DPs had declined. Six weeks after treatment was initiated, behavioral assessment indicated normal hearing in at least one ear in the frequency region 500–4,000 Hz, while DPs indicated further decline in outer hair cell function. Posttreatment, 18 months later, behavioral test results indicated a bilateral high-frequency sensorineural hearing loss. The OAEs gave an early indication of outer hair cell damage prior to changes in audiometric thresholds.

Auditory Brainstem Response The auditory brainstem response (ABR) is a measure of neural activity generated in the cochlea, auditory nerve, and brainstem, in response to acoustic stimuli (see ▶ Hearing Testing, Auditory Brainstem Response (ABR)). Sound is delivered to the ear via earphone (insert or circumaural) and responses are measured with surface electrodes. The ABR is a relatively small signal that must be detected against background EEG activity. The lower the EEG activity, the more efficient and accurate the test session and results are. Infants younger than 6 months of age can be tested under conditions of natural sleep. Between the ages of 6 months and 4 years, testing frequently requires sedation to ensure low EEG activity and sufficient time to collect data. ABR testing can be done under moderate sedation, usually with chloral hydrate or secobarbital, or under general anesthesia. Inhalation of some gases, such as nitrous oxide, however, can

Hearing Assessment in Infancy and Childhood, Fig. 4 TEOAE test results. The *upper panel* illustrates partially absent TEs in the right ear while the *lower panel* illustrates robust TEs in the left ear. The TE response is analyzed in frequency regions (far left column) and reproducibility of the response is calculated (second column). The TE response is indicated in the far right column

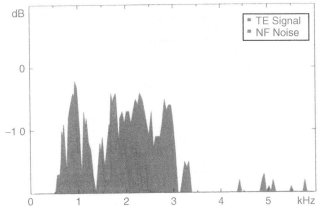

Right:	Stab: 99% :			
Frq(kHz)	Repro(%)	TE(dB)	NF(dB)	TE-NF(dB)
1.0	10	2.6	1.8	0.8
1.5	20	0.0	−1.5	1.5
2.0	37	4.7	−0.3	5.0
3.0	95	2.8	−7.0	9.8
4.0	53	−8.5	−13.0	4.5
1.2-3.4	46	7.7	2.6	5.1

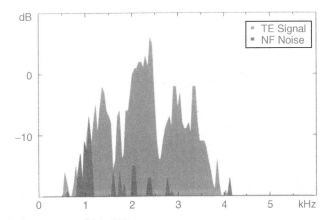

Left:	Stab: 99% :			
Frq(kHz)	Repro(%)	TE(dB)	NF(dB)	TE-NF(dB)
1.0	6	−2.3	−2.6	0.3
1.5	94	4.8	−8.2	13.0
2.0	98	13.0	−6.4	19.4
3.0	97	6.8	−6.7	13.5
4.0	73	−2.9	−10.8	7.9
1.2-3.4	97	14.4	−2.3	16.7

change middle ear pressure and subsequently affect acoustic reflexes and OAEs.

The ABR response is characterized by five waveforms, arising from activity in the cochlea up to the brainstem, which are analyzed in terms of latency. Wave latencies vary as a function of gestational age, stimulus intensity, and stimuli repetition rate, with longer latencies at younger ages, lower intensities, and faster repetition rates. ABR thresholds are determined by decreasing stimulus intensity in 10 dB steps until a response is no longer identifiable (see Fig. 7).

The use of frequency-specific stimuli using tone bursts is important to determine the degree and

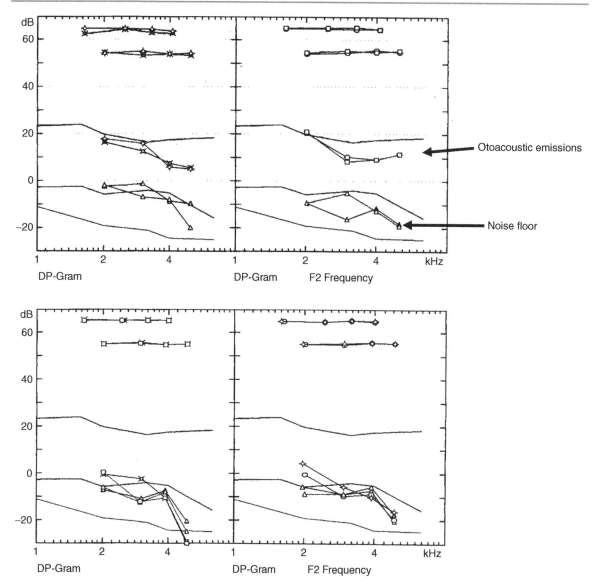

Hearing Assessment in Infancy and Childhood, Fig. 5 Illustration of DPOAEs when present (*upper panel*) and absent (*lower panel*)

configuration of hearing loss in each ear to facilitate appropriate intervention strategies (e.g., hearing aids, FM systems, cochlear implants). At a minimum, ABR thresholds should be measured for the low-frequency region (250 or 500 Hz) and the high-frequency region (2,000 Hz) using tone bursts. ABR thresholds corresponding to normal hearing are 30–40 dB nHL at 500 Hz, 20–30 dB nHL at 2,000 Hz, and 20–30 dB nHL at 4,000 Hz (American Speech-Language-Hearing Association (ASHA) 2004). When ABR thresholds by air-conduction are not within normal

limits, bone-conduction ABR measurements are indicated to determine the type of hearing loss.

Measurement of a click-evoked ABR is useful for determining neural integrity by evaluating interwave latencies, ear asymmetries and morphology and comparing with age-appropriate normative data. When the click-evoked ABR is abnormal or absent, click-evoked responses should be measured with both single-polarity condensation and rarefaction clicks to measure the cochlear microphonic (see Fig. 8) (Diefendorf 2009). Click-evoked ABRs correspond most closely to hearing

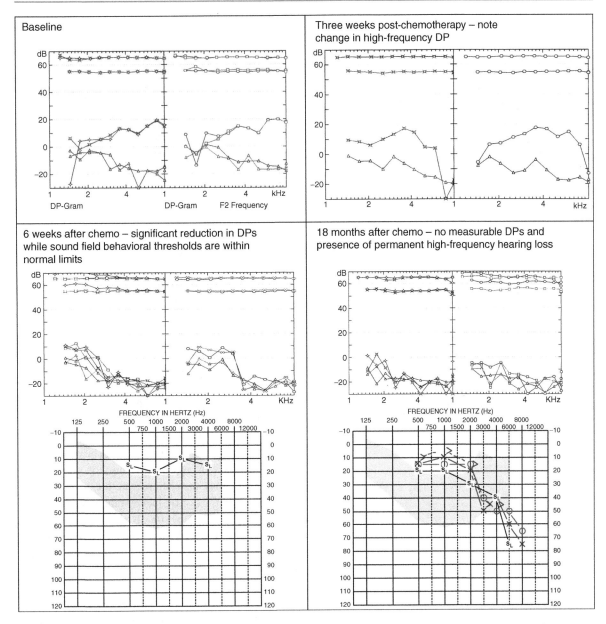

Hearing Assessment in Infancy and Childhood, Fig. 6 Example of early detection of hair cell damage from ototoxic treatment using distortion product otoacoustic emissions in a 13 month old child

sensitivity in the frequency region 2–4 kHz, except in cases of sharply sloping hearing loss. A click-evoked ABR is not sufficient for evaluating hearing status.

An emerging technique in the assessment of hearing is the auditory steady-state response (ASSR). This is a synchronized brain response to modulated tones. There is not yet sufficient evidence to support the use of ASSR as the sole measure of auditory

status (Joint Committee on Infant Hearing (JCIH) 2007).

Categorizing Hearing Loss and Assessing Impact
One of the objectives of a comprehensive audiological assessment is to establish the type, degree, and configuration of hearing loss in each ear. Hearing loss types include conductive, sensorineural, and mixed (Fig. 9).

Hearing Assessment in Infancy and Childhood, Fig. 7 Sample of a threshold ABR. As stimulus intensity is decreased, wave V latency increases. Earlier waveforms disappear more rapidly as stimulus intensity is decreased. During threshold ABR testing, stimulus intensity is decreased until wave V cannot be identified. The lowest level at which wave V is identified is the ABR threshold

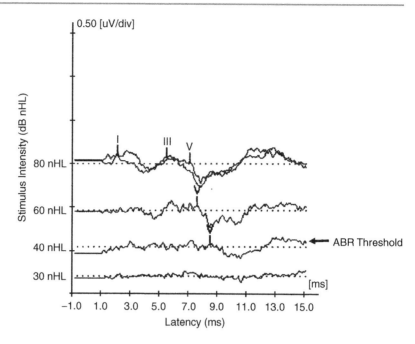

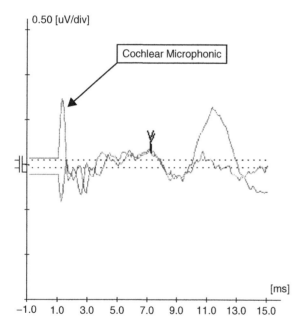

Hearing Assessment in Infancy and Childhood, Fig. 8 The cochlear microphonic, detected by measuring a click-evoked ABR with reversed polarity (i.e., rarefaction and condensation)

Conductive hearing loss is characterized by elevated air-conduction thresholds and bone-conduction thresholds that are within normal limits, resulting in air-bone gaps. With sensorineural hearing loss, both air- and bone-conduction thresholds are elevated; thresholds are interweaving and air-bone gaps are ≤10 dB. Both air- and bone-conduction thresholds are elevated with mixed hearing loss, but air-bone gaps are present and exceed 10 dB. The degree of hearing loss is defined as a function of air-conduction thresholds, as indicated in Table 3. Hearing loss configuration can be described as flat, downward- or upward-sloping, or cookie-bite. A flat hearing loss has audiometric thresholds that are ± 10 dB across the test frequency range, while sloping hearing loss changes by 10 dB or more per octave. A cookie-bite configuration is characterized by normal or near-normal hearing at the lowest and highest frequencies (e.g., 500 and 4,000 Hz) and hearing loss in the mid-frequencies (e.g., 1,000 and 2,000 Hz).

Physicians involved in the care of children with hearing loss should be cognizant of the possible impact of hearing loss on speech/language development, communication, and social interactions. Audiologists, speech/language pathologists, and other allied health professionals make recommendations and provide habilitation to minimize the impact of hearing loss. Infants and children with slight hearing loss may develop speech and language normally, but may encounter difficulty in the educational setting, when teachers are typically at a distance and competing noise is prevalent. The impact of hearing loss increases with greater degrees of hearing loss. Children with milder degrees of hearing loss may not encounter significant difficulty hearing in quiet

Hearing Assessment in Infancy and Childhood, Fig. 9 Audiograms illustrating different types of hearing loss. The *upper* audiogram illustrates a conductive hearing loss measured in a 5 year old child. Declining response reliability precluded assessment of masked bone-conduction thresholds. Tympanometry revealed no tympanic membrane/middle ear system compliance in either ear. The child had a confirmed diagnosis of bilateral otitis media. The *middle panel* is an audiogram obtained from a 7 year old child with a congenital gradually progressive bilateral sensorineural hearing loss. The *bottom panel* is an audiogram showing normal hearing in the left ear and a mixed hearing loss in the right ear

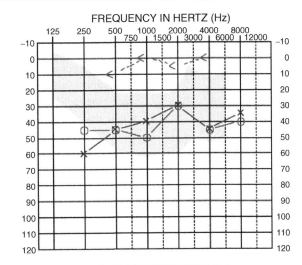

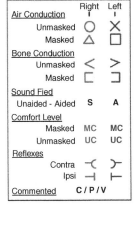

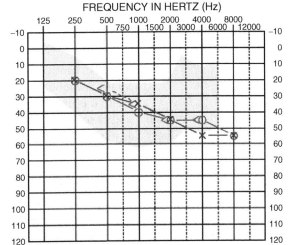

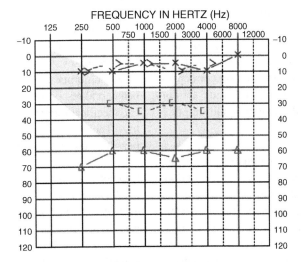

Hearing Assessment in Infancy and Childhood, Table 3 Degrees of hearing loss as a function of threshold

Degree of hearing loss	Classification of hearing loss
≤15 dB HL	Normal
16–25 dB HL	Slight
26–40 dB HL	Mild
41–55 dB HL	Moderate
56–70 dB HL	Moderately severe
71–90 dB HL	Severe
>91 dB HL	Profound

listening situations, but will likely have more difficulty when speech is at low volume levels or there is competing noise. Children with greater degrees of hearing loss will likely hear very little speech, even in quiet listening situations. Hearing loss can also have a major impact on reading skills and social development. Table 4 is a summary of the possible impact of various degrees and configurations of hearing loss on communication and social function.

Functional Auditory Status

When the comprehensive audiological evaluation reveals the presence of hearing loss and/or auditory dys-synchrony, assessment of functional auditory status is indicated (American Speech-Language-Hearing Association (ASHA) 2004). Functional assessments are used to evaluate how the child listens in real world settings, to determine not only what the child can hear but also how the child uses what is heard. The information from functional assessments can be used to determine the need for amplification (e.g., hearing aids or FM system) and/or environmental modifications, and to determine benefit from amplification. A summary of functional auditory assessment tools is available at http://www.oticonusa.com/eprise/main/SiteGen/Uploads/Public/Downloads_Oticon/Pediatrics/Inc_Functional_Measures_Guide.pdf.

Malingering

There is a higher incidence of malingering in children between the ages of 7 and 12 years. These children often present with a complaint of subjective hearing loss and a recent hearing screening failure. Parents sometimes report concern for hearing loss. Behavior during the test session is characterized by exaggerated listening behavior, an absence of false-positive responses (false-positive responses are normal), and/or significant variability in intra-test thresholds.

Frequently, there is a mismatch between SRT and PTA. Responses to pure tone stimuli are elevated, often to a degree that is inconsistent with the child's listening behavior during the case history and test instructions. More often than not, word recognition scores are >80% at subthreshold presentation levels. When malingering is suspected, modifications to the evaluation procedure can facilitate accurate assessment of hearing. For example, using an ascending method of presentation (rather than the conventional descending method), smaller step sizes (e.g., 2 dB rather than 5 dB), and longer interstimuli intervals can result in pure tone thresholds that are consistent with speech testing. Objective tests of auditory function, namely, acoustic immittance and OAEs, are necessary. In cases where behavioral responses cannot be accurately determined, a threshold ABR assessment is indicated.

The child who feigns hearing loss is seeking attention. The child may be experiencing significant stress related to family (e.g., a new baby in the family getting all the attention) or school (e.g., the child is not doing well). It is important to ensure that referrals for family and/or educational counseling, or to mental health professionals, are provided as needed based on case history information (Roeser and Clark 2004).

The Test Battery Approach

The assessment of children younger than 6 months of age consists almost exclusively of electrophysiological tests, namely, OAE, ABR, and tympanometry. The test battery for children between the ages of 6 months and 5 years includes developmentally appropriate behavioral assessment (e.g., VRA or CPA), tympanometry, and acoustic reflexes. OAEs are included when behavioral responses suggest hearing loss and tympanometry is within normal limits. ABR testing is indicated when behavioral responses are not reliable enough to provide ear-specific information and there is evidence of hearing loss. Table 5 illustrates the cross-check principle, with possible diagnostic outcomes based on test results.

Case Example of the Cross-Check Principle

An 18-month-old child was referred for an audiological evaluation by her pediatric otolaryngologist. The patient was accompanied by her mother, who reported concern for hearing loss because the child did not respond consistently to sound. The mother also reported that a recent evaluation at a different clinic indicated normal hearing in one ear and hearing loss in the other ear. According to the clinical report from the other clinic, OAEs were absent at all frequencies bilaterally, tympanometry revealed normal tympanic membrane/middle ear system compliance with normal pressure, and acoustic reflexes were absent bilaterally for ipsilateral stimulation. Behavioral testing was not attempted by clinician report. A click-evoked ABR test was conducted and the findings indicated a click-evoked ABR threshold of 30 dB nHL in

Hearing Assessment in Infancy and Childhood, Table 4 Effects of hearing loss on speech/language and social development as a function of degree and configuration of hearing loss (Modified with permission by K. Anderson). Separate pages for each hearing loss, including a section on the possible impact on education, are available to provide to families at http://kandersonaudconsulting.com/uploads/Relationship_of_Hearing_Loss__Listening__Learning_Need_1_per_pg.pdf

Possible impact on the understanding of language and speech	Possible social impact
16–25 dB HL (hearing loss)	
• Comparable to plugging ears with fingers. • Difficulty hearing faint or distant speech. • At 16 dB student can miss up to 10% of speech signal when teacher is at a distance of >3 ft. • At ≥20 dB hearing loss in the better ear can result in absent, inconsistent, or distorted parts of speech, especially word endings (s, ed) and unemphasized sounds. • Percent of speech signal missed will be greater when background noise is present (especially in elementary grades when instruction is primarily verbal and younger children have greater difficulty listening in noise).	• May be unaware of subtle conversational cues that could cause the child to be viewed as inappropriate or awkward. • May miss portions of fast-paced peer interactions that could begin to have an impact on socialization and self-concept. • Behavior may be confused for immaturity or inattention. • May be more fatigued due to extra effort needed for understanding speech.
26–40 dB HL (hearing loss)	
• Causes hearing difficulty greater than "plugged ear" loss. • Child can "hear" but misses fragments of speech leading to misunderstanding. • Degree of difficulty experienced in school will depend upon noise level in the classroom, distance from the teacher, and configuration of the hearing loss, even with hearing aids. • At 30 dB can miss 25–40% of the speech signal. • At 40 dB may miss 50% of class discussions, especially when voices are faint or speaker is not in the line of vision. • Will miss unemphasized words and consonants, especially when a high-frequency hearing loss is present. • Often experiences difficulty learning early reading skills such as letter/sound associations. • Child's ability to understand and succeed in the classroom will be substantially diminished by speaker distance and background noise, especially in the elementary grades.	• Barriers begin to build with negative impact on self-esteem as child is accused of "hearing when he/she wants to," "daydreaming," or "not paying attention." • May believe he/she is less capable due to difficulties understanding in class. • Child begins to lose ability for selective listening, and has increasing difficulty suppressing background noise causing the learning environment to be more stressful. • Child is more fatigued due to effort needed to listen.
41–55 dB HL (hearing loss)	
• Consistent use of amplification and language intervention prior to age 6 months increases the probability that the child's speech, language, and learning will develop at a normal rate. • Without amplification, child understands conversation at a distance of 3–5 ft, if sentence structure and vocabulary are known. • Amount of speech signal missed can be 50% or more with a 40 dB loss and 80% or more with a 50 dB loss. • Without early amplification the child is likely to have delayed or disordered syntax, limited vocabulary, imperfect speech production, and flat voice quality. • Addition of a visual communication system to supplement audition may be indicated, especially if language delays and/or additional disabilities are present. • Even with hearing aids, child can "hear" but may miss much of what is said if classroom is noisy or reverberant. • With personal hearing aids alone, ability to perceive speech and learn effectively in the classroom is at high risk; FM system necessary.	• Barriers build with negative impact on self-esteem as child is accused of "hearing when he/she wants to," "daydreaming," or "not paying attention." • Communication will be significantly compromised with this degree of hearing loss if hearing aids are not worn. • Socialization with peers can be difficult, especially in noisy settings such as cooperative learning situations, lunch, or recess. • May be more fatigued than classmates due to effort needed to listen.

(continued)

Hearing Assessment in Infancy and Childhood, Table 4 (continued)

56–70 dB HL (hearing loss)

- Even with hearing aids, child will typically be aware of people talking around him/her, but will miss parts of words said resulting in difficulty in situations requiring verbal communication (both one-to-one and in groups).
- Without amplification, conversation must be very loud to be understood; a 55 dB loss can cause a child to miss up to 100% of speech information without functioning amplification.
- If hearing loss is not identified before age of 1 year and appropriately managed, delayed spoken language, syntax, reduced speech intelligibility, and flat voice quality are likely.
- Age when first amplified, consistency of hearing aid use, and early language intervention strongly tied to success of speech, language, and learning development.
- Addition of visual communication system often indicated if language delays and/or additional disabilities are present.
- Use of a personal FM system will reduce the effects of noise and distance and allow increased auditory access to verbal instruction.
- With hearing aids alone, ability to understand in the classroom is greatly reduced by distance and noise.

- If hearing loss was late-identified and language delay was not prevented, communication/interaction with peers will be significantly affected.
- Children will have greater difficulty socializing, especially in noisy settings such as lunch, cooperative learning situations, or recess.
- Tendency for poorer self-concept and social immaturity may contribute to a sense of rejection; peer in service helpful.

71–90 dB HL and 91+ dB HL (hearing loss)

- The earlier the child wears amplification consistently with concentrated efforts by parents and caregivers to provide rich language opportunities throughout everyday activities and/or provision of intensive language intervention (sign or verbal), the greater the probability that speech, language, and learning will develop at a relatively normal rate.
- Without amplification, children with 71–90 dB hearing loss may only hear loud noises about one foot from ear.
- When amplified optimally, children with hearing ability of 90 dB or better should detect many sounds of speech if presented from close distance or via FM.
- Individual ability and intensive intervention prior to 6 months of age will determine the degree that sounds detected will be discriminated and understood by the brain into meaningful input.
- Even with hearing aids children with 71–90 dB loss are typically unable to perceive all high-pitch speech sounds sufficiently to discriminate them, especially without the use of FM.
- The child with hearing loss greater than 70 dB may be a candidate for cochlear implant(s) and the child with hearing loss greater than 90 dB will not be able to perceive most speech sounds with traditional hearing aids.
- For full access to language to be available visually through sign language or cued speech, family members must be involved in child's communication mode from a very young age.

- Depending on success of intervention in infancy to address language development, the child's communication may be minimally or significantly affected.
- Socialization with hearing peers may be difficult.
- Children may be more comfortable interacting with deaf or hard of hearing peers due to ease of communication.
- Relationships with peers and adults who have hearing loss can make positive contributions toward the development of a healthy self-concept and a sense of cultural identity.

Unilateral hearing loss

- Child can "hear" but can have difficulty understanding in certain situations, such as hearing faint or distant speech, especially if poor ear is aimed toward the person speaking.
- Will typically have difficulty localizing sounds and voices using hearing alone.
- The unilateral listener will have greater difficulty understanding speech when environment is noisy and/or reverberant, especially when normal ear is toward the overhead projector or other competing sound source and poor hearing ear is toward the teacher.
- Exhibits difficulty detecting or understanding soft speech from the side of the poor hearing ear, especially in a group discussion.

- Child may be accused of selective hearing due to discrepancies in speech understanding in quiet versus noise.
- Social problems may arise as child experiences difficulty understanding in noisy cooperative learning, or recess situations.
- May misconstrue peer conversations and feel rejected or ridiculed.
- Child may be more fatigued in classroom due to greater effort needed to listen, if class is noisy or has poor acoustics.
- May appear inattentive, distractible, or frustrated, with behavior or social problems sometimes evident.

(continued)

Hearing Assessment in Infancy and Childhood, Table 4 (continued)

Mid-frequency or reverse slope hearing loss

- Child can "hear" whenever speech is present but will have difficulty understanding in certain situations.
- May have difficulty understanding faint or distant speech, such as a student with a quiet voice speaking from across the classroom.
- The "cookie-bite" or reverse slope listener will have greater difficulty understanding speech when environment is noisy and/or reverberant, such as a typical classroom setting.
- A 25–40 dB degree of loss in the low to mid-frequency range may cause the child to miss approximately 30% of speech information, if unamplified; some consonant and vowel sounds may be heard inconsistently, especially when background noise is present.
- Speech production of these sounds may be affected.

- Child may be accused of selective hearing or "hearing when he wants to" due to discrepancies in speech understanding in quiet versus noise.
- Social problems may arise as child experiences difficulty understanding in noisy cooperative learning situations, lunch, or recess.
- May misconstrue peer conversations, believing that other children are talking about him or her.
- Child may be more fatigued in classroom setting due to greater effort needed to listen.
- May appear inattentive, distractible, or frustrated.

High-frequency hearing loss

- Child can "hear" but can miss important fragments of speech.
- Even a 26–40 dB loss in high-frequency hearing may cause the child to miss 20–30% of vital speech information if unamplified.
- Consonant sounds t, s, f, th, k, sh, ch likely heard inconsistently, especially in the presence of noise.
- May have difficulty understanding faint or distant speech, such as a student with a quiet voice speaking from across the classroom and will have much greater difficulty understanding speech when in low background noise and/or reverberation is present.
- Many of the critical sounds for understanding speech are high-pitched, quiet sounds, making them difficult to perceive; the words cat, cap, calf, and cast could be perceived as "ca," word endings, possessives, plurals, and unstressed brief words are difficult to perceive and understand.
- Speech production may be affected.
- Use of amplification often indicated to learn language at a typical rate and ease learning.

- May be accused of selective hearing due to discrepancies in speech understanding in quiet versus noise.
- Social problems may arise as child experiences difficulty understanding in noisy cooperative learning situations, lunch, or recess.
- May misinterpret peer conversations.
- Child may be fatigued in classroom due to greater listening effort.
- May appear inattentive, distractible, or frustrated.
- Could affect self-concept.

Fluctuating hearing loss

- Of greatest concern are children who have experienced hearing fluctuations over many months in early childhood (multiple episodes with fluid lasting 3 months or longer).
- Listening with a hearing loss that is approximately 20 dB can be compared to hearing when index fingers are placed in ears.
- This loss or worse is typical of listening with fluid or infection behind the eardrums.
- Child can "hear" but misses fragments of what is said. Degree of difficulty experienced in school will depend upon the classroom noise level, the distance from the teacher, and the current degree of hearing loss.
- At 30 dB can miss 25–40% of the speech signal.
- A child with a 40 dB loss associated with "glue ear" may miss 50% of class discussions, especially when voices are faint or speaker is not in line of vision.
- Child with this degree of hearing loss will frequently miss unstressed words, consonants, and word endings.

- Barriers begin to build with negative impact on self-esteem as the child is accused of "hearing when he/she wants to," "daydreaming," or "not paying attention."
- Child may believe he/she is less capable due to understanding difficulties in class.
- Typically poor at identifying changes in own hearing ability. With inconsistent hearing, the child learns to "tune out" the speech signal.
- Children are judged to have greater attention problems, insecurity, distractibility, and lack self-esteem.
- Tend to be non-participative and distract themselves from classroom tasks; often socially immature.

the left ear and no measurable ABR at the highest presentation level of 80 dB nHL in the right ear. Based on the click-evoked ABR, the child was judged to have normal hearing in the left ear. Using the table of cross-checks (Table 5), absent OAEs in the presence of normal tympanometry is not consistent with normal hearing. Recall that click-evoked ABR responses are limited to a restricted frequency region, usually 2–4 kHz. Based on the electrophysiological tests and parental report, there is an indication of hearing loss in both ears.

Hearing Assessment in Infancy and Childhood, Table 5 Illustration of the cross-check principle, with possible diagnostic outcomes based on the test battery outcome

Behavioral thresholds	OAE	Tympanometry	Reflexes	ABR thresholds	Possible diagnosis
Normal (<20 dB HL)	Present	WNL	Present	500 Hz = 30–40 dB nHL 2,000 Hz = 20–30 dB nHL 4,000 Hz = 20–30 dB nHL	Hearing is within normal limits
Elevated (20–35 dB HL)	Present	WNL	Present	500 Hz > 30–40 dB nHL 2,000 Hz > 20–30 dB nHL 4,000 Hz > 20–30 dB nHL	Slight/mild sensorineural hearing loss
Elevated (>30 dB HL)	Absent	Flat/negative pressure/low compliance	Elevated or absent	500 Hz > 30–40 dB nHL 2,000 Hz > 20–30 dB nHL 4,000 Hz > 20–30 dB nHL	Conductive hearing loss
Elevated (40–60 dB HL)	Absent	WNL	WNL	Normal wave V latency at high intensity 500 Hz > 30–40 dB nHL 2,000 Hz > 20–30 dB nHL 4,000 Hz > 20–30 dB nHL	Sensorineural hearing loss of mild/moderate degree
Elevated (>60 dB HL)	Absent	WNL	Absent	500 Hz > 30–40 dB nHL 2,000 Hz > 20–30 dB nHL 4,000 Hz > 20–30 dB nHL	Severe/profound hearing loss
Elevated (>30 dB HL)	Present	WNL	Absent	Poor morphology, delayed wave latencies	Auditory dys-synchrony

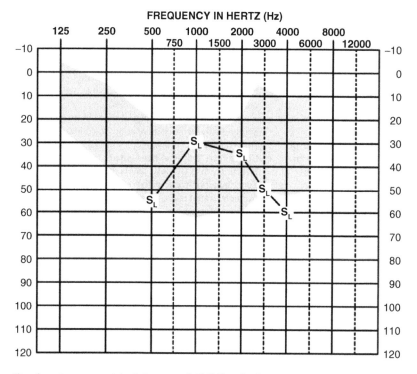

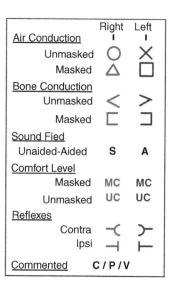

Hearing Assessment in Infancy and Childhood, Fig. 10 Audiogram from 18 month old patient who previously had been diagnosed with normal hearing in one ear based on a click-evoked ABR test

A behavioral audiologic assessment was conducted by conditioning the child using Visual Reinforcement Audiometry. Sound field test results indicated a hearing loss characterized by a moderate degree of loss at 500 Hz rising to a mild loss at 1,000 Hz, then sloping to a moderate loss at 4,000 Hz (see Fig. 10). Behavioral results were consistent with the electrophysiological test results from the other clinic and indicated the presence of significant hearing loss that would be expected to impact the child's speech, language, social, and educational development.

Conclusion

Assessment of hearing in infants and children is accomplished using a test battery approach and a combination of behavioral and electrophysiological tests. Hearing can be evaluated indirectly using electrophysiological tests, such as ABR, in infants who are developmentally younger than 6 months old while behavioral testing can be accomplished with infants who are developmentally 6 months of age and older. Electrophysiological tests (e.g., tympanometry, OAEs, and ABRs) are important cross-checks to assess hearing sensitivity and auditory system integrity. The expected outcomes of a comprehensive audiological assessment include: (1) identification of transient or permanent hearing loss, middle ear dysfunction, or auditory processing disorder; (2) evaluation of auditory system integrity; (3) quantification of hearing loss and expected impact on speech/language development, communication, social interaction, and education; (4) referrals for intervention and/or medical management; and (5) a monitoring plan when children are at risk for progressive or late-onset hearing loss (American Speech-Language-Hearing Association (ASHA) 2004). Early identification and intervention can minimize the potential impact of hearing loss and enable children to reach their full potential.

Cross-References

▶ Hearing (Sensorineural Hearing Loss – Pediatric)
▶ Hearing Testing, Auditory Brainstem Response (ABR)
▶ Sensorineural Hearing Loss-Congenital-Genetics

References

American Speech-Language-Hearing Association (2004) Guidelines for the audiologic assessment of children from birth to 5 years of age (guidelines). www.asha.org/policy. Accessed May, 2011

Anderson K, Matkin N (1991) Relationship of degree of long-term hearing loss to psychosocial impact and educational needs. http://kandersonaudconsulting.com/uploads/Relationship_of_Hearing_Loss__Listening__Learning_Need_1_per_pg.pdf. Accessed May, 2011

Diefendorf AO (2009) Assessment of hearing loss in children. In: Katz J, Medwetsky L, Burkard R, Hood L (eds) Handbook of clinical audiology, 6th edn. Lippincott Williams & Wilkins, Baltimore, pp 545–563

Hall JW III (2000) Handbook of otoacoustic emissions. Singular Publishing Group, Thomson Learning, San Diego

Joint Committee on Infant Hearing (2007) Year 2007 position statement: principles and guidelines for early hearing detection and intervention. Pediatrics 120:898–921

Madell JR (1998) Behavioral evaluation of hearing in infants and young children. Thieme, New York

NCHAM (National Center for Hearing Assessment and Management). www.infanthearing.org. Accessed Apr 2011

Northern JL, Downs MP (2002) Hearing in children, 5th edn. Lippincott Williams & Wilkins, Philadelphia

Prieve B, Fitzgerald T (2009) Otoacoustic emissions. In: Katz J, Medwetsky L, Burkard R, Hood L (eds) Handbook of clinical audiology, 6th edn. Lippincott Williams & Wilkins, Baltimore, pp 497–528

Roeser RJ, Clark JL (2004) Behavioral and physiological measures of hearing: principles and interpretation. In: Roeser RJ, Downs MP (eds) Auditory disorders in school children, 4th edn. Thieme, New York, pp 27–69

Hearing Exam

Brian J. McKinnon
Department of Otolaryngology-Head and Neck Surgery, Georgia Health Sciences University, Augusta, GA, USA

Synonyms

Anamnesis; Auditory system exam; Hearing assessment; Medical exam; Medical history; Physical assessment; Physical exam

Definition

Iatrotropic – that part of the medical history that the patient offers.

Non-iatrotropic – that part of the medical history that is elicited from the patient.

Eustachian tube dysfunction – alteration in middle ear gas exchange.

Tinnitus – the perception of sound that is not exogenous to the patient.

Vertigo – a perception of imbalance where there is the illusion of rotation.

Didactic – an activity related to classroom teaching or instruction.

Basic Characteristics

The Hearing Exam

About a quarter of the complaints encountered in the adult primary care setting involve areas of general otolaryngology, with the percentage of otolaryngology problems seen in a pediatric primary care setting being even higher. A recent study of undergraduate medical education in Canada is telling in this regard (Wong and Fung 2009), and likely reflects a similar training experience and exposure elsewhere, including the United States. Exposure to otolaryngology in Canadian undergraduate medical education varies considerably, with clinical skills sessions in particular being uncommon. Outside of formal otolaryngology residence training, such didactic and clinical skills training is also limited in Canadian primary care and emergency medicine residency training, with elective rotations either optional or not offered at all. However, when Canadian undergraduate medical students, postgraduate training primary care and emergency medicine residents, primary care physicians and community otolaryngologists were asked in this study, in aggregate they had high rankings for the importance of otolaryngology history taking, the otoneurologic exam, and the tuning fork exam.

The process of patient evaluation and diagnosis is begun with the taking of the medical history and performance of the physical exam. While the physical exam of the ear and hearing is limited, and augmented with audiology testing, history taking is extensive and detailed, requiring diligence and time to perform. Establishing the chief complaint, history of the present complaint, past and current medical concerns, previous surgeries and therapies, family medical history, medications, and allergies is an essential, and sometimes the critical step in determining the correct diagnosis or constellation of diagnoses that are causing the patient's

complaint (Hampton et al. 1975). In this respect, the more complex, technology focused evaluations should be consider as confirmatory of the differential diagnoses under consideration, and not the primary means of assessment. The critical and paramount importance of letting the patient speak whenever possible should be central to the patient-provider encounter.

Chief Complaint and History of the Present Illness

Gathering the patient information requires the collection of two forms of information, the presenting (iatrotropic) complaint or symptom, and the elicited (non-iatrotropic) symptom or history (Summerton 2008). Patient-centered interview techniques (letting the patient speak following the use of open-ended questions) should be followed by specifics elicited by close-ended questions. Queries into associated symptoms (hearing loss, Eustachian tube dysfunction, tinnitus, vertigo, or other forms of imbalance, for example), symptom frequency and constancy, timing of symptoms, actions that relieve or exacerbate the complaints, and association with symptoms in conjunction with others should be done for clarification if not mentioned or detailed by the patient.

Past and Current Medical and Surgical History

Collection and documentation of the past and current medical and surgical history often occurs during the presentation of the initial complaint, although further detailed information should be sought. Systemic diseases, such as arthrosclerosis, rheumatoid arthritis, and diabetes, can contribute to hearing loss as can therapies for these illnesses. Of particular importance is previous and current otologic diseases such as Meniere's disease or otosclerosis, and previous surgery such as tympanoplasty or stapedotomy, as these can be vital to assessing the current state of or the progression of disease. Documentation of previous treatments, and their success, or lack thereof, is useful in directing therapy, as well as may lead the diagnostician to consider other processes or disorders not previously noted.

Habits (use of tobacco products, alcohol, illicit drugs), occupational roles (military service, work noise exposure, communications issues), and recreational activities (firearms, hearing protection) may yield further information needed for diagnosis, prevention, and therapy. The use of portable audio players and the use of hearing protection in occupation and recreation are also important to document to assess possible actions that may increase or decrease the risk of noise-induced auditory trauma.

Family History

Both shared environment and shared genetics have roles in the diseases of the ear. Otosclerosis has an autosomal dominant inheritance, though variable penetrance, and history of hearing loss or surgery for otosclerosis in primary and distant relatives should be sought. Mitochondrial-linked sensorineural hearing loss has a maternal inheritance pattern, giving importance to the need to ask about siblings, and maternal relatives. Otitis media is linked to such environmental situations as daycare exposure, siblings in daycare, and second hand smoke exposure in caretakers, and their documentation can both influence medical and surgical therapy and behavior modification recommendations. Information regarding familial predecessors, current family relations, and in the case of older adults, their children and even grandchildren provides for improved diagnostic reasoning, and more focused clinical investigation

Medications and Treatments

Several medications can adversely impact the auditory system (aminoglycosides, diuretics, chemotherapy agents to name a few), and all medications, prescribed, over the counter, and alternative, should be carefully recorded and reviewed with the patient. It is often fruitful to ask about past therapies, particularly those with known potential for ototoxicity, as these may not be recalled unless prompted as the patient is not currently using the particular agent.

Physical Exam

As mentioned earlier, the ear and hearing physical exam is limited in scope due to the anatomy. Part of an overall head and neck exam, the general appearance of the auricles, patency of the meatus, and palpation of the mastoid and temporomandibular joint is documented. In patients with complaint of tinnitus, auscultation of the neck with a stethoscope, and the external auditory canal with a Toynbee tube may be revealing for a vascular cause of the patient's perception. The pinna should be examined for trauma, and deformity. As the pinna is easily exposed to sun, skins changes suggestive of cancerous or precancerous lesions are important details to document and act upon. Preauricular pits can suggest failures of branchial arch development. Microtia is suggestive of an atretic plate, middle ear ossicular

abnormalities, and variation in the anatomic position of the facial nerve. An ear lobe crease can indicate coronary artery disease (Hullar and Minor 2005).

The exam of the external auditory canal and tympanic membrane can be performed with either a handheld otoscope or a binocular microscope, although the binocular microscope has a number of advantages. The binocular microscope leaves the examiner's hands available to remove debris or cerumen, as well as provides a level of illumination and binocular magnification that is generally not available with a handheld otoscope. The improved magnification and illumination affords improved visualization of the tympanic membrane and its movement in autoinflation and patulous Eustachian tube dysfunction. Findings of exposed bone or granulation tissue on the canal or tympanic membrane, evidence of middle ear effusion, tympanic membrane mobility, protrusion, retraction, inflammation, perforation, loss of drumhead landmarks all provide further information in support or refutation of diagnoses under consideration.

Tuning Fork Exam

The tuning fork exam is a commonly performed element of the hearing physical exam, and as an adjunct to audiology testing is used to corroborate the audiogram findings (Glasscock and Shambaugh 1990).

The Weber test is performed with the 512 Hz tuning fork. After the tuning fork has been struck, it is placed either in the center of the forehead or bridge of the nose, and the patient reports either the sound is equal in both ears, or lateralized to one side. If the Weber test is normal on both sides, this suggests a sensorineural loss, if abnormal, then a conductive or mixed hearing loss.

The Rinne test is completed using 256 Hz, 512 Hz, and 1,048 Hz tuning forks. The testing is performed first by placing the struck fork adjacent (approximately two inches away) to and at the level of the ear, with the tines perpendicular to the side of the head, and then the stem of the fork is placed on the patient's mastoid about two inches behind the canal meatus. If the patient hears the sound louder by the meatus than when placed on the mastoid bone, the test is normal, and the exam is documented as air conduction greater than bone conduction (Rinne is positive). If the patient hears the sound louder on the mastoid than when placed by the meatus, the test is abnormal, and the exam is documented as bone conduction greater than air conduction (Rinne is negative). If the test is abnormal at 256 HZ, and normal in the remaining forks, that suggests the air-bone gap is 20–30 dB, if 256 Hz and 512 Hz abnormal, then the air-bone gap is 30–45 dB, and if 256 Hz, 512 Hz, and 1,024 Hz are abnormal, then the air-bone gap is 45–60 dB.

Cranial Nerve Exam

Testing of the cochlear nerve portion of cranial nerve VIII is already discussed with the tuning fork exam described above, and the vestibular nerve portion of cranial nerve VIII is described elsewhere in this work. The cochlear and vestibular portions of cranial VIII are certainly important to the discussion of the hearing exam, but should not be the exclusive focus. Dysfunctions of the hearing system not only can occur concurrently with vestibular dysfunction, but can involve the other cranial nerves as well. The nasal congestion or sinus infection that leads to disturbance of olfaction may also contribute to Eustachian tube dysfunction and its related middle ear concerns. Neurodegenerative processes such as multiple sclerosis and Alzheimer's disease can also impact olfaction and hearing. Exam findings of cranial nerve II can corroborate hearing complaints suggestive of autoimmune disease, increased intracranial pressure or mass effect, and systemic disease. Disruption of extraocular movements (cranial nerves III, IV, and in particular, VI) is seen in skull base trauma. Möbius syndrome is a congenital paralysis of VI (and VII). The paralysis of VI in a clinical picture of otitis media indicates progression to petrous apicitis, and when associated with pain (V_1) is known by the eponym of Gradenigo's syndrome.

Cranial nerve V provides motor innervations to the tensor tympani muscle, and the tensor veli palatine, as well as sensory innervation to the globe. Myoclonus of the tensor tympani muscle and the tensor veli palatine can be perceived as a fluttering tinnitus. The blink reflex (V_1) is part of the facial nerve exam. Cranial nerve VII passes through the internal auditory canal adjacent to cranial nerve VIII, and then passes through the middle ear. Dysfunction of the stapedial muscle (stapedial reflex), facial paresis and paralysis, can be due to cerebellopontine masses causing concurrent hearing complaints, temporal bone trauma, or progression of middle ear infection or masses. Cranial nerve IX (via Jacobson's nerve) provides sensory function to the middle ear, mastoid, and Eustachian tube, and the special sense of taste to the posterior third of the tongue; cranial nerve X (via Arnold's nerve) provides sensory function

for the area of the concha, external auditory canal, tympanic membrane, and postauricular skin. Irritative lesions of the larynx or base of tongue can cause referred pain to the ear, and noxious stimulation of the ear canal can cause cough and bradycardia. Cranial nerve XI and XII motor weakness can provide further supporting evidence of skull base trauma, intracranial mass, or neurodegenerative disease.

Exam

Cranial nerve I: Olfaction can be evaluated through the use of commercially available smell testing kits. If that is not available, then the use of a 70% alcohol wipe held gradually closer to the nose can be used as a challenge. If the aroma is not detected, or is detected at a distance of 5 cm or less, then anosmia should be suspected.

Cranial nerve II: Vision can be evaluated using either a hand held or wall mounted Snellen eye chart. Visual fields can be evaluated by the examiner confronting the patient from a close distance, and bringing in an object into the field of view, such as the examiner's fingers moving. Each eye is examined separately; the point at which the moving fingers are noted indicates the patient's visual field. Each eye is also examined for papillary reaction using a small light, with the examiner making note of both the ipsilateral and contralateral pupil movement.

Cranial Nerves III, IV, and VI: The movement of the globe is evaluated again by confronting the patient at a close distance, and either directing the patient to move the eyes in the vertical and horizontal direction, or having them follow the examiner's finger in the vertical and horizontal direction. Ptosis should be noted with the patient looking superiorly.

Cranial nerve V: Sensation of the face can be evaluated for light touch, sharp touch, and temperature. A wisp of cotton can be used to evaluate the corneal reflex, with the patient looking toward the examiner, and the wisp carefully drown from the sclera, which is not sensitive, on to the edge of the cornea, which should result in a bilateral blink. A cotton wisp can also be used to check touch on the skin, and a tin or freshly split wooden tongue depressor sharp. Cool and warm testing can be done with a warmed and cooled small laryngeal mirror.

Cranial nerve VII: The facial nerve can be evaluated by using the House-Brackmann facial nerve grading scale, which consists of 6 grades, with 1 being normal, and 6 being a complete paralysis. The House-Brackmann scale was initially developed as a common tool intended for use in assessing patients with idiopathic facial paralysis. Despite attempts at developing more sophisticated systems of evaluation and documentation, the House-Brackmann scale's simplicity and repeatability has led to its adoption and broad use in facial nerve dysfunction from other causes. In addition to documenting the overall grade, an examiner should comment on the specifics of the gross function, resting appearance, and dynamic appearance of the exam. In cases of incomplete paralysis, the involved branch or branches (temporal, zygomatic, buccal, marginal, and cervical) should be separately documented.

Cranial nerves IX and X: Cranial nerves IX and X are responsible for sensation of the external canal and middle ear and for swallowing and phonation. Cranial nerve IX can be tested by eliciting the gag reflex, though testing middle ear sensation is usually impractical. Cranial nerve X can be evaluated by checking sensation of the concha and external ear canal, observing palate elevation, and direct or indirect laryngeal exam for true vocal cord mobility.

Cranial nerve XI and XII: Cranial nerves XI and XII are both motor nerves. Cranial nerve XI function is assessed first by observing the sternocleidomastoid and trapezieus muscles for symmetry, then asking the patient to turn their head against resistance, raise their arm laterally above the shoulder (alternately, the patient may push against a solid vertical surface and look for evidence of scapula displacement). Shrugging may not adequately delineate cranial nerve XI dysfunction as the spinal muscles may compensate for cranial nerve XI weakness over time.

Cross-References

▶ Audiometry
▶ Disorders of Pinna, Relapsing Polychondritis
▶ ENG/VNG
▶ Eustachian Tube, Anatomy and Physiology
▶ Hearing Testing, Auditory Brainstem Response (ABR)
▶ Middle Ear Anatomy
▶ Middle Ear Physiology
▶ Physiology of Cochlea
▶ Rotary Chair
▶ Sensorineural Hearing Loss
▶ Temporal Bone Trauma
▶ Testing, Posturography

References

Glasscock ME, Shambaugh GE (1990) Surgery of the ear. Saunders, Philadephia
Hampton JR, Harrison MJG, Mitchell JRA (1975) Relative contributions of history-taking, physical examination and laboratory investigation to diagnosis and management of medical outpatients. BMJ 2:486–489
Hullar TE, Minor LB (2005) The neurotologic exam. In: Jackler RK, Brackman DE (eds) Neurotology, 2nd edn. Elsevier/Mosby, Philadelphia, pp 215–227
Summerton N (2008) The medical history as a diagnostic technology. Br J Gen Pract 58:273–276
Wong A, Fung K (2009) Otolaryngology in undergraduate medical education. J Otolaryngol Head Neck Surg = Le Journal D'oto-Rhino-Laryngologie Et De Chirurgie Cervico-Faciale 38(1):38–48

Conclusion

While complaints associated with hearing and the ear are common, formal education in this area outside of the specialty of otolaryngology is incomplete and uneven. As with any patient complaint, a carefully performed history, followed by a hearing exam as part of a comprehensive head and neck exam, is the essential approach of the careful and diligent clinician in caring for their patient. Hearing and ear complaints should not be thought of in isolation, but to be potentially part of a broader disease process or processes. An organized approach with attention to detail will facilitate, direct, and expedite the diagnostic and therapeutic course of action.

Hearing Loss in Inner Ear Malformations

Gonca Sennaroglu[1] and Levent Sennaroglu[2]
[1]Audiology Section, Department of Otolaryngology, Hacettepe University Medical Faculty, Ankara, Turkey
[2]Department of Otolaryngology, Hacettepe University Medical Faculty, Ankara, Turkey

Inner ear malformations (IEM) constitute approximately 20% of congenital hearing loss. In this entry, characteristics of hearing loss in different types of inner ear malformations are presented. Details of the radiological features and surgery of malformations are presented in the entry ▶ Surgical Devices (Cochlear Implantation-Pediatric-Congenital Malformations). IEM are classified according to the paper by Sennaroglu L published in 2010 (Sennaroglu 2010).

Labyrinthine Aplasia

The cochlea, vestibule, and vestibular and cochlear aqueducts are absent (Fig. 1a). As can be expected, majority of these cases demonstrate no response to pure tone or speech sounds. In spite of the fact that the inner ear is completely absent, sometimes these cases demonstrate profound hearing loss at 125, 250, and 500 Hz at maximum audiometric limits (Fig. 2). As they have no cochlear development, this finding shows that these patients receive these impulses as vibrotactile sensation. At the same time, these findings show that the response of children at these frequencies are outside the limits of hearing sensation and should not be considered during the process of candidate selection criteria.

Although it has not yet been universally accepted (Sennaroglu et al. 2011), auditory brainstem implantation (ABI) is the only possible option for hearing restoration in this group of patients. Ideally, the operation should be done between 1.5 and 3 years of age, but depending on the experience of the team it can also be done as early as 12 months of age (Sennaroglu et al. 2011). If ABI is done later than 4 years of age, audiological outcome is not expected to be as good as the younger implantees.

Cochlear Aplasia

This is the absence of the cochlea. The accompanying vestibular system may be normal (Fig. 1b) or there may be an enlarged vestibule (Fig. 1c). As it is indicated under labyrinthine aplasia, majority of these cases have total SNHL, but occasionally they may show profound hearing loss at 125 and 250 Hz, which should be accepted as vibrotactile sensation. Similar to cases with labyrinthine aplasia, ABI is the only option for restoring hearing in patients with cochlear aplasia.

Common Cavity

In this malformation, cochlea and vestibule are represented by a single compartment (Fig. 1d).

Theoretically, it has cochlear and vestibular neural tissue.

Common cavity patients also demonstrated similar audiological findings to labyrinthine and cochlear aplasia cases. They only had thresholds on low frequency with maximum audiometric limits. It is more appropriate to categorize this response as vibrotactile sensation rather than hearing sensation. Therefore, their hearing was accepted as total SNHL. No fluctuations or progressivity is observed in their hearing levels.

In this patient population, Hacettepe Cochlear Implant Group has a common cavity patient who developed excellent speech after cochlear implantation via transmastoid labyrinthotomy approach, which was first done by McElveen et al. (1997) and reported by Molter et al. (1993). This male patient had profound SNHL. After CI surgery, he developed near-normal speech and language. Therefore, it is possible to develop good audiological outcome in some patients with common cavity deformity. Majority of the common cavity cases have poor outcome with CI. One possible reason is the radiological similarity between cochlear aplasia and vestibular dilatation, which can be confused with common cavity. If the CI surgery is done in a patient with cochlear aplasia and vestibular dilatation, audiological outcome will be very poor.

Incomplete Partition of the Cochlea

According to the defect in the modiolus and the interscalar septum, three different types of incomplete partition cases are identified:

Incomplete Partition Type I (IP-I)

This is the type of the cochlea described in "cystic cochleovestibular malformation" (Sennaroglu and Saatci 2002). The cochlea looks like an empty cystic structure as it lacks the entire modiolus and interscalar septa (Fig. 1e). It is accompanied by large dilated vestibule.

Majority of IP-I patients had severe to profound SNHL, where cochlear implantation has been the method for hearing restoration after sufficient follow-up with hearing aids (Fig. 3). It was also observed that a minority of these patients presented with moderate hearing loss unilaterally, where the contralateral ear

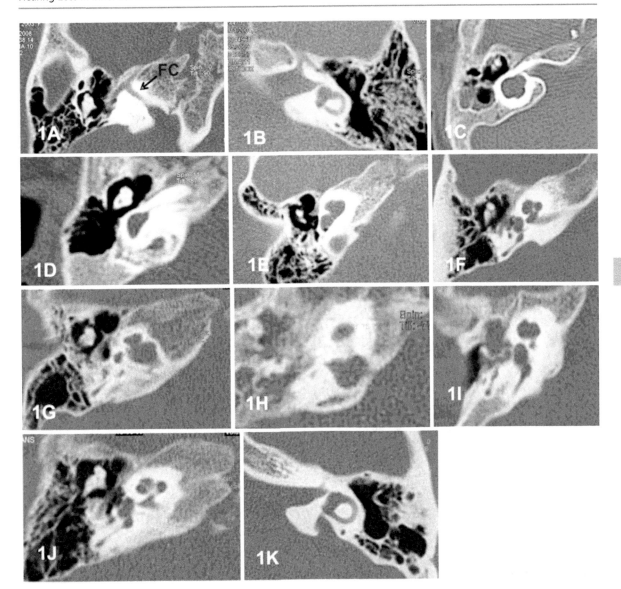

Hearing Loss in Inner Ear Malformations, Fig. 1 Radiological classification of inner ear malformations. 1A Complete labyrinthine aplasia (Michel aplasia) FC: facial canal. 1B Cochlear aplasia with normal vestibule. 1C Cochlear aplasia with dilated vestibule. 1D Common cavity. 1E Incomplete partition type I. 1F Incomplete partition type II. 1G Incomplete partition type III. 1H Cochlear hypoplasia type I (bud type). 1I Cochlear hypoplasia type II (Cystic hypoplastic cochlea). 1J Cochlear hypoplasia type III (Cochlea with less than 2 turns). 1K enlarged vestibular aqueduct

had profound sensorineural hearing loss. It is interesting to see that even though IP-I is a severe malformation of the cochlea, audiological examination may reveal moderate hearing loss. These three cases were rehabilitated with hearing aids. In our department, 32 patients with IP-I received CI.

In some patients with IP-I, cochlear nerve aplasia may also be observed. In this situation, CI surgery is contraindicated and ABI is the only option for hearing restoration. They may receive a cochlear implant in the contralateral ear if the cochlear nerve is present on that side. In case of bilateral cochlear nerve absence, ABI is the only option.

Incomplete Partition Type II (IP-II)

In a type II cochlea, only the basal part of the modiolus is present (Fig. 1f). The apical part of the modiolus and the corresponding interscalar septa are

Hearing Loss in Inner Ear Malformations,
Fig. 2 Profound hearing loss at 125, 250, and 500 Hz. This can be seen in patients with complete labyrinthine aplasia, cochlear aplasia, and common cavity

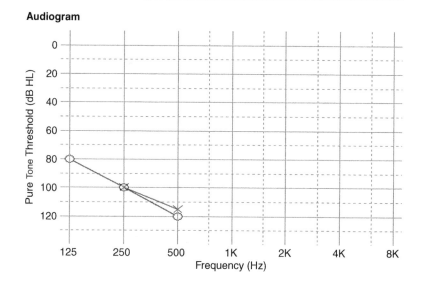

Audiogram

Audiogram

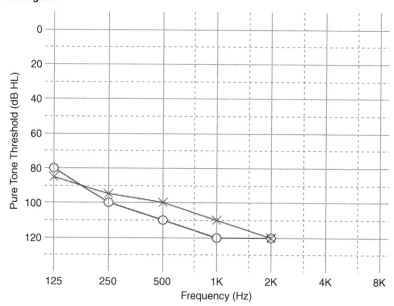

Hearing Loss in Inner Ear Malformations,
Fig. 3 Profound SNHL which can be seen in majority of IP-I patients

defective. The apex of the cochlea has a cystic appearance due to the confluence of middle and apical turns. As the basal part of the modiolus is normal and majority of the spiral ganglion cells are located there, they have better hearing levels than IP-I. Majority of IP-II patients can be rehabilitated with hearing aids at the beginning. When their hearing loss progresses to severe SNHL, they usually need CI. Theoretically, CI surgery should be able to provide considerable stimulation to the inner ear in a way similar to a cochlea with normal architecture. In addition to normal basal turn and cystic apex, these patients are accompanied by minimal vestibular dilatation and a large vestibular aqueduct.

It was observed that hearing level in these patients changes throughout the lifetime. There are patients with profound SNHL during birth or infancy and they undergo CI surgery very early in their life. Majority

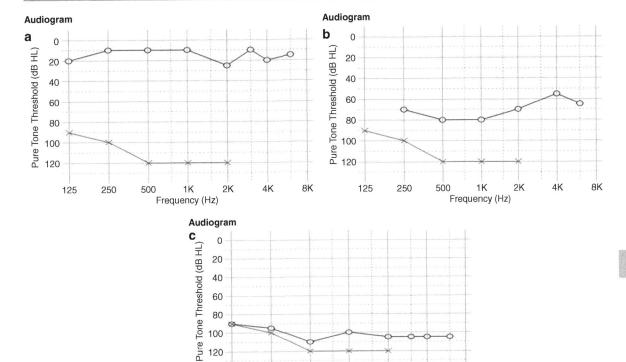

Hearing Loss in Inner Ear Malformations, Fig. 4 (**a**) Left side profound hearing loss. On the right side there was normal hearing until the age of 6. (**b**) Right side sudden SNHL. (**c**) Further progression of hearing loss on the right side

of IP-II patients have better hearing levels and they can develop near-normal speech with hearing aids. Hearing is usually not stable and usually shows progressive loss over time. The hearing level also shows fluctuations and sometimes sudden SNHL (Fig. 4a, b), but generally speaking, it usually progresses to profound hearing loss over time (Fig. 4c). They may also present the clinician with sudden SNHL. Therefore, it is not always possible to give a characteristic hearing level in patients with IP-II. One of the authors (Sennaroglu L.) explored the middle ear of three cases of LVA when they presented with sudden SNHL. All three patients had intense fluctuations in the round window membrane. Most possible explanation for the hearing loss in patients with large vestibular aqueduct based on these observations is that high unnatural CSF pressure exerted on inner ear structures causes sudden or progressive cochlear damage. This usually follows a progressive pattern. Recently, a 60-year-old female patient with unequal LVA on both sides developed sudden and progressive HL

after the age of 50 on the side with smaller vestibular aqueduct. The hearing loss on the larger side was lost in adolescence. This might indicate that the larger the size of the vestibular aqueduct the higher the chance of hearing loss.

They may also show an air-bone gap at low frequencies (Fig. 5).

Incomplete Partition Type III (IP-III)

This is the type of the cochlea observed in X-linked deafness (Sennaroglu et al. 2006). In this deformity, the interscalar septa are present but the modiolus is completely absent (Fig. 1g).

This anomaly is the rarest form of incomplete partition cases. So far, only three patients received CI. There may be two different forms of presentation:
1. The patients may apply with mixed-type hearing loss (Bento and Miniti 1985) (Fig. 6). Snik et al. (1995) reported that if the degree of hearing loss was not too much, stapedius reflex could be obtained in this group of patients. They explained

Hearing Loss in Inner Ear Malformations,
Fig. 5 Air-bone gap at low frequencies. This finding is observed in IP-II and large vestibular aqueduct patients

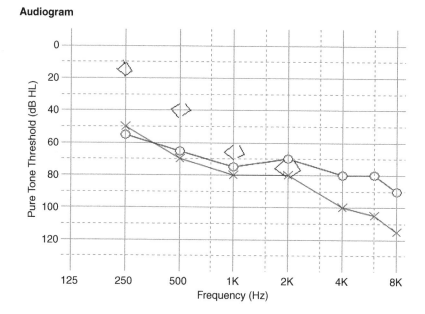

Hearing Loss in Inner Ear Malformations,
Fig. 6 Mixed-type hearing loss in IP-III case. The air-bone gap is usually larger than IP-II cases and involves high frequencies as well as low frequencies

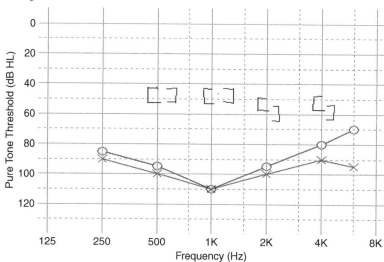

the air-bone gap with the third window phenomenon. Because of the air-bone gap, stapedectomy was attempted in these patients in the past, which resulted in gusher.

When compared with the air-bone gap of IP-II patients, the gap is usually larger than the one in latter group involving high frequencies as well as low frequencies (Fig. 6).

2. The other common form of presentation is profound SNHL. This is most probably due to the absence of the modiolus and in this situation CI surgery is the mode of treatment. All three patients followed in

our department had severe to profound SNHL and underwent CI surgery.

Cochlear Hypoplasia

This is the cochlea with dimensions less than normal. In smaller cochlea, it is usually difficult to count the number of turns with CT and/or MRI. But the definition "cochlea with 1.5 turns" should be used for hypoplasia (particularly type III), rather than for incomplete partition Type II cochlea.

Hearing Loss in Inner Ear Malformations, Fig. 7 Mild SNHL on the right side in a patient with hypoplastic cochlea

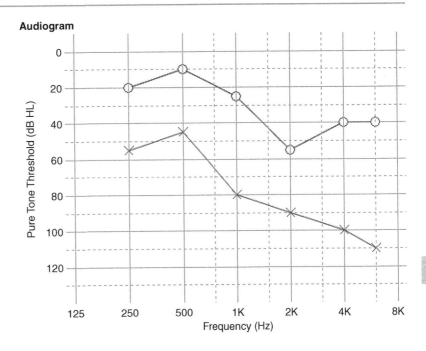

Three different types of cochlear hypoplasia can be identified:

Type I (Bud-like Cochlea)

The cochlea is like a small bud arising from the IAC (Fig. 1h). Internal architecture is severely deformed; no modiolus or interscalar septa could be identified.

Type II (Cystic Hypoplastic Cochlea)

The cochlea is smaller in its dimensions with no modiolus and interscalar septa, but its external architecture is normal (Fig. 1i). There is a wide connection with the IAC. The vestibular aqueduct may be enlarged and the vestibule is minimally dilated.

Type III (Cochlea with Less Than Two Turns)

The cochlea has a shorter modiolus, the overall length of the interscalar septa is less, resulting in a fewer number of turns (less than two turns). The internal and external architecture (modiolus, interscalar septa) is similar to that of a normal cochlea, but the dimensions are less and hence the number of turns is less (Fig. 1j). The vestibule and the semicircular canals are hypoplastic.

Patients with hypoplastic cochlea have different modes of audiological presentation. Some patients had mild SNHL who make use of hearing aids with normal language development (Fig. 7).

Some patients applied with severe to profound SNHL with very little benefit from hearing aids. In this situation, radiology is very important for further treatment options. If the cochlear aperture is normally developed and there is a cochlear nerve on MRI, CI is the mode of treatment. In the presence of cochlear nerve aplasia and cochlear aperture aplasia, ABI was indicated even though the cochlea is surgically accessible for CI surgery.

It was interesting to note that some patients had better hearing level at high frequencies than the low frequencies (Fig. 8). When the cochlea was examined on CT, it was seen that oftentimes the basal turn is developed. The apex of the cochlea might be underdeveloped. This may be the reason with better thresholds at high frequencies and almost total hearing loss at low frequencies.

Some patients demonstrated air-bone gaps.

Hypoplastic cochlear nerve is most commonly associated with this type of inner ear malformations. They usually present with profound SNHL. There is a dilemma whether CI or ABI should be the choice for hearing restoration. So far, the dilemma has not been solved. Electrical ABR results may look promising but so far a universally accepted protocol has not yet been developed. For the time being, audiological examination with hearing aid and 3–6 months of follow-up for language development by an experienced audiologist and speech pathologist may be the most important method for determination between CI and ABI.

Hearing Loss in Inner Ear Malformations,
Fig. 8 Better hearing levels at high frequencies than the low frequencies in a patient with hypoplastic cochlea consisting of only basal turn

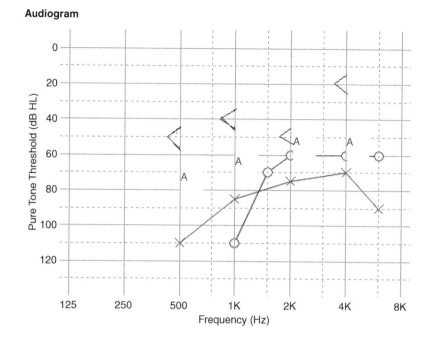

Some infants, who were diagnosed during hearing screening tests, demonstrate behavioral response to speech sounds during hearing aid trial, in spite of no response during objective test methods. They underwent cochlear implantation rather than ABI. One patient developed language acquisition similar to her age group. The remaining two patients are still being under follow-up.

Large Vestibular Aqueduct Syndrome (LVAS)

This is the presence of enlarged vestibular aqueduct (the midpoint between posterior labyrinth and operculum is larger than 1.5 mm) in the presence of normal cochlea, vestibule, and semicircular canals (Fig. 1k). Hearing patterns observed in this group of patients are similar to patients with IP-II.

References

Bento RF, Miniti A (1985) X-linked mixed hearing loss: four case studies. Laryngoscope 95(4):462–468

McElveen JT Jr et al (1997) Cochlear implantation in common cavity malformations using a transmastoid labyrinthotomy approach. Laryngoscope 107(8):1032–1036

Molter DW, Pate BR Jr, McElveen JT Jr (1993) Cochlear implantation in the congenitally malformed ear. Otolaryngol Head Neck Surg 108(2):174–177

Sennaroglu L (2010) Cochlear implantation in inner ear malformations – a review article. Cochlear Implants Int 11:4–41

Sennaroglu L, Saatci I (2002) A new classification for cochleovestibular malformations. Laryngoscope 112(12): 2230–2241

Sennaroglu L, Sarac S, Ergin T (2006) Surgical results of cochlear implantation in malformed cochlea. Otol Neurotol 27(5):615–623

Sennaroglu L et al (2011) Auditory brainstem implantation in children and non-neurofibromatosis type 2 patients: a consensus statement. Otol Neurotol 32(2):187–191

Snik AF et al (1995) Air-bone gap in patients with X-linked stapes gusher syndrome. Am J Otol 16(2):241–246

Hearing Preservation

Amir Ahmadian, Angela E. Downes and A. Samy Youssef
Department of Neurosurgery, University of South Florida, Tampa, FL, USA

Definition

Preservation of hearing within normal and social hearing classification, i.e., pure tone audiometry (PTA) ≤ 50 dB and speech discrimination score

(SDS) $\geq 50\%$, according to guidelines of the American Academy of Otolaryngology-Head and Neck surgery. AAO-HNS class A&B or Gardener-Robertson class II.

Cross-References

▶ Cranial Nerve Monitoring – *VIII, IX, X, XI*

Hearing Testing

▶ Audiometry

Hearing Testing, Auditory Brainstem Response (ABR)

Shruti N. Deshpande[1], Lisa Houston[2] and Robert W. Keith[1]
[1]Department of Communication Sciences and Disorders, College of Allied Health Sciences, University of Cincinnati, Cincinnati, OH, USA
[2]Department of Audiology, UC Physicians ENT, Cincinnati, OH, USA

Synonyms

Brainstem auditory evoked potentials (BAEP); Brainstem auditory evoked response (BAER); Brainstem evoked response (BSER); Brainstem evoked response audiometry (ERA); Early/fast response

Introduction and Definition

Auditory evoked potentials (AEPs) are small, changing electrical potentials that can be recorded from the auditory nervous system of an animal or human being (via surface electrodes typically placed on the forehead and ear lobe or mastoid process of the subject) as a result of acoustic stimulation.

ABRs are short-latency AEPs originating from the parts of the auditory pathway peripheral to the auditory midbrain. The first detailed description of the ABR was given by Jewett and Williston in 1971. The ABR response has seven peaks, of which the first five, labeled using Roman numbers – I, II, III, IV, and V – are considered clinically important. They occur within 15 ms of the onset of a high intensity (70–90 dB nHL) click stimulus in human adults. The amplitude of the wave (in microvolts) is plotted against time (in milliseconds). Tone bursts at 500, 1,000, and 2,000 Hz are sometimes used to determine hearing thresholds at various frequencies.

Purpose

ABR is an auditory electrophysiological test that is primarily used in the clinic for two purposes – estimation of hearing thresholds and for differential diagnosis of cochlear versus retrocochlear hearing pathology.

Principle and Description

Neural Generators

The neural generators of waves I and II of the ABR have been well studied. However, for the waves that follow, the anatomic generators are less precisely defined. That is, each wave could have more than one neural generator and each neural generator in the auditory pathway could potentially be responsible for evoking more than one wave.

As cited by Hall (2007, p. 41–46), often, an *inaccurate* mnemonic – "ECOLI" is nurtured by students of medicine, attributing the ABR waves to the following anatomical locations:

Wave I – *E*ighth cranial nerve distal and central to the internal auditory meatus
Wave II – *C*ochlear Nucleus
Wave III – Superior *O*livary Complex
Wave IV – *L*ateral Leminiscus
Wave V – *I*nferior Colliculus

This basic attribution has potential inaccuracies: the source of each potential was based on studies on smaller animals with experimental lesions. Due to anatomical and physiological differences between these experimental animals and humans, direct comparisons may not be valid. Experiments using intracranial measurements using near-field techniques (electrodes are not placed on the skull and ears but on the neural structures, intracranially) on human subjects

Hearing Testing, Auditory Brainstem Response (ABR), Fig. 1 A normal ABR showing ABR waves I through V. Waves VI and VII are also visible. The stimulus intensity was 80 dB nHL

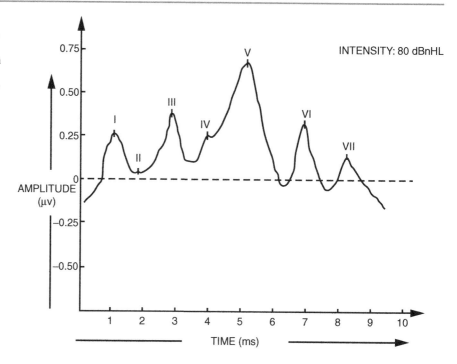

have been most accurate with respect to providing information about the anatomical generators of ABR.

To state correctly and simplistically, waves I and II of the ABR are compound action potentials of cranial nerve VIII and are generated from the distal and proximal parts of the nerve, respectively. Wave III in humans is generated from the caudal portion of the auditory pons, probably ipsilateral to the side of stimulation. Evidence suggests that the cochlear nucleus also contributes to the generation of wave III.

As a result of decussation of the auditory fibers beyond the level of the cochlear nucleus, determining the exact generators of waves IV and V is difficult (Hall 2007, p. 45). The pontine third-order neurons located primarily in the superior olivary complex contribute to wave IV of the ABR. Research by Møller et al. (1995) demonstrated parallel processing of multiple generators for the generation of wave IV in human beings.

Wave V of the ABR, considered to be the most robust and most frequently utilized in clinical diagnosis, is primarily generated at the junction where the lateral leminiscal fibers enter the inferior colliculus of the side contralateral to the side of stimulation.

In summary, there is a "one-neural-generator-to-many-waves" and "many-neural-generators-to-a-single-wave" kind of phenomenon that exists. Identification of these waveforms along with measurement of their

absolute and interwave/interpeak latencies is useful in describing auditory pathway transmission of neural energy. An example of a normal ABR response is shown in Fig. 1.

For diagnostic purposes, waves I, III, and V are the most important to identify. Wave I is often small in amplitude and sometimes difficult to identify without special recording techniques. Wave III is relatively robust and identifiable. Wave V of the ABR is considered to be the most robust and most frequently considered in diagnosis. In general, the interwave latencies between waves I, III, and V are used to describe pontomedullary transmission of the signal as it ascends the auditory system. The absolute measurement of amplitude is not typically used for diagnostic purposes.

Test Protocol

The ABR equipment consists of hardware and software for stimulation, waveform acquisition, and data analysis. Table 1 summarizes stimulus and acquisition parameters typically used for ABR measurement.

Testing Procedure

Testing is conducted in a sound-treated room with the participant lying down or sitting in a reclined position.

Hearing Testing, Auditory Brainstem Response (ABR), Table 1 Stimulus and response parameters commonly used in ABR measurement

Stimulus parameters	Preference	Comments/reasons
Transducer	Insert earphones	*Reduce*: ambient noise, ear canal collapse, chances of infection because they are disposable. *Increase*: interaural attenuation, precision of placement (as opposed to circum- or supra-aural headphones)
	Bone vibrator	For bone conduction ABR
Type	Click	The instantaneous onset of the click waveform is necessary to generate simultaneous firings of multiple neurons of the auditory nerve, resulting in a compound action potential
	Tone bursts	For frequency-specific ABR
Duration	0.1 ms	Facilitates synchronous neuronal firing
Intensity (dB nHL)	High-intensity stimulation is used for differential diagnosis of cochlear versus retro-cochlear lesions	
	ABRs are obtained at different intensities for threshold estimation	
Polarity	Rarefaction	Better wave morphology than "condensation." Results in larger amplitudes and shorter latencies
Rate	~21 clicks per second	Used for threshold estimation
	For example, 21.1 clicks per second	Results in enhanced waveform morphology as opposed to high-rate ABR
		Faster than ABRs at low rates and saves time
	~61 clicks per second	ABR at high rates increase the chances of detecting retro-cochlear pathologies by challenging the auditory nerve
	For example, 72.3 clicks per second	*Using odd number rates prevents interaction with 60 Hz electrical noise used in electrical currents of the USA and some other countries
Number of clicks presented	~2,000 clicks	The number may vary and the basic objective is to obtain adequate signal-to-noise ratio (SNR)
Mode	One ear is tested at a time (Monaural)	Facilitates acquisition of ear-specific information
Masking		Is typically not required when insert earphones are used
Acquisition parameters	Preference	Comments/Reasons
Electrodes		Different electrode configurations will enhance Waves I, III, and V in different ways
Noninverting/positive	Fz or Cz (high forehead or top of the head in the midline)	
Inverting/negative	Ai (ear lobe ipsilateral to the stimulating earphone or the contralateral mastoid)	
Ground	Fpz (low midline forehead)	
Filters		The low-pass filter is set to 1,500 Hz in case of excessive high-frequency artifact. The high-pass filter can be increased to 300 Hz in case of excessive muscle or other artifact
High pass (HP)	30 Hz	
Low pass (LP)	3,000 Hz	
Amplification	100,000 (100,000 times amplification is equivalent to sensitivity of ± 25–$50\ \mu V$)	
Analysis window	15 milliseconds (ms)	
Number of trials	At least two and if there is any question of repeatability run three trials	A valid ABR response is indicated by precise repetition of the waveform on repeated measures. A single trial is insufficient for clinical purposes

The skin surface to which electrodes are attached is cleaned with alcohol and an abrasive gel, and the electrodes are affixed to the skin using a conducting gel. The electrodes are plugged into the differential amplifier of an averaging computer that is programmed with ABR software. An acoustic stimulus is delivered to the patient's ears via insert earphones. The raw neural response is processed and averaged to obtain the required signal-to-noise ratio. This can be done while the test is in process, or the data can be saved for off-line analyses later.

Analysis and Interpretations

Although there is a general consensus with respect to ABR analysis, normative data for waveform latencies can vary from clinic to clinic. Collecting normative data for every clinic is, therefore, highly recommended.

ABR waveforms are plotted on the time domain – the amplitude of the ABR peaks (in micro-volts) is plotted against the time (in milliseconds). Various stimulus and subject factors affect ABR waveforms and, therefore, interpretations and diagnoses should be made with caution. An acoustic click tests only high-frequency hearing (>1,500 Hz), and therefore the ABR will be abnormal in cases of high-frequency hearing loss poorer than 65–70 dB HL, even if the hearing thresholds are within normal limits for frequencies 250–1,000 Hz.

The following factors are considered prior to arriving at a clinical interpretation based on ABR.

1. Waveform morphology
   Morphology is a subjective parameter. Generally, the clinician reviews an ABR waveform and makes a subjective judgment about its "appearance" in terms of the presence of the waves/peaks, their amplitudes, latencies, and repeatability. Based on that, the clinician classifies the ABR morphology as "good," "fair," or "poor." Wave morphology is one of the components that clinicians generally discuss in their interpretation and diagnosis.

   Wave morphology needs to be fair to good with repeatable responses on two to three trials in a normal ABR waveform. Poor wave morphology generally indicates the presence of a neuro-otologic pathology (e.g., multiple sclerosis or auditory neuropathy) or a severe-profound sensorineural hearing loss.

   The following is a case of a 63-year-old male with the chief complaint of hearing loss with tinnitus in the right ear. Audiologic testing revealed left hearing thresholds within normal limits with excellent word recognition a normal to moderate sensorineural hearing loss with 68% (fair) word recognition and positive rollover in the right ear. For the left ear, ABR revealed a fair to good wave morphology and absolute and interpeak latencies for waves I, III, and V within normal limits. ABR in the right was abnormal with poor wave morphology and no repeatable waves I, III, and V. Surgically a final diagnosis of right acoustic neuroma/vestibular ▶ schwannoma of 10×4 mm was made. Figure 2 demonstrates an abnormal ABR with poor morphology and poor repeatability.

2. Absolute latency
   Absolute latency is the time interval between the onset of the stimulus and appearance of the particular ABR peak (see Fig. 1). At high intensities (e.g., 80 dB nHL), the absolute latencies for peaks I, II, III, IV, and V are approximately 1.5, 2.5, 3.5, 4.5, and 5.5 ms, respectively. As stimulus intensity decreases, latency increases. Delayed absolute latency of wave I and subsequent waves indicates presence of a ▶ conductive hearing loss. In case of a ▶ sensorineural hearing loss (moderate to profound), wave I is generally absent, the other waves are delayed or absent, and waveform morphology is affected. In the case of an acoustic neuroma, a number of results occur, one of which is the presence of wave I (generated at the level of the auditory nerve) with absent or delayed responses for subsequent waves. Auditory nerve dys-synchrony caused by auditory neuropathy or demyelinating disease results in poorly repeatable or absent waveforms.

   Presence of waves I and II and severely delayed or absent waves III and V indicate normal peripheral auditory function but a severe brainstem dysfunction, a demyelinating condition (like multiple sclerosis), a brainstem bleed, a space-occupying lesion, or a hypoxic-ischemic brain insult. In fact, an abnormal ABR can identify the site of lesion but not the type.

3. Interwave latency
   Interwave latency (IWL), or interpeak latency, is the time interval between two ABR waves (see Fig. 1). Generally, the IWL for waves I–III, III–V, and I–V are considered for diagnosis. At high intensities (e.g., at 80 dB nHL), normal IWL values for

Hearing Testing, Auditory Brainstem Response (ABR), Fig. 2 ABR with poor morphology. The stimulus intensity was 80 dB nHL. However, poor repeatability and absent waves I through V are observed

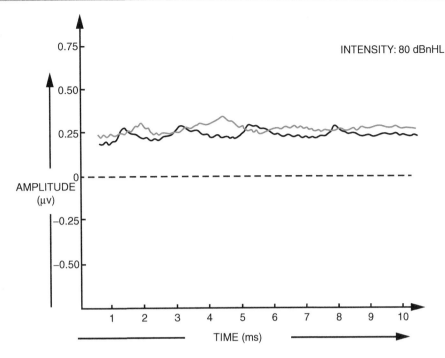

I–III, III–V, and I–V are 2, 2, and 4 ms, respectively.

A unilateral delay in wave I–III or I–V IWL is seen with cerebellopontine angle tumors. Bilateral ABR I–III or I–V latency delay is consistent with bilateral eighth nerve dysfunction (e.g., multiple sclerosis) or other brainstem (pons) dysfunction. A delay in IWL III–V is suggestive of a rostral brainstem (pons-midbrain) dysfunction of the auditory pathway. In patients with increased intracranial pressure, a delay in III–V IWL would indicate a supra-tentorial compression of the upper brainstem.

4. V:I Amplitude ratio

Wave V of the ABR is considered to be the most robust wave. In the same waveform, the amplitude ratio of wave V to I of 0.5:1 or lower is abnormal and indicates an auditory neuropathology. However, the V:I amplitude ratio is seldom used in clinical diagnosis.

Factors Influencing ABR

The outcome of the ABR is affected by certain factors that need to be kept in mind for accurate analysis and interpretation.

1. *Subject characteristics*: Subject characteristics including age, gender, body temperature, as well as certain drugs can affect the ABR.

(a) Age

The ABR waveform is not fully developed at birth, and it matures over the first 18 months of life. In the case of preterm infants, the time required for ABR maturation could be greater. From 18–24 months, ABR latencies and amplitudes reach adult values. Reports in the literature indicate an increase in the peak latencies after the age of 25 years, indicating that advancing age affects ABR. For children younger than 18 months, the ABR assumes different waveform morphology, in comparison to a healthy adult's ABR and this is important in identifying hearing loss during this age period.

(b) Gender

There are statistically significant differences in ABR latencies of male versus female adult subjects. Females have shorter peak latencies and larger amplitudes for ABR waves. The interwave latencies for waves III–V and I–V are shorter for females compared to males. The implication of this finding is that norms for a given clinic should be based on the average ABR findings for approximately equal number of males and females.

(c) Body temperature

ABR latencies increase as a result of low body temperature (hypothermia). With severe hypothermia (body temperature less than 14–20°C), the ABR disappears. This factor becomes important when acquiring ABR from patients under anesthesia, coma, or undergoing open heart surgery.

(d) Subject state

Patient movement and muscular contractions lead to ABR response artifacts and unstable responses. It is thus not possible to obtain a valid ABR from subjects who are moving or restless. Mild sedation may be needed for subjects who are unable to remain relaxed, e.g., those who are cognitively challenged or infants and children.

(e) Drugs

ABR has been shown to be resistant to numerous drugs, sleep, and attention, and is present in deeply comatose patients as long as brainstem function is intact. Ototoxic drugs lead to peripheral hearing loss and thereby affect ABR.

2. *Technical considerations*: ABR morphology is affected by stimulus-related factors including intensity, rate of stimulus presentation, polarity, and filter settings.

(a) Intensity

With increasing stimulus intensity, ABR amplitude increases and latencies (absolute and interpeak) decrease. Thus, wave morphology is generally better at higher stimulus intensities.

(b) Rate of stimulus presentation

At a given stimulus intensity, ABR amplitude decreases and latencies (absolute and interwave) increase with increasing stimulus rates. For example, at 80 dB nHL waveform morphology will deteriorate as click rates increase from 21 to 71 clicks per second. The first wave to disappear is Wave I, followed by disappearance of Wave III at more rapid rates. Wave V is maintained at high click rates in typically functioning individuals. However, in subjects with retrocochlear pathologies, wave V disappears at high stimulus rates. This phenomenon is important for the differential diagnosis of cochlear versus retrocochlear hearing dysfunction.

(c) Polarity

Stimulus polarity does not have major implications on the ABR morphology described in this chapter. Certain other responses are affected by stimulus polarity (e.g., cochlear microphonics and summating potentials) but that discussion is beyond the scope of this chapter. Research indicates that click-evoked ABR morphology is better with "rarefaction" as opposed to "condensation" (Hall 2007, p. 211). Clinically, alternating polarity is often used while acquiring click-evoked ABR in order to reduce stimulus artifact.

(d) Filter settings

Filters contribute to the elimination of unwanted "noise" during ABR acquisition. The filter settings typically used in clinical situations are 30–3,000 Hz (Hall 2007, p. 211). Changes in filter settings affect waveform morphology. It is essential that the clinician uses the same filter settings for testing as those that were used while collecting the normative data for the given clinic.

It is important to point out that the above-mentioned variables interact in a complex fashion to affect the ABR waveforms.

Advantages

There are two primary clinical applications of ABR testing. The first is an audiometric application to determine hearing loss and hearing levels. The second is a neuro-otologic application to determine the presence of lesions of the auditory pathway through the eighth nerve and brainstem. Below is a brief description of these applications (Glattke 1983; Hall 2007; Hooks and Weber 1984; Jacobson 1985; Russo et al. 2004).

1. Determination of the presence of hearing loss and estimation of hearing thresholds

Prediction of hearing loss (screening) and determination of hearing thresholds (diagnostic application) are two widely used applications of the ABR. Since ABR is not affected by sleep or mild sedation, it is a popular "objective" audiological tool that is used for neonatal hearing screening and diagnosing hearing acuity in infants, children and difficult to test patients (including adults and children with cognitive impairment).

ABR is also used in combination with other audiological tests in order to determine true, ear-specific hearing thresholds in cases of pseudohypacusis (functional hearing loss).

2. Neuro-otologic applications
   (a) Retro-cochlear pathologies

   The neuro-audiologic applications of ABR are extensive. As discussed earlier, certain characteristic ABR responses are indicative of a retro-cochlear site of lesion.

   (b) Auditory dys-synchrony/Auditory Neuropathy

   An atypical or absent ABR with robust otoacoustic emissions (OAE) and cochlear microphonics is suggestive of auditory neuropathy/auditory dys-synchrony. This describes a special group of patients with severe speech perception difficulties. Diagnosis of this condition is vital for further audiological rehabilitation of these patients.

   (c) Differentiating auditory nerve from brainstem involvement

   Auditory nerve and brainstem pathologies are both considered retro-cochlear. However, if one can clearly differentiate between an auditory nerve and brainstem lesion, differential diagnosis and treatment can be accelerated. An abnormal III–V interwave latency in the face of a normal wave I and II indicates a brainstem involvement. Absence of wave V (or IV/V) when the earlier peaks are present and normal indicates a brainstem abnormality. The absence of all waves of the ABR indicates auditory nerve dysfunction if peripheral hearing is intact.

3. Special applications

   A brief description of the special applications of the ABR is presented here. For detailed explanations and test protocols, the reader can review the references cited at the end of this chapter (Hall 2007; Jacobson 1985).

   (a) Bone conduction-ABR (BC-ABR)

   BC-ABR is an essential component of the hearing assessment of infants and children who are not able to adequately respond to behavioral tests that are important to infer the type of hearing loss (conductive vs. sensorineural vs. mixed). For example, BC-ABR can accurately determine the amount of air-bone gap in cases with atresia and microtia.

   (b) Electrical ABR (EABR)

   EABR is a technique that uses electrical stimulation to obtain an auditory brainstem response. Prior to ▶ cochlear implantation, this technique was used to assess neural survival and integrity, determine candidacy, and decide which ear to implant. Post cochlear implantation EABR is important for assessing the integrity and functioning of the cochlear implant, estimation of hearing thresholds, and setting cochlear implant (CI) parameters (e.g., most appropriate rate of stimulation through the CI). For additional information on the test protocol, the reader may refer to Hall (2007).

   (c) Intraoperative ABR for VIIIth nerve and brainstem function

   Preservation of neural structures is important during surgical procedures. In surgeries of the cerebro-pontine angle, for example, mechanical, ischemic, or thermal damage could affect the cochlea, auditory nerve, and brainstem, and this may result in hearing loss, speech discrimination problems, and tinnitus. To reduce the risk of these injuries, continuous monitoring of the auditory function is carried out using intraoperative ABR (Hall 2007; Burkard et al. 2007).

   (d) BioMARK

   Biological Marker of Auditory Processing or BioMARK™ needs a special mention. BioMARK™ is a noninvasive, electrophysiological technique that tests brainstem function using speech-syllable-like stimuli (King et al. 2002). The purpose of this special application is to identify brain-stem dys-synchrony. It is an audiological assessment tool that helps assess complex auditory-related problems in individuals with central auditory processing dysfunction/disorders, communication disorders, reading problems, and dyslexia.

   (e) Stacked ABR

   The stacked ABR is a special modification of the conventional ABR. It uses high-pass masking sequences to obtain ABR at different frequency regions. Research indicates that this technique is more sensitive compared to the traditional ABR in detecting small acoustic neuromas.

Disadvantages

Click-elicited ABR does not provide frequency-specific auditory thresholds. Tone burst ABR is a better test for acquiring frequency-specific hearing thresholds.

It is important to realize that although ABR is the most popular and frequently used auditory evoked potential test, it is not a "definitive" test of hearing. As such, ABR results must be interpreted after taking into consideration the findings of other clinical tests, including pure tone audiometry, speech audiometry, immittance audiometry, and otoacoustic emissions.

Although ABR provides estimates of hearing thresholds and/or the status of the auditory pathway, it does not provide any information regarding speech perception and understanding.

Acknowledgments The authors would like to acknowledge that the figures in this article were the work of Aniruddha Deshpande, Doctoral Candidate at the University of Cincinnati. We thank him for the artwork. We would also like to thank Dr Nael Shoman for reviewing our work and for his invaluable suggestions.

References

Burkard R, Don M, Eggermont JJ (2007) Auditory evoked potentials: basic principles and clinical application. Lippincott Williams and Wilkins, Baltimore, pp 229–253

Glattke TJ (1983) Short latency auditory evoked potentials. University Park Press, Baltimore

Hall JWIIIJ (2007) New handbook of auditory evoked responses. Pearson Education, Boston

Hooks RG, Weber BA (1984) Auditory brain stem responses of premature infants to bone-conducted stimuli: a feasibility study. Ear Hear 5:42–46

Jacobson JT (1985) The auditory brainstem response. College Hill Press, San Diego

King C, Warrier CM, Hayes E, Kraus N (2002) Deficits in auditory brainstem encoding of speech sounds in children with learning problems. Neurosci Lett 319: 111–115

Møller AR, Jho HD, Yokota M, Jannetta PJ (1995) Contribution from crossed and uncrossed brainstem structures to the brainstem auditory evoked potentials: a study in humans. Laryngoscope 105:596–605

Russo N, Nicol T, Musacchia G, Kraus N (2004) Brainstem responses to speech syllables. Clin Neurophysiol 115:2021–2030

Heavy Metals

Erika Woodson
Head and Neck Institute, Cleveland Clinic Foundation, Cleveland, OH, USA

Definition

Metallic elements with toxic properties. Many have ototoxic potential.

Cross-References

▶ Sensorineural Hearing Loss (Ototoxicity)

Hematologic Considerations in Pediatric Surgery

John Puetz
Department of Pediatrics, Division of Pediatric Hematology and Oncology, Cardinal Glennon Children's Medical Center, Saint Louis University, St. Louis, MO, USA

Clinical Features

The clinical features of hematologic diseases in childhood vary significantly with the underlying disorder and are best subdivided into disorders of white blood cells, disorders of red blood cells, disorders of platelets, and disorders of the hemostatic system. As disorders of platelets and the hemostatic syndrome are likely to have the greatest impact when considering surgical procedures in children with hematologic disorders, they will be discussed first.

Disorders of Platelets and the Hemostatic System

The properly functioning hemostatic system requires an orchestrated interaction between coagulation factors, Von Willebrand Factor, platelets, endothelial cells of blood vessels, and the extracellular matrix (Fig. 1). Dysfunctions of any step of this process can

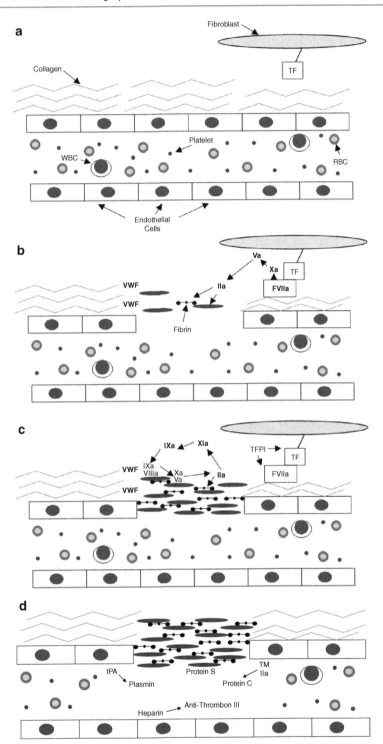

Hematologic Considerations in Pediatric Surgery, Fig. 1 (a) Under normal physiologic conditions, blood flows through the vasculature without forming intravascular thrombi. *TF* tissue factor, *WBC* white blood cell, *RBC* red blood cell. (b) Initiation of hemostasis: disruption of vascular endothelial cells causes blood to escape from the blood vessel. Von Willebrand Factor (*VWF*) binds to extravascular collagen. *VWF* and collagen receptors on platelets cause platelets to adhere to the extravascular space and become activated simultaneously, activated factor VII (*FVIIa*) binds to tissue factor. The

lead to recurrent abnormal bleeding, including abnormal surgical bleeding, or thromboembolic events.

Disorders Resulting in Abnormal Bleeding

1. Platelet Disorders: Platelet dysfunction can be subdivided into quantitative disorders and qualitative disorders (Buchanan 2005; Hayward et al. 2006). Both qualitative and quantitative deficiencies can be congenital or acquired (Table 1). The principal quantitative disorder encountered in the pediatric population is immune thrombocytopenia purpura (ITP). Other quantitative disorders include bone marrow diseases including leukemia or aplastic anemia, splenic sequestration, and congenital heritable disorders of platelet number. Qualitative disorders include those due to exposure to platelet-inhibiting drugs such as nonsteroidal anti-inflammatory drugs (NSAIDS), and congenital platelet function disorders involving receptor, signal transduction, and storage pool deficiencies. Although congenital qualitative platelet disorders are poorly described, they may be the most common. Recent investigations have revealed that up to one half of women with menorrhagia have a qualitative platelet disorder.

Although there are a wide variety of platelet disorders, they have similar clinical manifestations. Patients with platelet disorders suffer from recurrent abnormal mucocutaneous bleeding. The manifestations of their bleeding disorder include abnormal bruising, prolonged bleeding from minor cuts, epistaxis, gum and oral mucosal bleeding, gastrointestinal bleeding, menorrhagia, and abnormal surgical bleeding. Unfortunately, there is a great deal of overlap in bleeding symptoms between the normal population and patients with platelet disorders. For this reason, there is no clinical information one can gather to clearly delineate patients with platelet disorders from those without. Methods using clinical data to identify patients with mucocutaneous bleeding disorder such as the bleeding score are under investigation. A history of recurrent abnormal mucocutaneous bleeding, along with a laboratory evaluation is required to identify these patients.

2. Von Willebrand Disease: Von Willebrand factor has at least two roles in hemostasis. It is a carrier molecule for factor VIII, and it cross-links platelets to collagen, leading to platelet adhesion and activation. Von Willebrand disorders can be congenital or acquired, but the majority of patients have a congenital disorder. Von Willebrand disease has been divided into qualitative and quantitative disorders (Nichols et al. 2008). Von Willebrand disease is subcategorized into type 1, type 2, or type 3 disease depending on whether patients have a quantitative (type 1 and type 3) or qualitative (type 2) defect. Patients with qualitative disorders have abnormal functioning of their Von Willebrand factor leading to abnormal platelet or factor VIII binding. Patients with a loss of function mutation leading to reduced platelet binding have type 2A and 2M disease, while patients with a gain of function mutation leading to enhanced platelet binding (and thrombocytopenia) have type 2B disease. Patient with abnormal factor VIII binding (and factor VIII deficiency) have type 2N disease. Quantitative disorders include type 1 disease in which the patients have a mild to moderately reduced amount of Von Willebrand factor, and type 3 disease, characterized by a complete absence of Von Willebrand factor. With the advent of genetic analysis, it was

---

Hematologic Considerations in Pediatric Surgery, Fig. 1 (continued) tissue factor, factor VIIa complex, then activates factor X (*Xa*). Factor *Va* and Factor *Xa* form the prothrombinase complex on the cellular surface. The prothrombinase complex activates thrombin (*IIa*). Thrombin forms fibrin from fibrinogen. Thrombin can also activate platelets. (c) Propagation phase of hemostasis. Tissue factor pathway inhibitor (*TFPI*) rapidly inactivates the factor VIIa/tissue factor complex, halting the initiation phase of hemostasis. Additional thrombin is generated during the propagation phase. Thrombin formed during the initiation phase activates factor XI (*XIa*). Factor *XIa* then activates factor IX (*IXa*). Factor *VIIIa* (*VIIIa*) and *IXa* form the Tenase complex on the activated platelet surface. Tenase activates additional factor X. Additional prothrombinase is formed on activated platelet surfaces generating additional thrombin. The propagation phase leads to a burst of thrombin formation, which generates a sufficient amount of fibrin to form a stable clot. Thrombin also activates factor XIII (not shown). Factor XIII cross-links the fibrin monomers. (**d**) Hemostasis is extinguished. Heparin-like moieties on the endothelial surface activate anti-thrombin III. Anti-thrombin III then inactivates factor *IIa* and Xa. Thrombin (*IIa*) binds to thrombomodulin (*TM*), which then activates protein C. Protein S and activated protein C form a complex on platelet surfaces, which inactivates Va and VIIIa. Endothelial cells generate tissue plasminogen activator (*tPA*), which converts plasminogen to plasmin. Plasmin then cleaves fibrin

Hematologic Considerations in Pediatric Surgery, Table 1 Platelet disorders seen in children

Quantitative platelet disorders in children
Increased platelet destruction
Immune thrombocytopenia purpura
Neonatal alloimmune thrombocytopenia
Disseminated intravascular coagulation
Hemolytic uremic syndrome
Thrombotic thrombocytopenic purpura
Vascular malformations/Kasabach merritt
Heparin-induced thrombocytopenia
Drug reaction
Snake bite
Autoimmune lymphoproliferative syndrome
Lupus
Antiphospholipid syndrome
Abnormal heart valves
Splenic sequestration
Type 2B Von Willebrand disease
Decreased platelet production
Leukemia
Neuroblastoma and other cancers
Myelofibrosis
Myelodysplastic syndrome
Aplastic anemia
Fanconi anemia
Congenital amegakaryocytic thrombocytopenia
Thrombocytopenia absent radius syndrome
Infectious agents
Drugs/toxins
Wiskott-Aldrich syndrome
Giant platelet syndromes
Qualitative platelet disorders in children
Aspirin/NSAIDS/antiplatelet drugs
Bernard soulier
Glanzmann's Thrombasthenia
Other platelet receptor deficiencies
Signal transduction defects
Storage pool deficiencies
Abnormal release reaction
Giant platelet syndromes
Uremia

discovered that numerous patients previously thought to have type 1 disease have no mutations in their Von Willebrand gene. These patients have a Von Willebrand deficiency independent of their Von Willebrand gene. In light of this discovery, a new category of quantitative Von Willebrand deficiency has been recently proposed and called "low Von Willebrand levels." In contrast to the other forms of Von Willebrand disease, patient with "low Von Willebrand levels" do not have simple mendelian inheritance, such as the autosomal dominant inheritance for type 1, 2A, 2B, 2M, and 2N disease, or the autosomal recessive inheritance as seen in type 3 disease. Patients with "low Von Willebrand levels" generally have milder bleeding symptoms than the other types of Von Willebrand disease, but are still at an elevated risk for bleeding during surgical procedures.

Owing to the interactions between Von Willebrand factor and platelets during hemostasis, the bleeding manifestations of patients with Von Willebrand disease are identical to patients with platelet disorders, namely, recurrent abnormal mucocutaneous bleeding. As with patients with platelet disorders, there is a great deal of overlap between patients with Von Willebrand disease and the normal population. The diagnosis of these patients requires a detailed medical history and laboratory investigation. Unlike patients with platelet disorders, patients with Von Willebrand disease are more likely to have a family history of a bleeding disorder.

The otolaryngologist is often the first clinician to encounter patients with Von Willebrand disease or a platelet disorder because they oftentimes present with epistaxis or oral mucosal bleeding. Epistaxis lasting more than 10 min or occurring more than 10 times in a year is suggestive of a potential bleeding disorder. Any epistaxis requiring cauterization, packing, or a red cell transfusion should prompt an evaluation for an underlying bleeding disorder, especially if the patient has other bleeding symptoms, or a family history of a bleeding disorder.

3. Coagulation Factors: The coagulation cascade is an interaction of coagulation factor zymogens resulting ultimately in the generation of thrombin and fibrin. Deficiencies in any of the coagulation factors can lead to abnormal bleeding (Bolton-Maggs et al. 2004; Sharathkumar 2008). By far, the most common factor deficiencies are factor VIII and factor IX leading to hemophilia A and hemophilia B, respectively. Unlike patients with platelet disorders or Von Willebrand disease, patients with hemophilia have deep tissue bleeding in addition to mucocutaneous bleeding. The hallmark of hemophilia is hemarthrosis and myohematomas, but hemophiliacs are also at risk

for other deep tissue bleeding events including intracranial hemorrhage and retroperitoneal bleeding. Hemophilia is divided into mild, moderate, and severe deficiency based on coagulation factor levels. Patients with severe deficiency typically have no measurable factor activity. Patients with moderate deficiency have between 1% and 5% activity, while those with mild deficiency have between 6% and 60% activity. The bleeding manifestations vary greatly between those with mild deficiency and those with severe deficiency. Before the advent of factor replacement therapy, hemophilia patients with severe disease typically had spontaneous bleeding events occurring as often as weekly. In contrast, those with mild deficiency typically bleed only following significant trauma or surgery, with abnormal bleeding events occurring every few years. Hemophilia A and B are inherited in an X-linked recessive pattern, and occur with a prevalence of 1 in 10,000 people to 1 in 40,000 people, respectively. Patients with congenital hemophilia can generate an immune response to factor replacement resulting in allo-immunoglobulins directed against factor VIII or factor IX, known as an inhibitor. Rarely, patients without hemophilia can develop auto-antibodies to factor VIII or factor IX, known as acquired hemophilia.

Deficiencies of all the other coagulation factors have also been described, but occur much less frequently than hemophilia A or B. The prevalence of these disorders ranges from 1 in 500,000 to 1 in 1,000,000. The bleeding manifestations of the rare factor deficiencies is quite varied, and ranges from mostly mild mucocutaneous bleeding (factor XI deficiency) to mostly severe deep tissue bleeding (factor X deficiency). Unlike hemophilia in which the severity of bleeding is generally predictable based on the degree of factor deficiency, the severity of bleeding does not always correlate with the severity of the factor deficiency in several of the rare factor deficiencies.

Patients with severe factor deficiencies are generally diagnosed early in life because of their severe bleeding manifestations. Patients with mild coagulation factor deficiencies may present with abnormal epistaxis or mucosal bleeding, and the otolaryngologist must take this into consideration, especially if the patient has other bleeding manifestations, including abnormal surgical bleeding, or a family history.

Disorders Resulting in Abnormal Blood Clotting

The hemostatic system requires a delicate balance between factors promoting coagulation (procoagulants) and those limiting the size of the developing clot (anticoagulants). Deficiencies of the procoagulants lead to abnormal bleeding, while deficiencies of the anticoagulants lead to an elevated risk of thrombosis (thrombophilia). Children are generally diagnosed with thrombophilia either due to a thromboembolic event, or due to a family history (Roth 2011). Thrombophilic states can be inherited (protein C deficiency, protein S deficiency, antithrombin III deficiency, factor V Leiden, prothrombin gene mutation 20210, hyperhomocysteinemia), acquired (antiphospholipid syndrome), or of unclear etiology (elevated coagulation factors and lipoprotein (a)). The risk of thrombosis in children with thrombophilia varies from 50-to-100-fold (homozygous factor V Leiden or coinheritance of thrombophilic states) to 0.3 fold (hyperhomocysteinemia). Because the baseline risk of a thrombotic event in children is extremely low, even a high relative risk of a thrombotic event gives these children a low absolute risk of an event. For this reason, children with thrombophilia are generally not placed on anticoagulant medication, unless they have already had a thromboembolic event.

Unless the surgical procedure requires prolonged immobilization, prophylactic anticoagulation is not generally recommended for children with thrombophilia. Children who are receiving therapeutic anticoagulation will require bridging therapy and discontinuation of their anticoagulant during the perioperative time period.

Disorders of White Blood Cells

White cells are key components of the immunological, inflammatory, and tissue repair systems. It is imperative that white cells function properly for normal wound healing to take place. White blood cells include lymphocytes, neutrophils, eosinophils, basophils, monocytes, and macrophages. White cell disorder can be of quantitative or qualitative deficiencies (Table 2). Quantitative disorders resulting in an excess number of white cells include the leukemias or reactive leukocytosis due to infections or inflammation (Hutter 2010). Quantitative disorders resulting in a deficient number of white cells commonly seen in children include transient or permanent bone marrow aplasia due to drugs, toxins, infections, or heritable congenital

Hematologic Considerations in Pediatric Surgery,
Table 2 White cell disorders in children

Low white cell count
Decreased production
Leukemia
Other marrow infiltrative processes
Myelofibrosis
Infectious agents
Drugs/toxins
Kostmann's syndrome
Shwachman-diamond syndrome
Aplastic anemia
Fanconi's anemia
Chronic benign neutropenia
Increased destruction
Immune neutropenia
Autoimmune lymphoproliferative syndrome
Drugs/toxins
High white cell count
Leukemia
Leukemoid reaction
Steroids/drugs
Normal WBC count with abnormal function
Chronic granulomatous disease
Leukocyte adhesion defect
Severe combined immunodeficiency
AIDS
B-Cell immunodeficiencies
T-Cell immunodeficiencies
Common variable immune deficiency
Drugs/toxins

conditions (Tamary 2007). The qualitative disorders typically present with abnormal immunological dysfunction and recurrent infections (Fleisher 2006).

Patients with white cell deficiencies are frequently immunocompromised. As a result, they are prone to frequent infections involving the head and neck, including unusual organisms. The otolaryngologist is frequently called up to assist in the diagnosis of and management of infectious complications of patients with white cell deficiencies. The otolaryngologist should also keep in mind the immune state of the patient with white cell abnormalities when performing routine procedures on these patients.

Disorders of Red Blood Cells

The primary role of red blood cells is to deliver oxygen to tissues. Oxygen delivery is determined by the affinity and saturation of hemoglobin present in red cells, the quantity of red cells present, and the delivery of the oxygen and red cells by the cardiovascular system. The totality of red cells present is typically determined by the ratio of red cells to whole blood, the hematocrit, or the concentration of hemoglobin present. Red cell abnormalities can be categorized into red cell deficiencies (anemia) and red cell excess (polycythemia). Abnormal affinity of hemoglobin to oxygen typically presents as an anemia. Although polycythemia has been described, it is rare in children. The classification of red cell disorders can be divided into abnormal red cell production, abnormal red cell destruction, and blood loss (Segal et al. 2002a, b). An alternative form of classification is based on red cell size (Table 3). Microcytic anemias are typically due to insufficient red cell production and in children commonly include iron deficiency, thalassemia, and anemia of chronic disease. Macrocytic anemias in children also cause abnormal red cell production and are typically due to folate or vitamin B12 deficiency. Normocytic anemias can be caused by abnormal red cell production, abnormal red cell destruction, or blood loss from bleeding. The reticulocyte count is helpful in determining the presence of abnormal red cell destruction, and is elevated with these disorders. Common causes of normocytic anemias with a normal reticulocyte count in children include either congenital or transient red cell aplasia, bone marrow suppression from infectious or drug causes, or bone marrow infiltrative disorders such as leukemia, which typically have associated abnormalities in white cells and platelets. Normocytic anemias with elevated reticulocyte counts include antibody- or drug-induced destruction, membrane or cytoskeletal abnormalities such as hereditary spherocytosis, enzyme deficiencies including glucose-6-phosphate dehydrogenase (G6PD), hemoglobinopathies (sickle cell) and unstable hemoglobin, and microangiopathic causes including disseminated intravascular coagulation (DIC).

Tests

Tests Used to Evaluate for Abnormal Bleeding

1. History: Because there is a great deal of overlap in bleeding symptoms between healthy children and those with a bleeding disorder, the patient's history alone cannot be used to discriminate those deserving further laboratory testing and those who do not. However, certain symptoms will increase the

Hematologic Considerations in Pediatric Surgery, Table 3 Red cell disorders seen in children

Microcytic anemia
Iron deficiency
Thalassemia
Chronic disease
Refractory anemia (sideroblastic)
Macrocytic anemia
B12 deficiency
Folate deficiency
Myelodysplasia
Normocytic anemia with elevated reticulocyte count
Blood loss
Sickle cell disease
Hemoglobinopathies
Spherocytosis/cytoskeletal deficiency
G6PD
Red cell enzyme deficiencies
DIC/microangiopathic anemia
Autoimmune hemolytic anemia
Evans syndrome
Autoimmune lymphoproliferative syndrome
Neonatal alloimmune anemia
Drugs/toxins
Normocytic anemia with normal or low reticulocyte count
Infectious agents
Drugs/toxins
Transient erythrocytopenia of childhood
Diamond-blackfan anemia
Fanconi's anemia
Leukemia/cancer
Myelofibrosis
Aplastic anemia
Renal disease

likelihood of the patient having a bleeding disorder. The following symptoms are suggestive of a child with a bleeding disorder:

(a) Any abnormal bleeding requiring medical attention or a red cell transfusion.

(b) Any surgical procedure in the past with abnormal bleeding, especially if a red cell transfusion was required.

(c) Bruising: Spontaneous bruises greater than 1 cm in diameter, palpable bruises, or multiple bruises on multiple body sites at the same time.

(d) Epistaxis: Epistaxis requiring cauterization, packing, or a red cell transfusion; epistaxis

lasting greater than 10 min, or greater than 10 episodes in a year.

(e) Minor Cuts: Any minor cut lasting more than 10 min or requiring medical attention.

(f) Gum Bleeding: Episodes lasting more than 10 min or requiring medical attention.

(g) Tooth Extractions: Prolonged bleeding following a tooth extraction.

(h) Menorrhagia: Bleeding that necessitates changing pads or tampons more than once every 2 h, bleeding lasting more than 1 week, or the passage of clots greater than 2 cm in diameter.

(i) Intracranial Hemorrhage: Any episode of spontaneous intracranial hemorrhage.

(j) Hemarthrosis/Myohematoma: Any nontraumatic hemarthrosis or myohematomas.

(k) Umbilical Cord: any abnormal umbilical cord bleeding.

(l) Circumcision: Any abnormal bleeding following a circumcision.

(m) Family History: A family history of a known bleeding disorder, or a family member with recurrent abnormal bleeding.

(n) Although not used to diagnose a congenital bleeding disorder, the patient's medication intake is an essential part of the evaluation of the patient prior to considering an invasive procedure. Several medications, most notably NSAIDS, can interfere with coagulation and platelet function.

If the child meets all of the following criteria, the probability of this child having a bleeding disorder is very small, and no further evaluation is required.

(a) More than one invasive medical procedure without abnormal bleeding

(b) Epistaxis: None or trivial

(c) Bruising: None or trivial

(d) Gum Bleeding: None or trivial

(e) Menorrhagia: Changing pads or tampons every 6 h or less frequently, periods never lasting greater than 1 week

(f) Intracranial Hemorrhage: Never

(g) Hemarthrosis/Myohematoma: Never

(h) No abnormal bleeding following circumcision or abnormal bleeding from umbilical cord separation

(i) No family history of a bleeding disorder

2. Laboratory Tests: There are no laboratory tests or group of tests which can accurately predict abnormal bleeding during invasive medical procedures. There are also no laboratory tests which can accurately screen for the mucocutaneous bleeding disorders, that is, Von Willebrand disease or platelet disorders. Patients identified by historic criteria to have a high pretest probability of a bleeding or other hematological disorder deserve laboratory testing. The following tests can be used to diagnose children with a bleeding disorder:

(a) Complete Blood Count (CBC): The CBC is used to identify children with white cell, red cell, or quantitative platelet disorders. A normal platelet count does not rule out a qualitative platelet disorder. The presence of anemia may be used to provide a more objective measure of the amount of bleeding the patient may be having. It can also be used to guide red cell replacement if the bleeding is severe.

(b) Prothrombin Time and activated Partial Thromboplastin Time (PT and aPTT): The PT and aPTT are used to screen for coagulation factor deficiencies. The PT screens for extrinsic pathway factor deficiencies, while the aPTT is used to screen for intrinsic pathway factor deficiencies. The predictive power for the PT and aPTT in predicting surgical bleeding is very poor (<10%). The PT and aPTT should only be used to screen for patients identified by history to have a high pretest probability of a bleeding disorder. Some of the rare coagulation factor deficiencies do not present with an abnormal PT or aPTT and specific testing for these disorders will be required.

(c) Bleeding Time: The bleeding time has never been shown to be predictive of surgical bleeding or a bleeding disorder. It is also a technically difficult test to perform and can leave scars. For this reason, the bleeding time is no longer recommended as part of a routine evaluation for a bleeding disorder.

(d) PFA-100: This test was initially designed to be a replacement test for the bleeding time, and a screening test for mucocutaneous bleeding disorders. Initial investigations suggested the PFA-100 was a highly sensitive screening test for Von Willebrand disease. However, more recent analysis has shown a poor sensitivity and predictive power for patients presenting to hemostasis clinics with an unknown diagnosis. The PFA-100 is highly sensitive to recent NSAID intake. Because a positive PFA-100 is not diagnostic of Von Willebrand disease or a platelet disorder, and a negative test does not rule it out, the utility of the PFA-100 in the evaluation of a child with a potential bleeding disorder remains to be clarified.

(e) Von Willebrand testing: Testing for Von Willebrand disease includes testing for quantitative deficiencies by measuring the Von Willebrand antigen. Testing for qualitative deficiencies includes assays for the various functions of Von Willebrand factor including a factor VIII assay to test for abnormal factor VIII binding, the ristocetin cofactor or Von Willebrand assay to screen for abnormal platelet binding, and Von Willebrand collagen-binding assay to test for abnormal collagen binding. Because Von Willebrand factor is an acute phase reactant, Von Willebrand levels vary from day to day. Repeated testing of Von Willebrand levels may be required to diagnose patients with "low Von Willebrand levels." The history and pretest probability should drive the need for repeated Von Willebrand testing. Patients with positive testing for Von Willebrand disease may need analysis of their Von Willebrand multimers, factor VIII-Von Willebrand binding assays, or platelet aggregometry to clarify the exact subtype of Von Willebrand disease.

(f) Platelet Aggregometry: Platelet aggregometry measures the transmission of light following the administration of various platelet agonists to platelet rich plasma. It is a cumbersome, technically challenging test, and typically only performed in specialty hematology laboratories. Large volumes of blood are frequently required, and the need for age-matched controls makes platelet aggregometry impractical for infants and small children. The CBC can be used to identify patients with quantitative platelet disorders, and a careful review of the smear may identify patients with storage pool deficiencies. The PFA-100 can also be used as a screen for qualitative platelet disorder, but suffers from the same low sensitivity and specificity as it does for Von Willebrand disease. Platelet aggregometry remains the mainstay for diagnosing qualitative platelet disorders. Flow cytometry is sometimes used to identify certain receptor deficiencies, and electron microscopy can be used to identify storage pool deficiencies.

(g) Specific Coagulation Factor Levels: Patients identified by history with a high probability of a bleeding disorder and an abnormal PT or aPTT or both have a high likelihood of a coagulation factor deficiency. The presence of a lupus anticoagulant can also give an elevated aPTT, but a lupus anticoagulant typically does not cause abnormal bleeding. Some rare factor deficiencies, such as factor XIII, alpha 2 anti-plasmin, and tissue plasminogen activator inhibitor deficiency, cannot be screened for by the PT and aPTT. A clinical history consistent with these disorders along with a normal PT and aPTT will drive the necessity of testing for these disorders.

Because coagulation factor testing is expensive, the history and results of the PT and aPTT should guide the order of specific coagulation factor testing. Physicians with an expertise in the coagulation pathways should be sought out to guide specific coagulation factor testing.

Tests Used to Evaluate for Abnormal Blood Clotting

Children with a family history of a heritable thrombophilic state or children who have suffered a thromboembolic event may be considered for thrombophilia testing. Because the results of the thrombophilia testing may not ultimately alter the management of the child, it is unclear which children should or should not undergo thrombophilia testing.

There are no general screening tests available for a thrombophilic state, so when there is a suspicion of a thrombophilic state in a child, direct testing must be performed. Testing for heritable thrombophilic states includes measuring protein C and antithrombin III activity levels. Protein S activity levels are fraught with assay difficulties, and many experts recommend testing for protein S deficiency by measuring free and total protein S levels. Testing for Factor V Leiden and Prothrombin gene mutations are obtained by genetic assays. An activated protein C resistance (APCR) tests can be used to screen for Factor V Leiden mutations.

The most common acquired thrombophilic state in children is the antiphospholipid syndrome (APS). The etiology of this disorder remains to be clarified, but involves the generation of autoantibodies that interact with the hemostatic system leading to a high risk of thrombotic events. APS is diagnosed by the presence of a clinical event (thrombosis, pregnancy loss) and antiphospholipid antibodies. One of the more common antibodies seen in APS is a lupus anticoagulant. Although lupus anticoagulants frequently cause an elevation in the aPTT, they typically do not cause bleeding. Lupus anticoagulants are commonly seen in children who do not have APS. They can be seen following viral or streptococcal infections, are transient, and not clinically relevant. Other antibodies seen in APS include cardiolipin antibodies and beta 2 glycoprotein 1 antibodies.

Elevations in homocysteine, various coagulation factors, especially factor VIII, and lipoprotein (a) are associated with thrombophilic states in children, and assays for these substances can be considered when evaluating for a thrombophilic state in a child.

Tests Used for White Blood Cell Disorders

The principal diagnostic test used when evaluating for white cell disorder is the CBC. The total white cell number, as well as the differential count of the various types of white cells can provide invaluable information about the etiology of the white cell disorder. A careful review of the peripheral blood smear also provides essential diagnostic information.

When bone marrow disease is suspected, a bone marrow aspirate and/or biopsy may be required. The resulting specimen can be sent for total white cell and differential counts. The morphology of the cells should also be evaluated. Other potentially useful testing of marrow or peripheral blood specimens includes flow cytometry, cytogenetic, and other specific genetic testing.

Tests Used for Red Blood Cell Disorders

As with most hematologic disorders, the CBC is an essential test for evaluating children with red cell disorders. The CBC can not only determine the presence of an anemia, but the red cell indices are used to determine if the anemia is microcytic, normocytic, or macrocytic. A review of the peripheral blood smear is used to determine the red cell morphology, which can help direct additional testing. The reticulocyte count and haptoglobin can aid in determining if the anemia is due to abnormal production, increased destruction, or blood loss.

1. Microcytic Anemia: The most common cause for microcytic anemias in children is iron deficiency. Oftentimes, the CBC and history are sufficient to make this diagnosis. Serum iron, transferrin, and ferritin levels can also aid in the diagnosis of iron deficiency. The red cell morphology and hemoglobin electrophoresis are used to diagnose thalasemia and thalasemia traits. Occasionally, a marrow aspirate is needed to evaluate bone marrow iron stores, as well as determine the presence of a sideroblastic anemia.

2. Macrocytic anemia: B12 and Folate levels should be determined in children with a macrocytic anemia. Myelodysplastic syndromes may also present with a macrocytic anemia, and a review of bone marrow aspirate may be necessary for the diagnosis.

3. Normocytic Anemia with elevated reticulocyte count: In addition to a review of the peripheral smear, tests used to diagnose these anemias include direct and indirect coombs test, osmotic fragility, G6PD and other red cell enzyme tests, and hemoglobin electrophoresis.

4. Normocytic anemia with a normal or reduced reticulocyte count: In addition to a good medical history to determine the presence of bleeding, drug, toxin, and infectious exposures, testing for these anemias includes a review of the marrow aspirate and biopsy as well as cytogenetic and specific genetic testing.

Treatment

White Blood Cell Disorders

Patients who are neutropenic are at a particularly high risk of infections. Therapy aimed at the underlying disorder is the ultimate method of treating the neutropenia. A variety of chemotherapeutic agents, steroids, immunoglobulin, and colony stimulating factors have been used. However, on occasion, invasive procedures must be carried out in immunocompromised patients. Precautions to reduce the risk of infectious complications, including appropriate antibiotic use are required.

Red Blood Cell Disorders

Most anemias can be corrected acutely with red cell transfusions. Ultimately, therapy aimed at treating the underlying disorder will be most effective. The degree of anemia and anticipated bleeding risk will guide the need for and amount of red cell replacement. Steroids and other immunosuppressant are used to treat the disorders caused by an altered immune system. Iron, B12, and folate are used to treat nutritional deficiencies. Children with sickle cell anemia, thalasemia, red call aplasia, and bone marrow failure syndromes are oftentimes on chronic transfusion regimens.

Platelet Disorders

A platelet count below 50,000 per microliter is generally thought to place the patient at an increased risk for bleeding during invasive procedures, although this guideline is not evidence based. Quantitative platelet disorders due to insufficient platelet production can be corrected by a platelet transfusion. Platelet disorders due to platelet destruction, such as ITP, may show a transient rise in platelet count following a platelet transfusion, but this rise is typically not sustained. Additional therapies, such as steroids or intravenous immunoglobulins, may also be necessary.

Patients with qualitative platelet disorders may also benefit from a platelet transfusion for invasive procedures. DDAVP has also been recommended, but evidence demonstrating the benefit of DDAVP in treating patients with qualitative platelet disorders is lacking. Several case reports and small series have demonstrated the efficacy of recombinant factor VIIa (rFVIIa) in treating some qualitative platelet disorders. rFVIIa has been approved in some countries for treating Glanzmann's Thrombasthenia.

Platelets for transfusion can be derived from random donor units or pheresis units. Patients expected to require repeated platelet transfusions may benefit from pheresis units as this will reduce the risk of alloimmunization to platelets. Adjuvant therapies may also be used to achieve hemostasis in patients with platelet disorders.

Von Willebrand Disease

The therapy used to treat Von Willebrand disease varies depending on the type and severity of Von Willebrand disease, and the expected bleeding risk of the invasive procedure. Most patients with "low Von Willebrand levels" and type 1 Von Willebrand disease respond to DDAVP, and some patients with type 2 disease will also respond. However, because response cannot be accurately predicted, response to DDAVP should be demonstrated prior to its use for invasive procedures. The half-life of the rise in Von Willebrand levels is around 12 h, so dosing more frequent than every 12–24 h is not recommended. Because DDAVP causes the release of Von Willebrand factor stored in endothelial cells, tachyphylaxis can occur after 2–3 days of DDAVP use. DDAVP can be given intravenously or subcutaneously at a dose of 0.3 mcg per kg per dose. A nasal spray is also available at a concentration of 150 mcg per spray. One spray is given for patients between 20 and 50 kg, while two sprays are given for patients greater than 50 kg. A DDAVP spray with a lower concentration of DDAVP is used for other disorders and should not be confused with the high dose spray used for treating Von Willebrand disease or mild hemophilia A. Side effects of DDAVP include facial flushing, warm flashes, headaches, nausea, and vomiting. Hyponatremia can also occur if there is an excessive amount of free water intake. Monitoring of serum sodium levels may be required following invasive procedures, especially if the patient is receiving intravenous fluids.

Patients who do not respond to DDAVP, or those undergoing procedures with a higher risk of bleeding, should receive Von Willebrand containing coagulation concentrates. These are plasma-derived coagulation concentrates that contain Von Willebrand factor and factor VIII. They can only be given intravenously. They have undergone viral inactivation processes so that the risk of transmitting infectious agents is extremely small. Recombinant Von Willebrand concentrates are currently under investigation. Von Willebrand concentrates are dosed to achieve normalization of Von Willebrand activity and to maintain a hemostatic level until wound healing has occurred. It should be kept in mind that, during a tonsillectomy, the greatest risk for bleeding is during the perioperative period and during clot retraction approximately 10 days post operation. Additional dosing of DDAVP or Von Willebrand concentrates may be necessary at the time of clot retraction.

Coagulation Factor Deficiencies

Specific coagulation factor concentrates are available as replacement for Fibrinogen, factor VII, factor VIII, factor IX, factor XI, and factor XIII deficiency. However, not all concentrates are available and approved for use in all countries. Recombinant concentrates are

available for factor VII, factor VIII, and factor IX. Recombinant concentrates for other deficiencies are under investigation. Both plasma-derived and recombinant factor concentrates have undergone viral inactivation procedures to nearly eliminate the risk of transmission of infectious agents. Coagulation concentrates can only be given intravenously. Although there are not specific concentrates available for factor II and factor X deficiencies, prothrombin complex concentrates or activated prothrombin complex concentrates which contain factor II, VII, IX, and X can be used for these disorders. Fresh frozen plasma (FFP) can be used for factor V deficiency or for other deficiencies in which specific concentrates are not approved or available.

The dosing of concentrates varies with the concentrate used and the type of deficiency which needs to be corrected. In general, concentrates should be dosed to achieve normalization of factor levels for the perioperative period, and to maintain hemostasis until wound healing has occurred. A unit of factor activity is defined as the amount of activity present in 1 ml of normal plasma. For most concentrates, each unit per kilogram will increase the factors activity by 1%. Factor VIII is one exception to this rule in which each unit per kg will raise the level by 2%. If FFP is used, each ml per kg will only raise most factor levels by 1%. For this reason, large volumes of FFP may be required to achieve hemostasis.

Patients with mild hemophilia A may also respond to DDAVP. If the mild hemophilia patient's factor VIII level doubles or triples following DDAVP, they may achieve factor VIII levels sufficient for hemostasis. Tachyphylaxis to DDAVP will also occur in patients with mild hemophilia A.

Transfusion of Blood Products

Red Blood Cells: Red cells can be replaced from packed red cell transfusions or whole blood. Each 10 ml per kg of packed reed cells will raise the patient's hemoglobin by 3 g/dl. The decision on when to transfuse red cells is guided more by the patient's symptoms and need for improved oxygen-carrying capacity than an absolute level of hemoglobin. Packed cells are often given with leukodepletion filters to reduce the risk of CMV transmission and white cell HLA sensitization. Packed red cells can also be irradiated to reduce the risk of transfusion-associated graft versus host disease in immunocompromised patients. Whole blood is difficult to maintain for transfusion and generally reserved for massive blood loss.

Platelets: Platelets can be transfused from random donor platelets, or single donor pheresed units. Unless a qualitative platelet dysfunction is present, most surgeries can be safely performed if the platelet count is greater than 50,000 per microliter. Transfusion of a random donor unit of platelets per 10 kg should raise the platelet count by 50,000. Similar levels can be obtained by transfusing 1 pheresis unit per meter squared.

Fresh Frozen Plasma: although plasma contains all of the coagulation factors, specific coagulation factor concentrates are the most efficient method of replacing deficient coagulation factors. Fresh frozen plasma should be reserved for replacing factor deficiencies in which specific coagulation factor concentrates are not available. Although 10 ml per kg is a frequent recommended dose for fresh frozen plasma, this may not be sufficient to raise most coagulation factors to hemostatic levels. Higher doses may be required.

Patients with thrombophilia: Patients on anticoagulation will need to have their anticoagulation discontinued prior to undergoing invasive procedures. The anticoagulation will need to be discontinued for a sufficient period of time to allow for the resumption of normal hemostasis. Patients receiving Coumadin may require several days for this to occur. Vitamin K can be given to hasten this process. Emergent reversal of Coumadin can be achieved with vitamin K, rFVIIa, activated prothrombin complex concentrates, or FFP, although the optimal regimen and dosing have not been clearly established. Intravenous unfractionated heparin has a relatively short half-life and as a general rule only needs to be discontinued a few hours before surgery. Protamine can be used to acutely reverse unfractionated heparin. Patients receiving fractionated low molecular weight heparin should discontinue the medication 24 h prior to the procedure. Patients who cannot be off their anticoagulant, typically Coumadin, for prolonged periods of time may require bridging therapy. After discontinuing Coumadin, the patient begins either unfractionated or fractionated heparin until surgery occurs. The heparin is then resumed once hemostasis is achieved post operation and continues until a therapeutic Coumadin level is achieved.

Patients with thrombophilic states who are not receiving therapeutic anticoagulation do not require prophylactic anticoagulation unless the surgical procedure poses a significant risk of thrombosis. In these situations, prophylactic anticoagulation may be indicated, although evidence supporting this process is currently lacking.

Thrombolysis: Children with life or organ threatening thrombosis may benefit from thrombolysis. Because of the significant risk of bleeding with thrombolysis, clinicians with expertise in this area should be sought.

Adjuvant Therapy: Epsilon amino caprioc acid (AMICAR) and tranexamic acid are plasmin inhibiting agents which have been shown to stabilize clots following surgical procedures to mucosal surfaces. These agents are recommended as adjuvant therapy for all bleeding disorders. Topical hemostatic agents, such as fibrin glue or topical thrombin, can also be used successfully to achieve hemostasis in patients with bleeding disorders.

References

Bolton-Maggs P, Perry D, Chalmers E et al (2004) The rare coagulation disorders-review with guidelines for management from the United Kingdom Haemophilia Centre Doctor's Organisation. Haemophilia 10:593–628

Buchanan G (2005) Thrombocytopenia during childhood: what the pediatrician should know. Pediatr Rev 26:401–409

Fleisher T (2006) Back to basics: primary immune deficiencies: window into the immune system. Pediatr Rev 27:363–372

Hayward C, Rao A, Carraneo M (2006) Congenital platelet disorders: overview of their mechanisms, diagnostic evaluation and treatment. Haemophilia 12(Suppl 3):128–136

Hutter J (2010) Childhood leukemia. Pediatr Rev 31:234–241

Nichols W, Hultin M, James A et al (2008) von Willebrand Disease (VWD): evidence-based diagnosis and management guidelines, The National Heart, Lung and Blood Institute (NHLBI) Expert Panel report (USA). Haemophilia 14:171–232

Roth M, Manwani D (2011) Thrombotic disorders. Pediatr Rev 32:41–43

Segal G, Hirsh M, Feig S (2002a) Managing anemia in pediatric office practice: part 1. Pediatr Rev 23:75–84

Segal G, Hirsh M, Feig S (2002b) Managing anemia in pediatric office practice: part 2. Pediatr Rev 23:111–122

Sharathkumar A, Pipe S (2008) Bleeding disorders. Pediatr Rev 29:121–130

Tamary H, Alter B (2007) Current diagnosis of inherited bone marrow failure syndromes. Pediatr Hematol Oncol 24:87–99

Hemicranial Atrophy

▶ Parry-Romberg Syndrome

Hemifacial Atrophy

▶ Parry-Romberg Syndrome

Hemifacial Microsomia

Robert J. Tibesar
Pediatric Otolaryngology-Facial Plastic Surgery,
Pediatric ENT Associates, Children's Hospitals and
Clinics of Minnesota and University of Minnesota,
South Minneapolis, MN, USA

Synonyms

Auriculo-branchiogenic dysplasia; Facioauriculo-vertebral dysplasia; Facioauriculovertebral malformation complex; First and second branchial arch syndrome; First arch syndrome; Goldenhar syndrome; Goldenhar-gorlin syndrome; HFM; Lateral facial dysplasia; OAV; Oculoauriculovertebral spectrum or dysplasia; Otomandibular dysostosis; Unilateral craniofacial microsomia; Unilateral intrauterine facial necrosis; Unilateral mandibulofacial dysostosis

Definitions

According to Gorlin, hemifacial microsomia was originally defined as a disorder affecting primarily the ear, oral, and mandibular development (Gorlin et al. 2001). Manifestations of the disease range from mild to severe, and involvement is typically limited to one side in most cases. Bilateral involvement is also known to occur with more severe expression typically present on one side. Goldenhar syndrome is considered a variant of hemifacial microsomia characterized by the additional presence of vertebral anomalies and epibulbar dermoids. Hemifacial microsomia is now understood to be extremely complex and heterogeneous. Gorlin prefers the term oculoauriculovertebral spectrum (OAV) for the spectrum of anomalies, ranging from hemifacial microsomia, which denotes unilateral microtia or ear anomalies, mandibular hypoplasia, and macrostomia (Gorlin et al. 2001). As mentioned, this is distinguished from Goldenhar

syndrome, which also includes epibulbar dermoids and vertebral anomalies.

There are no universally accepted precise diagnostic criteria. Isolated microtia or auricular or preauricular skin tags or other abnormalities may represent the mildest manifestation. Some authors hold that unilateral microtia or ear abnormality is a mandatory feature (Tewfik and Der Kaloustian 1997). Suggested minimal diagnostic criteria for hemifacial microsomia are: (1) ipsilateral mandibular and ear defects or (2) asymmetric mandibular or ear defects in association with either (a) two or more indirectly associated anomalies or (b) a positive family history of hemifacial microsomia (Gorlin et al. 2001).

Of historical interest, this syndrome was first mentioned in the teratological tables written about the seventh century BC by the Chaldeans of Mesopotamia. More recently in 1654, Bartholinus reported on a child with the absence of an auditory orifice. Thompson in 1845 was credited as being the first to emphasize the etiologic relationship between the development of the first and second branchial arches with the malformations of the face (Stricker 1990).

Etiology and Epidemiology

Hemifacial microsomia occurs sporadically in most cases. It is the second most common facial birth defect after cleft lip and palate, with an incidence in the range of 1 in 3,500–4,500 live births. It can occur on one side of the face or both; approximately one third of cases demonstrate bilateral involvement, and the right side is involved in 60% of cases. Those with Goldenhar syndrome constitute only about 10% of cases. The male-to-female ratio is 3:2 (Tewfik and Der Kaloustian 1997). Inheritance patterns do not fit neatly into autosomal dominant or autosomal recessive categories; although, some families, probably about 1–2% of cases, clearly manifest an autosomal dominant form with variable penetrance. Wide variability of expression is characteristic of hemifacial microsomia (Vendramini-Pittoli and Kokitsu-Nakata 2009).

Theories of etiology for hemifacial microsomia include vascular disruption with expanding hematoma formation in utero, disturbance in branchial arches, and disturbance in neural crest cell migration that impede the development of adjacent medial or frontal nasal processes. The origin is approximately during

30–45 days of gestation. Another theory deals with the disturbance in chondrogenesis. A common pathway for CHARGE association (coloboma, heart disease, choanal atresia, retarded growth and retarded development and/or CNS anomalies, genital hypoplasia, and ear anomalies and/or deafness) and OAV spectrum has also been suggested (Hartsfield 2007). Infants exposed to thalidomide, primidone, and retinoic acid have been born with first and second branchial arch anomalies as well as facial palsy. Additionally the OAV phenotype has been noted in infants with diabetic embryopathy. According to Gorlin, several chromosomal anomalies have been associated with hemifacial microsomia (Gorlin et al. 2001).

Animal models demonstrate that vascular disruption and hematoma formation affect the developing structures of the jaw and the ear regions in utero. In a mouse model, focal hematomas arising from disruption of the stapedial artery were observed; however, a causative association between the bleeding and the subsequent deformities has not been made. Similarly, intermittent occlusion of the internal carotid artery system of fetal sheep late in gestation has been shown to result in deformities similar in appearance to hemifacial microsomia; therefore, the vascular disruption hypothesis cannot be excluded (McCarthy and Grayson 2006). In summary, the exact etiology of hemifacial microsomia is currently unknown. It likely involves numerous factors ranging from genetic abnormalities to external teratogens and environmental insults as well as vascular events.

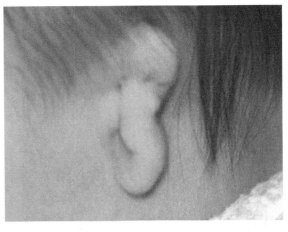

Hemifacial Microsomia, Fig. 1 Male infant with left-sided hemifacial microsomia and Grade III microtia

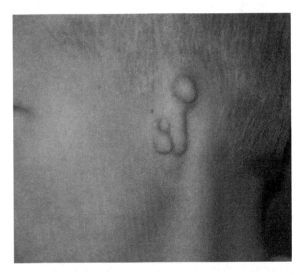

Hemifacial Microsomia, Fig. 2 Male of age 6 years with left-sided hemifacial microsomia and more severe Grade III microtia

Clinical Presentation

Mandible: There are numerous craniofacial physical abnormalities present in hemifacial microsomia. Examples are depicted in Figs. 1–6. The most notable physical manifestation is hypoplasia or aplasia of the mandibular ramus and condyle on the affected side. Mandibular malformations are less severe near the body and symphysis. The gonial angle is obtuse and the antigonial notch is accentuated (Figueroa and Pruzansky 1982). There are numerous dental and occlusal abnormalities that ensue from the mandibular deformity (Monahan et al. 2001).

Craniofacial: The maxillary, temporal, and zygoma bones on the affected side may also be hypoplastic and flattened. Hypoplasia of the maxilla on the affected

side is clearly demonstrated by the obliquity of the occlusal plane. This is demonstrated in Fig. 5. The zygomatic process of the temporal bone may be underdeveloped or absent causing an interrupted zygomatic arch and flattening of the malar eminence. A depression and recession of the inferior lateral angle of the orbit indicates involvement of the malar eminence with orbital dystopia observed. The floor of the maxillary sinus and the nasal base on the affected side is elevated (Vargervik 2002). In some patients, the skull base on the affected side is inclined in a more superior plane. The styloid process is frequently smaller and shorter on the affected side.

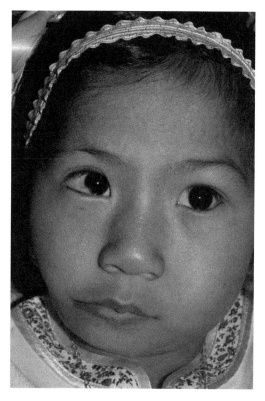 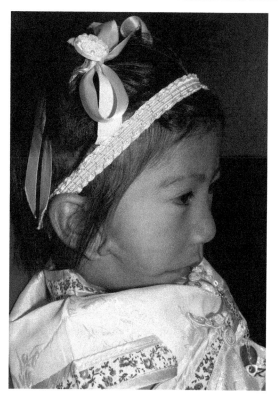

Hemifacial Microsomia, Fig. 3 Anterior view of a 3-year-old female with right-sided hemifacial microsomia with right epibulbar dermoid, right macrostomia, right mandibular ramus and condyle hypoplasia, and right facial soft tissue deficiency

Hemifacial Microsomia, Fig. 4 Right profile view of 3-year-old female with right-sided hemifacial microsomia with right epibulbar dermoid, right macrostomia, right mandibular ramus and condyle hypoplasia, right preauricular skin tag, right low set ear, and right facial soft tissue deficiency

Muscles of Mastication: The masticatory muscles (the temporalis, masseter, and pterygoids) may be differentially hypoplastic on the affected side. A fused mass of muscles may be observed on CT scans containing elements of each of these individual muscles. Underdevelopment of the lateral pterygoid muscle causes a limitation of mandibular opening and protrusion. Furthermore when the patient opens the mouth, the chin deviates toward the affected side. This causes the condyle on the opposite side to be displaced abnormally downward and laterally almost to the point of dislocating the condyle out of the temporomandibular joint (Patel and Sykes 2010). Meanwhile no discernible condylar movement is detected on the affected side. Additionally in many cases the coronoid process on the affected side is absent, and there is a reduction in size of the temporalis muscle. The associated masseter and medial pterygoid muscles are also deficient (Cousley and Calvert 1997).

Oral: There may be agenesis of the ipsilateral parotid gland. Often there is decreased palatal width on the

affected side. Palate and tongue musculature may be hypoplastic. Unilateral or bilateral cleft lip and/or cleft palate occur in approximately 7–10% of patients. Canting of the occlusal plane and malocclusion are very common. Aplasia of the ipsilateral levator veli palatini muscle resulting in concomitant velopharyngeal insufficiency occurs in a minority of patients. Macrostomia, or lateral facial cleft, ranging from a small muscular diastasis at the oral commissure to full thickness defects of the cheek is present in about 16% of cases as well.

Skin and Soft Tissue: The deficiency of soft tissues on the affected side in hemifacial microsomia is evidenced from a reduced distance between the mastoid process and the oral commissure or lateral canthus of the eye. The skin and subcutaneous tissue shows atrophy particularly in the parotid region.

Otologic: Auricular anomalies are present in approximately 65% of cases. This can range from mild microtia or preauricular skin tag to complete anotia. The auricle is typically displaced anteriorly

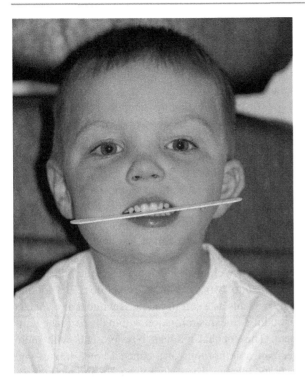

Hemifacial Microsomia, Fig. 5 Preoperative photo of a 4-year-old male with hemifacial microsomia and occlusal cant from left-sided mandibular hypoplasia

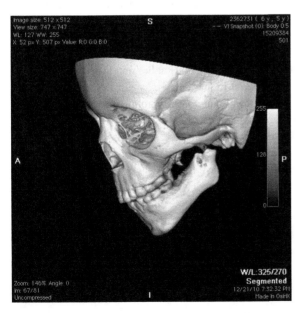

Hemifacial Microsomia, Fig. 6 Preoperative three-dimensional computed tomography scan depicting left-sided mandibular hypoplasia

and inferiorly. Preauricular tags of skin and cartilage are extremely common, and the supernumerary ear tags may occur anywhere from tragus to the oral commissure. They are more commonly seen in patients with macrostomia and aplasia of the parotid gland. External auditory canal stenosis or atresia also marks the spectrum. At times the auricle may be small but otherwise anatomically normal. Isolated microtia can be considered a microform presentation of hemifacial microsomia. The mastoid air cells typically lack pneumatization. Any part of the temporal bone other than the petrous portion may be affected. Conductive hearing loss is frequently present. There may be hypoplasia or middle ear ossicular anomalies with an aberrant course of the facial nerve. There is a correlation between the presence of external auditory canal stenosis and the severity of microtia or the severity of mandibular malformations. A similar relationship has been observed between the presence of ossicular malformations and the severity of microtia or the severity of mandibular anomalies. Congenital sensorineural hearing loss may be due to malformation of the inner ear, hypoplasia of the cochlear nerve, and brainstem auditory nuclei (Gordon and Hurwitz 2002).

Ocular: Narrowed palpebral fissure occurs in about 10% of cases. Epibulbar dermoid tumors are found in approximately 35% of cases. This is a solid yellowish or pinkish-white ovoid mass occurring most commonly in the inferotemporal quadrant of the globe at the limbus. However, they can occur at any location on the globe or orbit and can be dermoid or lipodermoid in histology. The surface of the dermoid tumor is usually smooth and may have fine hairs present. Encroachment of the dermoid tumor onto the pupillary axis can impair vision. Patients with epibulbar dermoids have a higher frequency of eyelid or extraocular and lacrimal drainage abnormalities. Unilateral coloboma is present in approximately 20% of patients. Blepharoptosis, microphthalmia, and retinal abnormalities have also been documented in hemifacial microsomia. Visual acuity is usually reduced.

Central Nervous System: Impairment of cranial nerve function is variably present. Facial nerve paralysis occurs in about 10–20% and this is the most common cranial nerve anomaly. It is most likely secondary to agenesis of the facial nerve in the temporal bone or hypoplasia of the intracranial portion of the facial nerve and facial nucleus in the brain stem. Intracranial neurologic abnormalities may include hypoplasia of the cerebrum, cerebellum, brain stem, and corpus callosum.

Hydrocephalus or intracranial lipoma may also be present. Mental retardation occurs in about 5–15% of cases. Children with anophthalmia/microphthalmia and cleft lip/palate seem to be at an increased risk for cerebral malformation and mental retardation.

Skeletal Malformations: Cervical vertebral fusions may occur in as many as 60%. Hemivertebrae or hypoplastic vertebrae are other possibilities.

Others: Congenital heart defects have been reported in 5–58% of the patients. Additionally, a variety of renal abnormalities have been reported including absent kidney, double ureter, and hydronephrosis.

Diagnostic Studies

While there is no specific genetic test for hemifacial microsomia, a variety of diagnostic tests are helpful in the evaluation of a suspected case. Cephalometric X-rays are a useful and repeatable examination technique for measuring facial asymmetry and monitoring facial growth. Reconstruction of the craniofacial skeleton requires careful preoperative planning. Three-dimensional computed tomography (3-D CT) has become an irreplaceable diagnostic and evaluation tool for patients with hemifacial microsomia. It provides valuable information about the integrity of the mandible and mandibulo-maxillary interface. A medical model can be made from the scan which is a useful surgical adjunct. Temporal bone CT scan is helpful in evaluating the middle and inner ear anatomy. Other systemic tests and examinations include echocardiogram, renal ultrasound, screening spinal X-rays, and dilated ophthalmologic examination.

Classification

There are multiple classification systems that have been described for hemifacial microsomia. The most inclusive and flexible classification is OMENS. The acronym represents each of the five major manifestations of HFM: O is for orbital distortion, M is for mandibular hypoplasia, E is for ear anomaly, N is for nerve involvement, and S is for soft tissue deficiency (McCarthy and Grayson 2006; Gougoutas et al. 2007). The term OMENS-plus is used to include the expanded spectrum: cardiac, skeletal, pulmonary, renal, gastrointestinal, and limb anomalies.

Typing or grading of the mandibular deformity, as first proposed by Pruzansky (Pruzanski 1969; Figueroa and Pruzansky 1982) and later modified, is as follows:

Type I is a miniature mandible with identifiable anatomy.

Type II is a functioning temporomandibular joint (TMJ) but with an abnormal shape and glenoid fossa.

Type II is subcategorized. Type IIA includes the glenoid fossa in an acceptable functional position (in reference to the opposite TMJ). In type IIB, the TMJ is abnormally placed and cannot be incorporated in the surgical construction.

Type III indicates an absent ramus and nonexistent glenoid fossa.

For better clinical understanding, microtia can be divided into two descriptive categories. The lobular type presents as a soft tissue mass without any concha or auditory meatus formation within the cartilage remnant. The conchal remnant type presents with more recognizable portions of a conchal bowl, tragus, and external meatus. The descriptive term auricular dystopia has been applied in cases associated with significant craniofacial microsomia.

Microtia can be classified as follows based on a gradient from less severe (Grade I) to total absence of the external ear (anotia):

Grade I: The pinna is malformed and is smaller than normal. Most of the characteristics of the pinna, such as the helix, triangular fossa, and scaphoid fossa, are present with relatively good definition.

Grade II: The pinna is smaller and less developed than in Grade I. The helix may not be fully developed. The triangular fossa, scaphoid fossa, and antihelix have much less definition.

Grade III: The pinna is essentially absent, except for a vertical sausage-shaped skin remnant. The superior aspect of this sausage-shaped skin remnant consists of underlying unorganized cartilage, and the inferior aspect of this remnant consists of a relatively well-formed lobule.

Grade IV/Anotia: Total absence of the pinna is observed.

Differential Diagnosis

The differential diagnosis for hemifacial microsomia includes temporomandibular joint ankylosis, Parry-Romberg syndrome, CHARGE syndrome, Townes-Brocks syndrome, Nager syndrome, branchio-oto-renal syndrome, hemifacial hypertrophy, and postradiation deformity. Treacher Collins syndrome or severe orbital-facial clefts can also be confused with bilateral hemifacial microsomia. Trauma or infection to the temporomandibular joint and condylar cartilage at a young age can also result in decreased mandibular growth with secondary effect on the growth of the surrounding craniofacial skeleton.

Treatment

The surgical reconstructive treatment of a patient with hemifacial microsomia is quite variable and dependent on the individual anatomic and functional deficiencies. Modern treatment protocols emphasize reconstruction of soft tissue deficiencies in addition to the skeletal framework (McCarthy and Grayson 2006). The timing of reconstruction has long been controversial. On the one hand, there are benefits to early reconstruction. For one, the child grows up with improved facial appearance and function. This has multiple benefits in oral-motor function, social interactions, and self-esteem and personality development (Kaban et al. 1986, 1988, 1998). Conversely, there are potential risks, in that performing osteotomies and large bone movements in the immature face can impede subsequent facial growth. Additionally revision surgery is often necessary to achieve proper occlusion in the adult. Early efforts at correction of the skeletal deficiency in hemifacial microsomia are focused on onlay techniques. Autogenous rib grafts, iliac crest bone grafts, or allografts of cartilage or bone have been used to augment the deficient craniofacial skeleton. These techniques, however, have limitations, in that they are unable to correct the malocclusion or the soft tissue contour deficiencies. A reasonable evaluation and management strategy as described below focuses on the needs of the patient during the progressive stages of development.

Evaluation of the newborn with hemifacial microsomia focuses on airway evaluation and feeding difficulties. An assessment of the mandibular position and glossoptosis alerts the clinician to potential airway difficulties. Some children with bilateral hemifacial microsomia and severe micrognathia have significant upper airway obstruction from glossoptosis. These children necessitate adjunctive airway maneuvers

such as prone positioning, nasopharyngeal airway insertion, consideration of tongue-lip adhesion, bilateral mandibular advancement with distraction osteogenesis, or even possibly tracheotomy. In more recent years, the need for tracheotomy has been lessened in some cases due to the ability to perform bilateral mandibular advancement with distraction osteogenesis (Singhal and Hill 2008). This technique, in which the mandible is slowly advanced after an initial osteotomy, relieves hypopharyngeal airway obstruction by bringing the tongue base forward.

However, if the child has severe micrognathia with the absence of a mandibular condyle, distraction osteogenesis is often unsuccessful in adequately advancing the mandible and tongue base. This is due to the fact that the distraction segment pushes the posterior mandible more posteriorly until it rides against the skull base. Often the surgeon is not able to achieve adequate mandibular advancement to open up the airway in these cases and tracheotomy is necessary until mandibular bony reconstruction has been performed. For these children, the author's practice is to perform neonatal tracheotomy and later, when the child is 3–5 years old, reconstruct the bilateral mandibular condyles with autogenous rib grafts. The surgeon can proceed after 6 months with bilateral mandibular distraction osteogenesis to advance the reconstructed mandible and tongue base and move toward tracheotomy decannulation.

These infants often have significant dysphagia and failure to thrive and often require gastrostomy tube placement for nutritional maintenance. The feeding difficulties are often exacerbated by the upper airway obstruction. If the upper airway obstruction is treated, the feeding difficulty invariably improves.

Closure of the lateral facial cleft with commissuroplasty is indicated in patients with macrostomia or a true lateral facial cleft. Reconstruction of the orbicularis oris muscle at the commissure is important to achieve oral competency in this procedure. This is usually performed at around 10–12 weeks of age. If children have ear tags or cartilaginous remnants in the cheek, removal can be scheduled electively anytime during the first year of life.

Around age 3–6 years, reconstruction of the hypoplastic mandibular ramus can be undertaken, traditionally with autogenous rib graft. It is wise to wait until this time for the growth and development of adequate stock of rib cartilage and bone for grafting.

The cartilage cap is used to recreate the temporomandibular joint, and the rib bone is used to lengthen the ramus. Through a parotid approach, the mandibular remnant and glenoid fossa are exposed in a subperiosteal plane. If necessary, a neo-glenoid fossa can be created by gently hollowing out the bone of the skull base with a drill. The cartilaginous end of the costochondral rib graft is placed into this neo-glenoid fossa, and the osseous portion is then rigidly fixated to the mandibular remnant. The key points of this procedure are highlighted in Figs. 7–10. Subsequent growth of the mandible is usually achieved. This growth is often unpredictable, and patients may need later corrective orthognathic surgery. The goal of surgery is to provide skeletal symmetry to the mandible, improve the occlusion, and set the stage for proper growth in the future. Figures 11 and 12 show the desired postoperative results.

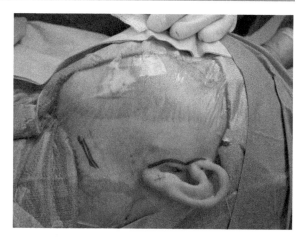

Hemifacial Microsomia, Fig. 7 Intraoperative photo showing the planned incisions for placement of rib bone and cartilage graft for reconstruction of left-sided hypoplastic mandibular ramus

Reconstruction of the mandibular ramus and condyle can alternatively be achieved with transport distraction osteogenesis of the small residual bone segment of the ramus to create a new condyle and temporomandibular joint. Maxillomandibular distraction osteogenesis has also been described in which complete mandibular osteotomy is performed and distraction device applied (McCarthy and Grayson 2006). The LeFort I corticotomy is then performed on the maxilla as an incomplete osteotomy. The teeth are then placed in maxillomandibular fixation. As the mandible device applies the distraction vector, the maxilla comes along with it to its new improved position while maintaining good occlusion.

More recently some surgeons have reconstructed the absent ramus and condyle with a microvascular free fibula flap (Santamaria et al. 2008). Advantages include robust blood supply ensuring more reliable graft survival, adequate availability of fibular bone stock, and predictable subsequent growth of the neo-ramus. Major disadvantages include the risk of flap loss and the bone-on-bone contact of the fibula flap with the glenoid fossa, which can sometimes lead to ankylosis.

During the childhood years, the patient undergoes the necessary orthodontic adjustments to optimize occlusion. It is during this time that auricular reconstruction is undertaken. Options for auricular reconstruction include bone-anchored prosthesis versus autogenous rib graft creation of an auricle. (Detailed discussion of auricular reconstruction is presented in

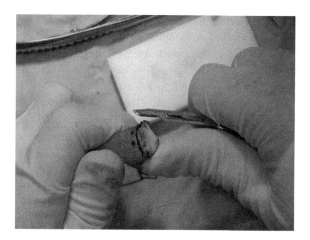

Hemifacial Microsomia, Fig. 8 Intraoperative photo demonstrating the custom carving of the rib cartilage with the scalpel so it will contour properly with the ipsilateral glenoid fossa

another chapter in this series.) It is also during the childhood and adolescent years that soft tissue augmentation can be considered. Soft tissue restoration can be achieved by transfer of vascularized free tissue, de-epithelialized skin, subcutaneous tissue, and fat. Muscle can also be incorporated; however, it tends to atrophy over time. Occasionally, a skin island is used to release and augment the skin deficiency. Dermis can also be used, but this frequently loses considerable volume over time. Lipoaspirated fat injection can be employed because it is a relatively safe and easy procedure, with minimal complications. Because of its

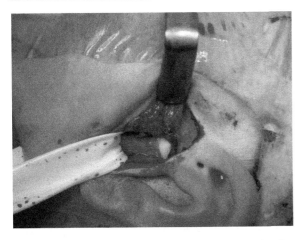

Hemifacial Microsomia, Fig. 9 Intraoperative photo showing the proper placement of the cartilage portion of the rib graft into the glenoid fossa with fascia interlayed to prevent ankylosis of the newly created temporomandibular joint

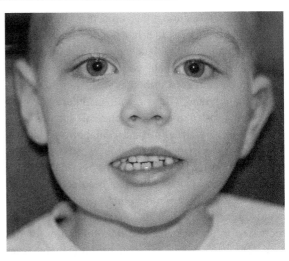

Hemifacial Microsomia, Fig. 11 Postoperative photo showing improvement in facial contour and symmetry after placement of rib graft

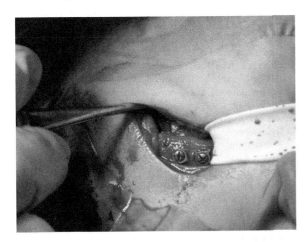

Hemifacial Microsomia, Fig. 10 Intraoperative photo showing the proper placement of the bony portion of the rib graft onto the existing hypoplastic mandible, with lag screws used for fixation to the ramus and angle of the mandible

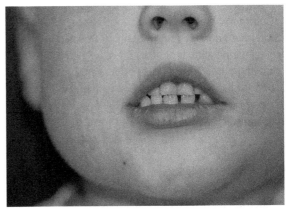

Hemifacial Microsomia, Fig. 12 Close-up postoperative photo showing the improvement in occlusion and alignment in the facial midline after placement of the rib graft

temporary nature due to fat resorption, most patients need to undergo multiple procedures. Microsurgical free tissue transfer techniques have become popular for soft tissue restoration of facial contour in hemifacial microsomia (Siebert and Longaker 1994). Free omentum has been used successfully for many instances of facial recontouring. It is highly pliable, flexible, and has excellent vascularity. The disadvantages, however, include intra-abdominal harvest and the difficulty of long-term flap fixation due to the lack of dermal or fascial attachments. Because of these

limitations with omentum, fasciocutaneous free flaps seem to have the best results with the ability to customize the contouring to fit the defect. Fasciocutaneous free flaps are readily available, can be contoured to various degrees of thickness, and hold their position well. Typically the superficial temporal vessels, the facial artery, or other branches of the external carotid artery system are of adequate size for microvascular anastomosis for facial recontouring.

When adolescence is reached (approximately an age of 15 years for girls and 17 years for boys), craniofacial growth and development are nearing completion. It is during this time that orthognathic surgery plays a major role. In a single surgical procedure, the craniofacial skeletal structure can be restored and optimal occlusion achieved. This is typically done by way of a combined orthodontic and surgical rehabilitation program. The surgical procedure involves a LeFort I osteotomy with bilateral sagittal split osteotomy of the mandible and genioplasty. This has been shown to be the therapeutic workhorse of the reconstruction of hemifacial microsomia. Distraction osteogenesis techniques have also been used successfully in the treatment of older children with hemifacial microsomia. The advantages include less morbidity, decreased infection rates, and the elimination of the need for intermaxillary fixation or autogenous bone graft harvesting.

Summary

In summary, hemifacial microsomia is an uncommon congenital anomaly that presents with various craniofacial manifestations. Following a systematic, developmental clinical approach, patients are best managed in a multidisciplinary team. Most patients will undergo various reconstructive procedures to achieve significant improvement in craniofacial form and function.

Cross-References

▶ Microtia and Atresia

References

Cousley RR, Calvert ML (1997) Current concepts in the understanding and management of hemifacial microsomia. Br J Plasti Surg 50(7):536–551
Figueroa AA, Pruzansky S (1982) The external ear, mandible and other components of hemifacial microsomia. J Maxillofac Surg 10(4):200–211
Gordon CB, Hurwitz DJ (2002) Principles and methods of management. In: Bluestone CD, Stool SE, Alper CM, Arjmand EM, Casselbrant ML, Dohar JE, Yellon RF (eds) Pediatric otolaryngology, vol 1, 4. Saunders, Philadelphia, pp 83–112
Gorlin RJ, Cohen MM, Hennekam RCM (2001) Syndromes of the head and neck, 4th edn. Oxford University Press, New York, pp 790–797
Gougoutas AJ, Singh DJ, Low DW, Bartlett SP (2007) Hemifacial microsomia: clinical features and pictographic representations of the OMENS classification system. Plast Reconstr Surg 120(7):112e–120e
Hartsfield JK (2007) Review of the etiologic heterogeneity of the oculo-auriculo-vertebral spectrum (Hemifacial Microsomia). Orthod Craniofac Res 10(3):121–128
Kaban LB, Moses MH, Mulliken JB (1986) Correction of hemifacial microsomia in the growing child: a follow-up study. Cleft Palate J 23(Suppl 1):50–52
Kaban LB, Moses MH, Mulliken JB (1988) Surgical correction of hemifacial microsomia in the growing child. Plast Reconstr Surg 82(1):9–19
Kaban LB, Padwa BL, Mulliken JB (1998) Surgical correction of mandibular hypoplasia in hemifacial microsomia: the case for treatment in early childhood. J Oral Maxillofac Surg 56(5):628–638
McCarthy JG, Grayson BH (2006) Reconstruction: craniofacial microsomia. In: Mathes SJ (ed) Plastic surgery, 2nd edn. Saunders Elsevier, Philadelphia, pp 521–554
Monahan R, Seder K, Patel P, Alder M, Grud S, O'Gara M (2001) Hemifacial microsomia. Etiology, diagnosis and treatment. J Am Dent Assoc 132(10):1402–1408
Patel KG, Sykes JM (2010) Craniofacial anomalies and deformities. In: Thomas J (ed) Advanced therapy in facial plastic and reconstructive surgery. People's Medical Publishing House, Shelton, pp 83–103
Pruzanski S (1969) Not all dwarfed mandibles are alike. Birth defects 1:1203
Santamaría E, Morales C, Taylor JA, Hay A, Ortiz-Monasterio F (2008) Mandibular microsurgical reconstruction in patients with hemifacial microsomia. Plast Reconstr Surg 122(6):1839–1849
Siebert JW, Longaker MT (1994) Microsurgical correction of facial asymmetry in hemifacial microsomia. Oper Tech Plast Reconstr Surg 1:94
Singhal VK, Hill ME (2008) Craniofacial microsomia and craniofacial distraction. In: Bentz ML, Bauer BS, Zuker RM (eds) Principles and practice of pediatric plastic surgery, vol 1. Quality Medical, St Louis, pp 755–797
Stricker M (1990) Classification of craniofacial malformations. In: Stricker M (ed) Craniofacial malformations. Churchill Livingstone, New York, pp 217–222
Tewfik TL, Der Kaloustian VM (1997) Congenital anomalies of the ear, nose, and throat. Oxford University Press, New York
Vargervik K (2002) Hemifacial microsomia: classification and management protocols. In: Papel I (ed) Facial plastic and reconstructive surgery, 2nd edn. Thieme Medical, New York, pp 865–872
Vendramini-Pittoli S, Kokitsu-Nakata NM (2009) Oculoauriculovertebral spectrum: report of nine familial cases with evidence of autosomal dominant inheritance and review of the literature. Clin Dysmorphol 18(2):67–77

Hemilaryngectomy

▶ Conservation Laryngeal Surgery

Hereditary Hearing Loss

Matthew Ng[1] and Drew M. Horlbeck[2]
[1]Department of Surgery, Division of Otolaryngology, University of Nevada School of Medicine, Las Vegas, NV, USA
[2]Department of Surgery, Division of Pediatric Otolaryngology, Nemours Children's Clinic, Jacksonville, FL, USA

Definition

Hearing loss conveyed by genetic inheritance, may be syndromic or non-syndromic, present at birth (congenital) or after birth (delayed onset).

Cross-References

▶ Sensorineural Hearing Loss-Congenital-Genetics

Heschl's Gyrus

Hinrich Staecker[1] and Jennifer Thompson[2]
[1]Department of Otolaryngology-Head and Neck Surgery, University of Kansas Medical Center, Kansas City, KS, USA
[2]University of Kansas Medical Center, Kansas City, KS, USA

Definition

Found in the primary auditory cortex in the superior temporal gyrus of the brain, occupying Brodmann areas 41 and 42. It is the first cortical area in the brain, processing the ascending auditory information.

Cross-References

▶ Central Auditory System, Anatomy
▶ Vestibular and Central Nervous System, Anatomy

Heterotopias, Teratoma, and Choristoma

Kenneth H. Lee[1] and Peter S. Roland[2]
[1]Department of Otolaryngology-Head and Neck Surgery, University of Texas Southwestern Medical Center at Dallas, Dallas, TX, USA
[2]Department of Otolaryngology-Head and Neck Surgery, UT - Southwestern Medical Center, University of Texas Southwestern, Dallas, TX, USA

Synonyms

Cystic teratomas; Dermoids; Hairy polyps

Definitions

1. Heterotopia: The presence of normal tissue in an abnormal location.
2. Teratoma: A tumor comprising of one or more of the three germinal layers and is composed of different kinds of tissue, none of which normally occur together or at the site of the tumor. By strict definition, a mature teratoma contains all three germinal layers.
3. Choristoma: A mass of histologically normal tissue in an abnormal location.

Basic Characteristics

Choristomas

Overview: Tissue that is classified as heterotopic is histologically normal, but presents in an abnormal location. A choristoma is a mass formed by heterotopic tissue. Thus, by definition, choristomas are benign tumors. While choristomas are frequently encountered in some parts of the body, such as in the case of endometriosis (ectopic ovarian tissue) in the pelvis, choristomas in the head and neck are relatively rare. The sites where choristomas present in the head and neck most commonly are the nasal region (gliomas) and the oral cavity (lingual thyroid and ectopic gastric or respiratory tissue).

The presentation of choristomas in the ear and temporal bone are extremely rare and are discussed in this entry. Choristomas in this region have been reported in the bony ear canal and the middle ear. In cases where these have presented in the bony ear canal, the masses have been found to be cartilaginous on histological examination (Lee 2005). When choristomas present in the middle ear, they are most commonly ectopic salivary gland tumors (Buckmiller et al. 2001). However, neuroglial choristomas of the middle ear have also been reported (Lee et al. 2004; Farneti et al. 2007).

Ear Canal Choristomas

The choristomas that have been reported in the bony ear canal are cartilaginous tumors. They were initially considered as chondromas, which are cartilaginous tumors that arise in most cases from bone or periosteum. However, in a review of 36 cases, the cartilaginous external ear canal tumors were found to be histologically separate from the bone and periosteum of the ear canal, supporting the conclusion that these tumors are choristomas and distinct from chondromas (Lee 2005). They present in both adults and children as small (1–4 mm) solitary masses, in the anterior medial bony canal wall, usually within 3 mm of the tympanic membrane (Fig. 1a). On otoscopic examination, they can appear similar to an isolated exostosis lesion. Histopathology reveals that these tumors consist of mature hyaline cartilage (Fig. 1b, c). In addition, 20% of cases present with an associated accessory ear lobe near the ipsilateral tragus suggesting an embryologic developmental error (Lee 2005).

In most cases, canal cartilaginous choristomas are asymptomatic and are found incidentally on routine otoscopy. However, patients with these lesions can present with recurrent episodes of external otitis. Differential diagnosis includes exostosis, osteoma, keratoma, and fibroma. In the largest published series of canal choristomas, 72% were surgically excised, and there were no local recurrences in these cases. However, as these tumors are benign and since no growth was noted in cases that did not undergo surgical resection, they can be managed with conservative observation unless they become symptomatic or a concern for malignancy develops (Lee 2005).

Middle Ear Salivary Gland Choristomas

While salivary choristoma is the most common type of heterotopia that presents in the middle ear, overall it is extremely rare. Since it was first described in 1961 (Taylor and Martin 1961), there have been less than 40 cases reported in the literature. A review of the first 25 cases revealed that patients with a middle ear salivary choristoma most commonly present with hearing loss since childhood, usually in the absence of chronic middle ear infections or other otologic symptoms (Buckmiller et al. 2001). The hearing loss in most cases is conductive (64%), but can be mixed (28%) or sensorineural (4%). The degree of hearing loss is most frequently moderate, but can range from mild to profound deafness. Middle ear salivary gland choristomas are unilateral, and interestingly, are more commonly found on the left side (el-Naggar et al. 1994). While it is a unilateral disease, there have been reported cases of middle ear salivary choristomas with bilateral hearing loss (Peron and Schuknecht 1975). In addition to hearing loss, otorrhea and tinnitus have also been reported as presenting symptoms (el-Naggar et al. 1994).

Most typically, on physical examination, a middle ear mass is seen behind an intact tympanic membrane (Buckmiller et al. 2001). In addition, middle ear salivary gland choristomas are associated with anatomical abnormalities of other ear structures. Most notable are facial nerves that are dehiscent in the tympanic segment or have an anomalous course through the temporal bone. In roughly one third of cases, the choristoma is found to be adherent to the facial nerve in the middle ear. Intraoperatively, ossicular abnormalities have also been found. The reported malleus abnormalities include fusion of the malleus and incus, bowing or hypertrophy, erosion or partial absence. Abnormalities found in the incus include short or absent long process, general malformation, and complete absence. The stapes is most commonly malformed, usually found with partial or complete absence of the suprastructure. In some cases, the stapes is completely absent, and there have even been reports of absence of the oval window. Other anomalies associated with these tumors include external ear malposition or malformation, absence of the stapedius muscle, asymmetry of the face, various branchial cleft anomalies, temporal swelling or alopecia, facial paresis, and inner ear anomalies. Consequently, Buckmiller and colleagues propose that salivary choristomas of the middle ear may represent a component of a syndrome that includes hearing loss, and anomalies of the ossicular chain, facial nerve, and branchial arch (Buckmiller et al. 2001).

The differential diagnosis includes paraganglioma, schwannoma, rhabdomyosarcoma, dermoid cyst, teratoma, lymphoma, and congenital cholesteatoma.

Heterotopias, Teratoma, and Choristoma, Fig. 1 Otoscopic view of bony ear canal cartilaginous choristoma in typical location in anterior superior canal with close proximity to the tympanic membrane (**a**). Low magnification (40×, **b**) and high magnification (200×, **c**) view of histopathology of ear canal cartilaginous choristoma showing mature hyaline cartilage on Hematoxylin-eosin stain (Reprinted from Lee 2005)

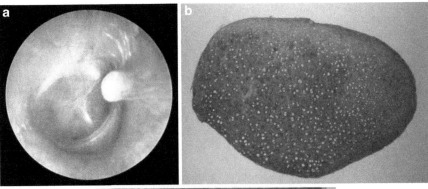

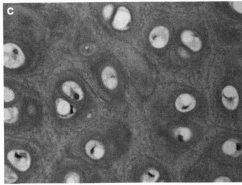

Imaging can be useful in narrowing down the differential diagnosis. While these masses can be visualized on both computed tomography (CT) and magnetic resonance imaging (MRI), high resolution CT is the modality of choice to identify and characterize these small middle ear masses. On CT, middle ear salivary gland choristomas are usually found to be intimately related to the facial nerve and ossicular chain and do not display overt bony erosion (Fig. 2). Intraoperatively, these tumors are most commonly found in the posterior superior quadrant and can appear white, yellow, or pink in color.

Salivary gland choristomas, when found in the middle ear, are most commonly managed by surgical resection. Definitive diagnosis is confirmed with histopathology which demonstrates serous and mucous glandular structures typical of normal salivary gland tissue (Fig. 3). However, because of the risk of postoperative facial paresis due to frequent facial nerve involvement, conservative excision is the recommended approach as these are benign tumors and there are no reports of recurrence in cases of subtotal resection. In addition, middle ear salivary gland choristomas have not been shown to grow over time and the associated hearing loss is stable and does not

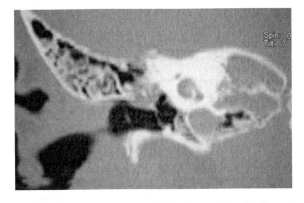

Heterotopias, Teratoma, and Choristoma, Fig. 2 Coronal CT of salivary choristoma in right temporal bone showing mass intimately surrounding the ossicles and adjacent to facial nerve (Reprinted from Toros et al. 2010)

progress (Buckmiller et al. 2001). Nevertheless, when the tumor is small, pedunculated, and can safely be removed completely without risk to surrounding ossicles and facial nerve, total excision is recommended (Lee et al. 2006) as there are rare reports of malignant transformation (Kartush and Graham 1984).

The exact etiology of this rare tumor is not completely understood. One hypothesis is that ectodermal cells intended to develop into salivary tissue

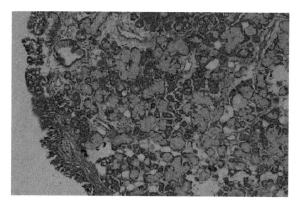

**Heterotopias,   Teratoma,   and   Choristoma,
Fig. 3** Histopathology of salivary choristoma showing normal mucus and serous glands under ciliated epithelium on Hematox-ylin-eosin stain (100×, Reprinted from Toros et al., 2010)

become trapped in the temporal bone similar in theory to the origin of congenital cholesteatomas (Peron and Schuknecht 1975). It has also been proposed that these tumors arise from expansion of aberrant parotid epithelium in the developing middle ear during the fourth month of gestation, which is a critical time period for development of the ossicles and facial nerve, explaining the intimate relationship of the facial nerve and middle ear ossicles with salivary choristomas (Ha et al. 2000).

Middle Ear Neuroglial Choristomas

Extracranial neuroglial choristomas are usually found along midline structures such as the nose, pharynx, lips, soft palate, tongue, and tonsils. The most common type of extracranial neuroglial choristoma found in the head and neck is the nasal glioma. Finding neuroglial tissue in heterotopic locations that are not in the midline, such as in the middle ear or mastoid bone, is extremely rare. Compared to midline neuroglial chorismas, which commonly present in young children, middle ear neuroglial choristomas are most often identified in older adults (Gyure et al. 2000). In addition, as opposed to the more common salivary choristoma of the middle ear, heterotopic neuroglial tissue in this location is frequently associated with chronic infection, inflammation, trauma, or previous surgery and patients often present with a history of recurrent ear infections and/or otorrhea (Lee et al. 2004), thus raising the hypothesis that middle ear neuroglial choristomas may potentially have originated from an acquired encephalocele.

In general, these tumors are evaluated and managed in the same manner as salivary choristomas of the middle ear. It is critical to obtain and carefully review a high-resolution CT of the temporal bone to confirm that the mass does not have continuity with intracranial contents through a defect in the tegmen. Such a finding would favor the diagnosis of an encephalocele and would alter the strategy and approach for surgical management. In addition, these tumors differ from their counterparts of salivary origin as they are most often found not to be associated with the facial nerve or ossicular abnormalities (Farneti et al. 2007), which attests to the different etiologies of neuroglial and salivary choristoma in the middle ear. The diagnosis of these tumors can be confirmed with positive staining for glial fibrillary acidic protein (GFAP) and S-100 (Lee et al. 2004), or immunolabeling of neuronal cells with anti-Neu antibodies (Farneti et al. 2007). These tumors are extremely rare and heterotopic glial or brain tissue cannot be differentiated on histopathology from the far more common encephalocele. Thus, to ensure proper surgical planning and intraoperative management, an accurate differentiation of the two must be made with careful review of imaging and operative findings.

Teratomas

In general, dermoids and teratomas are very similar. By strict definition, dermoids are comprised of ectoderm and mesoderm while true or mature teratomas contain all three germ layers. Approximately 7% of all dermoids and 6% of all teratomas are found in the head and neck. However, it is extremely rare to find either of these tumors in the temporal bone. In the temporal bone, these tumors have been reported to arise in the middle ear and Eustachian tube. Dermoids are three to four times more common than true teratomas in the middle ear. Dermoids in the middle ear are thought to arise when the ectoderm from the first branchial cleft anomalously becomes included in the endoderm of the first pharyngeal pouch before these two germ layers are separated by mesoderm. The pathogenesis of teratomas in the middle ear and Eustachian tube, on the other hand, is not well understood. There is a notable sixfold predominance of head and neck dermoids in females compared to males. When dermoids arise from the Eustachian tube, 11 out of 12 cases have been found on the left side (Sichel et al. 1999).

Teratomas of the middle ear most commonly present in young children who have had a history of recurrent middle ear infections or chronic otorrhea that has been refractory to standard medical and surgical treatment (Gourin and Sofferman 1999). Depending on the extension of the mass, other symptoms such as facial palsy, snoring, stridor, and airway obstruction have also been described (Forrest et al. 1993; Navarro Cunchillos et al. 1996). Findings on otoscopy can vary from a visible mass, to an inflamed tympanic membrane, to a completely normal examination. Imaging is recommended to assist with assessment and treatment planning. CT is the recommended study of choice as careful review of bony structures will assist in the diagnosis since these nonhomogeneous tumors often demonstrate local destruction of bone (Gourin and Sofferman 1999). However, MRI and angiography can assist in delineating the relationship of the mass to the internal carotid for surgical planning (Gourin and Sofferman 1999).

The diagnosis of a middle ear dermoid can be made during surgery based on gross appearance of the tumor or by histopathology revealing fibroadipose tissue with epidermis, skin appendages such as hair, sebaceous glands, cartilage, and muscle (Gourin and Sofferman 1999). The optimal treatment for dermoids and teratomas in the middle ear is complete surgical excision. The different surgical approaches that have been used for these tumors include postauricular with simple or modified radical mastoidectomy, preauricular incision and protympanic approach, as well as postauricular with modified neck dissection to access the parapharyngeal space (Gourin and Sofferman 1999). Often times, two procedures were required to achieve complete surgical excision due to limitations in exposure. Without complete excision, these tumors tend to recur. In the case of dermoids, if complete excision is achieved, prognosis is excellent as they are not known to undergo malignant degeneration. Unfortunately, teratomas have been reported to undergo malignant transformation in 20% of cases (Navarro Cunchillos et al. 1996). Thus, complete surgical excision is critical for patients with teratomas, and these patients need close follow-up for surveillance.

Cross-References

▶ Benign Sinonasal Neoplasms

References

Buckmiller LM, Brodie HA, Doyle KJ, Nemzek W (2001) Choristoma of the middle ear: a component of a new syndrome? Otol Neurotol 22(3):363–368
el-Naggar AK, Pflatz M, Ordóñez NG, Batsakis JG (1994) Tumors of the middle ear and endolymphatic sac. Pathol Annu 29(Pt 2):199–231
Farneti P, Balbi M, Foschini MP (2007) Neuroglial choristoma of the middle ear. Acta Otorhinolaryngol Ital 27(2):94–97
Forrest AW, Carr SJ, Beckenham EJ (1993) A middle ear teratoma causing acute airway obstruction. Int J Pediatr Otorhinolaryngol 25(1–3):183–189
Gourin CG, Sofferman RA (1999) Dermoid of the eustachian tube. Otolaryngol Head Neck Surg 120(5):772–775
Gyure KA, Thompson LD, Morrison AL (2000) A clinicopathological study of 15 patients with neuroglial heterotopias and encephaloceles of the middle ear and mastoid region. Laryngoscope 110(10 Pt 1):1731–1735
Ha SL, Shin JE, Yoon TH (2000) Salivary gland charistoma of the middle ear: a cafe report. Am J Otolasyngol 21(2):127–130
Kartush JM, Graham MD (1984) Salivary gland choristoma of the middle ear: a case report and review of the literature. Laryngoscope 94(2 Pt 1):228–230
Lee FP (2005) Cartilaginous choristoma of the bony external auditory canal: a study of 36 cases. Otolaryngol Head Neck Surg 133(5):786–790
Lee JI, Kim KK, Park YK, Eah KY, Kim JR (2004) Glial choristoma in the middle ear and mastoid bone: a case report. J Korean Med Sci 19(1):155–158
Lee DK, Kim JH, Cho YS, Chung WH, Hong SH (2006) Salivary gland choristoma of the middle ear in an infant: a case report. Int J Pediatr Otorhinolaryngol 70(1):167–170
Navarro Cunchillos M, Bonachera MD, Navarro Cunchillos M, Cassinello E, Ramos Lizana J, Oña EJ (1996) Middle ear teratoma in a newborn. J Laryngol Otol 110(9):875–877
Peron DL, Schuknecht HF (1975) Congenital cholesteatomata with other anomalies. Arch Otolaryngol 101(8):498–505
Sichel JY, Dano I, Halperin D, Chisin R (1999) Dermoid cyst of the eustachian tube. Int J Pediatr Otorhinolaryngol 48(1):77–81
Taylor GD, Martin HF (1961) Salivary gland tissue in the middle ear. A rare tumor. Arch Otolaryngol 73:651–653
Toros SZ, Egeli E, Kiliçarsian Y, Gümrükeü G, Gökçeer T, Noşeri H (2010) Salivary gland choristana of the middle era in a child with Situs inversus totalis. Aurs Nasus Larynx 37(3):365–368

HFM

▶ Hemifacial Microsomia

Hilger Test

▶ Nerve Excitability Test

Hirudo Medicinalis

▶ Medicinal Leeches

Hirudotherapy

▶ Medicinal Leeches

Histiocytosis X and its Variations

▶ Langerhans Cell Histiocytosis of Temporal Bone

History and Physical of Head and Neck

Seth Lieberman[1] and Richard A. Lebowitz[2]
[1]School of Medicine, Department of Otolaryngology,
New York University Langone Medical Center,
New York, NY, USA
[2]Department of Otolaryngology-Head and Neck
Surgery, New York University School of Medicine,
NYU Langone Medical Center, New York, NY, USA

History

As with most fields of medicine, the otolaryngologic history is essential in properly diagnosing diseases of the head and neck. Given the breadth of otolaryngology, the history will often begin broad and then become quite focused. However, given the immense variety of head and neck manifestations of systemic disease, it is important to take a complete history.

History of Present Illness

During this part of the history, the chief complaint is identified. Several mnemonics have been created to aid in eliciting the most important details of each symptom. One such mnemonic is "OPQRST." The patient is questioned about the details surrounding the **O**nset of symptoms include preceding events, illnesses, or medication. **P**alliative and **P**rovocative factors should be elicited with questions such as "what makes the symptom better" and "what makes the symptom worse." A description of **Q**uality of the symptom should be ascertained such as distinguishing whether pain is

burning, sharp, dull, aching, etc., or whether a ringing in the ear is pulsatile, nonpulsatile, high-pitched, whooshing, etc. **R**adiation refers to the movement of a symptom, such as a sore throat radiating to the ipsilateral ear as can often be seen with tonsillar and other pharyngeal pathology. The **S**everity of the symptoms is most easily described on a scale of 0 (symptom-free) to 10 (as severe as one can imagine). The **T**iming of the symptom includes when the symptoms first began, how long each episode lasts, and how frequently symptom occurs. This aspect of the history will evolve as the physician begins to formulate a differential diagnosis based on the acquired information.

Past Medical History
This part of the history focuses on the chronic illnesses that the patient has as well the medications he/she takes. Recent hospitalizations and doctors visits are often useful to document. Allergies should be documented.

Past Surgical History
This includes the past surgeries that the patient has undergone.

Family History
Illnesses of family members are recorded. Diseases specific to the chief complaint should also be elicited, e.g., hearing loss and thyroid cancer.

Social History
This includes smoking history, alcohol and substance abuse, betel nut use, sexual history, occupation and occupational exposure, and travel history.

Review of Systems
This part of the history assesses other systems that may be affected and prevents missing important diagnostic information. A review of systems includes questions about constitutional symptoms, skin, eyes, ears, nose, throat/mouth, neck, respiratory, cardiovascular, peripheral vascular, gastrointestinal, urinary, genital, musculoskeletal, hematologic, endocrine, neurologic, psychiatric, and sleep.

Physical Examination

General
The first seconds of a patient encounter can often provide a wealth of information. Simply watching

a patient walk to the exam room affords the examiner an opportunity to evaluate gait, body habitus, balance, and overall level of disability. Introducing oneself allows the examiner to evaluate the patient's voice, the presence of dysarthria or any upper respiratory sounds, and the odor of cigarette smoke or alcohol. Observing the patient's behavior will provide insight into the patient's level of depression, anxiety, pain, and distress. In a field where chief complaints relate to a wide variety of pathologies including head and neck cancer, thyroid disease, auditory and vestibular disorders, and sinus disease, such findings help the examiner make an overall initial assessment of the patient.

Cranial Nerve Examination

The following provides a basic overview of the cranial nerve examination.

I. Olfactory Nerve

A battery of tests may be used for formal olfactory testing, if indicated. Basic evaluation of olfaction can be performed using a substance with a distinct odor such as coffee or cinnamon, which is held under one nostril while the other nostril is occluded. The patient is asked to identify the odor. It is important to remember that certain noxious chemical smells, like ammonia, are sensed by the trigeminal nerve rather than the olfactory nerve.

II. Optic Nerve

A gross assessment of the optic nerve can be performed by evaluating visual acuity, pupillary reflexes, visual field testing, and examination of the fundi. Visual acuity should be tested using a Snellen chart, with one eye covered in order to test each optic nerve independently. The pupillary light reflex is actually testing both the optic nerve (afferent arc) and the oculomotor nerve (efferent arc). If abnormal, swinging the light from one eye to the other while observing for constriction of the pupil can help determine if there is an afferent pupillary defect. The diameter of each pupil at baseline and after constriction is reported in millimeters. A gross assessment of visual fields is performed with one eye covered at a time. The visual fields are assessed in each of the four quadrants by asking the patient to count the number of fingers the examiner is displaying in that quadrant. Ophthalmoscopic examination is performed to evaluate the retina and other structures at the back of the eye. It is best performed after dilation of the pupil, but a limited view can be obtained without dilation.

III. Oculomotor

Oculomotor nerve function is evaluated by assessing the patient's extraocular motility. The position of the eyelid is also evaluated, as ptosis may be caused by oculomotor nerve dysfunction. In addition, the oculomotor nerve provides the efferent limb of the pupillary light reflex.

IV. Trochlear Nerve

Trochlear nerve function is evaluated by assessing the patient's extraocular motility, specifically downward gaze of the adducted eye.

V. Trigeminal Nerve

The trigeminal nerve is responsible for innervating the muscles of mastication, providing sensory innervation to the face, and providing the afferent limb of the corneal reflex. To test the muscles of mastication, the examiner places his/her hands over the masseter muscle and temporalis muscle and asks the patient to clench his/her teeth. Sensation is tested over the distribution of each of the three divisions of the trigeminal nerve (V1 – forehead, V2 – malar eminence, and V3 – jaw) using light touch, temperature, and pain. The right and left sides are compared to determine if there are any differences. The corneal reflex is performed by touching a piece of cotton to the cornea, which should cause the patient to blink. The efferent limb of this reflex arc is provided by CN VII.

VI. Abducens Nerve

Abducens nerve function is evaluated by assessing the patient's extraocular motility, specifically abduction, or lateral movement.

VII. Facial Nerve

The facial nerve provides motor innervation to the superficial facial musculature, the platysma, the stylohyoid muscle, the posterior belly of the digastric muscle, and the stapedius muscle. The latter three cannot be tested with the physical examination. The face should be assessed at rest for symmetry, tone, and contracture. In order to assess each of the five branches of the facial nerve, the patient is then asked to raise the eyebrows, close the eyes tight, wrinkle the nose, smile, frown, and puff out the cheeks. The findings can be described specifically or reported using the House-Brackmann scale (See Table 1).

History and Physical of Head and Neck, Table 1 Facial nerve grading system

Grade	Description	Characteristics
1	Normal	Normal facial function in all areas
2	Mild dysfunction	Gross: slight weakness noticeable on close inspection; may have very slight synkinesis
		At rest: normal symmetry and tone
		Motion
		Forehead: moderate to good function
		Eye: complete closure with minimum effort
		Mouth: slight asymmetry
3	Moderate dysfunction	Gross: obvious but no disfiguring difference between two sides; noticeable but not severe synkinesis, contracture, and/or hemifacial spasm
		At rest: normal symmetry and tone
		Motion
		Forehead: slight to moderate movement
		Eye: complete eye closure with effort
		Mouth: slightly weak with maximum effort
4	Moderate severe dysfunction	Gross: obvious weakness and/or disfiguring asymmetry
		At rest: normal symmetry and tone
		Motion
		Forehead: none
		Eye: incomplete closure
		Mouth: asymmetric with maximum effort
5	Severe dysfunction	Gross: only barely perceptible motion
		At rest: asymmetry
		Motion
		Forehead: none
		Eye: incomplete closure
		Mouth: slight movement
6	Total paralysis	No movement

From House and Brackmann (1985)

The facial nerve also provides taste to the anterior two-third of the tongue and parasympathetic innervations to the lacrimal gland, palatal and nasal mucosa, submandibular gland, and lingual gland. These branches are generally not assessed during physical examination.

VIII. Vestibulocochlear Nerve

Auditory function is grossly assessed using a 512-Hz tuning fork. The Weber and Rinne tests are performed to help determine if a conductive or sensorineural hearing loss is present.

Vestibular function can be assessed by a variety of maneuvers as well as battery of formal testing including caloric testing and nystagmography. During the physical examination, the vestibular system can be grossly assessed by evaluating the patient's gait, observing for nystagmus at rest and upon lateral gaze (ideally while wearing Frenzel lenses), and performing the Dix-Hallpike maneuver, head-shake test, and Fukuda test.

IX. Glossopharyngeal Nerve

The glossopharyngeal nerve is difficult to evaluate in isolation as its functions include taste and sensation to the posterior one-third of the tongue, innervation to the stylopharyngeus muscle, sensory innervations to the carotid bodies, parasympathetic innervation to the parotid gland, and sensory innervation to the pharynx and tonsils. The last of these functions acts as the afferent limb of the gag reflex. The vagus nerve then supplies the efferent innervations for the gag reflex. The gag reflex is elicited by using a cotton tip applicator or tongue blade to touch the posterior pharyngeal wall.

X. Vagus Nerve

The vagus nerve is assessed by evaluating vocal fold mobility, palatal elevation, and gag reflex. Abnormality in vocal fold mobility can lead to hoarseness; however, this sign is not specific for vagal nerve dysfunction. Vocal fold mobility is best assessed with indirect mirror laryngoscopy or flexible fiberoptic laryngoscopy. The palate is inspected as the patient says "ahh." If there is vagal nerve dysfunction affecting the innervation to the palatal muscles, the ipsilateral soft palate will sag, and the uvula will deviate to the normal side. The vagus nerve acts as the efferent limb of the gag reflex, with the glossopharyngeal nerve providing the afferent limb.

XI. Accessory Nerve

Function of the spinal accessory nerve is easily assessed by having the patient raise his/her shoulders against resistance, or raising his/her hand above shoulder level. This maneuver tests the branch to the trapezius muscle. The sternocleidomastoid muscle is assessed by having the patient turn his/her head in each direction against resistance. Weakness suggests nerve dysfunction on the side contralateral to the side to which the patient is turning his/her head.

XII. Hypoglossal nerve

Function is assessed by having the patient protrude his/her tongue and move it from side to side. Unilateral dysfunction will result in deviation of the tongue to the side of the lesion on protrusion. Other signs of dysfunction may include dysarthria, atrophy, or fasciculations on one side of the tongue.

Head

Eyes

A complete examination of the eyes should include evaluation of cranial nerves II–VII as mentioned above. In addition to the cranial nerve exam, the position of the globes should be assessed. Proptosis may be found in Graves' disease, orbital trauma, and tumors involving the orbit or paranasal sinuses. This is best assessed by looking from above the patient as in a bird's eye view. If there is concern for elevated intraocular pressures as in the case of a retro-orbital hematoma after trauma, an ophthalmologist should be consulted immediately to evaluate intraocular pressures. Any hypophthalmos or enophthalmos should also be noted, as can be seen in facial trauma involving the medial wall or floor of the orbit, or in patients with chronic maxillary atelectasis (silent sinus syndrome). The orbital rim is palpated to assess for any stepoffs or crepitus. The conjunctiva is assessed for signs of chemosis, erythema, and injection, as can be found in allergic, inflammatory, and infectious diseases. Especially in children, the examiner should be vigilant for any congenital abnormality such as coloboma or heterochromia iridium. The area of the lacrimal gland in the superolateral aspect of the orbit is palpated to note any enlargement as can be seen in certain autoimmune, granulomatous, and infectious diseases. The upper and lower lids are evaluated for any signs of edema or venous congestion. If there is trauma near the eye, an ophthalmology consult to perform a dilated fundoscopic exam is prudent.

Ear

The ear exam can be divided into examination of the auricle or pinna, the external auditory canal (EAC), and the tympanic membrane (TM). If the patient has a unilateral ear complaint, the uninvolved ear should be examined first. For a proper ear exam, one should have a 512-Hz tuning fork, an otoscope with a working head as well as one that is able to perform pneumatic otoscopy, and any instruments that may be needed to debride the EAC or remove cerumen. Having a microscope available is ideal and will provide more detail than a handheld otoscope.

Auricle Prior to performing otoscopy, the pinna and periauricular structures should be evaluated, as these findings can often be overlooked.

Congenital anomalies such as preauricular pits, auricular deformities, and skin tags should be noted. Especially in syndromic children, the position of the auricle in relation to the head should be assessed. Proptosis of the ear should be noted and may be a sign of recent surgery or mastoiditis.

The skin of the auricle is assessed for dermatologic conditions such as eczema or the presence of any skin lesions. In the setting of trauma, the auricle should be palpated to assess for any underlying abscess or hematoma, which should be promptly drained. The mastoid tip is palpated for any tenderness or edema. The tragus is palpated for signs of tenderness as can be seen in otitis externa.

EAC The largest speculum that can be inserted into the EAC without causing trauma should be used for the otoscopic exam. The course of the EAC has varying degrees of tortuosity. The speculum should be inserted gently and with traction on the auricle in a posterosuperior direction in adults and posterior direction in children in order to better align the cartilaginous EAC with the bony EAC.

The EAC is a skin-lined canal and therefore is susceptible to dermatologic conditions such as eczema and skin cancer. The caliber of the EAC is noted, including any evidence of edema, stenosis, atresia, exostoses, or osteomas. Cerumen should be atraumatically removed if it is preventing a complete examination of the EAC or TM. This can be done using several techniques including using a curette, right angle pick, gentle suction, or irrigation with warm (body-temperature) water. Any discharge, debris, or foreign body should likewise be removed. The location and quality of any lesion should be accurately documented and may provide clues to diagnosis. For example, granulation tissue at the bony-cartilaginous junction may be a sign of necrotizing otitis externa. If the patient has had a canal-wall-down mastoidectomy, the mastoid bowl should be cleaned and properly inspected for any granulation tissue, infection, or cholesteatoma. It is important to remember that suctioning the ear of such patients can induce vertigo, nausea, and vomiting, which occurs when the horizontal semicircular canal is stimulated by the flow of air and local temperature change.

Tympanic Membrane (TM) The TM can be divided into four quadrants based on the trajectory of the handle of the malleus. The TM can also be divided into the pars tensa, which represents the lower four-fifth, and the pars flaccida, which lies above the malleolar folds and has a weaker middle fibrous layer than the pars tensa. The quality of the tympanic membrane should be described (dull, bulging, erythematous, presence of myringosclerosis, etc.). Effusions can be opaque, clear, or bloody depending on whether the fluid is infected, serous, or post-traumatic, respectively. Pneumatic otoscopy is performed to assess the mobility of the TM which may be immobile, hypomobile, have normal mobility, or be hypermobile. When performing pneumatic otoscopy, the patient may experience vertigo or display a few beats of nystagmus (Hennebert's sign) which may be a sign of perilymphatic fistula or a dehiscent semicircular canal.

If a retraction of the TM is present, it must be noted whether or not the base of the retraction can be visualized. If the depths of the retraction pocket cannot be visualized, a cholesteatoma should be suspected. The pars flaccida is more vulnerable to negative middle ear pressure because of the weak middle fibrous layer. Any keratin debris within a retraction pocket indicates the presence of a cholesteatoma.

Any perforation should be described in terms of size (e.g., 30% total), location (quadrant), and involvement of the annulus (marginal or central). Depending on the location of the perforation, the ossicles can be inspected for signs of erosion; the middle ear mucosa can be inspected for erythema, edema, granulation tissue, or epidermization; and the middle ear space can be inspected for signs of tympanosclerosis. A perforation without otorrhea (dry perforation) is a sign that there is currently no active disease. It is important to mention that any unilateral finding that suggests abnormal middle ear function (retraction, effusion, perforation) must be followed up with

nasopharyngoscopy to rule out nasopharyngeal malignancy obstructing the Eustachian tube orifice. Microtoscopy provides superior visualization in cases of TM and middle ear pathology.

Tuning Fork Test The tuning fork tests should be performed with a 512-Hz tuning fork. The Rinne test is performed by first placing the tuning fork over the mastoid tip (bone conduction) and then placing it next to the external auditory meatus (air conduction). The patient states whether air conduction (AC) is perceived as louder than bone conduction (BC) – a positive test – or vice versa – a negative test. In a normal ear, AC is greater than BC. A negative test suggests at least a 20-dB conductive hearing loss.

The Weber test is performed by placing a 512-Hz tuning fork in the center of the head or face, either over the vertex, the rhinion, or over the maxillary teeth. The patient is asked to identify on which side the sound is perceived or if it is perceived equally in both ears. If the sound "lateralizes" to one side, this suggests either a conductive hearing loss on that side or a sensorineural hearing loss on the contralateral side. Both tests must be used together to make a clinical assessment. Of course, an audiogram should be obtained to fully evaluate any patient with a hearing complaint (Table 2).

Nose/Nasopharynx
The examination of the nose can be divided into the external examination of the nose, anterior rhinoscopy, and nasal endoscopy (which will include the nasopharynx).

External Examination of the Nose The nose is inspected for any skin lesions, swelling, trauma, or congenital anomalies. A detailed analysis of the nose in preparation for rhinoplasty will not be discussed here. If trauma has occurred, the nose is inspected for dorsal deviation and asymmetry and is palpated to evaluate for mobility and crepitus.

The nares are also inspected for size and any evidence of collapse on inspiration as are the internal nasal valves, which may be pertinent for a patient complaining of nasal obstruction. The nasal vestibule is also inspected for evidence of lesions. A Cottle or modified Cottle maneuver is performed if indicated.

History and Physical of Head and Neck, Table 2 Tuning fork test examples

Rinne L	Rinne R	Weber	Diagnosis
AC > BC	AC > BC	Midline	Normal
AC > BC	BC > AC	R	CHL on the right
AC > BC	AC > BC	L	Right SNHL

CHL conductive hearing loss, *SNHL* sensorineural hearing loss, *AC* air conduction, *BC* bone conduction

Anterior Rhinoscopy A headlight or head mirror is used for illumination, and a nasal speculum is used to distend the nostrils. This exam is first performed without decongestion in order to evaluate the baseline state of the nasal mucosa. The mucosa of the head of the inferior turbinate is assessed for signs of hypertrophy and inflammation. The septum is assessed for perforations and deviations, especially caudal deviations which may not be appreciated on nasal endoscopy. Bony spurs as well as cartilaginous and bony deviations of the septum are common. Any finding must be taken in the context of the patient's complaints.

Nasal Endoscopy A $0°$ rigid scope or a flexible fiberoptic scope is used to evaluate the areas of the nasal cavity that cannot be seen on anterior rhinoscopy. Decongestion and topical anesthesia may be needed for this part of the exam. The scope is passed along the floor of the nasal cavity first to evaluate the patency of the nasal cavity into the nasopharynx. Once the nasopharynx is visualized, the torus tubarius, Eustachian tube orifice, and fossa of Rosenmuller are inspected. Again, this part of the examination is especially important in patients with middle ear findings such as a unilateral middle ear effusion or retraction. The adenoid tissue is evaluated for size, inflammation, and asymmetry. Adenoid tissue is generally much more prominent in children and is commonly a cause for sleep-disordered breathing among this population. In adults, there is generally minimal residual adenoid tissue, as there is normally involution of the adenoids in childhood. Causes of adenoid hypertrophy in an adult include infection and inflammation (e.g., adenoiditis secondary to chronic sinusitis), HIV, lymphoma, and nasopharyngeal cancer. With a flexible or angled rigid scope, both sides of the nasopharynx can be inspected through one nostril; however, a scope must be passed on both sides in order to adequately visualize the nasal passage on

each side. Velopharyngeal competence can be evaluated by having the patient say "Coca-Cola," which elevates the soft palate against the posterior pharyngeal wall.

The scope is then withdrawn and passed superior to the inferior turbinate in order to evaluate the middle turbinate and middle meatus. The middle meatus is the common drainage pathway for the frontal, maxillary, and anterior ethmoid sinuses. The middle meatus should be inspected for evidence of purulent drainage, polyps, edema, and masses. Accessory ostia into the maxillary sinus may be seen posterior to the natural ostium. Accessory ostia are round while the natural ostium is elliptical in shape. The sphenoethmoidal recess, which is located medial to the superior turbinate, is the site of drainage of the sphenoid sinus. This area should also be inspected for purulent drainage or polyps. The olfactory cleft which lies at the skull base between the superior attachment of the middle turbinate and septum is inspected for obstruction from polyps or other masses. Areas of the septum that cannot be well visualized on anterior rhinoscopy are inspected with endoscopy, noting the locations of any deviations. If a patient has had septal surgery in the past, a cotton-tipped applicator can be used to gently palpate the septum to determine where cartilage or bone may have been resected.

In patients who have undergone endoscopic sinus surgery, it may be possible to evaluate the condition of the sinus mucosa, depending on the size of the surgical sinusotomies and the position of the turbinates. This should be performed, if possible, to assess the patient for evidence of recurrent disease. Flexible fiberoptic or angled scopes are necessary for inspecting some of these areas such as the frontal sinuses and the anterior extent and floor of the maxillary sinus.

Oral Cavity/Oropharynx

Oral Cavity The oral cavity should be inspected in a stepwise fashion so as not to miss any areas. A headlight or head mirror is recommended for this part of the exam to allow for bimanual manipulation. The mucosa of the oral cavity can be affected by a variety of systemic disease processes, such as telangiectasias, petechiae, ulcers, watery edema, and pigmentary changes, as well as a variety of local disease processes, including leukoplakia, erythroplakia, candidiasis, and epithelial cancers.

The lips are examined for any evidence of swelling or lesions such as telangiectasias, ulcerations, nodules, and cysts. The patient is then asked to open his or her mouth. Any deviation of the jaw or trismus should be noted at this time. A tongue blade can then be placed against the buccal mucosa, and the patient is asked to relax his or her jaw. At this point, the buccal mucosa can be retracted away from the dentition in order to stretch out the mucosa and evaluate all of the surfaces. Similarly, this is done for the labial mucosa. The opening of Stensen's (parotid) duct can be found along the buccal mucosa just opposite the maxillary second molar tooth. With one hand in the oral cavity and the other externally, the duct can be milked to assess for any purulent drainage or flow of clear saliva.

While the buccal and labial mucosa are retracted, the gingiva and dentition can be inspected. The gingiva is inspected for lesions, signs of inflammation, and hyperplasia. In an adult, there are 32 teeth in the full dentition. The overall dental health is evaluated including hygiene and evidence of caries. This will often provide insight into the patient's attitude toward general hygiene. Especially in trauma patients, it is important to evaluate dental occlusion. In normal occlusion, the mesiobuccal cusp of the first maxillary first molar should rest on the buccal groove of the mandibular first molar. However, given the variability of occlusion, it is often more useful to look at the wear facts on the teeth to assess for any subtle changes in occlusion. In addition, the patient's subjective sense of occlusion should be noted.

The oral tongue is then inspected for evidence of swelling, mucosal lesions, atrophy, fasciculations, and normal tongue variants such as geographic tongue or black hairy tongue. The patient is then asked to lift the tongue to the roof of the mouth to inspect the ventral surface of the tongue and floor of mouth. The lingual frenulum can be seen in the midline of the ventral tongue with the opening of Wharton's (submandibular) ducts on each side. In the case of submandibular sialadenitis, the gland and ducts can be milked to assess for purulent drainage. The lateral tongue, glossomandibular sulcus, and retromolar trigone are inspected with the use of a tongue blade to retract the tongue to the contralateral side. The tongue is then palpated, which can be aided by holding the tip of the tongue with a gauze with one hand while palpating with the other. The floor of mouth and submandibular gland is palpated bimanually with one hand intraorally and the other providing pressure externally.

With a tongue blade used to depress the tongue inferiorly, the hard and soft palates and oropharynx are inspected. In the uncooperative adult or child, it is useful to use two tongue blades to depress the tongue. The uvula and soft palate are inspected for swelling, lesions, or asymmetry. A bulge of the soft palate can be a sign of peritonsillar abscess or a deeper parapharyngeal mass. The posterior border of the soft palate is then followed laterally to the tonsillar fossae. The size of the tonsils can be graded on a scale of 0–4 according to Brodsky: 0 = no enlargement, 1 = tonsils occupy less than half of the transverse diameter of oropharynx, 2 = tonsils occupy half of the transverse diameter of oropharynx, 3 = tonsils occupy more than half of the transverse diameter of oropharynx, and 4 = tonsils occupy the entire transverse diameter of oropharynx, i.e., kissing tonsils (Brodsky 1989). Asymmetry of the tonsillar size may be a sign of infection, neoplasm, or normal variant, but in an asymptomatic adult, neoplasm should always be considered. The posterior pharyngeal wall is inspected for evidence of postnasal drainage, erythema, and cobblestoning. After inspecting the mucosal surfaces, the oropharynx is palpated. This part of the exam will initiate the gag reflex, and the patient should be warned of this. The finger is slid back along the dorsum of the tongue down to the base of tongue to palpate for any mucosal irregularities or submucosal lesions. The finger can be slid from the tongue onto the tonsils or tonsillar fossae to assess for any palpable abnormalities or asymmetric findings. Visual inspection of the base of tongue can be performed with either a laryngeal mirror or fiberoptic exam as will be discussed.

Larynx/Hypopharynx

The larynx and hypopharynx can be inspected using a laryngeal mirror, a flexible fiberoptic laryngoscope, or a rigid, angled scope. Prior to inspecting the larynx, the base of tongue, lingual tonsils, and valleculae can be visualized. Having the patient protrude his or her tongue will open up the vallecula.

When inspecting the larynx, it is useful to initially get a global view of the larynx to get a general sense of airway patency prior to focusing on each individual structure. Angioedema, epiglottitis, or bulky tumor may suggest impending airway compromise and help to determine the acuity of the situation. The larynx is best inspected with the patient's head in sniffing position by having the patient lean forward with the neck slightly flexed and head extended.

The epiglottis is evaluated on both its lingual surface and laryngeal surface down to the petiole. The aryepiglottic folds are then inspected and followed back to the arytenoids cartilages, interarytenoid area, and postcricoid area. The piriform sinuses are inspected by having the patient puff out his/her cheeks as if playing the trumpet or having them phonate in a high-pitched "eeee." Any lesions, pooling of secretions, mucus, or effacement are noted. The true vocal folds are then assessed for evidence of lesions including nodules, cysts, Reinke's edema, or mucosal lesions. True vocal fold mobility is first assessed by inspecting the folds during quiet inspiration when abduction should reflexively occur with inspiration. Active abduction is further assessed by having the patient sniff in through the nose. True vocal fold adduction can be assessed by having the patient make a prolonged "eeee" sound. It is sometimes helpful to have the patient alternate between phonation and sniffing by having the patient perform an "eeee"-sniff-"eeee"-sniff maneuver when assessing mobility. By looking beyond the glottis from above the vocal folds, the subglottis can be inspected for stenosis and lesions. A patient with dysphonia and a seemingly normal exam can be further evaluated with stroboscopy.

Neck

Knowledge of the palpable landmarks of the neck is essential when performing this part of the physical examination. There are several bony and cartilaginous landmarks that can be used as reference points. The mastoid process represents the area of attachment of the sternocleidomastoid muscle. Just inferior to the mastoid process, the transverse process of the first cervical vertebra (atlas) can sometimes be palpated deep to the digastrics muscle in patients with a thin neck. The hyoid bone sits midline just below the mandible and is best palpated by rocking it back and forth between two fingers. Inferior to this is the thyroid cartilage followed by the cricoid cartilage. It is often easier to identify the cricoid cartilage by placing a finger on the sternal notch, then sliding onto the trachea and following the trachea superiorly to the prominent cricoid cartilage.

The neck is divided into anterior and posterior triangles. The posterior triangle is bounded by the posterior border of the sternocleidomastoid muscle anteriorly, the clavicle inferiorly, and the trapezius posteriorly. This triangle can be further divided into the supraclavicular triangle below the posterior belly of the omohyoid muscle and the occipital triangle above. The anterior triangle of the neck is bound by the posterior border of the sternocleidomastoid posteriorly, the midline medially, and the mandible superiorly. The anterior triangle can be further divided into the submandibular triangle (above the digastric muscle), the submental triangle (above the hyoid bone between the anterior bellies of the digastric muscle), the muscular triangle (anterior to the anterior belly of the omohyoid muscle and the anterior border of the sternocleidomastoid muscle), and the carotid triangle (posterior to the anterior belly of the omohyoid muscle and anterior to the sternocleidomastoid muscle). Knowledge of the underlying structures in these triangles is essential.

The neck is first inspected for evidence of skin lesions, masses, scars, and asymmetries. Palpation is performed with the patient's head in a neutral to slightly flexed position. Palpation is performed bilaterally in a pattern that will cover all areas of the neck including the parotid gland. When palpating the thyroid gland, one hand should be used to stabilize the thyroid, while the other assesses for nodules or enlargement of the lobe by rolling the fingers over the lobe on the other side. Having the patient extend his/her neck will make the thyroid gland more prominent. Having the patient swallow during thyroid examination will cause the thyroid gland to elevate and aid in identifying abnormalities.

The parotid gland and preauricular and retroauricular nodes are palpated noting any lymphadenopathy or parotid masses. The submandibular triangle is palpated, and the underlying submandibular gland is delineated. Bimanual palpation is performed with one finger palpating the floor of mouth and the other hand palpating the gland externally. The submental triangle can be palpated in a similar fashion.

In addition to lymph nodes, there are a variety of congenital and acquired neck masses that may be found during palpation. Any mass should be characterized by location, size, consistency, tenderness, mobility, and overlying skin changes. If a midline mass is found, the patient should be asked to swallow to evaluate for elevation of the mass which would suggest a thyroglossal duct cyst.

For lymphadenopathy, there is a classification system endorsed by the AAO-HNS that is used to denote the location of enlarged lymph nodes.

References

Brodsky L (1989) Modern assessment of tonsil and adenoid. Pediatr Clin North Am 36:1551–1569

House JW, Brackmann DE (1985) Facial nerve grading system. Otolaryngol Head Neck 93(2):146–147

HIV

▶ Head and Neck Manifestations of AIDS

Hoarseness

▶ Larynx, Neurological Disorders

Hoarseness and Pediatric Voice Disorders

Karen B. Zur
Department of Otorhinolaryngology-Head and Neck Surgery, The Children's Hospital of Philadelphia, Perelman School of Medicine, The University of Pennsylvania, Philadelphia, PA, USA

Synonyms

Dysphonia

Definition

A child is described as having a voice problem if the voice is distracting or unpleasant to listeners and is abnormal enough to interfere with communication (Wilson 1987).

Diagnosis

The evaluation of a dysphonic child is best done by a multidisciplinary team compromised of an otolaryngologist and a speech language pathologist (SLP) in the setting of a voice clinic. Additional input from the child's pediatrician, the child's parents, and possibly other specialists (gastroenterologist, pulmonologist, neurologist, allergist) prove to be invaluable in certain circumstances. Children are initially oriented to the entire voice clinic team and then are evaluated with a thorough history and physical by an advanced practice nurse or physician's assistant. A pediatric voice history including the onset and progression of symptoms, voice variability, developmental history, typical voice activities, and psychosocial environment is completed. Particular attention is focused on the functional, structural, and neurological aspects of the voice. Other factors such as allergies, medications, asthma, and reflux are important to explore during the evaluation process. At the Voice Clinic, the parents fill out a Pediatric Voice Handicap Index (pVHI), a recent adaption of the adult voice handicap index (VHI) (Appendix 1). It is a 23 question validated tool, created in 2005 for the dysphonic child to evaluate the functional, emotional, and physical impact of a voice disorder on their daily activities (Zur et al. 2007). It is a useful tool to follow the child's dysphonia through medical, surgical, and behavioral modifications. Other quality-of-life surveys used at other centers include the Pediatric Voice Outcomes Survey (PVOS) (Hartnick 2002) and the Pediatric Voice-Related Quality-of-Life Questionnaire (PV-RQOL) (Boseley et al. 2006).

An experienced speech language pathologist then performs subjective and objective evaluations of the voice, including an acoustic and perceptual evaluation. The objective data is obtained using a computerized system. Various programs exist to record and analyze the voice. Objective assessments of a child's voice include measurements of fundamental frequency (pitch); range, sound pressure (loudness); intensity perturbation (shimmer); and frequency perturbation (jitter). The combination of subjective and objective measures helps the speech pathologist generate a systemic and standardized way to evaluate and review patients' data and allow for a standardized means of communicating the findings to other specialists and care providers.

Voice recordings are noninvasive and well tolerated by the patients. An electroglottography (EGG) uses surface electrodes to measure the glottic cycle and assess basic objective measures such as pitch and jitter as well as vocal hyperfunction in the case of incomplete glottic closure. This test is less commonly performed in children.

Further, aerodynamic measurements can provide a more detailed understanding of the glottal airflow and subglottic pressure. Currently, aerodynamics equipment is available through Kay Pentax. It was developed for use in adults; however, standardization is underway for use in children as well. The aerodynamic measurements combined with the objective and subjective voice data give a useful picture of the nature of the voice pathology.

Once the speech language pathologist completes their evaluation, the otolaryngologist then performs a thorough history and physical, including video stroboscopy/laryngoscopy to best evaluate vocal fold pathology. Children more commonly have limitations in tolerating stroboscopy than adults. Both rigid video stroboscopy and flexible video stroboscopy/laryngoscopy provide valuable information. Rigid video stroboscopy allows for a very clear picture with a narrow depth of field, but it does lead to a higher gagging rate. Flexible stroboscopy causes less gagging and allows for better visualization of connected speech. In the past, images from the flexible laryngoscopes were poorer in quality than the rigid ones. However, with the recent advent of chip-in-tip technology (Kay Pentax, Olympus) the image quality obtained in the flexible laryngoscopes compared to the rigid scopes is nearly equal. Both flexible and rigid stroboscopy are important tools in the evaluation of a dysphonia.

Certain other specific tasks have been designed to accommodate children's shorter attention span while providing quick and accurate information. Oral-motor assessment of facial motion including range of motion, strength, speed, and coordination helps to assess neurologic involvement of the presenting voice disorder. Sampling of speech allows the speech pathologist to assess the voice quality with the GRBAS scale (Grade, Roughness, Breathiness, Asthenia, Strain) (Hirano 1981). Other perceptual assessments of speech such as child's alertness, muscle tone, temperament, emotional maturity, and social interaction are most easily assessed in interactions with the caregiver or sibling during free play (Stuart 2013). If the child is unwilling to play freely, then a structured activity such as reading a book or telling a story can be helpful in the evaluation process. Those noted to have poor attention or trouble socially interacting may need more directed behavioral therapy in conjunction with treatment of their voice disorder (or they may not be able to participate in

formal voice therapy – this capability is established during a voice clinic session as well).

Respiratory breathing patterns during speech can impact speech. Children naturally take more frequent breaths than adults but may not coordinate breathing with speech. History may note a child that "works" to finish their sentences or has increasing hoarseness as the day progresses. Maximum phonation time can help to measure the child's efficiency of speech. Pitch and volume measurements can help to map out the flexibility of the child's voice. Many with vocal disorders have certain inflexibility in their vocal range that negatively impacts their voice quality. This inflexibility can manifest as pitch inflexibility, volume inflexibility, or an inflection abnormality.

Differential Diagnosis and Management

Laryngopharyngeal Reflux

The incidence of gastroesophageal and laryngopharyngeal reflux in children is difficult to assess. Many infants "spit up," but a smaller proportion present to the otolaryngologist with dysphonia. Infants and children who do present with persistent dysphonia should be evaluated to ensure that reflux is not the cause or contributor to the symptoms. It has been reported that 71% of ex-premature children have resolution of reflux by 18 months of age (Khalaf et al. 2001). The higher prevalence of infantile reflux is multifactorial: anatomical (due to an obtuse angle of His), neurological (due to transient lower esophageal sphincter relaxation), and physiological (due to larger food bolus and supine feeding positioning).

Findings on laryngoscopy that are suggestive of laryngopharyngeal reflux include hyperemia and/or edema of the supraglottic larynx and interarytenoid regions; edema of the true vocal folds; and cobblestoning of the trachea and hypopharynx. Objective testing would be useful to support the notion of the effects of pathologic reflux on the larynx; however, a highly specific and sensitive test for children does not yet exist. Various testing modalities exist including milk scan, barium swallow, Ph/Impedance probe testing, esophagogastroduodenoscopy (EGD) with biopsy, and more recently introduced Pepsin assays in bronchoalveolar lavage. Restech probe, a nasopharyngeal probe, is currently being tested in children and has been utilized in adults with some promise. Its benefit is looking for active acidic reflux at the level of the upper aerodigestive tract.

Benign Lesions of the Vocal Folds

Benign lesions of the vocal folds, such as nodules, polyps, or cysts lead to dysphonia due to the physical impediments to good glottic closure and vibration. Vocal fold nodules are the most common cause of dysphonia in children and are more common in boys than girls (Shah et al. 2004) in a bimodal distribution (3–5 years old and 8–10 years old). They are composed of fibronectin deposits layered in the superficial lamina propria of the vocal folds. These lesions are associated with thicker collagen in the basement membrane and typically present at the midportion of the vocal fold. An initial insult leads to the inflammatory deposit, which is exacerbated by repeated strain on the voice to overcome the dysphonia. This "weighted mid-fold" causes further trauma with repeated use.

A study analyzing the outcome of children with nodules noted that 44% achieve normal voice in adolescence (De Bodt et al. 2007), with few proceeding to surgical intervention. In order to help improve the voice, the typical therapy includes voice and behavioral therapy. Shah and Nuss noted that 75% of patients exhibit muscle tension dysphonia, which improves with voice rest and worsens with repeated voice use (Shah et al. 2004). It is important to rule out laryngopharyngeal reflux as well, as the inflammatory effect of the reflux can exacerbate the size and character of the nodules. Surgical intervention is extremely rare and may result in scarring and poor outcomes.

Vocal fold cysts (congenital or acquired) present similarly to vocal fold nodules. Congenital cysts are either mucus retention cysts or epidermal cysts. Cysts may also occur following a course of intubation and may present on the vocal fold or in the subglottis, effecting vocal fold vibration and airflow through the glottis, thus leading to hoarseness. The cysts are typically unilateral but may cause a reactive lesion on the contralateral vocal fold. These are distinguished from vocal fold nodules by video stroboscopy and do not improve with voice and behavior therapy. Surgical excision with careful microlaryngoscopy is typically required, with careful removal of the entire cyst wall to prevent recurrence.

Vocal fold polyps are inflammatory lesions forming on the superficial layer of the vocal fold and, similar to vocal fold cysts, are not amenable to voice and behavior therapy. Surgical excision with careful microlaryngoscopy is typically required. Cold dissection is the standard surgical procedure.

Malignant lesions of the larynx are uncommon in children, but if any suspicion arises, an intraoperative endoscopic biopsy should be performed. In children, the most frequent malignant lesions are squamous cell carcinoma and rhabdomyosarcoma.

Laryngeal Webs

Laryngeal webs may be congenital or acquired and typically affect the anterior margin of the vocal folds. As a result, the vibration of the true margin of the vocal fold is lost affecting vocalization quality. The most common causes of acquired laryngeal webs are due to interventions at the anterior commissure, laryngotracheal reconstruction, and thermal injury from laser or fire.

Congenital airway webs, 75% of which are glottic, are formed due to a failure in recanalization of the glottis during development. A narrowed cricoid is associated with congenital glottic webs. Velocardiofacial syndrome, a genetic deletion of chromosome 22q, is associated with congenital webs. Therefore, all congenital webs should have a genetic workup (FISH testing for deletion 22q) in their treatment plan (Miyamoto et al. 2004). Laryngeal webs are difficult to treat, as the goal is to restore a normal vibrating vocal fold with proper propagation of the mucosal wave. Typically cold sharp dissection is used in an endoscopic fashion, with or without placement of a keel to try and prevent reformation of the glottis web. If the cricoid is severely narrowed, a laryngotracheoplasty may be indicated.

Juvenile Recurrent Respiratory Papillomatosis

Juvenile recurrent respiratory papillomatosis (RRP) is the most common neoplasm of the pediatric airway and is a more aggressive variant than the adult-onset type. RRP is caused by the human papilloma virus (HPV) (Derkay and Darrow 2006), with HPV-6 and HPV-11 as the most common RRP-related subtypes (Wiatrak et al. 2004). HPV-11 was noted to be a more aggressive subtype in RRP formation (Wiatrak et al. 2004). Control of HPV infectivity is important in treating further spread of disease, and the recent advent of the quadrivalent HPV vaccine for women addresses HPV serotypes 6, 11, 16, and 18. This vaccine will hopefully help eradicate this difficult-to-treat condition.

Dysphonia is often the initial presenting symptom of a child with RRP, and it may progress to stridor and respiratory distress if untreated. Seventy-five percent of children with juvenile RRP initially present before age 5 (Derkay and Darrow 2006).

Direct visualization of the larynx and airway is important, and a bedside flexible laryngoscopy can help assess the extent of disease and whether it is critically obstructing the airway. Those children with a compromised airway should be evaluated in the more controlled operating room setting since surgical treatment is the mainstay of therapy for RRP. The papillomas can vary from small sessile lesions to large bulky and obstructive lesions. The challenge of management is to provide good voice and swallowing while maintaining an excellent airway with a disease known to have a latent, recurrent component. Careful microscopic laryngeal dissection is the gold standard for RRP.

Currently, microscopic dissection with cold instrumentation is most commonly used, with the powered microdebrider the most preferred (Schraff et al. 2004). Other surgical tools used for removal of the papillomatous lesions include the pulsed-dye lasers and newer CO2 lasers devices. The goal is to remove the lesion without undue thermal injury to the underlying vocal fold.

While the mainstay of treatment is surgical debulking and removal of clinically significant lesions, adjuvant therapy helps to provide additional therapy targeted to prevent or manage distal spread and to increase the time needed between surgical procedures. This is typically recommended to children needing four or more surgical interventions a year, which accounts up to 20% of those with juvenile RRP (Schraff et al. 2004). Various intralesional and systemic therapies are being investigated, and to date, no ideal treatment for RRP has been established. Some of the therapeutic interventions include Cidofovir, Interferon alpha, retinoid acid, indole-3-carbinol, Celebrex (Cox 2 inhibitor), retinoic acid, acyclovir, heat-shock protein E7, and epidermal-growth factor receptor blocker.

Neurogenic Voice Disorders

Neurogenic voice disorders include vocal fold paralysis/paresis and spasmodic dysphonia. Vocal fold paralysis/paresis may be congenital or acquired in nature. Iatrogenic causes include birth trauma, cardiac surgery, and surgical excision of central nervous system (CNS) tumors. Nontraumatic etiologies include neurogenic, infectious, or idiopathic causes.

The nerve supply of the vocal fold musculature is from the vagus nerve, which supplies both the superior laryngeal nerve (SLN) and recurrent laryngeal nerve (RLN). The particularly long pathways of the recurrent laryngeal nerves – the right RLN traveling around the right subclavian artery and left RLN traveling around the aorta – make the nerves particularly vulnerable to surgical stretch, trauma-related stretch injury, and vascular abnormalities. Cardiac and vascular abnormalities, such as vascular rings, ventricular septal defects, and patent ductus arteriosus have been associated with concomitant vocal fold palsies (Dedo 1979); however, iatrogenic injury due to the surgical repair of cardiac lesions is a more likely etiology for paralysis.

Birth trauma–related vocal fold paresis is typically associated with a forceps delivery, which places a traction injury on the recurrent laryngeal nerve. About 21% of bilateral vocal fold pareses have been attributed to birth trauma (Emery and Fearon 1984).

Central neurogenic causes include structural abnormality, such as Arnold-Chiari malformation, cerebral palsy, tumors, or leukodystrophies. In the case of Arnold-Chiari, patients frequently present with bilateral vocal fold paresis due to the typical inferior cerebellar tonsil displacement and vagal rootlet traction, although unilateral paresis has also been reported (deGaudemar et al. 1996). Other causes of vocal fold paresis include infectious causes (tuberculosis, West Nile virus, Lyme, poliomyelitis, pneumococcus, other viral infections) (Amin and Koufman 2001), intubation, foreign bodies, and chemotherapy (Burns and Shotton 1998).

The incidence of idiopathic unilateral vocal fold paresis in children ranges from 7% to 41% depending on the study (Cohen et al. 1982; Zbar and Smith 1996).

Evaluation of vocal fold paresis involves a detailed birth, family, and surgical history. Exam should note the nature of the stridor and its correlation with respiration, the presence of suprasternal or substernal retractions, the presence of any craniofacial abnormalities, masses, or surgical scars. A cranial nerve exam is essential in picking up other subtle associated findings. Flexible fiberoptic laryngoscopy allows visualization of the vocal folds to assess the level of mobility (if any) and also helps to assess whether there is any decreased sensation in the supraglottis. The direct view allows the evaluation of pooled secretions in the case of a patient at risk of aspiration. If a flexible fiberoptic laryngoscopy is not tolerated, a rigid exam in the operating room yields excellent visualization and allows the surgeon to rule out vocal fold fixation by palpating the cricoarytenoid joint.

A swallowing evaluation should be performed in there is any history of feeding issues as well. The commonly used modalities in children include a bedside clinical evaluation, as well as utilization of a modified barium swallow and/or a functional endoscopic evaluation of swallowing (FEES).

Imaging should be considered if there is no clear iatrogenic etiology of the vocal fold immobility. Laryngeal electromyography (EMG) is another useful tool in distinguishing vocal fold fixation from neurogenic paresis. This is easily done in the awake, cooperative adult, but relies on percutaneous placement of EMG needles for monitoring. In children, it is rare for such cooperation, and general anesthesia is used if an EMG is deemed necessary.

Treatment of vocal fold paresis depends on the etiology of the paresis. Many mild cases only need observation, while the majority of more severe cases need surgical intervention. It is important to have an honest, open discussion of the potential interventions as the need for voice therapy and postoperative care is important to the success of the intervention. Injection laryngoplasty, in which a filler material is injected into the paraglottic space, help medialize the immobile vocal fold. This allows for better closure and better voicing but does potentially narrow the airway. Materials for injection include autologous fat, several formulations of hydroxylapatite, micronized alloderm, and absorbable gelatin foam. Teflon was a material used in the past but is rarely being used currently due to the risk of granulation formation (O'Leary and Grillone 2006).

The Isshiki type I medialization thyroplasty is a more permanent solution to the glottic insufficiency that results from unilateral vocal fold paralysis. It improves vocalization by directly placing a permanent implant in the paraglottic space through an open procedure. Implants materials include cartilage, silastic, and Gore-Tex. In children, it is important to note that the vocal folds lie more inferiorly within the thyroid cartilage compared to the adult larynx, and so the procedure needs to be modified to accommodate

this developmental difference. This procedure can be combined with an arytenoid adduction if deemed necessary by the anatomy. The author defers the use of this form of surgical intervention in young children due to the risks of migration and airway obstruction. Furthermore, since children are not good candidates for an awake open procedure (which is how adult medialization thyroplasties are performed), the precise placement of the graft material is more challenging.

For this reason, surgical procedures that help augment vocalization without disrupting the laryngeal framework may be more appealing. Laryngeal reinnervation through a primary neurorrhaphy can help to provide tone to the deinnervated laryngeal musculature. Multiple nerves have been brought to anastomose with the recurrent laryngeal nerve. The ansa cervicalis is the typical nerve of choice and it is identified just deep to the omohyoid muscle in the neck and anastomosed with the RLN proximal to the larynx. This anastomosis provides neurogenic signals to the laryngeal musculature, providing tone and bulk to the thyroarytenoid muscle, as well as improved interarytenoid strength which improves posterior glottis closure. It is important to note that vocal fold motion per se is not restored. This procedure is often done in combination with a temporary injection laryngoplasty (with a short-term agent) to provide immediate relief of dysphonia while the reinnervation begins to take effect months later.

Conclusion

The field of pediatric laryngology is an emerging area of otolaryngology that has been undervalued in the past. The significance of hoarseness in children cannot be understated. Families often describe social isolation and academic impact due to voicing issues, which can affect a child's intelligibility and communication. The evaluation of pediatric hoarseness is important, mostly to rule out an underlying neoplasm or surgically correctable lesion. The value of conservative management cannot be overlooked either. This is crucial in a child whose larynx is still undergoing development and has not yet reached its adult state (late teen years). Therefore, it is recommended to evaluate the larynx, assess for the feasibility of voice therapy/rehabilitation, and offer surgical management when necessary.

Cross-References

▶ Vocal Cord Surgery

References

Amin AR, Koufman JA (2001) Vagal neuropathy after upper respiratory infection: a viral etiology? Am J Otolaryngol 22:251–256

Boseley ME, Cunningham MJ, Volk MS, Hartnick CJ (2006) Validation of the pediatric voice related quality-of-life survey. Arch Otolaryngol Head Neck Surg 132(7):717–720

Burns BV, Shotton JC (1998) Vocal fold palsy following vinca alkaloid treatment. J Laryngol Otol 112:485–487

Cohen SR, Keller KA, Birns JW et al (1982) Laryngeal paralysis in children: a long-term retrospective study. Ann Otol Rhinol Laryngol 91:417–424

De Bodt MS, Ketelslagers K, Peeters T et al (2007) Evolution of vocal fold nodules from childhood to adolescence. J Voice 21(2):151–156

Dedo DD (1979) Pediatric vocal cord paralysis. Laryngoscope 89:1378–1384

deGaudemar I, Roudaire M, Francois M et al (1996) Outcome of laryngeal paralysis in neonates: a long term retrospective study of 113 cases. Int J Pediatr Otorhinolaryngol 34:101–110

Derkay CS, Darrow DH (2006) Recurrent respiratory papillomatosis. Ann Otol Rhinol Laryngol 115:1–11

Emery PJ, Fearon B (1984) Vocal cord palsy in pediatric practice: a review of 71 cases. Int J Pediatr Otorhinolaryngol 8:147–154

Hartnick CJ (2002) Validation of a pediatric voice quality-of-life instrument: the pediatric voice outcome survey. Arch Otolaryngol Head Neck Surg 128(8):919–922

Hirano M (1981) Clincial examination of the voice. Springer-VerlagWein, New York

Khalaf MN, Porat R, Brodsky NL, Bhandari V (2001) Clinical correlations in infants in the neonatal intensive care unit with varying severity of gastroesophagealrelux. J Gastroenterol Nutr 32:45–49

Miyamoto RC, Cotton RT, Rope AF et al (2004) Association of anterior glottis webs with velocardiofacial syndrome (chromosome 22q11.2 deletion). Otolaryngol Head Neck Surg 130(4):415–417

O'Leary MA, Grillone GA (2006) Injection laryngoplasty. Otorlaryngol Clin North Am 39:43–54

Schraff S, Derkay CS, Burke B et al (2004) American society of pediatric otolaryngology members' experience with recurrent respiratory papillomatosis and the use of adjuvant therapy. Arch Otolaryngol Head Neck Surg 130:1039–1042

Shah RK, Woodnorth GH, Glynn A, Nuss RC (2004) Pediatric vocal nodules: correlation with perceptual voice analysis. Int J PediatrOtorhinolaryngol 68(4):409–412

Stuart S (2013) Speech and language disorders. In: Batshaw ML, Roizen NJ, Lotrecchiano GR (eds) Children with Disabilities, 7th edn. Paul H. Brooks Publishing, Baltimore

Wiatrak BJ, Wiatrak DW, Broker TR et al (2004) Recurrent respiratory papillomatosis: a longitudinal study comparing severity associated with human papillomas viral types 6 and 11 and other risk factors in a large pediatric population. Laryngoscope 114:1–23

Wilson DK (1987) Voice problems of children, 3rd edn. Williams & Wilkins, Baltimore

Zbar RI, Smith RJ (1996) Vocal fold paralysis in infants twelve months of age or younger. Otolaryngol Head Neck Surg 114:18–21

Zur KB, Cotton S, Kelchner L, Baker S, Weinrich B, Lee L (2007) Pediatric voice handicap index (pVHI): a new tool for evaluating pediatric dysphonia. Int J Pediatr Otorhinolaryngol 71(1):77–82

Horizontal Partial Laryngectomy

▶ Supraglottic Laryngectomy

Hormone Replacement Following Thyroidectomy

Honey E. East, Shema Ahmad and Christian A. Koch
Department of Medicine/Endocrinology,
Division of Endocrinology, University of Mississippi Medical Center, Jackson, MS, USA

Synonyms

Postsurgical hypoparathyroidism; Postsurgical hypothyroidism

Definition

Postsurgical hypothyroidism: Need to replace thyroid hormone (levothyroxine and/or T3 = triiodothyronine) after the surgical attempt to remove the thyroid gland completely, subtotally, or partially. If thyroid surgery has resulted in additional permanent or temporary damage of parathyroid gland function, postsurgical hypoparathyroidism may ensue requiring the need to administer calcium.

Basic Characteristics

Epidemiology and Etiology

With improved imaging techniques, detection of thyroid or neck abnormalities requiring surgical intervention has become increasingly common. Dependent on factors including iodine sufficiency, known or unknown exposure to radiation, family history, and others, the prevalence of thyroid nodules varies and can be up 25% or more. Most thyroid nodules are benign and may require surgical intervention only if symptoms related to mass effect or thyroid dysfunction develop. Thyroid and parathyroid function must also be evaluated if neck tissue is removed or extensive damage is done to local tissues during neck surgery, for instance, because of head and neck sarcoma, squamous cell carcinoma, and other reasons. Parathyroid function inadequacy is suspected if the serum calcium becomes low after total/subtotal thyroidectomy or other surgery which may involve the parathyroid glands. In such cases, calcium and vitamin D are administered to combat symptoms of hypocalcemia. On experimental protocols, patients with permanent hypoparathyroidism may also receive parathyroid hormone injections.

Preoperative thyroid function, the presence of anti-TPO antibodies, and the extent of thyroid removal (if less than 6 ml/6 g of thyroid tissue are remaining, LT4 replacement is always necessary) are important factors in determining need and/or extent of thyroid hormone replacement, typically done with levothyroxine (LT4). Since the goal of total thyroidectomy is to remove all thyroid tissue, hormone replacement is necessary. By definition, subtotal thyroidectomy usually leaves only a few (approximately 3) grams of thyroid tissue remaining; therefore, thyroxine replacement is also necessary. After thyroid lobectomy, a minority of patients require replacement therapy while patients undergoing partial thyroidectomy or hemithyroidectomy (approx. 28% of cases) are also at risk for resultant postsurgical hypothyroidism. If replacement is needed, lower dosages of LT4 may be appropriate depending upon the amount of functioning thyroid tissue removed and left behind.

Replacement

The preferred replacement for thyroid insufficiency is levothyroxine. LT4 monotherapy provides T4 as well as T3 through peripheral deiodination at a normal or near-normal ratio of T3/T4. Generic hormone preparations have 80–125% bioequivalence to their parent drug. Therefore, a patient who is prescribed 100 mcg of LT4 could receive inconsistent dosages such as 80 mcg 1 month and 125 mcg the next. Name brand replacement is preferred to avoid this occurrence. Desiccated thyroid is no longer a preferred treatment as it provides more T3, resulting in an abnormal T3/T4 ratio in variable, inconsistent dosages. Triiodothyroxine is not a preferred treatment as it is quickly absorbed and blood levels are inconsistent. If intravenous replacement is necessary, then 50% of oral dose of levothyroxine is given as IV replacement. Adrenal function should always be evaluated before thyroid hormone replacement as cardiovascular collapse is possible if thyroid hormone is given to a patient who is adrenally insufficient. In the case of adrenal insufficiency, corticosteroids need to be administered before replacing thyroid hormone, especially when T3 is used instead or in addition to LT4.

Timing

The timing of initiating thyroid replacement is based on the 7-day half-life of LT4. If a euthyroid state exists before surgery, then satisfactory amounts of LT4 remain for days after surgery depending on the individual baseline free thyroxine level (i.e., 0.8–1.8 ng). Therefore, immediate initiation of replacement often is not necessary and may be held in cases when there are barriers to oral replacement, such as prolonged "nothing per mouth" status. It is advisable to ensure thyroid hormone is started before hospital discharge to avoid the possibility of inadvertent omission of LT4 replacement therapy. In thyrotoxic patients, the length of time before starting replacement should be based on preoperative (baseline) levels of thyroid hormone (free thyroxine, T3) as well as comorbid conditions (i.e., coronary artery disease, heart failure, and hypertension). For patients who were preoperatively hypothyroid and already on LT4, replacement with LT4 should be continued through the perioperative period, while the dose of LT4 should be adjusted based on the amount of functioning thyroid tissue removed.

After total thyroidectomy, a dosage of 1.6–1.7 mcg/kg of ideal body weight is generally recommended. In the current pandemic of obesity with many people being overweight or frankly obese, it often is not easy to achieve thyroid homeostasis as defined by a free T4 and TSH within normal range.

TSH should not be checked until at least 6 weeks on a stable dose of thyroid hormone replacement therapy. At 6-week follow-up for patients who are euthyroid prior to surgery, TSH should be 0.5–2.0 mIU/L. If TSH is not within normal range, then one should generally adjust by 25–50 mcg every 6 weeks until TSH is at goal level. If TSH levels are abnormal before surgery, then it may take longer than 6 weeks to reach steady state because of the resetting in the hypothalamic-pituitary-thyroid axis. In that case, at 6-week follow-up, free T4 values are used to evaluate adequacy of replacement instead of TSH levels. Measuring free T4 levels is preferred over total T4 or T3 because T4 levels are dependent on binding proteins and T3 has a half-life that is about 1 day with more fluctuant levels.

Preoperative Hyperthyroidism

Although current nonsurgical therapies such as radio-active iodine ablation and antithyroid medications are available for the treatment of thyrotoxicosis, clear indications exist for surgical removal of the thyroid. Regarding the most frequent cause of hyperthyroidism, Graves's disease, removal of the thyroid gland is indicated in patients with severe and moderate to severe Graves' orbitopathy or such patients who might have concomitant suspicious (for cancer) thyroid nodules. Thyroidectomy may stabilize or reverse Graves' associated ophthalmopathy and is the treatment modality for (radioactive iodine) resistant disease. Total thyroidectomy is more effective at improving Graves' ophthalmopathy than subtotal thyroidectomy.

Surgery is the preferred treatment for massive thyroid enlargement with compressive symptoms, a dominant nodule (quasi as open biopsy on grounds of a multinodular goiter), and patient preference. To prevent recurrence, near-total or total thyroidectomy is preferred over subtotal thyroidectomy. In cases of amiodarone-induced thyrotoxicosis where amiodarone must be continued, thyroidectomy is considered a relatively safe and sometimes life-saving option. In cases where thyrotoxicosis must be quickly resolved, such as pending cardiac transplantation, surgery should be considered. Certainly, thyroid cancer is an indication for thyroidectomy, sometimes performed with (central) lymph node dissection.

Adequate time should elapse before starting thyroid hormone replacement therapy in previously thyrotoxic patients. Keeping in mind that the half-life of LT4 is 7 days, this could be several days. In previously

thyrotoxic patients, TSH values within normal range are considered the goal of replacement therapy; however, as stated above, TSH may not return to normal values until months after thyroidectomy. In this case, free T4 levels should guide replacement adequacy. If comorbid conditions such as heart disease, cardiac arrhythmias, or osteoporosis exist, then one may adjust TSH and/or free T4 goals to patient needs.

Preoperative Hypothyroidism

Unless other conditions coexist, goal values for TSH in patients who are hypothyroid before thyroid surgery are within normal limit range. However, TSH takes significantly longer to equilibrate than free T4. Therefore, if there is a significant elevation of TSH prior to thyroid surgery, at 6-week follow-up appointments free T4 should guide accuracy of thyroid hormone replacement therapy.

Preoperative Euthyroidism

The most common indication for thyroid surgery in benign multinodular goiter is compressive symptoms. Total or near-total thyroidectomy is preferred over partial thyroidectomy because of the increased rate of the need for completion thyroidectomy due to incidentally diagnosed well-differentiated thyroid carcinomas. TSH levels should not be checked until at least 6 weeks after stable doses of LT4 have been administered. Approximately 17% of preoperatively (on LT4) euthyroid patients undergoing hemithyroidectomy and 42% of preoperatively (on LT4) euthyroid patients undergoing subtotal thyroidectomy require postoperative dose adjustments of LT4 (Schaeffer 2010).

Non-differentiated Thyroid Cancers

Anaplastic and medullary thyroid cancers are considered non-differentiated for which the goal of replacement therapy after surgery is a TSH within the normal range. Medullary thyroid cancer is frequently associated with multiple endocrine neoplasia type 2 (MEN2). MEN2 carriers often have a *RET* germline mutation and *RET* mutational testing is routinely used to diagnose the carrier state, even in patients with apparently sporadic medullary thyroid cancer. Genotype-phenotype correlations in patients with *RET* germline mutations can facilitate optimal timing of preventive thyroidectomy. In general, total thyroidectomy during childhood is recommended for almost all MEN2 carriers.

Well-Differentiated Thyroid Cancers

Papillary and follicular thyroid cancers are considered well-differentiated thyroid cancers. Total or near-total thyroidectomy is recommended for patients diagnosed with these cancers.

TSH may represent a growth factor and aggravate papillary or follicular carcinoma of the thyroid; thus, TSH suppressive therapy with levothyroxine is recommended. Goal TSH should be 0.1–0.5 mIU/L for low risk patients and <0.01 mIU/L for intermediate and high risk patients as well as for those with persistent disease after total thyroidectomy. For TSH suppressive therapy, the dose of LT4 treatment should be calculated by 2.1 mcg/kg/day of ideal body weight. After 5–10 years surveillance if serum thyroglobulin levels are undetectable, consideration is given to decreasing the dosage to reach a low normal TSH value in appropriate patients. Of note, we recommend individualization of TSH goals in patients with differentiated thyroid cancer, depending on individual risk factors, comorbidities, and age, i.e., heart conditions including atrial fibrillation, osteoporosis, and others.

Diagnostic and therapeutic interventions in patients with differentiated thyroid cancer often require elevated TSH levels. Therefore, recombinant TSH can be given or thyroid hormone replacement may be withheld. In the case of (whole body) uptake scans or radioactive iodine treatment, LT4 must be held for approximately 4 weeks. Since T3 has a shorter half-life than T4, it may be given until 2 weeks prior to the procedure (whole body scan and/or serum thyroglobulin level, radioactive iodine therapy) when withdrawal of treatment is deemed to be adverse to the patient. The T3 dose should be approximately one third of the appropriate LT4 dose.

Special Populations

Patients who undergo thyroid surgery for non-thyroid conditions such as trauma, laryngeal or pharyngo-laryngeal cancer including squamous cell cancer require LT4 replacement therapy to maintain normal physiologic levels (TSH within normal limits). Children who undergo thyroid surgery may need higher doses of LT4 replacement and doses up to 10 mcg/kg are used (Table 1). The elderly may require lower doses of thyroid hormone replacement since this population is at increased risk for treatment-related

Hormone Replacement Following Thyroidectomy, Table 1 Levothyroxine replacement dose in various populations

Population	Initial dose of levothyroxine/ ideal body weight
General	1.6–1.7 mcg/kg
Children (8 months–10 years)	4–10 mcg/kg
Elderly	1.0 mcg/kg
Known CAD or arrhythmia	25 mcg
Pregnancy	Increased dose 1.8–2.0 mcg/kg
Osteoporosis	Decreased dose

CAD coronary artery disease

complications including cardiac arrhythmias and bone loss, leading to osteoporosis. In elderly patients, one may initiate LT4 doses based on 1.0 mcg/kg rather than 1.6–1.7 mcg/kg of ideal body weight. Patients with known cardiac disease should be started at 25 mcg of LT4 per day and adjusted every 6 weeks. In patients with osteoporosis, TSH levels should be maintained at the upper end of normal. Pregnant patients require higher levels of LT4 replacement therapy and failure to maintain adequate replacement can lead to fetal abnormalities. TSH levels of 0.5–2 mIU/L with a free T4 in the upper third of normal should be achieved in pregnant patients. Also, in order to become pregnant, fertility may be improved by aiming at a TSH of 2.5 mIU/L and lower in women of childbearing age.

Multiple medications interfere with thyroid replacement and adjustments need to be made based on coadministration or addition of these medications. For patients with central hypothyroidism undergoing thyroid surgery, monitoring and adjustments to treatment should be done based on free T4 levels and not TSH levels because of their inability to produce TSH. In this case, free T4 should generally be in the upper third of the reference range.

Medication Interactions

Approximately 80% of LT4 is absorbed from the GI tract, mainly in the jejunum and upper ileum. Acidic pH is required for proper absorption. Therefore, any medication(s) that lower the GI tract pH may decrease absorption of LT4 replacement. Similarly, malabsorption syndromes or medications that interfere with GI tract absorption decrease absorption of

Hormone Replacement Following Thyroidectomy, Table 2 Medications interfering with levothyroxine absorption

Decrease absorption
Calcium
Iron (sulfate)
Orlistat
Bile acid sequestrants
Raloxifene
Sevelamer
Polystyrene sulfonate
Sucralfate
Simethicone
Kayexalate
Proton pump inhibitors
Aging
Malabsorption
Increase metabolism
Carbamazepine
Rifampin
Theophylline
Phenobarbital
Phenytoin
Inhibition of 5-deiodinase
Dexamethasone
Propanolol
Cytokines
Increased Thyroxine-binding globulin effect (requires increase in LT4 therapy)
Estrogen including oral contraceptives
Pregnancy
Genetic predisposition

LT4. Medications that interfere with LT4 absorption should be taken 4 h apart from LT4. Since food products block absorption, it is recommended that LT4 replacement be given 30 min prior to food intake. Levothyroxine is preferably administered at the same time each day. Traditionally, LT4 is given before breakfast but recent studies suggest that evening replacement may be preferable. If a patient is unable to comply with the above recommendations, then consistent dosing conditions are necessary and vital and TSH and free T4 levels should be followed closely with adjustments as needed. Multiple prescription and over-the-counter medications interfere with metabolism and excretion of thyroid hormone, making monitoring for effect on LT4 replacement therapy necessary (Table 2).

Noncompliance

Noncompliance with medications is a common problem. Laboratory results of noncompliant patients are similar to the laboratory in patients who are not on adequate thyroid hormone replacement doses with elevations in TSH levels and low free T4 levels. However, recent compliance in anticipation of lab work may show an elevated TSH level and a free T4 level (recent intake of LT4) within normal range. Continued noncompliance with thyroid hormone replacement puts patients at increased risk for complications including heart disease. One clue to noncompliance is unchanged lab results in the face of increased thyroid hormone replacement doses. Since the half-life of thyroxin is 7 days, it is acceptable to have the patient visit the office and have a provider administer LT4 for directly observed therapy if noncompliance persists.

Conclusions

Thyroid hormone replacement is complex and depends on many factors including the amount of functioning thyroid tissue remaining, the need for TSH suppressive therapy, comorbid conditions, and concurrent medications. Levothyroxine (LT4) is the preferred treatment. In most cases, appropriateness of therapy is based on steady state TSH levels or TSH levels at goal for the respective underlying condition, i.e., well-differentiated thyroid cancer, elderly above age 65 years, etc. TSH and in some cases free T4 levels should be routinely monitored and adjustments of LT4 made as needed.

Cross-References

▶ Neck Dissection, Complications
▶ Endoscopic Thyroidectomy
▶ Thyroid Nodules, Evaluation
▶ Hypopharyngeal Squamous Cell Carcinoma
▶ Medullary Thyroid Cancer
▶ Neck Dissection Indications
▶ Parathyroidectomy
▶ Thyroid Physiology
▶ Thyroidectomy
▶ Thyroiditis
▶ Well-Differentiated Thyroid Cancer

References

Abalovich M, Amino N, Barbour LA et al (2007) Management of thyroid dysfunction during pregnancy and postpartum: an endocrine society clinical practice guideline. J Clin Endocrinol Metab 92:S1–S47

Agarwal G, Aggarwal V (2008) Is total thyroidectomy the surgical procedure of choice for benign multinodular goiter? An evidence-based review. World J Surg 32:1313–1324

Ben-Shachar R, Eisenberg M, Huang S, Distefano JJ (2012) Simulation of post-thyroidectomy treatment alternatives for T3 or T4 replacement in pediatric thyroid cancer patients. Thyroid

Celi FS, Zemskova M, Linderman JD, Babar NI, Skarulis MC, Csako G, Wesley R, Costello R, Penzak SR, Pucino F (2010) The pharmacodynamic equivalence of levothyroxine and liiothyronine: a randomized, double-blind, cross-over study in thyroidectomized patients. Clin Endocrinol 72(5):709–715

Jensen E, Hyltoft PP, Blaabjerg O, Hansen PS, Brix TH, Kyvik KO, Hegedüs L (2004) Establishment of a serum thyroid stimulating hormone reference interval in healthy adults The importance of environmental factors including thyroid antibodies. Clin Chem Lab Med 42(7):824–832

Johner A, Griffith OL, Walker B, Wood L, Piper H, Wilkins G, Baliski C, Jones SJ, Wiseman SM (2011) Detection and management of hypothyroidism following thyroid lobectomy: evaluation of a clinical algorithm. Ann Surg Oncol 18(9):2548–2554

Jonklaas J (2010) Sex and age differences in levothyroxine dosage requirement. Endocr Pract 16(1):71–79

Jonklaas J, Davidson B, Bhagat S, Soldin SJ (2008) Triiodothyronine levels in athyreotic individuals during levothyroxine therapy. JAMA 299(7):769–777

Paschke R, Hegedüs L, Alexander E, Valcavi R, Papini E, Gharib H (2011) Thyroid nodule guidelines: agreement, disagreement and need for future research. Nat Rev Endocrinol 7(6):354–361

Schaeffler A (2010) Hormone replacement after thyroid and parathyroid surgery. Dtsch Arztebl Int 107(47):827–834

Stoll SJ, Pitt SC, Liu J, Schaefer S, Sippel RS, Chen H (2009) Thyroid hormone replacement after thyroid lobectomy. Surgery 146(4):554–558

Hounsfield Unit (HU)

Majid A. Khan and Todd A. Nichols
Division of NeuroRadiology, University of MS
Medical Center, Jackson, MS, USA

Definition

Hounsfield Unit is a density measurement tool utilized to differentiate between different tissues on the CT scan.

Cross-References

▶ Imaging Cystic Head and Neck Masses

HTLV-III

▶ Head and Neck Manifestations of AIDS

Human Nervous System

▶ Vestibular and Central Nervous System, Anatomy

Human Papillomavirus in Head and Neck Cancer

Alan R. Grimm
Department of Otolaryngology and Communicative Sciences, University of Mississippi Medical Center, Jackson, MS, USA

Definition

The human papillomavirus (HPV) is a diverse and ubiquitous DNA virus that has long been recognized as a cause of urogenital squamous cell malignancies. Although also theorized to play a role in head and neck malignancy, it is only relatively recently that a link to head and neck cancer has been identified. However, this development coincides with a noted increase in incidence of head and neck cancer of the oropharyngeal subsite at a time when overall tobacco consumption rates are declining in the United States. What is more, multiple studies now suggest that HPV status is a strong determinant of response to standard treatments and overall prognosis. It has even been proposed by some researchers that HPV-associated disease may indeed represent a unique and different disease process from traditional tobacco and alcohol-related head and neck squamous cell carcinoma (HNSCC). These facts only serve to heighten the imperative to better understand and define HPV's role in head and neck malignancy.

Pathophysiology

The human papillomavirus is an encapsulated double-stranded DNA virus with essentially 100 subtypes from the family Papillomaviridae. Viruses are categorized into high risk and low risk categories, based upon their propensity to undergo malignant transformation. Low risk variants such as HPV 6 and 11 are believed to cause benign papillomas, while HPV 16 and 18 are detected in malignant neoplasms. HPV infection takes place in proliferating basal epithelial cells. HPV gains access to the basal layer through breaks in the overlying epithelium. It is taken up by basal cells and eventually makes its way to the nucleus. It is here that viral replication takes place, and although the viral genome typically exists in an episomal state, it can eventually be integrated into host DNA. The viral genome can be divided into a coding and noncoding region, with the coding region being further subdivided into "E" (early) and "L" (late). The E region encodes for viral proteins E1-E7 which are involved in viral replication and gene expression, while L proteins are important in viral capsid formation.

Of particular interest in the study of malignant transformation are viral proteins E6 and E7. In HPV-associated tumors, the E6 and E7 proteins target critical cellular safeguards at multiple levels of control, thus allowing for aberrant cellular proliferation and immortality. E6, through enzymatic ubiquitination, tags the tumor suppressor gene p53, marking it for enzymatic degradation and preventing programmed cell death. Additionally, E6 may also activate telomerase, thus stabilizing the host cell chromosomes and allowing for continued progression through the cellular cycle. Meanwhile, E7 serves to tag and inactivate the pRb tumor suppressor gene. Rb participates in numerous gates of cell cycle control, including mitosis, cellular differentiation, and death. Further, E7 may be related to aberrant activity of some cyclin-dependent kinases involved in cell cycle progression, at least partly owing to an overexpression of p16. Although E6 and E7 are present in both high and low risk HPV strains, these viral oncogenes bind to their respective intracellular targets with much greater affinity in the high risk viruses. Another factor appears to be the inclusion of viral DNA into the host genome. Indeed, in cervical cancer, approximately 90% of tumors demonstrate viral DNA in an integrated form, and viral E6 and E7 proteins expressed from a source embedded in host DNA demonstrate greater ability for cellular transformation.

These mechanisms underlie a molecular distinction between non-HPV- and HPV-associated HNSCC. Unlike non-HPV-associated disease, wherein repeated and chronic alcohol and tobacco exposure causes DNA damage that commonly damages p53 and Rb, in HPV-associated tumors, these genes are still expressed and in fact may be expressed at higher levels. Their effects are simply blocked by the action of viral oncogenes. Similarly, a comparison between HPV-associated and non-HPV-associated HNSCC shows distinct differences in expression of certain tumor-related genes such as cyclin D and epidermal growth factor receptor as well as higher numbers of chromosomal alterations in non-HPV disease. For these reasons, as well as observed differences in prognosis to be discussed, HPV-associated HNSCC is increasingly viewed as a disease process distinct from non-HPV-associated disease.

Epidemiology

The overall incidence of HNSCC in the United States has declined over the past 40 years in concert with decreasing rates of tobacco use. However, the incidence of oropharyngeal SCC has increased, and this finding is echoed in several different countries. This rise is thought to be related to HPV. In Sweden, a review of banked tissue specimens has demonstrated increasing rates of HPV-associated oropharyngeal tumors. Indeed, although HPV DNA has been detected in tumors from all subsites of the head and neck, it is most commonly identified in oropharyngeal SCC, and it is most commonly the high risk HPV 16 subtype. Studies attempting to describe current rates of HPV association are highly variable and sometimes difficult to correlate, owing to different techniques for HPV detection. Nevertheless, a recent meta-analysis examining over 5,000 patients in 60 studies concluded that HPV prevalence in oropharyngeal cancers is approximately 35.6%. HPV is likely sexually acquired, and studies have shown that having a higher number of lifetime sexual partners does confer an increased risk of oropharyngeal cancer. In addition, patients with HPV-associated disease tend to be younger, herald from a higher socioeconomic background, and enjoy better dental and overall health. These patients also tend to have a less impressive history of alcohol and tobacco usage. Nevertheless, tobacco cannot be overlooked, as perhaps 10-30% of patients with HPV-associated disease report heavy usage.

Detection

In spite of the fact that several methods of detection for HPV have been described, some debate still remains as to the most effective practice. Various techniques, including measurement of HPV DNA, RNA, or protein products, have been studied. Polymerase chain reaction, or more familiarly PCR, is a sensitive tool used to detect and magnify HPV DNA when present in tumor cells. However, its specificity has been questioned in several studies. Furthermore, PCR is unable to provide the behavioral nature of the virus, i.e., whether the viral genome is episomal or integrated, or whether or not it is expressing its viral oncogenes. Quantitative PCR is an attempt to answer at least one of these questions by producing cDNA based upon copies of viral mRNA. The volume of cDNA is then quantified, thus giving one a proxy determination of the amount of viral transcription occurring in the cell. Both traditional and quantitative PCR share the common problem in that specificity is lacking as viral DNA from normal tissues surrounding the tumor will likewise be magnified when the specimen is analyzed.

Another test for viral DNA is in situ hybridization (ISH), wherein a DNA probe labeled with a radioactive or fluorescent marker is used to detect HPV DNA in a specimen. Then, using fine microscopy, HPV DNA can actually be visualized. This technique has the added benefit of being able to identify if the DNA is in an episomal or integrated form. However, successive application of this technique has shown deficiencies in sensitivity; further, it too fails to determine the biologic activity of the viral DNA.

A more ideal test would provide data regarding the biological activity of viral DNA, when present. Reverse transcriptase PCR, or RT-PCR, is a method in which viral mRNA is copied and then amplified. Although highly sensitive and specific, this test is currently very cumbersome and expensive, limiting its usage. Likewise, immunohistochemistry for detection of the p16 protein has been advocated, as this has been demonstrated to be elevated in tumors with HPV DNA. However, p16 is also elevated in some non-HPV-associated tumors, thus lowering specificity. Finally, similar techniques for detection of E6/E7 proteins have also been tried but at this time remain investigational. Therefore, current protocols call for some combination of the above techniques, with some combination of p16 and HPV ISH being most commonly advocated.

Clinical Relevance

Since the introduction and measurement of this new clinical variable, multiple retrospective and prospective studies have reported results mindful of HPV status. In keeping with its unique tumor biology and epidemiologic status, HPV-associated tumors respond differently to standard treatment regimens of chemotherapy and radiation. HPV positivity appears to confer a survival benefit to these patients. A recent study of over 400 patients with stage III or IV oropharyngeal SCC demonstrated significant differences in overall survival after three years in the subgroup of patients who demonstrated to be HPV-positive by p16 and ISH (82.4% vs. 57.1%, respectively). Several smaller studies highlight this finding. Moreover, this benefit seems to extend to locoregional control and progression-free survival and is not limited to patients treated only with nonsurgical therapies. Finally, several meta-analyses of studies containing reference to HPV status have confirmed this fact; importantly, though, this benefit appears to be limited only to oropharyngeal HPV-associated disease. In any event, given the improved performance and outcomes in patients with HPV-associated cancer, there is tremendous interest in studying whether treatment regimens can be de-intensified in these patients so as to save many of the short- and long-term toxicities of therapy. This matter awaits further study in future randomized control trials.

References

Allen CT (2010) Human papillomavirus and oropharynx cancer: biology, detection and clinical implication. Laryngoscope 120:1756–1772

Dayyani F et al (2010) Meta-analysis of the impact of human papillomavirus (HPV) on cancer risk and overall survival in head and neck squamous cell carcinomas (HNSCC). Head Neck Oncol 2:15

Doorbar J (2006) Molecular biology of human papillomavirus infection and cervical cancer. Clin Sci 110:525–541

D'Souza G et al (2007) Case-control study of human papillomavirus and oropharyngeal cancer. N Engl J Med 356(19):1944–1956

Du W, Pogoriler J (2005) Retinoblastoma family genes. Oncogene 25(38):5190–5200

Gillison ML, D'Souza G, Westra W et al (2008) Distinct risk factor profiles for human papillomavirus type 16-positive and human papillomavirus type 16-negative head and neck cancers. J Natl Cancer Inst 100:407–420

Kian Ang K et al (2010) Human papillomavirus and survival of patients with oropharyngeal cancer. N Engl J Med 363:24–35

Kreimer AR, Clifford GM, Boyle P, Franceschi S (2005) Human papillomavirus types in head and neck squamous cell carcinomas worldwide: a systematic review. Cancer Epidemiol Biomarkers Prev 14:467–475

Marur S, D'Souza G, Westra WH, Forastiere A (2010) HPV associated head and neck cancer: a virus-related cancer epidemic. Lancet Oncol 11:781–789

McLaughlin-Drubin ME, Münger K (2009) Oncogenic activities of human papillomaviruses. Virus Res 143:195–208

Näsman A, Attner P, Hammarstedt L et al (2009) Incidence of human papillomavirus (HPV) positive tonsillar carcinoma in Stockholm, Sweden: an epidemic of viral-induced carcinoma? Int J Cancer 125:362–366

Oxford Cancer Intelligence Unit (2010) Profile of head and neck cancers in England. http://library.ncin.org.uk/docs/100504-OCIUHead_and_Neck_Profiles.pdf

Perrone F, Suardi S, Pastore E et al (2006) Molecular and cytogenetic subgroups of oropharyngeal squamous cell carcinoma. Clin Cancer Res 12:6643–6651

Schiffman M, Castle PE, Jeronimo J, Rodriguez AC, Wacholder S (2007) Human papillomavirus and cervical cancer. Lancet 370:890–907

Sedaghat AR, Zhang Z, Begum S et al (2009) Prognostic significance of human papillomavirus in oropharyngeal squamous cell carcinomas. Laryngoscope 119:1542–1549

Uversky VN, Roman A, Oldfield CJ, Dunker AK (2006) Protein intrinsic disorder and human papillomaviruses: increased amount of disorder in E6 and E7 oncoproteins from high risk HPVs. J Proteome Res 5:1829–1842

zur Hausen H (2002) Papillomaviruses and cancer: from basic studies to clinical application. Nat Rev Cancer 2:342–350

Humoral Immunity

▶ Otolaryngologic Allergy/Immunology

Hyperparathyroidism

Steve C. Lee and Alfred Simental
Department of Otolaryngology-Head Neck Surgery, Loma Linda University School of Medicine, Loma Linda, CA, USA

Definition

Hyperparathyroidism is overproduction of parathyroid hormone (PTH) by the parathyroid glands. Release of PTH by the parathyroid glands regulates serum calcium and phosphorus levels, as well as vitamin D metabolism. As serum calcium drops, the parathyroid glands respond by producing PTH which aids in calcium absorption in the gut, recycling of calcium in the kidney, and release of calcium from the bones.

Classification

Hyperparathyroidism is subdivided into three types: primary, secondary, and tertiary hyperparathyroidism.

Primary hyperparathyroidism is caused by an intrinsic defect in the parathyroid glands that results in excessive production and release of PTH.

Secondary hyperparathyroidism results when the parathyroid glands appropriately produce large amounts of PTH in response to chronic abnormal stimuli resulting from low serum calcium levels.

Tertiary hyperparathyroidism is the persistence of long-standing secondary hyperparathyroidism despite correction of the abnormal stimuli.

Etiology

The etiology of hyperparathyroidism varies by type. Primary hyperparathyroidism is usually due to a parathyroid adenoma, a single benign tumor of the parathyroid gland, which autonomously produces PTH without regard to serum calcium levels or other feedback loops. Less commonly, hyperplasia of the several parathyroid glands results in increased cellularity and excretion of PTH. Rarely, parathyroid malignancy can also produce excessive PTH, resulting in primary hyperparathyroidism.

Parathyroid adenomas account for 85% of primary hyperparathyroidism. Recent studies have shown that parathyroid adenomas have monoclonal cell populations, which suggests a somatic mutation may be responsible for parathyroid adenoma formation (Nose and Khan 2010). Analyses of these clonal populations reveal that a single genetic derangement does not account for all adenomas but multiple pathways can lead to the development of parathyroid adenomas. One commonly found mutation is a reciprocal translocation between the PTH promoter and cyclin D1. This translocation between 11p15 and 11q13 results in overexpression of cyclin D1 which leads to loss of cell cycle regulation (Nose and Khan 2010). Additional mutations in various tumor suppressor genes have also been postulated to play a role in the formation of sporadic parathyroid adenomas. Some investigators have associated higher incidence of parathyroid adenomas to high parity (four or more live births), obesity, and vitamin D deficiency.

While most parathyroid adenomas are sporadic, several inherited syndromes include parathyroid adenomas in their constellation of clinical features. Two of these syndromes include familial isolated hyperparathyroidism and hyperparathyroidism-jaw tumor syndrome. Hyperparathyroidism-jaw tumor syndrome is caused by a dominant mutation at the HRPT2 locus which causes cystic parathyroid adenomas and ossifying fibromas of the mandible (Nose and Khan 2010). This condition is associated with Wilms tumor, renal hamartomas, and polycystic kidney disease. There is an increased rate of parathyroid carcinomas associated with this syndrome. Familial isolated hyperparathyroidism is closely related to hyperparathyroidism-jaw tumor syndrome with the same gene locus being implicated. These patients present with hyperparathyroidism secondary to parathyroid adenomas.

Parathyroid hyperplasia is the diffuse enlargement of multiple or all parathyroid glands and subsequent overproduction of parathyroid hormone. Hyperplasia is also most often a sporadic condition but can be associated with inherited syndromes such as MEN1, MEN2, neonatal severe hyperparathyroidism, and autosomal dominant mild hyperparathyroidism. The clinical feature of MEN1 is multi-glandular parathyroid hyperplasia, pituitary tumors, and pancreatic tumors. The gene implicated in the syndrome is MEN1 and the inheritance pattern is dominant. Neonatal severe hyperparathyroidism is caused by a dominant mutation in the calcium-sensing gene, CaSR, which leads to calcium insensitivity and severe hyperparathyroidism; this must be surgically treated. MEN2A is characterized by C cell hyperplasia, pheochromocytomas, and parathyroid hyperplasia. The genetic anomaly can be found in the RET proto-oncogene. Autosomal dominant mild hyperparathyroidism is caused by a dominant mutation in the cytoplasmic tail of CaSR and results in hypocalciuric hypercalcemia with normal or only mildly elevated parathyroid hormone. Surgery in this case can sometimes correct the hypercalcemia in the setting of normal parathyroid hormone levels.

Parathyroid carcinoma is the rarest etiology of primary hyperparathyroidism and accounts for about 1 % of cases of primary hyperparathyroidism. The etiology of parathyroid carcinoma is unclear, but there is an association with neck irradiation, end-stage renal disease, and

previous long-standing adenoma or hyperplasia. There is also a strong relationship between hyperparathyroidism-jaw tumor syndrome and parathyroid carcinoma. Molecular analysis of carcinomas indicated that mutations in tumor suppressor genes Rb and BRCA2 may play a role in the pathophysiology of the disease (Nose and Khan 2010).

Secondary hyperparathyroidism is the body's physiologic response to stimuli that normally stimulates parathyroid hormone production. In this instance, the hyperparathyroidism is a secondary response to an underlying primary pathology rather than an intrinsic problem in the parathyroid glands themselves. The stimuli that drive parathyroid hormone production are hypocalcemia, hyperphosphatemia, vitamin D deficiency, and chronic renal failure. Most commonly, secondary hyperparathyroidism is due to chronic renal failure. In chronic renal failure, the triad of hypocalcemia, hyperphosphatemia, and decreased renal production of calcitriol all drive PTH synthesis and secretion. Calcium and calcitriol are the primary inhibitory regulators of PTH whereas phosphate drives PTH synthesis by stabilizing PTH mRNA posttranscriptionally (Slatopolsky et al. 1999). As renal disease progresses, calcium and calcitriol receptors on the parathyroid glands decrease progressively making the gland more resistant to feedback inhibition and further driving PTH production. The other major, often overlooked cause of secondary hyperparathyroidism is vitamin D deficiency. Chronic hypocalcemia from inadequate dietary intake or malabsorption of calcium can also result in secondary hyperparathyroidism.

Tertiary hyperparathyroidism is merely the result of long-standing secondary hyperparathyroidism. Long-standing secondary hyperparathyroidism leads to diffuse hyperplasia which becomes autonomous in parathyroid hormone production and continues to overproduce parathyroid home despite correction of the primary pathology.

Clinical Presentation

In the developed world, the classic clinical presentation of "bones, stones, abdominal groans, and psychic overtones" is rarely seen. The most common modern clinical presentation of hyperparathyroidism is the incidental finding of hypercalcemia in an asymptomatic patient, with eventual discovery of elevated

Hyperparathyroidism, Table 1 Symptoms of hyperparathyroidism

Neuropsychiatric	Cognitive impairment, psychosis, confusion, headache, depression, nervousness, lack of concentration, memory dysfunction
Neuromuscular	Weakness, fatigue, proximal myopathy, leg movements in sleep, hypo-reflexia
Gastrointestinal	Anorexia, constipation, abdominal pain, nausea, vomiting, acute pancreatitis, peptic ulcer disease
Renal	Stones, polyuria, polydipsia, nocturia, renal colic, hypercalciuria, nephrocalcinosis
Cardiac	Hypertension, bradycardia, shortened QT, left ventricular hypertrophy
Skeletal	Osteoporosis, osteitis fibrosis cystica, bone and joint pain, pseudogout, chondrocalcinosis
Ocular	Conjunctivitis, band keratopathy
Dermatologic	Pruritis

parathyroid hormone levels. The symptoms of hyperparathyroidism can be categorized by organ systems (Gough and Pallazzo 2009) (Table 1).

Physical findings are rare in hyperparathyroidism. A palpable neck mass can be indicative of parathyroid carcinoma and soft tissue calcifications can occur in secondary hyperparathyroidism.

Diagnostic Workup

Laboratory Tests
Serum intact PTH – elevated.

Serum calcium – elevated in primary and tertiary hyperparathyroidism, low or normal in secondary hyperparathyroidism.

Serum phosphate – elevated in tertiary and in secondary as a result of renal disease. Low in primary and in secondary as a result of vitamin D deficiency.

Vitamin D levels – low in vitamin D deficiency in secondary hyperparathyroidism and tertiary hyperparathyroidism.

24-h urine calcium – normal or high in primary.

Radiographic Studies

Imaging studies have been used in the setting of primary hyperparathyroidism to help localize the site of single gland disease, thus directing surgical

exploration. Preoperative localization of abnormal glands dramatically decreases operative time and morbidity from unnecessary exploration.

Ultrasound is very cost effective, noninvasive, and can provide the anatomic location of abnormal glands. This resource remains highly operator dependent and the quality may vary greatly. The inability of ultrasound to penetrate bone makes discovery of mediastinal abnormalities difficult.

Sestamibi scan is a nuclear medicine imaging study that utilizes a coordination complex of a radioactive metal, technetium-99, and the ligand, methoxyisobutylisonitrile. Methoxyisobutylisonitrile is preferentially taken up and retained in the mitochondria of oxyphilic cells of abnormal parathyroid glands, but can also be absorbed by thyroid tissue. After injection of technium-99 m sestamibi, the abnormal glands will retain the radioactive signal which can be detected. This test can localize abnormal glands in 70–80% of patients. Variations on the sestamibi scan have been devised, utilizing dual isotope subtraction imaging, single photon emission computed tomography (SPECT), and SPECT/CT. SPECT utilizes a gamma camera taking multiple planar images which are fused into a true three-dimensional image. SPECT/CT fuses the SPECT image with standard CT to provide anatomic localization. In dual isotope subtraction imaging, radioactive sodium iodine-123 is administered orally before the administration of technium-99 m sestamibi and the iodine signal is subtracted out in the SPECT image (Neumann et al. 2008).

Computed tomography and MRI may be used in the localization of ectopic mediastinal parathyroid glands.

Bone mineral density scan is useful in determining the degree of osteoporosis and the subsequent need for surgical intervention in asymptomatic primary hyperparathyroidism.

Differential Diagnosis

Familial hypocalciuric hypercalcemia
Total parenteral nutrition
Malnutrition
Lactose intolerance
Malabsorption
Celiac sprue
Vitamin D deficiency
Vitamin D intoxication

Pancreatic insufficiency
Paget's disease
AIDS
Tuberculosis
Aluminum intoxication
Cystic fibrosis
Lithium treatment
Bisphosphonate treatment
Loop diuretics
Thiazide diuretics
Chronic renal failure
Adrenal insufficiency
Multiple endocrine neoplasias
Malignancy
Milk alkali syndrome
Calcium deficiency
Sarcoidosis
Heart block
Immobilization
Radiation

Therapy

Primary Hyperparathyroidism

Currently, there is only one curative treatment for primary hyperparathyroidism – parathyroidectomy. Once diagnosis is made, evaluation should be directed at determining if the patient is a surgical candidate.

The first set of guidelines were set in 1990 and then revised in 2002 and most recently in 2008. The guidelines for parathyroidectomy are outlined in Table 2 (Bilezikian et al. 2009).

Many physicians acknowledge that the guidelines are too stringent since parathyroid surgery results in measurable improvement in the majority of asymptomatic patients and suggest surgery should be utilized in the majority of patients (Eigelberger et al. 2004). Parathyroid surgery, when performed by experienced surgeons, provides successful results in approximately 95% of patients with minimal morbidity. The successful operation involves removal all hyperfunctioning parathyroid tissue.

Medical management consists of observation, routine surveillance workup, and symptomatic treatment of the sequelae of hyperparathyroidism. The 2008 consensus guidelines suggest surveillance of asymptomatic primary hyperparathyroidism is annual serum calcium, annual glomerular filtration rate, and bone density measurement every 1–2 years. Patients are encouraged to maintain a normal dietary intake of calcium and vitamin D, participate in regular weight bearing exercise, maintain good hydration, and avoid diuretics and lithium.

There are four classes of drugs that are used in the medical treatment of primary hyperparathyroidism: hormone replacement therapy, bisphosphonates, calcimimetics, and selective estrogen receptor modulators. Hormone replacement therapy with estrogen is effective in improving bone mineral density in normocalcemic postmenopausal women. Similarly, several studies using estrogen in postmenopausal women with primary hyperparathyroidism found increases in bone mineral density but no change in PTH or ionized calcium levels. Bisphosphonates are inhibitors of bone resorption that are primarily used to treat osteoporosis. Calcimimetics are allosteric modulators that sensitize the calcium-sensing receptor to extracellular calcium and result in blocking PTH production. Studies have shown calcimimetics to be effective in reducing serum calcium and PTH but do not alter bone turnover or bone mineral density. Selective estrogen receptor modulators are tissue-specific agonists or antagonists of the estrogen receptor and therefore have the potential to mimic estrogen's bone protective effects without estrogen's deleterious effects on breast and vascular tissue. Studies on raloxifene, the most studied of these modulators, found that its beneficial effects on bone mineral density, while measureable, are significantly less than those of hormone replacement therapy (Khan et al. 2009).

Secondary Hyperparathyroidism

The treatment of secondary hyperparathyroidism is correction of the underlying pathology. However, the most common underlying pathology, end-stage renal disease, is only correctable by kidney transplantation. Medical management of secondary hyperparathyroidism is the mainstay of treatment. Therapy is directed at maintaining anormal serum calcium, phosphate, and PTH levels. Active vitamin D analogs include calcitriol, doxercalciferol, and paricalcitol. Paricalcitol controls PTH levels without the same magnitude of hypercalcemia and hyperphosphatemia as the other two analogs and is preferred by some physicians (Andress et al. 2008).

Hyperparathyroidism, Table 2 Consensus guidelines for parathyroid surgery in primary hyperparathyroidism

Measurement	1990	2002	2008
Symptomatic hyperparathyroidism (kidney stones, overt bone disease, proximal myopathy, arrhythmia, etc.)			
Age	<50	<50	<50
Serum calcium above upper limit of normal	1–1.6 mg/dl	1.0 mg/dl	1.0 mg/dl
24-h urine calcium	>400 mg/day	>400 mg/day	Not a criteria
Glomerular filtration rate	Reduced by 30%	Reduced by 30%	<60 ml/min
Bone mineral density	Z-score < −2.0 in forearm	T-score < −2.5 at any site	T-score < −2.5 at any site

Surgery is indicated when pharmacotherapy can no longer adequately control secondary hyperparathyroidism or the patient becomes overtly symptomatic with bone pain, fractures, soft tissue calcifications, pruritis, or calciphylaxis. In these cases, the surgery consists of total parathyroidectomy with or without autotransplantation or 3.5 gland parathyroidectomy. In the first surgery, all parathyroid glands are removed and a portion of one gland is minced and reimplanted into the sternocleidomastoid or the forearm and the implantation site is marked with a hemoclip for later extraction. Cryopreservation of remaining parathyroid tissue may allow later implantation in patients with subsequent hypoparathyroidism. Implantation after total parathyroidectomy is controversial, as reoperative morbidity is not insignificant.

Tertiary Hyperparathyroidism

Tertiary hyperparathyroidism is almost uniformly treated with surgery as medical management is unfruitful. The surgical options for tertiary hyperparathyroidism usually include total parathyroidectomy with autotransplantation.

Prognosis

The prognosis for primary and tertiary hyperparathyroidism is linked to the success of surgery. Surgical cure rates in these diseases are very good with success rates in excess of 95%.

The prognosis for secondary hyperparathyroidism is dependent on the cause of secondary hyperparathyroidism. Secondary hyperparathyroidism caused by vitamin D deficiency is easily treated. The prognosis

for secondary hyperparathyroidism secondary to chronic renal disease depends on the prognosis of the renal disease. The prognosis for end-stage renal disease without transplantation is dismal and the prognosis with successful transplantation is good.

References

Andress DL, Coyne DW, Kalantar-Zadeh K, Molitch ME, Zangeneh F, Sprague SM (2008) Management of secondary hyperparathyroidism in stages 3 and 4 chronic kidney disease. Endocr Pract 14(1):18–27

Bilezikian JP, Khan AA, Potts JT Jr, Third International Workshop on the Management of Asymptomatic Primary Hyperthyroidism (2009) Guidelines for the management of asymptomatic primary hyperparathyroidism: summary statement from the third international workshop. J Clin Endocrinol Metab 94(2):335–339

Eigelberger MS, Cheah WK, Ituarte PH, Streja L, Duh QY, Clark OH (2004) The NIH criteria for parathyroidectomy in asymptomatic primary hyperparathyroidism: are they too limited? Ann Surg 239(4):528–535

Gough J, Pallazzo FF (2009) Presentation and Diagnosis of Primary Hyperparathyroidism. In: Hubbard JGH, Inabet WB, Lo CY (eds) Endocrine surgery: principles and practice. Springer, New York, pp 221–234

Khan A, Grey A, Shoback D (2009) Medical management of asymptomatic primary hyperparathyroidism: proceedings of the third international workshop. J Clin Endocrinol Metab 94(2):373–381

Neumann DR, Obuchowski NA, Difilippo FP (2008) Preoperative 123I/99mTc-sestamibi subtraction SPECT and SPECT/CT in primary hyperparathyroidism. J Nucl Med 49(12):2012–2017

Nose V, Khan A (2010) Recent Developments in the Molecular Biology of the Parathyroid. In: Lloyd RV (ed) Endocrine pathology: differential diagnosis and molecular advances, 2nd edn. Springer, New York, pp 157–180

Slatopolsky E, Brown A, Dusso A (1999) Pathogenesis of secondary hyperparathyroidism. Kidney Int 56(S14–S19): 1523–1755

Hypersalivation

▶ Salivary Gland Disorders, Sialorrhea

Hypertelorism

Michael M. Kim
Division of Facial Plastic & Reconstructive Surgery, Department of Otolaryngology-Head and Neck Surgery, Oregon Health & Science University, Portland, OR, USA

Definition

A condition of abnormally increased distance between the eyes characterized by both increased intercanthal distance (ICD) and interpupillary distance (IPD). This physical finding is associated with several congenital syndromes. Two syndromes, Crouzon's and Apert's syndrome, exhibit hypertelorism as a result of craniosynostosis. Craniofacial surgical techniques can be performed in order to correct hypertelorism.

Cross-References

▶ Craniofacial Surgery

Hypogeusia

Shelley Segrest Taylor
Department of Otolaryngology and Communicative Sciences, The University of Mississippi Medical Center, Jackson, MS, USA

Definition

The partial loss of taste resulting from radiation therapy to the head and neck.

Cross-References

▶ Dental Evaluation in Head and Neck Cancer Patient

Hypopharyngeal Squamous Cell Carcinoma

Mary G. Ashmead
Department of Otolaryngology and Communicative Sciences, University of Mississippi Medical Center, Jackson, MS, USA

Synonyms

Pharyngeal wall cancer; Postcricoid cancer; Pyriform sinus cancer

Definition

Hypopharyngeal cancer refers to any malignancy within the subsites of the hypopharynx, which is bounded by the oropharynx at the hyoid bone superiorly and the esophageal inlet inferiorly; this includes the pyriform sinus, lateral or posterior pharyngeal wall, and postcricoid region. The region surrounds the larynx and is the least common site for cancer in the upper aerodigestive tract. Hypopharyngeal cancer usually presents in an advanced stage and is associated with a worse prognosis than other head and neck cancers. Involvement of the mucosa and surrounding tissue is usually extensive, which adds to the complexity of treatment. Therefore, hypopharyngeal cancers are associated with increased morbidity and mortality when compared with other head and neck squamous cell cancers.

Etiology

These cancers arise from the mucosal lining of the hypopharynx and over 95% are squamous cell carcinomas. The etiology and tumor progression are similar to other head and neck cancers. The mucosal changes progress through stages of dysplasia to invasive malignancy with associated alterations in genetics and protein production. Many factors are involved with this transformation, and the cause is multifactorial.

Risk factors are similar to those of all aerodigestive tract malignancies. Use of tobacco and alcohol is directly related to development of head and neck cancer; tobacco users have a risk for head and neck cancer 13 times higher than nonsmokers (Andre and Schraub 1995). Those who use both tobacco and alcohol share a risk 34 times higher than non-users, which suggests that the two have a synergistic effect in causing dysplastic change. Nearly 100% of hypopharyngeal cancer patients use tobacco, and it is considered the primary risk factor in development of all head and neck cancers. A Canadian study showed that over 70% of the study patients had a history of heavy alcohol use (Hall et al. 2008). This rate of alcohol abuse is higher when compared to patients with cancer of other head and neck sites.

A risk factor unique to hypopharyngeal cancer is Plummer-Vinson, also called Paterson-Brown-Kelly syndrome. This syndrome is diagnosed by the triad of sideropenic anemia, dysphagia, and esophageal webs. The association of Plummer-Vinson syndrome to upper aerodigestive tract cancers was recognized in the early 1900s, and generally occurs in the postcricoid subsite or the esophageal inlet (Paterson 1919). Causation is believed to be irritation that results in webbing, which then progresses to malignancy (Uppaluri and Sunwoo 2010). Likely due to improved nutrition and supplementation, this syndrome is now rare in the United States.

Clinical Presentation

Because of the lack of limiting boundaries, the mass is able to grow substantially before causing any symptoms; thus, hypopharyngeal cancers often remain unnoticed by the patient until later stages of disease. This is in large contrast to cancers of the larynx or oral cavity which can quickly become symptomatic with very small lesions. Most patients with hypopharyngeal cancer present with stage 3 disease or higher, with less than 20% presenting with early stage disease (Hall et al. 2008).

There are many possible presenting symptoms. As far as general characteristics at presentation,

hypopharyngeal cancer patients present with malnourishment. This can be attributed both to the metabolic burden of the tumor itself, as well as a high incidence of dysphagia. Dysphagia is present in over 50% of patients at time of presentation, and it can be severe enough to require placement of surgical feeding access for nutrition at initial presentation (Hall et al. 2008). Because the posteroinferior boundary of the hypopharynx is the esophageal inlet, the mass can grow to cause mechanical obstruction of the esophageal opening. Also, the cancer can invade the nervous plexus of the esophagus and cause a functional dysphagia from poor muscular movement. Globus sensation, or the feeling of a "lump in the throat," is generally present in high numbers, sometimes even in the early stages of disease.

Because of the clinically silent course of hypopharyngeal cancer, many patients present with a neck mass from local metastasis via the lymphatic system. Approximately 50% of all patients will have involved lymph nodes at the time of diagnosis, with many of those having a neck mass as the presenting symptom. (Hoffman and Karnell 1997) While other symptoms will be present, the neck mass will be the sign that prompts medical attention. The delay in presentation is felt to be the main reason for increased nodal metastasis rather than any increased aggressiveness or invasive qualities of the tumor itself.

Pain is very common, either in the form of odynophagia or as otalgia due to referred pain from the auricular branch of the vagus nerve, also called Arnold's nerve or Alderman's nerve. Patients complain about a deep-seated pain inside the ear. Odynophagia can come both from mass effect onto other structures or involvement of nerves. Odynophagia, as well as globus sensation, gastroesophageal reflux, and otalgia, can occur early within the disease process. However, due to the vagueness of these complaints, they can be overlooked as benign symptoms.

Later symptoms include hemoptysis, continued weight loss and voice complaints, such as hoarseness or stridor. Vocal symptoms generally occur from direct extension into the laryngeal structures, such as into the surrounding musculature; however, recurrent laryngeal nerve involvement or mechanical interference from excessive tumor mass can also result in voice changes.

Diagnosis

When the patient presents with any of the symptoms mentioned above, a full head and neck exam must be performed. The general appearance of the patient is important to document. Initial impression may be of cachexia, pallor, and other findings consistent with malnutrition. The voice may be hoarse or breathy. Stridor can occur either from obstruction by tumor, from vocal cord compromise, or both. The neck should be thoroughly examined for any lymphadenopathy, as the majority of new hypopharyngeal cancers will have an advanced nodal stage at presentation. Neck masses should be examined for fixation within the neck, their size, their nodal level, and any overlying skin changes. Palpation of the neck for thyroid masses, lymph nodes, and mobility of the larynx can assist with evaluation, as well.

The mucosa of the upper aerodigestive tract should be inspected fully. In the oral cavity, the state of dentition should be noted, as many patients will need dental extractions prior to radiation therapy. The oral cavity is also the most common site for secondary malignancies and should be inspected for other masses, erythroplakia or leukoplakia. The remainder of the mucosa should be visualized with flexible endoscopy.

Diagnosis of cancer in the hypopharynx is generally made in the clinical setting by flexible laryngoscopy or mirror exam. On flexible laryngoscopy, the tumor is usually easily visible as a large, exophytic mass, usually involving more than one subsite of the hypopharynx, larynx, or supraglottis. Mucosal ulcerations, necrosis, and hyperkeratosis are common findings. Early stage tumors may have less obvious signs and can be easily missed. Findings such as pooling of secretions or submucosal fullness should prompt further evaluation by either direct laryngoscopy or radiographic imaging. More commonly, however, the tumor presents in a later stage and is recognized without issue. It may prove difficult to evaluate the full extent of tissue involvement in the clinic. Asking the patient to puff out his or her cheeks or perform a valsalva maneuver can assist with visualization of the pyriform sinuses. Opening the mouth and protruding the tongue can assist with visualization of the vallecula and base of tongue.

The larynx is often distorted by the growing mass or by direct invasion of the tumor into the laryngeal structure. Assessment of vocal cord function is important, both for airway evaluation and for staging purposes, as vocal cord fixation leads to at least a T3 stage in the current system. The entire airway itself can be obscured by the larger size of the tumor at presentation and can present with stridor. The physician must ascertain the safety of the patient's airway and whether a tracheotomy is indicated for airway protection, either as a planned or more immediate procedure.

There has been a recent shift toward using narrow band imaging to assist with diagnosing the degree of superficial or submucosal spread of the primary tumor. Hypopharyngeal cancers have a higher degree of submucosal spread than other head and neck sites, which cannot necessarily be visualized with traditional flexible or direct laryngoscopy. A study published in Laryngoscope in 2011 suggests that approximately half of patients with oro- or hypopharyngeal cancer have superficial spread of disease not perceived by traditional methods (Matsuba et al. 2011). However, upstaging of tumors occurred in only 2 of 45 patients. It is currently unclear how this should affect the staging of such tumors in general, as several studies have shown no difference in survival between patients with submucosal spread seen on pathologic evaluation and those without (Uppaluri and Sunwoo 2010).

Tissue sampling is required for definitive diagnosis and can be accomplished either by panendoscopy with biopsy of the primary site or by fine needle aspiration of an associated nodal mass. Direct laryngoscopy in the operating room will allow the physician to fully evaluate the pyriform sinuses and postcricoid region for the extent of their involvement. Treatment of these patients can vary based upon the subsites involved. Esophagoscopy is recommended because hypopharyngeal cancers—especially those of the pyriform sinus subsite—can invade into the esophageal wall. However, esophagoscopy can be difficult in advanced primary tumors due to mechanical obstruction. In these instances, either barium esophagram or computed tomography has been used to help visualize the extent of cancer invasion into the esophageal tissues. Bronchoscopy can evaluate for subglottic extension, which also affects treatment options, but is less common for hypopharyngeal cancers than for supraglottic or glottic sites.

Fine needle aspiration of a nodal metastasis is less invasive than panendoscopy and can be performed in clinic for more rapid diagnosis. A small gauge needle is inserted into the mass to aspirate malignant cells for cytopathology. Squamous cell carcinoma is readily identified on FNA. Cells will be immature with irregular shapes and can be divided into pathologic grades based on the stage of differentiation into squamous epithelium. Please see section on Fine Needle Aspiration for Head and Neck Malignancies for further details.

Imaging

Even if panendoscopy is performed, imaging is used to determine the extent of disease. Hypopharyngeal cancers often show submucosal spread, which is not seen by direct visualization of the mucosal surfaces. These tumors can also spread to nonpalpable lymph nodes. Other characteristics, such as spread to the thyroid tissues, involvement of the laryngeal skeleton, or metastasis to distant sites, can be seen best with radiologic studies. Upstaging has been shown to occur in up to 90% of cases due to radiologic findings, usually because of increased nodal involvement or cartilage invasion (Kim and Weber 2006).

Imaging, then, becomes an important adjunct to physical exam for full evaluation of the disease, staging purposes, and evaluation for any second primary tumor either of the head and neck or of the lungs. Scanning of the primary site and the neck lymph nodes is of principal importance. Computed tomography (CT) with use of intravenous contrast and magnetic resonance imaging (MRI) can be utilized. There have been many studies to evaluate the sensitivity and specificity of these modalities in regard to specific radiologic findings, most notably laryngeal cartilage invasion. Comparable rates have been found for sensitivity of diagnosis of invasion by CT and MRI, which can approach 90% (Uppaluri and Sunwoo 2010; Kim and Weber 2006). Specificity is higher in CT than MRI, as the increased signal on T2 and decreased signal on T1 can be indicative either of invasion or of other processes. CT is the most commonly used modality by most centers—scans are cheaper, faster, and generally easier to read for the common otolaryngologist.

The chest must also be evaluated for distant metastasis or for second primary malignancies. A chest radiograph can provide sufficient information in those with early stage disease and minimal to no lymph node involvement. Hypopharyngeal cancer, however, generally presents in advanced stage with increased incidence of distant metastatic disease. CT is the preferred method for chest imaging for this reason. Subcentimeter nodules can be identified and followed for growth. If suspicious for metastatic disease, positron emission tomography (PET) can help determine their significance. PET can prove to be a helpful tool in the preoperative as well as posttreatment periods. The most common use in hypopharyngeal cancer is to evaluate for distant metastatic spread. If lymph nodes or pulmonary nodules found on initial imaging are not clearly metastatic, PET can help discern their relevance for staging. It can be used in following patients after treatment as well, as traditional imaging is limited by the abnormal appearance of tissues after surgery or radiotherapy.

Differential Diagnosis

Hypopharyngeal squamous cell carcinoma is rarely confused with other disorders, especially once tissue diagnosis is confirmed. However, infectious etiologies should be considered, as well as lymphoproliferative disorders. Common pharyngitis can produce similar symptoms, such as odynophagia, dysphagia due to edema, hoarseness, and otalgia. Mucosal irritation as well as lymph node enlargement can mimic early stage cancers. However, the short duration and sudden onset of disease, as well as accompanying fever and other URI symptoms can help with diagnosis.

Diseases which result in cervical lymphadenopathy can suggest a hidden hypopharyngeal malignancy, especially when presenting in a patient with common risk factors of long-term tobacco and alcohol use. One must consider infectious lymphadenitis from cat scratch disease, Epstein-Barr infection, or other bacteria. Lymphoproliferative disorders can present with cervical lymphadenopathy, just as Hodgkin's and non-Hodgkin's lymphoma. A negative flexible laryngoscopy and findings of abnormal lymphocytes on FNA can suggest this diagnosis. Lymphoma can only be suggested but often not diagnosed by FNA, as pathologists require tumor architecture and cytometry for true diagnosis. Excisional lymph node biopsy would be preferred to confirm the diagnosis.

Also, while squamous cell carcinoma accounts for 95% of hypopharyngeal cancers, other types of malignancies must be contemplated. Undifferentiated carcinoma or adenocarcinoma can arise from the salivary tissue in the hypopharynx. Primary lymphoma must be considered, especially in HIV positive patients. Invasion into the hypopharynx from a thyroid malignancy is possible, as well as several forms of sarcomas.

Staging

Hypopharyngeal cancer is staged by the Tumor, Node, Metastasis (TNM) staging system put forth by the American Joint Commission on Cancer as detailed in Table 1. Physical exam and radiology findings should be used together to correctly stage the disease. It is not yet clear how information from biomarkers or narrow band imaging will affect staging. Currently, the extent of primary tumor involvement from flexible or direct laryngoscopy combined with information from CT scanning is used for staging. Please see the section on tumor staging for further information.

Therapy

Due to the rareness of cancers in the hypopharynx, there is little level 1 evidence from randomized, controlled trials regarding the appropriate treatment regimen. In addition to having minimal data, these patients are complicated, and the decision for the appropriate treatment is multifaceted. Generally, the three treatment modalities—surgery, radiation, and chemotherapy—are used in some combination and rarely alone. The classic therapy for hypopharyngeal cancer is full surgical excision via total pharyngolaryngectomy followed by external beam radiation. This is not appropriate for all tumors or all patients. The patient's stage, comorbid conditions, nutritional status, age, swallowing function, and other factors must be considered in determining the appropriate therapy.

Later stage tumors have better survival outcomes with surgery followed by radiation. Surgery generally consists of partial or total laryngopharyngectomy. Early stage tumors have more options for treatment than do late stage malignancies. Most T1 and T2 cancers can be treated either with surgery with adjuvant radiation or with radiation with or without chemotherapy and the possibility for salvage surgery.

Textbooks differ on the recommendations for early stage disease. Some show a preference for curative radiotherapy over surgery, especially for exophytic

lesions (Kim and Weber 2006). While no head-to-head study has been performed, anecdotal evidence suggests similar cure rates between surgery with adjuvant radiation and radiation as primary therapy for early stage tumors. Thus, the patient does not avoid radiation with either choice, making primary radiation a more attractive option. Other authors, however, suggest that no modality is necessarily preferable over the other (Uppaluri and Sunwoo 2010).

Surgery as the initial treatment may be laryngeal sparing, whereas salvage surgery nearly always results in total pharyngolaryngectomy. Laryngeal sparing options such as partial pharyngectomy or supracricoid hemilaryngectomy can avoid laryngeal excision as well as achieve local control rates reported to be nearly 90% (Uppaluri and Sunwoo 2010). However, the preoperative evaluation often excludes many patients from this option due to poor pulmonary status. Also, many of these patients will have postoperative and post-radiation laryngeal dysfunction, dysphagia, and aspiration, which would preclude the advantages of a laryngeal sparing procedure.

An article in the European Annals of Otolaryngology examined the quality of life issues of patients with hypopharyngeal cancer who were treated either with total pharyngolaryngectomy followed by radiation or a laryngeal sparing treatment of concurrent chemoradiation or induction chemotherapy followed by radiation. In this study, there was no significant difference of quality of life measures between chemoradiation and surgery followed by radiation therapy (Guibert et al. 2011).

Early Stage Therapy

In certain populations, laryngeal sparing procedures can be considered for early stage disease. Contraindications to a laryngeal sparing procedure, such as partial pharyngolaryngectomy or supracricoid laryngectomy, include tumor involvement of the pyriform apex, postcricoid space, or cartilages, abnormal ipsilateral vocal cord mobility, or poor performance on pulmonary function testing. Thus, there are several factors that may eliminate a patient from consideration for a laryngeal preservation surgery. It has already been discussed that the majority of patients will present with advanced stage disease, thus making only few patients of an already rare disease even eligible for these procedures. The tumor must fall within the superior portions of the pyriform sinus or

Hypopharyngeal Squamous Cell Carcinoma, Table 1 Staging of hypopharyngeal primary tumor

Primary tumor (T)		
TX	Primary tumor cannot be assessed	
T0	No evidence of primary tumor	
Tis	Carcinoma in situ	
T1	Tumor limited to one subsite of hypopharynx and/or $\leq$ 2 cm in greatest dimension	
T2	Tumor invades more than one subsite of the hypopharynx or an adjacent site, or measures > 2 cm but $\leq$ 4 cm in greatest dimension without fixation of the hemilarynx	
T3	Tumor $\geq$ 4 cm in greatest dimension or with fixation of hemilarynx or extension to esophagus	
T4a	*Moderately advanced local disease*	
	Tumor invades thyroid/cricoid cartilage, hyoid bone, thyroid gland, or central compartment soft tissue[a]	
T4b	*Very advanced local disease*	
	Tumor invades prevertebral fascia, encases carotid artery, or involves mediastinal structures	
Regional lymph nodes (N)		
NX	Regional lymph nodes cannot be assessed	
N0	No regional lymph node metastasis	
N1	Metastasis in a single ipsilateral lymph node, $\leq$ 3 cm in greatest dimension	
N2	Metastasis in a single ipsilateral lymph node > 3 cm but $\leq$ 6 cm in greatest dimension; or multiple ipsilateral lymph nodes, none $\geq$ 6 cm in greatest dimension; or bilateral or contralateral lymph nodes, none $\geq$ 6 cm in greatest dimension	
	N2a	Metastasis in a single ipsilateral lymph node > 3 cm but $\leq$ 6 cm in greatest dimension
	N2b	Metastasis in multiple ipsilateral lymph nodes, none > 6 cm in greatest dimension
	N2c	Metastasis in bilateral or contralateral lymph nodes, none > 6 cm in greatest dimension
N3	Metastasis in a lymph node > 6 cm in greatest dimension	
Distant metastasis (M)		
M0	No distant metastasis	
M1	Distant metastasis	

[a]Central compartment soft tissue includes prelaryngeal strap muscles and subcutaneous fat

lateral pharyngeal walls without inferior extension. Postcricoid cancers are generally bilateral and are very rarely appropriate for laryngeal sparing procedures.

If the above criteria have been met, the surgeon can consider several operative techniques for tumor excision. Partial pharyngotomy can be appropriate for lateral or posterior wall pyriform sinus tumors or for lateral or posterior pharyngeal wall tumors. Many different approaches exist and are tailored to the extent of the primary site. The lateral pharyngotomy approach consists of transection of the inferior constrictor musculature for access to the lateral or posterior pyriform sinus, which is separated from the thyroid cartilage. A transthyroid or transhyoid pharyngotomy will enter the upper aerodigestive tract through the vallecula. The hyoid and thyroid cartilage are transected for access to posteriorly based tumors, which lends a risk of swallowing dysfunction from interruption of the musculature and risk to the superior laryngeal nerves. Reconstruction is either by primary closure or by use

of a skin graft held in place by a bolster. A tissue flap is rarely needed for closure.

If the tumor is small and superficial, the CO_2 laser can be used for primary transoral excision, and the manipulation and swelling of tissues from open pharyngotomy can be avoided. The superior strap muscles are not compromised, theoretically resulting in better swallowing outcomes. Tracheotomy is often unnecessary, as the airway is not compromised. In this approach, the tumor is exposed with a laryngoscope and visualized with use of the operating microscope. The CO_2 laser incises the tissues for complete excision, which can be performed in a piecemeal fashion, if needed. When cutting through tumor, the edges are sealed by the laser lessening the risk of tumor spillage that accompanies cold knife dissection. Superficial defects can close by secondary intention or can be covered with a bolstered split thickness skin graft according to the surgeon's preference. However, if the depth of the tumor is more extensive, leaving a more sizeable defect or extension into surrounding fascial planes, a regional or free transfer flap might be indicated for closure.

Pyriform sinus tumors with involvement of the medial wall and limited laryngeal invasion may be considered for combined partial pharyngolaryngectomy. A partial pharyngolaryngectomy represents a combination of a supraglottic laryngectomy with the above-mentioned partial pharyngotomy. The medial wall of the pyriform sinus, ipsilateral hyoid, arytenoid, and superior thyroid cartilage, and a portion of the epiglottis are removed en bloc. The exclusion criteria are less strict for this procedure than for partial pharyngectomy alone. Some extension into the tongue base or vallecula is allowable, as these margins are resectable with the primary specimen. The ipsilateral hemilarynx can be partially invaded, but the lesion should not cross midline or cause vocal cord fixation. In this procedure, the suprahyoid strap muscles are transected and the vallecula entered contralateral to the tumor. The incision is extended around the superior portion of the tumor. The thyroid cartilage cuts are inferior to the anterior commissure on the ipsilateral side, and superior on the contralateral side. An interarytenoid incision is continued anteriorly in the ventricle to join with the thyroid cartilage cuts. After resection, the ipsilateral true vocal fold is sutured in the paramedian position to help prevent aspiration (Uppaluri and Sunwoo 2010; Kim and Weber 2006). For reconstruction, often the remaining mucosa can be reapproximated for primary closure. If less than 2 cm is available for closure, patch free flap reconstruction should be considered to prevent stricture, which is discussed further below. The pectoralis myocutaneous flap is generally avoided in laryngeal conserving procedures because of its increased bulk. A fasciocutaneous flap, such as the radial forearm or anterolateral thigh, is a more appropriate choice.

Advanced Stage Therapy

For advanced stage tumors, which comprise the majority of hypopharyngeal cancers, surgical excision and adjuvant radiation is the mainstay of treatment. T3 and T4 cancers do not qualify for a laryngeal sparing procedure, thus a total laryngectomy with partial pharyngectomy or total pharyngolaryngectomy is indicated. Primary goals are for full excision as well as restoring a functional swallow. The extent of pharyngectomy performed is dictated by the tumor and can involve complete excision of the pharyngeal walls if

needed. Uninvolved mucosa left in place will aid with closure. Please see chapter on total laryngectomy for further information on the laryngeal extirpation.

Reconstruction in these cases often requires a free flap or regional flap for reconstitution of the upper aerodigestive tract. Primary closure of the pharyngeal mucosa should only be attempted if more than 2 cm of normal mucosa is available because of concerns for stricture. There are multiple options available, including the pectoralis myocutaneous flap, fasciocutaneous flaps, gastric pull-up procedure, and jejunal interposition. The choice of reconstruction depends upon the extent of the resection.

Free tissue transfer has become the procedure of choice for reconstruction. A patch reconstruction is appropriate for a partial pharyngectomy defect. Fasciocutaneous flaps are gaining popularity, both for patch closure or tubing for circumferential reconstruction. The radial forearm and anterolateral thigh free flaps can be used for mucosal reconstruction without significant added bulk. For those in whom free tissue transfer is not an option, the pectoralis flap can be used. The pectoralis flap is a simple flap to perform and has a reliable blood supply, but often results in significant bulk and dysphagia. It can be considered in those who are poor candidates for free tissue transfer due to comorbidities or for salvage surgery. Tubing of the pectoralis flap for circumferential defects is not recommended.

Dysphagia is a concern with any patch technique for repair. Some authors suggest a complete resection of remaining pharyngeal tissue so that a circumferential reconstruction can be performed. As mentioned above, the fasciocutaneous grafts can be tubed for recreation of the pharynx. Another option is jejunal free tissue transfer, which has long been a method for circumferential reconstruction. Reported rates of stricture and fistula formation are lower than for tubed fasciocutaneous grafts, believed to be related to fewer incisions and anastamoses. However, with increasing number of otolaryngologic surgeons becoming comfortable with fasciocutaneous flaps, the acceptable rates of morbidity and mortality, and levels of speech and dysphagia after surgery, many believe that this method will replace intestinal free flaps for reconstruction (Richmon and Brumund 2007).

When total laryngopharyngoesophagectomy is required for resection, a gastric pull-up becomes the preferred procedure, which entails mobilization of the stomach on the right gastric and gastroomental arteries, followed by tunneling the stomach superiorly so that the gastroesophageal junction is anastamosed to the distal end of the pharynx. Esophagectomy has a known association with increased morbidity (50%) and mortality (10%); however, the surgeon can obtain excellent local control of cervical esophageal disease with total resection (Kim and Weber 2006).

Treatment of the Neck

The cervical lymph nodes should be addressed, whether by neck dissection, radiation therapy, or both. When there are clinically positive nodes, current treatment recommendations are for treating bilateral necks. The N0 neck can be treated only unilaterally. Neck dissection is generally performed at the time of primary surgery regardless of clinical N staging, as the rate of occult nodal metastasis is high. Primary lymphatic drainage is to levels II through IV; however, level V, retropharyngeal, and contralateral nodes can be involved. Hypopharyngeal cancers rarely involve level I (Takes 2010). When extracapsular spread or multiple nodes are involved, adjuvant radiation fields should include the cervical lymph node basin for improved regional control (Uppaluri and Sunwoo 2010).

Prognosis

Related to the delayed stage at presentation, prognosis for hypopharyngeal cancer is poor. According to the SEER database from 2001 to 2007, survival overall at 1 year is 66%, 5 years 30.2%. However, the range is wide when comparing early to late stage disease. For those tumors found early without regional metastasis, 5-year survival can be as high as 70%. When regional metastases are present, survival decreases accordingly, near 30% (Uppaluri and Sunwoo 2010). The patients who present with M1 disease share an even worse prognosis, with median survival of less than 1 year (Takes 2010). Other factors that negatively impact prognosis include increasing age, pathologic features like positive margins, perineural or vascular invasion, as well as increased T and N stages.

As mentioned above, stage 3 and 4 disease is reported to have better prognosis with surgery followed by adjuvant radiation than by radiation

alone with or without salvage surgery, regardless of the primary site. For posterior pharyngeal wall tumors, radiation has been shown to have failure rate of 49% at 1 year, compared with 25% for those treated with surgery and adjuvant radiation (Kim and Weber 2006).

Epidemiology

Hypopharyngeal cancer is the least common of all head and neck subsites. Historically, approximately 5% of head and neck malignancies occur within the hypopharynx, and this continues to be supported by SEER database information. Incidence is approximately 1.5 per 100,000 people but varies related to region and generally corresponds to the incidence of tobacco and alcohol use, with France having the highest incidence among reporting countries (Uppaluri and Sunwoo 2010). The most common subsite for the primary tumor is the pyriform sinus and accounts for 66–86% of hypopharyngeal tumors. This varies, however, according to region. The pharyngeal wall and postcricoid region share the remainder of primary tumors.

Cross-References

▶ Cervical Node Metastases from Squamous Cell Carcinomas, Patterns of
▶ Differential Diagnosis of Adult Neck Masses
▶ Facial Nerve Imaging, CT and MRI
▶ Fine Needle Aspiration for Head and Neck Tumors
▶ Free Tissue Transfer in Head and Neck
▶ Head and neck cancer staging
▶ Head and Neck Squamous Cell Carcinoma, Risk Factors
▶ Musculocutaneous Flap
▶ Salvage Surgery for Head and Neck Cancer
▶ Tobacco and Head and Neck Cancer
▶ Total Laryngectomy and Laryngopharyngectomy

References

Andre K, Schraub S (1995) Role of alcohol and tobacco in the etiology of head and neck cancer. Eur J Cancer B Oral Oncol 31B:301–309
Guibert M et al (2011) Quality of life in patients treated for advanced hypopharyngeal or laryngeal cancer. Eur Ann

Otorhinolaryngol Head Neck Dis. doi:10.1016/j.anorl.2011.02.010

Hall SF, Groome P, Irish J, O'Sullivan B (2008) The natural history of patients with squamous cell carcinoma of the hypopharynx. Laryngoscope 118:1362–1371

Hoffman HT, Karnell L (1997) Hypopharyngeal cancer patient care evaluation. Laryngoscope 107:1005–1017

Kim S, Weber R (2006) Hypopharyngeal cancer. In: Bailey B, Johnson J (eds) Head & neck surgery–otolaryngology. Lippincott, Philadelphia, pp 1691–1710

Matsuba H et al (2011) Diagnosis of the extent of advanced orophayrngeal and hypopharyngeal cancers by narrow band imaging with magnifying endoscopy. Laryngoscope 121:753–759

Paterson DR (1919) A clinical type of dysphagia. J Laryngol Otol 34:289–291

Richmon J, Brumund K (2007) Reconstruction of the hypopharynx: current trends. Curr Opin Otolaryngol Head Neck Surg 15:208–212

Takes R et al (2010) Current trends in initial management of hypopharyngeal cancer: the declining use of open surgery. Head Neck 34:270–281

Uppaluri R, Sunwoo J (2010) Neoplasms of the hypopharynx and cervical esophagus. In: Cummings otolaryngology head & neck surgery. Mosby, Philadelphia, pp 1421–1440

Hyposensitization Injections

▶ Otolaryngologic Allergy/Immunology

Hyposensitization Therapy

▶ Otolaryngologic Allergy/Immunology

Hypotympanum

Sébastien Schmerber[1,2,3], Arnaud Attye[1,2,4], Ihab Atallah[5], Cédric Mendoza[1,2,4] and Alexandre Karkas[1,2,6]

[1]Department of Otolaryngology-Head and Neck Surgery, Otology/Neurotology Unit, University Hospital of Grenoble, Grenoble, France
[2]Service ORL. Hôpital A. Michallon, Grenoble, France
[3]Otology, Neurotology and Auditory Implants Department, University Hospital of Grenoble CHU A. Michallon, Grenoble, France
[4]Department of Neuroradiology, University Hospital of Grenoble, Grenoble, France
[5]Department of Otolaryngology-Head and Neck Surgery, University Hospital of Grenoble, Grenoble, France
[6]Clinique Universitaire Oto–Rhino–Laryngologie, Centre Hospitalier Universitaire A. Michallon, Grenoble, France

Definition

The lower part of the middle ear (i.e., space below the lower part of the round window).

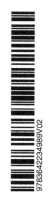